A TEXTBOOK OF
RADIOLOGY AND IMAGING

For Churchill Livingstone

Publisher: Simon Fathers
Project Editor: Clare Wood-Allum
Editorial Co-ordination: Editorial Resources Unit
 Copy Editor: Felicity Secretan
Design: Design Resources Unit
Production: Neil A. Dickson
Sales Promotion Executive: Caroline Boyd

A TEXTBOOK OF RADIOLOGY AND IMAGING

VOLUME 1

EDITED BY

DAVID SUTTON MD FRCP FRCR DMRD MCAR(Hon)
Consulting Radiologist, St Mary's Hospital and
The National Hospitals for Neurology and Neurosurgery,
London, UK

ASSOCIATE EDITORS

CT
Ian Isherwood MD FRCP FRCR FFRRCSI
W. St C. Forbes MA MB BCh DRCOG DRMD FRCR

MRI
Ian Isherwood MD FRCP FRCR FFRRCSI
Jeremy P. R. Jenkins MB BCh MRCP DMRD FRCR

Nuclear Medicine
E. Rhys Davies CBE FRCPE FRCR FFRRCSI FDSRCS

Ultrasound
William R. Lees MB BS FRCR

FIFTH EDITION

CHURCHILL LIVINGSTONE
EDINBURGH LONDON MADRID MELBOURNE NEW YORK AND TOKYO 1993

CHURCHILL LIVINGSTONE
Medical Division of Longman Group UK Limited

Distributed in the United States of America by Churchill
Livingstone Inc., 650 Avenue of the Americas, New York, N.Y.
10011, and by associated companies, branches and representatives
throughout the world.

First edition 1969
Second edition 1975
Third edition 1980
Reprinted 1983
Fourth edition 1987
Reprinted 1989, 1990
Fifth edition 1993

ISBN 0-443-04352-3

British Library Cataloguing in Publication Data
A catalogue record for this book is available from the British Library.

Library of Congress Cataloging in Publication Data
A catalog record for this book is available from the Library of
Congress.

The
publisher's
policy is to use
**paper manufactured
from sustainable forests**

Printed and bound in Great Britain by
William Clowes Limited, Beccles and London

PREFACE

The first edition of this textbook was published in 1969 and consisted of a single volume of 900 pages. The fourth edition published in 1987 had almost doubled in size and consisted of two volumes. This reflected the growth of the specialty as it changed from Diagnostic Radiology to Diagnostic Imaging. In 1969 radioisotopes were in established use but ultrasound was in its infancy, whilst CT and MRI were yet to be conceived. All four of these newer disciplines are now major subspecialties in their own right. At the same time other subspecialties such as Interventional Radiology have developed and the scope of Diagnostic Radiology continues to expand with technical advances such as digital imaging.

All the subspecialties based on techniques now have specialist journals devoted to their study and it is becoming increasingly difficult for the non-specialist radiologist to keep up to date with their constantly expanding scope. The fourth edition of this work still contained separate chapters dedicated to Radioisotopes, Ultrasound, CT and MRI. In the new fifth edition these have been replaced with the invaluable help of the Associate Editors by a more integrated approach based on clinical study of the various body organs.

This has been done both to keep the textbook within reasonable bounds of size and cost and to avoid unnecessary duplication. Since so many different imaging techniques are now available to investigate a particular clinical problem, the student must learn to choose between them, a choice which is sometimes difficult and controversial. Often a balance has to be struck between what is least invasive and provides least radiation and what provides most information and is most cost effective. It is our objective to provide the student with the most authoritative information on the methods currently preferred in centres of excellence. However the student should remember that this is a constantly expanding and changing field, and a book of this size can never be completely state of the art because of the inevitable time lag between writing and publication. Students with examinations in mind must also consult, and be familiar with, the current journals and be aware of the original papers presented at professional meetings and forums.

London, 1992   D.S.

CONTRIBUTORS

Graham R. Cherryman MB ChB FRCR
Professor of Radiology, University of Leicester,
Leicester Royal Infirmary, Leicester, UK

Roger Chisholm MA MB BChir MRCP FRCR
Consultant Radiologist, University of Manchester
School of Medicine, Hope Hospital, Salford, UK

E. Rhys Davies CBE FRCPE FRCR FFRRCSI FDSRCS
Professor of Clinical Radiology, University of Bristol;
Honorary Consultant Radiologist, United Bristol
Hospitals NHS Trust, Bristol; Civilian Consultant
Advisor to the Royal Navy, UK

Keith C. Dewbury BSc MB BS FRCR
Consultant Radiologist and Honorary Senior Lecturer,
Southampton University Hospitals, Southampton, UK

Robert Dick MB BS(Syd) FRACR FRCR
Consultant Radiologist, Royal Free Hospital; Dean
(Admissions), Royal Free Hospital School of
Medicine, London, UK

Claire Dicks-Mireaux BA MB BS MRCP DMRD FRCR
Consultant Radiologist, The Hospitals for Sick
Children, London, UK

Robert M. Donaldson MD FRCP FACC
Consultant Cardiologist, Royal Brompton National
Heart and Lung Hospital, London, UK

Stuart Field MA MB BChir DMRD FRCR
Consultant Radiologist, Canterbury and Thanet
Health Authority and Canterbury Hospital,
Canterbury, UK

W. St C. Forbes MA MB BCh DRCOG DMRD FRCR
Consultant Radiologist, Hope Hospital, Salford;
Lecturer, Department of Diagnostic Radiology,
University of Manchester, Manchester, UK

Joseph A. Gleeson FRCP FRCR
Consultant Radiologist, Westminster Hospital,
London, UK

I. H. Gravelle BSc MB ChB FRCPE FRCR
Consultant Radiologist, University Hospital of Wales,
Cardiff, UK

Roger H. S. Gregson BSc MB BS DMRD FRCR
Consultant Radiologist, University Hospital,
Nottingham; Clinical Teacher in Radiology, Queen's
Medical Centre, University of Nottingham,
Nottingham, UK

H. Highman MB FRCP FRCR
Consultant Radiologist, St Mary's Hospital;
Honorary Clinical Senior Lecturer, Imperial College of
Science, Technology and Medicine, (St Mary's
Hospital Medical School), London, UK

Ivan Hyde FRCPEdin FRCR DMRD DCH
Consultant Radiologist, Southampton General
Hospital, Southampton, UK

Ian Isherwood MD FRCP FRCR FFRRCSI
Professor of Diagnostic Radiology, University of
Manchester, Manchester, UK

Jeremy P. R. Jenkins MB BCh MRCP DMRD FRCR
Consultant Radiologist and Honorary Clinical Senior
Lecturer, Manchester Royal Infirmary, Manchester, UK

Simon N. Jones MB BS MRCP(UK) FRCR
Consultant Radiologist, Poole and Bournemouth
General Hospitals, Dorset, UK

Brian Kendall FRCP FRCS FRCR FFRRCSI(Hon)
Consultant Radiologist, National Hospitals for
Neurology and Neurosurgery, London; Consultant
Neuroradiologist, Hospitals for Sick Children and
Middlesex Hospital, London, UK

William R. Lees MB BS FRCR
Consultant Radiologist, Middlesex Hospital; Honorary
Senior Lecturer, University of London, London, UK

Glyn A. S. Lloyd MA DM FRCR
Consulting Radiologist, Radiology Department, Royal
National Throat, Nose and Ear Hospital, London, UK

Richard Mason FRCS MRCP FRCR
Consultant Radiologist, The Middlesex Hospital,
London, UK

Ivan Moseley BSc(Physiol) MD FRCP FRCR
Consultant Radiologist, National Hospital for
Neurology and Neurosurgery and Moorfields Eye
Hospital, London, UK

Janet Murfitt MRCP FRCR
Consultant Radiologist, The Royal London Hospital;
Teacher of the University of London, London, UK

Peter D. Phelps MD FRCS FRCR
Consultant Radiologist, Royal National Throat, Nose
and Ear Hospital, London and Walsgrave Hospital,
Coventry, UK

Maurice J. Raphael MA MD FRCP FRCR
Consultant Radiologist, Royal Brompton Hospital and
Middlesex Hospital, London, UK

Peter Renton FRCR DMRD
Consultant Radiologist, Royal National Orthopaedic
Hospital, University College Hospital, Hospital for
Tropical Diseases and University College Dental
Hospital; Honorary Senior Lecturer, University
College and Institute of Orthopaedics, University of
London, London, UK

David Rickards FRCR FFRDSA
Consultant Radiologist, The Middlesex Hospital and
St Peter's Institute of Urology, London, UK

Michael B. Rubens MB BS DMRD FRCR
Consultant Radiologist, Royal Brompton National
Heart and Lung Hospitals, London; Honorary Senior
Lecturer, Heart and Lung Institute, University of
London, UK

Donald Shaw MA MSc DMRD BM BCh FRCR FRCP
Consultant Radiologist, Hospitals for Sick Children,
London, UK

Keith C. Simpkins MB BS FRCP(Lond) FRCP (Edin) FRCR
FRACR(Hon)
Consultant Radiologist, The General Infirmary, Leeds.
Senior Clinical Lecturer in Diagnostic Radiology,
University of Leeds, UK

F. Starer FRCP(E) FRCR
Consulting Radiologist, Westminster Hospital and
Westminster Children's Hospital, London, UK

John M. Stevens MB BS DRACR FRCR
Consultant Neuroradiologist, St Mary's Hospital and
National Hospitals for Neurology and Neurosurgery,
London, UK

George Roberton Sutherland MB ChB FRCR FRCPEdin
FRCPGlas DMRD
Consultant Radiologist in Administrative Charge,
Royal Infirmary and Stobhill General Hospital;
Honorary Clinical Lecturer, University of Glasgow,
Glasgow, UK

David Sutton MD FRCP FRCR DMRD MCAR(Hon)
Consulting Radiologist, St Mary's Hospital and
National Hospitals for Neurology and Neurosurgery,
London, UK

Brian M. Thomas MB FRCP FRCR
Consultant Radiologist, University College Hospital
and St Mark's Hospital for Diseases of the Rectum
and Colon, London; Teacher in Radiology, University
College, London, UK

Iain Watt MRCP FRCR FFR
Consultant Radiologist, Department of Clinical
Radiology, United Bristol Hospitals NHS Trust;
Clinical Lecturer in Radiology, University of Bristol,
Bristol, UK

Peter Wilde BSc MRCP FRCR
Consultant Cardiac Radiologist, Bristol Royal
Infirmary and Bristol Royal Hospital for Sick
Children, Bristol, UK

Jeremy W. R. Young MA FRCR
Professor and Chairman, Department of Radiology,
Medical University of South Carolina, Charleston,
South Carolina, USA

CONTENTS

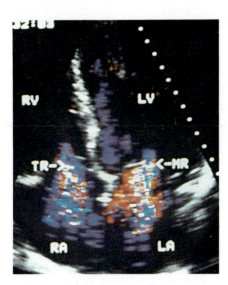

Fig. 23.10 Colour-flow Doppler in combined mitral and tricuspid regurgitation. The extensive red colouring in the left atrium indicates marked mitral regurgitation (MR), the lesser colouring in the right atrium indicates a lesser but still significant degree of tricuspid regurgitation (TR).

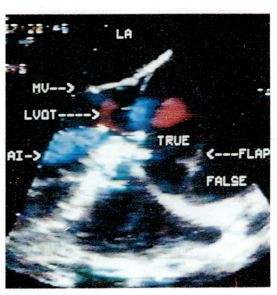

Fig. 23.21 Transoesophageal echocardiography in aortic dissection. True and false lumens, and the intimal flap, are all visualized. Colour-flow Doppler indicates significant aortic incompetence.

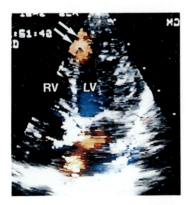

Fig. 24.11 Colour-flow Doppler study taken in an apical four-chamber view. The arrows indicate the orange flow pattern (towards the transducer) of an apical muscular defect. LV = left ventricle, RV = right ventricle.

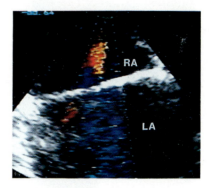

Fig. 24.13 Colour-flow Doppler study taken from the subcostal position in an adult with mitral valve disease. The patent foramen ovale is seen as an orange jet (towards the transducer). This was an incidental finding. LA = left atrium, RA = right atrium.

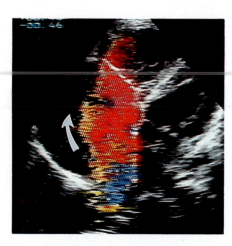

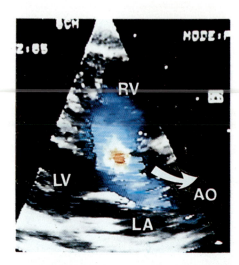

Fig. 24.17 Colour-flow Doppler study in a patient with a secundum atrial septal defect in the same orientation as Fig. 24.15. Flow through the defect towards the tricuspid valve is in red (towards the transducer).

Fig. 24.32 Colour-flow Doppler study in a child with tetralogy of Fallot. In this parasternal long-axis view there is right-to-left flow from the right ventricle (RV) to the aorta (AO). The majority of the flow is encoded blue (away from the transducer) but the fastest moving central flow shows aliasing (orange). LV = left ventricle, LA = left atrium.

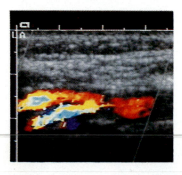

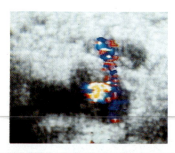

Fig. 25.74 Colour-flow study of a more than 50% stenosis of the common carotid bifurcation and internal carotid origin.

Fig. 25.75 False aneurysm of the femoral artery caused by arterial catheterization. High flow in the artery is shown in yellow and the jet into the aneurysm is largely red.

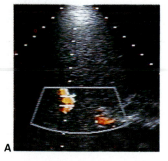
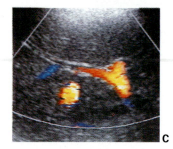

Fig. 25.78 **A**. Colour-flow map of portal vein flow. **C**. Flow in portal branches colour coded for direction. Yellow is high velocity flow.

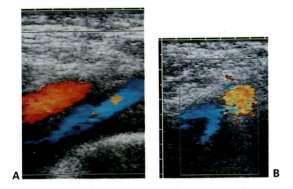

A | B

Fig. 26.35 **A**. Longitudinal CDI scan of the common femoral vein showing partially occluded flow (blue). **B**. Transverse scan.

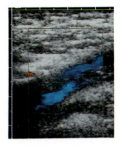

Fig. 26.36 Small amount of flow (blue) in an largely occluded popliteal vein. The vessel is incompressible and flow is only demonstrated after augmentation.

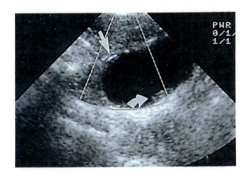

Fig. 45.33 Transvaginal study of a normal mature follicle showing the cumulus oophorus just prior to ovulation (curved arrow). Blood flow can be seen around the periphery of the follicle on colour Doppler imaging (CDI) (straight arrow).

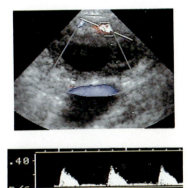

Fig. 45.34 Transvaginal duplex Doppler and CDI study of blood flow in the normal ovary (Day 14). The pulsatility index of 264% is calculated from the time velocity waveform.

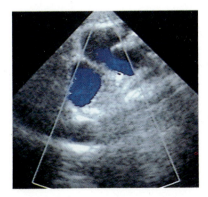

Fig. 45.35 Transvaginal CDI study of the pelvic veins showing distension and high flow. Pelvic venous congestion is now recognized as a cause of pelvic pain.

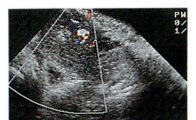

Fig. 45.62 CDI transvaginal scan of pelvic recurrence of an ovarian carcinoma showing characteristic hypervascularity.

PART 1

BONES AND JOINTS

CHAPTER 1

CONGENITAL SKELETAL ANOMALIES; SKELETAL DYSPLASIAS; CHROMOSOMAL DISORDERS

Peter Renton

CONGENITAL SKELETAL ANOMALIES

Very many congenital skeletal anomalies have been described. Some minor abnormalities are only discovered coincidentally or are never noticed. In many of these the skeleton is affected and often is the only system implicated. Many infective orthopaedic conditions acquired in childhood have been wholly or partially eradicated. Congenital abnormalities are therefore assuming increasing importance and present tremendous challenges to orthopaedic surgeons. However, only those of great importance to the radiologist will be dealt with in this section. Suggestions for further reading are given at the end of the chapter.

UPPER LIMB

Many congenital anomalies exist. A short glossary of descriptive terms in common use is presented here.

Adactyly — absence of fingers

Amelia — absence of limbs

Brachydactyly — short phalanges

Brachymesophalangy — short middle phalanges

Clinodactyly — incurving of a finger, usually the fifth, in the coronal plane

Hemimelia — absence of part of a hand

Hyper — or *hypophalangism* — the presence of a greater or lesser number of phalanges

Longitudinal defect — absence of part of the limb along its longitudinal axis. This may be pre-axial (radial), post-axial (ulnar) or central.

Macrodactyly — enlargement of a digit

Oligodactyly — absence of fingers

Phocomelia — absence of the proximal parts of a limb

Polydactyly — increased number of digits. May be pre- or post-axial

Symphalangism — fusion of phalanges in one digit

Syndactyly — fusion of adjacent digits. May involve soft tissues and/or bone.

(after Poznanski)

The lesions may be grouped into:

1. Failure of differentiation, e.g. syndactyly;
2. Failure of development, which may be transverse, e.g. aphalangy, or longitudinal;
3. Duplications;
4. Overgrowth — as in neurofibromatosis;
5. Generalized dysplasias;
6. Congenital (Streeter's) bands.

Some lesions are solitary and of no significance, i.e. isolated clinodactyly, while others occur in combination, so that clinodactyly is also seen as part of major syndromes, e.g. trisomy 21. Radial defects especially are associated with other anomalies, e.g. with atrial septal defects in the Holt-Oram syndrome. Some defects are attributable to drugs, such as thalidomide (Distaval) administered to the mother in the first three months of pregnancy. This may cause damage to the growing nerve, and it may be that the sensory nerve is the tissue organizer (McCredie 1975). Epanutin, used in the treatment of maternal epilepsy, may cause hypoplasia of distal phalanges *in utero*. Many lesions are genetically inherited so that the harmless *congenital broad thumb* may be seen in different generations of the same family. Other defects may represent sporadic mutations of the gene.

Sprengel's shoulder. This deformity consists of an abnormally high scapula. The deformity is due to failure of the shoulder girdle to descend from its embryonic position in the neck, a process which is normally completed by the end of the third fetal month. The lesion is usually unilateral though it may be bilateral. Other congenital anomalies are frequently associated.

Radiographs show the characteristic elevated scapula. The scapula may be normal in shape, but usually there is some shortening of its vertebral border with the result that its shape approaches that of an equilateral triangle. Rotation of the scapula may often be observed; gener-

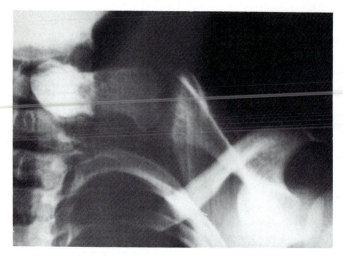

Fig. 1.1 The scapula is elevated and a large omovertebral bone is shown.

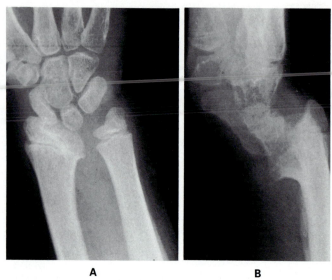

A   **B**

Fig. 1.2 A,B Madelung's deformity — defective development of the inner third of the radial epiphysis, increase in interosseous space, backward projection of the ulna and anterior displacement of the hand.

ally the inferior angle rotates towards the spine, though rotation in the opposite direction may occur.

From the upper part of the vertebral border or from the superior angle, an accessory bone — the omovertebral or suprascapular bone — may be found uniting this part of the scapula to the spine (Fig. 1.1). This structure may be represented only by fibrous tissue or cartilage and, if bony, may vary greatly in size and radiopacity.

Other anomalies which frequently co-exist include *cervical spina bifida*, the *Klippel-Feil anomaly*, *cervical ribs* and *other rib lesions*, *scoliosis* and *hemivertebrae*.

No difficulties in diagnosis should arise. In old *paralytic lesions* the scapula may be raised. If not evident from the history, the correct diagnosis should be suspected by noting the hypoplasia of bones typical of a paralytic lesion.

Radius and ulna. Radial defects are much more common than ulnar and may occur in isolation or as part of major syndromes, in which case they are usually bilateral.

Radial defects may occur with:
Ectodermal dysplasia
Holt-Oram syndrome
Fanconi syndrome
Thrombocytopenia — absent radius syndrome
Trisomy 18
Thalidomide embryopathy
Renal, ear and oesophageal anomalies

The defect may range from hypoplasia of the thumb to complete absence of radius, scaphoid, trapezium and thumb. The limb is shortened and a radial club hand results, with the hand deviated to the side of the absent bone.

Synostosis of the radius and ulna may be seen at the upper end and is usually associated with dislocation of the radial head. This lesion has marked hereditary tendencies.

Madelung's deformity. This lesion is much commoner in girls and it is generally bilateral. It usually presents during adolescence. The cardinal abnormality is defective development of the inner third of the epiphysis of the lower end of the radius. As a consequence the radial shaft is bowed, so increasing the interosseous space. The lower end of the ulna is subluxed backwards. The hand and carpus project forward at the wrist joint to produce a bayonet-like appearance in a lateral view (Fig. 1.2).

The lesion may be part of the *Leri-Weil syndrome* (dyschondrosteosis, see below) and *Turner's syndrome*. Similar appearances may follow trauma or infection to the growing epiphyseal plate (Fig. 1.3).

Hand and **wrist lesions**. Very many congenital abnormalities (and normal variants) may be found in the hands and feet. Specialist monographs should be consulted (see list at end of chapter).

Carpal fusions may occur in isolation or as part of a syndrome. In isolation they are usually transverse, e.g. lunate-triquetrum and capitate-hamate, and are much commoner in negroes. In syndromes, they are usually proximodistal and occur in *Apert's syndrome*, *dyschondrosteosis*, *chondroectodermal dysplasia*, *Holt-Oram syndrome* and *Turner's syndrome*. Similar appearances may follow trauma, infection and rheumatoid disease.

Polydactyly. Polydactyly is more common in negroes. It may be *postaxial* (ulnar) and may range from a minor ossicle to complete duplication of the little finger. *Preaxial* lesions (radial) range from minor partial duplication of the thumb distal phalanx to complete thumb duplication. On occasion the hand may be duplicated. Syndactyly may be associated with polydactyly.

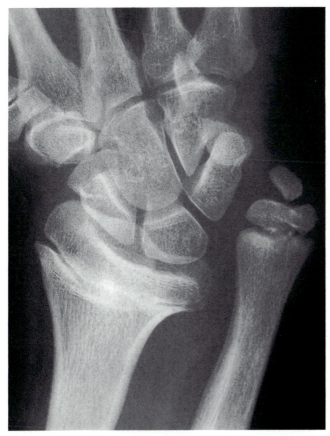

Fig. 1.3 Trauma to the distal radius has resulted in partial fusion of the epiphyseal plate and partial growth arrest. Avulsion of the ulnar styloid occurred at the same time.

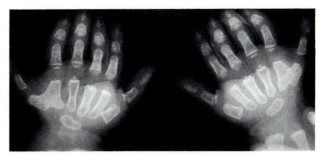

Fig. 1.4 Chondroectodermal dysplasia (Ellis–van Creveld syndrome). Polysyndactyly is demonstrated. In addition, the phalanges are abnormal in morphology.

Polydactyly may be associated with *Ellis–van Creveld disease* (chondroectodermal dysplasia) (Fig. 1.4), *Laurence-Moon-Biedl disease* (polysyndactyly, mental defect, obesity and retinitis pigmentosa), *trisomy 13*, and *asphyxiating thoracic dysplasia* — all postaxial — and with *Holt-Oram syndrome* and *Fanconi's anaemia* (preaxial).

Syndactyly occurs in *Apert's syndrome*, *Fanconi's anaemia*, *Laurence-Moon-Biedl syndrome*, *trisomy 13*, and *trisomy 18*. (For fuller list consult specialist texts; see references at end of Chapter).

THE LOWER LIMB

CONGENITAL DISLOCATION OF THE HIP

This is a very important condition because success in its treatment depends upon early recognition. The incidence of hip instability at birth is 5–10/1000, and of frank dislocation 1–1.5/1000. One-third of cases of congenital dislocation of the hip are detected late but these often have a family history of the disease.

Instability and dislocation is usually unilateral (L:R = 11:1) but both hips may be involved (unilateral: bilateral = 11:4). Females are more commonly affected (F:M = 5:1). Sixty per cent of affected children are first-born. These children are far more likely to have been breech presentations (breech:vertex = 6:1), possibly because the abnormal lie does not permit reduction in utero. Children born by caesarian section are thus also more likely to have associated instability and dislocation. A family or twin history is also common; a subsequent child has a 6% risk of involvement.

Congenital dislocation of the hip is more commonly found in the winter (winter:summer = 1.5:1), possibly because of tight swaddling of children in a position of dislocation in winter.

Imaging

Ultrasound (*W. R. Lees*) Using a high-frequency ultrasound transducer it is possible to image the anatomy of the infant hip joint. The bone of the acetabulum impedes the passage of the ultrasound beam, producing a highly echogenic interface. Cartilage allows through transmission, with its internal structure returning low-level echoes. Muscles and tendons also show characteristic echo patterns (Figs 1.5A,B).

The femoral head is seen as a spherical structure containing coarse low-level echoes. The triradiate cartilage presents similarly as an acoustic defect at the base of the acetabulum.

A stable hip joint does not permit posterior movement of the femoral head in the acetabulum. This defines the most commonly used scanning technique. The hip is scanned in the supine position with 90° flexion. Firm posterior pressure will result in subluxation of the unstable hip, which is best seen scanning in the transverse plane (Fig. 1.5C) Movement of 3–4 mm on the flexion stress manoeuvre is found with a loose joint. This corresponds to a slight click on clinical examination. Movement of more than 6 mm is significant subluxation.

The position of the limbic cartilage is important in complete dislocation, where it is interposed between the femoral head and the acetabulum (Fig. 1.5C).

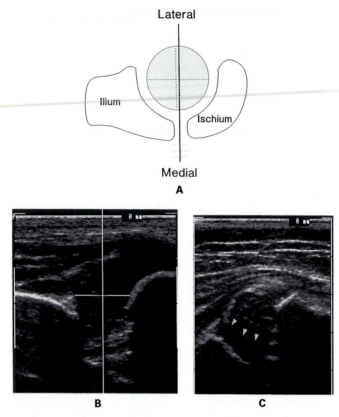

Fig. 1.5 A. Diagram of a transverse section through the infant hip showing the normal relationship of the ball of the femoral head to the acetabulum. **B.** A normal transverse section indicating the important axes, as in 5A. **C.** Inferior subluxation with interposition of poorly echogenic limbic cartilage (small arrows) between the moderately echogenic femoral head and the floor of the acetabulum.

of conventional radiology. The indications for conventional radiographs given below (taken from Catterall's work (personal communication, 1990)) of course apply also to ultrasound. Discussion of radiology is still necessary as access to ultrasound may be limited.

At the Royal National Orthopaedic Hospital, London, there are both absolute and relative indications for X-ray.

Absolute indications (If any one of these is present, the hips should be examined by imaging).

1. Family history of congenital dislocation of hip.
2. Neonatal hip instability.
3. Limb shortening.
4. Limitation of hip abduction in flexion.

Relative indications (If any two of these are present, the hips should be examined by imaging).

1. Breech presentation.
2. First-born child.
3. Caesarian section.
4. Other congenital anomalies.
5. Excessive fetal moulding.

At birth, neither femoral head is ossified but, occasionally, a notch above the acetabulum may be present (Fig. 1.6) and even in the absence of the femoral head, congenital dislocation of the hip can then be diagnosed.

The size, shape and symmetry of the femoral heads and acetabula can be monitored on treatment through windows cut in the hip spica. The ossification centre develops between 1 and 6 months and is seen as an echogenic focus within the poorly echogenic femoral head.

The acetabulum is best imaged in the coronal plane. If the acetabular cup accommodates less than one-third of the femoral head then acetabular dysplasia is definitely present and it must be suspected if one half to one-third only is accommodated.

Ultrasonography should be used whenever there is clinical suspicion of CDH. Conventional radiography has three shortcomings: cartilage is not directly visualized and its position has to be inferred from bony landmarks; the standard radiographic positions are those in which subluxation is least likely to occur; and the examination is static, with stress views rarely obtained. Ultrasonography is simple, rapid and free of hazard.

Plain film radiology. The advent of neonatal hip ultrasound, especially if it can be carried out as a screening test and again at three months, has limited the use

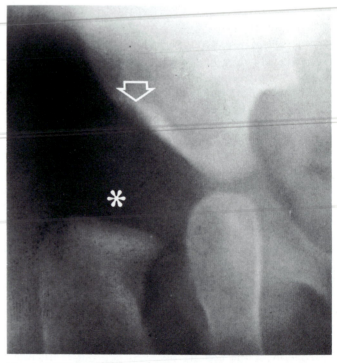

Fig. 1.6 A small defect with marginal sclerosis is seen above the acetabulum (arrow) in a neonate who later was shown to have a congenitally dislocated femoral head. The ★ marks the site of the projected femoral head.

Retarded ossification of the femoral ossific nuclei is a traditional sign of congenital dislocation of the hip. In some early cases, however, the femoral ossific nucleus may appear to be larger on the dislocated than on the normal side. Some incongruous findings are probably explicable by the lesion being bilateral.

Sometimes poor development of the acetabulum is obvious in cases of congenital dislocation of the hip. In our experience the acetabular angle is increased in congenital dislocations even in the neonatal period. The *acetabular angle* is the angle subtended by a line, drawn through the centres of both Y-cartilages (Hilgenreiner's line) and a line parallel to the acetabular roof.

The eventual position of the femoral head and its relationship to the acetabulum can often be inferred from a film of the hips in the neutral position. The site of the non-ossified epiphysis may be inferred as lying superior to the epiphyseal plate. This in turn lies at right angles and proximal to the femoral neck (Fig. 1.6).

Andren and von Rosen (1958) described an anteroposterior projection with the hips and knees fully extended, both legs abducted to 45° and the femora fully internally rotated. The baby must lie symmetrically on the table top and immobilization may be aided by a lightly applied compression band. The test may fail if the baby is grasped too firmly above the hips because reduction of the dislocation may occur.

Andren and von Rosen state that a line drawn through the shaft of an undislocated femur will point to the outer lip of the acetabulum and will, if extended, cross the spine at the level of the lumbosacral junction. On the other hand, if the hip is dislocated, a similar line will point outside the acetabulum and will cross the spine at a higher level (Fig. 1.7).

In an undislocated hip, the line through the long axis of an abducted femur will pass well within the acetabular contour.

Radiographically there is restricted abduction of the femoral shaft in congenital dislocation and abduction of 45° with the femur in internal rotation is difficult to attain or to maintain. It seems that the success of the Andren and von Rosen technique depends at least partially on this fact.

Seen later, from the age of 6 months onwards, the radiological diagnosis is usually easy (Fig. 1.8). The femoral head will be displaced upwards and outwards and delayed ossification of its epiphyses will be observed. The acetabulum will be shallower than that of the normal hip and its roof will not be set horizontally but will slope upwards and outwards. Use of the many lines and coordinates described in this condition is not necessary, provided heed is paid to the possibility of a bilateral dislocation.

During management the radiologist will be asked to decide whether reduction has been attained or maintained. This decision may be very difficult to make on radiographs taken through plaster. In such cases tomography may give the required information — three sections using a multisection box will suffice, or ultrasound may be available.

Reduction may be impossible to obtain or the hip may be unstable. In such cases *arthrography* may be used to study the disposition of soft tissue structures of the joint.

Possible abnormal findings are:

1. The fibrocartilaginous rim of the acetabulum, called the *limbus*, may become inverted into the joint and form a barrier to stable reduction. In an arthrogram of a normal

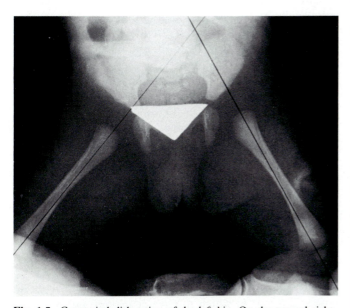

Fig. 1.7 Congenital dislocation of the left hip. On the normal right side a line through the long axis of the femur crosses the spine at the level of the lumbosacral articulation. On the dislocated side the spine is crossed at a higher level and the line through the long axis of the femur passes outside the acetabular rim. In practice it is unusual to find such a pronounced degree of dislocation in newborn infants.

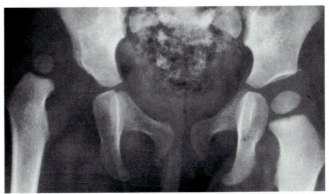

Fig. 1.8 Congenital dislocation of the right hip — note sloping acetabular roof, delayed ossification of the femoral capital epiphysis and false acetabulum formation.

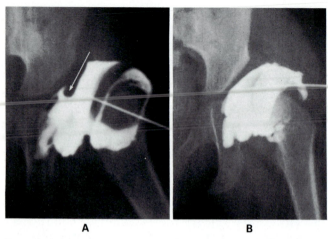

Fig. 1.9 A. Arthrogram of left hip shows filling defect caused by inverted limbus (arrow). **B.** Appearances following limbectomy. (Courtesy of Mr. A. C. Clark.)

hip a thorn-like projection marks a small gap between the outer part of the limbus and the capsular attachment. When the limbus is inverted, the 'thorn' is lost and the filling defect caused by the limbus is seen (Fig. 1.9).

2. The *ligamentum teres* may become so large that it may offer a barrier to reduction. A hypertrophic ligamentum teres may be visible on the arthrogram but estimation of its size by this means is unreliable.

3. The *psoas tendon* may become contracted and a notch for the tendon is seen inferiorly.

Arthrography is of particular service in deciding whether complete reduction of a dislocation has been achieved. There are times when it is not possible to obtain this information from examination of plain films — especially when the femoral ossific nucleus appears to be set eccentrically on the femoral neck.

The primary cause of unstable reduction of a dislocated femoral head has long been debated. Excessive anteversion of the femoral neck is often seen and the condition often necessitates a de-rotation osteotomy for reduction to be maintained. The femoral neck of a normal baby is usually anteverted to 35°; this diminishes to 15° in the adult. In congenital dislocation, the femoral neck may be anteverted to 70°–80°. Various specialized techniques are available for measuring the degree of anteversion.

In neglected dislocations, the misplaced femoral head may produce a depression on the side of the ilium above the acetabulum, constituting a *false acetabulum*. This may vary in size from a shallow depression to a deep socket. The original acetabular socket becomes progressively more shallow.

Osteochondritis may complicate a congenital dislocation of the hip, particularly after vigorous methods of reduction or surgery. Not all cases of osteochondritis are attributable to the complications of treatment, for there does appear to be a true association between congenital dislocation and Perthes' disease of the hip.

IDIOPATHIC COXA VARA OF CHILDHOOD: PROXIMAL FEMORAL FOCAL DEFICIENCY (PFFD)

Two types of idiopathic coxa vara are recognized:

1. A congenital form, generally present at birth, sometimes associated with other congenital lesions.

2. An infantile form, not present at birth, recognized around the age of 4 years and often bilateral (33%).

PFFD (congenitally short femur) consists of failure of normal development of a lesser or greater part of the proximal femur. Some distal femur, by definition, is always present, thus distinguishing it from femoral agenesis.

Coxa vara is included as part of the PFFD spectrum if the varus is associated with congenital femoral shortening present from birth, i.e. Type 1 above. If PFFD is severe, coxa vara cannot arise at all, even in congenital cases.

The mean angle of the neck on the shaft at one year of age is 148°, decreasing to 135° at 5 years, and 120° in the elderly. Coxa vara is present when the angle is less than normal, but certainly if below 110°.

Radiographic findings: Coxa vara. The lesion is usually bilateral, though it may be unilateral. Coxa vara will usually be obvious. The femoral head will be situated low in the acetabulum and its outline may appear woolly. Secondary deformity of the acetabulum may result. A triangular fragment of bone may be seen at the lower part of the femoral neck. This wedge of bone, commoner in the infantile cases, is bounded by two clear bands forming an inverted V (Fig. 1.10). The medial or inner band is the epiphyseal line. The outer one is, of course, abnormal. Some writers have regarded it as an area of osteochondritis, others as a stress fracture. In later cases the greater trochanter will be found to curve like a beak and it may articulate with the ilium. Not all these features are necessarily present in every case.

Acquired coxa vara may be found in conditions where bone is softened, e.g. in *rickets*, *fibrous dysplasia*, *osteogenesis imperfecta* and *cleidocranial dysplasia*, as well as in *Perthes' disease* and following *slipped epiphysis*.

In some cases which appear to have PFFD with no proximal femur in which to have coxa vara, arthrography of the hip may reveal a cartilaginous neck and head with varus deformity, as will ultrasound.

Radiographic findings: PFFD (Fig. 1.11). A short femur, which is laterally situated and proximally displaced, is demonstrated at birth. The distal femur is by

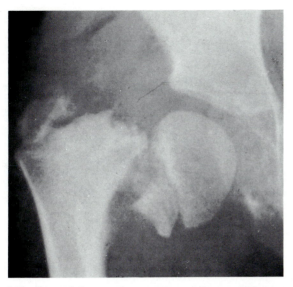

Fig. 1.10 Congenital coxa vara — extreme coxa vara with some slip of the epiphysis. A triangular fragment of bone is well shown.

definition present. Ossification of the proximal portion is delayed. A spectrum of proximal deficiencies exists.

ANOMALIES OF THE PATELLA

The patella is frequently *bipartite* and sometimes *multipartite*. The upper, outer part is always involved. The anomaly is often bilateral and well corticated all round, which helps to distinguish it from a fissure fracture. Not all cases, however, are bilateral.

In the *nail-patella syndrome* the patella may be rudimentary or hypoplastic and set laterally (see Fig. 1.17B).

The patella may be *dislocated* due to a variety of congenital causes, e.g. *hypoplasia of the lateral femoral condyle, external rotation of the tibia* and *malattachment of the iliotibial tract*. The displacement is invariably outwards.

CONGENITAL PSEUDARTHROSIS OF THE TIBIA AND FIBULA

The pseudarthrosis of the tibia is seen at the junction of the middle and lower thirds. Often a similar lesion is found in the fibula.

Radiological examination of early cases may show a sclerotic or radiolucent zone in the affected area. This bows, resorbs and fractures and the severed ends of the bone become sclerotic. Still later, the proximal part

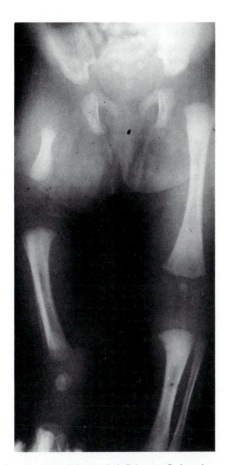

Fig. 1.11 Proximal focal femoral deficiency. Only a hypoplastic portion of the distal right femur is apparent.

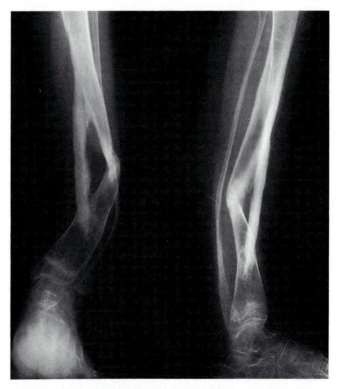

Fig. 1.12 Neurofibromatosis. Pseudarthroses are seen bilaterally. The fibulae are thin and bowed. Bony struts have been inserted at surgery.

becomes cupped and the distal part pointed, so forming a pseudarthrosis (Fig. 1.12). This uncommon lesion is notoriously resistant to treatment.

Neurofibromatosis is usually given as the most frequent cause of this condition. Other associations are with *fibrous dysplasia* and *idiopathic juvenile osteoporosis*. Occasionally, a similar lesion has been found affecting the *forearm bones*.

THE FOOT AND ANKLE

Accessory bones of the foot. Supernumerary centres of ossification are more common in the foot than in the hand. They should be identified to distinguish them from fractures. They may themselves fracture and be a cause of pain, or may be involved in arthritis, osteochondritis, infections and hyperparathyroidism. More than 50 have been described but most of them are rarities. As they become radiologically visible in adults, the incidence rises to 30%. The *os tibiale externum* is found in some 7% of feet, the *os trigonum* in 5% and the *os peroneum* in 8% but surveys differ as to their incidence. Two sesamoids are regularly seen at the head of the great toe metatarsal. The medial is bipartite in one-third of cases, the lateral in only 5%. A bipartite sesamoid is larger than its normal counterpart and corticated all round, while a fractured sesamoid shows non-corticated fracture parts. Pathology in metatarsal sesamoids can be demonstrated on axial views, and isotope bone scans will often be abnormal.

Congenital talipes equinovarus (*congenital club foot*). This condition is nearly always idiopathic but club foot is sometimes associated with other bony abnormalities.

The idiopathic type is of limited interest to the radiologist. The three cardinal abnormalities are: 1. adduction of the forefoot; 2. inversion of the foot; and 3. plantar flexion of the foot. Radiologically medial displacement of the navicular and cuboid in relation to the heads of the talus and calcaneum will be seen. The calcaneum will rotate medially under the talus. Plantar flexion will be seen by posterior displacement of the calcaneum.

Ossification of the talus and navicular may be retarded. Usually secondary hypoplasia of the bones of the tarsus and of the soft tissues is seen.

Ball and socket ankle joint. In this condition the ankle joint is abnormally shaped and its range of movement increased. It is usually found when the midtarsal and subtaloid joints are rigid, generally caused by tarsal fusions; in such cases inversion and eversion of the ankle compensate for the loss of these movements at the midtarsal and subtaloid joints.

Some cases are seen in patients with a short leg — in a few no underlying cause is seen.

Radiographic features are characteristic. The trochlear surface of the talus, normally convex anteroposteriorly and concave from side to side, loses this concavity and

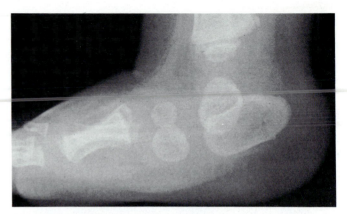

Fig. 1.13 Congenital vertical talus — note vertical position of the talus and elevation both of the calcaneum and of the forefoot.

approaches the shape of a sphere. The mortice of the talus becomes correspondingly moulded into a cup-like cavity to form a ball and socket articulation.

Congenital vertical talus. This is a rare cause of congenital flat foot in children. The radiographic appearances are diagnostic. The talus is vertical, its long axis following that of the tibial shaft. The vertical displacement of the talus remains constant whether the patient is standing or recumbent. The bones of the forefoot and the calcaneum are raised and produce the typical rocker-bottom foot (Fig. 1.13). When the navicular becomes ossified its shape will be seen to appear normal except for a little constriction of its waist. It will be seen obviously dislocated and lying in contact with the body of the talus.

Congenital fusions. Painful flat foot (the peroneal spastic flat foot) may be due to fusion of certain tarsal bones (Figs 1.14, 1.15). If the union is cartilaginous or fibrous, rather than bony, it is not seen radiologically. Flattening of the longitudinal arch of the foot is seen. Bony union is not directly demonstrable before adolescence but appears with ossification of the cartilaginous link between the bones. Fusion of the medial facet of the subtalar joint is the most common. It is well seen

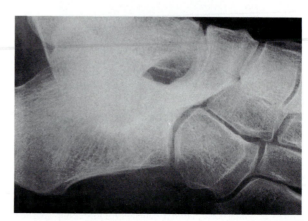

Fig. 1.14 Calcaneonavicular bar.

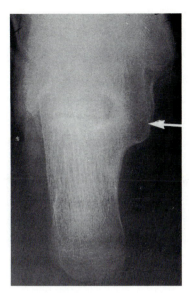

Fig. 1.15 Talocalcaneal synostosis.

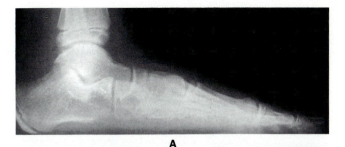

A

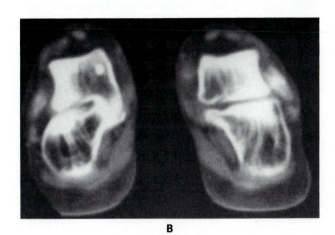

B

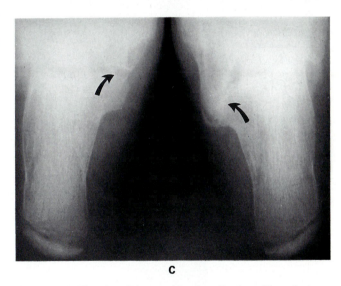

C

on an axial view of the foot. Calcaneo-navicular fusion is shown on oblique views of the foot (Fig. 1.14). Coalition has been described between all the bones of the hind foot. Restriction of movement at the subtalar joint causes abnormal movement, with lipping at the calcaneo-navicular joint, seen together with longitudinal arch flattening and obliteration of subtalar joints on the lateral view of the foot. These changes result in a local increase in uptake on *radionuclide bone scanning. CT scanning*, when available, will also show foot fusions (Fig. 1.16).

THE PELVIS

Iliac horns. These are bony processes projecting dorsally from the outer surface of the wings of each ilium. They may occur alone or be associated with the syndrome of rudimentary or absent patellae, deformity of the elbows (hypoplasia of capitellum and radial head) and dystrophy of the nails (*nail-patella syndrome — Fong's lesion*) (Fig. 1.17).

THE SPINE

Spinal anomalies range from gross defects, incompatible with life, to minor anomalies which are no more than anatomical variants. Some of these may be mistaken for fractures, e.g. the unfused accessory ossification centres at the tips of inferior articular facets or those related to the anterosuperior part of the margins of vertebral bodies. Fractures are rarely seen at such sites and have ragged rather than smooth edges.

Coronal cleft vertebra. This anomaly is seen in vertebral bodies of newborn infants and is due to failure of fusion of two ossification centres. In about half the cases

Fig. 1.16 **A**. Tarsal coalition resulting in a flat foot. The subtalar joints are no longer clearly visualized. **B**. CT scan of tarsal coalition showing right-sided fusion of the middle facet of the subtalar joint. **C**. Axial view showing unilateral coalition of the middle facet (arrows).

more than one vertebral body is affected. The abnormality has been seen on prenatal radiographs — it occurs more frequently in males.

The cleft is seen on a lateral radiograph as a linear or oval defect between a small posterior and larger anterior ossification centre (Fig. 1.18). The anteroposterior diameter of the affected vertebral body is often increased. The

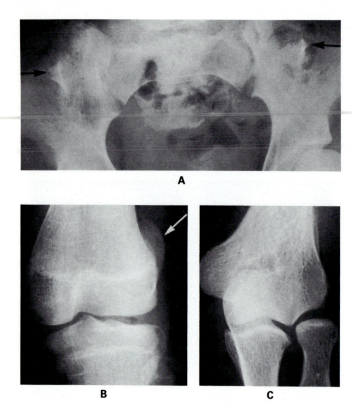

A

B   C

Fig. 1.17 Nail-patella syndrome. **A.** Iliac horns are seen (arrows). **B**. A small laterally placed patella is shown. **C.** Hypoplasia of the capitellum is shown.

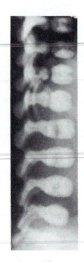

Fig. 1.18 Coronal cleft vertebra. (Courtesy of Dr. K. A. Rowley.)

cleft consolidates in a few months. These clefts are of no importance except that they are seen in some dysplasias (see *Chondrodystrophia calcificans congenita*).

Butterfly vertebra. In the affected vertebra, the upper and lower surfaces are deeply concave or V-shaped, so that the vertical dimension of the vertebral body in the midline is much reduced. In the frontal projection, it is

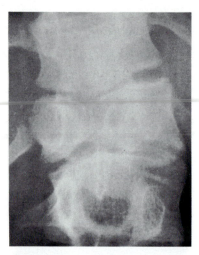

Fig. 1.19 Butterfly vertebra — upper and lower surfaces of affected vertebra are V-shaped, and contiguous vertebrae are moulded into the deficient centre.

seen that vertebrae above and below are moulded into the deficient centres of the affected vertebra (Fig. 1.19).

Malfusions of appendages. Epiphyses of the spinous processes, transverse processes and articular facets may remain unfused. The abnormality is without importance except that it may mimic a fracture.

Hemivertebra. They may cause scoliosis unless an equal number appear on each side. In the thoracic region, a hemivertebra will bear a rib. Multiple hemivertebrae may cause dwarfism.

Congenital vertebral fusions. Many forms of congenital vertebral fusion may be found. Complete fusion of the bodies and neural arches may occur, or the fusion may be limited to parts of the bodies or neural arches. At times it may not be possible to decide whether a fusion is developmental or post-inflammatory. Fusion of neural arches, however, is almost always a developmental anomaly. The anteroposterior diameter of congenital block vertebrae may be reduced and an anterior concavity may be found. These features may also be found in old postinfective fusions or after juvenile chronic arthritis. A posterior concavity in addition may indicate a congenital lesion. Complete vertebral fusions are often called 'block vertebrae'. They may be of no clinical significance, but frequently, disc degeneration develops above or below the fused vertebrae due to altered mechanics in the spine. Such lesions are relatively common in the cervical spine where a more severe anomaly, the *Klippel-Feil syndrome*, may be seen (Fig. 1.20). In this condition, many cervical vertebrae are fused, the neck is short and its movements limited, and hair grows low on the neck. Often there is torticollis and atrophy of facial musculature. Other congenital anomalies, such as spina bifida, rib lesions and Sprengel's shoulder, usually co-exist.

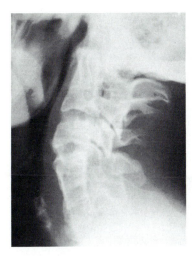

Fig. 1.20 Klippel-Feil syndrome. Cervical fusions are seen with a short neck.

Separate odontoid *(os odontoideum)*. The odontoid peg may sometimes be completely detached from the body of the second cervical vertebra, and be situated in the region of the foramen magnum (Fig. 1.21). Posterior fossa symptoms may result.

It has been shown that in some cases at least the separate ossicle results from a fracture in childhood of the base of the odontoid peg, with subsequent failure to unite. The lesion is thus not always 'congenital'.

Cervical rib. This is a common anomaly. The supplementary rib usually arises from the seventh cervical vertebra, rarely from the sixth and very rarely from the fifth.

The diagnosis is straightforward, though it may be necessary to count all the ribs in order to distinguish a rudimentary first thoracic rib from a cervical rib. Cervical ribs arise from cervical transverse processes. These slope downwards from the neural arch in the cervical spine but upwards in the thoracic spine. Cervical ribs vary greatly in size and shape, and clinical symptoms bear little rela-

tion to the radiographic abnormality. A very small cervical rib element may have a fibrous attachment to the first thoracic rib which causes much disability, whereas a large cervical rib may be asymptomatic.

Sacralization and lumbarization. It is often difficult to give a definite level to a particular vertebral body in the lumbar region, especially if the lumbosacral region is transitional. Again, it may be necessary to count all the vertebral bodies from C1 down. It has been said that the transverse processes of L3 are the lowest (most caudal) which lie truly transversely, while those for L4 are inclined upwards. Various permutations occur. Small, or absent, ribs on T12 may occur with large transverse processes on L5 which fuse with the sacrum (sacralization of L5). This is known as cranial shift. Caudal shift implies the presence of ribs on L1 and lumbarization of S1, that is, it comes to bear free-floating transverse processes. A rudimentary disc is then seen between S1 and S2.

The sacralized transverse process may form a pseudarthrosis with the ilium and degenerative sclerosis may appear around the false joint. This may be a site of low back pain. In addition, the free disc above the pseudarthrosis shows early degeneration.

Anomalies of lumbosacral facets *(trophism)*. The facet joints in the lumbar spine may be clearly seen in the anteroposterior projection. They should be symmetrical. With degeneration, the lower lumbar facet joints cease to be symmetrical, so that often one joint is seen and the other at that level is not (Fig. 1.22A). This rotational change is associated with much new bone around narrowed facet joints and adjacent laminae, often with symptoms of nerve root impingement. The changes are well demonstrated with CT scanning (Fig. 1.22B), when the acquired asymmetry of the entire neural arch is seen as well as the local new bone formation.

Spina bifida. Incomplete fusion of neural arches is a common finding. In most cases only a minor midsagittal defect in the neural arch is seen. The rather misleading term 'spina bifida occulta' is applied to this condition. There is no true breach in such cases; the radiolucent area represents merely non-ossified cartilage. In children many of these areas become ossified as growth progresses.

True breaches in the neural arch do, of course, occur, and they may be accompanied by a meningocoele protruding posteriorly and usually in the lumbar region. Occasionally, in the thorax and in the sacral region, the sac may protrude laterally and anteriorly through the intervertebral foramina and sacral foramina respectively. Other vertebral and rib anomalies are very frequent in the severe forms of spina bifida. The presence of hydrocephalus is a common feature in marked spina bifida.

Foot deformities, such as *pes cavus*, may be associated with spina bifida. Likewise, *perforating ulcers* causing absorption of metatarsal heads, *neuropathic joints* and *spontaneous fractures* accompanied by excessive callus may

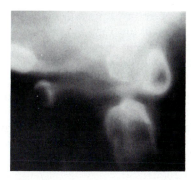

Fig. 1.21 Os odontoideum. The odontoid peg is clearly separate from the body of C2 but retains a normal relationship with the arch of the atlas. These lesions usually follow trauma in childhood.

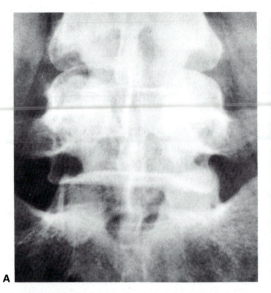
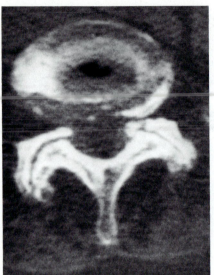

Fig. 1.22 **A**. The facet joints are no longer symmetrical and show features of degeneration. **B**. The CT scan shows gross new bone formation around narrowed facet joints. There is marked bony encroachment upon the exit foramina, especially the left. Gas is seen in the disc (vacuum phenomenon).

all occur. *Metaphyseal fractures* are sometimes seen in this condition.

In cases of alimentary reduplications, the possibility of associated malformations of the spine should be borne in mind. The reduplications or *neurenteric cysts* may be associated with severe anterior and posterior *spina bifida*, *hemivertebra*, *absent vertebra* or *diastematomyelia*. In some cases no vertebral deformity is demonstrable.

DYSPLASIAS OF BONE

The diagnosis of these lesions is mainly radiological and often entirely so. The radiologist will observe such features as alteration in bone density and in the size and shape of the bones. He will also observe the distribution of the lesion and the parts of the bones affected.

Accurate diagnosis is now of prime importance and not merely an academic exercise. Genetic counselling is, of course, a well-established speciality depending on accurate diagnosis. In other fields such as the *mucopolysaccharidoses* new lines of therapy such as bone marrow transplants are being evaluated.

CLEIDOCRANIAL DYSPLASIA (CCD)
(synonym: *cleidocranial dysostosis*)

This is a benign hereditary condition which is inherited as an autosomal dominant and which is recognized during childhood. The disease has considerable variation of expression.

Radiological features. Changes are widespread.

Clavicles. There may be total (in 10% of cases) or partial absence of the clavicle (Fig. 1.23A). The outer end is absent more frequently than the inner, but both to an extremely variable extent. Central defects also occur. The clavicles may also be normal. The scapulae tend to be small and high, and the glenoid fossae are small.

Thorax. The thorax is usually narrow, the ribs are short and directed obliquely downwards. Respiratory distress may occur in the newborn. The sternum is incompletely ossified. Failure of fusion of neural arches occurs, with delay in maturation of vertebral bodies, which retain an infantile biconvex shape. Supernumerary or bifid ribs also occur.

Skull. In the newborn, mineralization is delayed. The facial bones are small but the mandible is normal in size. The fontanelles remain open late and the sutures are widened. The bodies of the sphenoids are hypoplastic. Many Wormian bones are seen and frontal and parietal bossing may be present. Basilar invagination may also occur (Fig. 1.23B).

Pelvis. Delayed and imperfect ossification of the pubic bones is a recognized finding (Fig. 1.23C) and congenital coxa vara is frequently seen.

Teeth. See Chapter 50.

Hands. Anomalies of the hand are very common. The second and fifth metacarpals are long and have super-

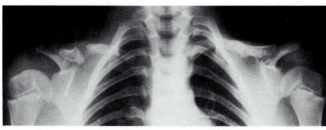

A

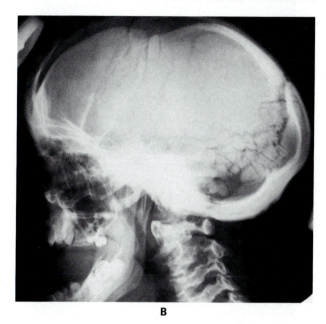

B

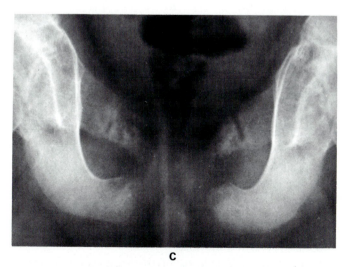

C

Fig. 1.23 Cleidocranial dysplasia. **A**. Clavicular defects are demonstrated, especially on the right side. **B**. Note delayed mineralization in the frontoparietal region and Wormian bones posteriorly. Facial bones are small but the mandible is normal. Delayed dentition is also seen. **C**. Failure of ossification of the symphysis pubis is demonstrated.

numerary ossification centres at their bases. The middle phalanges of the second and fifth phalanges are short. Cone epiphyses and distal phalangeal tapering are found.

Short fibulae, congenital pseudarthrosis of the femur, genu valgum and *obliquity of the articular space of the ankle joint* are among many reported associations.

PYCNODYSOSTOSIS

This condition has been confused with cleidocranial dysplasia (because of some similar clavicular and skull changes) and osteopetrosis (because of the generalized increase in diffuse bone density). It is inherited as an autosomal recessive disease, and parents may be closely related. The patients are short (below 150 cm) which is not a prominent feature of CCD. The skeleton is susceptible to fractures. The disease is rare and found in all races. The French painter Toulouse-Lautrec is believed to have suffered from this disease.

Radiographic features. *Skull*. There is brachycephaly with wide sutures and persistence of open fontanelles into adult life (Fig. 1.24A). Wormian bones are seen. The calvarium, base of skull and especially the orbital rims are very dense. The facial bones are small and the maxilla hypoplastic (Fig. 1.24A). The mandible has no angle — it is obtuse (see Ch. 50).

Limbs. Normal modelling of long bones is usually seen. The cortices are dense but the medullary canals not completely obliterated.

Thorax. Hypoplasia of the lateral ends of the clavicles is present to a varying degree. The ribs are dense overall.

Spine. Failure of fusion of the neural arches and spondylolisthesis are found. In adults the vertebral bodies resemble spools, with large anterior and posterior defects. The bones are uniformly dense (Fig. 1.24B).

Hands. Acro-osteolysis occurs, often with irregular distal fragments of the distal phalanges.

ACRO-OSTEOLYSIS
(eponym: *Hajdu-Cheney syndrome*)

Acro-osteolysis means disintegration of bone of the tips of the fingers and toes. This specific syndrome is inherited as an autosomal dominant. Other features include spinal osteoporosis, Wormian bones in children and basilar invagination causing posterior fossa symptoms. Other types of inherited phalangeal resorption exist.

There are many *other causes* of resorption of distal phalanges (Table 1.1). In some, resorption has a characteristic pattern and is accompanied by other features of the disease. Thus, in hyperparathyroidism, tuft resorption is accompanied by subperiosteal bone resorption around the cortices of middle phalanges.

Some patients have neurological lesions, e.g. in *syphilis*, *syringomyelia* and *diabetes*. In some conditions, such as

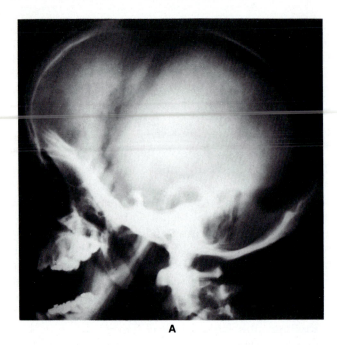

A

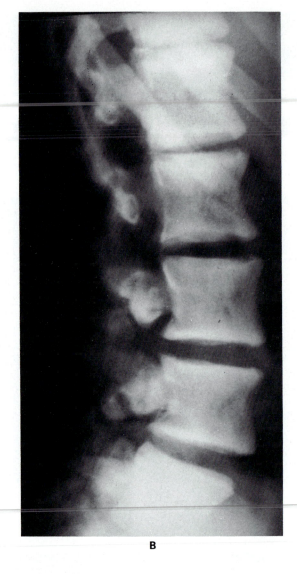

B

Fig. 1.24 Pycnodysostosis. **A**. The skull shows failure of sutural fusion and sclerosis of the base. The angle of the mandible is obtuse and the maxilla hypoplastic (see Ch. 50). **B**. Increased density of spool-shaped vertebral bodies with multiple pars fractures. (Courtesy of Dr. A. Thomas.)

Table 1.1 Atrophic changes in distal phalanges

Atrophy of distal phalanges may be seen in disorders due to many causes:

Congenital	Many forms of phalangeal agenesis may be found as congenital familial disorders.
Dysplastic	Cleidocranial dysplasia. Pycnodysostosis. Acro-osteolysis.
Infective	In acute infections usually only one digit affected — diagnosis obvious. Leprosy — neurotrophic factors contributory. Sarcoid.
Trauma	Frostbite. Electrical injuries.
Poisons	Ergot — peripheral arterial spasm and gangrene. Polyvinyl tank cleaners.
Metabolic	Hyperparathyroidism.
Vascular	Scleroderma with secondary Raynaud's phenomenon. Occlusive vascular disease. Pseudoxanthoma elasticum.
Neurotrophic	Tabes syringomyelia. Diabetes — vascular and infective changes may be contributory.
Neoplastic	Kaposi's sarcoma, where diffuse cutaneous and visual lesions are seen.
Miscellaneous	Psoriasis, pityriasis rubra, epidermolysis bullosa, reticulohistiocytosis. Ainhum. Neurofibromatosis. Progeria.

rheumatoid arthritis and *psoriasis*, peripheral vascular deficiency has been shown to occur in the region of tuft resorption.

OSTEOGENESIS IMPERFECTA
(synonym: *fragilitas ossium*; eponyms; *Vrolik = congenital recessive form*; *Lobstein = dominant form*)

This is a relatively rare disorder manifested by increased fragility of bones and osteoporosis, as well as dental abnormalities (see Ch. 50), lax joints and thin skin. Collagen is defective, so that the sclera, cornea, joints and skin are also abnormal.

Recessive form. Diagnosis of the more severe form of the disease, the congenital recessive form, has been made in utero. The children may be stillborn or die shortly after birth; only rarely do less severely affected patients survive into adult life. These patients often have blue sclerae.

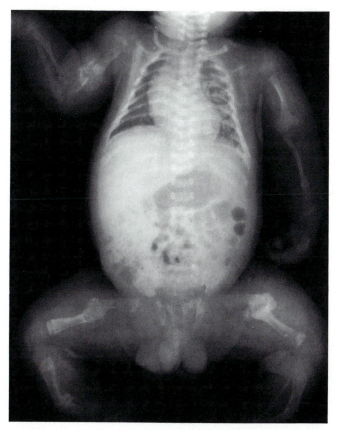

Fig. 1.25 Osteogenesis imperfecta congenita. Multiple fractures are seen at birth in this severely affected child.

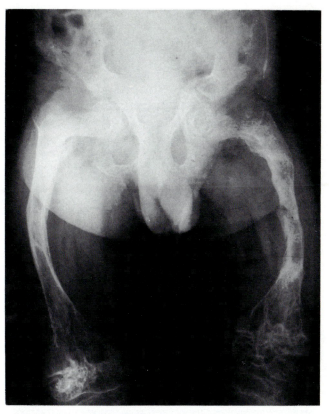

Fig. 1.26 Osteogenesis imperfecta — marked deformities, diminished bone density and recent and old fractures.

Overall the bones are grossly demineralized with thin cortices. Numerous healed or healing fractures are seen at birth despite the protection of amniotic fluid. Fractures also occur during delivery. Ribs and long bones are especially affected (Fig. 1.25), and hyperplastic callus may form.

Skull. Mineralization may be so severely retarded that only the petrous bones are calcified, and the vault is barely distinguishable from soft tissues. This may also occur in hypophosphatasia. Numerous Wormian bones are present.

Spine. Compression of vertebral bodies with demineralization is seen.

Limbs. Multiple fractures of soft bones in utero result in short, thick and bowed long bones with gross callus formation but non-union is also sometimes present. Fairbank (1951) commented on this 'thick bone type', distinguishing it from the 'thin bone type' which is probably not the recessive form even if present at birth. He also described a 'cystic type'. A cystic, grossly honeycomb appearance of bone is found in those recessive patients who survive birth.

Dominant form. This type is more frequent and varies greatly in its expression. Not all of the described changes need to be present.

Fractures may present at any age, but usually in the first five years of life. Some patients, however, develop multiple fractures in adult life; they clearly have a benign form of the disease. The fractures occur especially in the long bones of lower limbs and may be incomplete or transverse (Fig. 1.26). Healing again is by the formation of excessive callus, possibly because the periosteum is very loosely attached, and the appearance may simulate osteogenic sarcoma. A sarcomatous degeneration is indeed described but is extremely rare. If the callus does not organize properly, the bone ends up broad. Pseudarthroses are also found. Depending on the severity of the disease, however, the long bones are usually slender, deformed and bowed (Fig. 1.27). These changes, with demineralization and thin cortices, are characteristic of *osteogenesis imperfecta tarda*. Bowing results from softening and fractures. Metaphyseal softening results in invagination of the epiphysis into the metaphysis, often with premature fusion.

Skull. Wormian bones persist and the vault is thinned. The base of the skull is indented by the cervical spine so that the temporal and occipital bones bulge (Fig. 1.28). Basilar invagination may give rise to hydrocephalus. Deafness is found in adults and may be due to ankylosis of ossicles as well as to a form of osteosclerosis.

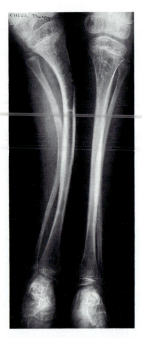

Fig. 1.27 Osteogenesis imperfecta. The long bones are gracile and bowed. Marked osteopenia is also present.

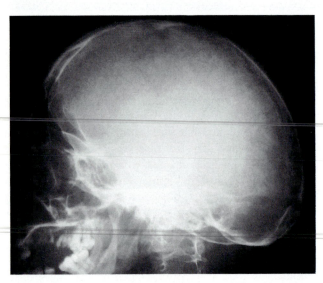

Fig. 1.28 Osteogenesis imperfecta. Persistence of Wormian bones and basilar invagination are shown.

Axial skeleton. Vertebral bodies are either flattened or have the appearance of 'cod fish' vertebrae. The pelvis shows protrusio acetabuli, and further compression hinders childbirth. The ribs are so soft and thin that the downward pull of the intercostal muscles makes their posterior portion convex *downwards*.

Teeth. Dentinogenesis imperfecta is an associated change (see Ch. 50).

Differential diagnosis.

Battered baby syndrome. In osteogenesis imperfecta the fractures are often diaphyseal rather than metaphyseal, and the urinary hydroxyproline is often elevated. The differentiation is often of medico-legal significance.

Idiopathic juvenile osteoporosis starts just before puberty and is usually self-limiting. Vertebral compression (Fig. 1.29) and characteristically *metaphyseal* fractures, especially of the lower limb long bones, occur (Fig. 1.30). The calcium balance is negative only in severe cases, otherwise the biochemical findings are normal.

FIBROGENESIS OSSIUM IMPERFECTA

This is a rare condition which affects elderly patients and usually presents with pathological fractures. *Radiologically,* a gross coarsening of trabeculae is present so that the

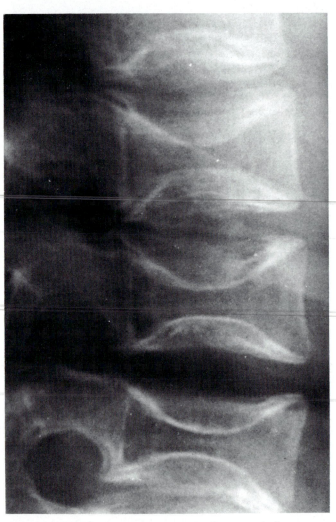

Fig. 1.29 Idiopathic juvenile osteoporosis. Gross vertebral compression affects mainly the central portions of the vertebral bodies.

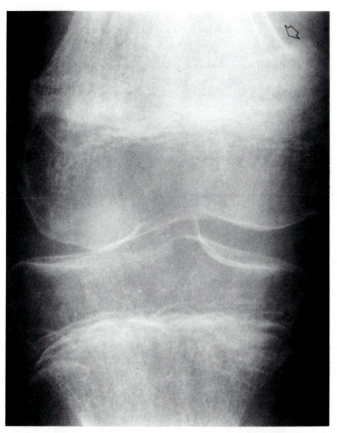

Fig. 1.30 Metaphyseal fractures around the knee in idiopathic juvenile osteoporosis distinguish this condition from osteogenesis imperfecta.

disease looks like Paget's disease (Fig. 1.31). All the bones are affected except the skull. Unlike Paget's disease, the bones retain their usual contour.

OSTEOPETROSIS

(synonym: *marble bones*; eponym: *Albers-Schonberg's disease*)

As with osteogenesis imperfecta and many other dysplasias, it is helpful to classify this disease into two forms.

1. A severe, often fatal, early form, manifest in infancy or childhood and inherited in an autosomal recessive form. This has been diagnosed in utero.

2. A more benign, tarda form, later in onset, inherited as a dominant.

Histologically there is failure of resorption of the primary primitive fetal spongiosa by the vascular mesenchyme. This primitive bone has a higher calcium content on ashing, and appears denser on radiology. The bone is brittle and fractures easily, but heals normally.

Normal bone may be laid down in episodes so that zones of normal and of denser bone may be seen, but the marrow is encroached upon and extramedullary haemopoiesis occurs (Fig. 1.32).

In the severe forms of the disease, anaemia and hepatosplenomegaly are found within months of birth and life expectancy is poor.

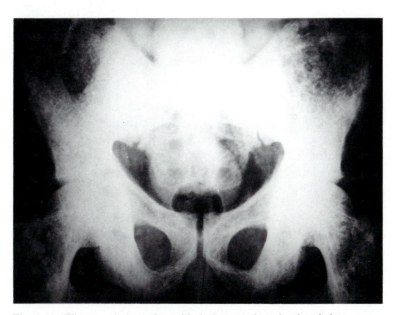

Fig. 1.31 Fibrogenesis imperfecta. Marked coarsening of trabeculation occurs throughout the skeleton but the bones retain their contour.

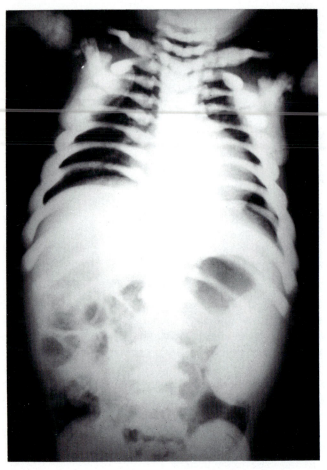

Fig. 1.32 Osteopetrosis. Bone density is uniformly increased apart from a small curved zone of normal bone at the iliac crest metaphysis. The spleen is the site of extramedullary haemopoiesis.

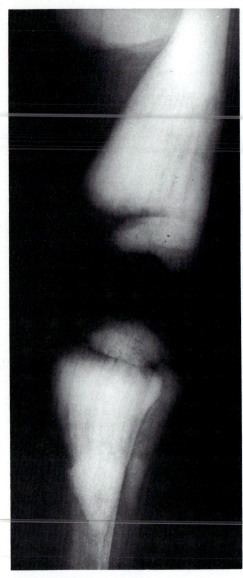

Fig. 1.33 Osteopetrosis — fine vertical lucencies are seen extending to the metaphyses, together with a 'bone within a bone' appearance at the tibial and fibular diaphyses.

In the tarda form of the disease, the diagnosis is often made fortuitously when 2–3 fractures occur, perhaps in the space of a year, in an adult patient. The bones may be slightly dense. Modelling abnormalities are seen in both forms with metaphyseal undertubulation.

Dental disease is common (see Ch. 50) with osteomyelitis occurring in the rather compact bone.

Radiological features. Increased density and thickening of long bones, especially metaphyses, can be seen in utero. The presence of a 'bone within a bone' differentiates osteopetrosis from the other sclerosing dysplasias. This is due to the cyclical nature of the disease, so that the dense shadow of, say, the tibia at the time of formation of abnormal bone is seen within the outline of the current normal or abnormal shadow. The timing of intrauterine onset of disease can thus be assessed. This 'bone within a bone' may be vertical in the long bone shafts and digits, transverse at the metaphyses or arcuate beneath the iliac crests.

Long bones. Besides the *'Erlenmayer flask'* deformity due to failure of metaphyseal remodelling, giving gross distal

undertubulation, and the presence of dense bone, vertical fine lucencies extending to the metaphyses are also present (Fig. 1.33), probably due to vascular channels being better seen against dense bone.

Fractures are usually transverse (Fig. 1.34) and heal with normal callus. Residual varus results from proximal femoral fractures. Some diaphyseal remodelling is to be expected. Skeletal maturation is normal.

Skull. (For dental abnormalities, see Ch. 50). The bones of the skull base are initially affected with sclerosis and thickening, prominent in the floor of the anterior cranial fossa. The cranium is affected to a lesser degree. The sphenoid and frontal sinuses and mastoids are underpneumatized or not at all. Neural foramina are

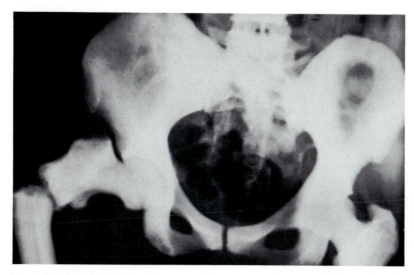

Fig. 1.34 Osteopetrosis — spontaneous fracture of upper end of right femur.

encroached upon and blindness results in serious cases. Bone softening with hydrocephalus does not appear to be a problem.

Spine. Platyspondyly does not seem to occur, but spondylolisthesis does. In vertebral bodies, an appearance like a 'rugger-jersey' spine may be seen due to the inserted shadow of an earlier, more dense body (Fig. 1.35).

In the adult form of the disease, the bones are roughly normal in shape. The medulla in the proximal skeleton is primarily involved and the periphery spared.

MELORHEOSTOSIS
(eponym: *Leri's disease*)
This is a very rare lesion affecting both sexes; no familial trend has been reported. Though the condition has not

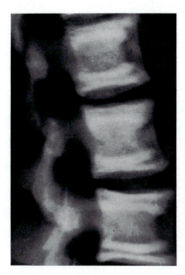

Fig. 1.35 Osteopetrosis — note inset of an earlier vertebra within each vertebral body.

been observed in a child under the age of 3 years, there is strong presumptive evidence that it is present at birth.

Patients may complain of pain and of restricted movements of joints but the condition is often asymptomatic. Some cases are associated with skin lesions, such as scleroderma, and with vascular anomalies; joint contractures may be found in some patients.

The condition is characterized by the presence of dense irregular bone running down the cortex of a long bone. Both the internal and external aspects of the cortex may be affected. Dense areas tend to be overgrown and bowing may result. Murray and McCredie (1979) have pointed out that the distribution of the new bone corresponds to a sclerotome, the segmental root nerve innervation of a bone.

The new bone has been likened to molten wax running down the side of a burning candle (Fig. 1.36). The lesions tend to be segmental and unilateral, though both limbs on one side of the body may be affected. Occasionally the condition is bilateral but never symmetrical. Some lesions are progressive. The lower limbs are most commonly affected. Premature epiphyseal fusion may result, so that an affected limb may be larger or smaller than normal.

The skull, spine and ribs are rarely affected. Ectopic bone may be found in soft tissues around joints between affected bones.

OSTEOPOIKILOSIS
(synonym: *osteopathia condensans disseminata*)
This is usually an incidental radiological finding but some patients have associated skin nodules. The lesions are familial. It affects both sexes equally and is characterized by the presence of multiple dense radiopaque spots which are round, oval or lanceolate, and tend to be situated

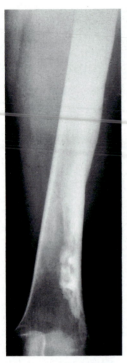

Fig. 1.36 Melorheostosis. New bone is applied both on the inside and outside of the femoral cortex. The bone as a whole is widened.

This lesion must be differentiated from serious conditions such as tuberous sclerosis and metastases, but their distributions around joints, and the fact that the nodules rarely increase in size or number under observation, distinguish this benign condition from metastases.

OSTEOPATHIA STRIATA
(eponym: *Voorhoeve's disease*)

In this asymptomatic disorder sclerotic striations are found in the long bones, especially of the lower limbs, affecting both bone ends and diaphyses (Fig. 1.38).

FIBROUS DYSPLASIA

This is a disease of unknown aetiology. It is probably more common in women. The disease is found in two

parallel to the axis of the affected bone. They are usually uniform in density but may have relatively clear central zones. Any bone may be affected. They occur especially frequently in the ends of long bones and around joints, in the carpus and tarsus, and in the pelvis (Fig. 1.37).

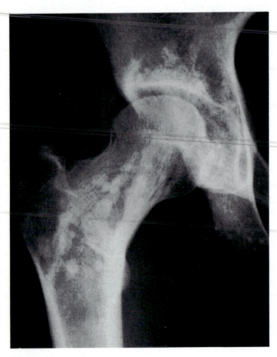

Fig. 1.37 Osteopoikilosis.

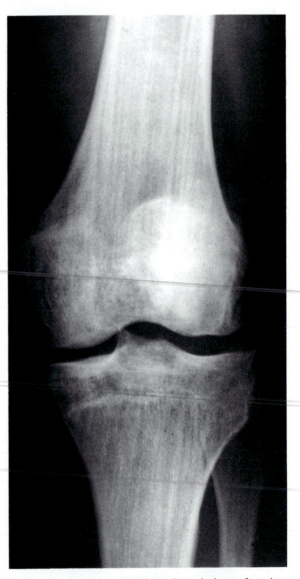

Fig. 1.38 Vertical striation extends to the articular surfaces in osteopathia striata.

forms, monostotic and polyostotic. With polyostotic disease, over 50% of the skeleton may be involved, but symmetry is unusual and the lesions tend to be unilaterally distributed. The lesions are usually found incidentally or following pathological fracture. Deformity may occasionally be marked. The alkaline phosphatase is elevated but does not correlate with the extent of the disease. The age of onset is usually between 10 and 30, but polyostotic disease may present in the first decade. The lesions often cease growing with skeletal maturity but may be seen in old age. Monostotic lesions are more likely to enlarge in adult life. Prognosis is worse when the lesions occur early in life.

Pathologically, medullary bone is replaced by well-defined areas of fibrous tissue, and cysts containing blood or serous fluid. These appear similar on radiographs. The fibrous tissue then undergoes varying degrees of abnormal ossification so that some of the lesions show an increase in density, dependent on the extent of ossification. This increase in density may thus be patchy, giving a cottonwool appearance, or homogeneous giving a ground glass appearance.

Radiologically, the lesions have a smooth dense margin of varying width, often so wide as to resemble the rind of an orange. The bone is expanded and the cortex scalloped and thinned but intact. Lesions tend to be multilocular and expand down the medulla rather than cause great cortical expansion (Fig. 1.39). Unlike Paget's disease, the bone ends are not necessarily affected and lesions tend to be diametaphyseal. Bone ends may be involved after fusion and epiphyses may be involved in the child.

Any bone may be affected, though involvement of the spine is uncommon and vertebral collapse is unusual. Lesions do not really need to be diagnosed by biopsy as the appearances are usually characteristic.

The pelvis (Fig. 1.40), femur and ribs are commonly involved. In the skull, the frontal, sphenoid parietal and maxillary bones and mandible are often affected (Fig. 1.41). In the *femur*, deformity due to softening, expansion and fracture give an appearance likened to a 'shepherd's crook' (Fig. 1.42) and discrepancies in limb length result. Lesions are well defined and may be expanded with well-defined margins. These may be lucent, dense or a mixture of the two, with small flecks of density due to ossification.

In the *skull*, a grossly expanded sclerotic hyperostosis of the sphenoid may resemble a meningioma. Orbital fissures may be encroached upon and proptosis may result. Obliteration and bony expansion of the facial sinuses make the face appear grotesque and mask-like. In the vault, lesions tend to be grossly expansile, sclerotic, but localized (blister lesion).

The lesions show increased uptake on *radionuclide scans*.

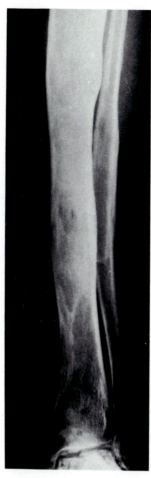

Fig. 1.39 Fibrous dysplasia — tibia and fibula showing irregular expansion, ground-glass appearance in upper part of the tibia and cystic changes in the lower end.

Complications. — a. Fractures, deformity and irregularity of limb length have been mentioned. Nerve palsies may occur in the skull.

b. Endocrine complications. *Albright's syndrome* consists of skin pigmentation, usually on the side of the bone lesions, fibrous dysplasia (usually polyostotic) and precocious puberty. This occurs usually in girls, and only rarely in boys. Most patients with skin pigmentation and polyostotic disease do not have associated endocrine disease and, in girls, only 50% have precocious puberty.

Hyperthyroidism, acromegaly, Cushing's syndrome, gynaecomastia and *parathyroid enlargement* have all been reported in association with polyostotic fibrous dysplasia.

c. Sarcomatous degeneration occurs in less than 1% of patients, usually to *fibrosarcoma* (Fig. 1.43). Some, but not all, of these patients give a history of previous irradiation.

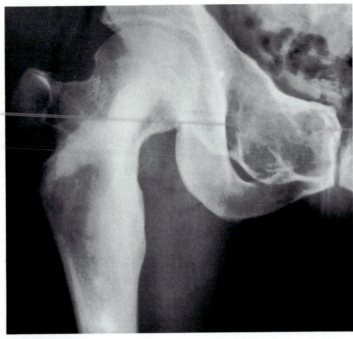

Fig. 1.40   Fibrous dysplasia — large expanding lesion in superior pubic ramus and sclerosis in upper end of the femur.

CHONDRODYSTROPHIA CALCIFICANS CONGENITA

(synonyms: *dysplasia epiphysealis punctata: stippled epiphyses*)

This disease exists in two forms.

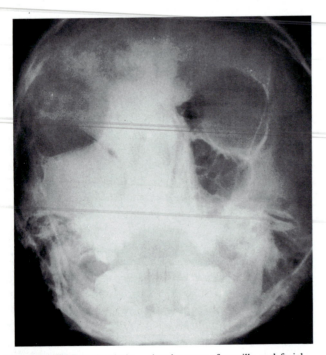

Fig. 1.41   Fibrous dysplasia — involvement of maxilla and facial bones on right side.

1. The less severe *dominant* form. Even in this form, early fatal disease may occur. The condition is characterized in infancy by stippling or punctate calcification of the tarsus and carpus, long bone epiphyses, vertebral transverse processes and the pubic bones. The resulting epiphyses in later life are often misshapen, and deformities with asymmetric limb shortening result. The spine often ends up scoliotic but if the infants survive, life expectancy is normal.

2. The more severe *recessive* form usually results in death in the first year; survivors are likely to be mentally defective. Stippling is present as above but is if anything more gross, also occurring in the trachea. Long bones show gross symmetrical shortening and metaphyseal irregularity. In this form the vertebral bodies show a vertical radiolucency on the lateral view which does not occur in the dominant type (Fig. 1.44). In survivors, there is marked retardation of epiphyseal development.

MULTIPLE EPIPHYSEAL DYSPLASIA

(synonym: *dysplasia epiphysealis multiplex*)

This condition, which is transmitted as an autosomal dominant, primarily affects epiphyses. Dwarfism of the short-limb type may be seen. The condition may express itself in various ways, so much so that some writers subdivide the disease into a severe form (*Fairbank*) characterized by small epiphyses, and a mild type (*Ribbing*) characterized by flat epiphyses.

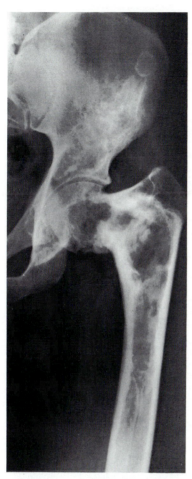

Fig. 1.42 Fibrous dysplasia — marked coxa vara secondary to cystic changes in the femoral neck. Sclerotic changes also in left ilium.

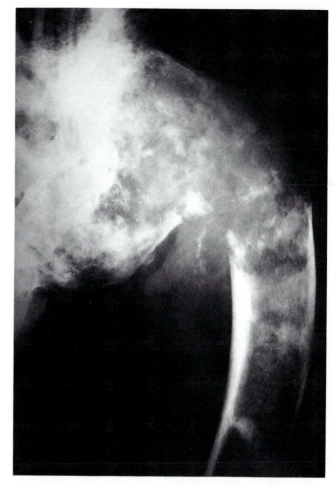

Fig. 1.43 A pathological fracture with irregular bone destruction due to malignant degeneration is superimposed upon fibrous dysplasia.

In order of frequency, the epiphyses affected are those of the hips, shoulders, ankles, knees, wrists and elbows. Epiphyses tend to appear late and are fragmented and flattened (Figs 1.45–48); the deformities persist throughout life and cause premature osteoarthritis. No characteristic changes are found in the metaphyses but they may be widened to conform to the deformed contiguous epiphyses. Secondary changes in contour are often seen in the glenoid and acetabular fossae. The carpal and tarsal bones may be affected and digits and toes may be 'stubby'. The skull is not affected. Some features may be characteristic but none are constant.

a. *Lower tibial epiphysis* — the lateral part of the lower tibial epiphysis is thinner than the medial part; the trochlear part of the talus is shaped to conform to the abnormal mortice. A tibiotalar slant results (Fig. 1.46).

b. *The double layered patella* (Fig. 1.47) is characteristic but is found in few cases.

c. *The femoral and tibial condyles* may be hypoplastic and the intercondylar notch shallow (Fig. 1.48). Flattening of the femoral and tibial condyles makes the joint look widened.

Spinal changes are seldom pronounced and may be absent. The appearances in the spine, if present, resemble osteochondritis. Some cases of chondrodystrophia calcificans congenita may survive and their pattern may later resemble that of multiple epiphyseal dysplasia.

DYSPLASIA EPIPHYSEALIS HEMIMELICA
(synonym: *tarsoepiphyseal aclasis*; eponym: *Trevor's disease*)

In this rare condition irregular overgrowth of part of an epiphysis or epiphyses lying on one side of a single limb is seen (Fig. 1.49). The leg is commonly affected but the arm may be. Sometimes both an arm and a leg may be involved and bilateral lesions have been recorded. If more

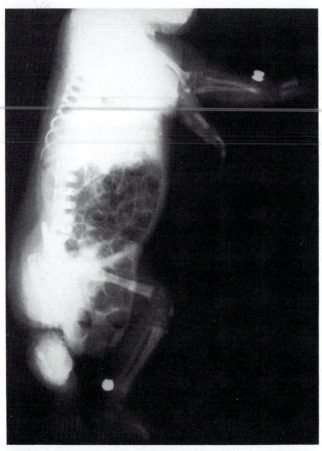

Fig. 1.44   Chondrodysplasia calcificans congenita. Clefts of the vertebral bodies are prominent in this case, together with stippled epiphyses and punctate calcifications around the joints and in the tracheal cartilages.

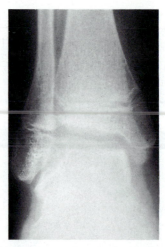

Fig. 1.46   Dysplasia epiphysealis multiplex, showing thinning of the outer part of the lower tibial epiphysis; this is seen in about half of all cases.

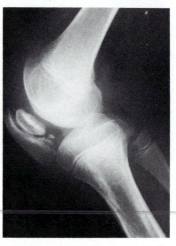

Fig. 1.47   Knee of same patient as Fig. 1.46. Marked fragmentation of the patella.

than one epiphysis is affected then the same parts, i.e. the medial or lateral, of the other epiphyses are abnormal.

Hyperplasia of the affected epiphysis may lead to a lesion that is indistinguishable radiologically and histologically from an osteochondroma. The lesions may be

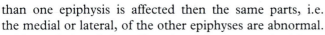
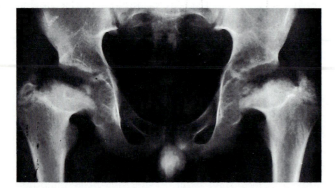

Fig. 1.45   Dysplasia epiphysealis multiplex. Both femoral heads are hypoplastic and fragmented. The femoral necks are irregular and broad. Similar changes are seen at the greater trochanteric apophyses. Dysplastic acetabula are demonstrated.

easily palpable. Such a feature is relatively common in the lower end of the fibula and adjacent talus (Fig. 1.49).

METAPHYSEAL CHONDRODYSPLASIA
(synonym: *metaphyseal dysplasia, metaphyseal dysostosis*)

1. *Schmid* described a mild type that is relatively common (Fig. 1.50). Metaphyses of long bones are cupped and resemble rickets. No biochemical changes are found. The patient may be wrongly diagnosed as suffering from vitamin D-resistant rickets and consequently and injudiciously given large doses of vitamin D.

2. *Jansen's metaphyseal chondrodysplasia*. Grossly irregular mineralization is seen in the metaphyses of tubular bones (Fig. 1.51). A large gap is also seen between the epiphyses and disordered metaphyses.

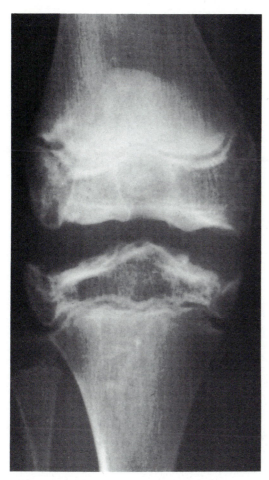

Fig. 1.48 Dysplasia epiphysealis multiplex — angular condyles and flat intercondylar notch. This is a characteristic appearance though not always present.

3. Other types named after *Pena* and *Vaandrager* show intermediate involvement of metaphyses, less than in the Jansen type but more than in the Schmid type. Such lesions may resemble Ollier's disease.

4. Some cases of metaphyseal chondrodysplasia are associated with *pancreatic insufficiency* and *neutropenia*.

5. *McKusick* described a syndrome of sparse hair, metaphyseal lesions and dwarfism in Amish families — *cartilage-hair hypoplasia*.

6. Sometimes metaphyseal changes are associated with lesions of the spine — such conditions should be designated *spondylometaphyseal dysostosis*.

DIAPHYSEAL ACLASIS
(synonym: *hereditary multiple exostoses*)

This disease is inherited and familial. Sixty per cent of those affected have an involved parent. The remainder are presumably mutants to the gene. The sex incidence is equal and lesions within the family are not necessarily of the same severity.

The bones chiefly affected are the long bones, especially in the *metaphyseal* regions of the shoulders, hips, knees and ankles, which become irregularly expanded and club-shaped. Upon these local enlargements of the shaft are projected osseous excrescences — *exostoses* — which are round or pointed. Their cortex merges with that of the shaft and their cancellous bone merges with the cancellous bone of the shaft, that is, they do not lie upon the cortex. Exostoses are also found on the vertebral bodies and on the medial border of the scapula. The epiphyses are not involved.

Exostoses may be seen as small metaphyseal projections in infants and their growth may be observed. With growth, they come to point away from the adjacent joint (Fig. 1.52). During skeletal growth, the bony exostoses are covered by a cartilage cap which undergoes spotty calcification, and with increasing maturity the cartilaginous mass becomes increasingly dense and a smooth margin can be discerned. By the time growth ceases, the cartilage has usually completely ossified. The exostoses and the metaphyseal clubbing are separate lesions though the former may be superimposed on the latter.

Increase in transverse width is often accompanied by shortening so that deformities result. These changes are especially common at the radius and ulna so that Madelung deformity results (Fig. 1.53). Metacarpal bowing, radioulnar synostosis and radial head dislocation may also be found. Ollier's disease gives a similar appearance.

Lesions may be apparent early in life, especially if it is known that one parent is affected or a lesion may affect a subcutaneous bone such as the tibia. Nerve compression may occur and paraplegia may result if the vertebral column is affected (Fig. 1.54.) Some lesions may present with a dull ache, but pain and rapid growth raise the possibility of malignant degeneration. The incidence of *chondrosarcoma* in diaphyseal aclasis is said to be about 10%, and these are often around the hip.

ACHONDROPLASIA

This is the most common type of disproportionate dwarfism. In sufferers, one part of a limb shows relatively greater shortening. If proximal, *rhizomelia* is present; if medial, *mesomelia*; if distal, *acromelia*. In recent years many conditions, such as *thanatophoric dwarfism*, have been split off from achondroplasia so that a truly homogeneous picture now emerges. Inheritance is autosomal dominant but most cases (85%) seem to be due to mutation of the gene, probably in older fathers. The patients have normal intelligence though a lack of muscle tone at birth suggests retardation.

The children have characteristic features at birth. *Trident hands* with short stubby fingers, a *depressed nasal bridge* with a prominent forehead and a disproportionally *large skull*, and *prominent buttocks* due to lumbar lordosis

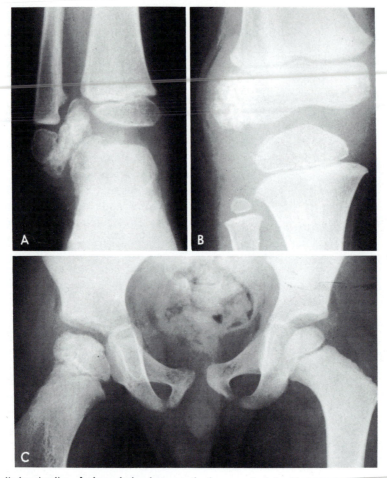

Fig. 1.49 Dysplasia epiphysealis hemimelica. **A** shows lesion between the lower end of the fibula and the talus; **B** and **C** show involvement of outer part of the lower femoral and femoral capital epiphyses respectively.

are all seen. The large head can obstruct labour. Limb bones are short with a rhizomelic pattern.

Radiological findings. *Long bones*. The tubular bones are short, appear relatively widened and have prominent muscle insertions. The humeri and femora are affected more than distal bones (rhizomelia). The fibulae are long and bowed. The epiphyses are deformed by their insertion into V-shaped defects at the metaphyses. The epiphyses themselves have V-shaped distal ends with deep inter-condylar notches. The appearances are similar to those

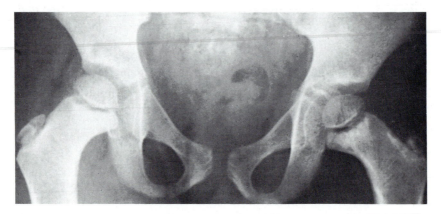

Fig. 1.50 Metaphyseal chondrodysplasia, type Schmid; mild changes only in upper femoral metaphyses. Other metaphyses were similarly affected.

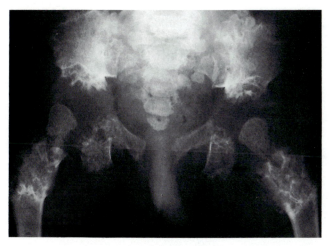

Fig. 1.51 Metaphyseal chondrodysplasia, type Jansen. Here a much more severe form of metaphyseal irregularity is seen than the type described by Schmid.

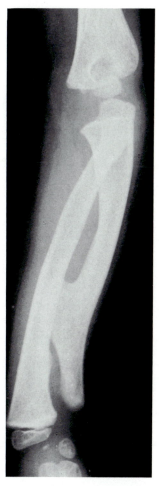

Fig. 1.53 Diaphyseal aclasis — typical deformity of bones of the forearm.

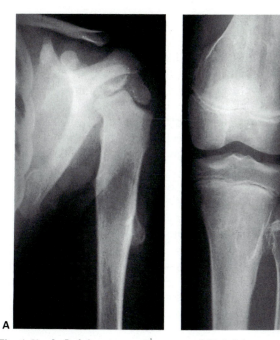

Fig. 1.52 **A**. Left humerus at 3¼ years, and **B**, left knee at 10 years, of the same child with diaphyseal aclasis. Films of the same areas taken in infancy seemed normal.

seen with local premature fusion after infection, trauma or irradiation. The joint spaces appear widened owing to the proximity of epiphyses and metaphyses.

Retardation of ossification and a reduced anteroposterior diameter cause the upper ends of the femora of babies to appear relatively radiolucent. A defect is present in older children at the site of the epiphysis of the tibial tubercle due to an excess of uncalcified cartilage at this age.

Pelvis. The pelvis is small and its diameters reduced. The iliac blades are particularly small and rather square

— the 'tombstone' appearance. The acetabula are set posteriorly and the acetabular roofs are horizontal (Fig. 1.55). L5 is deeply set and excessive pelvic tilt causes prominence of the buttocks and an illusion of lordosis. The sacrosciatic notch is narrow, with a prominent medially directed spur. The pelvic inlet resembles a champagne glass.

Spine. The anteroposterior diameters of vertebral bodies are often short but the height of vertebral bodies is insignificantly reduced. In the thoracolumbar region a vertebral body or two may appear wedged or bullet-nosed. In some a thoracolumbar vertebral body may resemble that found in Hurler's syndrome. Scalloping at the back of vertebrae may be seen (Fig. 1.56).

The spinal canal in the lumbar region tapers caudally so that the interpedicular distances decrease from L1 to L5 (Figs 1.55 and 1.56). The lateral view will also show the small spinal canal. Severe symptoms from disc protrusions are liable to develop in later life — the spinal stenosis in the lumbosacral region is an important predisposing factor and can be confirmed by radiculography or CT.

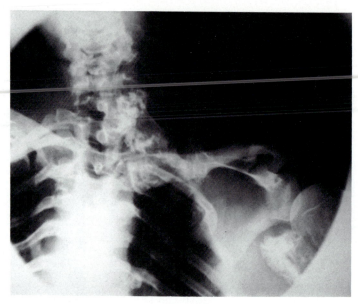

Fig. 1.54 Diaphyseal aclasis. Exostoses are seen associated with the spine in this patient who developed paraplegia.

Skull changes are mandatory to the diagnosis of achondroplasia. The calvarium is large but the base is shortened. The sella may be small. The foramen magnum is characteristically small and funnel-shaped — hydrocephalus may occur and has been attributed to this mechanical cause.

Chest. The ribs are short, the anterior ends widened and the sternum short and broad. The scapulae have peculiar shapes, losing their sharp angles; the glenoid fossae are small in relation to the humeral heads.

Hands and feet. Tubular bones of the hands and feet appear short and wide, but carpal and tarsal bones are little affected (Fig. 1.57). The *trident hand*, in which all the fingers are almost of equal length and diverge from one another in two pairs plus the thumb, is often found.

HYPOCHONDROPLASIA

This is a condition which has been separated from classical achondroplasia, though there are some features in common. The skull is never affected, and the patients are either normal or mildly reduced in height. The disease is inherited as a dominant. The abdomen and buttocks are prominent, as in achondroplasia, and the legs are bowed in childhood.

Radiologically, there is rhizomelia with a short, broad femoral neck. The distal fibula is overgrown compared with the distal tibia (Fig. 1.58). The iliac bones are smaller than normal but not as markedly reduced as in achondroplasia. The interpedicular distances narrow from L1 to L5 and the pedicles are short, so that spinal stenosis results (Fig. 1.59). The lumbar lordosis is increased.

PSEUDOACHONDROPLASIA

This condition is a short-limbed dwarfism occurring in both recessive and dominant forms of mild or marked severity, so that some patients are barely affected and some are grossly deformed. In all patients, however, the skull is normal, distinguishing this condition from achondroplasia. Also, no changes are seen in the first year of life.

Spine. Vertebral bodies may be flat and irregular with central anterior 'tongues' (Fig. 1.60A). In adult life appearances vary from near normal to platyspondyly and scoliosis. The spine in multiple epiphyseal dysplasia is barely affected.

Long bones. The epiphyses are delayed in appearance and markedly irregular (Fig. 1.60B), again differing from achondroplasia. Metaphyses are broad and spurred. After fusion, epiphyseal dysplasia of varying degrees of severity is found.

Pelvis. The acetabulum is irregular and premature osteoarthritis of the hips occurs. The ilia are large and the pubes and ischia short.

Hands. In severe cases, the tubular bones are short and stubby with delay in ossification of irregular epiphyses and carpal bones (Fig. 1.60C). In the adult the metacarpals end up shortened. Shortening of radius and ulna may be marked and both bones at the wrist may be hypoplastic centrally, giving a 'V' appearance.

THANATOPHORIC DWARFISM

This has only relatively recently been separated from achondroplasia and is the commonest fatal neonatal dysplasia.

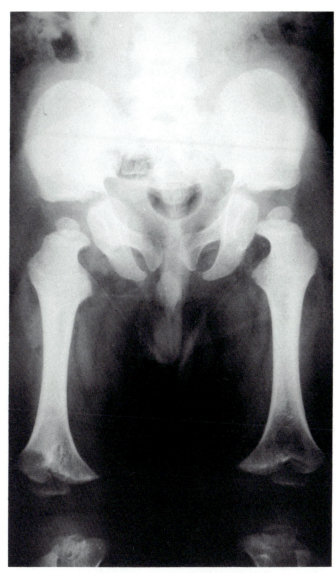

Fig. 1.55 Achondroplasia. Square iliac blades with horizontal acetabular roofs. Note also the narrow interpedicular distances in the lumbosacral region and the defects at the distal femoral metaphyses into which the epiphyses insert.

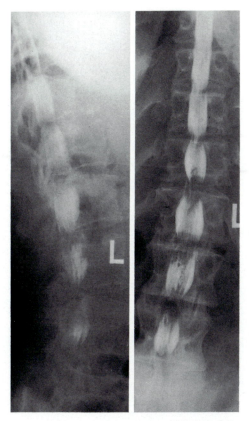

Fig. 1.56 Achondroplasia. Canal stenosis is demonstrated at radiculography. Posterior scalloping of vertebral bodies is shown between areas of discal indentation upon the opacified theca.

Radiological findings. *Limbs*. There is rhizomelic dwarfism but the long bones are bowed. The metaphyses are irregular. Epiphyses of the knee are absent at birth. Short, wide metacarpals and phalanges are shown.

Axial skeleton. There is marked platyspondyly but the posterior vertebral elements are normal, so that on an anterior view the vertebral bodies resemble the letter H (Fig. 1.61). The pelvis shows poor mineralization of ischium and pubis, and small square iliac blades. The skull often shows lateral temporal bulging (cloverleaf skull) due to craniostenosis.

The ribs are short and flared anteriorly.

The infants are stillborn or die shortly after birth.

ASPHYXIATING THORACIC DYSPLASIA
(eponym: *Jeune disease*)

Most, but not all, patients with the disease die in infancy from respiratory distress. In contradistinction to thanatophoric dwarfism, the spine is normal and the long bones are not curved and only a little shortened.

The thorax is stenotic. The ribs are short and horizontal and the clavicles highly placed (Fig. 1.62).

Polydactyly is present in many cases and epiphyses are present at the knee.

Inheritance is autosomal recessive. In those patients who survive, renal failure may result, even if bone changes revert to normal.

CHONDROECTODERMAL DYSPLASIA
(eponym: *Ellis–van Creveld disease*)

Fifty per cent of patients have congenital cardiac defects which may be fatal.

Radiographic features. *Limbs*. In the limbs, the paired long bones are short and the metaphyses dome-shaped (Fig. 1.63). At the proximal tibia the developing epiphysis is situated over the abnormal medial tibial plateau and is defective laterally so that valgus deformity

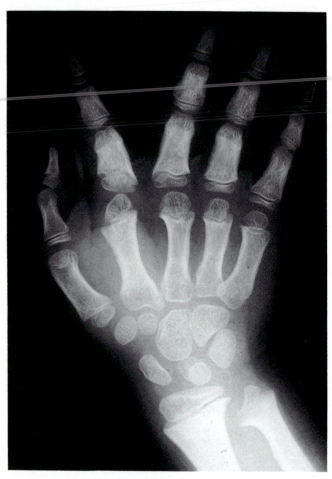

Fig. 1.57 Trident hand in achondroplasia.

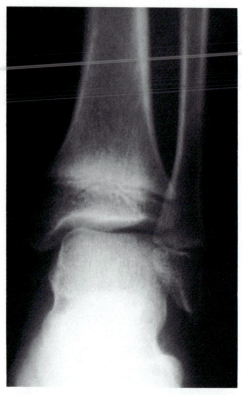

Fig. 1.58 Overgrowth of the distal fibula in hypochondroplasia.

results. Postaxial polysyndactyly is also present (Fig. 1.64).

Axial skeleton. The skull and spine are normal. The rib cage resembles that seen in asphyxiating thoracic dystrophy. The acetabulum has a medial spur in the region of the triradiate cartilage.

The ectodermal dysplasia, with partial or total absence of teeth, and abnormal hair and nails, is not seen in asphyxiating thoracic dystrophy.

DYSCHONDROSTEOSIS
(eponym: *Leri-Weil disease*)

Inherited as an autosomal dominant, the patients are short in stature with a mesomeric type of dwarfism. There is hypoplasia of the inner aspect of the distal radius and the ulna is therefore prominent. It is subluxed dorsally (Madelung deformity). The carpal bones herniate proximally into the deficiency caused by the hypoplastic radius (Fig. 1.65).

The medial aspect of the proximal/distal tibia is similarly defective.

MUCOPOLYSACCHARIDOSES AND MUCOLIPOIDOSES

The above terms embrace an extremely complex group of disorders. All members of the group are associated with an abnormality in mucopolysaccharide or glycoprotein metabolism. The most that can be expected of the radiologist is to suggest a diagnosis of mucopolysaccharidosis (MPS), and niceties of nosology are the province of the clinician, geneticist and biochemist. The same considerations apply to the mucolipoidoses.

Types of mucopolysaccharidoses are:

1. MPS I-H (Hurler syndrome; gargoylism)
2. MPS II (Hunter syndrome)
3. MPS III (Sanfilippo syndrome)
4. MPS IV (Morquio-Brailsford syndrome)
5. MPS I-S (Scheie syndrome)
6. MPS VI (Maroteaux-Lamy syndrome)

The *Hunter* type is inherited as an X-linked recessive, the rest as autosomal recessives. Some are severe, others relatively mild. Sufferers have various degrees of mental retardation, corneal clouding and skeletal changes.

MPS I-H
(synonym: *gargoylism*; eponym: *Hurler syndrome*)

Radiological features: Changes include macrocephaly,

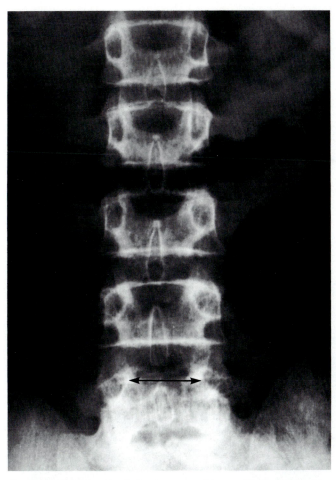

Fig. 1.59 Hypochondroplasia. A narrowed interpedicular distance at L5 in the same patient as Fig. 1.58.

J-shaped sella, thickened calvaria, oar-shaped ribs and hook-shaped vertebral bodies (Fig. 1.66). The ilia are widely flared, the femoral ossific nuclei fragmented and coxa valga is usual. The proximal ends of the metacarpals taper and in older children the distal ends of the radius and especially the ulna slope towards each other (Fig. 1.67).

MPS IV
(eponym: *Morquio-Brailsford disease*)

This condition presents with dwarfism, due mainly to shortness of the spine and to a marked kyphosis. The tubular bones are also widely affected. The lesion may be familial. Intelligence is unimpaired.

Radiographic features. Spinal changes are the dominant feature. The vertebrae are flat, and in childhood tend to have a characteristic form. The upper and lower surfaces of the vertebral body are defective and a central tongue of bone protrudes forwards (Fig. 1.68). This appearance is seen best in the lower dorsal and upper lumbar region. Later, as growth proceeds, the defect

becomes repaired. One dorsolumbar vertebra may be smaller than its fellows and displaced posteriorly, causing a marked kyphosis.

As a rule, tubular bones are not markedly affected but may be short and rather wide with somewhat irregular metaphyses. The epiphyses are markedly irregular and fragmented, notably those of the femoral heads. The joint spaces are increased and the joint surfaces, e.g. of the acetabulum and glenoid, are shallow and irregular.

The pelvis tends to be narrow, or shaped like that of an ape (Fig. 1.69). In the hands and feet the tubular bones are short and stubby, and some irregularity of the carpal and tarsal bones is also found.

SPONDYLOEPIPHYSEAL DYSPLASIA

The term 'spondyloepiphyseal dysplasia' (SED) is used to embrace a group of conditions characterized by platyspondyly and dysplasia of other bones. The degrees of spinal and tubular bone involvement and the amount of dwarfism vary between the different groups.

1. *X-linked variety — SED tarda*. This type has a distinctive spinal lesion. Mounds of dense bone are found on the superior and inferior surfaces of the posterior parts of the vertebral end-plates (Fig. 1.70). The tubular bones are not much affected and may resemble those in mild cases of dysplasia epiphysealis multiplex. The iliac wings are characteristically small. Hip degeneration frequently occurs prematurely (Fig. 1.71).

2. *Dominant variety — SED congenita*. In these the platyspondyly is maximal in the thoracic spine. Lesions of tubular bones are severe and early osteoarthritis may be expected. The hands are unaffected. Retinal detachment is common.

3. *Recessive variety*. — The platyspondyly is generalized and the severe wedging of the dominant form is not found.

HYPOPHOSPHATASIA

This is a genetically determined metabolic disease, included in this section on account of its manifestations. Several subgroups have been described, dependent on the age of onset and severity of symptoms. They are characterized by; 1. low or absent serum alkaline phosphatase; 2. phosphoethanolamine in the urine and plasma; 3. hypercalcaemia in severe forms.

In the severe type, gross general failure of ossification of the skeleton is seen (Fig. 1.72). These babies do not survive. Some less severe forms present as severe rickets. If they survive, the radiographic picture may resemble that of Ollier's disease. An adult form of this condition is characterized by osteoporosis and a tendency to fractures.

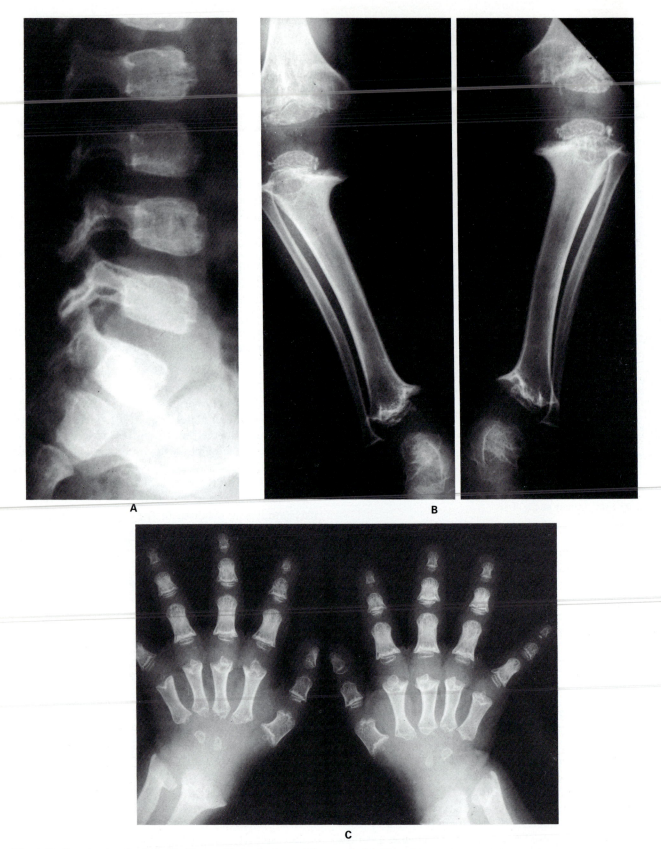

Fig. 1.60 Pseudoachondroplasia. **A**. Tongue-like projections of the vertebral bodies with superior and inferior defects. **B**. Long bones — irregular epiphyses and metaphyses with tilt deformities. **C**. Hands — the radius and ulna are flared at the metaphyses, the carpal bone epiphyses delayed and irregular, and the metacarpals short. The phalanges are stubby and the epiphyses angular and irregular.

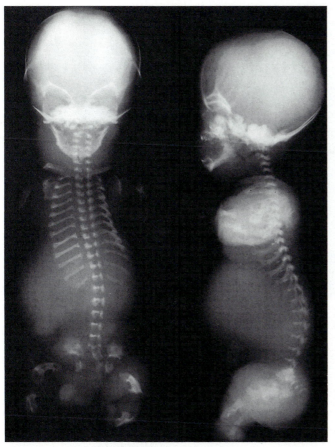

Fig. 1.61 Thanatophoric dwarfism. A cloverleaf skull is present. The scapulae are hypoplastic and the clavicles high. Platyspondyly is shown, resulting in H-shaped vertebral bodies. The bones are short and bowed.

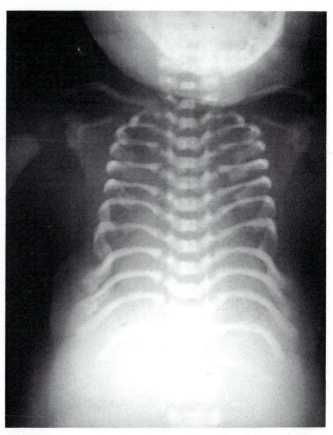

Fig. 1.62 Asphyxiating thoracic dystrophy — short horizontal ribs with high clavicles but a normal spine. The scapulae are hypoplastic.

ARACHNODACTYLY
(eponym: *Marfan's syndrome*)

This condition is inherited as an autosomal dominant. Clinically, the long bones are lengthened and muscle weakness, hypermobility and lens dislocations are found. A high arched palate, depressed sterum and scoliosis also occur. Cardiovascular lesions include aortic dissections, atrial septal defects and mitral valve lesions.

Radiographic features. The tubular bones are elongated and slender, the distal bones being much more affected than the proximal ones. The hands and feet are especially elongated (Fig. 1.73) and occasionally their bones have extra epiphyses. Kyphosis and scoliosis are frequent findings. Some scalloping of the back of vertebral bodies may be seen.

The diagnosis is usually straightforward. Estimation of the *metacarpal index* will aid the diagnosis in doubtful cases. This index is estimated by measuring the lengths of the second, third, fourth and fifth metacarpals and dividing by their breadths taken at the exact mid-points. The

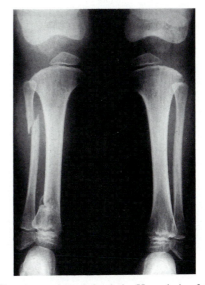

Fig. 1.63 Chondroectodermal dysplasia. Hypoplasia of the lateral portion of the upper tibial epiphyses is present and the metaphysis is dome-shaped. Incidental fractures are demonstrated.

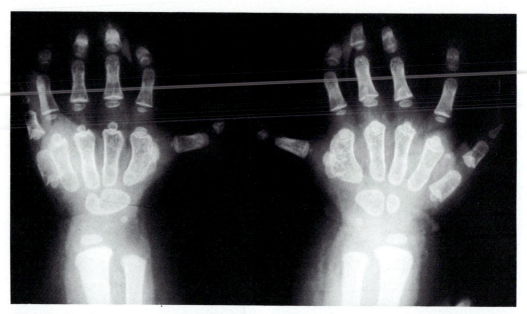

Fig. 1.64 Chondroectodermal dysplasia. Polysyndactyly is present together with anomalies of carpal segmentation.

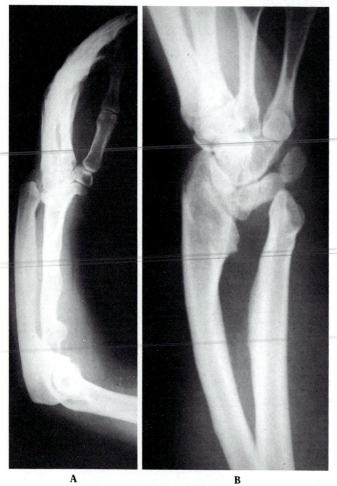

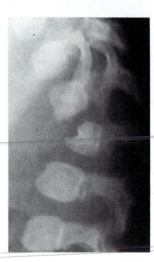

Fig. 1.66 MPS I-H (Hurler's syndrome). Hypoplasia of L2 body with a pronounced inferior beak and a resulting angular kyphosis.

A   **B**

Fig. 1.65 Dyschondrosteosis. **A**. There is separation of the hypoplastic distal radius and ulna with proximal herniation of the carpus. **B**. The lateral view shows the posterior situation of the ulna and hypoplasia of the proximal radius.

resulting figures, from each of the four metacarpals, are added together and divided by four. In normal adult subjects the metacarpal index varies from 5.4 to 7.9; in arachnodactyly the range varies from 8.4 to 10.4.

HOMOCYSTINURIA

This lesion has some similarity to Marfan's syndrome but is inherited as an autosomal recessive. A definite biochemical abnormality has been demonstrated. Absence of the enzyme cystathionine synthesase results in an excess of urinary homocystine. The most important feature is that thrombosis of arteries and veins is liable to occur,

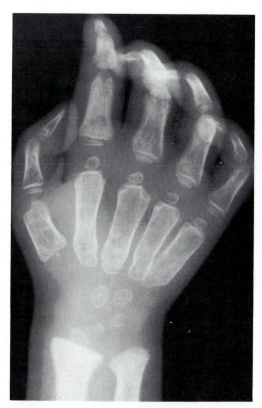

Fig. 1.67 MPS I-H (Hurler's syndrome). Undertubulation is associated with demineralization. The metacarpals are pointed proximally. The distal radius and ulna are angulated.

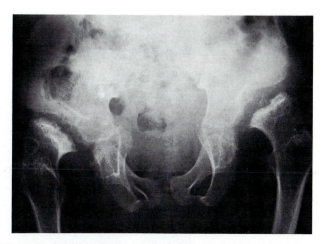

Fig. 1.69 MPS IV. Simian pelvis, fragmented maldeveloped femoral capital epiphyses with associated metaphyseal irregularity. Shallow acetabula with dislocation of both femoral heads shown also — a feature sometimes seen in this condition.

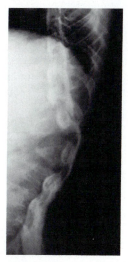

Fig. 1.68 MPS IV (Morquio's disease). At radiculography, multiple stenotic levels are demonstrated in the lower thoracic and lumbar regions, with scalloping of the posterior aspects of the vertebral bodies. Hypoplasia of an upper lumbar vertebral body is demonstrated. The 'beak' is central; a kyphos results.

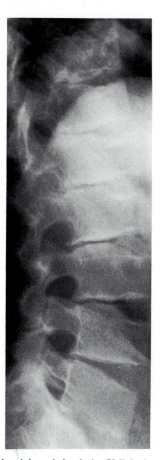

Fig. 1.70 Spondyloepiphyseal dysplasia (X-linked recessive form) showing characteristic platyspondyly. Mounds of bone are seen on the superior and inferior parts of the posterior parts of the vertebral bodies. Gas is seen in the prematurely degenerate discs.

especially after catheterization and fatalities have been reported.

Osteoporosis in the spine, with posterior scalloping of the vertebral bodies (Fig. 1.74), differentiates this con- dition radiologically from Marfan's syndrome. Epiphyses and carpal bones tend to be enlarged and metaphyses broadened (Fig. 1.75), but arachnodactyly is less marked. Also these patients tend to have pes cavus and grosser

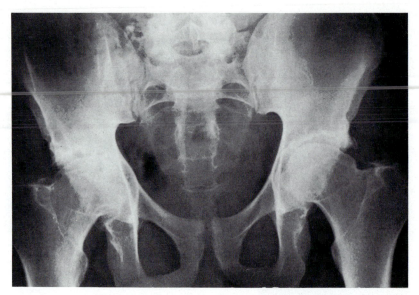

Fig. 1.71 Pelvis of patient in Fig. 1.70. Some (but not gross) osteoarthritis is seen, with some bilateral acetabular protrusion. The iliac wings are characteristically small in this condition.

sternal lesions than in Marfan's syndrome. Cardiac and aortic lesions are less common.

ACHONDROGENESIS

This is an uncommon lethal form of infantile dysplasia characterized by a large deformed head with gross under-development of the limbs and a large squat abdomen.

Radiologically, the long bones are extremely short, irregular and grossly undermineralized (Fig. 1.76). The

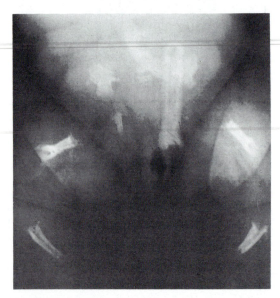

Fig. 1.72 Hypophosphatasia in newborn, gross failure of ossification of bones of the legs and of the pelvis.

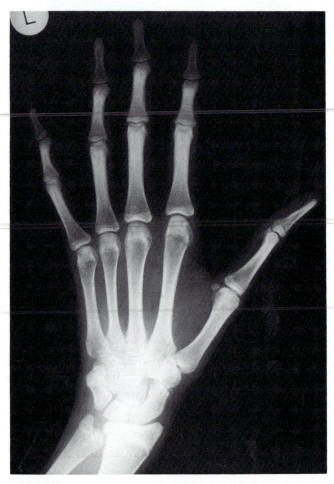

Fig. 1.73 Marfan's syndrome — elongation of metacarpals and phalanges is demonstrated.

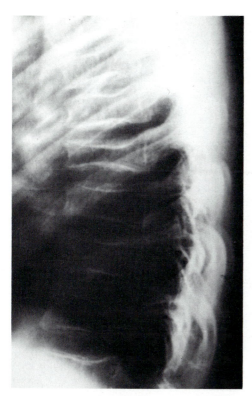

Fig. 1.74 Homocystinuria. Osteoporosis is associated with platyspondyly of the thoracic spine.

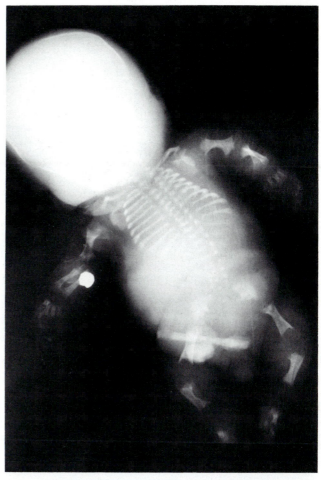

Fig. 1.76 Achondrogenesis. Gross shortening of the long bones is seen. The metaphyses are irregular and the epiphyses around the knee delayed in appearance. Poor mineralization of the caudal vertebral bodies, sacrum and pubic bones characterize Type II achondrogenesis.

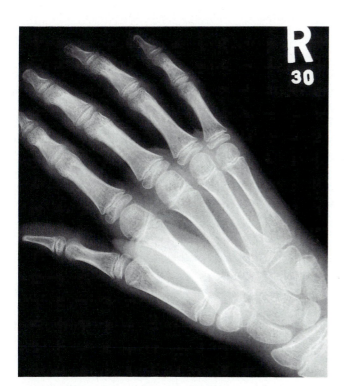

Fig. 1.75 Homocystinuria. Overgrowth of carpal epiphyses is present.

pelvis is barely visualized at birth or in utero (Type I). In Type II, the limb bones are still short and metaphyses irregular, but slightly better mineralized. The vertebral bodies, however, may not be mineralized, especially caudally.

The diseases are both inherited as autosomal recessives.

FIBRODYSPLASIA OSSIFICANS PROGRESSIVA
(synonym: *myositis ossificans progressiva*; eponym: *Munchmeyer's disease*)

The disease process primarily involves the connective tissues rather than muscle fibres. Soft tissue swellings begin in utero or early in life. These painful swellings affect the neck and upper trunk. *Ossification* commences in the lumps within months and is aggravated by surgical biopsy. Large masses of bone form in voluntary muscles which may extend to the normal skeletal structures and resemble exostoses (Figs. 1.77). Movements become restricted.

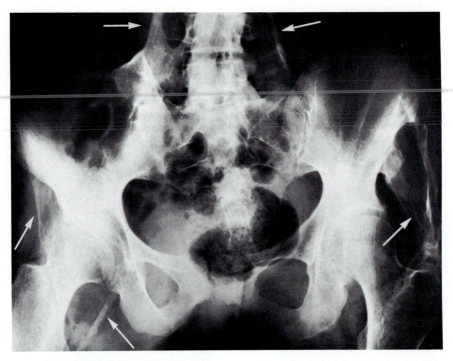

Fig. 1.77 Fibrodysplasia ossificans progressiva — soft tissue ossification (arrows).

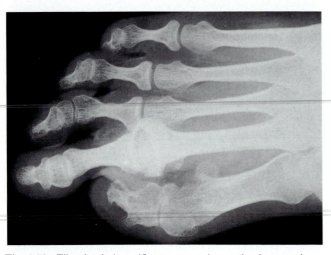

Fig. 1.78 Fibrodysplasia ossificans progressiva — developmental anomaly of the great toe. (Osteochondritis of the second metatarsal is also present).

A skeletal dysplasia is present at birth. Seventy-five per cent have involvement of the *great toe*, with fusion and microdactyly or hallux valgus (Fig. 1.78), and 50% have thumb hypoplasia and little finger clinodactyly. The femoral necks and mandibular condyles are broad and the cervical vertebral bodies are hypoplastic and fused.

Inheritance is probably autosomal dominant but most cases are sporadic as few patients survive to reproductive age.

CHROMOSOMAL DISORDERS

DOWN'S SYNDROME
(synonyms: *mongolism*; *trisomy 21*)

This condition is associated with an extra chromosome in the 21–22 group. The clinical diagnosis of older children suffering from mongolism is usually easy. In a baby the diagnosis may not be evident clinically, but it is, of course, of great human importance. The newborn Down's syndrome baby has a large ilium with a flat acetabular roof; an elongated tapering ischium develops after a few months. Caffey and Ross (1956) expressed these features quantitatively. They described the *iliac index* obtained by adding the 'iliac angle' to the 'acetabu-

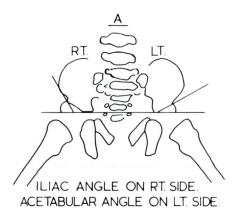

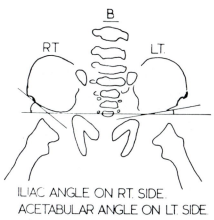

Fig. 1.79 Normal neonatal pelvis (**A**) and neonatal pelvis of a Down's syndrome baby (**B**). Note the protruberant ilium and flat acetabulum and consequent reduction in the iliac and acetabular angles compared with the normal.

range. Between 68 and 78 Down's syndrome is unlikely, but 6% of afflicted persons do occur in this range.

Many other skeletal and visceral anomalies have been described in this disease, though none of them is invariably present. Some of the following anomalies have been recognized relatively recently:

1. Brachycephaly, hypoplasia of the nasal bones, maxillae and sphenoids, and absent frontal sinuses. Instability of the atlantoaxial joint and abnormalities in the upper cervical spine may be found.

2. The interorbital distance is decreased in most cases, indicating orbital hypotelorism.

3. Extra ossification centres for the manubrium sterni are found in 90% of cases between the ages of 1 and 4 years; this sign is seen in 20% of normal children of the same age group.

4. Many Down's syndrome children have only eleven pairs of ribs.

5. The middle and distal phalanges of the fifth digits are often hypoplastic and curve inwards.

6. The lumbar vertebrae are often greater in height than in width, a reversal of the normal ratio, and they show concave anterior surfaces. Thus a lateral view of the lumbar spine may be of diagnostic help. This is not diagnostic of Down's syndrome but may be found in many children with delayed motor development.

7. Congenital heart disease is frequently found in Down's syndrome children, as is an aberrant right subclavian artery.

8. An increased incidence of duodenal stenosis and atresia and of Hirschsprung's disease may be found.

lar angle' (Fig. 1.79). These angles are obtained by first drawing a horizontal line through corresponding points of the articulation at the centre of each acetabulum. A line is then drawn between the most lateral part of the ilium and the outer part of the acetabular roof. The angle between this line and the horizontal is called the iliac angle. The acetabular angle is given by the intersection of a line between the outer and the inner lips of the acetabulum with the same horizontal line.

Caffey and Ross and, later, Astley concluded that the iliac index affords a useful though not infallible means of diagnosis of Down's syndrome in the first few weeks of life. Astley suggests the following criteria:

1. If the iliac index is under 60, Down's syndrome is very probable.

2. If the index is over 78, Down's syndrome is probably absent.

3. If the iliac index lies between 60 and 78, only a qualified report can be given. Between 68 and 60, Down's syndrome is probable, but 10% of normals occur in this

TURNER'S SYNDROME

Not all patients with Turner's syndrome have an abnormal sex chromosome pattern, nor do all individuals with the characteristic chromosomal pattern have Turner's syndrome. The essential components of this condition are: *agenesis of the gonads, webbing of the neck* and *cubitus valgus*. The syndrome is confined to females. Mental deficiency, congenital cardiac and aortic lesions and anomalies of the kidneys such as malrotation are often associated. Sometimes males are found with a similar body configuration, *viz.,* short stature and a webbed neck. However, these boys have a normal chromosomal pattern and they tend to get auricular septal defects and pulmonary stenosis rather than coarctation of the aorta which may be associated with Turner's syndrome.

Radiological findings. The skeletal features are inconstant and nonspecific. Density of the skeleton, especially of the hands and feet, is reduced. General osteoporosis is frequent in older patients. The metacarpals may be short, especially the fourth (Fig. 1.80) and accelerated fusion of the epiphysis may be found. The

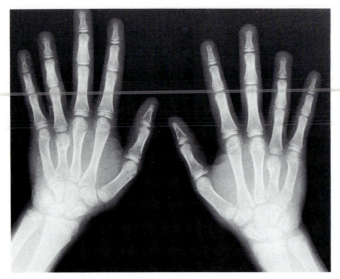

Fig. 1.80 Turner's syndrome — typical shortening of fourth metacarpals.

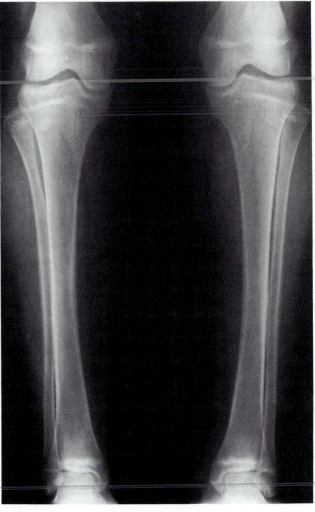

Fig. 1.81 Turner's syndrome. The medial tibial plateau is depressed and the adjacent femoral condyle enlarged.

so-called 'metacarpal sign' is an expression of gross shortening of the fourth metacarpal. Minor shortening may be seen in some normal subjects.

The increase in the carrying angle of the elbow is better assessed clinically than radiologically. The medial tibial condyle is depressed and beak-like and the medial femoral condyle may project downwards (as in Blount's disease) (Fig. 1.81).

Maldevelopment of the clavicles and slender ribs is often seen. Kyphosis and scoliosis are frequently found. Hypoplasia of the atlas and odontoid peg may be seen. In many females the pelvic inlet is android, the pubic arch narrowed and the sacrosciatic notches small.

REFERENCES AND SUGGESTIONS FOR FURTHER READING

Amstutz, H. C., Wilson, P. D. (1962) Dysgenesis of the proximal femur. *Journal of Bone and Joint Surgery*, **44A**, 1–23.

Andren, L., Von Rosen, S. (1958) The diagnosis of dislocation of the hip in newborns and the primary results of immediate treatment. *Acta Radiologica, Stockholm*, **49**, 89–95.

Astley, R. (1963) Chromosomal abnormalities in childhood. *British Journal of Radiology*, **36**, 2–10.

Baker, S. L., Dent, C. E., Friedman, M., Watson, L. (1966) Fibrogenesis imperfecta ossium. *Journal of Bone and Joint Surgery*, **48B**, 804–825.

Barlow, T. (1962) Early diagnosis and treatment of congenital dislocation of the hip. *Journal of Bone and Joint Surgery*, **44B**, 292–301.

Beighton, P., Cremin, B. J. (1980) *Sclerosing Bone Dysplasias*. Berlin: Springer Verlag.

Blockley, N. J. (1969) Observations on infantile coxa vara. *Journal of Bone and Joint Surgery*, **51B**, 106–111.

Boyd, H. B. Sage, F. P. (1958) Congenital pseudarthrosis of the tibia. *Journal of Bone and Joint Surgery*, **40A**, 1245–1270.

Caffey, J., Ross, S. (1956) Mongolism (mongoloid deficiency) during early infancy — some newly recognized diagnostic changes in the pelvic bones. *Paediatrics*, **17**, 643–651.

Fairbank, T. (1951) *An Atlas of General Affections of the Skeleton*. Livingstone, Edinburgh.

Fielden, P., Russell, J. G. B. (1970) Coronally cleft vertebra. *Clinical Radiology*, **21**, 327–328.

Houang, M. T. W., Brenton, D. P., Renton, P., Shaw, D. (1978) Idiopathic juvenile osteoporosis. *Skeletal Radiology*, **3**, 17–23.

Jacobs, P. (1966) Detection of early congenital dislocation of the hip. *Proceedings of the Royal Society of Medicine*, **59**, 1225–1229.

James, A. E., Jr., Merz, T., Janower, M. L., Dorst, J. P. (1971) Radiology of the most common autosomal disorders. *Clinical Radiology*, **22**, 417–431.

Kaufmann, H. J. (1973) Progress in pediatric radiology. In: *Intrinsic Diseases of Bones*. Basel: Karger.

Levinson, E. D., Ozonoff, M. B., Royen, P. M. (1977) Proximal femoral focal deficiency. *Radiology*, **125**, 197–203.

McCredie, J. (1975) Congenital fusion of bones — radiology, embryology and pathogenesis. *Clinical Radiology*, **26**, 47–57.

McCredie, J., McBride, W. G. (1973) Some congenital abnormalities possibly due to embryonic peripheral neuropathy. *Clinical Radiology*, **24**, 204–211.

Murray, R. O., Jacobson, H. G., Stoker, D. J. (1990) *The Radiology of Skeletal Disorders*. 3rd edn. Edinburgh: Churchill Livingstone.

Murray, R. O., McCredie, J. (1979) Melorheostosis and the sclerotomes. *Skeletal Radiology*, **4**, 57–71.

Neuhauser, E. B. D., Wittenborg, M. H., Dehlinger, K. (1950) Diastematomyelia. *Radiology*, **54**, 659–664.

Poznanski, A. K. (1984) *The Hand in Radiologic Diagnosis*. 2nd edn. Philadelphia, Saunders.

Renton, P. (1990) *Orthopaedic Radiology: Pattern Recognition and Differential Diagnosis*. London: Dunitz.

Rubin, P. (1964) *Dynamic Classification of Bone Dysplasias*. Chicago: Year Book Medical Publishers.

Singleton, E. B., Rosenberg, H. S., Yang, S. J. (1964) The radiographic manifestations of chromosomal abnormalities. *Radiologic Clinics of North America*. Vol. 2, pp. 281–295. Philadelphia: Saunders.

Spranger, J. W., Langer, L. O., Wiedemann, H.-R. (1974) *Bone Dysplasias*. Philadelphia: Saunders.

Warrick, C. K. (1973) Some aspects of polyostotic fibrous dysplasia. *Clinical Radiology*, **27**, 125–138.

Wynne-Davies, R., Fairbank, T. J. (1976) *Fairbank's Atlas of General Affections of the Skeleton*. 2nd edn. Edinburgh: Churchill Livingstone.

Wynne-Davies, R., Hall, C. M., Apley, A. G. (1985) *Atlas of Skeletal Dysplasias*. Edinburgh: Churchill Livingstone.

CHAPTER 2

PERIOSTEAL REACTION; BONE AND JOINT INFECTIONS; SARCOID

Peter Renton

PERIOSTEAL NEW BONE FORMATION
(periosteal reaction)

New bone is laid down in many conditions with different aetiologies (Table 2.1). In some the periosteum is physically elevated by tumour, haemorrhage or infection. Vascular abnormalities, viruses and autoimmune diseases may all cause new bone deposition. New bone may be deposited locally, around a solitary focus of disease, or may be generalized. In some systemic conditions, new bone is laid down in characteristic sites.

In its simplest form the new bone is seen as a linear density separated from the bony shaft by a clear zone, often later obliterated as the new bone merges with the cortex. Difficulty is caused by bones such as the fibula which have naturally irregular outlines. Insertions of interosseous membranes, ligaments and tendons in other bones also cause confusion.

There is a wide variety of types of periosteal reaction and often certain patterns can be discerned. However, the type of periosteal reaction cannot always be correlated with the underlying disease.

Tumours and periosteal new bone

A tumour, having broken through the cortex, elevates the periosteum and new bone forms beneath it. If the tumour grows slowly, the elevated periosteal new bone may remain intact and even take over the function of the destroyed cortex. If tumour growth is cyclical, as in Ewing's sarcoma, successive layers of periosteal new bone are laid down, giving a lamellated or onion-skin appearance. If tumour growth is rapid, the periosteal new bone becomes disorganized and remains intact at the tumour margins only. Buttressing and elevation of periosteal new bone at tumour margins leads to a so-called Codman's triangle which is usually indicative of a malignant tumour, though in an aneurysmal bone cyst Codman's triangle really indicates rapidity of progression.

In Ewing's sarcoma and in hypertrophic osteoarthropathy (see Ch. 4) the layers of new bone are characteristically fine, and thinner than the spaces between them. New bone in osteogenic sarcoma, parosteal sarcoma and secondary deposits tends to be coarser and

Table 2.1 Causes of periosteal new bone formation

Physiological	In neonates, especially in prematurity
Congenital	Tuberous sclerosis
Dysplastic	Melorheostosis, Engelmann's disease
Traumatic	Local subperiosteal trauma; fractures, including march fracture. Unrecognized skeletal trauma (Caffey's 'battered baby syndrome')
Infective	Acute: osteomyelitis — staphylococcal, streptococcal, pneumococcal, etc. Chronic — Brodie's abscess, tuberculosis, syphilis (congenital and acquired), yaws; also from nearby infection, e.g. varicose ulcer; ribs in pulmonary and pleural infections.
Hypo- and hypervitaminosis	Rickets, scurvy, hypervitaminosis A
Endocrine	Thyroid acropachy, hyperparathyroidism in healing phase; secondary hyperparathyroidism in renal osteodystrophy.
Vascular	Haemophilia and other bleeding diseases. Myeloid metaplasia probably due to associated thrombocytopenia. Erythroblastic anaemias. Leukaemias. Varicose veins (before ulceration occurs). Hypertrophic pulmonary osteoarthropathy (probably of vascular aetiology) and pachydermoperiostosis.
Collagen diseases	Polyarteritis nodosa.
Reticuloses	Hodgkin's disease, etc.
Neoplastic	Primary: benign — meningioma, angioma, osteoid osteoma. malignant — osteogenic sarcoma, fibrosarcoma, Ewing's tumour, etc. Secondary: any metastatic bony deposit may be associated with periosteal reaction.
Primary joint lesions	Ankylosing spondylitis, juvenile chronic arthritis (Still's disease), Reiter's syndrome, rheumatoid arthritis, osteoarthritis (femoral neck only).
Miscellaneous	Infantile cortical hyperostosis (Caffey), histiocytosis.

Trauma and *inflammation* are the commonest causes of periosteal reaction both in adults and in children. *Primary malignant neoplasms* are rare but nearly always cause periosteal reaction. Periosteal reaction is occasionally seen in *metastases*. In adults, less common causes such as *reticuloses, hypertrophic pulmonary osteoarthropathy* and *varicose ulceration* may cause diagnostic difficulty. In neonates, *congenital syphilis* and *infantile cortical hyperostosis* must be remembered. Later, *scurvy, leukaemia* and *erythroblastic anaemias* (in immigrants) are possible causes. *Ewing's tumour* and *metastases from neuroblastoma* are other childhood causes which may prove diagnostically elusive.

less well defined, so that the spicules are thicker than the intervening spaces. In osteogenic sarcoma, also, new bone may be perpendicular to the shaft and, originating from a finite focus of disease, resembles a sunray — so-called 'sunray spiculation'. This may also be found with angioma and thalassaemia, but is then generally more orderly and better organized. Meningioma may resemble osteogenic sarcoma more closely, but the site is characteristic. Vertical spicules ('hair-on-end') are also found in Ewing's sarcoma but, in keeping with the more diffuse nature of the underlying tumour, are not usually 'sunburst' but extend for a considerable distance along the bone, and are more delicate. Vertical spiculation may result from bony deposition along the elevated and stretched fibres connecting periosteum to bone, the Sharpey fibres.

Vascular insufficiency and periosteal new bone

Venous stasis causes changes in the lower limb, especially at the diaphysis and distal metaphysis of the tibia and fibula. The periosteal new bone which is formed may be lamellar or irregular. Changes may be seen in the presence of chronic ulceration (Fig. 2.1), but also in its absence, so that an ulcer is not essential. Indeed, the periosteal new bone often extends far proximally from an ulcer. Phleboliths may be present and varicosities may also be seen in subcutaneous tissues, which appear thickened and oedematous.

A florid and exuberant periosteal reaction occurs infrequently in polyarteritis nodosa. Arterial occlusion and skin ulceration are found and the periosteal reactions often occur around affected parts and in relation to skin lesions.

Thyroid acropachy

Literally, 'thickening of the extremities', this occurs in patients who have been treated for thyrotoxicosis and end up myxoedematous. The hands are more commonly affected than the feet. The distal ends of paired long bones are less often affected. The distribution is similar to that of hypertrophic osteoarthropathy but the new bone is more likely to be shaggy, spiculated and perpendicular to the shaft rather than lamellar. The overlying soft tissues are often grossly thickened (Fig 2.2).

INFECTION

OSTEOMYELITIS

An invading organism may attack bone by direct invasion from an infected wound, or from an infected joint, or it may gain access by haematogenous spread from distant foci, usually in the skin. Haematogenous osteomyelitis usually occurs during the period of growth, but all ages may be affected and cases are even found in old age. In

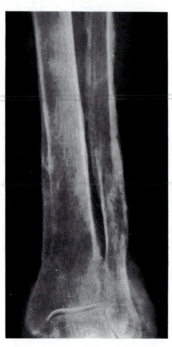

Fig. 2.1 Irregular periosteal new bone is demonstrated in a patient with varicose veins.

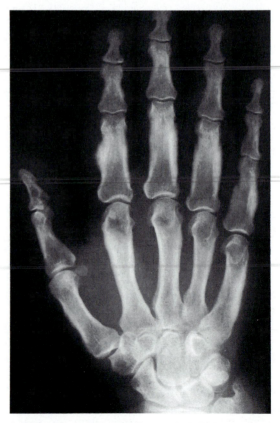

Fig. 2.2 Thyroid acropachy. Marked cortical thickening is demonstrated at the midshafts of the tubular bones of the hand (see Ch. 8).

infants, *Streptococcus* usually causes osteomyelitis. In adults, *Staphylococcus* is more common.

It is important to understand the blood supply to bone before describing blood-borne infection. The blood supply to a long bone is via:

1. **The nutrient artery**. This is the major source of blood supply throughout life. It supplies the marrow and most of the inner cortex.

2. **Periosteal vessels**. These supply the outer cortex.

3. **Metaphyseal and epiphyseal vessels**.

In the *infant*, vessels penetrate the epiphyseal plate in both directions. Metaphyseal infections can thus pass to the epiphysis and then the joint. Acute pyogenic arthritis is therefore a relatively common sequel of osteomyelitis in infants. The periosteum in infants is very loosely attached to underlying bone. Pus easily elevates periosteum and so can extend to the epiphyseal plate along the shaft. In situations where the metaphysis is intracapsular, such as the hip, metaphyseal infection also results in septic arthritis.

In *childhood*, between 2 and 16 years, few vessels cross the epiphyseal plate though the periosteum is still relatively loosely attached. The epiphysis and joint are thus less frequently infected. The metaphyseal vessels terminate instead in slow-flowing sinusoids which promote blood-borne infective change (Figs 2.3, 2.4).

In the *adult*, after the epiphyseal plate has fused, metaphyseal and epiphyseal vessels are again connected so that septic arthritis can occur again. Periosteum, however, is well bound down and articular infections via a metaphyseal route are less likely.

The formation of pus in the bone deprives local cortex and medulla of its blood supply. Dead bone is resorbed by *granulation tissue*. Pieces of dead bone, especially if cortical or surrounded by *pus*, are not resorbed and remain as *sequestra* (Fig. 2.5). As sequestra are devitalized they remain denser than surrounding vital bone, which

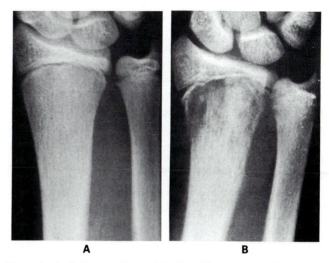

Fig. 2.4 **A**. Early metaphyseal infection. There is very minimal focal bone destruction at the distal radial metaphysis. **B**. With progressive bone destruction, metaphyseal abnormality is now very evident.

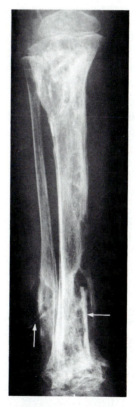

Fig. 2.5 Advanced osteomyelitis involving the whole of the right tibia and lower end of the fibula. Note sequestrum in tibia (arrow) and further sequestrum being extruded from the fibula (arrow).

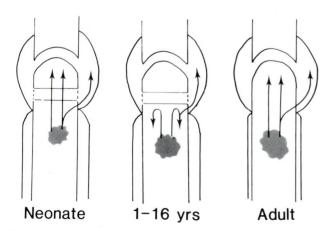

Neonate   1–16 yrs   Adult

Fig. 2.3 Osteomyelitis. The three ages of infection and how change involves the joint.

becomes demineralized due to hyperaemia and immobilization. Absorption of sequestra is also facilitated by the presence of an *involucrum*. The involucrum forms beneath vital periosteum which has been elevated by pus. As periosteum is poorly attached in infants, involucrum formation is greater and so is the resorption of dead bone, and healing.

In areas of dead periosteum, defects in the involucrum occur. These *cloacae* allow pus and sequestra to escape, sometimes to the skin via a sinus. The track and its deep connection to bone can then be demonstrated by sinography using water-soluble contrast medium.

Radiological findings. These depend to some extent on the age of the patient.

Soft-tissue changes may be immediately apparent, especially in infants, and on CT scanning. Swelling, with oedema and blurring of fat planes is seen — in distinction to the soft-tissue masses around tumours, where the displaced fat planes are preserved. Osteoporosis may be visualized within 10–14 days of onset of symptoms. In children this is usually metaphyseal.

An involucrum is usually visualized after 3 weeks and is more prolific in infants and children than in adults (Fig. 2.6). The rapid escape and decompression of pus which results prevents vascular compression and infarction, and promotes healing. Computed and conventional tomography is invaluable in detecting sequestra. These are seen as fragments of dense bone within areas of local bone destruction. Treatment by antibiotics and/or surgical decompression affects the course of the disease so that

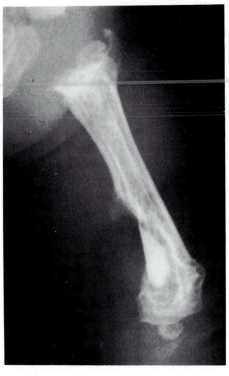

Fig. 2.6 Osteomyelitis of femur and septic arthritis of the hip in neonate. Note dislocation of hip, involucrum, cloaca and sequestrum.

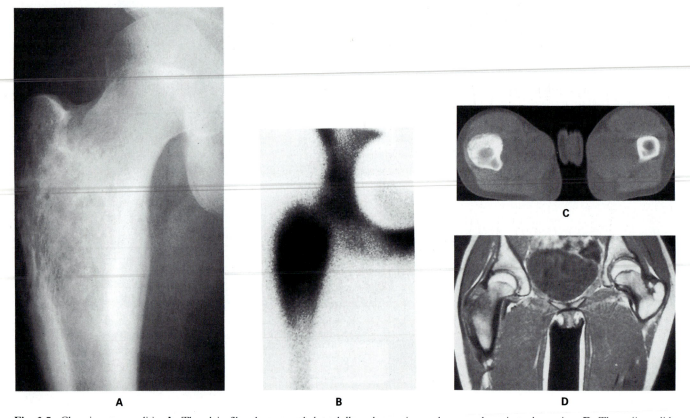

A   B   D

Fig. 2.7 Chronic osteomyelitis. **A.** The plain film shows mottled medullary destruction and a smooth periosteal reaction. **B.** The radionuclide bone scan shows gross increase in uptake locally. **C.** On CT scanning, gross periosteal reaction is demonstrated, causing considerable enlargement and sclerosis of bone. **D.** The MR scan shows the grossly altered signal in the affected femoral neck and greater trochanter, with replacement of the normal bright marrow.

often little apart from new bone may be found during the course of the disease.

With adequate treatment in infants and children, a return to more or less normal appearances with growth is to be expected, unless the epiphyseal plate and epiphysis have been damaged, in which case growth abnormalities may result. In adults the affected bone often remains sclerotic and irregular in outline (Fig. 2.7). Should chronic sepsis persist, tomography may reveal persistent cloacae and sequestra. The radiographic picture never returns completely to normal in cases discovered late (Table 2.2).

Table 2.2 Haematogenous osteomyelitis of tubular bones

	Infant	Child	Adult
Localization	Metaphyseal with epiphyseal extension	Metaphyseal	Epiphyseal
Involucrum	Common	Common	Not common
Sequestration	Common	Common	Not common
Joint involvement	Common	Not common	Common
Soft-tissue abscess	Common	Common	Not common
Pathological fracture	Not common	Not common	Common*
Fistulae	Not common	Variable	Common

* In neglected cases
(Reproduced from *Diagnosis of Bone and Joint Disorders*, by courtesy of Drs. D. Resnick and G. Niwayama, and W. B. Saunders, publishers)

SPECIAL FORMS OF OSTEOMYELITIS
Sclerosing osteomyelitis of Garré. This condition is manifested by gross sclerosis in the absence of apparent bone destruction (Fig. 2.8). True examples of this condition are found occasionally, but some of the cases described in the past were probably examples of *osteoid osteoma*.

Brodie's abscess. This localized form of osteomyelitis is usually found in the cancellous tissue near the end of a long bone. A well-circumscribed area of bone destruction has a surrounding zone of reactive sclerosis, sometimes accompanied by a periosteal reaction. It may have a finger-like extension into neighbouring bone towards the epiphyseal plate, which, when present, is pathognomonic of infection ('tunnelling') (Fig. 2.9). If a sequestrum is present an osteoid osteoma may be simulated.

OSTEOMYELITIS IN SPECIAL SITES
Skull. Lesions occur secondary to scalp infection or frontal sinus suppuration (Fig. 2.10).

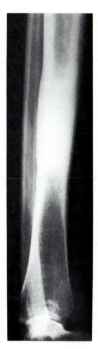

Fig. 2.8 Garré's type of osteomyelitis.

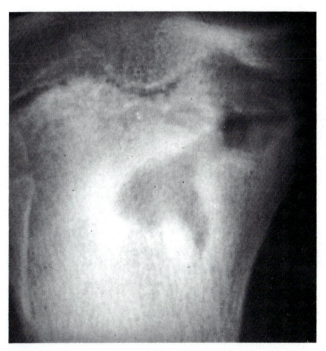

Fig. 2.9 A finger-like process of osteomyelitic bone destruction extends from the main focus. This is tunnelling, which usually indicates the presence of chronic infection.

Mandible. Infection may complicate a fracture into the mouth, or it may follow dental extraction. Infection via the pulp canal is probably most common and follows poor oral hygiene and dental decay.

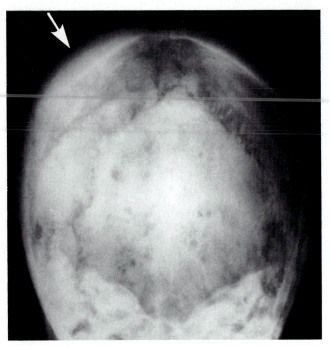

Fig. 2.10 Multiple areas of bone destruction and reactive sclerosis (arrow) are seen in a patient with chronic osteomyelitis.

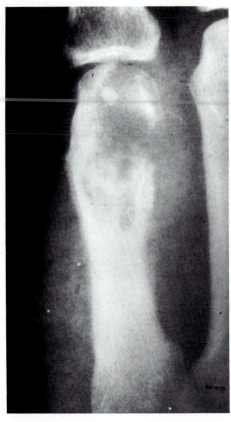

Fig. 2.11 Bone destruction, sequestrum formation and periostitis follow implantation of oral organisms after a bite.

Pelvis. The sacroiliac joint is occasionally affected. It may be difficult radiologically to differentiate pyogenic from tuberculous lesions. Ankylosis of the sacroiliac joint may result from either cause.

Osteitis pubis is a low-grade infection round the symphysis pubis which may complicate operations on the prostate and bladder or, occasionally, other pelvic operations.

Hands. Bone infections may follow perforating injuries to the pulp space. The distal phalanx may be involved by osteomyelitis or local pressure may cause ischaemia and avascular necrosis.

A bizarre form of osteomyelitis, often due to oral organisms, follows bite wounds on hands or after punching the face and teeth, with resulting perforations and implantation (Fig. 2.11).

Feet. Puncture wounds of the feet are common in children and in those societies where walking barefoot is common. Soft-tissue infections may lead to osteomyelitis, often with destruction of joints. In the tropics, direct implantation by mycetoma results in 'Madura foot' (see below under Mycetoma). Implantation by thorns leads to a particular lesion.

Complications of osteomyelitis

1. *Amyloid disease* infrequently complicates chronic osteomyelitis.

2. *Malignant changes* can follow longstanding suppurative osteomyelitis with draining sinuses. Increasing severity of symptoms with rapid osteolysis raises the possibility of a tumour, either an *epithelioma* of the sinus tract or, less frequently, an *osteosarcoma*.

The spine

Spinal osteomyelitis is not common, comprising less than 10% of bone infections (Epstein 1976) and can occur at any age. Patients often have a history of skin or pelvic infections. Spread of infection is usually to the vertebral body rather than to appendages and is mainly blood-borne, though osteomyelitis may follow spinal surgery. Spread of disease from the pelvis is facilitated through Batson's vertebral venous plexus which is a valveless system of veins joining the pelvis with the rest of the axial skeleton via the spinal canal. Flow in this valveless system ebbs back and forth with changes in intra-abdominal pressure. Vertebral bodies are very vascular, especially below endplates where large sinusoids with a sluggish blood flow potentiate infection. Spinal osteomyelitis is most common in the lumbar region and least common in the cervical and sacral spines.

Infective discitis Perforating blood vessels still supply the disc in children and young adults so that in these age groups a primary infection of the discs can occur. Changes are most common in the lumbar spine.

Radiological findings. Infection usually starts anteri-

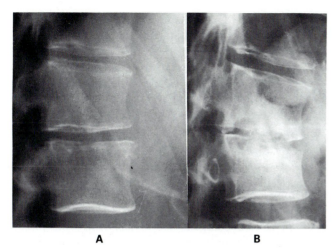

Fig. 2.12 A,B Infective spondylitis. **A**. The initial film shows early bone destruction beneath the end-plates around a narrowed disc. **B**. The later film shows progressive destruction of disc and bone with surrounding reactive sclerosis.

orly beneath the endplate. Plain film changes lag behind symptoms by 2–3 weeks, when a focus of osteolysis becomes visible and the cortex becomes blurred or vanishes. Infection may be beneath the anterior longitudinal ligament, facilitating vertical spread, or into the disc which is then rapidly destroyed and loses height (Figs 2.12, 2.13). The adjacent endplate then also loses density and vertebral destruction begins in the body above or below.

In most patients only two bodies are involved, and only rarely is the infection confined to one vertebral body.

Collapse of a vertebral body is accompanied by soft-tissue masses which are easily seen against air in the larynx, trachea or lung (Fig. 2.14). Blurring or displacement of the psoas shadows also occurs. Kyphosis and cord compression may also follow.

Reparative processes can begin as early as 4–6 weeks after the onset of radiological change if treatment is effective. Sclerotic new bone is formed around the disc, in the bodies and at vertebral margins (Fig. 2.15). Dense spurs bridge discs peripherally. Ankylosis across discs may result in fusion of bodies. If this occurs after skeletal maturity, the sagittal diameters of vertebral bodies are not likely to be reduced. 'Ivory' vertebrae and soft-tissue calcification are occasionally found.

OSTEOMYELITIS IN DIABETES
Infection occurs in both soft tissue and bone. Soft-tissue infection may follow a puncture through anaesthetic skin and presents with swelling and loss of fat planes due to oedema. In the presence of gas-producing organisms, spherical lucencies are seen extending proximally. Anaesthetic ulcers show as soft tissue defects, usually over pressure points such as the metatarsal heads, and over the tips and proximal interphalangeal joints of the commonly associated claw toes. Initially painless, the ulcers

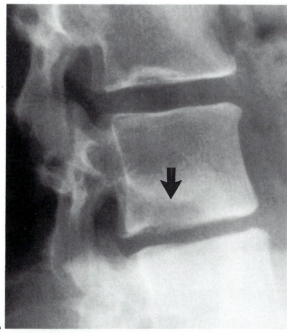

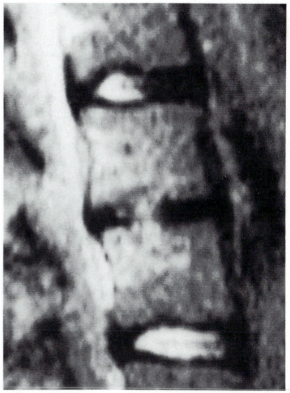

Fig. 2.13 Infective spondylitis. **A**. Another case showing destruction of disc and adjacent bone on the plain film. **B**. The MR scan shows discal narrowing, loss of the normal bright nuclear signal and its replacement by a rather diffuse abnormality involving the adjacent vertebral bodies due to infection.

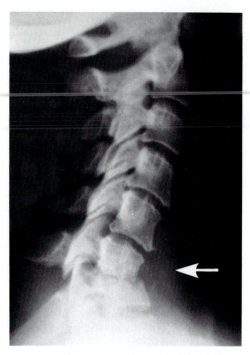

Fig. 2.14 End-plate destruction with discal loss and a kyphosis is associated with facet subluxation and a large anterior soft tissue mass (arrow).

involve underlying bones with the development of osteomyelitis. Sepsis may be superimposed on a neuropathic lesion, so that osteoporosis and destruction are accelerated (Fig. 2.16). If skin ulceration is absent, osteomyelitis is unlikely to be seen.

CHRONIC GRANULOMATOUS DISEASE OF CHILDHOOD

This is a group of disorders in which the leucocytes are unable to respond normally to infections, especially to those organisms which cause chronic low-grade infections. Leucocytes are able to engulf bacilli but cannot

destroy them so that toxins are still produced. A chronic inflammatory process results. Bones are commonly affected. Widespread small foci of osteolysis may be found, often abutting on to epiphyseal plates (Fig. 2.17). The lesions heal with florid formation of new bone, both end-osteally and superficially, so that sclerosis and expansion result, often resembling malignant tumours (Figs 2.18). The lesions are usually multifocal.

SEPTIC ARTHRITIS

Joint infections occur at any age, but especially in children. *Staphylococci, Streptococci* and *Pneumococci* are common causative organisms. Usually only one joint is affected. If more than one joint is infected, an immune defect should be suspected or the possibility of steroid administration queried.

A joint may be contaminated by:

1. Direct intervention — following surgery, aspiration or perforating injury.
2. Spread from adjacent bone (see above).
3. Haematogenous spread. Direct infection of synovium by septic emboli.

Radiological features. Initially synovial thickening and effusion distend the joint. Fat lines are displaced but may be blurred by oedema. Demineralization follows hyperaemia and immobilization. When infection begins to destroy cartilage, joint narrowing becomes apparent (Fig. 2.19). The articular cortex becomes blurred and then eroded, both peripherally and centrally, and subarticular bone is later destroyed. Severe cases are characterized by massive destruction, separation of bone ends, subluxation and dislocation.

During recovery, bones recalcify and in severe cases fibrous and bony ankylosis may result. Dystrophic calcification may be seen on occasion following pyogenic arthritis. Marginal erosions persist but their outlines become well demarcated and sclerotic.

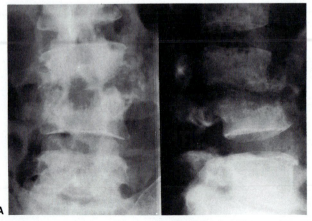
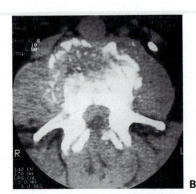

Fig. 2.15 Reparative sclerosis following infective discitis. New bone formation is seen, both on plain films (**A**) and CT scan (**B**).

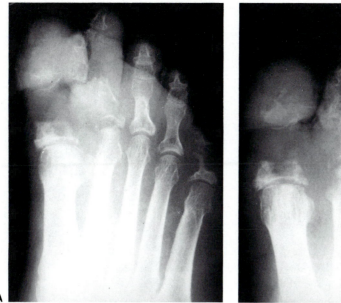
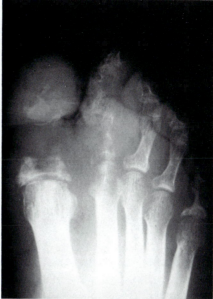

Fig. 2.16 A,B Osteomyelitis in diabetes. The changes at the little toe are those of neuropathic bone resorption. The cloudy resorption of bone with osteoporosis and soft tissue swelling at the first and second toes indicate superimposed osteomyelitis.

Arthritis of the hip in infants (Tom Smith arthritis). The hip joint in infants is especially susceptible to infection as explained above. In neonates sepsis may be transmitted via the umbilical vessels, often due to the

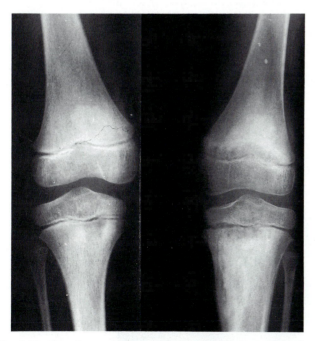

Fig. 2.17 Chronic granulomatous disease. Multifocal metaphyseal areas of destruction are demonstrated with surrounding reactive sclerosis.

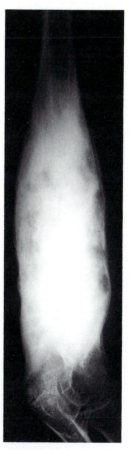

Fig. 2.18 Gross reactive sclerosis with new bone formation at multiple sites is found in chronic granulomatous disease.

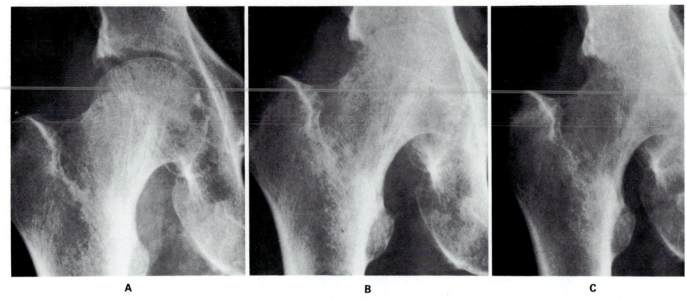

Fig. 2.19 A,B,C Pyogenic arthritis of the hip — rapid progression of the lesion during a period of 1 month.

streptococcus, but infection may be directly introduced following blood sampling at the groin. In infants, because of lax muscles around the hip and the cartilaginous nature of the acetabulum, an effusion may dislocate the hip (Fig. 2.20). This can be assessed even if the ossific nucleus has not appeared. In any case, gross metaphyseal destruction is soon apparent with cortical and medullary erosions. Gross sequestration rapidly occurs and an involucrum may involve the entire femur. The femoral shaft generally heals, but the femoral head and neck may be totally destroyed, never to appear. Deformity and shortening inevitably result. In older children, such change is less likely as the epiphyseal plate is not crossed by vessels. The femoral head, even if severely affected, then reconstitutes with a flattened mushroom-like appearance similar to old Perthes' disease or slipped epiphysis. Be-

cause of vascular compression, osteonecrosis may actually complicate infection.

TUBERCULOSIS OF BONES AND JOINTS

Though the incidence of skeletal tuberculosis has fallen markedly in recent years, the disease has not yet been eradicated. One-third of our present-day patients are immigrants to Britain; they tend to produce unusual disease patterns which will be described later.

Haematogenous spread of infection to the skeleton is assumed to be from the lung and may occur at the time of primary infection or later from post-primary foci. Chest radiography, however, shows active disease in less than 50% of cases, the organism presumably having lain dormant and become active later. The bacillus lodges in the

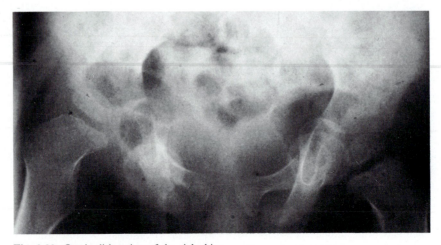

Fig. 2.20 Septic dislocation of the right hip.

spongiosa of the metaphysis of long bone, but the vertebral column is affected in 50% of cases. Lesions are usually single, though multifocal cystic osseous tuberculosis is described.

Certain features are relatively common. The tuberculous reaction is destructive and accompanied by pus which may later become calcified. Calcification of abscesses is rarely seen currently if antibiotic treatment is adequate. In contradistinction to pyogenic osteomyelitis, neither sequestration nor periostitis is a prominent feature. Abscesses often point to the skin and a sinus track may be demonstrated after injection of contrast medium.

Radiographic appearances. The diagnosis is usually made after considerable delay and radiographic changes are seen at presentation, in contrast to pyogenic infections where radiographic changes occur 2–3 weeks after clinical presentation.

The *metaphysis* is the site of election; an oval or rounded focus will be found which soon crosses the epiphyseal line (Figs 2.21, 2.22). No surrounding sclerosis is to be expected. Sequestra are small and are absorbed by granulation tissue. Though slight periosteal reaction may be found if the local lesion is subcortical, this is not a prominent feature. The initial focus may sometimes be sited in the epiphysis.

Lesions of the diaphysis are rare, and even rarer is the multiple cystic type of lesion.

LESIONS OF INDIVIDUAL BONES

Greater trochanter. This is a common site, particularly in adolescents and young adults. The lesion may start in the bone or in the overlying bursa. The erosion may be

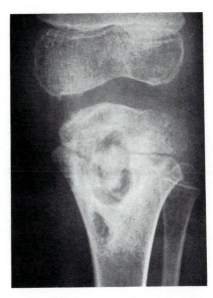

Fig. 2.22 Tuberculosis of knee — the metaphyseal lesion has extended across the epiphyseal line. The sequestrum is more prominent than usual but it was absorbed completely during healing.

deep, but often it is superficial and difficult to detect; sometimes it may be cystic (Fig. 2.23).

The spine. Roughly half the cases of osteoarticular tuberculosis seen in this country occur in the spine. Most lesions occur in or below the mid-dorsal spine and involvement of the cervical and upper dorsal spine is uncommon. All ages may be affected.

Radiographic appearances. (Figs 2.24, 2.25, 2.26). Vertebral bodies may be first affected in three places — at the upper or lower disc margin, in the centre, and anteriorly under the periosteum. The disc substance is often eroded. Two or more vertebrae may be attacked.

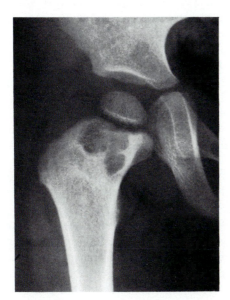

Fig. 2.21 Tuberculosis of femur — large metaphyseal focus.

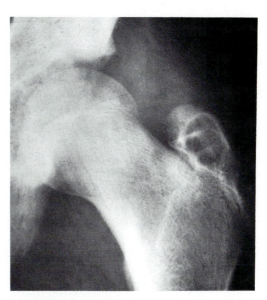

Fig. 2.23 Tuberculous focus in greater trochanter. This type is less common than a surface erosion.

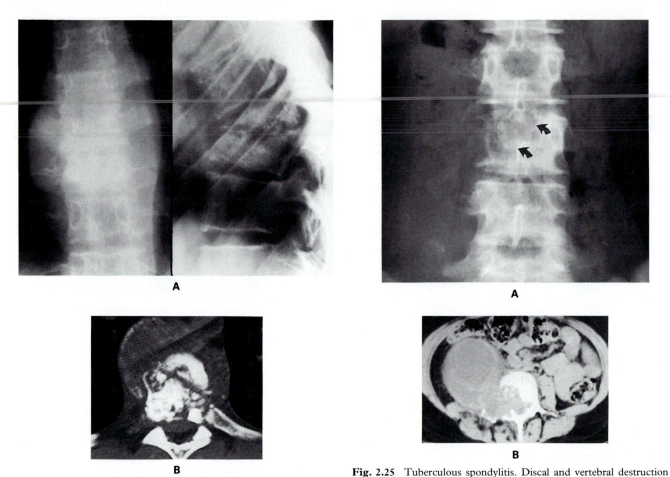

Fig. 2.24 Tuberculosis of spine. **A**. Discal and vertebral body destruction is associated with a large paraspinal mass. The change affects vertebral bodies above the abnormal disc. An anterior destructive lesion is seen associated with an anterior soft tissue mass. **B**. The CT scan shows the extensive destructive process as well as the surrounding soft tissue swelling.

Fig. 2.25 Tuberculous spondylitis. Discal and vertebral destruction is associated with a large right-sided paraspinal abscess. **A**. Plain film shows bone destruction (arrows). **B**. CT shows large paraspinal abscess.

Tomography may show the lesion to be more extensive than it appears from examination of routine films. Since the anterior parts of the vertebrae are most affected, a local *kyphos* or *gibbus* will appear, and some scoliosis may also occur. Abscesses form early and are easily seen in the dorsal region in contrast to the radiolucent lungs. In the lumbar region, lateral bulging of the psoas outlines may be demonstrable. Abscesses may track widely and may become calcified. They may sometimes be intraosseous and subsequently calcify (Fig. 2.27). Rib crowding may be seen, even on a chest radiograph, if vertebral bodies collapse.

It is often difficult to differentiate between tuberculous and pyogenic spondylitis, especially if the patient is white. Clearly, tuberculosis must always be suspected if the patient is of African or Asian origin. Reactive new bone formation is much less pronounced in tuberculous disease, so that sclerotic osteophytes are unusual. Discs are destroyed early with simple infections and later, or infre-

quently not at all, in tuberculosis. Calcification, where present, indicates tuberculosis.

The lesions generally respond rapidly to antibiotics, but before antibiotics were introduced, gross destructive lesions were common and the affected vertebral bodies frequently became fused.

The subperiosteal type of infection begins anteriorly under the periosteum and spreads under the anterior common ligament. Disc destruction may be late, and the anterior erosions may be difficult to detect.

Aortic pulsation, transmitted through an anterior paraspinal abscess between D4 and D10, may cause the vertebral bodies to become deeply concave anteriorly (Fig. 2.28). This process does not affect the intervertebral discs. An *aneurysm* causes similar changes by direct pulsation.

In black patients, tuberculous spondylitis has a somewhat different presentation. Often, only one vertebra is involved, with conspicuous preservation of adjacent discs, even if the body is totally destroyed or flattened. Occasionally, *vertebra plana* results (Fig. 2.29). Sclerosis and new bone formation is a feature of the disease in

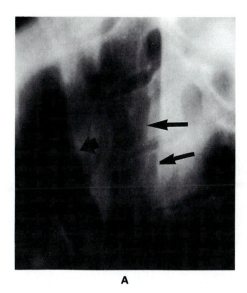

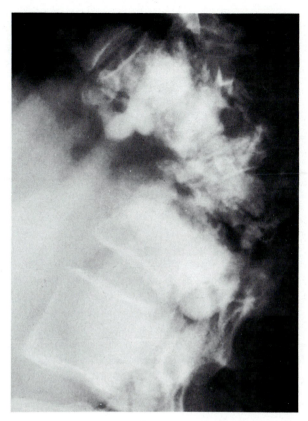

Fig. 2.27 Tuberculous spondylitis has healed with calcifying psoas abscesses and angular kyphos.

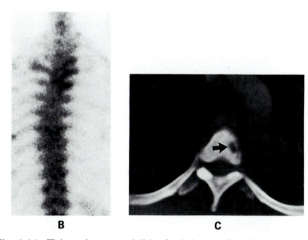

Fig. 2.26 Tuberculous spondylitis. **A.** A large soft tissue mass indents the trachea from behind (thick arrow). Anterior erosive lesions are shown on the adjacent vertebral bodies (arrows). There is early discal narrowing. **B.** The radionuclide scan confirms the presence of bone change affecting at least three levels. **C.** The CT scan confirms the destructive lesion of the vertebral body on the left side and the associated paraspinal mass.

black patients, as in pyogenic spondylitis. More importantly, the posterior elements are frequently involved, especially in the lumbosacral and thoracolumbar junctions, often with huge abscesses (Fig. 2.30). The cervical spine is also more frequently involved than in white patients, with dysphagia or paraplegia as complications. Multiple lesions are also more common. Involvement of the spinal column also follows gibbus formation or extrusion of granulation tissue into the canal.

Tuberculous dactylitis. This lesion is sometimes seen in our immigrant population. The affected phalanx is characteristically widened by medullary expansion (spina ventosa), whereas in syphilitic dactylitis the bone is widened by the production of cortical new bone (Fig. 2.31).

The skull. Tuberculous lesions are rare in the skull,

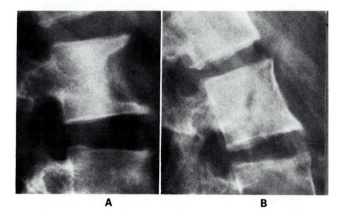

Fig. 2.28 A,B Anterior subperiosteal type of Pott's disease.

except in immigrants. They may be localized and well-defined, resembling eosinophilic granuloma, or they may be more diffuse (Fig. 2.32). Overlying cold abscesses are generally associated.

JOINT LESIONS

Tuberculous arthritis usually affects major joints — the hip and knee especially. Multifocal infection is rare. Infection may be synovial or secondary to bony disease.

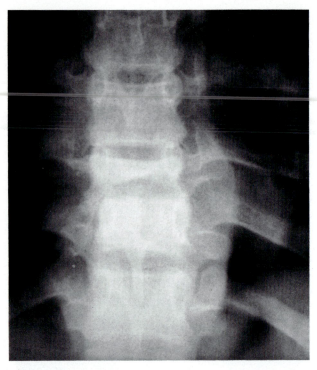

Fig. 2.29 Tuberculosis. Flattening of the vertebral body is accompanied by a paraspinal swelling but the discs are relatively spared. Adjacent end-plates are also relatively intact.

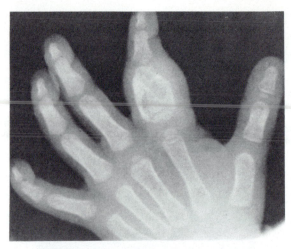

Fig. 2.31 Typical spina ventosa of the proximal phalanx of the forefinger. (Courtesy of Dr. D. J. Mitchell.)

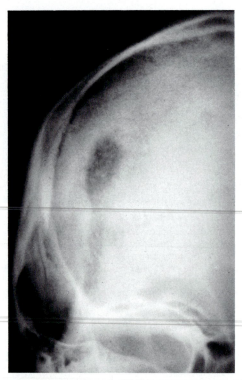

Fig. 2.32 Tuberculosis of the skull vault. The fairly well-defined lytic lesion was a solitary finding but these changes are often multiple. Note the gross tunnelling.

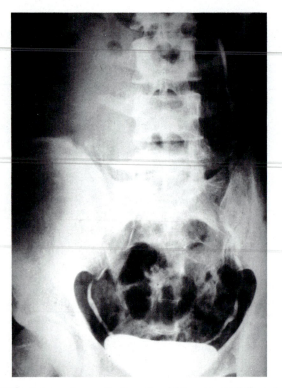

Fig. 2.30 A large abscess displaces the right ureter medially and destroys the right transverse process and adjacent part of the body of L5. Two and a half pints of tuberculous pus were removed at operation.

The latter is facilitated as the epiphyseal plate apparently offers little resistance to tuberculosis.

Early radiographic signs in synovial lesions are non-specific and will be manifested by capsular thickening, synovial effusion and surrounding osteoporosis. Later, continued hyperaemia will cause accelerated maturation of bone ends and epiphyses if the infection occurs in children. Bony trabeculae become blurred and the cortex thinned (Fig. 2.33).

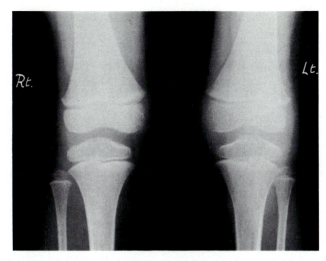

Fig. 2.33 Synovial tuberculosis of left knee — note synovial effusion, osteoporosis, blurring of trabeculae and accelerated maturation of bone ends (normal right knee for comparison).

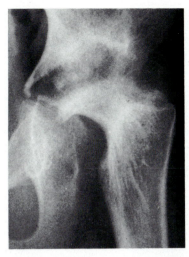

Fig. 2.35 Late tuberculosis of hip — 'bird's beak' appearance.

The bone ends eventually become affected. Local marginal or surface erosions may appear (Fig. 2.34). Loss of joint space will ultimately occur, but this is not as prominent a feature as it is in pyogenic arthritis. Sometimes one-half of a joint will be affected and bony erosions seen on contiguous bony surfaces.

The advent of antibiotics has changed the picture considerably. Patients usually respond well to treatment so that only the earlier phases are now seen. Formerly such sequelae as subluxation and ankylosis of joints, severe bone atrophy and tracking abscesses were common.

Hip. This is a common site; lesions may arise in the acetabulum, synovium, femoral epiphysis or metaphysis. Sometimes infection spreads to the hip from foci in the greater trochanter or ischium. All degrees of bone loss of the femoral head and neck could be found. A frequent finding was the pointed 'bird's beak' appearance (Fig. 2.35) with intrapelvic protrusion.

Knee. With synovial infection in childhood, effusion, osteoporosis and accelerated skeletal maturation are seen (Fig. 2.33). Overgrowth leads to modelling abnormalities, with big bulbous squared epiphyses, so that the appearance resembles that seen in juvenile chronic arthritis and haemophilia.

Shoulder. The humeral head, the glenoid, or both may be affected (Fig. 2.36). Sometimes a lesion in the humeral head is large and cystic in appearance and may resemble an osteoclastoma.

Some tuberculous shoulder lesions run a relatively benign course without pus formation — *caries sicca*. In such cases a relatively small pitted erosion is seen on the humeral head. These may resemble degenerative changes.

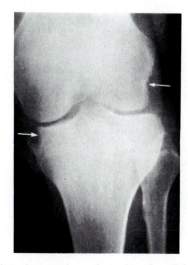

Fig. 2.34 Tuberculous erosions of margins of medial tibial condyle and lateral femoral condyle (arrows).

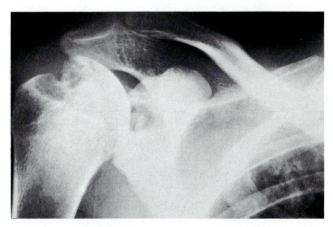

Fig. 2.36 Tuberculosis of shoulder — note lesions of humerus and glenoid and also lung.

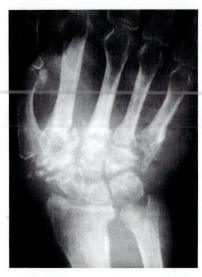

Fig. 2.37 There is soft-tissue swelling around the wrist with evidence of a widespread synovial abnormality. Bone and cartilage are destroyed. Osteoporosis is seen at the metacarpophalangeal joints. The metacarpal shafts however remain normal in density. The fifth metacarpal shaft has a periosteal reaction.

Wrist and carpus (Fig. 2.37). All carpal bones tend to be attacked in the adult, whereas more localized lesions are the tendency in children. This is possibly due to the relatively thicker articular cartilage in the latter. With cartilage destruction the carpal bones become crowded and even if initially one bone is the focus of irregularity, the destructive process soon involves adjacent bones. Intense demineralization is found throughout the carpus and distal radius and ulna, within the confines of synovium. Demineralization is often also pronounced at distal small

joints of the hand, with relative preservation of metacarpal and phalangeal shaft density. However, these joints are not eroded as in rheumatoid arthritis.

Sacroiliac joints (Fig. 2.38). This joint is affected more often in young adults than in children. Only occasionally is the condition bilateral. Subarticular erosions cause widening of joint space. The infection is usually associated with abscess formation over the back of the joint and, later, pus may calcify. Tuberculous infection of the spine is a frequent accompaniment.

SYPHILIS OF BONES AND JOINTS

Very few cases of syphilis of bone are now seen in Britain. Yet up to the time of the last war it was a condition that merited serious consideration in the differential diagnosis of most conditions of bone. In this section merely a summary of the findings is presented and illustrations are selected with a view to emphasizing the protean pattern of the lesions.

CONGENITAL SYPHILIS

Lesions may be found in infants whose serological reactions are negative, especially when the mother is receiving treatment. They may appear early, i.e. from birth to 4 years, or later, i.e. between the ages of 5 and 15 years.

Radiographic appearances. The lesions may be widespread and are usually symmetrical. Generally they

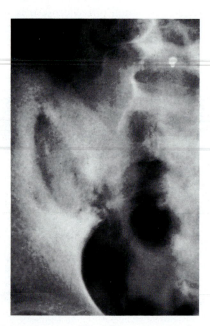

Fig. 2.38 Tuberculous sacroiliac joint — extensive destructive lesion.

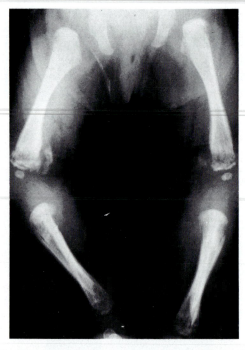

Fig. 2.39 Congenital syphilis — some increased density with subjacent translucent zones of lower ends of femora. Metaphyseal fractures are shown.

are best shown in the lower ends of the radius and ulna and around the knee. Changes are:

1. *Periostitis*. This is the commonest feature and is seen either as a thin layer or as more marked laminated layers. Marked thickening on the convexity of a diaphysis may be seen in later cases as, for example, in the so-called 'sabre tibia'.

2. *Metaphysitis*. There may be irregularity of metaphyses and metaphyseal fractures may occur (Fig. 2.39).

3. *Osteitis or osteomyelitis*. Erosions on the upper medial surfaces of the tibiae are very characteristic of congenital syphilis. Sometimes more diffuse osteomyelitis of single bones is seen. Syphilis is a productive lesion, so sclerosis will be found frequently in such lesions.

4. *Syphilitic dactylitis* is rare; it resembles tuberculous dactylitis.

5. *Skull lesions* may be purely sclerotic or may present as a combination of sclerosis and osteolysis. In purely sclerotic lesions, new bone may be laid down in the frontal and parietal regions, so producing the 'hot cross bun' skull.

ACQUIRED SYPHILIS

Any bone may be affected by this condition. Radiological manifestations comprise periostitis and osteomyelitis.

Periostitis. This sign may be seen as a simple laminated periosteal reaction or as a more exuberant lace-like appearance. Bony spiculation at right-angles to the shaft is rare but, when it occurs, it may mimic a neoplastic lesion.

Osteomyelitis. This may occur as a localized or as a diffuse lesion. The localized lesion is termed a gumma (Fig. 2.40), but a more diffuse lesion is often referred to as 'gummatous osteitis' (Figs 2.41, 2.42). Sclerosis is generally found; irregularity of bone trabeculation is often apparent. Syphilis causes a combination of destruction and proliferation of bone.

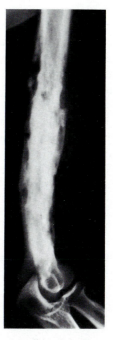

Fig. 2.41 Syphilitic osteomyelitis of the humerus. (Courtesy of Dr. W. Fowler.)

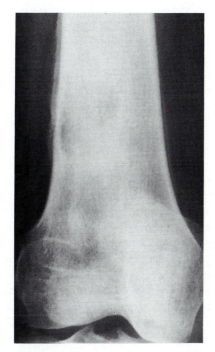

Fig. 2.40 Gumma of the lower femoral shaft. Note bone destruction and periosteal reaction.

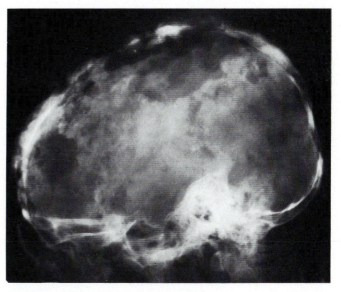

Fig. 2.42 Gummatous osteomyelitis of the skull.

It is important to remember the possibility of syphilis when presented with an atypical bony lesion.

RADIONUCLIDE SCANNING IN BONE INFECTION

Skeletal scintigraphy in infection should rightly precede plain film examination. Plain radiographic changes cannot be seen for up to 10–14 days with simple infections, though in tuberculous disease changes are usually present at first presentation. Using scintigraphy, however, the diagnosis of osteomyelitis can be confirmed as early as 48 hours after the onset of the disease, even if clinical signs are equivocal. Early aggressive treatment may prevent gross bone destruction and, indeed, if given early enough on the basis of a positive scan, need never develop.

Standard techniques involve the use of technetium-99m-labelled phosphonate and phosphate compounds. The accretion of radionuclide in bone is related to blood flow as well as to local bone turnover. This allows two separate sets of images to be obtained in osteomyelitis:

1. A 'blood pool' image of the painful area immediately after injection. This shows increased local radioactivity, if positive, in areas of increased blood flow.
2. Delayed skeletal scintigraphic images at 3–4 hours. By this time the radionuclide has been absorbed onto bone crystal. This gives a skeletal image with local accentuation in areas of increased blood flow and bone turnover. This also differentiates osteomyelitis from cellulitis.

Using these techniques it can safely be said that not only is scanning more sensitive in detecting infective foci earlier, but it is nearly always accurate — positive or negative. It is however nonspecific, since tumours and infection may give similar appearances. Technetium uptake is, however, limited if blood vessels are occluded in the infective process by tamponade or thrombus.

Gallium-67-labelled citrate scans may be used when the technetium scan is negative in patients with clinical osteomyelitis, or even in conjunction with a technetium scan. Gallium concentrates avidly at a site of infection following local accumulation of leucocytes and proteins which are labelled in vivo. The radiation dose is higher however and the image poorer. Gallium scans are also probably more helpful in follow-up of active osteomyelitis, as such scans are negative earlier than technetium scans when disease becomes quiescent. Technetium scans remain positive for some time even in inactive disease, as the mode of uptake depends on a different physiological process. Gallium scans cannot distinguish with accuracy between cellulitis and osteomyelitis.

Similar results may be obtained with in-vitro indium-labelled leucocytes which are reinjected into the patient.

BONE BIOPSY IN INFECTION

This heading can be extended to malignant disease, since bone biopsy by needle is performed in the diagnosis of both infections and tumours. Generally in our radiological practice the spine is most frequently biopsied; open biopsy for tissue and bacteriological diagnosis is clearly a much more serious procedure and is generally not the first technique to be used.

As far as infection is concerned, the results of a successful biopsy are: 1. to confirm the presence of infection and exclude tumour or other causes of a radiological lesion; 2. to distinguish the organism, both by direct microscopic examination of the aspirate and after culture; and 3. to allow correct antibiotic treatment after appropriate sensitivities have been established.

General anaesthesia is unnecessary except in infancy, or if noncooperation is expected. Sedation and analgesia are adequate. Analgesia should be both intravenous and local, including infiltration of local anaesthesia down to the periosteum.

Biopsy is best performed using biplane fluoroscopy. The use of plain films for one plane delays the procedure considerably. Many types of biopsy needle are available. Some are of very large bore and consist of pointed trochars in a cannula which are used to enter bone, when the pointed trochar is replaced by a trephine with a cutting edge. Certainly hard bone needs a rigid biopsy needle. Infections of bone or disc, however, tend to be soft, and in practice a fine aspiration needle is often all that is needed. Complications using a fine needle are usually minor. Pneumothorax and bleeding in the chest, or bleeding from abdominal organs, are not usually a serious problem. Usually the preference of the histologist governs the size of the sample the radiologist needs to obtain.

SARCOIDOSIS

This disease is a non-caseating granulomatous disorder commoner in young adult males and especially in patients of black African descent. Changes in the skeleton are moderately common, occurring in up to 15% of cases. The hands and feet are far most commonly affected but any bone may be involved. Lesions in the skull, vertebrae and long bones have all been described. Though the granulomas usually cause lysis of bone, often resembling tuberculosis, sclerosis occasionally results. Radionuclide scanning detects early bone lesions with greater sensitivity than plain radiographs.

Radiological findings. The changes in the bones include:

1. Punched-out, well-defined areas of lucency in the phalanges (Fig. 2.43). These are probably due to deposition of sarcoid tissue but, as in granulomatous leprosy (see below), the nutrient foramina are also said to be enlarged.

2. A more diffuse reticular lace-like pattern of resorption permeating the bone, described as a lattice-like appearance (Fig. 2.44).

3. Resorption of distal phalanges (Fig. 2.43) and of cortical bone along phalangeal shafts. Cortical resorption vaguely resembles that seen in hyperparathyroidism.

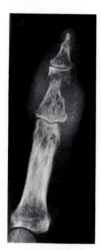

Fig. 2.43 Sarcoid — coarsened trabeculation of middle phalanx with marked bone resorption and spontaneous fracture. Absorption of the tuft of the distal phalanx is also seen.

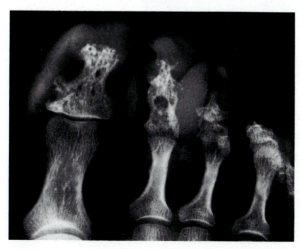

Fig. 2.44 Sarcoid — foot of same patient as Fig. 2.43, showing typical pseudocysts and absorption of tufts of distal phalanges.

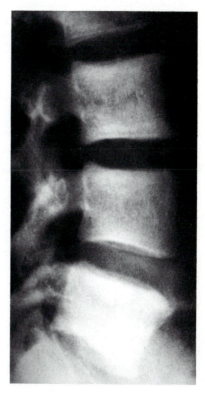

Fig. 2.45 Multiple foci of sclerosis are a recognized, if uncommon, feature of sarcoid.

4. Sclerosis, which may be widely disseminated (Fig. 2.45).

5. Periosteal reaction.

6. Soft-tissue nodules — far commoner than bone changes.

7. Periarticular calcification due to hypercalcaemia, which occurs in 20–45% of cases of sarcoid.

Sarcoid arthritis. An arthritis is a common manifestation of sarcoid, occurring in up to 37% of patients, most commonly in females. In the acute form joint destruction does not occur but in chronic disease a destructive arthropathy of large joints does rarely occur due to local granulomas.

RARE BONE INFECTIONS

BRUCELLOSIS

(synonyms: *undulant fever, Malta fever*)

This disease is more prevalent in Britain than was once thought. Transmission is from unpasteurized milk or by direct contact with affected animals. *Brucellus melitensis* infects sheep, *Br. abortus* infects cattle and *Br. suis* pigs.

The bones are affected in 10% of cases, most often the spine and especially in the lumbar region. Widespread granulomatous lesions may be present.

1. *Spinal lesions.* These bear a marked resemblance to other forms of osteomyelitis. Focal sclerosis develops to

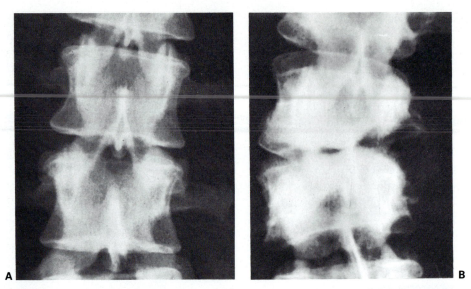

Fig. 2.46 Brucellosis. **A**. Reduction of disc space at L2–L3 — no bony involvement. **B**. Three months later. Destructive changes L2 and L3, sclerosis and lipping between L2 and L3 seen on original radiograph. (Courtesy of Dr. O. Bauerova.)

a marked degree around the end-plate (Fig. 2.46). The disc is rapidly destroyed and adjacent vertebrae rapidly affected. Healing is by the production of extremely large, coarse and shaggy bridging osteophytes.

2. *Changes in other bones*. The radiographic appearances resemble those of subacute osteomyelitis.

3. *Changes in joints*. These resemble the changes of synovial tuberculosis. In advanced cases erosive lesions may be seen.

In obscure and atypical bone infections, it is always advisable to test samples of the blood and of the synovial fluid of affected joints for the agglutination reaction for brucellosis, and also for the typhoid and paratyphoid group of bacilli.

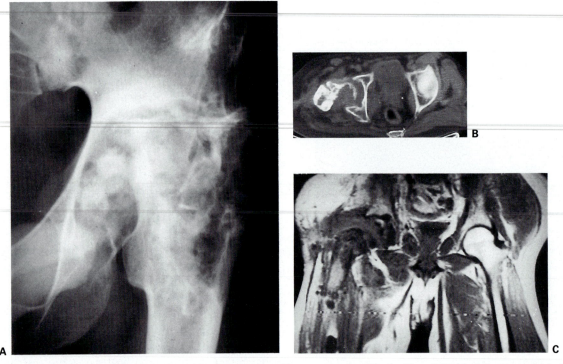

Fig. 2.47 Hydatid disease. **A**. Bone destruction with the formation of large cysts around both sides of the hip joint are a classic feature of osseous hydatid. Sequestra can be seen. At CT scanning. (**B**) and MRI (**C**) the cystic nature of the lesions is demonstrated, together with destruction fo the hip joint from both sides.

ACTINOMYCOSIS

Bony lesions due to this disease are rarely seen. They usually result from direct extension of soft tissue lesions. Manifestations may be seen in the following sites:

1. *Mandible*. Chronic osteomyelitis arises by direct spread from oral infections and infected cervical glands. The lesion appears to be irregularly destructive.

2. *Ribs and thoracic spine*. Destructive foci and periosteal reaction in these bones arise from pleuropulmonary lesions.

3. *Right side of the pelvis and lumbar spine*. Infection spreads to these bones from ileocaecal foci. Spinal lesions are usually accompanied by paravertebral abscesses. The disc is usually spared.

Very rarely destructive metastatic foci are found in other bones.

HYDATID (ECHINOCOCCUS) DISEASE

Hydatid disease is rare in Britain and in less than 2% of affected patients is bone involved. The pelvis, spine and proximal long bones are usually involved. The disease is found in sheep-farming areas.

The enlarging cysts in bone absorb trabeculae and spread along the medulla, thinning the cortex and expanding the bone. Later the cystic lesions become well defined so that fibrous dysplasia may be simulated in long bones.

Around the hip joint both the acetabulum and femoral head and neck are destroyed by large cystic lesions (Fig. 2.47). Fusion may result.

In the spine the cysts break out of the cortex, forming large paraspinal masses which do not calcify but do cause paraplegia (Fig. 2.48). The appearance may resemble dumb-bell tumours in neurofibromatosis.

TROPICAL CONDITIONS

YAWS (*treponematosis*)

This disease, which has more or less been eradicated, may still be seen in chronic cases. It is prevalent in the Caribbean, Indonesia and parts of tropical Africa and South America, and is due to a non-venereal infection by *Treponema pertenue*. As the disease is not transmitted to the fetus, congenital yaws does not occur but children become infected. Infection usually occurs through a cut or abrasion. Bony changes are seen in the secondary and tertiary stages; these are usually indistinguishable radiologically.

Any bone may be involved. The distribution may be random, but there is a tendency to symmetry. In the early stages, multiple small rarified areas of bone destruction are shown with overlying periosteal new bone (Fig. 2.49). The hand may be especially affected. Larger areas of

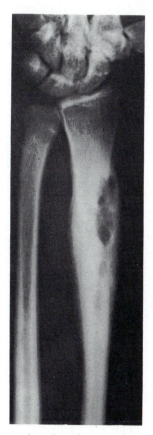

Fig. 2.49 Yaws — moderately early stage, showing destructive areas and much periosteal new bone formation. The appearances of the small destructive foci in yaws have been likened to the effects of a borer beetle. (Courtesy of Dr. A. G. Davies.)

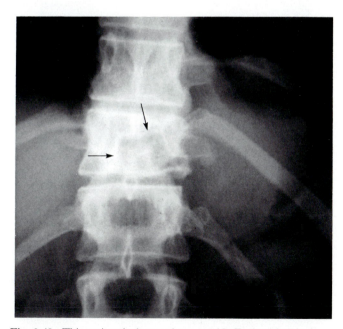

Fig. 2.48 This patient had never been outside England but had hydatid disease of the spine. Note the large paraspinal soft-tissue mass.

destruction occur in the skull and long bones, often with marked surrounding reactive sclerosis and new bone formation. Periostitis along the shaft, and softening of bone due to osteitis, lead to the sabre tibia deformity.

In the skull gummatous lesions cause foci of osteolysis while slowly growing masses arising from the premaxilla produce a dense hyperostosis known as *goundou*. *Gangosa*, another manifestation of yaws, is an ulceration of the face causing severe necrosis of subjacent bone.

LEPROSY

This disease has a widespread geographical distribution, occurring in Egypt, Africa, Asia, the Caribbean and Pacific islands. It is also seen in Britain's immigrant population. The lesions seen radiologically mostly affect the hands, feet and face, and are caused by infection by *M. leprae*. This bacillus is of low infectivity and prolonged exposure is needed. The nature of the disease depends on host resistance. The incidence of bony change in leprosy may be around 15%.

Three types of bony lesions are found:

1. *Specific changes of osteitis leprosa* (15%). Granulomas cause areas of focal cortical or medullary bone destruction. The lesions may be rounded or may infiltrate, giving a lacy pattern just as in sarcoid. In addition, medullary nutrient foramina enlarge (Fig. 2.50).

2. *Non-specific leprous osteitis* (50%). In these patients Hansen bacilli are rarely found in the marrow. Neuropathic resorption gives a 'licked candy stick' appearance with bone loss both longitudinally and circumferentially (Fig. 2.51). In addition, Charcot-like changes take place in the tarsus. These patients have abnormal, thickened nerves and arterial occlusions. Abnormal stance potentiates this bone resorption in the denervated weight-bearing foot.

With anaesthesia, plantar ulceration and bone and soft tissue infections are superimposed, so that pyogenic osteomyelitis is common in these patients. These changes are superimposed upon those of the neuropathic osteopathy.

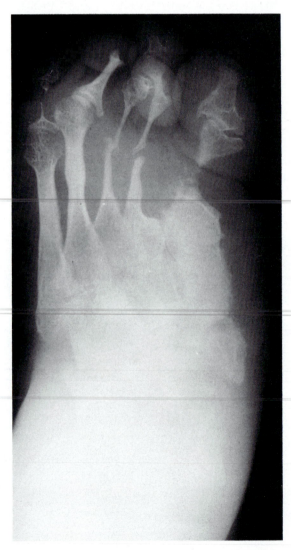

Fig. 2.51 Well-defined longitudinal and circumferential bone resorption with no evidence of superadded osteomyelitis in leprosy. Charcot-like changes are evident in the tarsus.

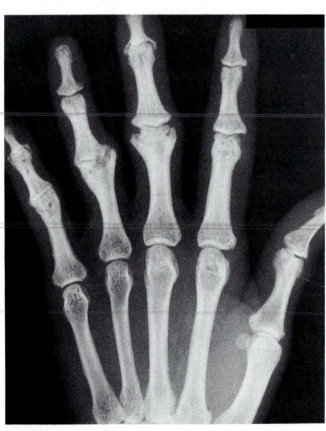

Fig. 2.50 Leprosy. Some small 'cysts' are seen, e.g. in the head of the proximal phalanx of the fifth finger — this condition is sometimes called 'osteitis multiplex cystica leprosa'. The end-results of lepra granulomata are seen in the heads of the proximal phalanges of the third and fourth fingers. (Courtesy of Dr. D. E. Paterson.)

3. *A diffuse osteoporosis* in seen which is non-specific. Nerve calcification is occasionally seen.

TROPICAL ULCER

This common lesion found throughout the tropics may also be seen in immigrants to Britain. Chronic indolent skin ulcers cause secondary bone changes, usually in the tibia or fibula. Periostitis is seen early in various forms, e.g. linear, onion-layer, lacework and spicular. In very chronic cases, much dense cortical new bone is deposited and the final picture resembles that of an ivory osteoma (Figs 2.52, 2.53).

COCCIDIOIDOMYCOSIS

This is a chronic granulomatous condition caused by a fungus and found in the south-western parts of the USA. The lesions are multiple and are most commonly found

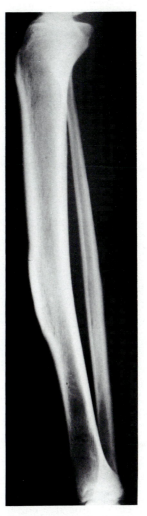

Fig. 2.53 Tropical ulcer — osteoma-like lesion on the front of the tibial shaft, a late sequel of tropical ulcer.

in the spine, pelvis, hands and feet. The bone lesions have the appearances of acute and chronic osteomyelitis; the joint lesions are similar to those found in tuberculous arthritis. The more frequent intrathoracic lesions of coccidioidomycosis are described in Chapter 15.

MYCETOMA

Mycetoma implantation occurs mainly in the (bare) feet in semi-desert regions throughout the tropics. The skull and knees may also be implanted, usually by thorns. Different organisms are found in different regions — *M. mycetoma* in the Middle East, Africa and India, and *S. somaliensis* and *pelletieri* in the Sudan. Lesions due to *M. mycetoma* are usually localized as large, well-defined black fungus balls which can be seen on soft-tissue radiographs. These erode the cortices and cause cystic defects in the medulla. Madura foot results (the lesions were first described in that region of India). With super-

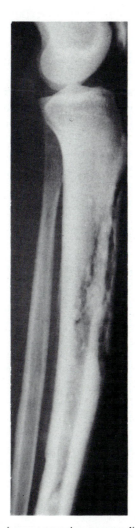

Fig. 2.52 Tropical ulcer — extensive osteomyelitis is seen in the underlying tibia.

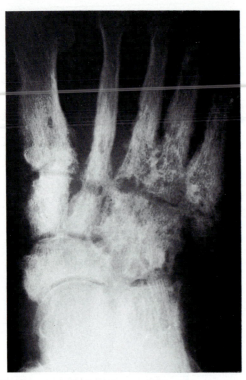

Fig. 2.54 Mycetoma: Madura foot — diffuse infiltrating destruction affecting the whole tarsus and proximal ends of the metatarsals.

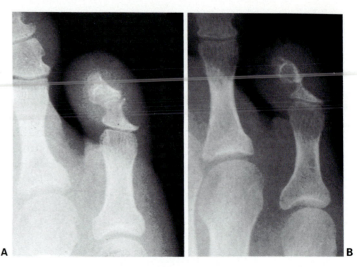

Fig. 2.55 Ainhum, showing progression of the lesion in an African immigrant. **B** was taken two years after **A**.

added infection via the implantation track, gross bone destruction results (Fig. 2.54). Reactive sclerosis and a shaggy periostitis with bone resorption give an appearance likened to melting snow. With *S. pelletieri*, diffuse infection occurs earlier but the end-stage appearances after secondary infection are usually similar.

AINHUM (dactylosis spontanea)
This is seen in 2% of the Nigerian population. The local word *ayun*, from which ainhum is derived, means to saw or file and a pointed fifth, or less commonly, fourth toe is found (Fig. 2.55).

A groove begins on the medial side of the base of the toe which deepens. This can be identified radiologically. As the constriction deepens, auto-amputation occurs, leaving a pointed proximal phalanx of the little toe.

Constriction rings (Streeter's bands) cause similar congenital lesions of hands and feet, often in association with clubfoot.

REFERENCES AND SUGGESTIONS FOR FURTHER READING

Bjarnson, D. F., Forrester, D. M., Swezey, R. L. (1973) Destructive arthritis of large joints. A rare manifestation of sarcoid. *Journal of Bone and Joint Surgery*, 55A, 618–622.

Chapman, M., Murray, R. O., Stoker, D. J. (1979) Tuberculosis of the bones and joints. *Seminars in Roentgenology*, 14(4) 266–282.

Cockshott, P., Middlemiss, J. H. (1979) *Clinical Radiology in the Tropics*. Churchill Livingstone, Edinburgh.

Cremin, B. J., Fisher, R. M. (1970) Lesions of congenital syphilis. *British Journal of Radiology*, 43, 333–341.

Edeiken, J. (1978) Infections of bones and joints. In: Feldman, F. (ed.) *Radiology, Pathology and Immunology of Bones and Joints*. Appleton Century-Crofts, New York.

Enna, C. D., Jacobson, R. R., Rausch, R. O. (1971) Bone changes in leprosy: correlation of clinical and radiographic features. *Radiology*, 100, 295–306.

Epstein, B. S. (1976) *The Spine*. 4th edn. Lea & Febiger, Philadelphia.

Gohel, K., Dalinka, M. K., Edeiken, J. (1973) The serpiginous tract: a sign of subacute osteomyelitis. *Journal of the Canadian Association of Radiologists*, 24, 337–339.

Griffiths, H. J. (1979) Interventional radiology: the musculoskeletal system. *Radiologic Clinics of North America*, 17(3) 475–485.

Jacobs, P. (1964) Osteo-articular tuberculosis in coloured immigrants. *Clinical Radiology*, 15, 59–69.

Kido, D., Bryan, D., Halpern, M. (1973) Haematogenous osteomyelitis in drug addicts. *American Journal of Roentgenology and Radium Therapy*, 118, 356–363.

Kolawole, T. M., Bohrer, S. P. (1970) Ulcer osteoma: bone response to tropical ulcer. *American Journal of Roentgenology and Radium Therapy*, 109, 611–618.

Lodwick, G. S. (1971) *The Bones and Joints*. Year Book Medical Publishers, Chicago.

Murray, R. O., Jacobson, H. G., Stoker, D. J. (1990) *The Radiology of Skeletal Disorders*. 3rd edn. Churchill Livingstone, Edinburgh.

Renton, P. (1982) Radiology of the foot. In: Klenerman (ed), *The Foot and its Disorders*, 2nd edn. Blackwell Scientific, Oxford.

Resnick, D., Niwayama, G. (1988) *Diagnosis of Bone and Joint Disorders*. 2nd edn. W. B. Saunders, Philadelphia.

CHAPTER 3

AVASCULAR NECROSIS OF BONE; OSTEOCHONDRITIS; MISCELLANEOUS BONE LESIONS

Peter Renton

OSTEONECROSIS

(synonyms: *aseptic necrosis, avascular necrosis, bone infarction*)

The term 'osteonecrosis' implies that a segment of bone has lost its blood supply so that the cellular elements within it die. The phrase 'aseptic necrosis' indicates that infection generally plays no part in the process, though a sequestrum is also necrotic and avascular.

Pathology. Ischaemia of bone follows occlusion of arteries or veins and is therefore dependent on the anatomy of the blood supply to a given bone (a rise in venous pressure eventually arrests arterial supply). Ischaemia results in death of haemopoietic tissue within 6–12 hours; of the osteoclasts, osteoblasts and osteocytes within 12–48 hours; and of marrow fat in 2–5 days. Empty osteocyte lacunae indicate death of bone. Dead bone at this stage is radiologically normal since the trabecular framework remains intact.

Revascularization is seen at the live marrow–dead marrow interface. The necrotic zone is invaded by capillaries, fibroblasts and macrophages. Fibrous tissue replaces dead marrow and in turn may calcify. New osteoblasts lay down fresh woven bone on the devitalized trabeculae. This advancing front of neo-vascularization and ossification has been termed 'creeping substitution' (Phemister).

At bone ends, cartilage receives nutrition from synovial fluid. Cartilage and subcartilaginous bone are not therefore necessarily affected.

Radiological changes are thus:

1. *Acute stage.* No changes are visible.

2. *Intermediate stage.* Disuse, for instance following immobility, leads to a generalized osteoporosis, except in devitalized avascular bone which is now devoid of osteoclasts and osteocytes. Avascular areas therefore remain normal in density while immobile but vascular bone loses density. The avascular proximal pole of the scaphoid thus remains dense after waist of scaphoid fractures.

3. *Late stage.* At large joints — hip, shoulder, knee — structural failure in subarticular bone at areas of maximal stress results in cortical microfractures followed by collapse and trabecular compression. This results in a flattened articular surface with increased subarticular density as trabeculae are compressed into a smaller space.

In the diametaphysis and subarticular regions, the infarcted area is surrounded by a serpiginous line of sclerosis, representing the advancing front of new bone laid down on the old trabecular framework. The central area within the infarct may look relatively lucent, or may actually be the site of osteoclastic resorption, but may also contain foci of added density representing dystrophic calcification in débris.

In some diseases following infarction, a 'bone-within-a-bone' or 'split cortex' is seen as a linear density lying within and parallel to the healthy cortex. This probably represents the old infarcted cortex left behind by processes of growth and remodelling beneath the vital periosteum. This change is seen in Gaucher's and in sickle-cell disease, and following osteomyelitis.

Epiphyseal abnormalities. Infarcts at growth plates, for instance in the hands and at the vertebral end-plates in sickle-cell disease, cause local arrest of growth or may result in 'cone' epiphyses or premature fusion. The latter also occurs after irradiation, infection or trauma.

Infarcted bone, e.g. following irradiation, is susceptible to fractures. This is seen in the ribs following irradiation for breast cancer and in the femoral necks after pelvic irradiation, though less commonly nowadays.

Causes of osteonecrosis (Table 3.1)

Vascular insufficiency to bone is of three types.

1. *Interruption to the flow of blood* to bone most commonly follows trauma with tearing of blood vessels.

2. *Emboli or sludging.* This occurs in *sickle-cell disease* where abnormal red cells aggregate; in *pancreatitis* where fat emboli obstruct vessels; and in *decompression disease* where possibly gas bubbles occlude small vessels. Vasculitis, in collagen disorders and following irradiation, also occludes small vessels.

3. *Intraosseous compression of vessels* occurs in Gaucher's disease where masses of Gaucher cells pack marrow spaces.

Table 3.1 Conditions associated with spontaneous aseptic bone necrosis

**Alcoholism	*Hypercorsticism
Arthropathy	Hypercholesterolaemia
**Rheumatoid arthritis	**Hyperlipaemia
Psoriasis	Hypertension
Neuropathic	**Hypertriglyceridaemia
Osteoarthrosis	**Hyperuricaemia
Clotting defects	Immobilization
Convulsive disorders	*Immunosuppressive therapy
*Cushing's syndrome	*Irradiation
*Decompression syndrome	Microfractures
**Diabetes	Mitral insufficiency
Endocarditis	Myxoedema
**Fat embolism	Obesity
Giant cell arteritis	**Pancreatitis
Gonorrhoea	Peripheral neuropathy
**Gout	Peripheral vascular disease
*Haemoglobinopathy	Periarteritis nodosa
*Haemopoietic disorders	Pregnancy
Haemophilia	**Systemic lupus erythematosus
Gaucher's disease	*Thermal injuries
Histiocytosis	Burns
Polycythaemia	Electrical
	Frostbite
	*Trauma

 * Generally accepted contributory factor
** Commonly reported associated factor
(Reproduced from J. K. Davidson (ed.), *Aseptic Necrosis of Bone*, by kind permission of Excerpta Medica, Amsterdam)

Table 3.2 Types of eponymous osteochondritis

Disease	Cause	Site
Legg-Calvé-Perthes	Primary aseptic necrosis	Femoral head
Köhler	? primary aseptic necrosis ? necrosis following fracture	Tarsal navicular
Freiberg	? primary aseptic necrosis ? necrosis following fracture	Metatarsal head
Kienböck	? necrosis following fracture ? primary aseptic necrosis	Lunate
Osgood-Schlatter	Necrosis following partial avulsion of patellar tendon	Tibial tubercle
Sinding-Larsen	Necrosis following partial avulsion of patellar tendon	Lower pole of patella
Sever	Necrosis following partial avulsion of tendo achilles	Calcaneal apophysis
Calvé	Eosinophil granuloma	Vertebral body epiphysis
Scheuermann	Disc herniation through defective end-plate	Ring-like epiphysis of vertebra

(Reproduced from J. K. Davidson (ed.) *Aseptic Necrosis of Bone* by kind permission of Dr. Mary Catto, and Excerpta Medica, Amsterdam)

The role of drugs in avascular necrosis. Steroids and non-steroidal anti-inflammatory drugs are associated with bone necrosis.

Pain relief and euphoria associated with prolonged dosage lead to overuse of often already damaged joints and a Charcot-type lesion results with bone loss and eburnation. Similar changes may follow alcohol abuse. In addition, steroids cause vasculitis and marked subcortical osteoporosis which further potentiates bone collapse.

OSTEOCHONDRITIS (Osteochondrosis)
Osteochondritis is a disease of epiphyses, beginning as necrosis and followed by healing. The term 'osteochondritis' is used to describe the lesions but is a misnomer, as: 1. there is no inflammation; and 2. cartilage is not primarily involved. Over 40 sites have been described and all have eponyms which are too closely associated with the lesions to be currently abandoned (Table 3.2).

The mechanism of pathological change is not identical at all sites. Some changes, such as in Perthes' disease, are generally regarded as being due to vascular occlusion. The mechanism for this is not clearly understood, especially as in some patients an osteochondritis affects more than one epiphysis. At other sites — the tibial tubercle and the lower pole of patella — tendons avulse bone which subsequently necroses. Vertebra plana follows eosinophil granuloma. Adolescent kyphosis may follow discal herniation into end-plate defects.

Epiphyseal areas of necrosis eventually heal and are converted into normal bone. In some sites, especially at the femoral head, prominent metaphyseal changes are also present.

OSTEOCHONDRITIS OF THE FEMORAL CAPITAL EPIPHYSIS
(synonym: *coxa plana*; eponyms: *Waldenström (1909), Legg (1910), Calvé (1910), Perthes (1910)*)
This condition is commoner in boys than girls (M : F = 4 : 1) and most cases present between 4 and 9 years of age. The age of onset is earlier in girls and the prognosis worse.

Bilateral disease is even more common in boys (M : F = 7 : 1) but the disease is rarely symmetrical. If symmetry is present, hypothyroidism or multiple epiphyseal dysplasia should be excluded. There is no increased familial incidence, but parents of affected children are often elderly. Many of the affected children have a below-average birthweight and, at presentation, show skeletal growth retardation in the hands. This is especially seen in boys. There is an increased incidence of associated congenital anomalies, including congenital heart disease, pyloric stenosis, hernia, renal anomalies and undescended testes.

Following ischaemia, the ossific nucleus of the epiphysis necroses, causing growth arrest. The overlying cartilage, which is supplied by synovial fluid, survives and thickens, especially in the non-weight-bearing regions, medially and laterally. Creeping substitution eventually occurs in the ossific nucleus which thus becomes denser, the process usually reaching the dome from the peripheral and deep parts of the epiphysis.

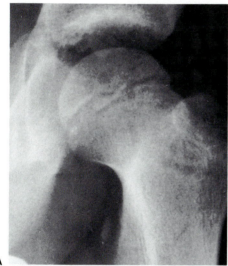

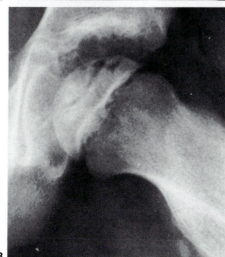

Fig. 3.1 **A**. Perthes' disease, showing increased joint space in AP view. **B**. Fissures in the femoral head are shown well in the frog view.

Radiological features

1. *Lateral displacement of the femoral head.* Early on, and in the irritable hip syndrome, displacement of the femoral head (Waldenström's sign) is seen (Fig. 3.1), possibly due to effusion or to thickening of the ligamentum teres. Later, the superior part of the joint may also be widened. These changes may be seen on ultrasound.

2. *A subcortical fissure in the femoral ossific nucleus.* This sign is seen early in the disease but is transient. It is best seen in the 'frog' lateral view.

3. *Reduction in size of the ossific nucleus of the epiphysis.* This is found in some 50% of cases and is due to growth retardation. The medial joint space then seems wider.

4. *Increase in density of the femoral ossific nucleus.* This is due to trabecular compression, dystrophic calcification in débris and creeping substitution (see above) (Fig. 3.2).

Catterall (1971) has grouped Perthes' disease according to the degree of epiphyseal involvement as assessed radiologically (Fig. 3.3). Prognosis depends on the degree of radiological involvement.

Stages of the disease occur within each group.

There is an *initial* phase of onset, with widening of the joint space and increased density of all or part of the ossific nucleus, which is followed by collapse of part or all of the nucleus, according to group. *Repair* removes the fragmented, crushed, necrotic bone. *Healing* shows as an increase in size and re-ossification (Fig. 3.2). *Remodelling* then occurs and is aided when the femoral head is completely contained within the acetabulum. Uncovering of the lateral margin of the femoral head has a bad prognosis.

The metaphyseal lesion leads to an abnormal femoral neck. The most severely involved cases have a broad, short neck, that is, the neck length/width ratio is lower than normal (Fig. 3.2).

Prognosis. The prognosis in untreated disease is proportional to the degree of epiphyseal involvement. Thus, Group I and Group II patients have a good prognosis.

The irritable hip syndrome

A few patients with this syndrome (up to 7%) develop changes of Perthes' disease. The affected children present with acute hip pain and often fever and a raised ESR. Most cases resolve with simple bed rest, but prolonged immobilization and traction may be necessary. Other causes of acute hip pain — infection or juvenile arthritis — must also be excluded.

RADIONUCLIDE BONE SCANNING IN ASEPTIC NECROSIS OF THE FEMORAL HEAD

Technetium scan images of bone depend in part on blood flow to bone. Avascular areas, therefore, are seen as scan defects. Nuclide scanning of a painful hip distinguishes a 'cold' area in infarction from an area of increased uptake

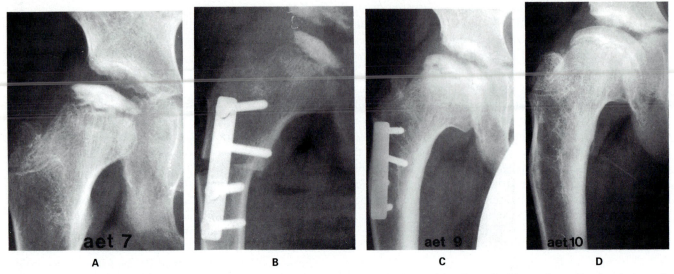

A	B	C	D

Fig. 3.2 Perthes' disease. A series of radiographs showing the stages of healing. **A**. The initial radiograph shows a flattened, sclerotic femoral head. **B**. An osteotomy is performed. **C, D**. Later films show resorption of the sclerotic dead bone and its replacement with vital bone, resulting in a mushroom-shaped femoral head.

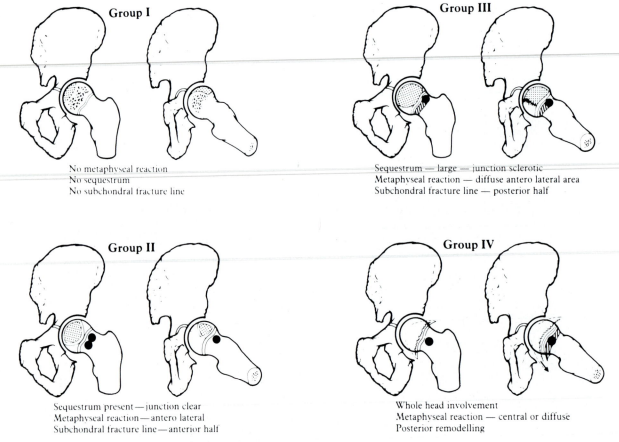

Group I

No metaphyseal reaction
No sequestrum
No subchondral fracture line

Group III

Sequestrum — large — junction sclerotic
Metaphyseal reaction — diffuse antero lateral area
Subchondral fracture line — posterior half

Group II

Sequestrum present — junction clear
Metaphyseal reaction — antero lateral
Subchondral fracture line — anterior half

Group IV

Whole head involvement
Metaphyseal reaction — central or diffuse
Posterior remodelling

Fig. 3.3 Catterall classification of Perthes' disease. (Reproduced by courtesy of Mr. A. Catterall F.R.C.S.; see list of Further Reading.)

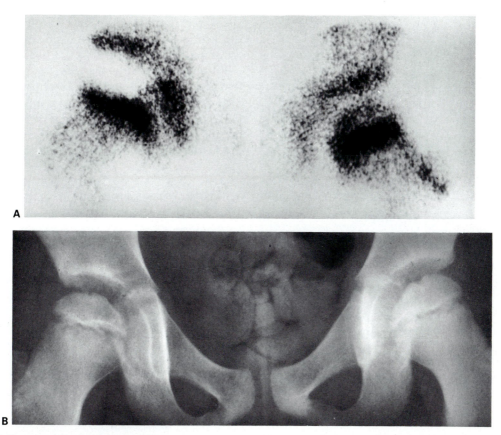

Fig. 3.4 Perthes' disease. **A**. The lateral aspect of the right femoral head does not show up on radionuclide scanning. **B**. On X-ray, the involved area looks smaller than on the scan.

in infective or inflammatory disease. It seems logical to scan all children with acutely painful hips.

In the early stage, when no radiological abnormality is yet visible in the child with an avascular lesion, a defect is seen in the femoral head image on radionuclide scanning. In the early case, the size of the defect on the scan correlates well with the eventual size of the defect on the radiograph, which only becomes assessable some 6–9 months after the initial nuclide scan (Fig. 3.4).

In cases of established disease, correlation of the scan defect with radiological change is less helpful, as revascularization gives a local increase in activity, so that the defect size is underestimated.

Prognosis in an early case can be assessed from the defect size on the early scan, so that a small defect has a good prognosis.

OSTEOCHONDRITIS OF THE TIBIAL TUBERCLE
(eponyms: *Osgood's disease, Schlatter's disease*)
The diagnosis is essentially clinical and is confirmed radiologically by a soft-tissue lateral film of the area. This demonstrates local soft-tissue swelling over an often fragmented and dense tuberosity (Fig. 3.5). The other knee

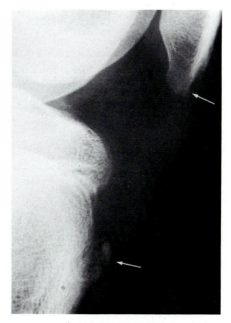

Fig. 3.5 Osgood-Schlatter disease. Note also some osteochondritis of the epiphysis of the lower pole of the patella.

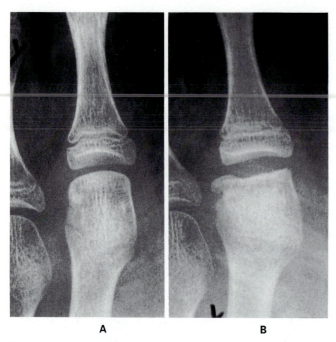

Fig. 3.6 Osteochondritis of second metatarsal head: **A.** minimal change of increased density of the epiphysis; **B.** later stage of flattening of the epiphysis, increased joint space and loose body separation.

should also be examined radiologically, especially to compare the soft tissues. The condition is usually self-limiting and rest brings relief of symptoms.

The tubercle fuses to the shaft at 15 years, but occasionally remains unfused and fragmented. Examination of soft tissues will rule out ongoing disease.

OSTEOCHONDRITIS OF THE METATARSAL HEAD
(eponyms: *Freiberg's infraction, Köhler's disease*)

The second metatarsal head is most frequently involved. The condition is commoner in girls. Its usual incidence is between 10 and 15 years. There is a history of chronic trauma, e.g. girls wearing high heels for the first time.

Radiographic appearances. Condensation, increased density (Fig. 3.6) and fragmentation of the epiphysis are seen. The joint space may be increased in size and the opposing bone surfaces greatly splayed. Gradual thickening of the metatarsal neck and shaft occurs.

OSTEOCHONDRITIS OF THE TARSAL NAVICULAR
(eponym: *Köhler's disease*)

As in Osgood-Schlatter's disease, the combination of pain and radiological change is needed for the diagnosis to be made. The disease is much more common in boys. Age incidence is 3–10 years, with the peak between 5 and 6

years, and the disease appears earlier in girls — as does the ossific nucleus itself. The process is thought to be ischaemic in origin. 15–20% are bilateral.

Radiographic appearances. Irregularity of the outline of the navicular and fissure formation are early signs. The bone may appear later as a mere dense disc (Fig. 3.7). No loss of cartilage on either side of the bone occurs. The onset of regeneration is shown by the production of new bone round the compressed disc.

OSTEOCHONDRITIS OF THE VERTEBRAL BODY
(eponym: *Calvé's disease;* synonym: *vertebra plana*)

This condition is manifested by collapse and increased density of a vertebral body; the adjacent disc spaces are normal or increased in width (Fig. 3.8). Recovery to normal shape follows, but it may be incomplete.

Most cases may be shown to be a manifestation of histiocytosis. Regeneration is expected but histiocytosis may be associated with paraplegia. Leukaemia, Ewing's sarcoma, metastases, tuberculosis etc. may cause similar appearances and should always be excluded before a diagnosis of Calvé's disease is accepted.

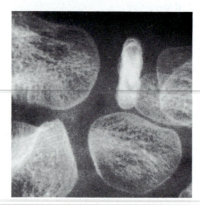

Fig. 3.7 Osteochondritis of the tarsal navicular.

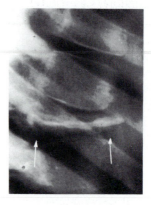

Fig. 3.8 Calvé disease (vertebra plana) of a mid-thoracic vertebral body. Complete regeneration occurred. No evidence of histiocytosis was found on biopsy.

ADOLESCENT KYPHOSIS

(synonyms: *vertebral epiphysitis, osteochondritis of vertebral epiphyseal plates;* eponym: *Scheuermann's disease*)
The condition affects both sexes; it usually begins at puberty, having a peak incidence from 15 to 16 years. The mid and lower thoracic spine is the region most commonly affected and usually several adjacent vertebrae are involved (Fig. 3.9). Less frequently the lesion may be found in the lumbar spine (Fig. 3.10) and in the upper thoracic spine. Sometimes changes are confined to a single vertebra.

Radiographic appearances. Irregularity is seen affecting the superior and inferior parts of the vertebral bodies. Later, wedging of vertebral bodies and kyphosis appear. Some scoliosis may also be present. Schmorl's nodes are seen and disc spaces become narrowed. Sometimes a small paraspinal bulge is observed at the level of the lesion.

The radiographic picture tends to remain static for a while. Improvement is slow and consolidation may take several years. Radiographic recovery is often incomplete: various degrees of irregularity and wedging of thoraco-lumbar vertebrae may be permanent. Indeed, evidence of old adolescent kyphosis is one of the most frequent abnormalities seen in spinal radiographs.

No constitutional effects are found in adolescent kyphosis and the vertebral defects are bounded by sclerotic rims, which are not seen in tuberculous lesions.

Residual wedging in late cases may be indistinguishable

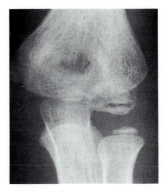

Fig. 3.11 'Osteochondritis' of the capitellum. (Reproduced with permission of the Editor of *Clinical Radiology*.)

from that caused by a previous compression fracture. The ring apophysis may be displaced by discal herniation, never to unite. It is then seen as a triangular fragment of bone adjacent to the end-plate. Discography shows a disc filled with contrast medium which extends between the vertebral body and the detached fragment of bone.

OSTEOCHONDRITIS AT OTHER SITES

Most osteochondritis is found in the hip or spine. Other sites include:
1. *Capitellum* (Fig. 3.11).
2. *Patella — primary centre* (Köhler's disease).
3. *Patella — Secondary centre* (Sinding-Larsen's disease).

Some cases are associated with Osgood-Schlatter's disease. This condition is also almost always due to an avulsion strain by the patellar ligament.

4. *Tibia vara* (osteochondritis of the medial tibial condyle — Blount's disease). This change may be seen from the first to the 12th year of age, but is most common in the earlier age group. As the name implies, the abnormality is usually to be seen on the medial aspect of the knee joint. An irregular defect is often present on the medial aspect of the proximal tibial metaphysis beneath which a large and prominent spur sticks out, almost at right angles. The adjacent aspect of the tibial epiphysis may be defective, and a local femoral spur may also be seen. The overall effect is a varus deformity. The lateral aspect of the proximal tibial metaphysis is straight, and not bowed as in physiological bow-legs.

The changes are possibly related to early onset of walking.

OSTEOCHONDRITIS IN ADULT BONES

Often a closer link with trauma is seen in adult osteochondritis than in juvenile cases, but this is not always so. Sites subject to trauma include the *scaphoid*, the *carpal lunate* (Kienbock's disease) (Fig. 3.12), the *tarsal navicular* and the *medial sesamoid bone of the great toe.*

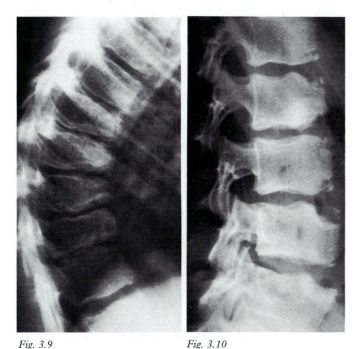

Fig. 3.9   *Fig. 3.10*

Fig. 3.9 Adolescent kyphosis (advanced case).

Fig. 3.10 'Osteochondritis' of lumbar vertebral bodies.

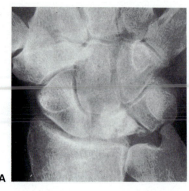
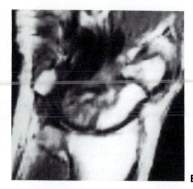

Fig. 3.12 A. Osteochondritis of the lunate bone (Kienbock's disease).   **B**. Avascular necrosis of the lunate. On MR scanning the lunate shows a mixed signal, with patchy areas of low and high intensity. Compare with the normal signal coming from the scaphoid.

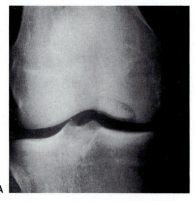
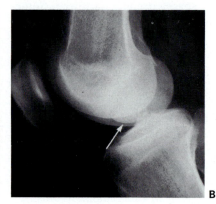

Fig. 3.13 A,B Osteochondritis dissecans of the medial femoral condyle.

OSTEOCHONDRITIS DISSECANS

In this condition fragments of articular cartilage, with or without subchondral bone, become partially or completely detached at characteristic sites. The separated fragment is avascular, in contradistinction to that at an osteochondral fracture, and the 'bed' of the defect remains vital, in contradistinction to avascular necrosis.

Sites of election are the medial femoral condyle, the capitellum of the humerus and the trochlear surface of the talus. The lesion is twice as common in males as females and about one-third of all cases are bilateral. In some patients several epiphyses are affected. The condition is not always symptomatic. The lesion characteristically occurs in adolescence and early adult life. It is the commonest cause of a loose body in the joint of a young adult. The present tendency is to emphasize the role of trauma in the aetiology of this lesion.

Radiographic features. In early cases it may be necessary to take several views of the joint in different degrees of obliquity in order to demonstrate the lesion adequately. Conventional and computed tomography are often helpful, and arthrography is sometimes useful.

When separation of the fragment is being established, one will see a radiolucent ring surrounding the bony fragment when viewed from the front; the loosening fragment may be seen opposite a pit in the bone when viewed in profile (Figs 3.13, 3.14). The loose fragments are usually small and ovoid in shape though they may be larger and irregular.

The fragment may become completely separated and form an intra-articular loose body. If entirely cartilaginous in content, the image of the loose body will not be seen on routine radiographs but it may be demonstrable by arthrography. If not removed surgically, the loose body may grow and calcify later; it is able to obtain adequate nourishment from synovial fluid even when it is completely detached from its parent bone. On the other hand, the fragment may not become free, but may become incorporated in the parent bone or may become absorbed leaving a residual gap in the underlying bone.

CAISSON DISEASE

(synonym: *dysbaric osteonecrosis*)

Exposure to a hyperbaric atmosphere may result in decompression sickness — 'the bends' — and in the late

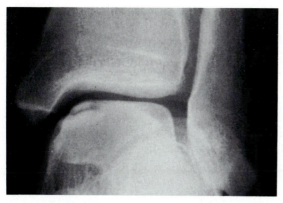

Fig. 3.14 Osteochondritis dissecans of the medial part of the articular surface of the talus.

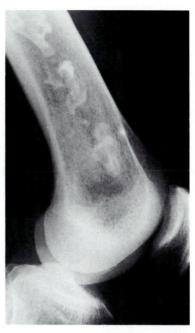

Fig. 3.16 Caisson disease.

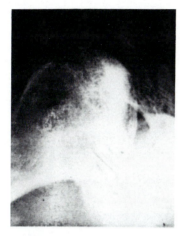

Fig. 3.15 Caisson disease. The humeral head shows a subcortical band of radiolucency with underlying sclerosis. The articular surface is collapsing.

complication of osteonecrosis. The lesions are liable to appear if the worker is too rapidly decompressed. It is thought that nitrogen becomes liberated from bone marrow and causes bone infarcts by occluding small blood vessels.

A history of previous decompression sickness is not necessary for the occurrence of osteonecrosis.

Radiographic findings. 1. *Juxta-articular lesions*. They are recognized as:

a. A transradiant subcortical band that may underlie as much as two-thirds of the articular cortex (Fig. 3.15).

b. Collapse of part of the articular cortex.

c. Sequestration of part of the cortex.

d. Secondary osteoarthritis.

2. *Neck and shaft lesions*. They cause the following appearances:

a. Dense areas — small, multiple, bilateral, ill-defined opacities resembling bone islands in the upper ends of the femoral and humeral shafts and in the femoral neck.

b. Irregular calcified areas — typically in the distal part of the femoral shafts (Fig. 3.16) and in the proximal parts of the shafts of the humeri and tibiae.

c. Malignant changes have occasionally been reported in such infarcts, usually in the form of malignant fibrous histiocytoma (Fig. 3.17).

INFANTILE CORTICAL HYPEROSTOSIS
(Caffey's disease)

The cause of this disease is unknown. Many affected children have high fever, most have raised sedimentation rates and occasionally pleural exudates are found. However, an infective agent has never been identified. Occasionally the disease has been reported in siblings, cousins and twins.

The condition has been diagnosed in utero. Usually, however, the babies are well for several weeks before the onset. The average age of onset is 9 weeks and cases do not apparently start after the age of 5 months.

Three features common to all these patients are hyper-irritability, soft-tissue swelling and bony cortical thickening. The soft-tissue swellings may be very painful, but are deeply situated and not accompanied by surface warmth or discoloration. Such swellings appear before bony changes are demonstrable and they disappear long before the bone lesions resolve. Sometimes the swellings may recur at their original site or new swellings may appear at other sites. The disease is characterized by the patchy distribution of the lesions and by remissions and relapses.

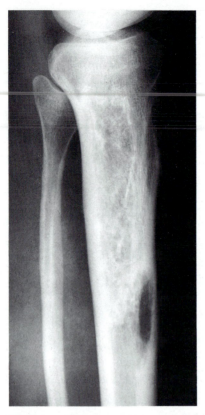

Fig. 3.17 Changes of medullary infarction are associated with an area of osteolysis due to fibrosarcoma.

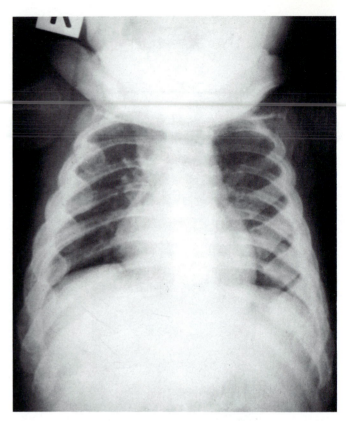

Fig. 3.18 Caffey's disease. Gross periostitis affects the ribs and the mandible is also thickened. (Courtesy of Dr. Ann Barrington, Sheffield.)

Bones commonly affected are the *mandible, ribs* (Fig. 3.18), *clavicle, scapula* (Fig. 3.19) and the *ulna,* but any tubular bones except the phalanges may be affected. The condition may also be found in the *skull* and *pelvis* but not in the spine. Lesions are confined to the shafts of the bones, and the epiphyses and metaphyses are not affected. This distribution affords a ready differentiation from rickets, scurvy and congenital syphilis.

Radiologically, marked periosteal proliferation and cortical thickening are seen in bones beneath the soft tissue swellings. The cortical hyperostosis may be massive. Patients usually recover after several weeks or months; in about 12 months, bones will usually have returned to normal.

PAGET'S DISEASE
(synonym: *osteitis deformans*)

Sir James Paget first described this disease in 1876. Its origin is not definitely known. Nonetheless, current thinking is that a 'slow' virus may be the initiating factor. Though no virus has been isolated, histological changes are seen that are present in viral infections.

There is variation in the distribution of the disease. It is common in the United Kingdom, parts of the United States, Australia and New Zealand, but uncommon in

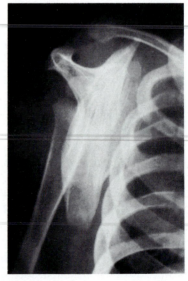

Fig. 3.19 Infantile cortical hyperostosis — massive cortical thickening of the scapula. (Courtesy of Mr. T. McSweeney.)

the Far and Middle East and Scandinavia. Within Britain there appear to be some regional differences in the incidence.

The incidence of the disease as judged by pathological and radiological surveys is 3–4% of the population.

Slightly more men are affected than women. Paget's disease is predominantly found in the elderly. Monostotic disease is not common (10–20%). Overall, the condition is found most commonly in the sacrum and lumbar spine, followed by the skull, pelvis and right femur. Apart from the skull, the weight-bearing and persisting red marrow areas are most commonly involved, though multiple rib and upper limb lesions are uncommon. No bone is exempt. Lesions of the fibula are very rare.

The radiographic appearances are explained by the underlying pathological processes.

1. An initial phase of increased osteoclastic activity results in bone resorption. This early phase is osteolytic and is not commonly seen radiologically, still less in established disease. It may persist in the skull, as osteoporosis circumscripta (Fig. 3.20).

2. Mixed phase (spongy type with coarse irregular trabeculation). Increased resorption of bone is followed by increased formation of abnormally coarsened trabeculae of increased volume (Figs. 3.21, 3.22). Haversian systems are destroyed and replaced by new bone with a characteristic mosaic pattern. The margin between cortex and medulla is lost.

3. Sclerotic phase (amorphous appearance) (Fig. 3.23). Osteoclastic activity declines and osteoblastic activity proceeds, so that disorganized new bone of increased density replaces lytic areas. Eventually the disease becomes quiescent.

Radionuclide bone scanning is of value during early activity, when it will pick up lesions which may not be radiologically detectable, while in the quiescent phase the presence of disease is best shown by conventional means.

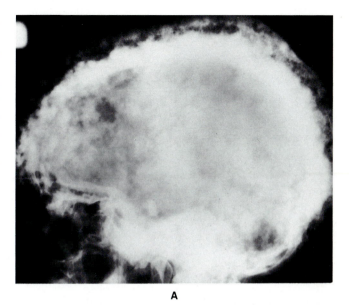

A

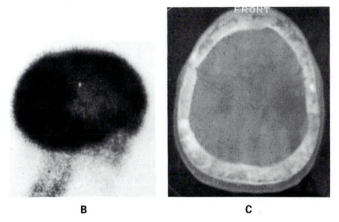

B   C

Fig. 3.21 A. Paget's disease of skull. Marked thickening of calvarium. Note the well-demarcated intracranial border of the inner table. Marked sclerosis of the base of the skull is also present. **B,C**. Paget's disease demonstrated by radionuclide and CT scanning. The vault is thickened and there is increased isotope uptake.

The total body scan detects disease in sites not routinely examined, such as the foot, but such sites are not commonly affected. The scan does however provide a quick overview of the skeleton and is useful in assessing change or malignant degeneration, so that follow-up is probably best performed by scanning.

Radiological features. *Long bones*. Paget's disease starts at a bone end and, as it extends to the other bone end, it is demarcated from normal bone by a V-shaped zone of transition (Fig. 3.23).

Long bones increase in cortical width and the femur and tibia may be bowed. Bones also increase in length and this may result in bowing if only one of a pair of long bones is affected. Paget's disease may cause more bony enlargement than is seen in any other disease.

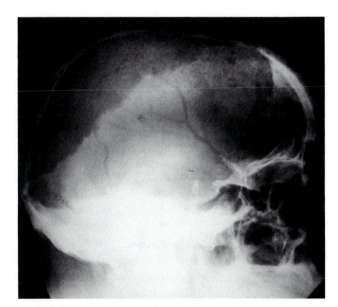

Fig. 3.20 Osteoporosis circumscripta. A well-defined osteolytic lesion affects most of the skull vault.

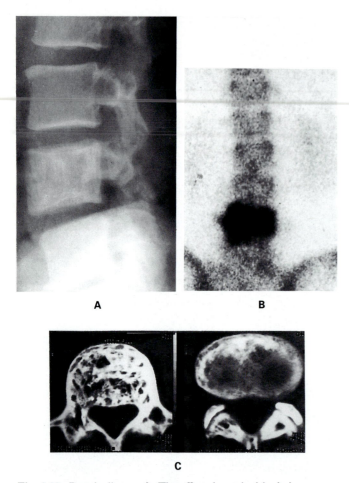

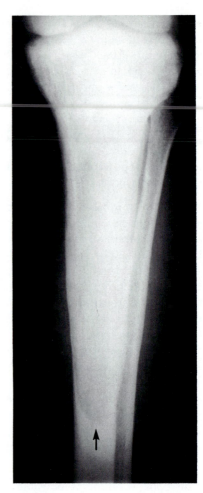

Fig. 3.22 Paget's disease. **A**. The affected vertebral body is expanded as well as showing abnormal texture. **B**. The bone scan confirms the increase in uptake in the expanded vertebral body. **C**. The CT scan shows the rather spongy texture of the abnormal body, extending into the pedicles and laminae.

Fig. 3.23 Paget's disease. Changes are seen extending downwards from the proximal tibia, ending with a flame-shaped border (arrow).

Pelvis. In early stages loss of some trabeculae with coarsening of those remaining may be seen. Thickening and loss of clarity of the ileopectineal line and the teardrop also indicate the disease. Narrowing of the hip joint space, especially in a medial direction, leads to protrusio with deformity of the pelvic brim. Secondary osteoarthritis then develops (Fig. 3.24).

Vertebrae. All three forms of the disease may be found in the vertebrae. The neural arch and pedicles may be involved as well as the vertebral body, and all parts are enlarged. The width of the body is increased so that the interpedicular distance is also increased, even if the pedicles are enlarged. A characteristic, if infrequent, finding is a picture-frame appearance with condensed thickened end-plates and vertebral margins enclosing a cystic spongiosa (Fig. 3.25). The condensed end-plates are not seen with haemangiomas and involvement of posterior elements is also less common. Enlargement is unusual in both haemangiomas and metastatic disease.

Collapse is common and may cause spinal nerve com-

pression. Vertebral enlargement distinguishes this from osteoporotic or malignant disease.

Skull. In the skull the disease begins as a destructive process affecting the outer table and sparing the inner table (Fig. 3.20). The full picture of osteoporosis circumscripta is rarely seen. In the reparative stage, sclerosis of the inner table is pronounced, and later the diploic spaces and the outer table become thickened. A classic, widespread cotton-wool effect results (Fig. 3.21A). The cranial cavity is not encroached upon.

Dental abnormalities include loss of lamina dura and hypercementosis (see Ch. 50).

Complications of Paget's disease

1. *Marginal (incremental) or incomplete transverse fractures.* These fractures are usually found on the thickened convex surface of the bowed bone where they may be multiple (Fig. 3.26). Occasionally such a fracture may become complete (see below).

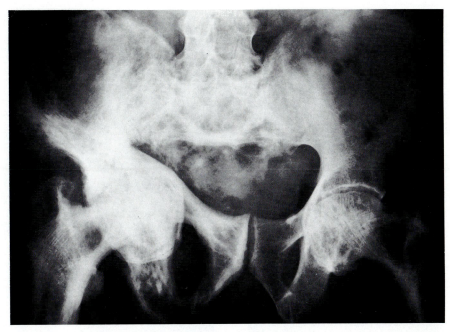

Fig. 3.24 Pelvis in Paget's disease. There is a combination of spongy and amorphous bone. Note the striated appearance of the left femoral head and neck. Marked deformity of the pelvic inlet and acetabular protrusion on the right side are shown. There is enlargement of the right pubis and ischium.

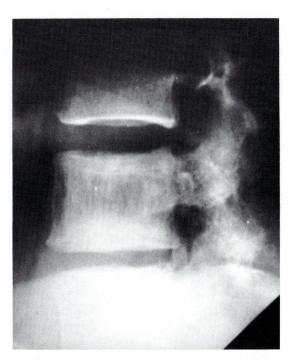

Fig. 3.25 Picture-frame appearance in a vertebral body of a patient with Paget's disease. The appendages are also enlarged.

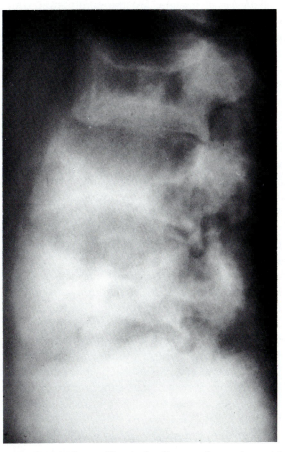

Fig. 3.26 Paget's disease. Vertebral collapse *and expansion* together with abnormal bone texture.

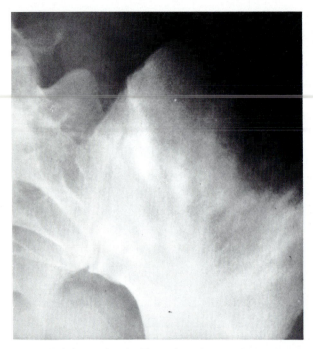

Fig. 3.27 Tuberous sclerosis. Flame-shaped areas of sclerosis in the iliac blades.

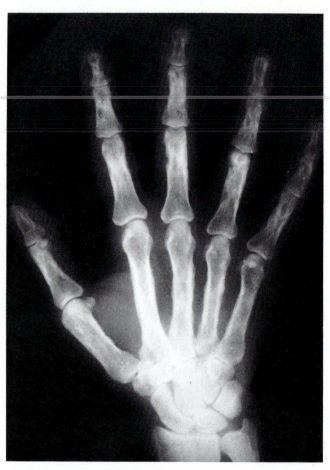

Fig. 3.28 Tuberous sclerosis in the hands. Cyst-like defects are seen in the bones, both beneath the fingernails and more proximally. Cortical defects and periostitis are also present.

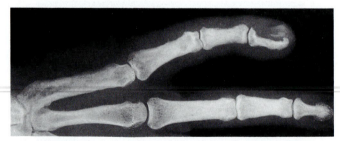

Fig. 3.29 Tuberous sclerosis. Note periosteal thickening of fifth metacarpal, cysts in head of proximal phalanx and pressure erosion of distal phalanx by subungual tumour. (Courtesy of Dr. L. Langton.)

2. *Pathological fractures* are the commonest complication of Paget's disease and are most often seen in the early stages of the disease. Usually transverse, they are more common in women. Often multiple, they are most common in the upper femur and upper tibia. Healing is poorer in Paget's disease than in normal bone. Sarcoma may follow a pathological fracture.

Bone may also be avulsed at sites of muscle insertions.

3. *Osteoarthritis* occurs at major joints (see above).

4. *Skull complications.* Cranial nerve palsies result when foramina are encroached upon. Vascular compromise also causes blindness. Deafness may result from involvement of the ossicles or cochlea or compression of the 8th nerve.

Basilar invagination may cause brain-stem compression. CSF obstruction can lead to hydrocephalus. Stretching of vertebral arteries may give rise to vertebrobasilar insufficiency.

5. *Cardiovascular complications.* Cardiac output is increased and, if much of the skeleton is actively involved, cardiomegaly, cardiac ischaemia and high output failure result. Systemic hypertension and calcification of the media of the arteries also result, not purely due to age but related to the extent of the disease and its activity.

6. *Malignant degeneration.* Osteogenic sarcoma and, to a lesser extent, fibrosarcoma, chondrosarcoma and malignant fibrous histiocytoma may arise as complications of Paget's disease (see Ch. 5).

Differential diagnosis. Most difficulties arise in monostotic cases. Sometimes a full bone survey will reveal evidence of Paget's disease elsewhere. A solitary dense vertebra or vertebra nigra may cause diagnostic difficulties because osteosclerotic metastases and reticuloses can cause identical appearances. The amorphous type of Paget's disease in the pelvis may be difficult to differentiate from prostatic secondaries, especially if little bone enlargement is evident. Elevation of the serum acid phosphatase will be found in the latter lesion.

An angioma of a vertebral body may resemble Paget's disease, but an angioma will not produce the typical widening of the bone seen in Paget's disease.

LEONTIASIS OSSEA

This term is used in two senses: *specifically* for an isolated progressive sclerosing hyperostosis of the skull, and *descriptively* when such diseases such as Paget's disease and fibrous dysplasia affect the skull and facial bones. Whether or not the condition is ever a specific entity is debatable. It could well be that the isolated lesion is really a form of fibrous dysplasia.

TUBEROUS SCLEROSIS

(synonym: *epiloia*; eponyms: *von Recklinghausen (1862), Bourneville (1880)*)

The classical clinical manifestations are a triad of epilepsy, mental retardation and adenoma sebaceum. The disease is inherited as an autosomal dominant condition but most cases are sporadic. Pathologically, hamartomas are formed in many of the body tissues — brain, eyes, lungs, kidneys and gastrointestinal tract.

In the skeleton, the commonest finding is that of poorly defined areas of sclerosis, affecting the skull, spine and pelvis. In the skull, woolly areas of density may be due to osteosclerosis, or to tuberous calcifications within the brain. CT scanning rapidly differentiates between the two. Sclerosis also affects vertebral bodies. In the pelvis, the iliac blades are the sites of flame-shaped densities which do not resemble metastases (Fig. 3.27), or more nodular densities which do simulate malignancy.

Periostitis may be found on long bones, metatarsals and, to a lesser extent, metacarpals. In the hands, rather than the feet, cysts occur in phalanges (Fig. 3.28). These may be related to subungual fibromas and are well demarcated (Fig. 3.29).

REFERENCES AND SUGGESTIONS FOR FURTHER READING

Aichroth, P. (1971) Osteochondritis dissecans of the knee — a clinical survey. *Journal of Bone and Joint Surgery*, **55B**, 440–447.

Catterall, A. (1971) The natural history of Perthes' disease. *Journal of Bone and Joint Surgery*, **53B**, 37–53.

Catterall, A. (1982) *Legg-Calvé-Perthes' Disease.* Churchill Livingstone, London.

Davidson, J. K. (ed) (1975) *Aseptic Necrosis of Bone.* Excerpta Medica, Amsterdam.

Edeiken, J., Hodes, P .J., Libshitz, H. L., Weller, M. H. (1967) Bone ischaemia. *Radiologic Clinics of North America*, 5(3), 515–529.

Fisher, R. L., Roderique, J. W., Brown, D. C., Danigelis, J. A., Ozonoff, M. B., Sziklas, J. J. (1980) The relationship of isotopic bone imaging guiding the prognosis in Legg-Perthes' disease. *Clinical Orthopaedics*, **150**, 23–29.

Hamdy, R. C. (1981) *Paget's Disease of Bone.* Praeger, New York.

McCallum, R. I., Walder, D. N. (1966) Bone lesions in compressed air workers. *Journal of Bone and Joint Surgery*, **48B**, 207–235.

Murray, R. O., Jacobson, H. G., Stoker, D. J. (1990) *The Radiology of Skeletal Disorders*. 3rd edn. Churchill Livingstone, Edinburgh.

Resnick, D., Niwayama, G. (1988) *Diagnosis of Bone and Joint Disorders*. 2nd edn. Saunders, Philadelphia.

CHAPTER 4

DISEASES OF JOINTS; ARTHROGRAPHY

Peter Renton

LESIONS OF JOINTS

RHEUMATOID ARTHRITIS

This disease is seen at all ages, but especially from 20–55 years, with smaller peaks in childhood and in the elderly. Women are more commonly affected (M : F=1 : 3).

The joints most typically involved are the small joints, especially the metatarsophalangeal and metacarpophalangeal and carpal joints, but any joint, including the temporomandibular and cricoarytenoid, may be affected. The axial skeleton is later and less often affected, with the exception of the cervical spine. Sites of ligamentous and tendinous insertions (entheses) are also infrequently involved. The tendency at the peripheral joints is to symmetry and often identical digits on either side of the body are affected. Asymmetry of distribution may follow unilateral paralysis or weakness, when under-utilization of a limb may prevent the onset of rheumatoid disease in that limb. Conversely, asymmetry may follow over-use of a limb which often is more severely involved. This is seen especially in men and in those performing heavy manual work. In general, excess physical activity leads to more severe forms of joint disease.

Radiological findings

Joint changes may be summarized as follows:

1. Soft-tissue changes
2. Osteoporosis
3. Joint space changes and alignment deformities
4. Periostitis
5. Erosions
6. Secondary osteoarthritis

Changes 1, 2, 4 and 5 may be seen at entheses, that is, metabolically active sites of ligamentous and tendinous insertions into bone. Rheumatoid arthritis is a systemic disease, and other body systems may be involved, e.g. lung parenchyma and pleura.

1. SOFT-TISSUE CHANGES. These changes are best as-sessed clinically but may also be shown radiologically in the hand (Fig. 4.1), knee or foot and other joints. Soft tissue swelling is due to oedema of periarticular tissues and to synovial inflammation in bursae, joint spaces and along tendon sheaths. Joint distension also follows an increase in synovial fluid.

In the hand, fusiform swelling due to capsular distension and local oedema may be seen over interphalangeal and metacarpophalangeal joints. Soft-tissue swelling over the third and fourth metacarpophalangeal joints is seen as a local increase in density and occasionally as a soft-tissue projection into adjacent web spaces. Soft-tissue swelling over the ulnar styloid can be due to local involvement of the extensor carpi ulnaris tendon sheath. Changes at the radial styloid are related to local radiocarpal joint synovial hypertrophy.

Soft-tissue changes are less well demonstrated in the foot. Changes over the first and fifth metatarsophalangeal joints reflect synovitis in the bursae over the first and fifth metatarsal heads, but swelling over the remaining metatarsophalangeal joints may be seen as fusiform increases in density.

The Achilles tendon inserts into the back of the calcaneum below its upper margin. It is sharply demarcated anteriorly by the pre-Achilles fat pad and more inferiorly, by the retrocalcaneal bursa. Local synovitis thickens the bursa and oedema obliterates the fat and blurs out the tendon, which also thickens. Similar changes occur inferiorly, at the plantar fascial origin at the base of the calcaneum.

Distension of the capsule of the knee joint is shown on the anteroposterior radiograph as a lateral bulging of the normally poorly seen fat lines over the distal femur. On a lateral view of the knee the supra-patellar pouch is distended and its surrounding fat lines blurred. Posteriorly, a distended joint capsule may give a local increase in density and in this way a Baker's cyst is often identified. This can be confirmed by ultrasound or arthrography.

On the lateral view of the elbow, the anterior and posterior fat planes are displaced in a direction vertical to

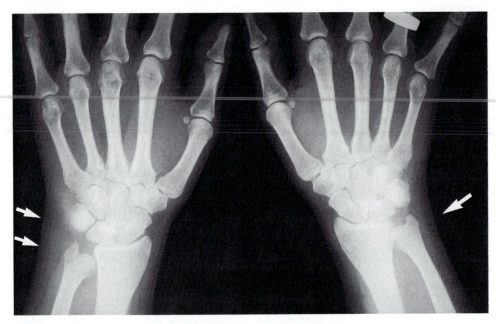

Fig. 4.1 Marked soft-tissue swelling is present over the right ulnar styloid and adjacent carpus in an early case of rheumatoid arthritis with no local erosion.

the long axis of the joint, but may be obliterated by local oedema.

Swelling around an affected joint is symmetrical while in gout the swelling is eccentric. In rheumatoid arthritis, however, a rheumatoid nodule may cause a localized eccentric swelling, and these often occur at pressure points.

2. OSTEOPOROSIS. Assessment of osteoporosis depends in part on film quality, and comparison between normal and abnormal joints in the same patient may be helpful. Interpretation is subjective and changes are seen only after loss of 25–50% of mineral. Differences in assessment of osteoporosis may exist, both between different observers and between the same observer at different times.

Osteoporosis in rheumatoid arthritis is of two types:

Generalized. This may be due to steroids or limitation of movement due to pain, or muscle wasting. This type is uncommon and occurs late in the course of the disease. It may also reflect coincidental bone loss in post-menopausal woman, commonly affected by this disorder.

Local osteoporosis around joints occurs earlier and is due to synovial inflammation and hyperaemia.

Osteoporosis increases in incidence with the duration of the disease and the age of the patient. Some 30% of patients show it at presentation but two years after, 80% are affected.

Osteoporosis is a precursor of erosive disease and may mask early erosions. Generalized or solitary *sclerosis* of one or more distal phalanges (terminal phalangeal sclerosis) is often rendered more prominent because of osteoporosis elsewhere. This occurs in some 35% of patients with

rheumatoid arthritis and other arthropathies and may be present before any other abnormality. In a woman, especially, it may prognosticate future disease, but is seen in some normal patients.

3. JOINT SPACE CHANGES AND ALIGNMENT DEFORMITIES. In the early stage a joint space may be widened by synovial hypertrophy and an effusion. Later in the disease, joint spaces narrow due to cartilage destruction by pannus (Fig. 4.2). Narrowing of joint spaces may, however, be apparent rather than real in the presence of flexion deformities, so that an oblique view is needed to assess the space. Alignment abnormalities at joints may result from local synovitis weakening the capsule and tendinitis preventing normal musculotendinous action. Tendons may also rupture in the region of roughened bone. Thus, rotator cuff tears allow upward subluxation of the eroded humeral head.

The classic changes of alignment in the rheumatoid hand are irreversible. Subluxations at metacarpophalangeal joints lead to ulnar deviation (Fig. 4.2) which occurs in up to 50% of those with chronic disease. This is also associated with increasing palmer flexion. This change may result from ulnar deviation of extensor tendons.

The boutonnière deformity (Fig. 4.2) results from proximal interphalangeal joint flexion and distal interphalangeal joint extension, and the swan-neck deformity from the reverse (proximal interphalangeal joint extension and distal interphalangeal joint flexion). The boutonnière deformity is the more common.

Similarly, lateral deviation of the toes may be found. Hallux valgus is especially common. The hallux sesa-

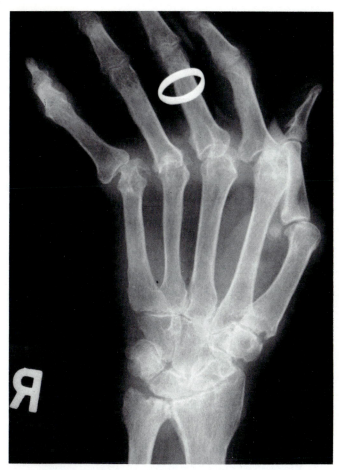

Fig. 4.2 Gross rheumatoid arthritis at the carpus with ulnar deviation, subluxation and joint narrowing at the metacarpo-phalangeal joints. Boutonnière deformities are present at the index and little fingers.

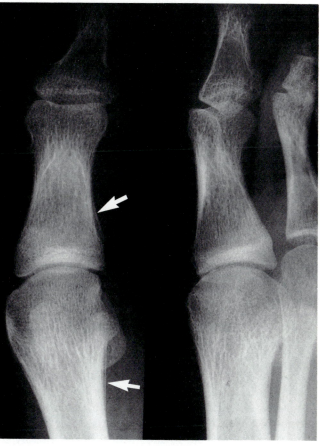

Fig. 4.3 Rheumatoid arthritis with narrowing of the metatarsophalangeal joint of the great toe and a fine periostitis on the adjacent shafts (arrows).

moids sublux between the first and second metatarsal heads and the transverse arch flattens as local inflammation causes ligamentous laxity.

4. PERIOSTITIS. Local periosteal reactions occur either along the midshaft of a phalanx or metacarpal as a reaction to local tendinitis, or at the metaphysis near a joint affected by synovitis. Such changes are less common in rheumatoid arthritis than in the sero-negative arthropathies. They are difficult to identify, may be mistaken for lumbrical impressions and are commoner in the feet (Fig. 4.3). Periostitis in the form of fluffy calcaneal spurs, plantar and posterior, is also less common in rheumatoid arthritis than in the seronegative arthropathies (Fig. 4.4). When present, they are larger and more irregular than the normal small well-corticated spurs of the elderly. Spurs may arise ab initio or may follow healing of erosions.

5. EROSIONS. These are the most important diagnostic change but are not necessarily present when the patient first attends. Their incidence rises from less than 40% of

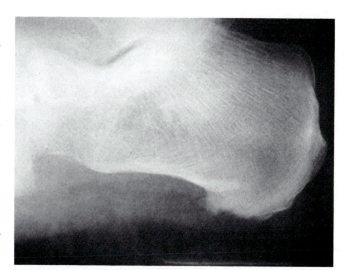

Fig. 4.4 Irregularity and erosion in the region of the plantar spur distinguishes this painful lesion from the normal benign spur, which is seen in around 20% of the population.

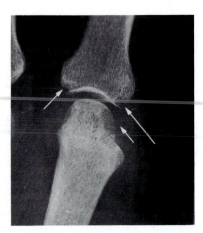

Fig. 4.5 Early rheumatoid arthritis showing marginal erosions (arrows).

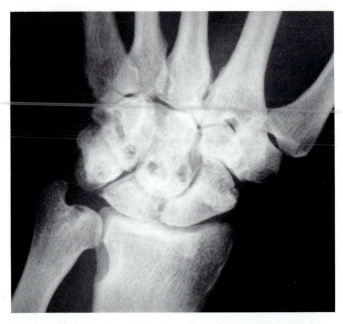

Fig. 4.6 Rheumatoid arthritis. Apart from the carpal changes, there are also erosions at the distal radioulnar joint, proximal to the triangular cartilage at the distal ulna, and at the ulnar styloid tip.

patients at three months to up to 90% or 95% at ten years.

Classical periarticular erosions occur at the so-called 'bare areas' of bone between the edge of the articular cartilage and the attachment of the joint capsule (Fig. 4.5).

Erosions in rheumatoid arthritis should be sought for at the common sites. Supplementary views, such as the Norgaard 'ball-catcher' view (supine 25° oblique view), may be needed. Erosions appear earlier and are more often seen in the feet, 90% of which will eventually be affected, than in the hands (75%), and most often at the fifth metatarsophalangeal joint. The hallux metatarsophalangeal is the least often involved. Erosions affect typically the lateral side of the fifth metatarsal but the medial side of the others.

The metatarsal head erodes before the base of the distal phalanx. In the hand, the second and third metacarpophalangeal joints are the earliest affected, initially on the radial aspects. More distal erosions are inconstant. Erosions occur at the ulnar styloid, at the radial styloid and at the proximal compartment of the distal radio-ulnar joint (Fig. 4.6). Carpal erosions occur throughout the wrist. An erosion is, for example, commonly seen on the lateral scaphoid at its waist. Carpal disease may be followed by fusion, but this is uncommon elsewhere in adult rheumatoid arthritis. On occasion, massive carpal destruction may be found in the presence of virtually normal peripheral joints.

Tarsal erosions, other than at the posterior and inferior surfaces of the calcaneum, are uncommon and are also less common in rheumatoid arthritis than in the seronegative spondyloarthropathies (Fig. 4.7). In rheumatoid arthritis, erosions are usually seen at or above the insertion of the tendo achillis into the back of the calcaneum.

Erosions are first seen as an area of local demineralization beneath the cortex which eventually vanishes, leaving irregular underlying trabeculae. The destroyed

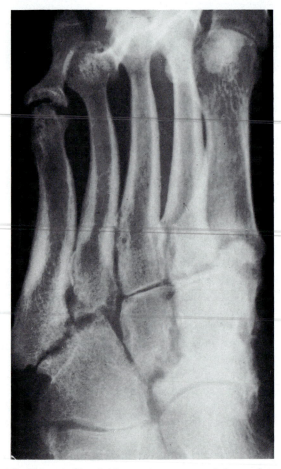

Fig. 4.7 Rheumatoid arthritis — very pronounced destructive changes in the tarsus and in metatarsal heads.

area increases in size and, as pannus spreads over articular surfaces, the entire articular cortex may be destroyed, leaving a pointed bone end. Chronic trauma, in weight-bearing or due to abnormal tendon alignment, may further collapse articular surfaces. Steroids and analgesics also modify the disease so that neuropathic-type destructive changes may result. Healing rarely reverses erosions and so it is not often that a normal appearance returns. Usually the margins of healed erosions become corticated and they do not enlarge on follow-up.

Erosive change is less common at the larger joints but often bone destruction is greater owing to the greater stresses placed on knees, elbows and shoulders. On occasion, intraosseous defects — *cysts* or *geodes* — up to 2–3 cm in diameter, may be seen beneath joint surfaces (Fig. 4.8). An alternative form of change at large articular surfaces is a superficial surface irregularity with a little reactive sclerosis in the presence of much joint narrowing. This change is seen at the elbow, knee and hip. In the hip joint it is characteristically the medial joint space which is narrowed and eroded (as opposed to the superior in osteoarthritis). Muscle pull on adjacent irregular articular surfaces leads to medial migration of the femoral head and acetabular resorption, causing protrusio acetabuli. This is classical, but not pathognomonic of rheumatoid arthritis, as it also occurs in osteoarthritis, in conditions with bone softening, and in an idiopathic inherited form. Gross loss of bone, especially at the femoral head, may result in a 'bird's beak' appearance (Fig. 4.9). Marked loss of bone around articular surfaces is also common at the elbow (Fig. 4.10) and shoulder, and deformities of alignment follow. Bone loss at the acromioclavicular joint may often be seen on a chest radiograph, with pointing of adjacent bone ends and scalloping of the undersurface of the acromion (Fig. 4.11). Erosions of the superior aspects of the upper ribs are seen in patients with long-standing disease and muscle wasting, and are probably due to the adjacent scapula rubbing on the rib.

RHEUMATOID CHANGES IN THE AXIAL SKELETON.

Sacroiliac joints: Changes are less common and less severe than in seronegative disease but may be seen in up to 30% of those with long-standing disease. The changes are more common in women (cf. ankylosing spondylitis) and rarely end in fusion.

Spinal changes: Rheumatoid changes are common in the cervical spine but uncommon in the thoracic and lumbar regions.

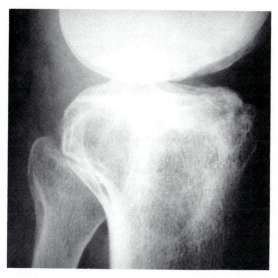

Fig. 4.8 A large cyst is seen beneath the articular surface of the tibia — rheumatoid arthritis.

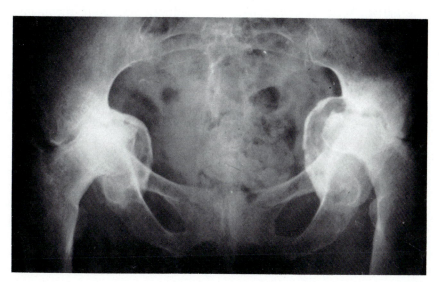

Fig. 4.9 Rheumatoid arthritis — extreme protrusio with medial migration and erosion of the femoral heads. Compare this film with Fig. 4.36B (protrusio in osteoarthritis).

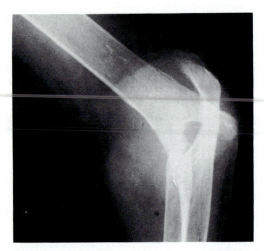

Fig. 4.10 Rheumatoid arthritis — marked bone absorption shown. At this stage the patient was free from pain.

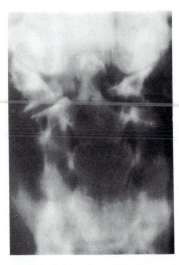

Fig. 4.12 Rheumatoid arthritis of cervical spine — tomographic section showing erosions of the left atlantoaxial articulation. Similar changes affect the right side and also the occipito-atlanto joints and the odontoid peg.

Osteoporosis, disc narrowing and end-plate irregularity are seen (Fig. 4.12) with only a little reactive new bone formation at the *upper* cervical vertebrae. Osteoarthritis, in distinction, is seen more inferiorly. Facet joint erosions may result in subluxation (Fig. 4.13), so that nerve entrapment follows. Subluxation and erosion also occur at the synovial joint between the odontoid peg and arch of atlas, and are potentiated by laxity of ligaments around the peg. Separation in flexion of more than 2.5 mm in adults or 5 mm in children is held to be abnormal. This instability can be seen in up to 30% of patients with chronic rheumatoid arthritis. The eroded odontoid may also fracture.

Resorption of bone at non-articular surfaces occurs in the cervical spine at the spinous processes which become short, sharp and tapered in patients with chronic disease (Fig. 4.13).

6. SECONDARY OSTEOARTHRITIS. Weight-bearing joints affected by rheumatoid arthritis often develop secondary osteoarthritis. Indeed, at the hips, osteoarthritic change may be superimposed on a previously unrecognized rheumatoid arthritis. Reactive sclerosis and new bone formation in osteoarthritis is not marked in those whose underlying disease has characteristic features of osteoporosis and bone destruction.

ARTHRITIS IN CHILDREN

There are many causes of polyarthritis in children, the most common being viral infections. It is now recognized that chronic childhood polyarthritis is a heterogenous group of disorders, the generic term for which is '*juvenile chronic polyarthritis*' (Table. 4.1). Some 10% of the total eventually have a *seropositive* form of disease similar to, or identical with, adult rheumatoid arthritis, that is, an essentially peripheral erosive polyarthritis. The remaining

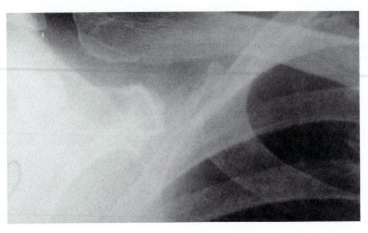

Fig. 4.11 Widening of the right acromioclavicular joint with well demarcated margins distinguishes rheumatoid arthritis from hyperparathyroidism. The erosion of the third and fourth ribs superiorly may be seen in both conditions.

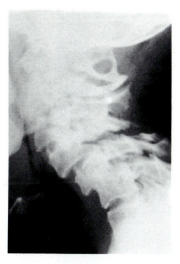

Fig. 4.13 Rheumatoid arthritis of the cervical spine — gross bizarre destruction. Subluxation of C4 on C5 and of C5 on C6 is seen. Note gross destruction in the spinous processes and posterior arches.

Table 4.1 Classification of juvenile chronic polyarthritis

1. Adult-type rheumatoid arthritis (with IgM rheumatoid factor)
2. Polyarthritis with ankylosing spondylitis-type sacroiliitis
3. Still's disease
   a. systemic
   b. polyarticular
   c. pauciarticular, with or without chronic iridocyclitis
4. Psoriatic arthropathy
5. Arthritis associated with ulcerative colitis or regional enteritis (as in adults)
6. Polyarthropathies associated with other disorders, such as systemic lupus erythematosus or familial Mediterranean fever, etc.

(Reproduced by kind permission of Dr. B. M. Ansell)

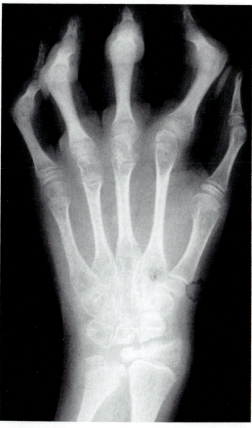

Fig. 4.14 Juvenile chronic arthritis. Accelerated skeletal maturity with modelling abnormalities of the carpal bones and metacarpal heads together with osteoporosis and soft-tissue wasting. At the distal radius and ulna the epiphyses are fragmented and overgrown.

patients have *seronegative* juvenile chronic arthritis for which definite clinical and histological diagnostic criteria exist.

Children with seronegative juvenile chronic arthritis may be further subdivided:

1. Acute systemic onset type (true Still's disease) with constitutional symptoms and hepatosplenomegaly, but little or no joint involvement.

2. Pauci-articular (not more than four joints involved) affecting especially the knees, wrists and ankles. This usually ends up as:

3. Polyarticular disease, which may also present at the onset. Radiological changes are late and the disease in non-erosive.

In the carpus and tarsus the bones show accelerated maturation due to hyperaemia, crowding of bones with joint space narrowing and an abnormal angular shape (Fig. 4.14). In general, early overgrowth of epiphyseal centres (Fig. 4.15) with squaring or angulation (Fig. 4.16) leads to premature fusion and eventual hypoplasia.

This occurs at metacarpal and metatarsal epiphyses and around the knees, hips, elbows and shoulders. The abnormally modelled bone ends cannot easily be distinguished from the similar changes of synovial tuberculosis or haemophilia. Osteoporosis may result from hyperaemia or steroid administration which, in large doses, also causes undergrowth. Pathological fractures may result. Residual trabeculae along lines of stress are rendered very prominent. At the elbow, marked radial head enlargement may be seen and the paired long bones may bow. The cervical spine is often affected and indeed is the cause of presentation in 2% of cases. Diminution of neck movement is followed by apophyseal joint changes, maximal at C2–3, where erosions lead to ankylosis. The associated vertebral bodies fail to develop. Atlantoaxial subluxation is said to occur only rarely in those patients with seronegative disease, and neurocentral joint lesions do not occur in seronegative disease.

Juvenile ankylosing spondylitis has a characteristic onset at about 10 years of age. It is five times more common in boys and presents initially with an asymmetric peripheral arthropathy. Sacroiliac changes develop some 5–15 years later.

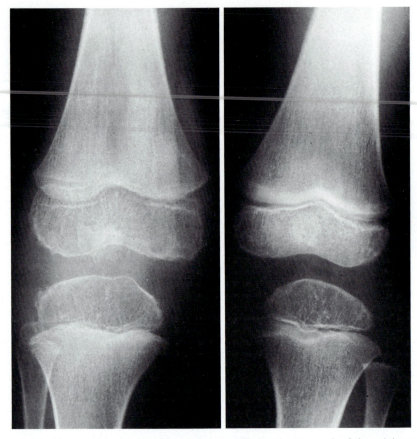

Fig. 4.15 Juvenile chronic arthritis. Monarticular arthritis with soft tissue swelling and overgrowth of the epiphyses at the right knee. Normal left knee.

SERONEGATIVE SPONDYLOARTHROPATHIES

This is a group of non-rheumatoid seronegative disorders which have clinical, radiological and familial inter-relationships. There are definite criteria for their diagnosis. These features include:

1. Absence of rheumatoid factors;
2. Peripheral arthropathy;
3. Sacroiliitis with or without ankylosing spondylitis;
4. Clinical overlap, including two or more of the following features — psoriatic skin or nail lesions, conjunctivitis, ulceration of mouth, intestines or genitals, genitourinary infections, erythema nodosum.
5. Increased incidence of the same or any other of these disease in families.

The diseases which fit into these categories are:

1. Ankylosing spondylitis
2. Psoriatic arthritis
3. Reiter's syndrome
4. Ulcerative colitis
5. Crohn's disease
6. Whipple's disease
7. Behçet's syndrome

The inter-relationships between the diseases are seen in Fig. 4.17. Chronic inflammatory bowel disease can for instance be seen to be linked to spondylitis and uveitis, while spondylitis is further linked to aortitis, seronegative arthritis and psoriasis.

This genetic and clinical overlap accounts for the marked radiological overlap of these syndromes, so that spondylitis is seen in many of these conditions. Nonetheless, differences in the type of spondylitis seen in these diseases also exist.

PSORIATIC ARTHRITIS

An association between psoriasis and arthritis was described as long ago as 1822. Some 10% of patients develop arthritis before the skin lesions appear, in 25% the two develop simultaneously, and in 65% psoriasis precedes arthritis, often by up to 35 years. It seems that about 5% of patients with psoriasis develop an arthritis but 15–30% of these are seropositive and have a radiological appearance identical with that of rheumatoid disease. The remainder have a 'pure' pattern of psoriatic arthropathy, or a mixture of the two types. Normal bone mineralization is regarded as a solid diagnostic criterion

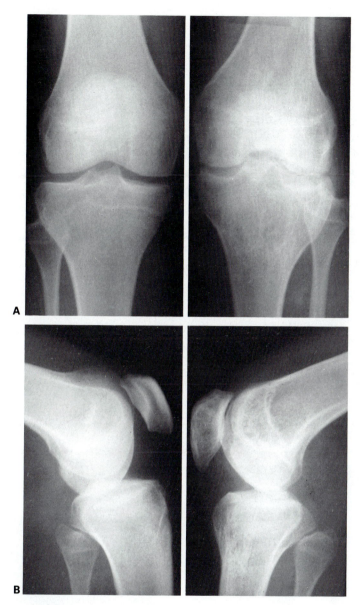

Fig. 4.16 A,B Juvenile chronic arthritis (left knee). After five years, modelling abnormalities and osteoporosis are seen, but erosive change is not present.

for psoriatic arthritis, but is not in fact particularly common, especially in chronic or severe disease.

The hands are as frequently affected by erosive change as are the feet in psoriatic arthropathy, in contradistinction to the patterns of Reiter's disease. Nail changes are related to resorption of the distal phalanges but no definite correlation exists between nail lesions and interphalangeal joint erosions. Erosions have a predilection for the distal interphalangeal joints (Fig. 4.18), and especially the interphalangeal joint of the great toe. Erosive changes are asymmetrical, even late in the disease, unlike rheumatoid arthritis, and especially if the metacarpophalangeal joints are involved. Joint narrowing may never occur.

Erosions are modified by proliferation of adjacent new bone at the interphalangeal joints and especially around erosions on the calcaneum, where large, irregular fluffy painful spurs form both posteriorly and inferiorly. Such erosions are not found as often as in Reiter's syndrome (these changes are uncommon in rheumatoid arthritis). Late changes in the hands include osseous fusion of the interphalangeal joints, and a 'cup-and-pencil' appearance at affected joints, leading to arthritis mutilans, but not ulnar deviation.

Periostitis in psoriatic arthritis occurs along the shafts of the tubular bones on hands and feet (Fig. 4.19), which become sclerotic and expanded.

Involvement of the larger joints is not common, but

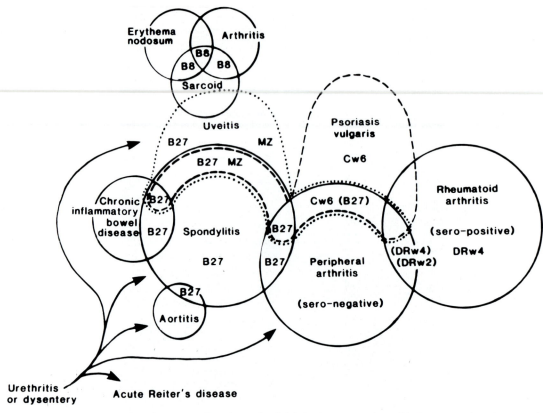

Fig. 4.17   The relationship between the different manifestations of arthritis is shown, together with the appropriate tissue markers. (Reproduced by kind permission of Dr. D. A. Brewerton, Westminster Hospital, London.)

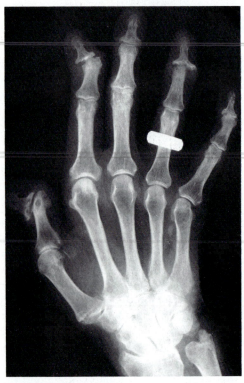

Fig. 4.18   Psoriasis. Erosive changes with overlying soft tissue swelling are found predominantly at the distal interphalangeal joints. The erosions are initially peripheral, and splaying of the distal phalangeal, bases results.

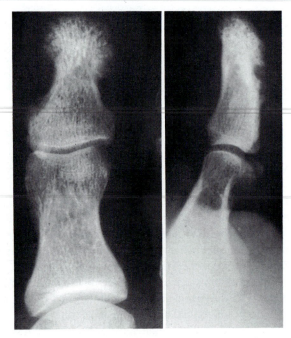

Fig. 4.19   Periostitis in psoriatic arthritis results in irregular expansion of the bone which now shows an increase in density.

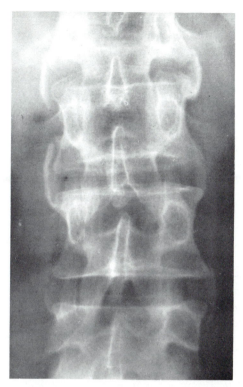

Fig. 4.20 Psoriatic spondylitis. Non-marginal vertical floating syndesmophytes are more typical of psoriasis and are less often seen in ankylosing spondylitis. (Courtesy of Dr. J. T. Patton, Manchester.)

sacroiliitis may be seen in up to 50% of those with psoriatic arthritis. Usually symmetrical, erosions, joint widening and sclerosis are seen but fusion is less common than in ankylosing spondylitis.

Paravertebral ossification may be the only feature of an osteopathy, even occurring in the absence of sacroiliac or digital disease. These *syndesmophytes*, which may be vertically directed and are not always attached to vertebral margins, should be distinguished from the more horizontally directed degenerative osteophytes. Vertebral squaring is uncommon in psoriatic spondylitis (Fig. 4.20).

REITER'S SYNDROME
This occurs most commonly in young men and is usually sexually transmitted. The classic triad in Great Britain consists of a male patient with arthritis, urethritis and conjunctivitis. Gonococcal arthritis may thus cause confusion, especially if the classic three features of Reiter's syndrome are not all present. In continental Europe, the similar syndrome, originally described by Reiter in 1916, occurs in association with bacillary dysentery in both sexes.

Skeletal abnormalities will eventually be found in up to 80% of patients. Initial attacks of pain subside, but later recur, leaving progressive change at joints and entheses (the sites of musculotendinous insertion into

bone). Reiter's syndrome affects the feet rather than the hands, and also in a more severe form. In the foot, erosions occur at the metatarsophalangeal joints and the interphalangeal joint of the great toe. Osteoporosis is not a prominent feature of the disorder. It can be asymmetric, unlike rheumatoid arthritis.

Irregular erosions occur at entheses. Periostitis may be fine and lamellar in acute cases (Fig. 4.21), or fluffy and irregular in chronic disease. Painful erosions (Fig. 4.22) and reactive spurs are very common around the calcaneum, probably more so than in any other arthropathy, occurring in 20% of patients. In contrast to ankylosing spondylitis, the feet are severely affected. Sacroiliitis develops late in Reiter's syndrome but may be seen in about half of all cases (Fig. 4.23). The changes are often asymmetrical. Fusion is also less frequent than in ankylosing spondylitis. Spinal non-marginal syndesmophytes, identical to those seen in psoriatic arthritis, occur, especially around the thoracolumbar junction, but less frequently than in psoriatic arthritis.

ANKYLOSING SPONDYLITIS
Ankylosing spondylitis (Marie Strumpell arthritis, Bechterew disease) is a seronegative spondyloarthropathy.

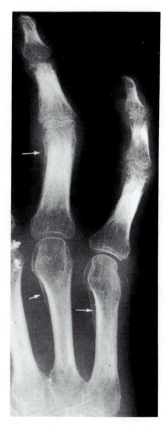

Fig. 4.21 Reiter's syndrome — acute form, showing marked osteoporosis and periosteal reaction (arrows).

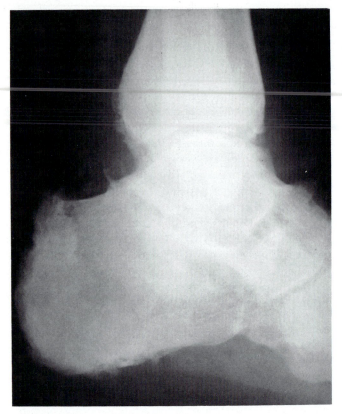

Fig. 4.22 Reiter's syndrome. Periostitis and erosive changes on the plantar and posterior aspects of the calcaneum and of the distal tibia.

Some 90% of patients with this disease have the HLA-B27 antigen or, to put it another way, an individual with this antigen is 300 times as likely to have ankylosing spondylitis as is a person without the antigen. Sixty-five per cent of patients with psoriasis and spondylitis, or inflammatory bowel disease and spondylitis, have HLA-B27 but

in psoriasis with a peripheral arthropathy there is only a weak association if spondylitis or sacroiliitis are not present. Thus the antigen is essentially related to the presence of spinal changes.

Histologically, the synovitis of ankylosing spondylitis is identical with that of rheumatoid arthritis; the enthesopathy consists of destruction of ligaments and local bone with subjacent inflammatory infiltrates. The destructive lesion heals by deposition of new bone which joins the eroded ligament, causing healing with bone proliferation at non-articular sites, syndesmophytes at vertebral margins and ossification of joint capsules.

Though the disease may affect children, it is said to occur more often in young men in their late teens and twenties, but recently it has been realized that women may be affected in equal numbers. The onset is often insidious so that sacroiliitis is usually seen at presentation. Spondylitis need not be present but develops subsequently, often at the thoracolumbar region initially, but sometimes affecting the cervical spine in females. Spinal changes without sacroiliac changes are very rare in this disease.

Sacroiliac joints. Symmetrical change is almost inevitable (Fig. 4.24). Erosions, often worse on the iliac side, widen the joint and its hazy margins may resemble the normal adolescent joint. The erosions later show considerable sclerosis, and the joint narrows as irregular new bone bridges the joint space, so that fusion eventually occurs. Joint changes are assessed using the *prone* view of the sacroiliac joint, though oblique views and CT are helpful.

Spinal changes. Erosions of vertebral margins heal by proliferation of sclerotic bone, which stands out in marked contrast to the rest of the vertebral body (Fig. 4.25). These healed erosions of vertebral margins may account for vertebral 'squaring'; an alternative cause is the laying down of new bone anteriorly beneath the

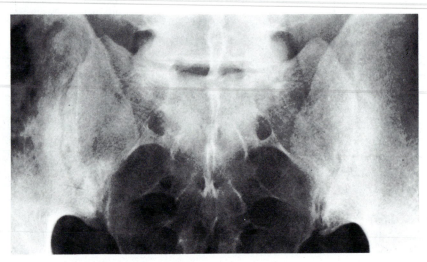

Fig. 4.23 Sacroiliitis in Reiter's syndrome.

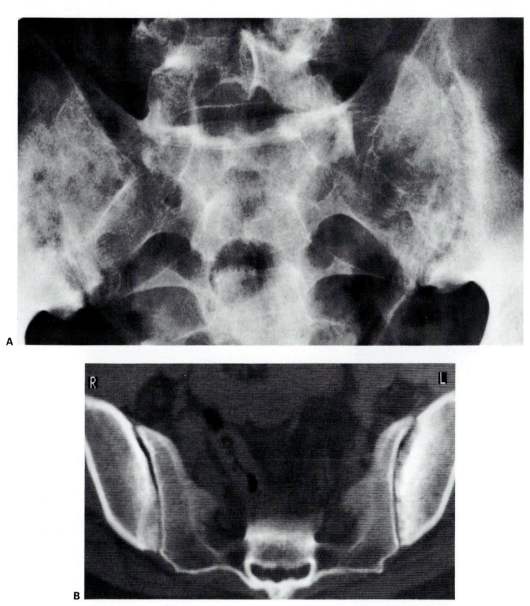

Fig. 4.24 Ankylosing spondylitis — early. **A.** Serrated margins of sacroiliac joints and periarticular sclerosis. **B.** CT scanning demonstrates bilateral sacroiliitis.

longitudinal ligament. Both mechanisms may be operative (Fig. 4.26).

Further bony outgrowths in a later stage of healing lead to neat, vertically disposed marginal syndesmophytes which may extend all the way up the spine (Fig. 4.27). The ossification lies in the annulus. Similar well-defined bands of ossification may be seen in the interspinous ligaments and around minor and major joints. If the intervertebral disc is intact at the time of syndesmophyte formation, it often never narrows, but may undergo central calcification. This phenomenon often follows vertebral fusion from any cause. Should the disc bulge, the syndesmophytes may be displaced. Syndesmophytes give the spine a knobbly appearance (Fig. 4.27), likened

to a bamboo stick. Erosions at costotransverse and apophyseal joints also end in fusion. A cauda equina syndrome may result from arachnoiditis when large posterior dural diverticula are occasionally seen at radiculography, with osseous defects in the laminae.

If the patient falls forward onto the head or chest, the rigid spine may snap, often through the porotic bone just beneath the end-plate. Hypermobility may be demonstrated on fluoroscopy. Fractures may also occur through discs (Fig. 4.28).

Occasionally localized destructive lesions of adjacent end-plates are seen, with disc narrowing and marked reactive sclerosis (Fig. 4.29). This lesion resembles infective discitis and neuropathy but is probably post-traumatic.

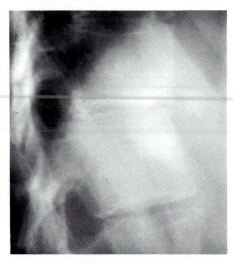

Fig. 4.25 Ankylosing spondylitis. Discal narrowing and adjacent erosions heal with prolific new bone formation. Sclerosis and vertebral squaring result.

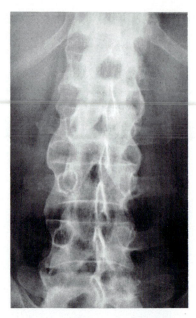

Fig. 4.27 Ankylosing spondylitis — 'bamboo spine' with marginal syndesmophytes.

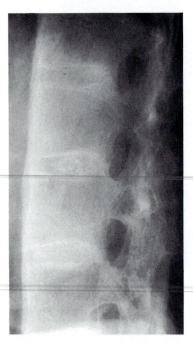

Fig. 4.26 Ankylosing spondylitis. Squaring of vertebral bodies is demonstrated, much of which is due to ossification in the line of the anterior longitudinal ligament. Long-standing fusion has resulted in calcification of the discal nucleus. There is also quite marked ankylosis of the posterior spinal elements.

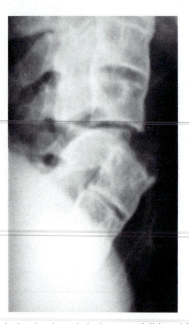

Fig. 4.28 Cervical spine in ankylosing spondylitis, with fractures through the C4-5 and C5-6 discs.

An associated pseudarthrosis is usually present at the neural arch at the same level.

Peripheral joints. Osteoporosis, erosions and joint space narrowing are less prominent than in rheumatoid arthritis, but shaggy periostitis and ankylosis are more common. At the hip, a prominent fringe of new bone may form at the capsule–bone junction. Bony ankylosis may precede or follow prosthetic joint replacement (Fig. 4.30).

Enthesopathies at iliac, ischial and calcaneal sites of ligamentous and tendinous insertions cause erosions followed by marked sclerotic periostitis.

ENTEROPATHIC SPONDYLOARTHROPATHIES
Ulcerative colitis, regional enteritis and Whipple's dis-

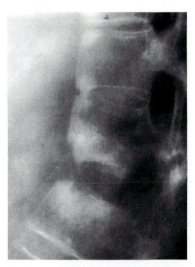

Fig. 4.29 Ankylosing spondylitis. Vertebral squaring is demonstrated. This is associated with reactive sclerosis at the sites of marginal erosions rather than new bone apposition. In addition, there is a posterior pseudarthrosis associated with instability and end-plate reactive sclerosis at that level.

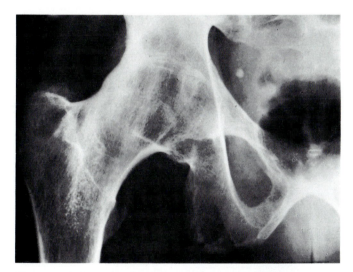

Fig. 4.30 Ankylosing spondylitis — note bony ankylosis across joint cartilage. Irregularity of the surface of the ischium is also shown.

eases may be associated with joint disease of two distinct types.

1. *Peripheral arthropathy*. Episodes of fleeting asymmetric peripheral arthritis follow the cyclic course of the gut disease and its severity is also proportional to the extent of the lesion. Radiographic change is usually confined to soft-tissue swelling and local periostitis. These patients are seronegative and HLA-B27 negative.

2. *Sacroiliitis and spondylitis*. Pelvic and spinal changes identical to those of ankylosing spondylitis are seen. These do not correlate with gut disease activity but may precede its onset and continue to worsen even if, for

instance, the colon is totally removed. These patients (usually male) have a high level of HLA-B27 antigen.

DIFFUSE IDIOPATHIC SKELETAL HYPEROSTOSIS (DISH)
(*Forestier's disease, senile ankylosing spondylitis*)

This condition was originally thought to affect the spine only. The current title clearly indicates that the condition is a generalized one, in which extensive ossification is found at many sites. It is usually seen in elderly men (M : F = 3 : 1). Some studies show an increased incidence of HLA-B27 in patients with DISH.

In the spine, dense ossification is found in the cervical (Fig. 4.31) and especially the lower thoracic regions. Bone is laid down often in continuity anteriorly and, in the thoracic region, on the right side, as the left-sided aortic pulsation presumably prevents its deposition. The thick, flowing, corticated plaques may indent the oesophagus. This florid exuberance is grosser than that seen in degenerative change. While continuity might also be seen following spinal infections, in DISH it is superimposed on a background of normal vertebrae and discs. On the other hand, osteoarthritis shows underlying bone and disc disease. In contradistinction to ankylosing spondylitis, the sacroiliac joints show neither erosions nor ankylosis. The patients may, however, complain of spinal stiffness and low back pain. Florid neo-ossification is also seen at

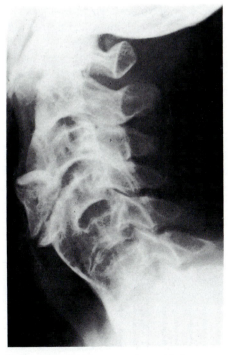

Fig. 4.31 Senile ankylosing hyperostosis — this is an extreme example of this common lesion. A tremendous amount of new bone has formed. The outlines of the original vertebral bodies and disc spaces are preserved.

extraspinal sites, around the iliac crests, ischia and above the acetabulum, and at the sites of ligamentous or tendinous insertions into bone.

Similar changes are found in the foot, especially on the calcaneum, where florid spur formation is sometimes seen. The new bone is generally well defined and not related to local erosive or degenerative change. Fusion between the paired long bones may occasionally occur.

Rarely posterior ligamentous ossification encroaches on the theca and produces cord compression.

OSTEOARTHRITIS (OSTEOARTHROSIS, DEGENERATIVE ARTHRITIS, HYPERTROPHIC ARTHRITIS)

Osteoarthritis is a degenerative condition affecting articulations, especially those which bear weight or those subjected to much 'wear and tear'. The disease may be considered *primary* when no underlying cause can be discerned, or *secondary* if the joint is abnormal in form ab initio or is subjected to unusual stresses. In terms of end-stage appearances and treatment, the difference is probably academic.

Though there may be differences in the radiological appearances of osteoarthritis at different joints, degenerative disease has a number of specific features wherever it occurs.

Joint space narrowing
The width of a joint space seen radiologically is due to the radiolucent cartilage; joint space narrowing is therefore the result of cartilage destruction. Often in a given joint a predictable pattern of joint narrowing may be expected. This change characteristically occurs in areas of excessive weight-bearing.

Joint space remodelling
Joint narrowing due to cartilage destruction is followed by loss of underlying bone in stressed areas, and formation of new bone and cartilage in non-stressed areas and at joint margins, so that joint alignment alters (Fig. 4.32).

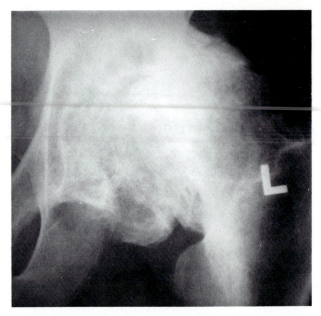

Fig. 4.32 Osteoarthritis of the hip. Lateral migration of the femoral head with loss of bone superiorly and marked new bone formation, both on the medial aspect of the head and at the adjacent part of the acetabulum. A superior acetabular cyst is present.

Beneath areas of cartilage destruction, eburnation results (Figs 4.32, 4.33). Localized increase in density is presumably due to: 1. stress-induced new bone formation; and 2. trabecular collapse. Flattening and sclerosis result. New bone is formed in areas of low stress, at joint

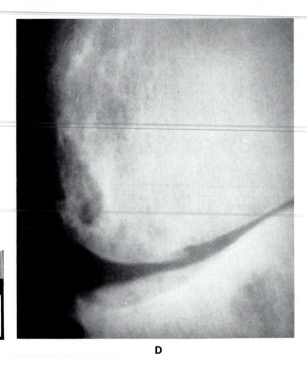

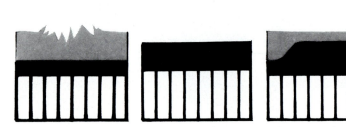

A Fibrillation   **B** Eburnation   **C** Reduplication   **D**

Fig. 4.33 A,B,C Patterns of degeneration (see text). Key: gray = cartilage; black = cortex; stripes = medulla. **D**. Reduplication with new bone laid down on the articular surface.

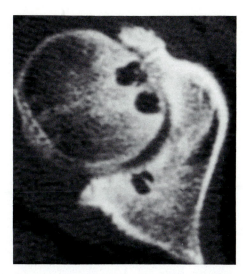

Fig. 4.34 CT scan of osteoarthritis showing new bone formation within the acetabulum and cyst formation at the articular surfaces.

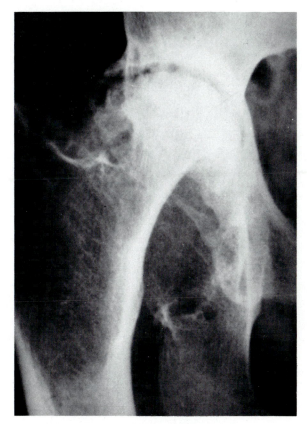

Fig. 4.35 Loss of the femoral head and deepening of the acetabulum may be the end-stage of osteoarthritis.

margins — peripheral osteophytosis — or within the joint — central osteophytosis. Osteophytic new bone is formed in response to new lines of force and prevents further malalignment. Buttressing osteophytes may thus be seen on the narrower side of a degenerate disc.

Cyst or geode formation in subarticular regions occurs in osteoarthritis as well as in rheumatoid arthritis and is found in the weight-bearing areas, often associated with joint narrowing, eburnation and collapse of bone (Fig. 4.34).

Loose bodies
These are formed by detachment of osteophytes, crumbling of articular surfaces or ossification of cartilage débris. Osteoporosis and bony ankylosis are not manifestations of degenerative disease. Indeed, hypertrophic new bone is seldom seen in patients who are osteoporotic. Osteoporotic patients often fracture their femoral necks, but do not form masses of new bone about their hips. Conversely, patients with florid osteophytosis tend to have good bone density and fewer femoral neck fractures. When osteoarthritis results in pain and immobility, osteoporosis and soft-tissue wasting may result secondarily.

OSTEOARTHRITIS IN PARTICULAR JOINTS

The hip joint
Murray (1965) has shown that only 35% of cases have no underlying radiologically determinable abnormality. Many patients who develop premature osteoarthritis — in their 40s — are found to have a pre-existing abnormality. Some result from childhood — congenital dysplasias, congenital dislocation of the hip, acetabular dysplasia, Perthes' disease or slipped epiphysis. The

underlying cause is often recognizable. Others occur later — Paget's disease, scoliosis, rheumatoid arthritis and variants and aseptic necrosis from any cause.

There is no 'typical' appearance for osteoarthritis of the hip; rather, groups of different patterns may be defined. The appearances are complicated by analgesic therapy which may result in a neuropathic-type appearance with eburnation and rapid loss of bone (Fig. 4.35).

Patterns of osteoarthritis of the hip
These depend on the direction of migration of the femoral head which may be displaced superiorly (78%) (Fig. 4.36A), or medially (22%) (Fig. 4.36B). Superior migration may occur laterally (Fig. 4.32), medially, or in an intermediate direction with narrowing of the appropriate segments of the joint.

Medial migration may lead to protrusio acetabuli (Fig. 4.36B), lateral migration to lateral acetabular restraining osteophytes and new bone within the medial aspect of the acetabulum (Fig. 4.32). Capsular traction leads to buttressing new bone formation, usually on the medial, rather than the lateral, aspect of the femoral neck (Fig. 4.32).

The end result is often a femoral head which shows bone loss in weight-bearing areas and bone proliferation

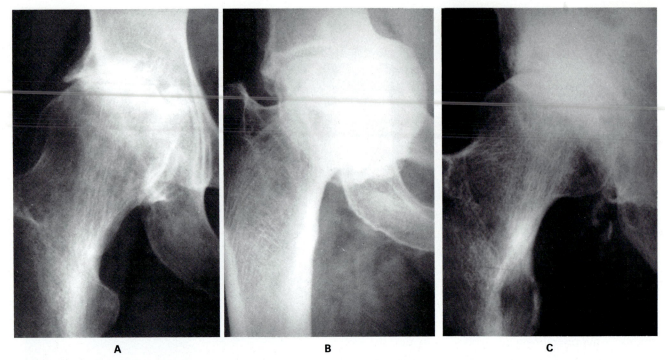

A   B   C

Fig. 4.36 A,B,C Patterns of osteoarthritis. **A**. Superior migration of the femoral head. There is new bone on the medial aspect of the acetabulum. **B**. Osteoarthritis associated with protrusio acetabuli. **C**. Migration of the femoral head is in a superomedial direction.

in non-weight-bearing areas (Fig. 4.32). The acetabulum may be deepened following medial migration or show new bone medially and superolaterally following lateral migration of the femoral head.

The shoulder joint

Osteoarthritis does not usually occur at the glenohumeral articulation in the absence of a predisposing factor, e.g. the use of crutches, or secondary to acromegaly, or with the malalignment that follows a chronic rotator cuff tear. Golding (1962) has shown that degenerative changes in the shoulder joint are closely linked with soft-tissue degeneration. Radiological manifestations include cupping and sclerosis of the greater tuberosity, cysts or irregular sclerosis along the anatomical neck (at the site of the capsular insertion) (Fig. 4.37); later, atrophy of the tuberosities and upward subluxation of the humeral head occur. Occasionally, however, examples of the more classical type of osteoarthritis are seen in the shoulder, manifested by osteophytosis, sclerosis and marked loss of cartilage space (Fig. 4.38). Changes are commonly seen at the acromioclavicular joint, with irregularity, sclerosis and cyst formation at the articular surfaces.

The knee joint

This is the most commonly affected joint found in clinical practice. It consists of three compartments — a medial and lateral tibiofemoral, and the patellofemoral. The bone

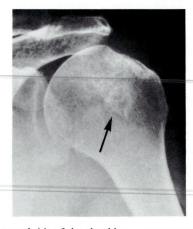

Fig. 4.37 Osteoarthritis of the shoulder — note excavation of the upper part of the anatomical neck with local sclerosis, and cysts seen en face (arrow).

most commonly involved in osteoarthritic change is the *patella*, which is especially subjected to large loads when the knee is flexed in a squatting position. Joint narrowing, osteophytosis and articular irregularity can be seen at the patellofemoral compartment on the lateral and skyline views, especially at the lateral facet of the patella, and the patella often migrates outwards. The lateral view also shows a scalloped defect of the anterior distal femur, especially in severely affected women (Fig. 4.39).

Spiking of the tibial spines and osteophytes on the

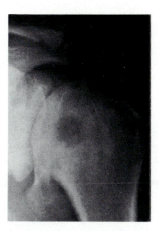

Fig. 4.38 Osteoarthritis of the shoulder, classic type — loss of joint space, eburnation, cyst formation and osteophytosis shown.

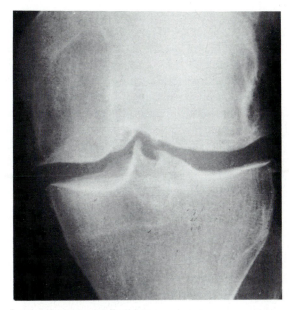

Fig. 4.40 Early osteoarthritis of the knee. Note spiking of the tibial spines and marginal osteophytic formation.

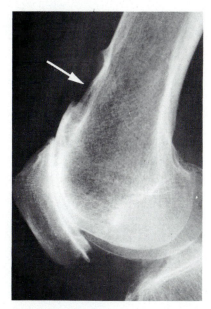

Fig. 4.39 Osteoarthritis of the patellofemoral joint. There is a groove on the lower anterior part of the femoral shaft (arrow).

in rheumatoid arthritis. In osteoarthritis, in contrast to the changes in rheumatoid arthritis, the distal interphalangeal joints are most commonly affected, but any joint may be involved. Narrowing may affect all, or a few, distal interphalangeal joints, with large osteophytes on the distal phalangeal bases and overlying soft-tissue swelling. There may be small periarticular ossicles in the adjacent soft tissues (Fig. 4.42).

articular margins are seen in early disease (Fig. 4.40). Joint narrowing affecting one or other compartment results in valgus or varus deformity, best seen in erect anteroposterior views, with gross buttressing osteophytosis on the side of the narrowing. The opposite compartment may then be widened. Varus deformity is more common and is possibly related to the more common medial meniscus abnormalities. Osteoarthritis of the knees is also more common in the obese. The *fabella* may also be enlarged and irregular in osteoarthritis.

The hands

The carpometacarpal joint of the thumb and the trapezioscaphoid joint are commonly affected, especially in women (Fig. 4.41). These joints are seldom involved

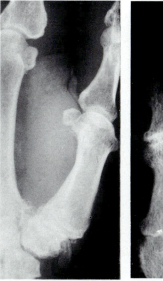 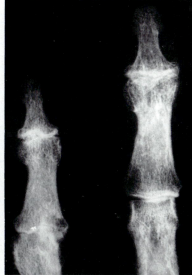

Fig. 4.41   *Fig. 4.42*

Fig. 4.41 Severe osteoarthritis of the carpometacarpal joint of the thumb.

Fig. 4.42 Osteoarthritis. Joint narrowing and osteophyte formation, with broadening of the joint underlying the Heberden's nodes.

EROSIVE OSTEOARTHRITIS

Patients are typically seronegative and complain of episodic pain due to a symmetric arthritis of the interphalangeal joints and, less commonly, metacarpophalangeal and carpometacarpal joints. Bone density remains good but the joints show a mixture of marked joint narrowing and erosion with florid base-of-phalanx new bone formation. The erosions spread across the entire joint surface, which then collapses (Fig. 4.43). Fusion at interphalangeal joints or marked deformity may result. Pathologically, the synovium is inflamed and some patients seem to develop rheumatoid arthritis later.

SPINAL DEGENERATIVE DISEASE

Though the structure of a disc and its surrounding vertebral end-plates differs anatomically from that at a synovial articulation, the radiological appearance of degeneration at both sites is similar. The space between two opposing bones becomes narrowed and marginal new bone formation, 'articular' irregularity and sclerosis appear. Later, malalignment may result. In the spine the marginal new bone results from elevation of the paraspinal ligaments following disc narrowing. New bone forms beneath the displaced and elevated ligaments. The outgrowths — osteophytes — are generally laterally directed. Osteophytes also develop on the concavity of a

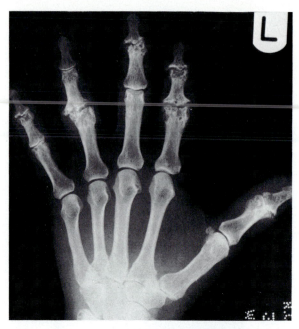

Fig. 4.43 Erosive osteoarthritis of the interphalangeal joints. Appearance of destruction around some proximal and distal IP joints.

scoliosis, no doubt also secondary to ligamentous redundancy, but act as a buttress, similar to the restraining osteophytes in hip degeneration.

Disc degeneration alters mobility at the apophyseal

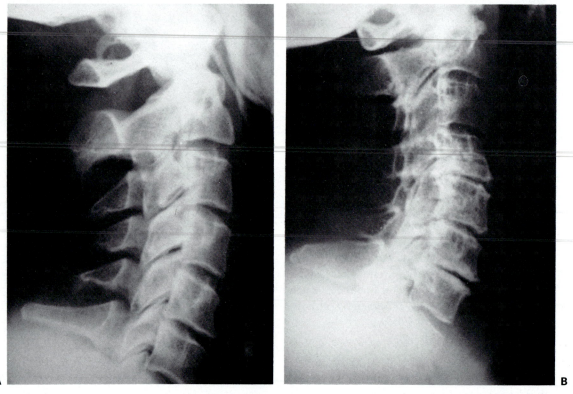

Fig. 4.44 Cervical spondylosis. **A.** There is early narrowing of the C5-6 disc and the beginnings of anterior osteophytosis. **B.** Disc degeneration is now pronounced, with both anterior and posterior osteophytes.

joints, where degenerative changes become manifest by joint space narrowing and sclerosis. Facet slip at these joints results in encroachment on exit foramina, and new bone around them may narrow the spinal canal. Compressive symptoms result. Degenerative instability, scoliosis and spondylolysis may also result.

Cervical spine. Additional synovial joints, the uncovertebral or neurocentral joints of Luschka, are found from C3 down and are easily recognized on the anteroposterior view. As elsewhere, disc degeneration results in narrowing of these joints with osteophytic lipping. In the adult, maximal movement between flexion and extension occurs around the level of the disc between the fifth and sixth cervical vertebral bodies and it is here that the earliest and also most severe degenerative changes are to be found. The next most common site of changes is around the C6–7 disc, but degeneration is less common superiorly.

Oblique views confirm the level of degeneration, and show encroachment on exit foramina at levels affected by disc narrowing (Figs 4.44, 4.45).

Posterior vertebral body osteophytosis, disc narrowing and longitudinal ligament laxity may all cause cord compression.

Thoracic spine. Degeneration in the thoracic spine is not usually severe or significant, though girdle type pain may result, or even long tract signs if disc material herniates posteriorly.

Minor disc narrowing and osteophytosis is usually present anteriorly, especially in the elderly, often in association with a smooth kyphos.

Lumbar spine. Disc narrowing most commonly affects the L4/5 and L5/S1 discs. When the radiograph is initially inspected the number of lumbar type vertebral bodies should be noted. The first sacral body may be totally or partially lumbarized, with a narrow disc between S1 and S2. A unilateral pseudarthrosis between S1 transverse process and the iliac crest may be the seat of degeneration, and the disc above it degenerates early on. Facet joint degeneration may cause osteophytic encroachment into the spinal canal and exit foramina (trophism). Slip at the facets narrows the exit foramina further. Disc degeneration may result in fissuring and gas is seen in the disc space — a 'vacuum' phenomenon — as well as calcification on occasion.

Facet and disc degeneration may result in vertebral slip without pars defects. With an excessive lordosis, contact between 'kissing' spinous processes may result in soft tissue entrapment and local pain (Fig. 4.46).

Discography — the insertion of opaque contrast medium into the nucleus of the disc — is used to demonstrate the integrity of the nucleus and annulus. Pain reproduction during injection confirms the level of abnormality prior to surgery (Fig. 4.47).

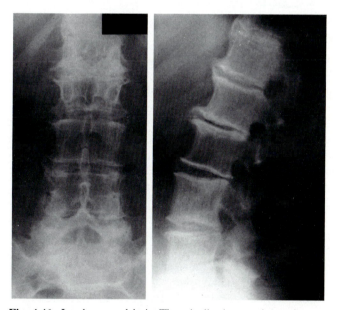

Fig. 4.46 Lumbar spondylosis. There is discal narrowing and a vacuum phenomenon is present in the degenerate discs. Marginal osteophytes are present. Inferiorly the facet joints show features of degeneration and, with the increase in lordosis, the spinous processes are in contact.

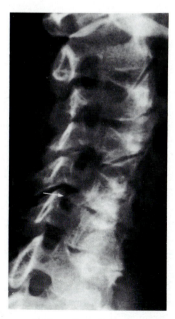

Fig. 4.45 Oblique projection of cervical spine showing large osteophytic protrusions into the C5-C6 intervertebral foramen (arrow).

RADIONUCLIDE SCANNING IN ARTHRITIS

Radionuclide scans using technetium-99^m phosphate compounds will usually be positive in diseased joints. Exceptions are seen in joints in which the disease is inactive, as in fused sacroiliac joints, and, surprisingly, in some

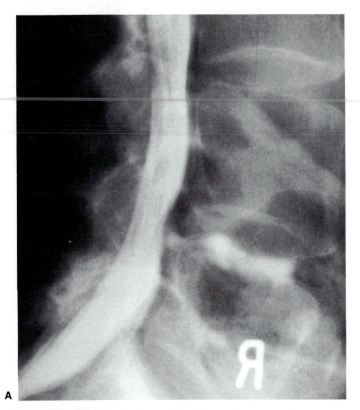

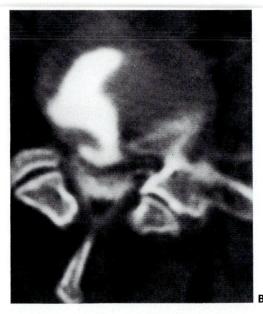

Fig. 4.47 A. Simultaneous discography and radiculography demonstrate a torn annulus, through which contrast medium escapes and impinges upon the opacified theca. **B**. The CT scan shows, in the axial plane, the site of the annular tear and the displacement of the nucleus. Indentation of the opacified thecal sac is demonstrated.

cases of osteoarthritis. Because of their sensitivity, positive scans antedate even clinical activity as well as radiological change, and indicate further sites of involvement in patients with established joint disease elsewhere. Using high-resolution gamma cameras, even the smallest joints can be successfully imaged. The areas of increased uptake indicate a joint abnormality but not the type of lesion. The distribution of the disease may indicate the underlying process and, in rheumatoid arthritis, scanning is probably more helpful than conventional radiography, especially in the early case where bone changes are minimal. Changes are maximal in the appendicular skeleton, especially at the wrist.

Rheumatoid variants may usually be distinguished from true rheumatoid arthritis by their different distribution pattern. Again, scanning is probably more sensitive than radiography. It is less specific than radiography in distinguishing subgroups of seronegative arthritis, possibly because of overlap of syndromes, and also because inactive burnt out disease is not registered. Scanning is probably also of value in long term follow-up of patients in recording response to therapy. Nonetheless, it is likely that scanning will remain an adjunct to conventional radiology. It cannot stage disease processes as other than active or inactive, whereas the conventional radiographs show the degree of anatomical change. Taken in corre-

lation with clinical assessment, scanning is theoretically more effective than conventional radiology.

GOUT

Radiographic findings. 1. *Erosions*. These are caused by deposition of *sodium biurate* and are typically punched out in appearance. They tend to appear near joint margins. As they enlarge, they tend to involve more of the cortex of the shaft rather than the articular surface (Fig. 4.48). Large erosions extend to the articular cortex and diffusely in the shafts (Fig. 4.49).

Cartilage destruction is a relatively late manifestation. Usually much bony destruction is seen before cartilage loss supervenes. In the hand, gout tends to attack the distal and proximal interphalangeal joints, whereas rheumatoid arthritis affects the metacarpophalangeal and proximal interphalangeal joints.

2. *Osteoporosis* is not seen except in advanced cases which have been immobilized.

3. *Tophi*. These are shown as soft-tissue swellings eccentric in distribution, in contradistinction to the fusiform soft-tissue swellings of rheumatoid arthritis (Fig. 4.49).

Eventually, both soft-tissue and intraosseous tophi may become calcified (Fig. 4.50) but this is uncommon.

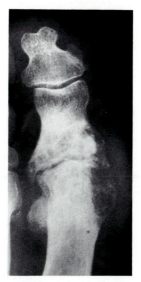

Fig. 4.48 Gout — erosion on medial part of first metacarpal extends away from the joint surface.

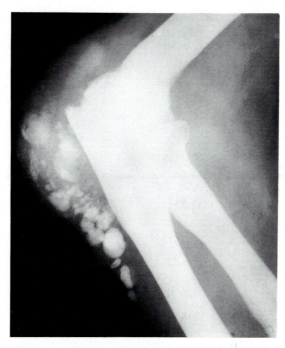

Fig. 4.50 Gout — large calcified tophi in olecranon bursa.

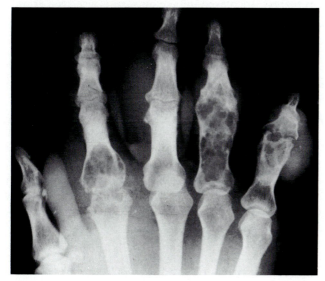

Fig. 4.49 Very advanced gout. Note eccentric soft tissue swellings, intraosseous tophi extending to bone ends and lack of osteoporosis.

Differential diagnosis. Differentiation between gout and *multiple enchondromas* may be difficult radiographically. The tendency of multiple enchondromas to spare bone ends is an important diagnostic point. The clinical findings and history readily differentiate the two conditions.

In practice, the most frequent difficulty is in differentiating gout from *rheumatoid arthritis*. Important points are: the longer latent period of gout; its eccentric, often gross soft-tissue swellings; and tendency to attack distal interphalangeal joints. Osteoporosis is found much more frequently in rheumatoid arthritis. Rheumatoid erosions are not so sharply defined as those of gout. Calcified tophi

are, of course, diagnostic of gout. In difficult cases, differentiation will be made by laboratory tests revealing a raised uric acid level in blood.

HYPERTROPHIC (PULMONARY) OSTEOARTHROPATHY

This condition was originally thought to be associated solely with intrathoracic disease, but it is now known to be associated with intra-abdominal and other diseases. The word 'pulmonary' is best avoided in the title. The vast majority of cases are associated with intrathoracic neoplasms, mainly bronchogenic carcinoma, up to 12% of which have hypertrophic osteoarthropathy, with the exception of oat-cell carcinomas. Hypertrophic osteoarthropathy is also associated with secondary lung tumours. Its highest incidence is found with fibrous mesothelioma of the pleura. Hypertrophic osteoarthropathy is more common with peripherally seated tumours.

Hypertrophic osteoarthropathy is also observed with bronchiectasis, rarely with tuberculosis, and congenital cyanotic heart disease, and may also be found with chronic liver and gut inflammatory disorders. Even though hypertrophic osteoarthropathy is usually accompanied by clubbing, the latter should be separated on clinical, radiological and pathological grounds.

Periostitis is seen earliest at the distal third of the radius and ulna (Fig. 4.51), then the tibia and fibula, and then the humerus and femur, metacarpals, metatarsals and proximal and middle phalanges (Fig. 4.52). Distal phalanges and the axial skeleton are rarely affected.

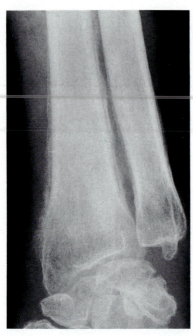

Fig. 4.51 Hypertrophic pulmonary osteoarthropathy — exuberant periosteal reaction of the radius and ulna. In this patient, changes in the bones of the hands were minimal.

Radiologically, soft-tissue swelling may be seen over distal phalanges if clubbing is present, but the underlying bone is normal. In the long bones, periostitis affects the distal diaphyses but the bone ends are uninvolved. A single fine layer, or multiple layers, of periosteal new bone, giving an onion-skin appearance, may be seen. On occasion the periostitis may be shaggy. The new bone merges with the cortex in long-standing cases. Endosteal new bone is not seen.

Occasionally joint pain and swelling are related to an underlying arthritis, usually of larger joints. Radiologically, osteoporosis and effusions may be recognized but erosions do not apparently occur.

Radionuclide scanning in hypertrophic osteoarthropathy
Hypertrophic osteoarthropathy is a disease in which blood flow to the limb is increased and new bone is formed. As expected, scanning is an accurate and sensitive means of detecting disease, and the changes are seen before those on the plain films. Increased uptake is seen symmetrically along the shafts of affected long bones paralleling the cortices and thus differing from focal or widespread metastatic foci. With treatment of the underlying condition, the changes evident on both film and scan regress. Increased uptake on scan is also seen around affected joints.

PACHYDERMOPERIOSTOSIS
In this condition radiological changes identical with those seen in hypertrophic osteoarthropathy present early in life, often after puberty. Though the periosteal new bone is similar to that seen in hypertrophic osteoarthropathy, it is often coarser and may extend further along the shafts to the epiphyses. A familial history is present in over 50% of cases and males are said to be more commonly affected. No related chest disease is found. The skin of the face, especially the forehead, becomes thickened and greasy with acne and hyperhydrosis.

SYSTEMIC LUPUS ERYTHEMATOSUS
This disorder is more common in young females and in black Africans. It is associated with a 'butterfly' skin rash over the cheeks, with pleurisy, pericarditis, glomerulonephritis and psychiatric disorders. It may be precipitated by drugs.

Systemic lupus erythematosus may present with a symmetrical peripheral arthropathy in which erosive change is infrequent. Soft-tissue swelling and osteoporosis are seen, but erosive change is minimal and uncommon. Soft-tissue calcification also occurs around joints and in blood vessels. Alignment deformities of the hands are more typical, so that ulnar deviation and swan-neck deformities are seen, which are reversible, voluntarily and involuntarily.

Avascular necrosis is common, being found in the hips, knees and shoulder joints. It probably follows steroid therapy but, in view of the high incidence (10%), may

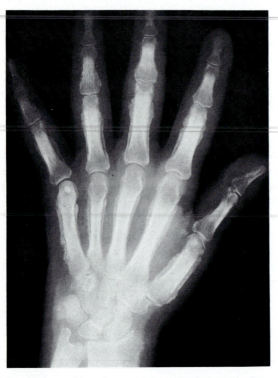

Fig. 4.52 Hypertrophic pulmonary osteoarthropathy secondary to pulmonary neoplasm.

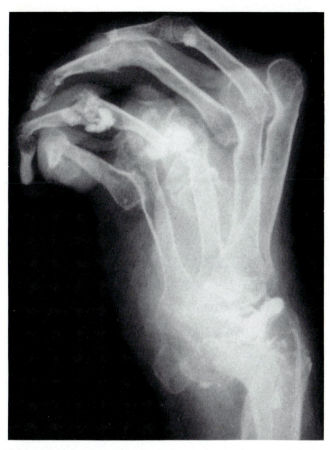

Fig. 4.53 Scleroderma. Contractures result in pressure resorption of bone at metacarpal necks. Para-articular calcification is prominent, as is distal phalangeal sclerosis.

be due to the disease alone. C1/C2 subluxation may be found.

PROGRESSIVE SYSTEMIC SCLEROSIS

This is a widespread disorder of connective tissue which often presents with Raynaud's phenomenon due to small vessel occlusion. Fibrosis of the skin, especially over distal phalanges, leads to resorption of the distal phalanges and then progressively of the middle and proximal phalanges. Soft-tissue calcification is seen, especially over distal phalanges and around joints. Fibrosis may lead to contractures (Fig. 4.53). These changes may be preceded or accompanied by a polyarthritis similar to rheumatoid arthritis in at least 10% of patients. Osteoporosis, joint-space narrowing, erosions and subluxations may be seen. Changes of an erosive arthropathy in association with calcification should suggest the presence of progressive systemic sclerosis.

JACCOUD'S ARTHROPATHY

This arthropathy does not involve synovium but causes capsular fibrosis. Deformities of the hands and feet, that are initially reversible, occur. Lateral deviation of the hands and feet may be seen when these parts are examined without weight-bearing. When pressed down onto the cassette surface the deformities vanish. The joint spaces are mainly preserved. True erosions are not found, but so-called 'hook' erosions of the metacarpal heads are produced, possibly because of local capsular pressure (see Fig. 4.53). The patients are seronegative for rheumatoid arthritis.

MIXED CONNECTIVE TISSUE DISEASE

This is a so-called 'overlap syndrome' comprising a mixture of features of rheumatoid arthritis, dermatomyositis, systemic lupus erythematosus and progressive systemic sclerosis.

Osteoporosis, soft tissue swelling and joint-space narrowing are found at affected joints. The distribution also may mimic rheumatoid arthritis, but distal interphalangeal joints may be affected and the peripheral arthropathy may be asymmetrical. Erosive change is not inevitably present at these sites, which are a mixture of the sites of rheumatoid arthritis and psoriasis. The distal phalanges may show soft-tissue loss, distal tuft bone resorption and calcification suggesting progressive systemic sclerosis. Ulnar drift as in systemic lupus erythematosus or rheumatoid arthritis is also seen. Pericardial and pleural effusions may be shown by chest radiography.

ARTHROGRAPHY

Radiological visualization of intra-articular structures is achieved by the injection of iodine-based water-soluble contrast media, or a suitable gas, or both, into the joint.

KNEE JOINT

Arthrography of the knee is of most value in the diagnosis of meniscal lesions. It is as accurate as arthroscopy in experienced hands and requires neither hospitalization nor anaesthesia. The examination takes 15 minutes and the patient walks away.

Technique. Single-contrast techniques using a water-soluble medium, such as Conray 280, or air or carbon dioxide alone may be used. Gas alone is used if there is a history of major allergic reaction. A double-contrast technique is more aesthetically satisfying, though recent work indicates that it is not necessarily more accurate than a single-contrast technique using a water-soluble medium.

The normal arthrogram

The meniscus is seen to be triangular in cross-section and

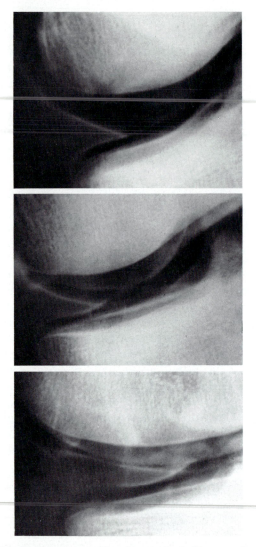

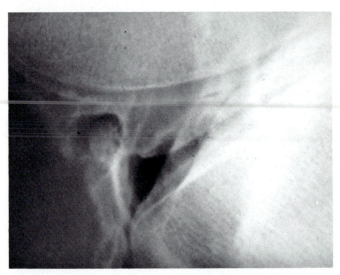

Fig. 4.55 Posterior horn of the lateral meniscus shows a peripheral defect through which runs the popliteus tendon sheath. The superior and inferior struts around the defect are intact.

meniscus. Thus this region must be very carefully examined (Figs 4.57, 4.58, 4.59).

Defects in articular cartilage and chondromalacia patellae may occasionally be confirmed, the latter by using skyline views.

Baker's cysts may be associated with congenital plicae (septa) in the suprapatellar pouch, but they are also seen with joint disease. Should they rupture, synovial fluid is released into the calf muscles which become painful and swollen, giving a clinical picture resembling deep-vein thrombosis. Rupture of a Baker's cyst may be diagnosed by injecting 20 ml of contrast medium into the joint, which is then exercised. Leak of contrast medium confirms rupture (Fig. 4.60).

Following attempted meniscectomy, symptoms refer-

Fig. 4.54 Medial meniscus from front to back. The posterior horn is larger than the anterior horn. The normal meniscus is triangular in shape. (Reproduced by kind permission of Dr. D. J. Stoker, and Chapman & Hall, publishers.)

its surface smooth (Fig. 4.54). The local articular cartilage and underlying bone are clearly shown. The joint space can also be assessed for loose bodies, and lateral stress may demonstrate collateral ligament laxity.

The lateral meniscus has, from the midline of the knee posteriorly, a smooth peripheral crescentic defect representing a tunnel, the superior and inferior margins of which are fairly mobile. In this synovium-lined tunnel runs the popliteus tendon sheath (Fig. 4.55). Failure of meniscal involution in utero leaves an abnormally large discoid meniscus (Fig. 4.56).

Tears are seen as interruptions in the normal meniscus that fill with air, contrast medium, or both. They are potentiated by contralateral stressing of the joint. Tears are three times as common in the medial meniscus as in the lateral, especially in the posterior horn of the medial

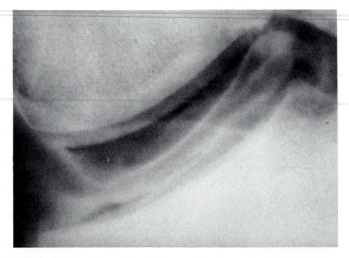

Fig. 4.56 Discoid meniscus. The meniscus extends medially to the midline of the joint and has a bulbous internal aspect.

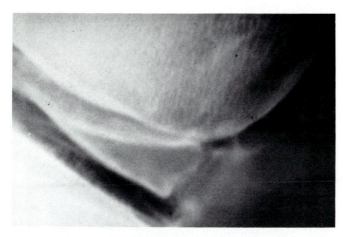

Fig. 4.57 Vertical peripheral tear of the medial meniscus. (Reproduced by kind permission of Dr. D. J. Stoker, and Chapman & Hall, publishers.)

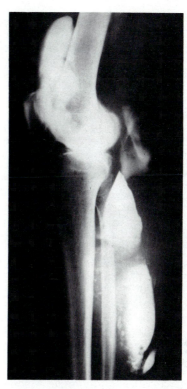

Fig. 4.60 Rupture of a Baker's cyst is demonstrated. This is probably chronic, as the cavity in the calf has a smooth margin. (Courtesy of Dr. A. R. Taylor.)

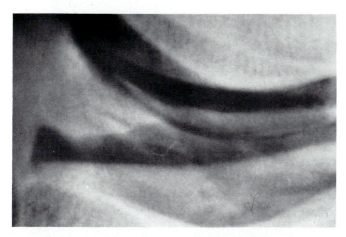

Fig. 4.58 A complex tear which has horizontal and oblique components. The internal portion of the meniscus is no longer present but may be intact 'on the horizon', indicating a local defect. (Reproduced by kind permission of Dr. D. J. Stoker, and Chapman & Hall, publishers.)

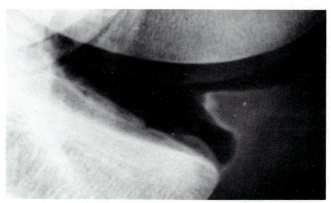

Fig. 4.61 A posterior horn remnant is seen after meniscectomy. Its internal aspect is irregular. (Reproduced by kind permission of Dr. D. J. Stoker, and Chapman & Hall, publishers.)

able to a torn meniscus may recur. Arthrography is of value in showing how much meniscus remains. The posterior horn of the medial meniscus is the part most frequently left behind, and it may suffer further tears (Fig. 4.61).

SHOULDER JOINT

Arthrography is used especially to demonstrate tears of the rotator cuff and the long head of biceps, but also to

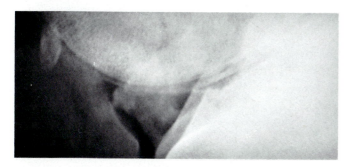

Fig. 4.59 Peripheral detachment of the lateral meniscus. The struts seen in Fig. 4.55 are no longer visible and the meniscus is hypermobile.

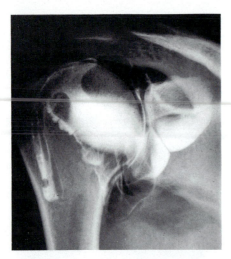

Fig. 4.62 A normal shoulder arthrogram showing the extent of the glenohumeral synovium. There is no contrast beneath the acromion. The synovial reflection around the long head of biceps tendon is shown.

demonstrate loose bodies and to assess joint volumes in restrictive capsulitis.

The normal shoulder has an intact Mahoney's line (cf. Shenton's line) and a space of 1–1.5 cm between the humeral head and the acromion. This space consists, (from above downwards) of the subacromial bursa, the rotator cuff, the long head of biceps and the shoulder joint space proper. The two synovial spaces are thus separate (Fig. 4.62). With chronic rotator cuff tears, the defect in the tendon allows the humeral head to sublux upward and contrast medium fills the subacromial bursa from the glenohumeral joint, that is, it comes to lie beneath the acromion, which may be scalloped by the elevated humeral head (Fig. 4.63) (see also Fig 9.31A).

On an axial view, contrast medium is shown to extend inferiorly, below the line of the anatomical neck.

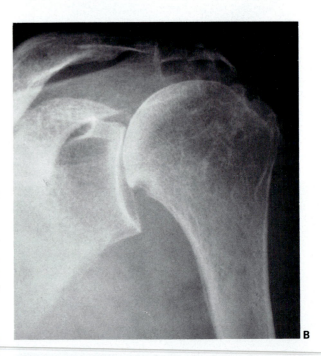

B

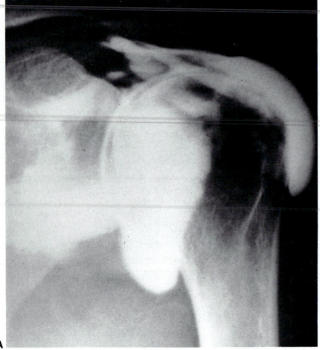

A

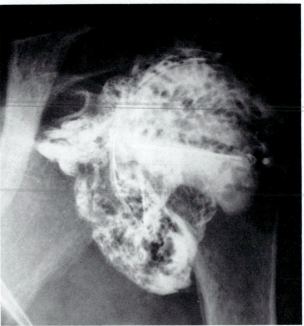

C

Fig. 4.63 Abnormalities at shoulder arthrography. **A**. A rupture of the rotator cuff is seen at shoulder arthrography, with contrast medium filling the subacromial space. **B**. Rheumatoid arthritis. Erosions and upward subluxation of the humeral head. **C**. Arthrogram of Fig. 4.63B. Numerous 'millet seeds' float freely within the joint. There is also a rotator cuff tear.

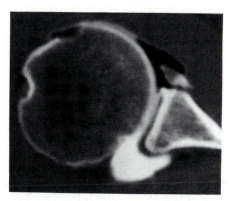

Fig. 4.64 CT arthrotomography showing a labral and glenoid fracture.

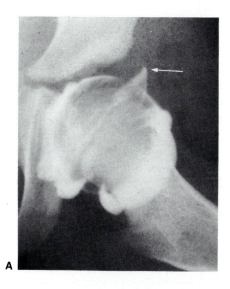

The normal joint also shows a normal subcoracoid recess and an axillary recess.

Double-contrast arthrography may be combined with axial tomography. This especially demonstrates the presence or absence of articular cartilage at the glenoid labrum and humeral head, as well as showing the presence or absence of a hatchet defect following recurrent dislocation (Fig. 4.64). In addition, the long head of biceps tendon is well demonstrated in its sheath.

Foreign bodies are especially easily shown in the shoulder.

ANKLE JOINT

Investigation of ligamentous injuries is the main indication, but arthrography is seldom used in practice in studying this joint.

In the normal arthrogram, contrast medium may extend upwards for 1 cm into the inferior tibiofibular joint. In ligamentous and capsular ruptures, contrast medium will seep into adjacent tissues and into tendon sheaths.

ELBOW JOINT

Arthrography of the elbow is usually performed in the search for loose bodies.

Capsular ruptures are shown by spreading of contrast medium into adjacent soft tissues. Intra-articular loose bodies are outlined by contrast medium.

HIP JOINT

Indications

1. Evaluation of hip dysplasias — congenital dislocation of the hip, proximal focal femoral deficiency, epiphyseal dysplasias.
2. Evaluation of Perthes' disease.

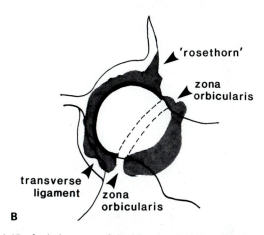

Fig. 4.65 **A.** Arthrogram of the hip, showing 'rose thorn' appearance of normal limbus (arrow). The 'rose thorn' is larger than usual. **B.** Diagrammatic representation of the normal hip arthrogram (see text).

3. Assessment of synovial infection, inflammation or tumours.
4. Localization of loose bodies.
5. The assessment of pain following total hip replacement.

Anatomy of the infant hip. The plain radiograph may show a shallow acetabulum and a small, or no, ossific nucleus for the proximal femoral epiphysis. The rest of the 'lucent' joint space is, of course, taken up by articular cartilage, and this is demonstrated after contrast medium has been injected. The ossific nucleus lies centrally within the spherical cartilage (Fig. 4.65).

The acetabular cartilaginous labrum deepens the acetabulum and has a triangular, sharply-pointed prominence on its superolateral aspect, the *limbus*. This is covered by synovium and is lax. If medially displaced into the joint, it prevents normal location of the femoral head.

The cartilage of the head should fit congruously within that of the acetabulum and contrast medium should be parallel with, and evenly distributed between, them, indicating that the joint space is even throughout (Fig. 4.65A).

Hip arthrography in children should be performed under fluoroscopic control and, if possible, videotape recordings should be made during manipulation of the hip, as well as taking static films. The head should be contained at all times within the congruous acetabulum and its movement not restricted.

Congenital dislocation of the hip. With partial dislocation, or subluxation, movement is excessive and the lateral aspect of the head is uncovered. The limbus and 'rose thorn' are elevated and laterally displaced. Contrast medium pools medially with distension of the medial joint space. Manipulation of the hip under screen control in congenital dislocation of hip shows the positions in which the femoral head and acetabular fossa are congruous (Fig. 4.66A) and incongruous (Fig. 4.66B). This information aids the surgeon in planning the operation required to facilitate joint development.

With total dislocation, the cartilaginous femoral head is totally uncovered, the limbus is medially and posteriorly displaced and may prevent reduction (Fig. 1.8). Contrast medium again pools medially. Lateral subluxation of the head and medial displacement of the limbus narrows the capsule, giving a so-called 'hour-glass' constriction.

Perthes' disease. It must be understood that the ossific nucleus is not the entire femoral head and, in Perthes' disease, the cartilaginous outline of the femoral head is essentially normal and not flat, irregular and fragmented, as the ossific nucleus may be. Arthrography does not diagnose Perthes' disease but determines: 1. the size and shape of articular cartilage; 2. the presence or absence of congruity (Fig. 4.67).

Hip arthrography in adults: indications. Most adult hip arthrograms are performed to assess either loosening or infection of a prosthesis. These patients complain of pain of increasing severity, often years after hip replacement. Such complications arise in up to 20% of patients, and 5% are infected.

Methyl methacrylate cement causes thermal necrosis of bone. A 1-mm zone of lucency is thus to be expected at the cement-bone interface, especially around the cup of the acetabular prosthesis. Lucency between cement and metal or bone and metal is less prominent and may result from movement during insertion of the prosthesis, pressure on weight-bearing or osteoclastic stimulation. Excessive or progressive widening of the interface lucency, or settling of the prosthesis into bone or cement, may indicate loosening or infection with resorption of bone.

Loosening is shown at arthrography by tracking of contrast medium between interfaces (Fig. 4.68). This is especially seen at the femoral component, but a thin (less than 1 mm) smear of contrast medium around the cup does not necessarily indicate loosening, especially if it does not cover the entire cup.

Infection also causes bone resorption at interfaces, but occasionally sinuses develop. Sinograms then show a connection with the prosthesis (Fig. 4.69). Bone resorption is usually more severe and focal.

Synovial lesions or loose bodies may also be demonstrated by arthrography (Fig. 4.70). The needle is again inserted vertically over the central part of the femoral neck.

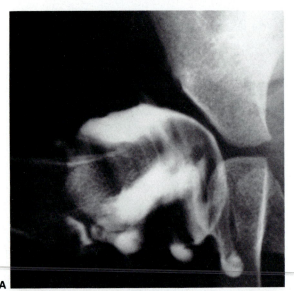

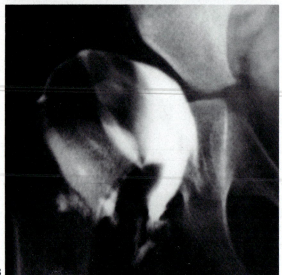

Fig. 4.66 Hip arthrogram in a child. The acetabulum is dysplastic. The ossific nucleus is seen within the largely cartilaginous head. **A**. In abduction the femoral head is congruous with the acetabular cartilage. **B**. In the neutral position the femoral head is incongruous, with pooling of contrast agent medially.

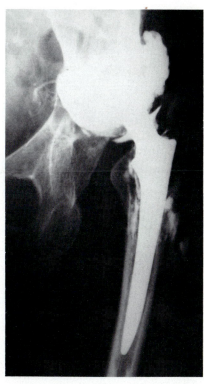

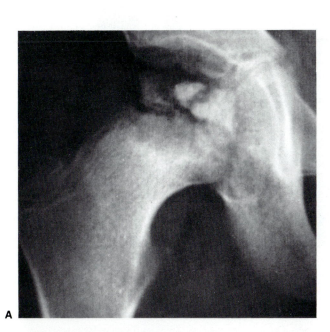

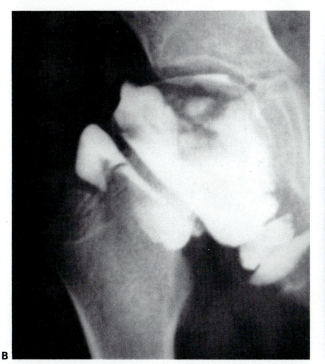

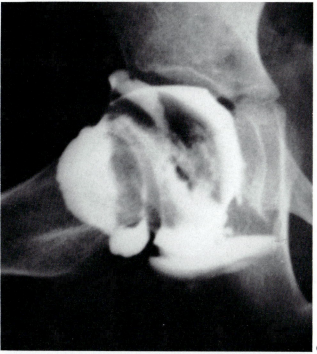

Fig. 4.68 Loosening of the hip prosthesis is demonstrated at arthrography. Contrast medium surrounds the acetabular component and tracks down the femoral stem. There is also a defect in the bone through which contrast medium escapes into the soft tissues.

Fig. 4.67 **A**. Gross Perthes' disease of the femoral head. **B**. The outline of the cartilaginous epiphysis is somewhat dome-shaped with slight flattening and broadening laterally. The lateral aspect of the femoral head is uncovered but in the neutral position is in congruity. **C**. In abduction there is pooling of contrast agent medially within the joint.

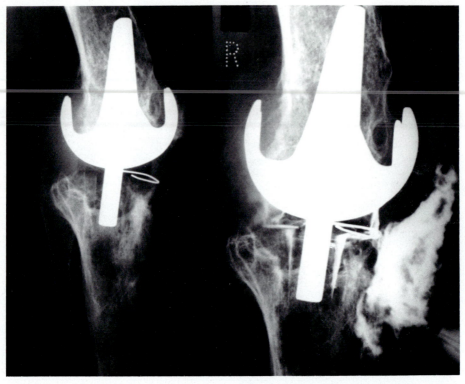

Fig. 4.69 Sinogram following total knee replacement demonstrates the track extending from the skin through to the joint, and contrast medium outlines the tibial portion of the prosthesis, indicating loosening probably associated with infection.

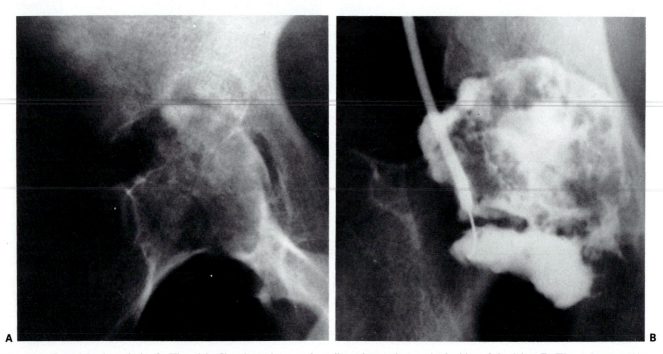

Fig. 4.70 Synovial tuberculosis. **A**. The plain film shows bone and cartilage destruction on both sides of the joint. **B**. The arthrogram shows gross irregular synovial hypertrophy. The geode does not fill.

RADIONUCLIDE BONE SCANNING AND PROSTHETIC LOOSENING

Following insertion of a prosthesis, increased uptake of tracer is to be expected in the surrounding bone. This is uniformly distributed and lasts for up to one year, after which no increase is seen. No conclusion as to abnormality can be drawn in this early stage. After this time, *focal* increase in uptake using technetium-99^m-labelled phosphate tracers can be assumed to represent infection or loosening or both. Such uptake is most commonly found at the tip of the femoral prosthetic stem and along its lateral margin (Fig. 4.71).

Differentiation between loosening and infection cannot be made using TC 99^m scans, though a negative technetium scan probably rules out these factors as a cause of hip pain. Differential scanning using gallium-67 citrate in addition to technetium is said to differentiate between loosening and infection. Gallium localizes well in leucocytes at the site of infection. This change is best seen 24 hours after injection, when the vascular phase of increased local uptake is over. A positive technetium but negative gallium scan indicates loosening alone, while if both are positive, infection is probably present.

MRI OF JOINT LESIONS
Ian Isherwood and Jeremy P. R. Jenkins

The advent of MRI has provided the opportunity for new imaging strategies in the diagnosis of joint disorders. Current and projected technical developments, particularly in specially designed surface coils and three-dimensional data acquisition, suggest that the full potential of MRI has yet to be realized. MRI has a number of advantages over other imaging techniques in joint disorders. These advantages include an exquisite soft-tissue contrast definition and discrimination, a high spatial resolution in any scanning plane and the ability to image in the presence of a joint effusion without the need for joint manipulation. In addition it is non-invasive, painless and uses no ionizing radiation. MRI demonstrates morphological detail of both normal and disease processes more clearly, allowing new insights into the pathogenesis of existing disease and the identification of new disease.

Knee. Attention to procedural detail is important to obtain high-resolution images, with a requirement for special surface coils and a facility to image small (i.e. less than 15 cm) off-centre fields of view. MR scans in the sagittal and coronal imaging planes are required particularly for the demonstration of *meniscal 'bucket handle' tears*, *discoid menisci*, *degenerative tears* at the free edge of menisci, and *collateral ligamentous tears*. T$_2$-weighted images are useful to demonstrate *cysts* and *effusions* around the knee but similar information can be obtained with gradient echo RF sequences in a much shorter data acquisition time. Three-dimensional gradient echo imaging, in which each RF pulse excites the entire imaging volume instead of just one slice, has advantages over conventional two-dimensional spin echo imaging. These include reconstruction in any plane (i.e. orthogonal and non-orthogonal), allowing the complex internal anatomy of the knee joint to be well delineated, an improved spatial resolution with section thicknesses of 1 mm or less, a better discrimination between intra-articular fluid, fibrocartilage and hyaline cartilage, and the demonstration of meniscal and ligamentous tears, bone marrow disease and osteochondral defects. MRI is a painless

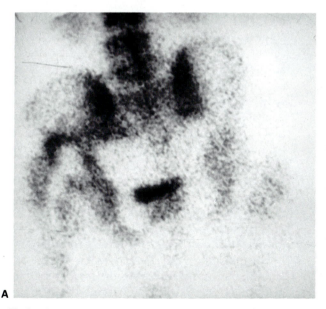
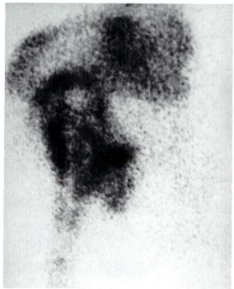

Fig. 4.71 Technetium bone scan. **A**. Anterior scan of pelvis. **B**. Oblique scan of right hip. The prosthesis can be seen as a defect on the scan, and there is increased uptake around it, especially at the femoral component.

procedure even in the acutely injured patient, and internal derangements of the knee can be depicted on MRI with an accuracy comparable with arthroscopy.

Menisci have a homogeneous low signal intensity on all RF pulse sequences. With advancing age areas of high signal, due to *mucoid degeneration*, typically occur in menisci. Both degenerative abnormalities and frank *tears of menisci* demonstrate a high signal. In an attempt to separate meniscal tears from degenerative changes a grading system has been devised. A Grade 1 meniscus contains a globular high signal, whilst a Grade 2 demonstrates a linear high signal of any size, neither of which extend to the articular surface. A Grade 3 meniscus shows areas of high signal which extend to the articular surface of the meniscus. Both Grades 1 and 2 represent internal degenerative changes, whilst a Grade 3 signal depicts a frank meniscal tear (Fig. 4.72). The latter MR diagnosis correlates with surgical findings of a tear in over 90% of patients studied. Discrepancies between reported findings on MRI and arthroscopy have been caused by difficulty in the MRI evaluation of the free meniscal edge and in the interpretation of normal structures which can mimic meniscal tears. These latter structures include the *transverse ligament*, the *lateral inferior genicular artery* and the *popliteus tendon*, all of which have an inherently low signal. Correct interpretation of normal structures with three-dimensional imaging should overcome this problem. Evaluation of the knee following moderate or extensive meniscal surgery can be difficult, as the presence of a Grade 3 signal in the meniscus often does not indicate a re-tear but represents post-operative change.

Ligaments are bands of paucicellular fibrous tissue that connect two or more bones and have a low signal intensity on all RF pulse sequences (Figs 10.71 and 10.73). The anterior cruciate ligament is the most frequently torn knee ligament, the majority of tears being interstitial. The MR criteria for a *torn cruciate ligament* include disruption and irregular contour of the ligament associated with a high signal within the ligament on either T_1- or T_2-weighted images. Tears are more obvious on T_2-weighted images, due to the higher signal intensity of fluid within the tear. The MRI appearance, however, does depend on the age and degree of disruption. The accuracy rate for demonstration of anterior cruciate ligament tears is 95–97%, particularly if T_2-weighted images are obtained. In a recent reported series of 202 patients who underwent arthroscopy or arthrotomy, MRI correctly depicted 11 posterior cruciate ligament tears with no false positive or false negative results. Marrow abnormalities of low and high signal on T_1- and T_2-weighted images respectively have been demonstrated in patients with internal derangement of the knee and are thought to represent either oedema or occult fractures. The significance of this finding is uncertain but its presence in the tibia on MRI can be used as an indicator of a torn or avulsed posterior cruciate ligament close to its tibial attachment, which can otherwise be difficult to diagnose. (See Figs 10.71 and 10.73.)

Cartilage abnormalities are best shown on gradient echo imaging where normal articular cartilage has a high signal. Disruption of the high-signal articular cartilage associated with *osteochondral loose bodies* and low-signal *subchondral defects (osteochondritis dissecans)* are readily detected (see Fig. 9.34). *Meniscal and popliteal cysts* can also be demonstrated, together with associated intra-articular anomalies (see Fig. 10.72). MRI can be employed in the investigation of *bone ischaemia* when both marrow changes and associated meniscal and articular cartilage pathology can be shown. Both knees can be studied simultaneously, an important feature in the detection of bilateral disease in patients with unilateral symptoms. *Pigmented villonodular synovitis* has characteristic findings on MRI due to the deposition of haemosiderin within synovium producing a very low signal (a superparamagnetic effect from preferential T_2 shortening). Haemosiderin is also deposited in the synovium in *haemophilia* and *rheumatoid arthritis*.

Hip. In the diagnosis of *bone ischaemia* (avascular necrosis) MRI is the most sensitive diagnostic technique, allowing early detection, staging and monitoring of treatment. Currently CT is superior to MRI, however, in the diagnosis of fractures associated with bone ischaemia; knowledge of the presence or absence of associated fractures, together with the total area of the femoral head involved, can help determine whether conservative treatment is possible.

A chronological pattern of segmental MRI signal fea-

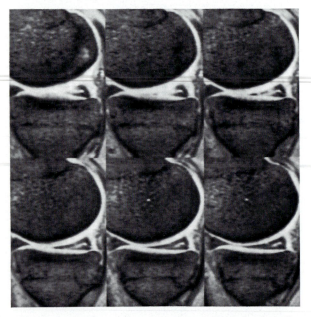

Fig. 4.72 A meniscal tear demonstrated on 3-dimensional gradient echo sagittal scans (slice thickness 3 mm). Area of high signal extends to the articular surface of meniscus. (Courtesy of IGE.)

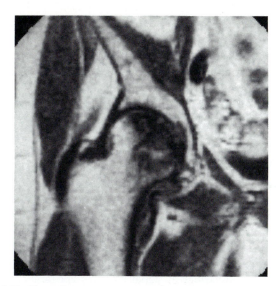

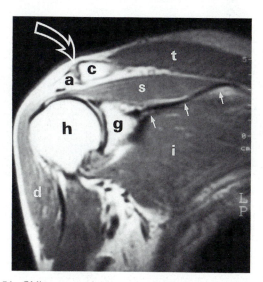

dislocation of the hip MRI provides anatomical information that cannot be obtained on arthrography. The excellent visualization of soft tissues and the cartilaginous structures of the hip enables the identification and differentiation of an everted and inverted limbus, iliopsoas invagination, acetabular dysplasia, and true femoral head containment. MRI is also particularly useful in the presurgical assessment of patients with irreducible congenital dislocation of the hip.

Shoulder. To obtain high-resolution images of both shoulders, oblique-coronal plane imaging, small off-centre fields of view and paired surface coils are required. The normal morphology can be well demonstrated on MRI (Fig. 4.74). Capsular and labral abnormalities can be depicted (Fig 10.46). *Inflammation* (tendonitis) can be demonstrated as areas of increased signal, on all RF sequences, within the low signal from normal tendons. Irregularities and complete *tears of the rotator cuff* can be shown (Fig. 9.31B). Difficulty occurs, however, in differentiating a partial tear from degeneration/tendinitis as these conditions are manifest by an increased signal intensity within the tendon. Fluid within the joint and in the subdeltoid and subacromial bursae has a conspicuous high signal on T_2-weighted images. Atrophy and retraction of muscle as well as fatty infiltration, features indicating chronicity and with prognostic significance, can also be shown (see Fig. 9.31B).

Changes in the *impingement syndrome* (i.e. compression of the supraspinatus tendon between the head of the humerus and the undersurface of the acromion),

Fig. 4.73 Extensive non-traumatic bone ischaemia of the right hip on a conventional T_1-weighted image (spin echo 740/40).

tures may allow staging of *bone ischaemia* although the appearances can be variable. *Early change* is characterized by retention of normal fat signals throughout the lesion, except for a low signal rim, usually in the anterior portion of the femoral head. *Advanced disease*, including associated fractures, has a low signal throughout the lesion on both T_1- and T_2-weighted images (Fig. 4.73). This latter effect is presumed to be due to replacement of fat by sclerosis and fibrosis. Occasionally a low signal area extends beyond the crescentic margin of the lesion into the femoral neck. The area within this low signal rim may contain high, low or intermediate signals on T_2-weighted images. The high signal within the low signal margin on T_2-weighted images, suggestive of vascular congestion or oedema, has thus far only been noted in symptomatic lesions. Following core decompression, both the high signal intensity and pain resolve, which is consistent with the proposed mechanism of reducing intramedullary pressure by the surgical treatment. Premature changes in the distribution of marrow signal have been demonstrated in patients with bone ischaemia, with early conversion to fatty marrow in the majority. This is presumed due to reduced vascularity in the proximal femur and may allow early detection of patients at risk. Occasionally patients with apparently typical MRI changes of regional or transient osteoporosis of the hip may proceed to frank bone ischaemia.

In the study of paediatric hip disorders, MRI is useful in providing important clinical management information. In *Perthes' disease* MRI not only allows delineation of hyaline cartilage around both the femoral head and the acetabulum, but also permits the early detection of cartilage and synovial thickening, together with an assessment of femoral head containment. In *congenital*

Fig. 4.74 Oblique-coronal proton density-weighted (spin echo 2000/25) image of the shoulder showing minor degenerative change in the acromioclavicular joint (curved arrow) indenting the subacromial fat pad. No abnormal signal noted in the supraspinatus tendon excluding significant impingement.
Key: a = acromion; c = clavicle; d = deltoid; g = glenoid; h = humeral head; i = infraspinatus; s = supraspinatus; t = trapezius; small arrows = spine of scapula.

which include damage to supraspinatus tendon, sub-acromial and subdeltoid bursal compression, acromio-clavicular joint hypertrophy and bony spur formation, can be demonstrated. Calcification is, however, difficult to evaluate on MRI and the requirement for plain radiographs is important.

Elbow and Ankle. The ligaments, articular cartilage, tendons and surrounding muscles are well delineated. Experience at present is limited but, as in other joints, tendon and cartilage abnormalities, loose bodies, cysts and tumours can be demonstrated (see Figs 9.33 and 9.47).

Wrist. Disruption of the triangular fibrocartilage of the wrist, which previously could only be demonstrated on arthrography, can be shown particularly well on coronal MRI scans. Transverse sections are important in the demonstration of associated radio-ulnar subluxation or disruption. Evaluation of the intercarpal ligaments, especially the scapholunate ligament, can be made. A variety of pathologies involving the bone marrow and soft tissues of the wrist have been differentiated. Lesions studied have

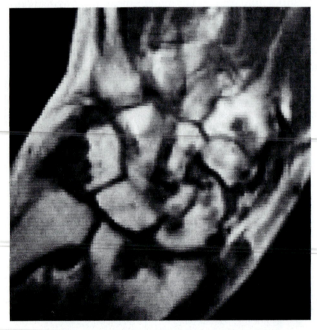

Fig. 4.75 Rheumatoid arthritis of the hand, showing extensive erosions as areas of low signal in the radius, carpus and base of the second metacarpal on T_1-weighted image. (Reproduced courtesy of Dr John Stack.)

included ganglions, carpal fractures, osteochondritis of the lunate, carpal tunnel syndrome, tendinitis and tendon rupture. In rheumatoid arthritis, synovial lesions including pannus formation and effusions have been demonstrated (Fig. 4.75).

Gadolinium-DTPA. The role of gadolinium-DTPA, a contrast agent used in MRI, has yet to be fully exploited in the assessment of joint disorders. Preliminary work has shown that the intravenous administration of gadolinium-DTPA improves detection and evaluation of neoplastic, infective and inflammatory conditions. In rheumatoid arthritis, synovial proliferation with or without a joint effusion precedes narrowing of the joint space due to cartilage destruction and bony erosion. The distinction between synovial proliferation and joint effusion can be difficult on MRI using conventional spin echo sequences because of similarities in signal intensity appearances. Synovial proliferations exhibit a low signal on T_1-weighted images and a variable heterogeneous signal on T_2-weighted scans. This latter effect is due to varying amounts of fibrous tissue and haemosiderin producing a low signal, with an increased fluid content of active inflammation leading to a high signal. A recent study of 34 joints in 31 patients with rheumatoid arthritis and related disorders has shown that intravenous injection of gadolinium-DTPA, combined with a gradient echo sequence, can improve discrimination between markedly enhancing synovial proliferation of pannus and essentially non-enhancing effusion and surrounding normal tissue, including ligaments. There was no correlation between disease activity and degree of enhancement after administering gadolinium-DTPA, the latter representing a non-specific response to inflammatory tissue. A potential role for gadolinium-DTPA in these disorders could be in the selection of patients for synovectomy and in the monitoring of response to medical therapy.

MRI arthrography in vivo has been performed using intra-articular injection of gadolinium-DTPA. In the evaluation of MRI arthrography of the shoulder, the glenoid labrum, capsular anatomy and glenohumeral ligaments were better defined after gadolinium-DTPA than with conventional MRI scans. It has also been noted that following intra-articular injection of gadolinium-DTPA, the contrast agent diffuses into the articular cartilage, an appearance which may allow assessment of cartilage function to be made.

REFERENCES AND SUGGESTIONS FOR FURTHER READING

Ansell, B. M. (1980) *Rheumatic Disorders in Childhood.* Butterworths, London

Ansell, B. M., Kent, P. A. (1977) Radiological changes in juvenile chronic polyarthritis. *Skeletal Radiology*, **1**, 129–144

Ball, J. (1979) Spondyloarthritides: aspects of pathology. *Rheumatology and Rehabilitation*, **18**, 210–213

Bergs, H., Remans, J., Drieskens, L., Kiebooms, L., Polderman, J. (1978) Diagnostic value of SI joint scintigraphy with 99 m technetium pyrophosphate in sacro-iliitis. *Annals of the Rheumatic Diseases*, 37, 190–194

Boriazon, G. S., Seigel, R., Kuhns, L. R., Good, A. E., Rapp, R., Martel, W. (1981) CT in the evaluation of SI arthritis. *Radiology*, 139, 437–440

Brewerton, D. A. (1967) A tangential radiographic projection for demonstrating involvement of metacarpal heads in rheumatoid arthritis. *British Journal of Radiology*, 40, 233–234

Brewerton, D. A. (1979) Symposium on the spondyloarthritides — genetic aspects. *Rheumatology and Rehabilitation*, 18, 204–209

Copeman, W. S. C. (1986) *Copeman's Textbook of the Rheumatic Diseases.* 6th edn. J. T. Scott, ed. Churchill Livingstone, Edinburgh

Curry, H. L. F., Key, J. J., Mason, R. M., Swettenham, K. V. (1966) Significance of radiological calcification of joint cartilage. *Annals of the Rheumatic Diseases*, 25, 295–305

Golding, F. C. (1962) The shoulder — the forgotten joint. *British Journal of Radiology*, 35, 149–158

Goldman, A. B. (1981) Hip arthrography. *Radiologic Clinics of North America*, 19, 329–348

Goodman, N. (1967) The significance of terminal phalangeal sclerosis. *Radiology*, 69, 709–712

Grech, P. (1977) *Hip arthrography.* Chapman & Hall, London

Greenfield, G. B., Schorsch, H., Shkolnick, A. (1967) The various roentgen appearances of pulmonary hypertrophic osteoarthropathy. *American Journal of Roentgenology*, 101, 927–931

Lawson, J. P. (1982) Connective tissue diseases. *Seminars in Roentgenology*, 17, 25–28

Lazarus, J. H., Galloway, J. K. (1973) Pachydermoperiostosis. *American Journal of Roentgenology*, 118, 308–313

Martel, W., Stuck, K. J., Dworin, A. M., Hyland, R. G. (1980) Erosive osteoarthritis and psoriatic arthritis: a radiologic comparison in the hand, wrist and foot. *American Journal of Roentgenology*, 134, 125–135

Moll, J. M. H., Haslock, I., Wright, V. (1986) Seronegative spondyloarthritides. In: *Textbook of the Rheumatic Diseases*, 6th edn. Ed. J. T. Scott. Churchill Livingstone, Edinburgh

Murphy, W. A., Staple, T. W. (1973) Jaccoud's arthropathy reviewed. *American Journal of Roentgenology*, 118, 300–307

Murray, R. O. (1965) The aetiology of primary osteoarthritis of the hip. *British Journal of Radiology*, 38, 810–824

Norgaard, F. (1970) The earliest radiological changes in polyarthritis of the rheumatoid type. In: *Symposium Ossium*, pp. 72–74 Livingstone, Edinburgh

Patton, J. T. (1976) Differential diagnosis of inflammatory spondylitis. *Skeletal Radiology*, 1, 77–85

Peter, J. P., Pearson, C. M., Marmor, L. (1966) Erosive osteoarthritis of the hands. *Arthritis and Rheumatism*, 9, 365–387

Reing, C. M., Richin, P. F., Kenmore, P. I. (1979) Differential bone scanning in the evaluation of a painful total joint replacement. *Journal of Bone and Joint Surgery*, 61A, 933–936

Resnick, D., Shaul, R., Robins, J. M. (1975) Diffuse idiopathic skeletal hyperostosis: Forestier's disease with extraspinal manifestations. *Radiology*, 115, 513–524

Resnick, D., Niwayama, G. (1988) *Diagnosis of Bone and Joint Disorders.* 2nd edn. W. B. Saunders, Philadelphia

Ropes, M. W., Bennett, G. A., Cobb, S., Jacox, R., Jesser, R. A. (1959) 1958 revision of diagnostic criteria for rheumatoid arthritis. *Bulletin of the Rheumatic Diseases*, 9, 175–176

Sholkoff, S. D., Glickman, M. G., Steinbach, H. L. (1970) Roentgenology of Reiter's syndrome. *Radiology*, 97, 497–503

Simon, M. A. (1981) Radioisotope evaluation of skeletal disease. *Journal of Bone and Joint Surgery*, 63A, 673–681

Solokoff, L. (1969) *The Biology of Degenerative Joint Disease.* University of Chicago Press, Chicago

Stoker, D. J. (1980) *Knee Arthrography.* Chapman & Hall, London

Weissberg, D. R., Resnick, D., Taylor, A., Becker, M., Alazraki, N. (1978) Rheumatoid arthritis and its variants. Analysis of scintigraphic, radiographic and clinical examinations. *American Journal of Roentgenology*, 131, 665–673

M. R. I.

Bassett, L.W., Gold, R. H., Seegar, L. L. (eds) (1988) *MRI Atlas of the Musculoskeletal System.* Martin Dunitz, London.

Burk, D. L., Dalinka, M. K., Kanal, E., Brunberg J. A. (1988) High resolution MR imaging of the knee. In: Kressel, H. Y. (ed), *Magnetic Resonance Annual*, pp. 1–36.

Dalinka M. K., Kricun M. E., Zlatkin, M. B., Hibbard, C. A. (1989). Modern diagnostic imaging in joint disease. *American Journal of Roentgenology*, 152, 229–240.

Deutsch, A. L., Mink, J. H. (1989). Magnetic resonance imaging of musculoskeletal injuries. *Radiologic Clinics of North America*, 27, 983–1002.

Grover, J. S., Bassett, L. W., Gross, M. L., Seeger, L. L., Finerman, G. A. M. (1990) Posterior cruciate ligament: MR imaging. *Radiology*, 174, 527–530.

Herman, L. J., Beltran, J. (1988) Pitfalls in MR imaging of the knee. *Radiology*, 167, 775–781.

Holt, R. G., Helms, C. A., Steinbach, L., Neumann, C., Munk, P. L., Genant H. K. (1990) Magnetic resonance imaging of the shoulder: rationale and current applications. *Skeletal Radiology*, 19, 5–14.

Kneeland, J. B., Hyde, J. S. (1989) High-resolution MR imaging with local coils. *Radiology*, 171, 1–7.

Middleton, W. D., Lawson, T. L. (eds) (1989) *Anatomy and MRI of the Joints: A Multiplanar Atlas.* Raven Press, New York.

Mink, J. H., Deutsch, A. L. (1989) *MR of the Musculoskeletal System. A Teaching Atlas.* Raven Press, New York.

Mitchell, D. G. (1988) MR of the normal and ischaemic hip. In: Kressel, H. Y. (ed), *Magnetic Resonance Annual*, pp. 37–39.

Mitchell, D. G. (1989) Using MR imaging to probe the pathophysiology of osteonecrosis. *Radiology*, 171, 25–26.

Munk, P. L., Helms, C. A., Genant, H. K., Holt, R. G. (1989) Magnetic resonance imaging of the knee: current status, new directions. *Skeletal Radiology*, 18, 569–577.

Reiser, M. F., Bongartz, G. P., Erlemann, R. et al (1989) Gadolinium-DTPA in rheumatoid arthritis and related diseases: first results with dynamic magnetic resonance imaging. *Skeletal Radiology*, 18, 591–597.

Stoker, D. J. (Ed) (1989) Musculoskeletal radiology. *Current Opinion in Radiology*, 1, 309–371.

Turner, D. A., Templeton, A. C., Selzer, P. M., Rosenberg, A. G., Petasnick, J. P. (1989) Femoral capital osteonecrosis: MR finding of diffuse marrow abnormalities without focal lesions. *Radiology*, 171, 135–140.

CHAPTER 5

TUMOURS AND TUMOUR-LIKE CONDITIONS OF BONE (1)

Iain Watt

INTRODUCTION

Bone tumours present problems which vary from simple to impossible. Whilst benign and innocuous lesions such as fibrous cortical defects are common, being said to occur in about 30% of normal children, primary malignant tumours of bone are relatively rare and are responsible for only about 1% of all deaths from neoplasia. Consequently most radiologists will see comparatively few cases and, even in referral centres, considerable difficulty often arises in making a differential diagnosis.

Three important questions require to be answered: *First*, is the lesion neoplastic or infective? *Second*, is it benign or malignant? *Third*, is it a primary or secondary neoplasm? In many cases these problems can be resolved without hesitation. In others, notably those in which cartilaginous tissue is involved, great difficulty may be experienced. It must never be forgotten that it is much more common for malignancy in bones to be metastatic rather than primary. It is important that a radiological diagnosis should be made prior to biopsy. An apparently simple radiological diagnosis may not be confirmed histologically and vice versa. Biopsy itself may significantly alter radiological features. It is also important to remember that although the pathologist may be regarded as the final arbiter, fully representative material must be available for opinion, and this may require sectioning the whole lesion. In some benign conditions, such as non-ossifying fibroma or an osteochondroma, it may be considered unnecessary to resort to pathological confirmation, and a conservative attitude or treatment by a minor surgical procedure may be adopted. On the other hand, if a more radical course is being considered, radiology serves not only to provide a diagnosis but also to delineate soft tissue and bony involvement, thereby permitting procedural planning. Inadequate investigations have occasionally been responsible for erroneous diagnoses of benign lesions as malignant, resulting in unnecessary surgical procedures, including especially such iatrogenic disasters as amputation.

Many different types of bone tumour are now recognized, varying greatly in their mode of clinical presentation, pathology and behaviour. Their aetiology remains obscure. Some seem superimposed upon pre-existing disease such as Paget's disease and bone infarctions. An accepted incidence of both benign and malignant neoplasms is known to follow radiation therapy.

Classification of bone tumours

It would be convenient to classify bone tumours according to their cell of origin or histogenesis. However, histologically the exact cell of origin of a tumour is not always certain and typing may depend only on the cell or cells which predominate in the developed lesion. In some cases a single tumour may produce several major different types of cell line (for example, osteosarcoma); in others, undifferentiated small round cells may be a predominant histological feature, permitting only a broad collective diagnosis of malignant round-cell tumour. A number of inter-related connective tissue cells are present in bone and from this skeletal connective tissue the majority of bone tumours appear to arise. Other bone tumours are related to nonosseous components of the skeleton, including blood vessels and nerves. Those associated with haematopoietic and lymphoreticular elements are discussed elsewhere (Ch. 7).

A classification of bone tumours is suggested in Table 5.1. Non-neoplastic tumours (the word tumour is literally synonymous with a swelling), abscess, haematoma and so forth, have been included since they must feature in the differential diagnosis. Never forget that a radiologically unusual metastasis is commoner, particularly with older patients, than a primary tumour.

GENERAL PRINCIPLES OF RADIOLOGICAL DIAGNOSIS OF BONE TUMOURS

Before attempting to interpret the radiological features of a bone tumour, consider the *age* of the patient and the *clinical history*. Many tumours are found in fairly constant age groups. The history may be less useful, since many lesions present with nonspecific features of pain, swelling or pathological fracture. However, lesions are not infre-

Table 5.1 Classification of primary tumours of bone

	Benign	Malignant
A. Presumed to arise from skeletal tissue		
Bony origin?	Bone island	Osteosarcoma
	Ivory osteoma	Parosteal
	Osteoid osteoma	osteosarcoma
	Osteoblastoma	
Cartilaginous?	Chondroma	Chondrosarcoma
	Chondroblastoma	Dedifferentiated
		chondrosarcoma
	Chondromyxoid fibroma	Mesenchymal
		chondrosarcoma
Fibrous?	Fibrous cortical defect	Fibrosarcoma
	Non-ossifying fibroma	
	Desmoplastic fibroma	Fibrous histiocytoma
	Fibromatosis	
	Atypical Paget's disease	Paget's sarcoma
Giant-cell	Giant-cell tumour	Malignant giant-cell
containing?	Aneurysmal bone cyst	tumour
	Hyperparathyroid brown	
	tumour	
B. Presumed to arise from other tissues in bones		
Blood vessels?	Haemangioma	Angiosarcoma
	Cystic angiomatosis	
	Haemangiomatosis	
	[Massive osteolysis/	
	vanishing bone	
	disease]	
	Glomus tumour	
	[Haemangiopericytoma]	
Nerves?	Neurofibroma	Neurofibrosarcoma
	Neurilemmoma	Neuroblastoma
Fat?	Lipoma	Liposarcoma
	[Intraosseous and	
	parosteal]	
Notochord?	—	Chordoma
Epithelium?	Implantation dermoid	Adamantinoma
Lymphoid/	—	Leukaemias
haematopoietic?		Lymphomas
(see Ch. 7)		Plasmacytoma
		Myelomatosis
C. Presumed to arise from joints		
	Intraosseous ganglion	Synovioma
	Pigmented villonodular	
	synovitis	
	Synovial chondromatosis	
	[Differentiate from:	
	Osteoarthritic cyst	
	Rheumatoid geode]	
D. No known origin		
	Solitary bone cyst	Malignant
		round-cell
		tumours
		(including
		Ewing's,
		neuroblastomas,
		reticulosarcoma)
E. Non-neoplastic tumours		
(a tumour is a	Brodie's abscess	
swelling!)	Haematoma	
	Infarction	
	Histiocytosis	

quently discovered by chance. The sex incidence in primary bone tumours is of little diagnostic value, although of relevance in skeletal metastasis.

The basis of diagnosis will be plain X-ray films and these will be supplemented as necessary by computerized tomography, scintigraphy, angiography and magnetic resonance imaging.

1. Is the lesion solitary or multiple? With the exception of multiple osteochondromas of diaphyseal aclasia and multiple cartilage tumours in dyschondroplasia, most primary bone tumours are solitary.

In the first instance technetium-99m-HDP bone scan is the investigation of choice to establish whether or not the lesion is unifocal (Fig. 5.1). Other abnormal foci may then be subjected to radiographic examination. Difficulties will be experienced in myelomatosis when most lesions are photon-deficient, or with metastasis from some primary carcinomas, such as cholangiocarcinoma or primary pelvic lesions, including cervix uteri. The high false-negative detection rate in these tumours may justify the more time-consuming and expensive radiographic skeletal survey. Never forget to take an X-ray of the chest, whether or

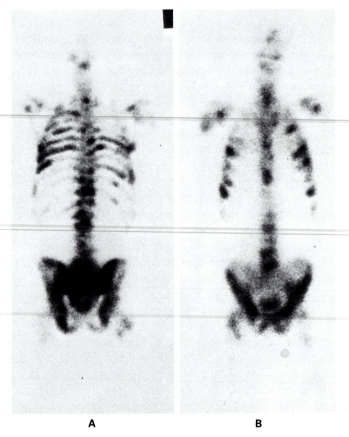

A   B

Fig. 5.1 Multiple skeletal metastases are demonstrated on a whole-body radionuclide bone scan. The primary tumour was carcinoma of the breast in a middle-aged woman. Note the predominantly axial distribution of the lesions, many of which were not apparent on plain X-rays. **A**. PA view. **B**. AP view.

not a plain film skeletal survey has been undertaken. The diagnosis becomes easier if a bronchial carcinoma or an obvious metastasis can be detected.

2. What type of bone is involved? It is of some value to differentiate between flat bones and tubular bones since, for example, lesions in the axial skeleton or proximal ends of long bones are in the sites of persistent haematopoietic tissue and should always raise the possibility of a metastasis or a reticulosis. Osteoid osteoma is very rare in membrane bone. A radiolucency in the mandible is more likely to be myeloma than metastasis. Although no part or the skeleton is exempt from involvement by a primary bone tumour, a large proportion are found in the pelvis and in the long bones, particularly around the hips and knees.

3. Where is the lesion within the bone? Many benign tumours tend to appear in characteristic sites: for example, nonossifying fibroma and fibrous cortical defects are by definition in the cortex, eccentrically towards the metadiaphysis of a long bone. Chondroblastoma occurs in an epiphysis or apophysis. Giant-cell tumour is almost invariably immediately subarticular and eccentric in location. Most tumours of cartilaginous origin, except those which are associated with an osteochondroma, have a medullary location.

4. Plain film features. Never settle for anything less than perfect plain films. It is important that soft tissue detail is not lost on an overexposed film, because a soft-tissue tumour extension typically presents a well-defined margin, whereas soft-tissue swelling associated with inflammation is ill-defined. Similarly, soft-tissue calcification or ossification may be overlooked. Do not settle for underpenetrated films since the inner texture of a tumour, for example the ground-glass quality of fibrous dysplasia, may be overlooked, or the radiolucent focus of an osteoid osteoma may not be visualized. Take films 'around the clock'. Simply because periosteal new bone cannot be visualized on a standard AP and lateral film does not mean that it will not be present on an oblique. Is the pattern of bone change destructive, proliferative or both? Correlating the size of the lesion with the length of history may be a guide as to its rapidity of growth, and similarly, follow-up films permit an assessment of its aggressive potential or malignancy. Tumours of osteoblastic origin are commonly, but not always, bone-producing. Consequently areas of increased density and/or surrounding new bone formation extending into soft tissue are likely to be evident. Cartilaginous tumours are mainly radiolucent but small foci of calcification represent an important hallmark.

5. What do the margins of the lesion look like? Is there a narrow or wide zone of transition between apparent tumour and normal bone? A wide zone of transition suggests an aggressive tumour or infection. Is the zone of transition marked with bone reaction or not? A thin rim of sclerosis is present characteristically around a non-ossifying fibroma, whereas extensive sclerosis is typical of a cortical osteoid osteoma. These findings are, of course, not constant and ill-defined sclerosis with a widened zone of transition may occur in such benign conditions as histiocytosis. Examine the cortex: is it resorbed from within, indicating medullary lesions as cartilaginous tumours or myelomatosis? Peripheral cortical lesions, on the other hand, with the exception of 'saucerization' of Ewing's sarcoma, are caused more commonly by pressure or direct invasion from abnormalities in adjacent soft tissues. If the margins of such a defect are smooth the lesion is usually benign, e.g. a neurofibroma, or non-neoplastic, as in the case of anterior erosions of the vertebral bodies by an aortic aneurysm. Conversely an irregular margin may suggest invasion by a malignant soft-tissue lesion, e.g. metastasis, or direct invasion by carcinoma of the antrum or lymphoma. Finally is there an associated soft-tissue mass? The presence of a soft tissue mass can frequently be shown in relation to malignant bone tumours, although oblique views may be necessary to delineate the masses. An ill-defined soft-tissue mass is almost invariably associated with an inflammatory lesion. Examine the margin of the soft-tissue lesion to see whether or not there is a thin shell of bone as occurs in some aggressive types of aneurysmal bone cysts, particularly those arising in the spine.

Further imaging investigations

Tomography. All further investigations are performed in order to delineate or elicit differential characteristics of a lesion already demonstrated by plain films. Tomography has been largely superseded by computerized tomography (CT). The object of a tomogram is either to delineate the characteristic radiological features summarized above or to assist demarcation of the intra- and extra-osseous extent of the abnormality.

Scintigraphy may be performed as the first additional investigation in most instances, depending on the availability of MR or CT. High-resolution gamma camera images using Tc^{99m}-labelled diphosphonate compounds provide the optimal images. Two phases of the bone scan should be recorded. Firstly, by counting the first 300 000 events after the injection a blood pool scan is obtained whilst the radiopharmaceutical is still largely in the intravascular or perivascular extracellular fluid space. Two to three hours later the skeleton is imaged, when the radiopharmaceutical has localized in bone and is in the delayed or bone-scan phase. The blood-pool phase is vital and should never be overlooked. Scintigraphy may be used to assess the primary presenting lesion and also to detect whether it is monostotic or accompanied by other skeletal lesions, such as metastasis.

Examine the blood-pool phase: is the lesion vascular, as in an aneurysmal bone cyst, or avascular, as in most cartilage tumours? Does the lesion itself accumulate radio-pharmaceutical, suggesting that it is being bound into a fibrous, cartilaginous or bone-forming matrix, or is the lesion essentially photon-deficient with increased activity surrounding it, suggesting either a heterogenous tumour or a host reaction? Does the lesion extend beyond the confines demonstrated by plain film, remembering that the apparent extent of intraosseous involvement can be slightly greater because the scan may not distinguish between bone-forming tumour and a rim of reactive host response? If the lesion is photon-rich, **check the lungs** since metastases from an osteosarcoma are frequently detectable by bone scanning. Finally, are there any lesions elsewhere? If so, radiograph them.

Computerized tomography has a most important part to play both in the assessment of the primary presenting lesion and in the detection of potential metastatic dissemination. CT will give an impression of the predominant variety of tissue present, particularly if there is fat or calcification. It will not, however, necessarily indicate whether or not those tissues are benign. Examine the intra-osseous extent of the tumour, looking for subtle changes in medullary fat. Examine also extra-osseous extent and soft-tissue relationships. Contrast-medium enhancement is of little value, since most tumours do not helpfully enhance. However, the vascular nature of a tumour may be detected and the relationship of the soft-tissue component of the tumour to blood vessels be assessed. More metastases are detected by CT, or whole-lung tomography, than is possible with routine plain film examinations.

Angiography has been the subject of fashion but in recent years has fallen into disrepute. The initial hope that it would, in isolation, distinguish reliably between benign and malignant lesions has foundered. No characteristic angiographic feature of malignancy exists. However, two signs — encasement and tumour vessels — occur with much greater frequency in malignant tumours. Encasement results from the vessel being surrounded by tumour and hence is shown by a localized segment of narrowing. Tumour vessels are defined as structures pursuing a random course with an irregular branching pattern.

Angiography should be used in the differential, rather than in the absolute, diagnosis of a lesion, as for example, to distinguish between tumour and infection. A malignant round-cell tumour has an intrinsically abnormal vascular pattern, whereas osteomyelitis is characterized by an increased number of normal arterial branches and enlarged periosteal veins. Similarly, angiography may be used to distinguish between tumours, since osteosarcomas are highly vascular, whereas most chondrosarcomas are hypovascular. It is arguable, however, whether angiography now contributes significantly to the assessment of primary tumours and their extent, since much of the information obtainable on angiogram may be obtained by scintigraphy, CT and MRI.

Angiography, however, may still be necessary in order to delineate involvement of major vessels by extension of a tumour into soft tissues when prosthetic or other limb conservation surgery is being considered. Interventional angiography has also enjoyed a vogue. Very vascular tumours may be infarcted prior to resection or intra-arterial chemotherapy given.

Magnetic resonance imaging. Magnetic resonance images have come to be of prime importance in the assessment of bone and soft-tissue contrast, with the ability to distinguish between various soft tissues by altering pulse sequences. Not only is a superb delineation of intra- and extra-osseous extent of tumour possible but also the flexibility of imaging planes permits advantageous visualization for tumour staging and planning of surgery. Intra-osseous oedema and extra-osseous inflammatory response may also be demonstrated. The relationship between tumour masses, inflammatory response, blood vessels and other important structures such as joints may be gauged very accurately. This information is of prime importance in planning limb salvaging procedures and assessing whether or not soft-tissue compartments are breached. Calcification, fibrous tissue and cortical compact bone are not distinguishable however. CT remains valuable for this purpose. Similarly, current images of the lung fields are not yet of high enough resolution to confidently detect the presence of a small metastasis. Again, CT is recommended for this purpose. Some sense of tumour aggressiveness may be gauged by measuring T_2 values, and the rate of enhancement following intravenous contrast medium and from strength of signal on some pulse sequences, for example STIR (short tau inversion recovery).

Other investigations. On occasions virtually the whole spectrum of radiological investigations will be necessary to differentiate between tumours or to gauge their extent. For example, lymphography may be necessary in order to detect local nodal involvement or arthrography to demonstrate the degree of synovial involvement in synovial chondromatosis or pigmented villonodular synovitis.

SECONDARY NEOPLASTIC INVOLVEMENT OF BONE

The later stages of many malignant neoplasms are associated almost inevitably with metastasis and the skeleton is very commonly affected. The radiographic presence of such lesions very often lags behind their detectability by scintigraphy, CT or MR (Fig. 5.2). Bony metastases are present in approximately 25% of all deaths from malignant disease. Any primary tumour may metastasize to bone, but in women the most important carcinoma is

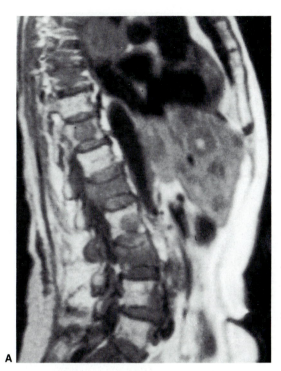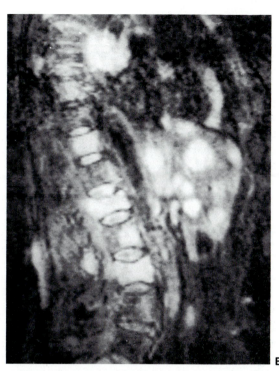

Fig. 5.2 Metastatic carcinoma of the bronchus. Sagittal T₁-weighted (**A**) and STIR (**B**) MRI sequences demonstrate extensive metastases throughout the thoracolumbar spine and also in the liver. The primary bronchial carcinoma is also demonstrated.

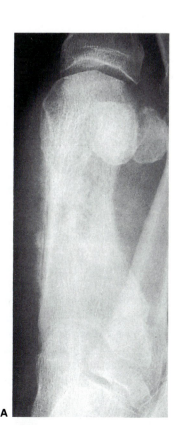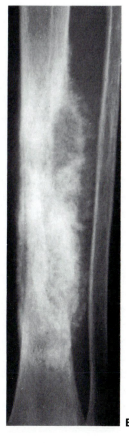

breast, from which secondary deposits develop in about two-thirds of cases. In men, approximately 80% of cases of carcinoma of the prostate and a quarter of tumours of the lung and kidney may be expected to produce bone metastases. A metastasis, indeed, may be the presenting feature of the disease.

Clinical features. Whilst a bone metastasis may present as a pathological fracture, usually they produce only vague pain or are entirely occult. Biopsy of a metastasis may indicate the site of origin of a previously unsuspected primary tumour. Usually the more malignant the primary tumour, the more rapidly does secondary spread occur. Some tumours, however, may present with a metastasis years before the primary lesion is clinically apparent and indeed the metastasis itself may remain virtually unchanged radiologically for a long time. This may be observed particularly with carcinoma of the thyroid or kidney. A latent period often separates the removal of a primary tumour, particularly from the breast, and the subsequent development of skeletal metastases.

The *spine*, *pelvis* and *ribs* are the most common sites of involvement together with the proximal ends of the *humeri*

Fig. 5.3 Two examples of solitary metastases producing bone in the adjacent soft tissues. **A**. Carcinoma of the colon in a great toe metatarsal and **B**. transitional cell carcinoma of the bladder in the mid tibia.

and *femora* and, less often, the *skull* (Fig. 5.1). These areas correspond to sites of persistent haematopoiesis in the adult, malignant spread usually occurring by a haematogenous route. Local spread to the lumbar spine and pelvis may be expected from tumours arising in the pelvis, notably carcinoma of the cervix. Some metastases have a predictable distribution, the majority of renal cell carcinoma metastasis occurring in the lumbar spine and pelvis. They have a rather characteristic radiological appearance (see below). Metastasis distal to the knee and elbow is rare and usually arises from a primary tumour of the bronchus or pelvic organs, particularly colon and bladder.

Blood chemistry studies may be of some value. The *serum alkaline phosphatase* is always raised in the presence of multiple bony metastasis, but remains normal in myelomatosis. With widespread osteolytic destruction the *serum calcium* is usually elevated and in the case of carcinoma of the prostate a marked rise in the *serum acid phosphatase* level is characteristic.

Some metastases respond to treatment with, for example, hormone therapy. Under these circumstances both radiography and scintigraphy are needed to monitor the progress of such lesions. Remember that it is inadequate simply to document the number and extent of metastasis; it is a radiologist's duty to draw the clinician's attention to those which may be considered hazardous — for ex-

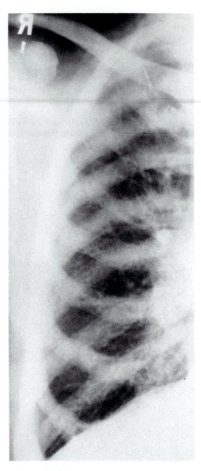

Fig. 5.5 Carcinoma of prostate — extensive sclerosis is present in the ribs and clavicle due to widespread metastasis in an elderly man.

ample, associated with significant vertebral body collapse (and the possible development of cord compression) or in long bones of the lower limb (with the potential for disabling fracture). In the latter circumstance prophylactic nailing of the femur is more acceptable than protracted recumbency in a Thomas splint to a patient with a limited life expectancy.

Radiological features. The majority of metastases are predominantly osteolytic. Typically they arise in the medulla and progressively extend in all directions, destroying the cortex, usually without the development of much periosteal reaction. Soft-tissue extension is relatively uncommon. Some metastasis, particularly from bronchial carcinoma, may appear eccentric and primarily destroy cortex, especially in the femur. Others are predominantly osteoblastic, including those derived from the prostate, stomach and carcinoid. They produce dense and often well-circumscribed areas of increased radiopacity. Such lesions are less subject to pathological fracture. A small group of metastases is accompanied by tumour bone formation; this includes osteosarcoma, liposarcoma, transitional cell carcinoma (of either bladder or kidney) and some adenocarcinomas of the colon (Fig. 5.3).

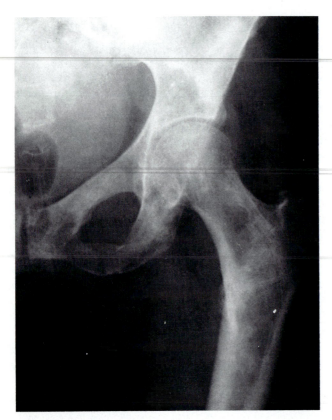

Fig. 5.4 Mixed skeletal metastases from carcinoma of the breast in a middle-aged woman.

The diagnosis of metastases is usually simplified by the multiplicity of lesions. Difficulty may arise when a lesion is apparently solitary. Unusual primary tumours are often responsible for unusual metastases and, further, a metastasis can simulate closely almost any known primary bone tumour!

Breast. Not only is this the most common primary tumour in women but its metastases show an unusual affinity for bone. Bone scanning demonstrates a significant incidence of bone metastases at the time of diagnosis, roughly in proportion to the degree of malignancy. The lesions are usually osteolytic and commonly multiple. Diffuse infiltration, however, may cause an apparently coarse trabecular pattern without an obvious area of bone destruction. The condition should be suspected in the presence of vertebral compression fractures in older women. Differentiation of these from osteoporotic collapse may be difficult, although in the latter, evidence of focal areas of bone destruction is usually lacking. MRI may be extremely helpful in the difficult case. Multiple lytic lesions also may resemble myelomatosis, but in that condition the margins of the lucencies are sharply defined with endosteal scalloping and the serum alkaline phosphatase is usually normal. About 10% of metastases from carcinoma of the breast produce osteoblastic lesions and in another 10% the lesions are mixed (Fig. 5.4). Sclerosis may occur in lytic lesions following successful hormone or radiation therapy. Difficulty may be experienced in dif-

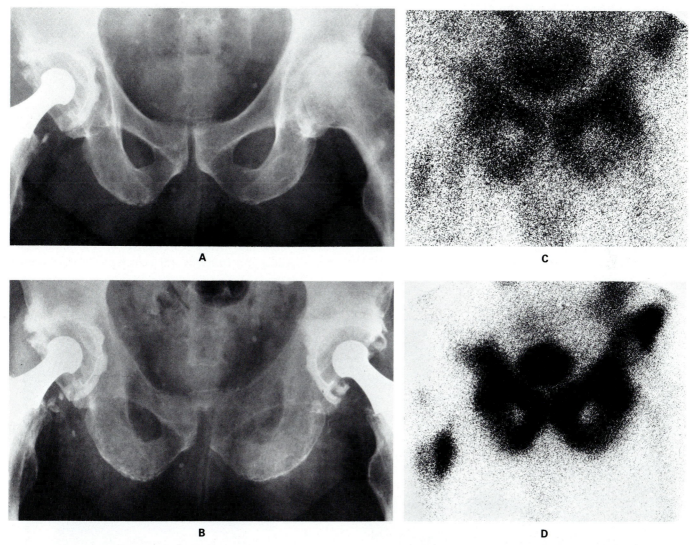

A

B

C

D

Fig. 5.6 Carcinoma of the prostate with expansile lytic metastases. **A**. A view of the pelvis before the onset of symptoms reveals no abnormality in the pubic rings. **B**. 5 years later the patient was complaining of severe pain in the groin. Note the ill-defined trabecular pattern, expansion of bone and ill-definition of cortex which has developed since the previous picture. **C**. Blood-pool phase of a bone scan and (**D**) delayed image reveals a marked increase in activity. Note the abnormality in the lesser trochanter of the right femur. These features could not be distinguished from active aggressive Paget's disease on purely scintigraphic grounds except that the lesion in the right femur has not started at a joint. The diagnosis was established by biopsy and the presence of a very high acid phosphatase level in the blood.

ferentiating between intense disuse osteoporosis following radiotherapy and metastatic disease. This problem arises particularly around the shoulder where the bones inevitably have been included in the radiation field. The lesions of intense disuse osteoporosis, however, tend to be sharply defined and ellipsoid in the long axis of bone. Similarly, multiple rib fractures secondary to radiation therapy should not be mistaken for metastases. The fractures often occur at the edge of the radiation field and consequently tend to be in a line, a distribution observed also in osteomalacia.

Prostate. This is the commonest secondary bone tumour in men and, in contrast to breast deposits, almost all these metastases are osteoblastic (Fig. 5.5). They appear as round or oval areas of increased density, particularly in the pelvis and spine, growing slowly and merging so that widespread and diffuse increase in bone density may ensue. Periosteal new bone formation and/or apparent expansion of bone may occur, so that the differentiation from Paget's disease may be difficult. The deposits may be shown to regress with hormone therapy. In some patients metastases from the prostate may be osteolytic and expansile (Fig. 5.6). They may even be solitary. If the carcinoma involves the base of the bladder some metastases may be associated with new bone formation in the adjacent soft tissue, resembling an osteosarcoma.

Kidney. Renal cell carcinoma is characteristically responsible for solitary bone metastases, with a marked predeliction for the pelvis and lumbar spine. Even when multiple their number seldom exceeds six. These lesions are typically expansile with a crenellated margin and usually have a typical radiological appearance (Fig. 5.7).

They are richly vascular, as demonstrated scintigraphically or angiographically. Since these tumours grow slowly, renal cell carcinoma is often associated with a relatively good prognosis, particularly following excision of the affected kidney and a solitary deposit. Transcatheter embolization may prove a useful addition to management.

Lung. In men this tumour is second only to the prostate in causing a high proportion of cases which develop skeletal metastases, such bone lesions occurring eventually in about a third. These metastases are almost always osteolytic and can be unusual, occurring in the small bones of the hand or eccentrically in the cortex of a long bone.

Alimentary tract. Carcinoma of the stomach and colon, and carcinoid, may metastasize to bone in both sexes. Metastases from the stomach and carcinoid are often osteoblastic and may be multiple. The bone-forming characteristic of colonic metastases has been already emphasized.

Other primary tumours often produce bizarre and atypical radiological patterns. In particular the metastases from thyroid carcinoma are classically expansile, osteolytic and often solitary (Fig. 5.8).

INVASION AND DESTRUCTION OF BONE BY EXTRAOSSEOUS PRIMARY MALIGNANT TUMOURS

Lesions of this type are rare compared with skeletal metastases, but may be observed in association with direct spread of such lesions as carcinoma of the cervix or bladder, and also from carcinoma of the paranasal sinuses. Malignant tumours adjacent to bone may cause

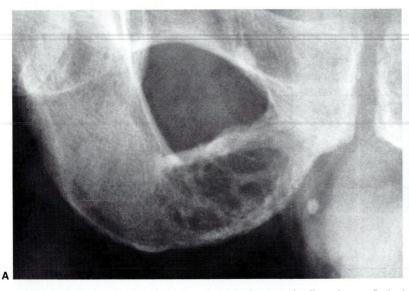
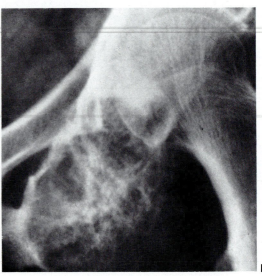

A   B

Fig. 5.7 A,B Two examples of solitary metastases from renal cell carcinoma. In both cases these metastases were the presenting abnormality. Both are expansile and have crenellated margins, with trabeculation in the lesion.

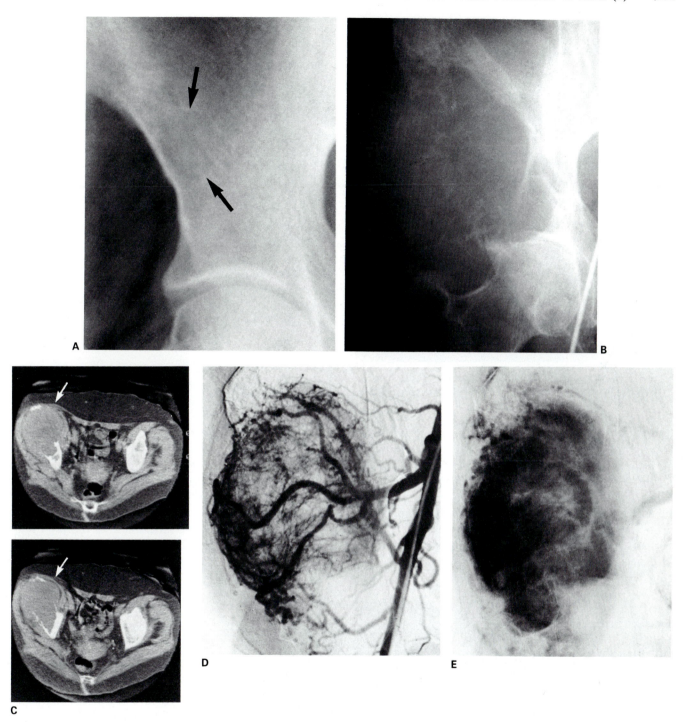

Fig. 5.8 Metastasis from carcinoma of thyroid. **A.** A localized view of the anterior inferior iliac crest shows a small radiolucent defect with a faint sclerotic margin (arrows). **B.** 5 years later a very large destructive bone lesion is present with relatively well-defined margins and apparent strands of calcification within the lesion. **C.** CT scan confirms the very extensive nature of the tumour and shows soft-tissue planes to be preserved (arrow). The strands of calcification are shown to be residual bone anteriorly and posteriorly and not new bone in the metastasis. **D.** and **E.** Common iliac arteriography (subtraction images) demonstrates the very vascular nature of this metastasis. Note the increase in number of abnormal vessels with changing calibre, the dense tumour blush and early venous filling.

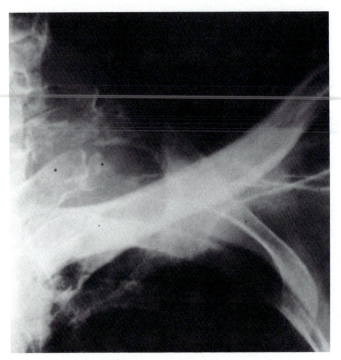

Fig. 5.9 Pancoast tumour — carcinoma of the apex of the lung — invading and destroying the first and second ribs.

resorption of the cortex with a permeative pattern, but lower-grade malignancies, including tendon sheath abnormalities, may produce well-defined cortical defects suggesting pressure erosion. Destruction of adjacent bones should suggest a lesion originating in soft tissues. An important example is involvement of the upper ribs by bronchial carcinoma (Pancoast tumour) in patients being assessed for neck, brachial plexus or shoulder pain (Fig. 5.9).

BONE TUMOURS PRESUMED TO ARISE FROM SKELETAL TISSUE: BONE-FORMING

BONE ISLAND (also known as *enostosis*)

Although no evidence exists to suggest that this is a true bony neoplasm, confusion may arise on occasions. The lesions may be single or multiple, are always medullary in location and consist of normal, compact lamellar bone. The lesion is uniformly dense but the margins may be ill-defined, showing radiating spiculation into the surrounding medullary cavity with a narrow zone of transition (Fig. 5.10). Bone islands may grow up to the age of skeletal maturity and occasionally thereafter. Exceptionally they may regress. Periosteal new bone and cortical expansion do not occur. On a radionuclide bone scan they may show a slight increase in activity, the degree being related to their size. No blood-pool abnormality becomes evident. In elderly patients it may be necessary to differentiate these sclerotic lesions from osteoblastic metastases.

OSTEOMA

True osteomas are rather rare, arising principally from skull, paranasal sinuses and mandible (Fig. 5.11). They are benign, slow growing tumours consisting entirely of well-differentiated bone. They have a broad base with a smooth well-defined margin. Two types are recognized: the dense variety, the so-called ivory osteoma; and the trabeculated or spongy variety more commonly occurring in the cranial vault. Whilst varying in size few are larger than 2.5 cm in diameter. The tumour itself is asymptomatic, but growth from the inner table of the skull may produce raised intracranial pressure or other symptoms similar to those of a meningioma. Growth within the

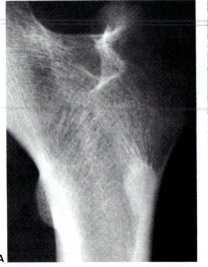
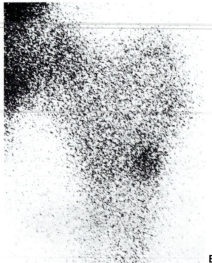

Fig. 5.10 Bone island — enostosis. **A.** A dense area of endosteal sclerosis present in the upper femoral shaft, discovered by chance following injury. **B.** A bone scan reveals slight increase in activity localized to the area of sclerosis. Biopsy confirmation.

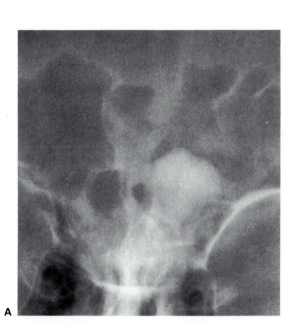 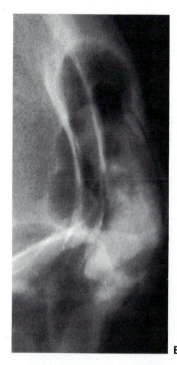

Fig. 5.11 Ivory osteomas of the frontal sinus. A typical, compact, rounded, dense opacity is demonstrated on (**A**) the frontal view. **B**. In another patient a larger lesion has moulded to the shape of the sinus.

paranasal sinuses may interfere with nasal drainage, causing a mucocoele. The rarer, spongy variety is shown histologically to contain moderate quantities of fibrous tissue and may be a variant of fibrous dysplasia.

Further investigation is rarely necessary apart from documenting the secondary effects of the lesion. Scintigraphically the increased activity reflects the size of the lesion as in the case of a bone island.

When craniofacial osteomas are detected, the possibility of Gardner's syndrome should be considered, particularly if lesions are present in the mandible. The presence of osteomas elsewhere in the skeleton, soft-tissue tumours of connective tissue origin and polyposis coli establish the diagnosis.

OSTEOID OSTEOMA

Unlike other bone tumours this lesion has a definite male preponderance of the order of three to one. The majority of cases present in the second and third decades. The typical history is of localized, intermittent bone pain of several weeks' or months' duration, occurring especially at night with dramatic relief by aspirin. Pain may be sufficient to provoke muscle wasting from limitation of movement. Growth disparities may develop in the immature skeleton, including failure of tubulation and leg length discrepancy. Difficulty in diagnosis sometimes causes these patients to be referred to psychiatrists in the belief that their symptoms are functional. The natural his-

tory of this tumour is uncertain since most cases are treated by immediate surgical excision but it appears probable that untreated lesions eventually undergo spontaneous involution.

The diaphyses of long bones are the sites of predeliction with at least half of all cases occurring in the femur, especially its proximal end, and the tibia, although virtually any bone may be affected. When the spine is involved the tumour is almost always situated in the neural arch and not the vertebral body. The symptoms of spinal involvement may mimic those of an adolescent disc protrusion, and indeed painful scoliosis in a child or adolescent demands careful scrutiny of the neural arches at the apex of the concavity to exclude the presence of this tumour.

Radiological features. The lesion comprises a round or oval area or radiolucency with a sclerotic margin. This radiolucency usually contains a small dense opacity known, on this side of the Atlantic, as the nidus (Fig. 5.12). In North America the word nidus (meaning nest) is employed more correctly for the radiolucency itself. While the overall size of the lesion varies up to about 2.5 cm in diameter the width of the central density rarely exceeds 1 cm. The lesion is surrounded by a variable degree of dense sclerosis. The extent of this density depends on the actual site of the tumour within the affected bone. It is minimal when the tumour lies in the spongy bone of the medulla, particularly close to joints (Fig. 5.13). Occasionally no peripheral density may be

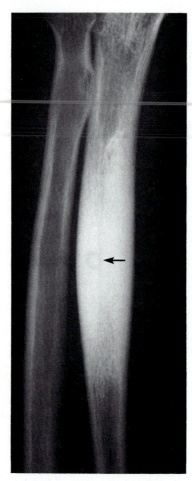

Fig. 5.12 Osteoid osteoma of the ulna in a 13-year-old boy. The appearances are typical, with a well-defined area of radiolucency (arrow) containing a dense nidus. Extensive cortical sclerosis is present around the lesion.

evident and the small central opacity appears to lie within an area of radiolucency. More commonly, the lesion is sited in relation to cortical bone and is surrounded by dense sclerosis which may be extensive and extend into the medulla. When the lesion is adjacent to the periosteum in children new bone formation is particularly florid. The reactive new bone may be so dense that the lesion itself is obscured on plain radiographs.

Provided that the essential features of the radiolucency and its central density are demonstrated, the diagnosis is usually established radiologically with little difficulty. When the lesion is surrounded by dense sclerosis further investigation is necessary, requiring overpenetrated films, tomography (either conventional or CT) and bone scintigraphy. Because of the extensive sclerosis it is important not to overcount the bone scan since the focal area of increased activity due to the osteoid osteoma may be obscured. In the case of a medullary osteoid osteoma with little or no radiological abnormality on conventional films, bone scintigraphy remains the most important means of detecting the presence of a lesion. An intense focal abnormality is evident in the blood pool image and intense activity persists in the delayed image. *Scintigraphy* should be undertaken in any young person with bone pain and apparently normal radiographs. These scintigraphic abnormalities correspond to the highly vascular nature of the neoplasm which may be demonstrated by angiography, particularly by the tumour blush evident in the late venous phase. The presence of the lesion and its exact site may require localization with *computerized tomography.*

The pain produced by these tumours is relieved immediately by surgical excision and the reactive new bone slowly undergoes remodelling. If, however, removal of the tumour is incomplete, not only will the pain persist but the lesion will recur. On rare occasions, osteoid osteoma may be multifocal, more than one opacity being contained within a single area of radiolucency. Some lesions near joints in childhood may be associated with synovitis, with resulting diffuse hyaline cartilage thinning and disuse osteoporosis.

Osteoid osteoma must be differentiated from osteoblastoma (described below) and other causes of chronic cortical thickening. These include chronic sclerosing osteomyelitis, foreign body granulomas ('blackthorn'), polyarteritis nodosa and subperiosteal haematoma, particularly along the shin. In general the distinction between osteoid osteoma and chronic osteomyelitis is straightforward. In osteomyelitis the area of radiolucency tends to be more irregular, although a sequestrum may be confused with a nidus. Whereas the central opacity of an osteoid osteoma is almost always round or slightly oval, the majority of osteomyelitic sequestra are irregular and often linear in shape. Scintigraphy shows a diffuse increase in activity both in the blood pool and the delayed phases. MRI may demonstrate considerable bone oedema in both cases but a fluid collection clearly indicates infection.

OSTEOBLASTOMA

This tumour is now accepted as a distinct entity, although a considerable overlap undoubtedly exists with osteoid osteoma. Indeed the situation is confused by the occasional osteoid osteoma which is larger than usual and may be referred to as giant osteoid osteoma. Both osteoblastoma and osteoid osteoma superficially have similar histological characteristics. The tumour is, in almost all circumstances, benign, but may be aggressive (see below). It is accompanied often by a long insidious history of pain, one in ten patients suffering worsening of the pain at night. Aspirin relief is not a feature. No definite sex incidence has been recognized but at least 80% of the patients are under the age of 30. Whilst any bone may be involved, the majority of lesions occur in the spine and flat bones, particularly the vertebral ap-

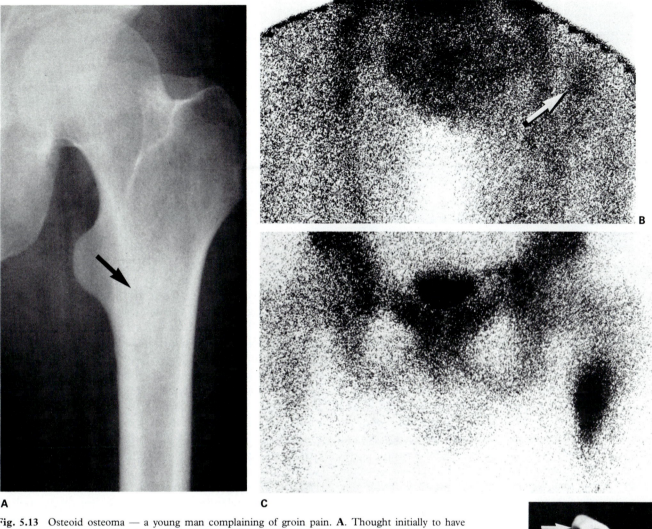

Fig. 5.13 Osteoid osteoma — a young man complaining of groin pain. **A**. Thought initially to have normal X-rays; however, in retrospect, a small radiolucency (arrow) is present. A bone scan was performed in order to detect any occult cause of pain. **B**. A localized focus of increased vascularity is shown on the blood pool film (arrow). **C**. Extensive abnormality on the delayed film. **D**. Computerized tomography demonstrates clearly the radiolucent defect anteriorly (closed arrow) with associated, consolidated periosteal new bone. A nutrient artery is demonstrated posteriorly (open arrow) and is an incidental finding.

pendages. Again, as in the case of osteoid osteoma, the last location may stimulate a scoliosis; indeed in one series as many as 50% of the patients had a scoliosis, some with positive neurological signs.

Pathologically the lesion is larger than an osteoid osteoma, irregular in shape, friable and haemorrhagic. Abundant osteoid tissue is present with broad, widely spread trabeculae, in relation to which are numerous osteoblasts and osteoclasts. Many thin-walled capillaries account for the marked vascularity of the tumour.

Radiological features. An area of radiolucency is typical, being considerably larger than that of an osteoid osteoma and of the order of 2–10 cm in diameter (Fig. 5.14). Difficulty may arise on occasions in distin-guishing this appearance from an exceptionally large osteoid osteoma. The margins of the radiolucency show considerable irregularity, even though they are usually sharply demarcated. This margin, however, may sometimes be ill-defined and not easily distinguishable from a malignant lesion, particularly an osteosarcoma. A giant-cell tumour may be considered when the lesion is subarticular in location. Cortical expansion and exquisite thinning is common so that only a fine opaque shell may remain. This appearance simulates the cortical expansion caused by an aneurysmal bone cyst, but may be distinguished easily by the total absence of bone reaction and the poorly defined margin of the latter tumour. The majority of osteoblastomas enlarge slowly, with consequent

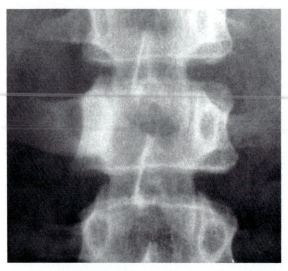

Fig. 5.14 Osteoblastoma of the right transverse process and pedicle of L3. An ill defined radiolucency is shown within a sclerotic and expanded transverse process and pedicle.

remodelling of bone around the lesion. The degree of associated bone sclerosis varies considerably but may be profound. Calcification or ossification of osteoid tissue within the tumour may cause a punctate increase in density (Fig. 5.15), best appreciated on *tomography* or *CT*. Calcification is never annular as in a cartilage tumour. *Scintigraphically* these lesions are extremely active both in the blood-pool and delayed phases of a bone scan. On the delayed phase the lesion may seem very extensive, reflecting the secondary bone sclerosis. If *angiography* is undertaken the radiolucency may be shown to contain an increased number of vessels with a blush and small lakes of contrast

medium, but encasement and other features suggestive of malignancy are not present. As with osteoid osteoma, *MRI* demonstrates considerable bone oedema surrounding a lesions.

In the vast majority of patients the prognosis is excellent once total excision of the tumour has been achieved. On some occasions, however, an osteoblastoma behaves in an aggressive fashion, particularly after incomplete removal. Not only is the lesion radiographically aggressive, with soft-tissue masses containing ill-defined calcification and ossification, but a similar pattern of aggression is visible also under the microscope. On rare occasions the lesion behaves frankly as an osteosarcoma with pulmonary metastasis (Fig. 5.16).

OSTEOSARCOMA

Osteosarcoma is the commonest primary malignant bone tumour. Characteristically it is histologically pleomorphic, but two diagnostic features are: firstly, its ability to produce osteoid tissue, without necessarily the development of a cartilaginous precursor; and, secondly, the presence of abundant alkaline phosphatase histochemically within the tumour cells. The osteoid tissue may undergo some degree of ossification. However, because of the pleomorphic nature of the sarcoma a dominant cell line may modify the appearance. If osteoblasts predominate, tumour bone formation will result, whereas, if cells of cartilage origin are present, extensive calcification may be a presenting feature. Terms such as osteoblastic (Fig. 5.17), chondroblastic (Fig. 5.18), fibroblastic, and anaplastic or telangectatic (Fig. 5.19) are often applied. No convincing evidence has been established that these

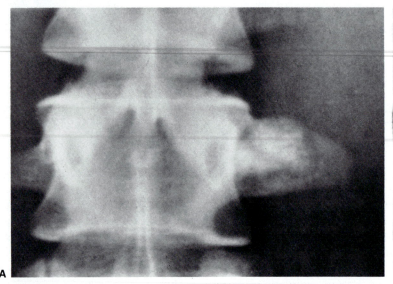
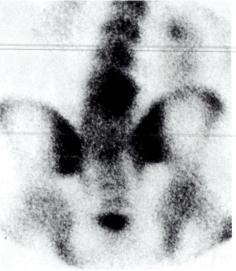

Fig. 5.15 Osteoblastoma of the left transverse process of L3. **A**. In this example the central area exhibits calcification. Expansion is present with diffuse sclerosis. **B**. Note on the bone scan (which has been reversed for ease of comparison) the extensive area of increased activity corresponding to the whole of the osteoblastoma on the plain film. Note also the scoliosis with which these patients may present.

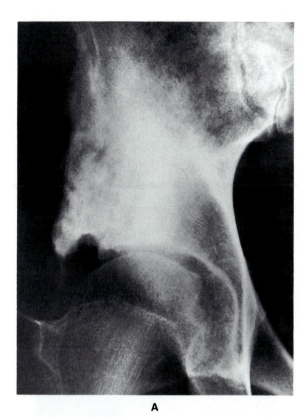

A

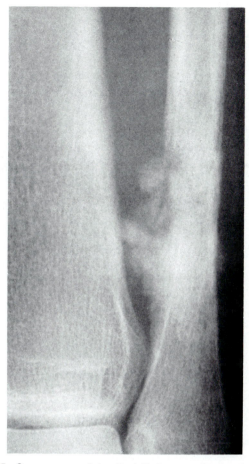

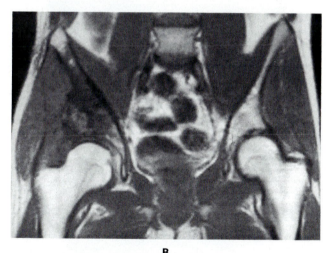

B

Fig. 5.16 Aggressive osteoblastoma. Plain film (**A**) demonstrates a large area of ill-defined bone sclerosis extending into the soft tissues above the acetabular roof. This had been previously biopsied. A vague ill-defined zone of radiolucency is demonstrated within the proliferative new bone. A T_1-weighted coronal MR image (**B**) demonstrates extensive low-signal abnormality throughout the whole of the right iliac blade down to the acetabular roof. A soft-tissue component is also demonstrated. This scan also illustrates how difficult it is to assess sclerotic lesions using MRI.

Fig. 5.17 Osteosarcoma of the distal fibula — predominantly osteoblastic. Amorphous calcification/ossification is present in the soft tissues with cortical destruction and a little periosteal new bone formation.

pathological subgroups have much influence on prognosis. Nonetheless, each has slightly different radiological characteristics. Osteosarcoma arising in relation to the periosteum and secondary to other conditions is considered below.

Osteosarcoma presents usually with localized pain or swelling, particularly around the knee in an adolescent or young adult. Not infrequently the lesion may present with a pathological fracture (Fig. 5.20). A slight male preponderance exists, the peak incidence occurring between 10 and 25 years of age. Many of the tumours occurring in older age groups are associated with Paget's disease (see below). Although any bone may be involved, rather more than half of all osteosarcomas are located around the knee, involving the metadiaphyses of the distal end of the femur and the proximal end of the tibia. Indeed the vast majority of osteosarcomas arise in those sites in long bones which are exhibiting the greatest longitudinal growth. About 10% of tumours arise in the diaphysis. These have a similar age and sex incidence to ordinary osteosarcoma (see below). Orthodox teaching suggested that epiphyseal involvement occurs late, metaphyseal cartilage acting as a temporary barrier to spread of the tumour. Although this appears supported by the evidence of plain films, investigation by scintigraphy, angiography and MR has indicated that in many cases epiphyseal involvement occurs earlier.

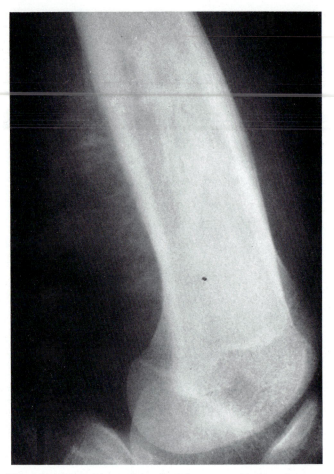

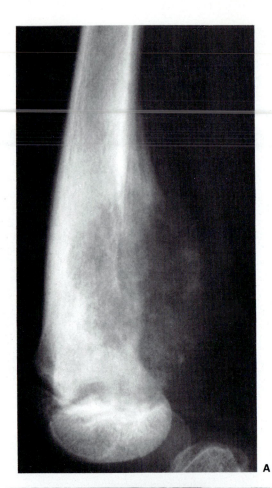

Fig. 5.18 Osteosarcoma of the distal femur — predominantly chondroblastic. Note the well-defined soft tissue mass and radiating spiculation of calcification within it. Sclerosis and lysis are present within the medullary cavity which is slightly expanded.

The lesion commonly arises eccentrically in the medullary cavity, with ill-defined cortical destruction and soft-tissue involvement. The pleomorphic nature of the histology may cause misleading biopsy results, since if the sample is taken from areas rich in cartilaginous elements, a misdiagnosis of chondrosarcoma may occur. Metastatic spread occurs by the haematogenous route so that a search for pulmonary metastasis should be undertaken. Pulmonary metastasis is associated with an unusually high incidence of pneumothorax (Fig. 5.21). Any lung lesion arising in a patient with osteosarcoma should be regarded with suspicion (Fig. 5.22). Lymphatic spread is relatively rare. In the later stages metastasis may develop in bone; population surveys have suggested that these deposits are themselves metastatic from the pulmonary lesions.

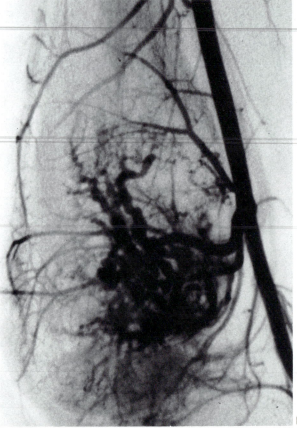

Fig. 5.19 Telangectatic osteosarcoma of the distal femur.
A. A predominantly radiolucent defect is shown on plain film which (**B**) angiographically is shown to contain large, tortuous, pathological vessels. Well-marked Codman's triangles are present together with sclerosis in the shaft of the bone, surrounding the lesion.

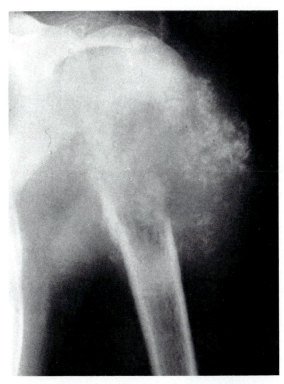

Fig. 5.20 An advanced osteosarcoma of the proximal humerus presents with a pathological fracture. A large well defined soft tissue mass contains calcification and ossification. Codman's triangles are present. Extensive tumour in the medulla has caused both bone destruction and bone formation.

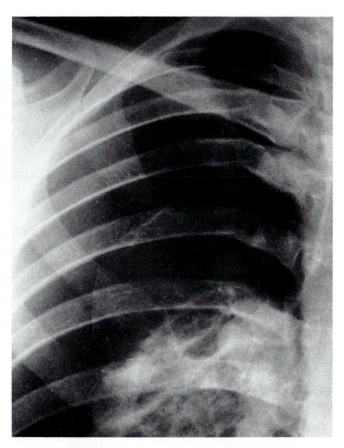

Fig. 5.21 Osteosarcoma — metastasis in the lungs presents with a pneumothorax.

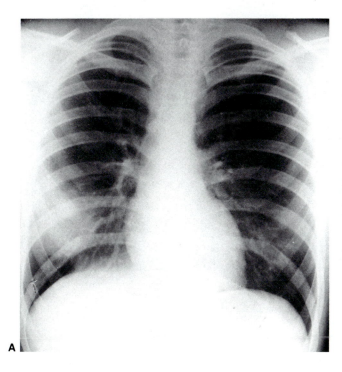

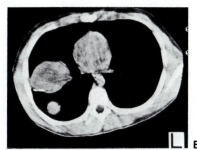

Fig. 5.22 Metastasis from osteosarcoma presents with (**A**) an encysted pleural effusion on the right after several months apparently disease-free after amputation. **B**. A CT scan demonstrates the encysted effusion in the horizontal fissure with calcification dorsally due to metastasis. This feature had not been appreciated on conventional tomography. A second metastasis is shown in the right lower lobe, again not obvious on plain films. (W 200, L + 16).

Imaging features. On *plain films* an eccentric area of bone destruction is usually present in the metadiaphysis adjacent to the knee joint, being associated typically with cortical destruction and a well-defined extension of the lesion into soft tissues. Elevation of the periosteum is associated with new bone formation, the so-called Codman's triangles. The epiphysis usually appears normal radiologically. The soft-tissue mass may contain calcification which may show either an amorphous or a spiculated appearance. A mixture of sclerosis and bone destruction is usually present within the bony lesion. It is unusual for a lesion to be purely lytic. *Scintigraphically,* increased vascularity is constant in the blood-pool phase of a bone scan with an extensive abnormality on the delayed images (Fig. 5.23). The extent of the tumour, as delineated by a bone scan, may be greater than that shown on plain film, being due to a surrounding rim of reactive bone. Scintigraphy may confirm epiphyseal spread of the tumour, but an apparent increase in activity in an adjacent joint should not be mistaken for synovial involvement. Scintigraphy also may detect the presence of lung metastasis, although this procedure is not reliable if purely fibroblastic lesions are present or if the metastases have been treated. A cerebral metastasis may not be observed with a bone scan. *Computerized tomography* demonstrates to advantage those features on the plain films and is particularly useful for delineating the intra- and extra-osseous extent of tumour (Figs 5.22C, 5.24D). It is the most sensitive means of detecting pulmonary metastases (Fig. 5.23B). The *angiographic features* suggest an aggressive tumour and again may be used to establish the extent of tumour, if treatment by prosthetic replacement is being considered (Figs 5.24, 5.25).

Magnetic resonance imaging is the prime investigation of choice for osteosarcoma, if available, following plain X-ray films. An obvious heterogenous tumour is

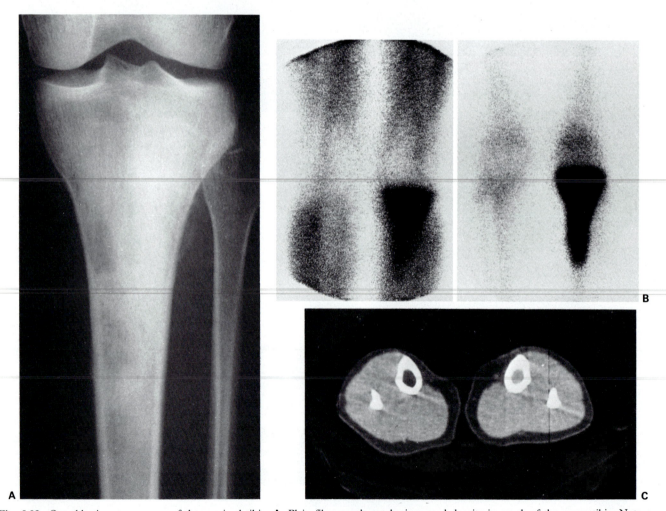

Fig. 5.23 Osteoblastic osteosarcoma of the proximal tibia. **A**. Plain film reveals patchy increased density in much of the upper tibia. Note a little new bone laterally. **B**. A scan in the early blood-pool (left) and delayed phases (right) demonstrates an extensive abnormality. Note the activity is more uniform and extensive than the apparent involvement shown on the plain film. The distal extent of the tumour is confirmed however by (**C**) a CT scan which shows a subtle change in marrow attenuation below the level of the apparent tumour on plain film. An example of how CT may be used to gauge the extent of marrow involvement.

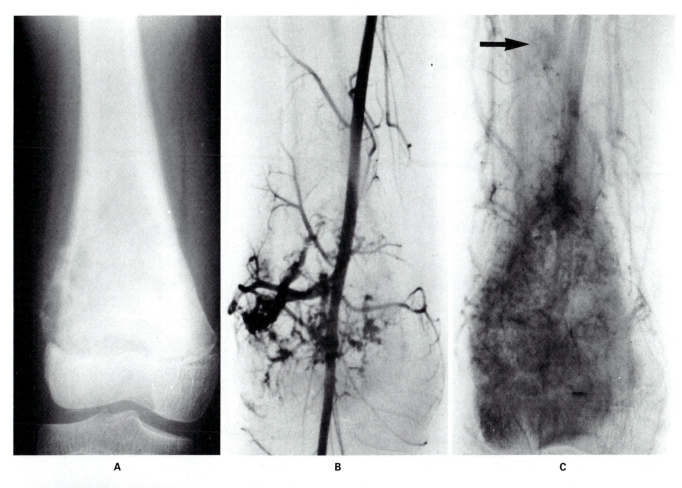

A   B   C

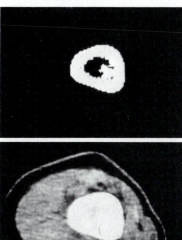

D

Fig. 5.24 Osteosarcoma of the distal femur of a young woman. **A**. The full intraosseous extent is difficult to assess on the plain film. **B**. An arteriogram demonstrates a very extensive pathological circulation and (**C**) on the late capillary phase note that the tumour extends into the epiphysis, almost to the articular surface, and that there is a satellite or 'skip' lesion in the proximal femoral shaft (arrow). This latter lesion is confirmed by (**D**) CT and is shown to be bone- forming (the upper image shows an attenuation of 94 EMI units in the lesion, the lower image is at L12, W200).

demonstrated with surrounding bone and usually a soft tissue mass. Areas of calcification and ossification are shown as low signal but even within the sclerotic component within the medullary canal there is usually high signal associated with tumour bulk. Careful delineation of the lesion and assessment of relationships between it and adjacent blood vessels and joints are essential in pre-operative planning (Fig. 5.26).

Differential diagnosis is either from other neoplasms, including malignant round-cell tumours and metastases, or from chronic bone infections, including tuberculosis and mycetoma. In the case of infections the aetiology may be suggested by diffuse swelling of soft tissues, disproportionately extensive new bone formation and widespread photon activity on a bone scan.

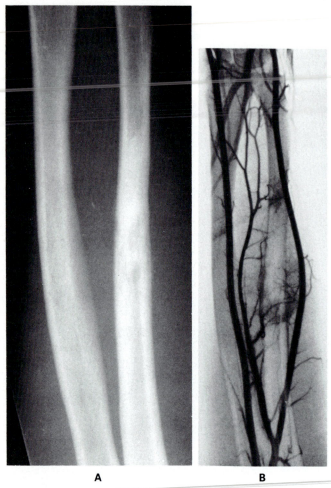

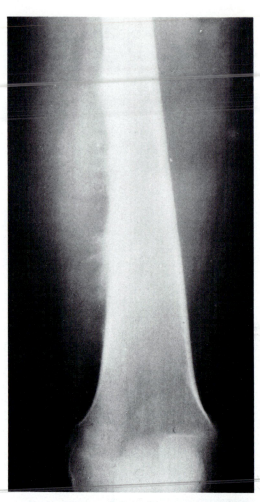

Fig. 5.25 Osteoblastic osteosarcoma. A middle-aged woman presented with pain and swelling in the mid-ulna. **A**. A radiograph shows ill-defined sclerosis and cortical destruction. **B**. An angiogram demonstrates an egg-shaped soft-tissue mass with displacement of both the ulnar and interosseous arteries. The extraosseous extent of the tumour was thereby delineated.

Fig. 5.27 Diaphyseal osteosarcoma of the midshaft of the femur. Note the radiating speculation of bone, Codman's triangles and well-defined soft tissue mass.

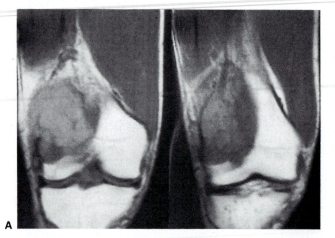

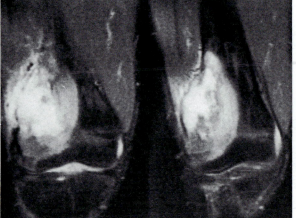

Fig. 5.26 Osteosarcoma. Coronal T_1-weighted (**A**) and STIR sequences (**B**) demonstrate an extensive osteosarcoma of the lateral femoral condyle. The pleomorphic nature of the tumour can be appreciated by the more superficial main neoplasm with subadjacent marrow oedema. Note the overlying abnormal vessels shown as a signal void and the joint effusion on the STIR sequence. Clear extension across the metaphysis is also shown. These features confirm an extracompartmental osteosarcoma.

Special types of osteosarcoma

Diaphyseal. Approximately 10% of tumours arise in the diaphyses of long bones and may cause diagnostic confusion. Whilst most resemble those of osteosarcoma elsewhere (Fig. 5.27), others are purely lytic or indeed purely sclerotic (Fig. 5.28) and an accurate pre-biopsy diagnosis may not be possible.

Central osteosarcoma. Similar difficulty may arise when a lesion presents in the metadiaphysis as an area of dense sclerosis which may be thought to represent a large bone island. Specific characteristics on plain films to suggest malignant disease are absent. Scintigraphy, MR and angiography, however, will demonstrate much more aggressive features.

Multifocal osteosarcoma is extremely rare and occurs only in childhood. The condition is rapidly fatal, with pulmonary metastases and is characterized by a marked elevation of serum alkaline phosphatase. Radiologically symmetrical and densely sclerotic lesions have a predilection for metaphyses and flat bones. Unlike ordinary osteosarcoma, epiphyseal and soft tissue involvement occurs early.

Soft-tissue osteosarcoma. On rare occasions the tumour arises purely in soft tissue (Fig. 5.29). Various sites of origin have been described, including breast and kidney. Usually, however, the lesion is para-articular. The ill-defined amorphous nature of the soft-tissue opacification may suggest tumour bone rather than calcification. The differential diagnosis is from post-traumatic myositis ossificans which can also produce markedly abnormal features with scintigraphy and angiography, particularly early in its evolution. Histological examination of both entities also is fraught with diagnostic pitfalls in inexperienced hands.

Radiation-induced sarcoma

Radiation therapy. Sarcomas arise in bone following radiation typically when the total dose has exceeded 30 Gy (3000 rad), often after a latent interval of 7–10 years. Whilst most are fibrosarcomas, a few osteosarcomas occur. The diagnosis is not difficult radiologically but they often have a predominantly lytic nature and are markedly aggressive. They arise in predictable sites, based on radiation fields, for example in the pelvis following treatment of gynaecological cancer (Fig. 5.30).

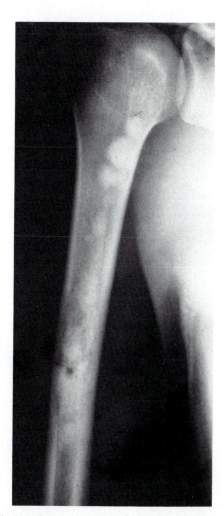

Fig. 5.28 Diaphyseal osteosarcoma. A pathological fracture is present in the mid humerus with extensive endosteal sclerosis and cortical destruction from the medullary aspect. Tumour is present to the neck of the humerus with areas of dense sclerosis and surrounding faint radiolucency. These 'skip' lesions do not represent isolated tumour; the shaft was involved continuously. This variety carries a poor prognosis.

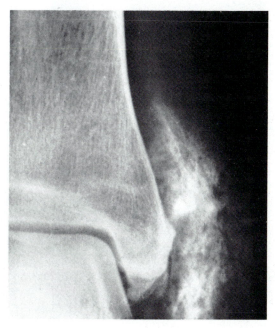

Fig. 5.29 Soft-tissue osteosarcoma. An elderly vicar complained of an enlarging soft-tissue mass adjacent to the medial malleolus of his right ankle. Note the amorphous soft-tissue ossification and calcification and normal bone underlying the lesion.

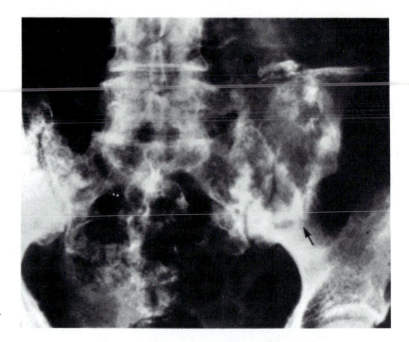

Fig. 5.30 Radiation sarcoma arising in the posterior iliac crest on the left, in an elderly woman treated 6 years previously for carcinoma of the cervix. The lesion is purely osteolytic with ill-defined surrounding sclerosis (arrows).

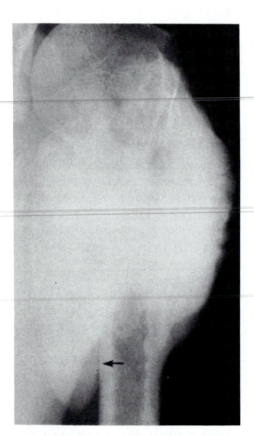

Fig. 5.31 Parosteal osteosarcoma of the proximal humerus. A well-defined mass of dense tumour bone surrounds the humeral shaft. A typical radiolucent line is present between the tumour bone and the proximal shaft inferomedially (arrow). The underlying bone seems normal.

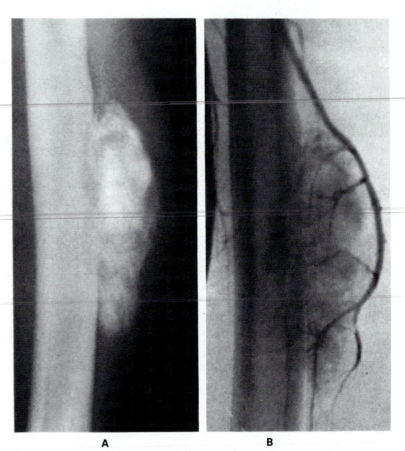

A   B

Fig. 5.32 Parosteal osteosarcoma arising from anterior aspect of the femur (**A**) is shown (**B**) angiographically to be unremarkable apart from a slight increase in number of branches going into the tumour. The lesion was found at biopsy, to be of very low-grade malignancy.

The ingestion of radioactive material. Radium and radiomesothorium were introduced in America in 1914 in the preparation of luminous paint. In applying this to watch dials, ingestion of the radioactive material occurred through pointing the paint brush with the lips. The subsequent development of osteosarcoma was first reported in 1931 although more usually areas of bone destruction and sclerosis are due to infarction. A long latent interval between ingestion and tumour development is typical. Thorium is, of course, associated with abdominal neoplasia (see Ch. 25).

Parosteal osteosarcoma

Some confusion in nomenclature relates to osteosarcomas arising in or near the periosteum. For practical purposes these may be divided into two groups: *parosteal osteosarcoma* which will be described; and periosteal osteosarcoma which is similar in most ways to an ordinary osteosarcoma except that it arises close to the periosteum.

Parosteal osteosarcoma comprises some 1% of all malignant primary bone tumours and about 4% of osteosarcomas. Clinically it occurs in older patients, at least 50% being over the age of 30. The tumour is slow-growing by comparison and has a much better prognosis. In low-grade lesions the histology may not immediately suggest a neoplasm at all.

Radiological features. Typically a dense tumour surrounds a long bone, particularly a femur or a tibia. The tumour bone may be extensive, ranging between 2 and 10 cm in length and as much as 5 cm in breadth. The margins are sharply defined but tend to undulate. Whilst the peripheral margin may be clear-cut, it may be difficult to demonstrate separation of the lesion from underlying bone. This feature is important since the characteristic radiological sign is a zone of radiolucency between the tumour and the host bone (Fig. 5.31). Penetrated films, tomography or CT may be required in order to demonstrate this sign. The tumour appears usually to be attached to bone by a broad pedicle. Endosteal sclerosis may occur. Scintigraphically the blood-pool image is usually unremarkable although considerable increase in activity is evident in the delayed phase. Some evidence suggests that the malignancy of this tumour is reflected by the degree of abnormal vascularity on an angiogram (Fig. 5.32).

The condition must be differentiated from subperiosteal haematoma and other benign causes of periosteal new bone formation.

Sarcoma in Paget's disease

Malignant tumours are said to arise in bone affected by Paget's disease in about 1% of cases. It is difficult to gauge the exact incidence, since many cases of Paget's disease are asymptomatic or diagnosed by chance. The possibility of a sarcoma arising in Paget's disease should be considered when alteration occurs in the character of bone pain, either an increase in severity or more precise localization; or if a pathological fracture develops. The presence of a soft-tissue mass and a further rise in the serum alkaline phosphatase may be observed. Sarcomas may occur in the polyostotic or monostotic disease, though there seems to be a particular predilection for the humerus in the latter. Overall the skull, pelvis and long bones are typical sites (Fig. 5.33). Men are more com-

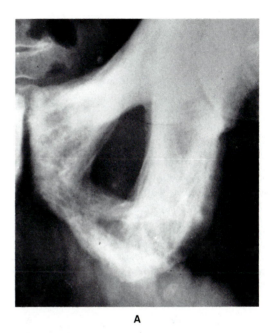

A

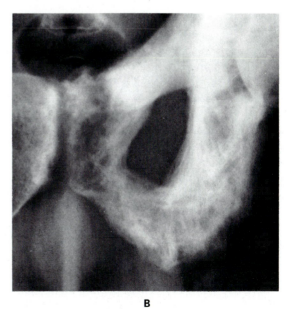

B

Fig. 5.33 Paget's sarcoma of the body of the pubis. **A**. No malignancy was seen in this man at initial presentation with polyostotic Paget's disease. **B**. 3 years later, however, he complained of local pain with the development of a purely lytic destructive lesion involving the body of the pubis.

monly affected, even allowing for the increased male incidence of Paget's disease. Histologically the tumours may be classified as osteosarcoma, fibrosarcoma and chondrosarcoma. However, the tumour is very aggressive and the outlook is very poor. Radiologically, in order of frequency, the lesion is lytic, mixed or sclerotic and the tumour grows rapidly with an extensive soft-tissue mass. The margins of the lesion within bone are usually ill-defined, frequently with extensive cortical destruction. Periosteal new bone formation is relatively uncommon.

BONE TUMOURS PRESUMED TO ARISE FROM SKELETAL TISSUE: CARTILAGE-FORMING

Benign cartilage lesions divide into two main groups, central and peripheral. The former includes chondroma (with which must be considered the generalized dysplasia of bone — dyschondroplasia), benign chondroblastoma and chondromyxoid fibroma. The malignant counterpart of chondroma is a central chondrosarcoma. There are no reports of the malignant transformation of chondroblastoma and chondromyxoid fibroma. The peripheral lesion to be considered is an osteochondroma, or cartilage-capped exostosis, which in its multiple form also constitutes a general bone dysplasia (diaphyseal aclasis). The cartilage cap of these lesions is a potential site for the development of chondrosarcoma. The majority of chondrosarcomas, however, arise with no evidence whatever of a pre-existing benign tumour.

CHONDROMA

Nearly all of these tumours are benign in their clinical presentation and in their radiological and histological appearances, yet all must be regarded as the site of potential malignancy. It is very unusual for the common chondromatous lesions which occur in the hands and feet to become malignant but every flat or long bone cartilage tumour should be regarded as a potential risk if the patient survives long enough. The development of increasing pain, the demonstration, on serial films, of alteration in the radiological appearances or the late development of a pathological fracture are in themselves sufficient to justify anxiety. The transition from benign to malignant in the histological spectrum may be very difficult and contentious. These tumours are notoriously insensitive to therapy. Local recurrence is very high unless there is meticulous surgical removal and cartilage tumours have the habit of becoming more aggressive with each subsequent episode of surgical or therapeutic interference. It must be emphasized that the exact time of change from benign to malignant is extremely hard to establish and it is possible that those which are frankly malignant have been so since their inception. Whilst most

cartilage tumours arise in conjunction with bone it is important to note that they may occur in soft tissues, particularly tendon sheaths and in relation to synovium. They may even occur intracerebrally, and when present at the base of the skull should be considered in the differential diagnosis of chordoma.

Single tumours are common. Approximately half are found in the hands, in the medullary cavity of the phalanges, less commonly in metacarpals. About 10% occur in the small bones of the feet. Long bones, particularly the femur, humerus and tibia, are involved in 20% of cases, the remainder occurring in flat bones, particularly the pelvis, scapula and vertebral bodies. It is in these areas that the potential danger of malignant transformation is greatest.

Clinical features. The age of onset is usually later than with bone-forming tumours. Since these lesions grow slowly, they are rarely symptomatic and are often uncovered through examinations for other indications, particularly trauma. However, on direct questioning the patient may admit to having noted a localized hard swelling for many years. Pathological fracture is not uncommon. To restate, low grade pain or swelling of recent onset should cause the possibility of chondrosarcoma to be considered.

Radiological features. Cartilaginous tissue is not radiopaque. The characteristic feature is of a single well-defined demarcated zone of radiolucency in the medulla. In the small bones of the hand and feet tumours are particularly likely to expand and thin the overlying cortex (Fig. 5.34), but without its destruction or the development of a periosteal reaction other than that following a fracture. The zone of transition is narrow and sclerotic. The endosteal margin may be scalloped. As in all neoplasms of cartilaginous origin, flecks of calcification are frequently present within the tumour, especially as they become more mature and may assume a pathognomonic 'popcorn' or annular configuration. Calcification also may be observed, together with ossification, in healing callus following a pathological fracture. Lesions rarely extend to the ends of the affected bones and are often situated in the distal portions. Very few other osteolytic lesions in the bones of the hands are likely to cause diagnostic difficulty, apart from the rare implantation dermoid cyst in a terminal phalanx or perhaps fibrous dysplasia. These cartilaginous tumours are unremarkable scintigraphically or angiographically and their low vascularity is readily demonstrated. The high water content may be demonstrated by MRI. This technique also does not distinguish between benign and malignant with certainty (Fig. 5.35). Unless they have fractures they are unlikely to be striking on the delayed phase of a bone scan. A marked increase of photon activity should raise the possibility of a chondrosarcoma.

Less commonly chondromas develop in the medullary

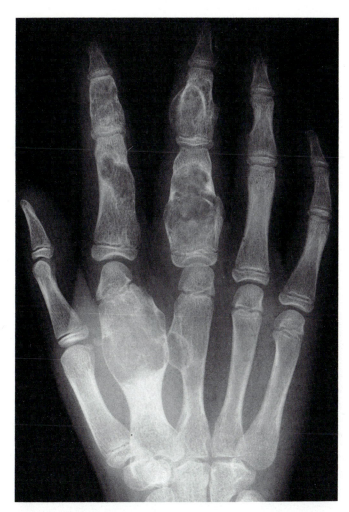

Fig. 5.34 Multiple chondromas in the hand. This child presented with painless swelling. Note the cortical expansion and thinning, well-defined defects, patchy amorphous calcification and moulding abnormalities indicating slow growth.

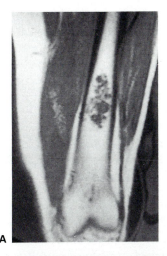

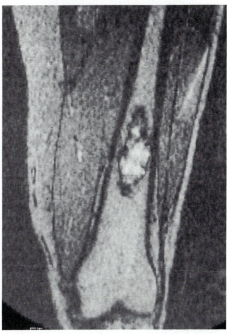

Fig. 5.35 Cartilage tumour. This patient presented with a long-standing ache in the thigh. Coronal T_1 (**A**) and STIR (**B**) sequences demonstrate a mixed lesion within the femoral shaft. Note that the cartilage has high signal on the STIR sequence. A surrounding rim of sclerosis is shown by deficient signal on both images. Histologically, this tumour was considered benign, in spite of giving rise to symptoms and to increased activity on a radionuclide scan and showing a high water content on MRI.

cavities of long bones and must be distinguished from other medullary osteolytic lesions. Here again the presence of calcification is a great help, but is not entirely specific. The tumour margin is usually sharply defined and accompanied by some evidence of sclerosis. The tumour erodes the cortex from within with a clear cut edge. The cortex, however, remains intact and the development of an enlarging lesion may cause eccentric expansion of bone due to organized periosteal new bone. Most of these tumours are discovered in adult life and therefore differentiation from other osteolytic lesions, such as bone cysts and non-ossifying fibromas, offers less difficulty because of the patient's age. Evidence of extension of the lesion or irregularity of the margin (particularly in the presence of periosteal new bone formation or a soft tissue mass) will immediately suggest a chondrosarcoma. Further investigation is unrewarding, although computerized tomography or MR may serve to delineate the extent of the intramedullary lesion.

It is necessary to distinguish the central variety of chondroma from unimportant areas of amorphous calcification arranged in a roughly linear fashion in the medullary canal, often described as 'cartilage rests'. The localized stippled nature of these opacities and the absence of any other radiological abnormality indicates the latter diagnosis. These lesions are scintigraphically inert. On the other hand, differentiation of a central chondroma from a medullary bone infarct may be more difficult. A helpful feature is the curvilinear peripheral calcification around the infarct rather than the annular calcification with a true cartilage tumour. Both lesions may be associated with subsequent malignant complications, dedifferentiated chondrosarcoma from chondroma (see below) and fibrosarcoma or malignant fibrous histiocytoma from the wall of an infarct.

Special types of chondroma

Juxtacortical chondroma is a rare benign cartilage tumour usually arising in young adults, related to the cortex of a long bone, most commonly the humerus or femur. The presenting complaint is of a slowly enlarging hard mass which may not be tender (Fig. 5.36). Radiologically a well-defined soft tissue mass may contain calcification and be bordered by a thin, but usually incomplete, shell of overlying bone. Pressure erosion of the underlying cortex usually provokes a variable sclerotic reaction. The presence of calcification within the lesion makes the diagnosis of a cartilage-containing tumour relatively easy. On the other hand, if calcification is absent the mass may have to be distinguished from non-ossifying fibroma, periosteal lipoma or neurofibroma.

Multiple enchondromas. The individual lesions of the bone dysplasia described by Ollier are now known as dyschondroplasia and are essentially neoplastic in type, corresponding to the descriptions already given. Cartilage tumours found in dysplasias may be extremely gross and cause complete destruction of the bones of the hand. In addition to the multiple cartilage tumours, columns of dysplastic cartilage frequently cause considerable tubulation anomalies and growth deformities of limbs. Although recognized in the literature to be subject to chondrosarcomatous change, this complication has been uncommon in the experience of the author.

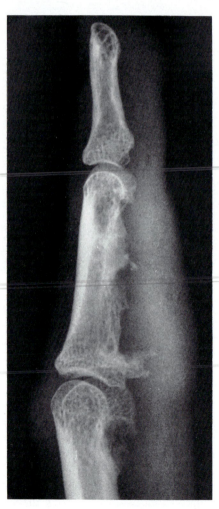

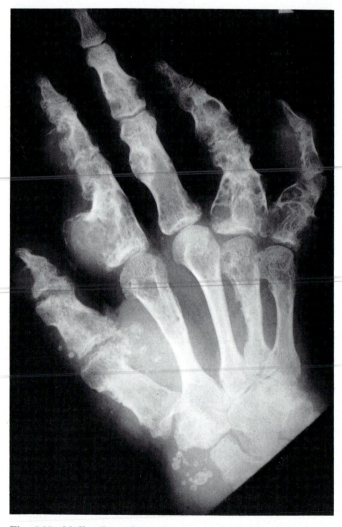

Fig. 5.36 Juxtacortical chondromas arising on the volar aspect of the proximal and middle phalanges of the index finger. Obvious pressure defects are present with new bone formation at the margins. Punctate calcification is present in the middle of the proximal lesion.

Fig. 5.37 Maffucci's syndrome (woman aged 23). Numerous chondromas in this case of dyschondroplasia are accompanied by soft-tissue swelling which contains phleboliths indicating haemangiomas. These skeletal lesions are more liable than ordinary chondromas to undergo malignant transformation.

Maffucci's syndrome is the rare association of dyschondroplasia with cavernous haemangiomas in the soft tissues, the latter being characterized by soft tissue masses containing phleboliths (Fig. 5.37). Chondrosarcomatous metaplasia is a recognized hazard of this entity and probably develops in about 20% of cases.

CHONDROBLASTOMA

This relatively rare tumour arises almost always in an epiphysis or apophysis, 50% occurring in the second decade of life. Presentation is of pain around the joint, usually of mild proportions and of months or even years duration. Joint movement often is limited. Most of these tumours occur in epiphyses of long bones, especially around the hips, knees or shoulders, but some have been observed in apophyses. Histologically the appearances are distinctive, cartilage cells being interspersed with foci of calcification and giant cells. This lesion has been considered as a giant-cell tumour variant.

Radiologically a well-defined, radiolucent, oval lesion within an epiphysis is characteristic, often with a thin rim of sclerosis and cortical expansion (Fig. 5.38). The endosteal margin is well defined. Not infrequently the tumour involves the metaphysis. Stippled calcification occurs in about a quarter of examples and in a smaller number an adjacent periosteal reaction may be present. The extreme vascularity of these lesions is confirmed by the blood-pool phase of the bone scan or by angiography. The delayed phase of a bone scan is not helpful. Computerized tomography or MR may be of value in assessing the extent of those few lesions which expand rapidly into the soft tissues. No incidence of spontaneous malignant transformation, however, has been recorded (Fig. 5.39).

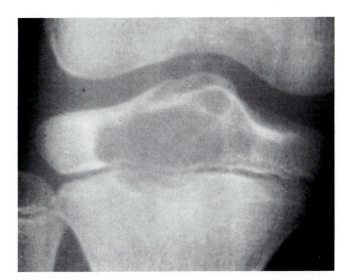

Fig. 5.38 Chondroblastoma in the proximal epiphysis of the tibia. The tumour has thinned the overlying cortex and extends across the growth plate into the upper metaphysis.

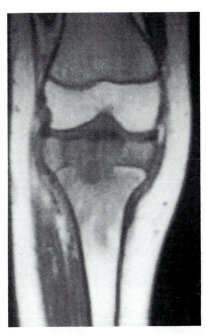

Fig. 5.39 Chondroblastoma. A chondroblastoma is demonstrated on a T$_1$-weighted coronal MR image rising in the upper tibial epiphysis and extending through the metaphysis. Note the extensive marrow oedema in the proximal tibia.

CHONDROMYXOID FIBROMA

This tumour is predominantly chondroid, but contains myxomatous tissue and giant cells. Histologically it may be mistaken for a chondrosarcoma. The presenting complaints are non-specific, usually localized pain and swelling, often of many months' duration. The peak age incidence is between 20 and 30, with no particular sex incidence. Typically the lesion occurs around the knee joint in two-thirds of cases, with an especial affinity for the proximal end of the tibia. Flat bones and short bones have been affected.

Radiologically the predominant feature is a radiolucent, eccentric, space-occupying lesion which is situated in the metaphysis. The margin within bone is usually well defined, with surrounding sclerosis (Fig. 5.40). The sharpness of the margin between the lesion and the sclerosis contrasts with the rather ill-defined margin between the sclerosis and host bone. In many cases the cortex is expanded considerably (Fig. 5.41), the peripheral bony margin often becoming hazy and poorly defined. This aggressive appearance may be so marked that the possibility of malignant change may be considered. Unlike other cartilaginous neoplasms, calcification within the lesion is very uncommon. Whilst scintigraphy in the blood-pool phase of a bone scan, or angiography, may reveal a slight increase in perfusion to the lesion, the vascular pattern is unremarkable. When the bone scan does show increased activity it is usually localized to the reactive sclerosis rather than to the lesion itself. CT may be necessary to

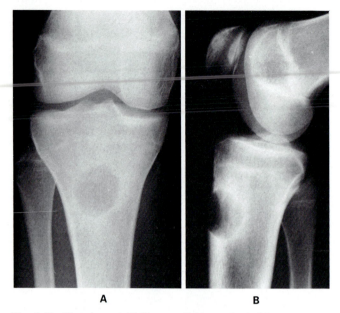

Fig. 5.40 Chondromyxoid fibroma of the proximal tibia. Note the extremely well-defined radiolucent defect with a sclerotic margin on the endosteal aspect. **A**. AP view. **B**. Lateral view.

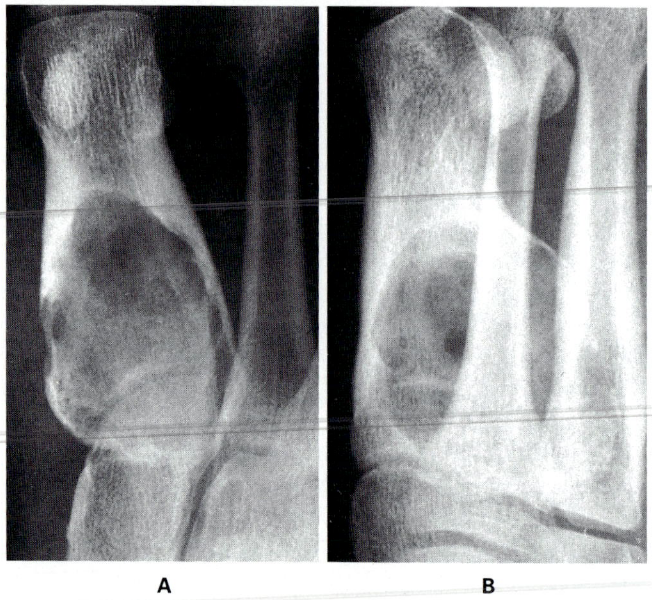

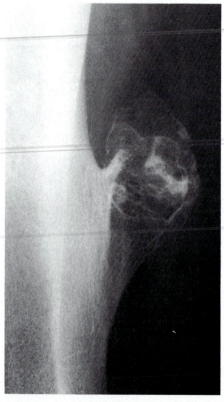

Fig. 5.41 **A,B** Chondromyxoid fibroma — great toe metatarsal. The tumour is eccentric in position with extreme cortical expansion and thinning. The endosteal margin is well defined and faintly sclerotic. No calcification is present.

delineate a cortical margin in the expanded soft tissue mass.

This tumour is undoubtedly very closely related to benign chondroblastoma and indeed aneurysmal bone cyst, since all three contain giant cells. Histological differentiation is reasonably well established, but unrepresentative biopsy material may create confusion. Radiologically,

confusion will only occur when these lesions occur in childhood, although the site of chondroblastoma and the ill-defined endosteal margin of an aneurysmal bone cyst will normally suggest the correct diagnosis.

OSTEOCHONDROMA (CARTILAGE-CAPPED EXOSTOSIS)

This lesion is essentially an osseous outgrowth arising from bony cortex. Usually it grows slowly during childhood and adolescence with endochondral ossification, the central spongiosa merging with that of the bone from which it is derived. Very occasionally the lesion involutes with increasing age and finally results only in a minor abnormality of tubulation. It is usual for growth to cease with skeletal maturity. Although commonly solitary the tumours may be multiple, when the condition is recognized as the deforming congenital bone dysplasia known as diaphyseal aclasia (Ch. 1). The importance of this relatively common benign tumour, and its place among bone tumours, relates to the cartilage cap with which it is covered. This structure may be very prominent and in this tissue lies the very small risk of malignancy in the form of chondrosarcoma. This risk is probably less than 1%,

Fig. 5.42 Osteochondroma of the distal femur. The cortex is continuous with that of the underlying bone and trabecular bone merges with that of the femur. A well-defined cartilage cap contains calcification and is directed away from the joint.

but may be significantly higher (of the order of 10%) in diaphyseal aclasia.

These tumours arise mainly in tubular bones near the metaphyses related to the sites of tendinous attachments. They are particularly common around the knee and the proximal end of the humerus. They may be either sessile or pedunculated. The latter type always grow away from the metaphysis, being directed towards the diaphysis. Flat bones also may be affected, the pelvis and scapula being equally involved. In the pelvis these lesions are almost invariably of the sessile type. Rare lesions related to the laminae of vertebral bodies may produce neurological signs.

Both types occur equally in the sexes and may be entirely asymptomatic, apart from their cosmetic effect. Presentation usually follows minor trauma. They may interfere with footwear comfort and can cause localized neural or vascular compression. Such symptoms are unlikely to develop until the later stages of growth, at or around puberty. Surgical removal should be undertaken if any increase in pain or size of the lesion occurs, particularly after growth has ceased. Features of this type may indicate chondrosarcomatous change in the cartilage cap.

Radiological features. Osteochondromas have a characteristic appearance. With a pedunculated tumour it is particularly easy to identify the continuation of its cortex with that of the underlying bone from which it arises and the merging of its trabecular pattern into the medullary cavity through the cortical defect (Fig. 5.42). In young adults the cartilage cap may not be visualized on plain films, although seen clearly on CT. As age progresses calcification becomes apparent within the cartilaginous element of the tumour, causing an increase in punctate or curvilinear radiodensity. Thus the developed lesion in the adult is likely to show irregular calcification. Growth of osteochondromas usually occurs until skeletal maturation is complete (Fig. 5.43), ceasing thereafter. Rarely osteochondromas may be shown to regress (Fig. 5.44). Pedunculated tumours vary in size, but may be up to 8 or 10 cm in length and are typically directed away from the nearest joint. Flat and sessile types are more commonly related to flat bones, particularly the pelvis, and may grow to a substantial size, be of considerable irregularity and become very dense. In such cases the resemblance to a cauliflower may be striking! Provided that the sharply defined peripheral margin is preserved, and serial examinations reveal no increase in size, their benign nature may be assumed. Any change in radiological appearance, particularly with the development of poor definition of the margin, even in one part of the lesion, is highly suggestive of chondrosarcoma, particu-

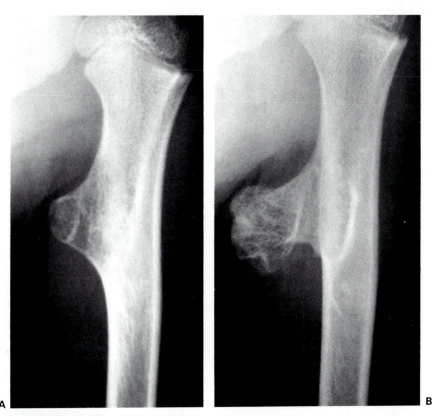

Fig. 5.43 A,B A pedunculated osteochondroma exhibits growth over a 2-year period in the humerus of a child. Such growth is common and stops usually at, or soon after, puberty.

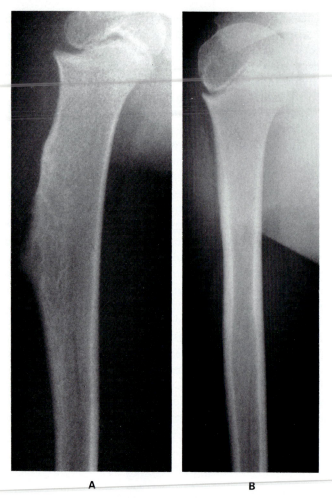

A   B

Fig. 5.44 A,B Osteochondromas may rarely be shown to regress, remodelling resulting in normal appearances. Here an osteochondroma of the proximal humerus cannot be visualized 6 years later.

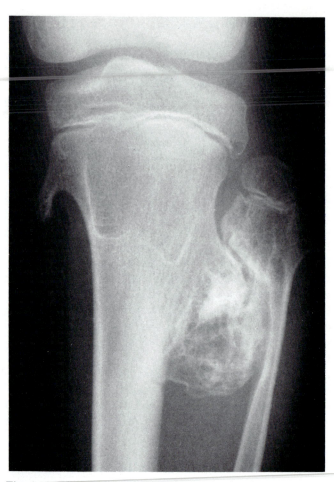

Fig. 5.45 Diaphyseal aclasia — multiple osteochondromas are present in the proximal tibia and fibula. A large sessile lesion of the proximal tibia has caused widening of the interosseous space and secondary moulding abnormalities of both the tibia and fibula.

larly if accompanied by a history of an insiduous increase in local pain. Local resection and histological studies then become essential because of the shortcomings of further radiological investigation in detecting chondrosarcoma (see below). The individual lesions of diaphyseal aclasia are those of any osteochondroma. However, their multiplicity results in considerable moulding abnormality and deformity (Fig. 5.45).

CHONDROSARCOMA

Differentiation of this malignant member of the group of cartilage-forming tumours is to be made from osteosarcoma with which it may be confused. Chondrosarcoma forms a spectrum of malignancy, but usually develops later in life than osteosarcoma and carries a much better prospect of survival because metastases often occur very late. A high-grade (aggressively malignant) chondrosar-

coma, however, behaves in a fashion very similar to an osteosarcoma.

The **clinical problem**, therefore, is not so much that of metastatic dissemination but of local recurrence. Failure to provide adequate and early excision is attended by the subsequent necessity of further and more difficult surgical procedures. Some evidence, indeed, exists that each surgical insult causes the tumour to become even more aggressive. Certain pleomorphic osteosarcomas demonstrate cartilage formation, but the established chondrosarcoma is associated with cartilage which is mature in its development. Although some of this cartilaginous tissue may ossify, no direct ossification (unlike an osteosarcoma) takes place in the absence of a chondroid precursor. In addition these cells are histochemically negative for the production of alkaline phosphatase.

Chondrosarcomas may develop in a cartilaginous lesion previously thought to be benign. Malignancy may arise in the cartilage cap of an osteochondroma or in a long or flat bone (Fig. 5.46). Chondrosarcoma of the hand or

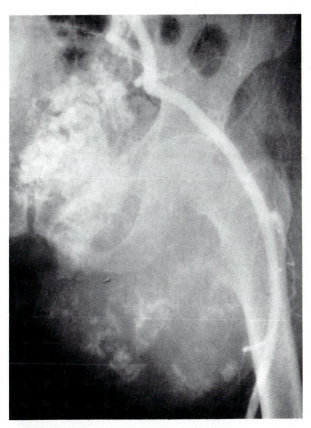

Fig. 5.46 Chondrosarcoma arising from the superior pubic ramus on the left. A huge mass is present containing extensive calcification. The femoral artery is displaced by the mass but note the absence of any pathological circulation. This is typical of a low-grade chondrosarcoma.

recurrence, it may be necessary to undertake amputation. The histological spectrum of chondrosarcoma varies widely. Difficulties with differentiation arise, at the benign end of the spectrum, from a benign chondroma, and at the aggressive end, from an osteosarcoma. In consequence, the interpretation by a highly skilled pathologist is essential. Particularly in case of less aggressive chondrosarcoma, situated in sites of easy access, such as the proximal end of the femur, prosthetic replacement is an effective and cosmetic surgical treatment.

Radiological features. When a chondrosarcoma arises from a previous cartilaginous lesion the diagnosis is usually straightforward. In the case of osteochondroma particular attention should be paid to areas of local cortical destruction with ill-defined margins. In addition, it may be possible to demonstrate an associated soft-tissue mass representing abnormal cartilage growth. These features are demonstrated more clearly by CT. The radiological demonstration of cartilage within such a mass by punctate or curvilinear calcification may be absent, as this characteristic feature tends to occur in the more mature parts of these tumours. Similarly the central

foot is distinctly unusual. The lesions of dyschondroplasia, particularly if associated with the haemangiomas of Maffucci's syndrome, are also subject to malignant change. Nonetheless the incidence of what might be called secondary chondrosarcoma is far less common than those apparently arising de novo. Indeed only 10% of these neoplasms arise from a recognizable precursor, usually the cartilage cap of an osteochondroma, especially in patients suffering from diaphyseal aclasia.

Primary chondrosarcoma occurs mainly between the ages of 30 and 70 years and is relatively rare distal to the elbow and knee joints, the pelvis and ribs being the most common sites, followed closely by the proximal end of the femur. Because of this distribution, virtually all chondromas arising in flat and long bones should be regarded as potentially malignant ab initio. Diagnosis may be delayed on account of slow growth or relatively mild symptomatology. The tumour, therefore, may be very large when it is first recognized.

Prognosis for chondrosarcoma is relatively good if complete surgical excision is possible before dissemination, metastases only occurring in the later stages by the haematogenous route. Because of the risks of local

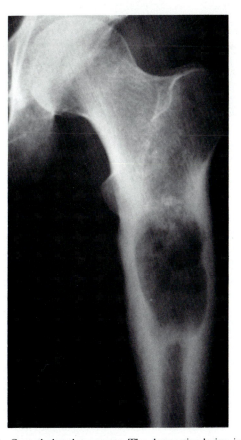

Fig. 5.47 Central chondrosarcoma. The destructive lesion in the femoral shaft has smooth well-defined margins, but in the upper portion, some characteristic punctate calcification is visible. The tumour is of a slow-growing type since organized periosteal new bone has thickened the cortex around the lesion.

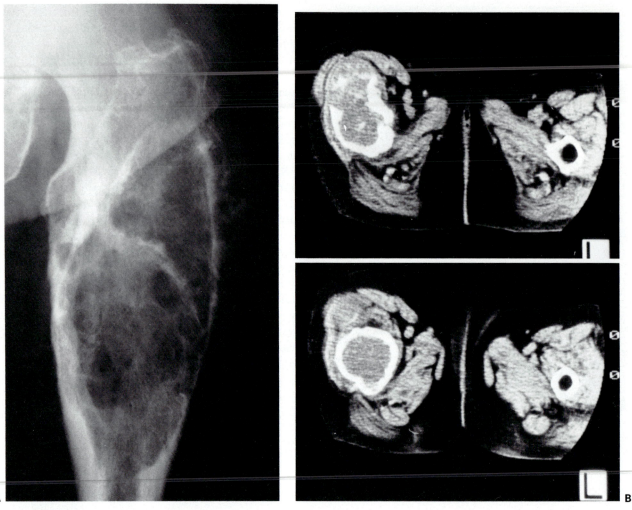

Fig. 5.48 A,B Central chondrosarcoma. **A.** The tumour is more aggressive than that in Figure 5.47, and has extended into soft tissues. This is confirmed by CT (**B**) showing extension anterior to the femoral shaft (W200, L25). Calcification is present both in the soft tissue mass and within the shaft lesion.

chondroma which becomes malignant tends clinically to grow silently, spreading within the medullary cavity to produce irregular medullary destruction. Uneven infiltration makes it difficult to determine the margin between normal and abnormal tissue. Irregular calcification is likely to be present in the older and central parts of the tumour. These more organized zones may be destroyed by newer malignant infiltration indicating the dedifferentiated form of chondrosarcoma.

As growth proceeds slowly, the tumour causes smooth, scalloped erosions on the endosteal aspect of the cortex. An overlying lamellar periosteal reaction is not rare, especially if the malignancy is low-grade. In consequence, the ultimate thickness of the cortex around the tumour may exceed that in the unaffected portion of the bone, the appearance then being that of a localized fusiform expansion (Fig. 5.47). Pathological fractures are quite common and may draw initial attention to these tumours.

The malignant nature of the lesion is unequivocal when actual penetration of the cortex occurs, with the development of an associated and clearly defined soft-tissue mass, within which calcification, or even ossification, may occur (Fig. 5.48).

Primary chondrosarcoma, particularly in its early stages, presents difficult diagnostic problems as the presenting symptoms of minor pain or discomfort may be accompanied by only minimal radiological change. This may be a poorly defined area of medullary translucency with possibly a little periosteal reaction or the presence of an abnormal soft-tissue mass. The acetabulum is sometimes the site of the development of these rather nebulous and difficult lesions (Figs 5.49, 5.50). The first radiological evidence of its presence may be a soft-tissue mass projecting into the pelvic cavity. The cortex of flat bones tends to be thinner than that of long bones and chondrosarcomas of the ribs or the pelvis penetrate it at an

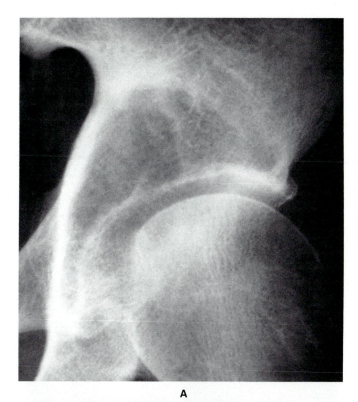

A

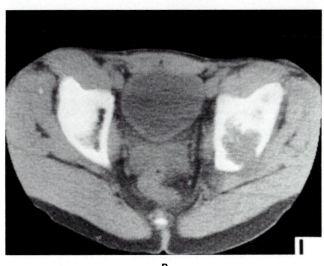

B

Fig. 5.49 Chondrosarcoma arising in the acetabulum of a 45-year-old man.
A. The tumour is purely lytic. Cortical thickening is shown medially.
B. CT demonstrates disruption of the cortex posteriorly, with a localized soft-tissue mass beneath the glutei and faint calcification within the lesion (W400, L20).

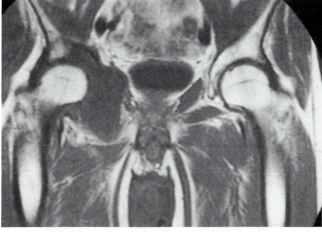

A

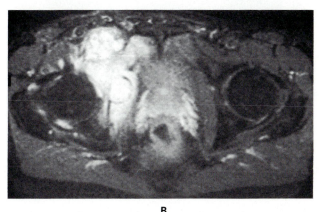

B

Fig. 5.50 Chondrosarcoma. A chondrosarcoma arising primarily in the region of the acetabulum. A coronal T_1-weighted (**A**) and axial STIR sequence (**B**) demonstrate a large lobulated mass occupying the floor of the acetabulum and extending through into the pelvis and the obturator foramen. Note the high signal on STIR, suggesting aggressive tumour, with also some increased signal surrounding the lesion due to oedema (secondary response). There is clear involvement of the hip joint.

As may be expected, the more mature cartilage elements frequently progress to calcification and ossification and larger tumours are frequently lobulated or cauliflower-like. Very rarely a chondrosarcoma may arise in soft tissues, including tendon sheath and meninges. Cranial lesions also can arise from the sphenoid (Fig. 5.51) and clivus.

Radiologically no criteria of malignancy are absolute. The demonstration of increase in size and ill-defined margins on plain film is highly suggestive. Destruction of organized existing cartilage calcification is indicative also of local infiltration. The demonstration of cortical disruption is helpful. Scintigraphically most of these neoplasms tend to have a slight increase in activity only on the delayed phase of a bone scan, but high-grade

early stage. This feature may be demonstrated more clearly by CT. Hence these tumours are especially liable to grow to a substantial size over a prolonged period, particularly if in a clinically occult area. Rapid growth naturally indicates a more aggressive type of malignancy.

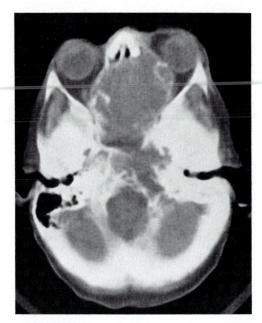

Fig. 5.51 Chondrosarcoma arising in the sphenoid bone of an adult woman. A large soft-tissue tumour extends from the nasal cavity to the middle fossa. A thin sclerotic margin outlines the mass, which contains faint punctate calcification. Note the displacement of the eyeballs (W400, L40).

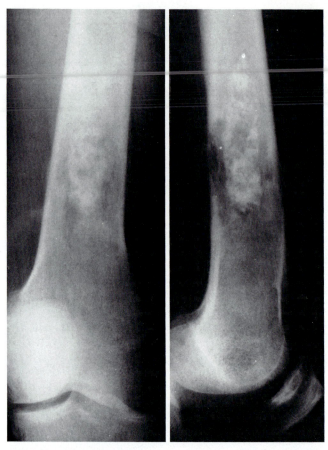

Fig. 5.52 Dedifferentiated chondrosarcoma. A chondrosarcoma is present centrally within the distal femoral shaft, characterized by slight expansion and amorphous calcification. In addition an area of osteolysis is present with cortical destruction around the lower half of the tumour. The latter represents a high-grade malignancy arising in conjunction with a pre-existing relatively low-grade tumour.

chondrosarcomas may demonstrate an increase in the blood-pool image. Angiographically, minor vascular displacement is usually evident, with scanty new vessels in the majority. Only when the tumour is of particularly high-grade malignancy is the type of increased perfusion and new vessel formation similar to that associated with an osteosarcoma. Whilst MRI may infer a cartilage tumour, by virtue of high water content, only a very bright T_2-weighted image of evidence of surrounding oedema will definitely suggest malignancy (Fig. 5.50). Reference has been made above to malignant cartilaginous tumours of relatively low grade malignancy undergoing relatively rapid deterioration. In such instances the radiological diagnosis may be suggested when an area of osteolytic destruction develops adjacent to the chondrosarcoma (Fig. 5.52) and which may, indeed, destroy part of the calcified portion of the original tumour. The age, sex and clinical features otherwise are comparable to those of an orthodox chondrosarcoma. These dedifferentiated forms may exhibit the microscopic appearance of a frank osteosarcoma, fibrosarcoma or, not uncommonly, malignant fibrous histiocytoma with its characteristic storiform pattern of the tumour cells (see below).

Mesenchymal chondrosarcoma

This malignant cartilage tumour is rare. Histologically it is characterized by the presence of more or less differentiated cartilage together with highly vascular spindle-cell or round-cell mesenchymal tissue. About a third of these tumours arise in the soft tissues, especially in the extremities (thigh and calf). The soft-tissue mass frequently shows irregular calcification (Fig. 5.53).

Fig. 5.53 Mesenchymal chondrosarcoma. A hard mass had been present in this middle-aged man's calf for 8 years. Recently it had increased in size. A soft-tissue radiograph (**A**) shows extensive calcification in a well-defined tumour mass. **B.** The blood-pool phase of a bone scan reveals a marked increase in vascularity throughout the lesion which is intensely active on (**C**) the delayed images (top right). Note also the presence of multiple metastases, particularly in vertebrae and the pelvis. **D.** A femoral arteriogram confirms the markedly abnormal vascularity with pathological vessels throughout the tumour mass. The similarity between the extent of the abnormality shown angiographically and on the blood pool phase of the bone scan is striking.

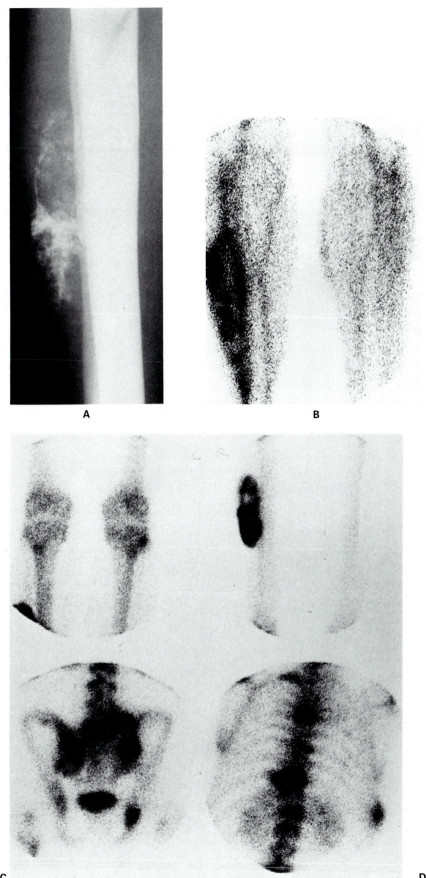

A

B

C

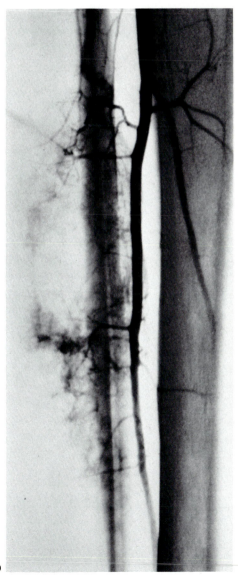

D

Radiologically this lesion shows a rapid increase in size with highly aggressive features and the early detection of metastases. The condition affects adults at an earlier age than most chondrosarcomas although in general the age group is older than that of osteosarcoma.

REFERENCES AND SUGGESTIONS FOR FURTHER READING

See end of Chapter 7.

CHAPTER 6

TUMOURS AND TUMOUR-LIKE CONDITIONS OF BONE (2)

Iain Watt

BONE TUMOURS PRESUMED TO ARISE FROM SKELETAL TISSUE — FIBROUS TUMOURS

1. FIBROUS CORTICAL DEFECT

Fibrous cortical defects are extremely common, occurring in up to a third of normal children between the ages of 2 and 15 years. Characteristically they occur around the knee, especially in the distal posteromedial femoral cortex. They are almost always discovered by chance and are not known to be symptomatic.

Radiologically they are blister-like expansions of the cortex with a thin shell of overlying bone (Fig. 6.1). They may be slightly lobulated, but are always sharply defined

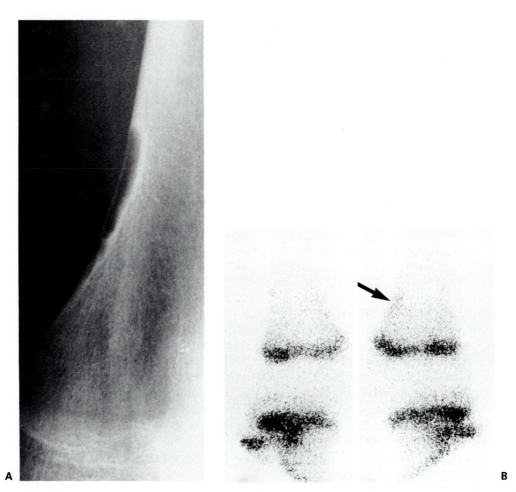

Fig. 6.1 Fibrous cortical defect arising in posteromedial aspect of the distal medial femur. **A.** The abnormality is confined to the cortex with very fine shell of overlying bone and a sharply defined endosteal margin. **B.** A bone scan demonstrates a slight increase in activity (arrow) at the site of the lesion.

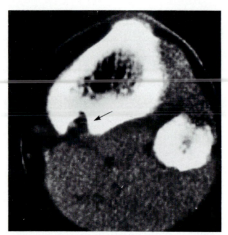

Fig. 6.2 Fibrous cortical defect in the upper medial tibia is shown on CT. Note the purely cortical position of the defect and its sharply defined margin. The thin shell of overlying bone is not seen completely because of the partial volume effect.

(Fig. 6.2) and have a fine sclerotic margin, particularly when seen in profile. Because of their characteristic site they are radiolucent when observed in a frontal view of the knee. An oblique projection will always show its cortical situation and these lesions fill in as the skeleton matures. Bone scans are unremarkable, revealing only a minimal increase in activity on the delayed phase in proportion to the size of the lesion.

The differential diagnosis, when the lesion occurs in its typical site, is from adductor trauma (cortical avulsion syndrome). This abnormality is attributed to chronic low-grade traction on the adductor tubercle, corresponding to the insertion of the adductor magnus muscle. It causes irregularity of the femoral cortex, sometimes with a radio-lucency, but often with irregular calcification. Because these lesions are almost certainly of traumatic origin, an abnormal increase in activity is evident on a bone scan and a slight increase in vascularity on an angiogram. The typical site and lack of endosteal abnormality should prevent the misdiagnosis of a sarcoma.

2. NON-OSSIFYING FIBROMA

The lesion is similar to a fibrous cortical defect except that it is much larger and characteristically occurs in a slightly older age group, between 10 and 20 years. The vast majority occur around the knee joint, the distal end of the femur being the most common site. The lesion occasionally presents with a pathological fracture (Fig. 6.3). Usually it is not symptomatic.

The radiological findings reveal an area of increased radiolucency which is sharply defined in the metadiaphysis, the margins are smooth and sharp, with a rather lobulated appearance, and are defined by a thin zone of reactive sclerosis. In larger bones such as the tibia and fibula the lesion may be eccentric and appropriate oblique

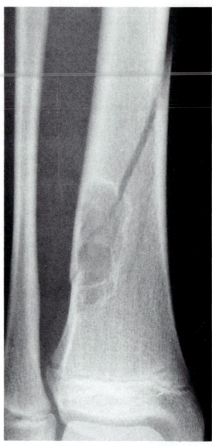

Fig. 6.3 Non-ossifying fibroma of the distal tibia presenting with a fracture. The well-defined outline and eccentric position of the tumour are demonstrated together with sharply defined sclerotic margins.

views will show its relationship to one of the cortices. However, in more slender bones, such as the fibula, the whole width of the bone may be involved. On the outer margin the cortex is usually slightly expanded but remains intact and thinned. Scintigraphically only a minimal increase in activity can be detected on the delayed phase scan, the degree of increased activity solely reflecting the size of the lesion, unless there has been a pathological fracture. As in fibrous cortical defect, the natural history is for the lesion to regress, initially by an increase in the surrounding zone of sclerosis and latterly by replacement with normal bone.

The differential diagnosis, particularly when the whole width of the bone is involved, is from a solitary bone cyst or monostotic fibrous dysplasia. Differentiation from the former may be very difficult on all radiological grounds whereas distinction from monostotic fibrous dysplasia is relatively straightforward, due to the avidity of the latter for bone-seeking radiopharmaceuticals.

3. DESMOPLASTIC FIBROMA

This rare tumour exhibits dense fibrous tissue, simulating

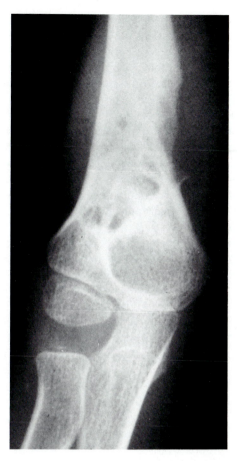

Fig. 6.4 Desmoplastic fibroma. A destructive, lobulated lesion is present in the distal metadiaphysis of the humerus. Bone expansion is present with sclerotic margins around the tumour. A soft-issue component has caused consolidated periosteal new bone formation.

4. FIBROSARCOMA

Although this is the least common of the malignant primary tumours arising in skeletal connective tissue, representing about 5% of all, individual lesions vary widely in their appearances and to this extent can create diagnostic difficulties. This variation corresponds to a wide range of histological characteristics, but the degree of malignancy and the radiological features correlate reasonably well. Many of the characteristics lie between those of osteosarcoma and chondrosarcoma.

Presentation is usually due to low-grade pain, sometimes swelling, usually present for less than a year. In many the precipitating factor may be a pathological fracture (Fig. 6.5). Whilst a few of these tumours arise primarily in soft tissue and cause secondary bony changes, the majority develop primarily in bone and may be either medullary or periosteal in location. A medullary lesion is considerably more common and usually arises in the metaphyseal area. Approximately 80% occur around the knee. It is less usual for a flat bone to be involved. The rarer periosteal type has a more widespread distribution, but still has a predilection for long bones, where any portion of the shaft may be affected. This type tends to develop a clinically palpable mass in the earlier stages.

desmoid tumours of the abdominal wall. Relatively few occur in bone and then usually in young adults. Pain is a constant presenting feature. The lesion is often tender. The majority arise in the metadiaphysis of long bones (Fig. 6.4), although the pelvis and spine are other sites of predilection.

Radiologically they tend to be large, solitary and destructive, with an expanded and irregular sclerotic margin. There may be a slight increase in density within the lesion, so that superficially it may resemble monostotic fibrous dysplasia. Slight irregularity of the margin may suggest an aneurysmal bone cyst when the lesion is purely osteolytic.

Multiple fibromatous tumours are present in **congenital generalized fibromatosis**, in which half the patients have associated bony abnormalities. This rare childhood condition demonstrates multiple, rounded, corticated, cystic metaphyseal lesions, often with sharply defined sclerotic margins. These fibromatous foci tend to regress with increasing age and have an excellent prognosis. However, some patients have associated involvement of skin, muscle, heart and lungs; the outlook in this group is poor.

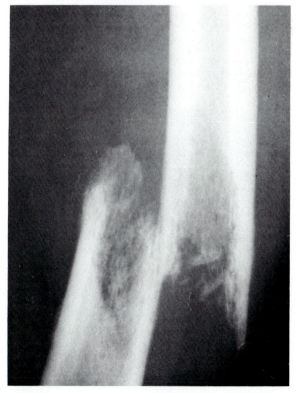

Fig. 6.5 Fibrosarcoma — presenting with pathological fracture of the femur in a woman of 50. Ill-defined bone destruction, particularly of the medulla, is associated with very minor periosteal new bone formation and no sclerosis. The cortex has been thinned on the endosteal surface.

Radiological features. The tumour is essentially osteolytic, provokes little new bone formation and usually lacks calcification or ossification. The medullary variety is characterized usually by an irregular area of radiolucency. The zone of transition may vary from being relatively narrow, indicating a well-differentiated tumour, to being diffuse and permeative, suggesting a highly aggressive tumour (Fig. 6.6). With very low grade tumours a minimal degree of sclerosis may surround the radiolucency. Slowly growing tumours may thin and expand the cortex, but with a diffuse infiltrative pattern it is more usual for actual destruction to occur. The subsequent soft tissue extensions are without calcification or ossification

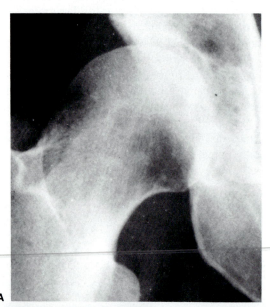

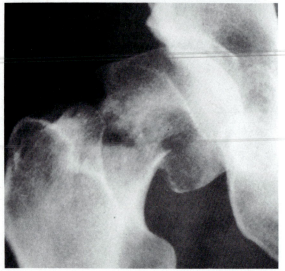

Fig. 6.6 Fibrosarcoma arising in the medulla of the femoral head and neck. This 35-year-old man presented with poorly localized pain in the hip. **A**. At presentation an ill-defined area of bone destruction on the medial aspect of the femoral head and neck. The cortex is preserved with no new bone formation; **B**. 3 months later a pathological fracture has occurred through the destructive lesion.

and periosteal new bone formation is unremarkable. This feature may differentiate the tumour from osteosarcoma or chondrosarcoma. The periosteum, on the other hand, frequently does exhibit shaggy ill-defined periosteal new bone arising from the underlying cortex. Destruction of the outer side of the cortex frequently takes place, but the erosion is usually clearly defined, almost as though a piece of bone has been removed surgically. In this respect considerable variance is shown from the poor definition of the edge of most malignant tumours. Consequently the impression may be gained of a benign periosteally related tumour, such as a lipoma. Secondary involvement of bone may result also from a fibrosarcoma arising in soft tissue.

As with the plain film appearances, angiography roughly mirrors the degree of malignancy of the tumour. Arteriography remains necessary, where MRI is not available, to assess soft-tissue lesions in order to delineate, with CT, not only the extent of the tumour but also evidence of major vessel involvement. The success of a bone scan is variable, as it depends on the degree of bone response and the amount of periosteal new bone formation. Metastatic dissemination from fibrosarcoma is not usually detectable with a bone-seeking agent.

Fibrosarcoma may also arise in the fibrous wall of a medullary infarct and is one of the histological patterns associated with Paget's sarcoma. To differentiate fibrosarcoma of bone from other malignancies is by no means straightforward. The major differential is from osteosarcoma and chondrosarcoma. Moreover, the more aggressive, ill-defined varieties may be indistinguishable from malignant round-cell tumours, particularly non-Hodgkin's lymphoma.

5. MALIGNANT FIBROUS HISTIOCYTOMA

A group of tumours have been separated, mainly from fibrosarcomas, on the basis of histological and clinical findings. These aggressive, often metastasizing, tumours are probably of histiocytic origin. They occur in an older population, usually around 55 years of age, affected individuals complaining chiefly of pain, swelling or of a slowly enlarging mass. The majority develop in soft tissues. The relatively small number arising in bone have a predilection for the femur and the ends of the tibia and humerus. Others arise in the pelvis and ribs.

The radiological features are primarily those of an ill-defined, purely osteolytic lesion with early cortical destruction, frequently in a permeative fashion, often with some expansion. To this extent they resemble fibrosarcomas of an aggressive type. Occasionally punctate, soft-tissue calcification is present and a small proportion exhibit periosteal reaction and endosteal sclerosis (Fig. 6.7). A soft-tissue mass often develops early. Angiographically, areas of avascularity and hypervascular-

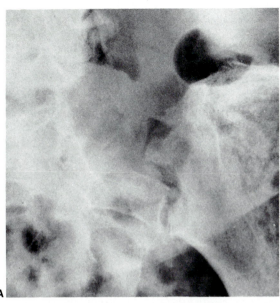
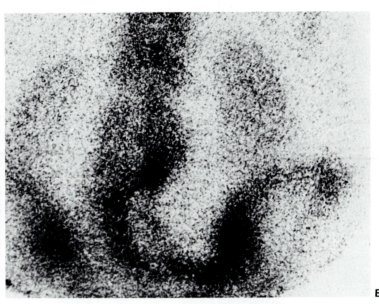

Fig. 6.7 Malignant fibrous histiocytoma arising in the sacral ala of a 60-year-old woman. **A**. A purely destructive, lytic lesion is present with slight sclerosis around its margins. Note that the lower border of L5 has also been destroyed together with part of the iliac wing. **B**. A radionuclide bone scan shows the tumour to be photon-deficient but a rim of increased activity corresponds to reactive bone sclerosis.

ity are typical, including the demonstration of new vessels and encasement. Scintigraphy is not typically informative. Many cases present with multiple skeletal lesions and the initial impression is the likelihood of skeletal metastases rather than of a primary or multifocal bone tumour. As with fibrosarcoma, malignant round-cell tumours require consideration in differential diagnosis.

6. ADAMANTINOMA OF LONG BONE

This rather unusual neoplasm is almost invariably located in the tibial shaft. **Clinically**, localized pain and swelling have usually been present for several years. The age range varies from 15 to 55 years. On examination a soft-tissue, possibly cystic, swelling is palpated. Histologically, difficulty may arise in differentiating this lesion from metastatic adenocarcinoma or squamous-cell carcinoma, since the glandular and fibrous component of the tumour may suggest an epithelial derivation.

Radiologically an eccentric area of destruction usually involves the anterior portion of the tibial shaft. Slight expansion and cortical thinning, with a cystic or multiloculated appearance, are usual (Fig. 6.8). Periosteal reaction is not marked, but cortical destruction may be extensive. The margin of the tumour varies from being sharply and clearly defined, with a slight sclerotic margin, to a hazy zone of transition several millimetres in width, comparable to that observed in giant-cell tumours. Some of these tumours may be 15 cm long or more, with satellite lesions.

Adamantinoma probably has a relationship to ossifying fibroma, which may be itself a localized form of fibrous dysplasia, in which it has been observed to develop as a

late complication. Whilst the radiological appearances of adamantinoma are not pathognomonic, the location and the clinical history suggest the diagnosis. The tumour continues to grow at a slow rate, but is characterized by local recurrence and eventual metastasis to lung. Extensive local resection is the usual form of treatment.

BONE TUMOURS PRESUMED TO ARISE FROM SKELETAL TISSUE: GIANT-CELL-CONTAINING

A group of tumours rich in giant cells, formerly confused in the literature, has now subdivided, on histological and radiological grounds, into giant-cell tumour ('osteoclastoma') and the giant-cell tumour variants. The latter include chondroblastoma (Ch. 5), chondromyxoid fibroma (Ch. 5) and aneurysmal bone cyst (see below). However, all these variants exhibit some areas which are histologically identical. In consequence, whilst broadly clear-cut radiological and histological categorization is possible, a definite overlap exists. The 'brown' tumours of hyperparathyroidism have also been included in this category.

1. GIANT-CELL TUMOUR (OSTEOCLASTOMA)

These tumours conform to a fairly constant clinical and radiological pattern. As with many other tumours, the initial presentation is of localized pain and swelling, some presenting following trauma or as an incidental finding. Histologically, richly vascular tissue contains plump spindle cells and numerous giant cells containing 50 to 100 nuclei. The tumour forms neither bone nor cartilage.

The majority of patients present between the ages of 20 and 40 years. Only about 3% of cases develop in immature skeletons, distinguishing these patients from those with aneurysmal bone cysts, in whom the tumour maximally occurs prior to epiphyseal fusion. Giant-cell tumours are multifocal in about 0.5% of cases, often in the hands. The solitary lesion shows a predilection for bones adjacent to the knee joint and the distal end of the radius. Histological review of a number of cases in which spinal lesions have been detected has indicated that the correct diagnosis is much more commonly an aneurysmal bone cyst. Facial bones appear to be exempt.

Radiological features. A zone of radiolucency is typically situated immediately beneath the articular cortex, sited eccentrically at the end of a long bone (Fig. 6.9). The exception to this rule is when the lesion arises in a former apophysis, notably the greater trochanter. Unless complicated by a fracture, the lesion does not contain calcification or ossification, although in about 40% of cases it is characterized by a 'soap-bubble' pattern of trabeculation. The margins are purely osteolytic; a sclerotic margin is rarely evident. Characteristically, therefore, the margin is hazy and ill-defined with no bone reaction (Fig. 6.10). More aggressive lesions are associated with widening of the zone of transition. The overlying cortex may be expanded and exquisitely thinned, usually without

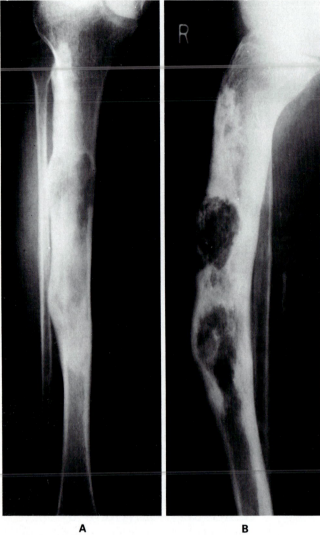

A   **B**

Fig. 6.8 Adamantinoma of the tibia. Eccentric areas of bone destruction are present anteriorly with thinning of the cortex. The cortex is expanded. In addition to this abnormality, sclerosis and ill-defined cortical thickening are present throughout the whole of the tibia, which is also bowed. These features are due to associated fibrous dysplasia (or a close variety sometimes known as ossifying fibroma which occurs only at this site). **A**. AP view. **B**. Lateral view.

It is locally aggressive and likely in more than half of instances to recur in spite of extensive curettage or excision with or without radiotherapy.

A small proportion are malignant. Malignancy may be mistaken in those which are initially extremely aggressive and others that become so following surgical or therapeutic intervention. Sometimes confusion arises because the extreme aggressiveness of the tumour, histologically and radiologically, does not correlate with the subsequent development of actual distant metastases to lung. A small group of undoubtedly malignant, metastatic giant-cell tumours has been recognized, often with a dominant fibrosarcomatous stroma. Attempts at histological and radiological grading have had only limited prognostic value.

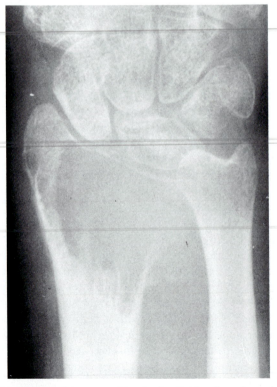

Fig. 6.9 Giant-cell tumour arising in the distal radius of an adult man. A characteristic, eccentric, immediately subarticular position makes this diagnosis very probable. The margins are ill-defined with no sclerotic reaction.

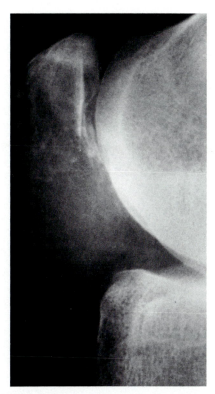

Fig. 6.10 Giant-cell tumour of the patella. Giant-cell tumours can arise in almost any bone but those around the knee are particularly affected. Note the immediately subarticular, eccentric position of the tumour which is purely osteolytic with no sclerotic reaction. The epiphyses have fused.

the development of periosteal new bone formation, except as a response to a pathological fracture. The tumour may produce a well-defined extension into the adjacent soft tissues, without evidence of calcification or new bone formation. The presence of such a soft tissue mass does not, of necessity, indicate a sarcoma. This complication is inferred by a rapid change in size or character of the tumour on sequential radiographs.

Angiographically, and on the blood-pool phase of a bone scan, vascularity is markedly increased, typically with an increased number of vessels, arteriovenous shunting and tumour staining. Many exhibit encasement. These features do not correlate with either clinical aggressiveness or sarcomatous change and may be extremely difficult to distinguish from those observed in other giant-cell-containing tumours, particularly aneurysmal bone cysts. The delayed phase of a bone scan is usually normal. CT or MRI (Fig. 6.11) may be necessary to delineate fully the soft tissue extent of the tumour.

Many of the rather more aggressive giant-cell-containing tumours in the younger age group may in fact be giant-cell-rich osteosarcomas (Fig. 6.12). It is possible that some of the reported metastasizing malignant giant cell tumours may be of this type. Usually, however, little difficulty arises in differential diagnosis, the eccentric, purely lytic and subarticular location of the tumour being characteristic. Differential diagnosis includes aneurysmal bone cysts and chondroblastoma. The 'brown' tumours

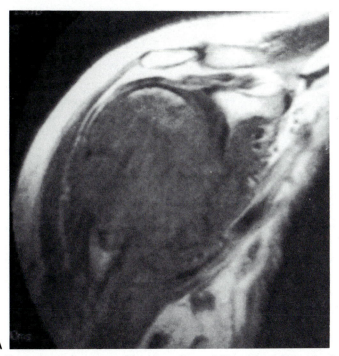

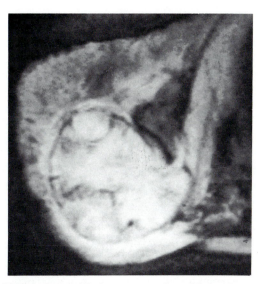

A   **B**

Fig. 6.11 A giant cell tumour of humerus. Coronal T₁-weighted (**A**) and axial STIR sequence (**B**) demonstrate a large lobulated mass in the humeral head and neck replacing all normal bone structures. Note the close approximation both to the articular surface and the displaced axillary vessels.

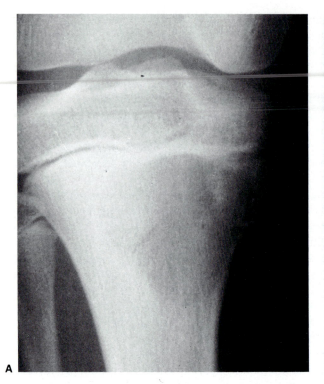

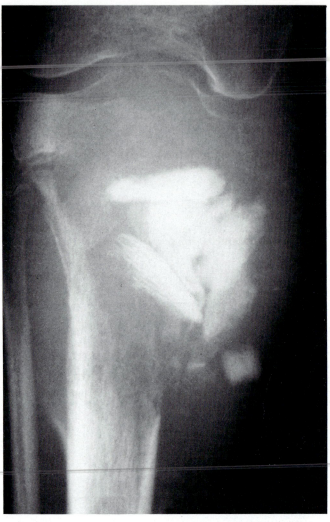

Fig. 6.12 Giant-cell-rich osteosarcoma **A**. A radiograph of this boy at presentation demonstrates an eccentric, purely osteolytic lesion in the upper tibial metaphysis. The cortex has been breeched but there is no periosteal new bone and only very faint surrounding sclerosis. **B**. 6 months later, following curettage and packing with bone chips, the flagrantly aggressive nature of this tumour is obvious. Note now the Codman's triangle on the lateral aspect of the tibial shaft and a substantial soft-tissue mass that contains ossification.

of hyperparathyroidism and monostotic fibrous dysplasia require consideration.

In spite of apparently successful curettage and packing with bone chips, these tumours have a tendency to recur, even years after initial treatment, and plain film follow-up is necessary. Secondary sarcomatous change may also occur following radiotherapy after intervals of several years. Treated tumours may be difficult to judge radiologically because of regression in the form of sclerosis on the one hand and continued evolution on the other. Total excision is the preferable means of therapy. On rare occasions the tumour may cross a joint or extend from one bone to another.

2. ANEURYSMAL BONE CYST

The exact aetiology of this tumour is unknown, but the descriptive name is derived from the macroscopic appearances of a blood-filled, expansile, sponge-like tumour containing numerous giant cells. Aneurysmal bone cyst

has been shown to arise in association with other abnormalities of the skeleton, particularly non-ossifying fibroma, fibrous dysplasia and chondromyxoid fibroma. Such lesions have been described as 'secondary' aneurysmal bone cysts. They have also been recorded following a fracture.

These tumours present in childhood or early adolescent life, with a predilection for the long bones and the lumbar spine. Those arising in the spine occur slightly later, between 10 and 20 years of age. The neural arch is more commonly involved than the body, half of these cases involving more than one vertebra. The prognosis is entirely benign apart from secondary neurological lesions due to spinal canal compression.

Radiological features. Typically an area of bone resorption occurs with slight or marked expansion (Fig. 6.13), the size of the lesion varying between 2 and in gross examples as much as 20 cm in diameter. The overlying cortex is thinned and may be expanded (Fig. 6.14) to such a degree that in places it can be identified only

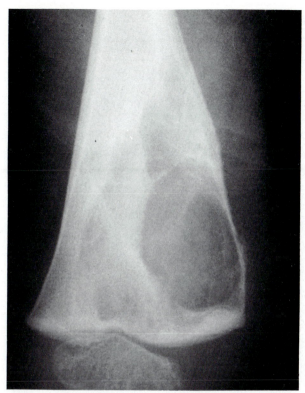

Fig. 6.13 Aneurysmal bone cyst (boy aged two). This film was taken because of an asymptomatic swelling and shows the characteristic features of metaphyseal involvement, cortical expansion and thinning, with a relatively well-defined endosteal margin.

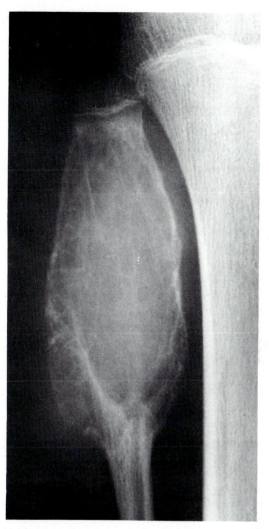

Fig. 6.14 Aneurysmal bone cyst of the proximal fibula. Considerably greater expansion has occurred in this example. The cortex is now very thin though apparently intact. The zone of transition between the lesion and adjacent bone is narrow but ill-defined. Note apparent multiple septa with the lesion.

by tomography or CT. The endosteal margin is relatively well-defined against cortex, and an ill-defined zone of transition is usual between the lesion and medullary bone, occasionally with slight sclerosis. A margin of this type is similar to that observed in giant cell tumour. Sometimes it is scalloped or irregular. Angiographically many features are common to giant cell tumour, in particular a rich increase in vessels with diffuse opacification and early venous filling. This appearance may be shown in the blood pool phase of a bone scan. Both CT and MRI may show fluid levels in the vascular spaces.

Most lesions evolve slowly. However a few show a highly aggressive radiological pattern and may increase alarmingly in size, even doubling in a few weeks. The possibility of a very malignant vascular tumour such as an angiosarcoma may then be entertained.

Differentiation from giant-cell tumour is aided by the age of the patient, as three-quarters of aneurysmal bone cysts occur before epiphyseal fusion has occurred, and their widespread anatomical distribution contrasts with the majority of giant-cell tumours occurring around the knee and wrist. Therefore difficulty is likely to arise only when the abnormality occurs after epiphyseal closure or

when it is situated at the end of a long bone. Aneurysmal bone cyst rarely extends to the articular surface and is often central, compared to the subarticular eccentric nature of giant-cell tumour. The spinal lesions need to be differentiated from osteoblastoma and osteoid osteoma. The bone-forming nature of these latter two tumours, together with their associated sclerotic reactions, provides valuable differential diagnostic signs.

Aneurysmal bone cysts are treated by curettage or radiotherapy, the latter being particularly valuable in spinal lesions where surgery may be considered hazardous. An increasing role, however, has developed for transcatheter embolization in the management of these tumours. Aneurysmal bone cyst is a particularly good example of the importance of radiological investigation being complete before biopsy is undertaken, since these lesions, not surprisingly, bleed considerably and the pre-operative demonstration of the vascular nature of this tumour may save some embarrassment!

TUMOURS PRESUMED TO ARISE FROM OTHER TISSUES IN BONE: BLOOD VESSELS

1. HAEMANGIOMA

Intraosseous haemangiomas are benign and slow-growing. Malignancy is virtually unknown. Many of these benign vascular neoplasms are asymptomatic, their presence being detected incidentally.

They are not infrequently shown on MR studies of the spine, particularly lumbar (Fig. 6.15). The autopsy incidence is about 10%. A few cause swelling and mild pain. Occasionally, significant neurological deficits may occur secondary to the collapse of an involved vertebral body with or without an extraosseous soft-tissue tumour component. The age of presentation is between 10 and 45 years.

Haemangiomas are either cavernous, with large thin-walled vessels occurring particularly in vertebrae and the skull, or capillary, tending to spread in a sun-burst pattern. Typically the tumour is solitary, the commonest site being a thoracic or lumbar vertebral body.

Radiologically, plain films show increased translucency with a characteristic fine vertical striation (Fig. 6.16). Half the lesions involve purely the vertebral body, the other half extending into the posterior elements. A small proportion have an associated soft-tissue mass. The overall size of the vertebral body is often within nor-

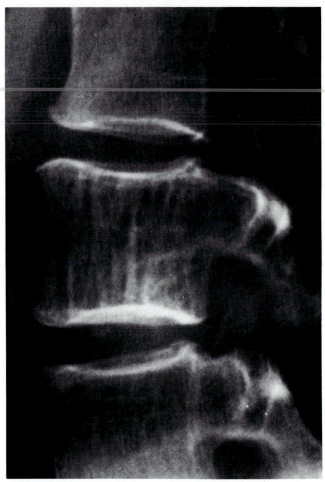

Fig. 6.16 Haemangioma of the vertebral body of L3. The whole body is marked by the characteristic vertical striation, which in this example does not extend into the pedicles.

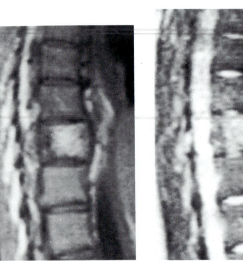
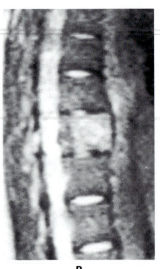
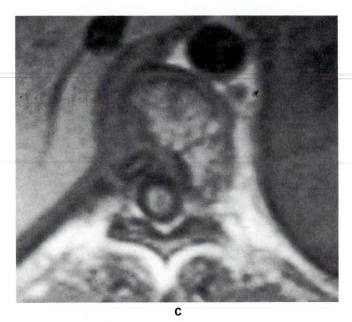

Fig. 6.15 Sagittal T$_1$-weighted (**A**), T$_2$ MAST (**B**) and T$_1$-weighted axial images (**C**) demonstrate a high signal abnormality occupying most of a mid-thoracic vertebral body extending back into the posterior elements on the left. High signal lesions both on T$_1$ and T$_2$ are usually benign in the spine. This particular case subsequendy required surgery because of compression fracture. Note expansion of the vertebral body which is relatively unusual in benign haemangioma.

mal limits, a helpful differential feature from Paget's disease.

The remainder of the skeleton is affected in approximately half of cases, the skull and long bones being sites of predilection. Although these tumours may present a striated appearance in long bones and ribs, as in the vertebral lesions, the radiological changes in these other areas are usually very different, tending to be osteolytic with sclerotic margins and often causing some cortical expansion. The osteolytic component has a soap-bubble appearance within which a sun-burst or stippled radiodensity may be evident, possibly extending into the soft tissues with radiating spicules of bone. This pattern may be encountered with a capillary haemangioma, particularly in the skull and pelvis (Fig. 6.17). In some cases localized cortical thickening, from which peripheral bone spicules may extend, simulates an osteosarcoma. However, closer scrutiny and appropriate further investigation resolves any difficulty.

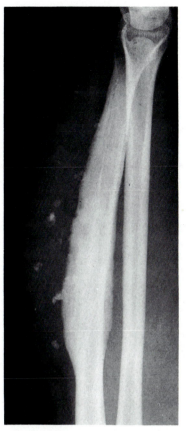

Fig. 6.18 Cavernous haemangioma of the soft tissues of the forearm is diagnosed by the presence of soft-tissue swelling within which there are phleboliths. The presence of extensive consolidated periosteal new bone and bowing of the ulna suggest an intimate relationship with the periosteum.

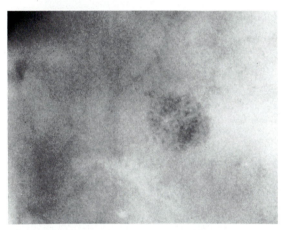

Fig. 6.17 Haemangioma of the skull is shown on a localized view of the temporal fossa. Note the purely osteolytic lesion with stippled radiodensities.

Soft-tissue cavernous haemangiomas may be recognized by well-defined circular calcifications due to phleboliths (Fig. 6.18). This is one component of Maffucci's syndrome, the other being multiple chondromas (see Fig. 5.34).

Scintigraphically, the bone lesion shows increased activity on the delayed phase of a bone scan (Fig. 6.19). Both bone and soft-tissue lesions may be detected by a blood-pool scan (Fig. 6.20). The appearance of increased activity in a vertebral tumour cannot therefore be used to distinguish between Paget's disease, a sclerotic metastasis or a haemangioma. On occasions the soft-tissue mass arising from a vertebral lesion may require delineation with spinal angiography if surgical resection is considered. It may be important to demonstrate the artery of Adamkiewicz in order that surgical excision or transcatheter embolization does not result in paraplegia. Some

lesions respond well to radiotherapy, particularly those in vertebrae.

2. VANISHING BONE DISEASE
(*Gorham's disease*)

This relatively rare syndrome is a variant of *angiomatosis* of bone in which vascular proliferation predominates. Its origin is unknown. It is recognized usually in childhood, but more than one third of patients are over the age of 35. Progressive weakness and limitation of movement of the affected area characterize the onset. Pain is not an early feature, although obviously occurring with a pathological fracture. After a period of months or years the limb becomes useless or flail. The course is unpredictable, either stabilizing or progressing fatally with the development of chylothorax.

Radiologically an ill-defined area of radiolucency may be observed in a single bone, but this destructive process progresses slowly to involve adjacent bones without respect for intervening joints (Fig. 6.21). Symptoms, however, may be so insidious that extensive absorption of many adjacent bony structures may be revealed at

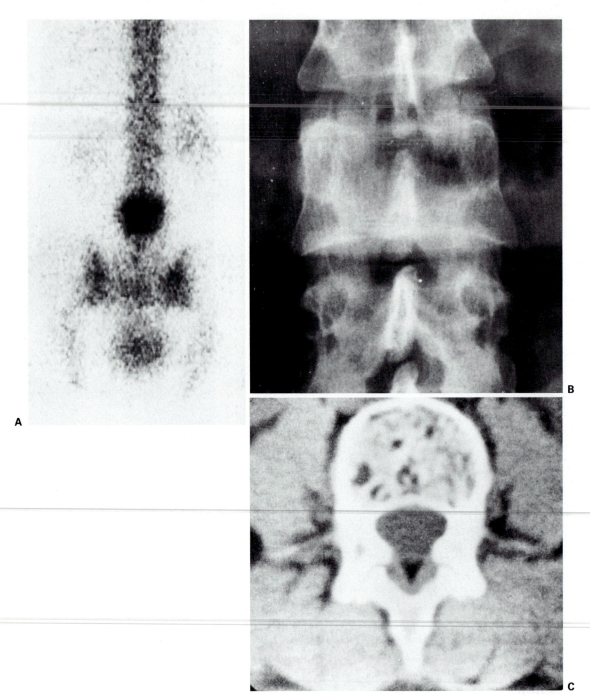

Fig. 6.19 Vertebral haemangioma was detected initially (**A**) on a whole-body radionuclide bone scan in this middle-aged woman with carcinoma of the breast. A marked increase in activity is present throughout the whole of L3. **B.** A radiograph demonstrates fine striation within an enlarged vertebral body. The pedicles, particularly that on the right, are enlarged. **C.** Computerized tomography confirms multiple radiolucencies throughout the vertebral body. This patient remained free of metastasis on annual follow-up for 5 years.

the initial examination. Arteriography and lymphography have shown no connection of these lesions to either the vascular or lymphatic circulations.

The radiological appearance is consequently that of a diffuse increase in translucency with progressive absorption of the affected structures. In the course of the

process, deformity is likely to develop and may be crippling. Although local recurrence is a major hazard, slow progression is the rule.

Similar massive osteolysis may occur with tumorous masses of lymphatic origin (**lymphangiomatosis**). Histological differentiation of the cavernous spaces that are

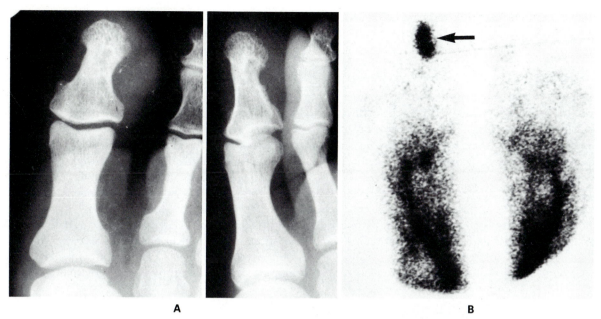

Fig. 6.20 Soft-tissue haemangioma of the great toe. This patient complained of a swollen great toe with a purple area of discoloration **A**. A plain film reveals soft-tissue swelling and pressure erosion of the plantar aspect of the distal phalanx. **B**. A blood-pool scan confirms an intense focus of activity (arrow) corresponding to the cavernous haemangioma.

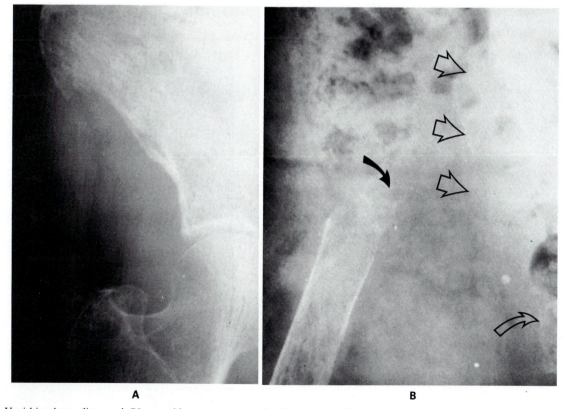

Fig. 6.21 Vanishing bone disease. A 70-year-old woman presented with poorly localized pain in her right hip. **A**. A radiograph at presentation reveals ill-defined destruction at the anterior inferior iliac spine. **B**. 9 months later there is total destruction of the whole of the hemipelvis and hip joint. Note the faint outline of the residual femoral head (arrow), pathological fracture of the femoral neck and the articular surfaces of the sacrum and symphysis pubis which no longer articulate with bone (open arrows).

found may be difficult and the radiological features are virtually identical.

3. CYSTIC ANGIOMATOSIS OF BONE

This rare entity is probably due to a hamartomatous malformation of primitive vessels. It may be difficult to distinguish the tissue of origin. Some lesions are clearly related to blood vessels, others to lymphatics. Among numerous synonyms, *cystic angiomatosis* is the most descriptive.

The condition may be recognized in childhood or adolescence in the virtual absence of symptoms, other than mild bony swellings or, occasionally, a pathological fracture. The diagnostic radiological abnormalities may be discovered incidentally. Broadly, two groups of patients are affected, those with and those without visceral and/or cutaneous involvement. The former have multiple angiomatous lesions in abdominal viscera, brain, muscle, lungs and lymph nodes, and although these lesions are histologically innocent, death may be caused from anaemia or bleeding. The prognosis in the latter group is excellent.

Radiologically, multiple sharply defined radiolucent lesions involve both cortex and medulla (Fig. 6.22). An initial impression of myeloma may be given. The skull, flat bones and proximal ends of long bones are affected particularly. Scintigraphically, activity may be increased around the lesions. Angiography is usually normal, but in those cases which have differentiated more closely along lymphatic lines a connection with deep lymphatics may be demonstrated by lymphography.

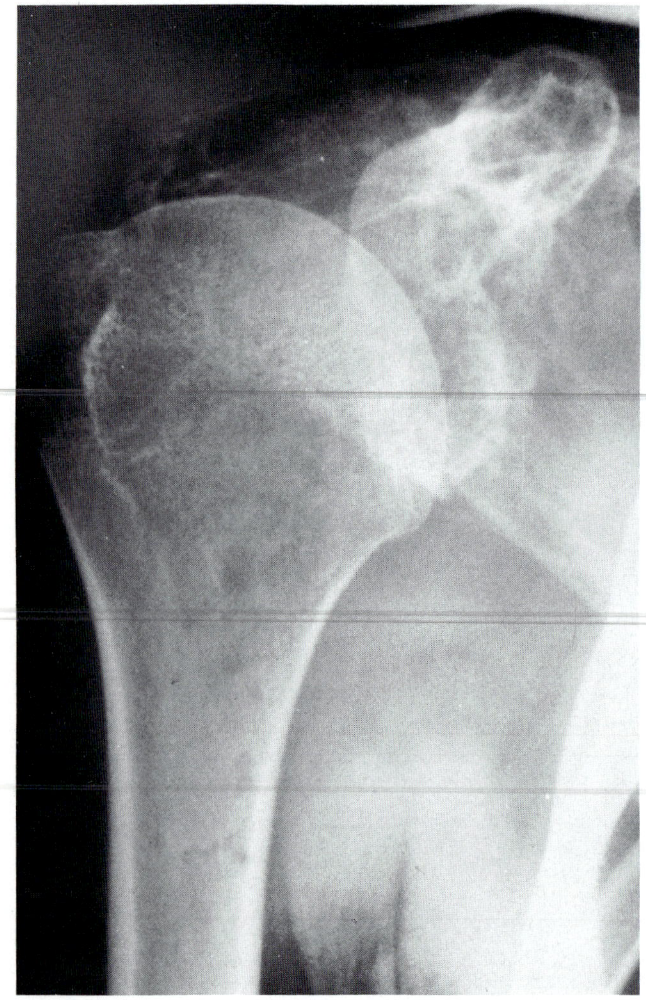

4. GLOMUS TUMOUR

This rare, highly differentiated, benign vascular tumour affects soft tissues more than bone. It creates, however, pressure erosion, usually of a terminal phalanx, particularly the subungual portion (Fig. 6.23). A few lesions may originally arise in bone. Typically an extremely sharp margin is associated with a well-marked sclerotic rim.

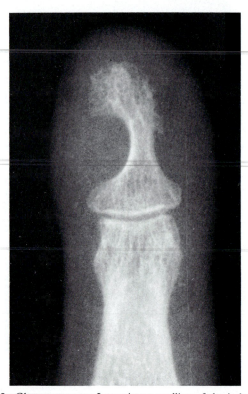

Fig. 6.22 Cystic angiomatosis of bone. Shortly before taking his university entrance examination this young man complained of a vague discomfort in his right shoulder. Note multiple well-defined radiolucencies involving the acromion, coracoid, glenoid and upper humeral shaft. The latter has a rather 'woodworm'-like appearance. Lesions were present elsewhere in the skeleton but he had no soft-tissue abnormality.

Fig. 6.23 Glomus tumour. Intermittent swelling of the index finger had been present for many years and had, intermittently, been exquisitely painful. A discrete soft-tissue mass caused a pressure erosion on the radial side of the terminal phalanx.

Clinically the tumours are exquisitely tender and have many episodes of stabbing pain, particularly with the rarer and less differentiated haemangiopericytoma. Angiographically, the lesion is richly vascular, and so may be detected on a blood-pool scan or on the early phase of a bone scan. The correct clinical diagnosis is usually established with little difficulty by the classic triad of pain, tenderness and sensitivity to cold.

5. ANGIOSARCOMA
(haemangioendothelial sarcoma)

Primary malignant vascular tumours in bone are rare. None have been observed to arise from a benign precursor.

Radiologically the lesions are purely lytic and rapidly fatal, with metastatic spread to the lungs often being present at the time the diagnosis is made. The destructive areas have irregular endosteal margins with slight expan-

sion or coarse loculation occasionally giving a rather soap-bubble appearance. Distinction of this lesion from a highly vascular (telangectatic) osteosarcoma may be very difficult. A clue may be derived from the sometimes multifocal nature of angiosarcoma, occurring in about one-third of cases.

TUMOURS PRESUMED TO ARISE FROM OTHER TISSUES IN BONE: NERVE TISSUE

1. NEUROFIBROMA AND NEURILEMMOMA

There is no clear distinction between these two tumours. It is thought that neurilemmoma or Schwannoma arises from a specific cell, the Schwann cell, whereas neurofibromas come from non-specific cells in nerve sheath. When these lesions enlarge in intimate relation to bone, the latter undergoes pressure erosion resulting in an os-

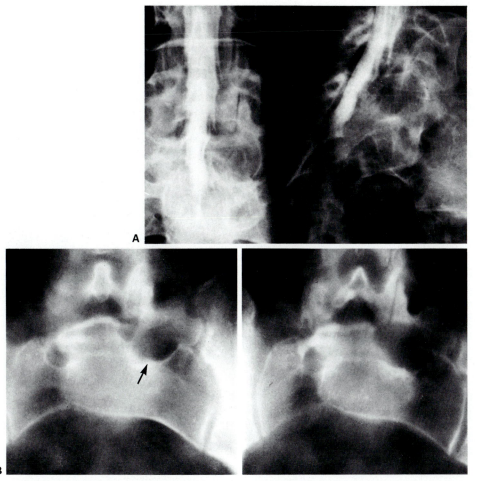

Fig. 6.24 Neurofibroma arising in the exit foramen of the first sacral segment. The patient presented with sciatic pain and (**A**) two views from a water soluble radiculogram reveal amputation of the S1 nerve root sheath, displacement of the S1 and S2 roots and a large well-defined rounded radiolucency with sclerotic margins in the exit foramen. **B**. Frontal tomograms confirm a large bony defect (arrow), compared with the normal right foramen.

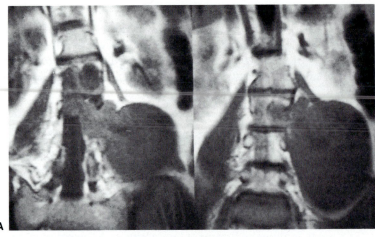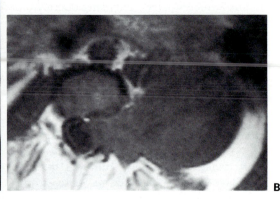

A   B

Fig. 6.25 Neurofibroma demonstrated by MRI coronal T$_1$-weighted (**A**) and axial (**B**) images. A typical dumbbell tumour is shown with large extra-neural component. Note however there is extension into the exit foramen and also intrathecal abnormalities.

seous defect. Radiological differentiation between such lesions is not possible. However there is some histological importance since neurilemmomas are usually solitary and never undergo malignant change, whereas neurofibromas are often multiple and may become sarcomatous. Tumours arise at any age, and in either sex, usually giving rise to symptoms only as the result of nerve pressure or occasionally pathological fracture. Nerve pressure arises typically when the tumour is located within an osseous canal. Neurilemmomas have a predilection for the mandible whereas neurofibromas are more closely related to the spinal canal.

Radiological features. The presence of a benign lesion within the spinal canal may be evident from erosion of a pedicle or widening of an exit foramen (Figs 6.24, 6.25). The width of the interpedicular distance may also be increased. A soft-tissue mass projecting through the enlarged foramen is typical of the so-called dumb-bell

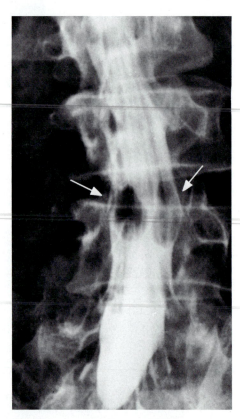

Fig. 6.27 Multiple neurofibromas in the cauda equina. This middle-aged patient was investigated for low back pain by radiculography. Two large ovoid neurofibromas are shown in close relationship to the L4 and L5 roots.

Fig. 6.26 Neurofibroma arising in the obturator ring has caused considerable pressure erosion of both right pubic rami, particularly the superior one. The margins of the pressure defect are sharply defined.

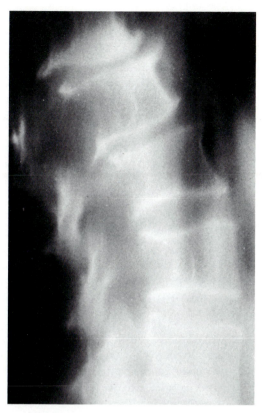

Fig. 6.28 Neurofibromatosis. A lateral tomogram of the lumbar spine demonstrates typical posterior scalloping, part of the general dysplasia of the neural canal and its contents found in this condition.

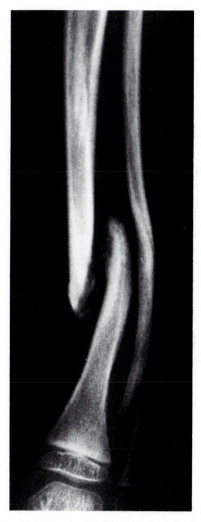

Fig. 6.29 Neurofibromatosis. Pseudoarthroses of the tibia and fibula shown in an infant. Bowing of bone and absence of any evidence of bone repair are typical.

tumour. Discrete pressure erosions on the surface of bone may be observed elsewhere in the skeleton (Fig. 6.26), but as these tumours are able to grow away from bone they are usually not symptomatic. Neurofibromas cause notches at the inferior surface of ribs but should not be confused with those in coarctation of the aorta, since they vary both in size and in distribution, not principally affecting the fourth to eighth ribs. All erosive lesions are rounded and clearly defined with a discrete sclerotic margin. An axial view or CT, however, may be necessary to demonstrate that they have predominantly a soft-tissue origin. Because of the predilection of neurofibromas to arise in nerve roots, many appear in the sacrum and are detected during the investigation of low back pain and sciatica (Figs 6.27, 6.24).

2. NEUROFIBROMATOSIS

Neurofibromatosis is often noticed at birth or soon after. Typical clinical manifestations are café-au-lait spots and multiple cutaneous tumours. Larger soft-tissue masses or growth disparities may also become apparent. These include scoliosis, pseudoarthrosis of long bones (particularly the tibia) and hemihypertrophy. Scoliosis, usually of short

segment distribution, often occurs in the thoracic spine. In addition numerous abnormalities arise related to the neural canal, including generalized dilatation with scalloping of vertebral bodies (Fig. 6.28), internal meningocoeles and dysraphic anomalies (see Ch. 58). Abnormal rib tubulation results in a 'ribbon-shaped' appearance. A particularly common abnormality is defective ossification of the posterior superior wall of the orbit. Pseudarthrosis of the tibia is characterized by marked absorption of the fracture margins, so that they become pointed (Fig. 6.29). Similar lesions may occur in the radius or clavicle. A number of published reports suggest that malignant sarcomatous change is relatively common, of the order of 5–12% of affected patients. The radiological appearances then become that of an infiltrating diffuse destructive process.

Many extraskeletal manifestations of neurofibromatosis

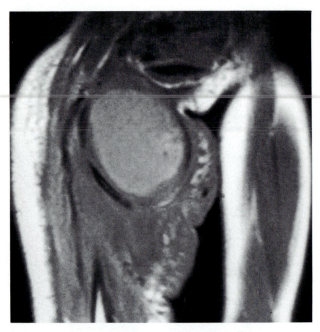

Fig. 6.30 A coronal T$_1$-weighted sequence of the thighs demonstrates an obvious abnormality on the right. In addition to a solitary neurofibroma displacing the femoral vessels (shown by a signal void), there is clear mesenchymal dysplasia, with extensive abnormalities of subcutaneous tissue and hemihypertrophy.

occur because of the neuroectodermal and mesodermal derivation of the tissue (Fig. 6.30). Gliomas of the optic nerves, phaeochromocytomas, aneurysms of cerebral and renal arteries, and acoustic neurilemmomas are well recognized. Similarly the incidence of fibrous tumour of bone is increased, particularly around the knee where radiologically they seem identical to non-ossifying fibromas and fibrous cortical defects.

TUMOURS PRESUMED TO ARISE FROM OTHER TISSUES IN BONE: FATTY TISSUE

LIPOMA AND LIPOSARCOMA

Although fat represents one of the normal connective tissue elements within bone, **intra-osseous lipomas** are exceedingly rare. The few that have been observed usually cause an oval lytic lesion within a long bone and bear a distinct resemblance to non-ossifying fibroma. A sharply defined discrete sclerotic margin is associated with bone expansion and trabeculation. Periosteal new bone formation is not a feature.

Parosteal lipomas on the other hand present a much more characteristic appearance with strands of ossification forming around the radiolucent fatty lobules of this rare tumour (Fig. 6.31). They tend to be very slow in growth and produce minor symptoms. Marked periosteal new bone formation does occur, with an obvious, but well-defined, soft tissue mass.

A more aggressive nature, however, must be considered when the soft-tissue element fails to contain fatty lucencies, possibly indicating the presence of a **parosteal liposarcoma. Intraosseous liposarcoma** has been described but is exceeding rare and produces an ill-defined lytic area usually in the femur or tibia, which is extremely vascular. Rapid extension into the soft tissues, and early pulmonary metastasis, is usual.

The characteristic radiolucencies of soft-tissue **lipomas** are discussed in Chapter 51, and **lipomas in the lumbar canal** are considered in Chapter 54. **Macrodystrophia lipomatosa** is a rare form of localized gigantism of a hand or foot accompanied by an overgrowth of the associated mesenchymal elements, particularly fat.

TUMOURS PRESUMED TO ARISE FROM OTHER TISSUES IN BONE: NOTOCHORD

CHORDOMA

The notochord extends, during embryological development, from the coccyx to the buccopharyngeal membrane and is the precursor of the vertebrae and intervertebral discs. Chordoma is a destructive bone tumour believed to arise from notochord cell rests. All are locally malignant with a strong tendency to recur after attempted excision. The lesions are slow growing and become apparent due to pressure symptoms, with or without localized pain. The extreme ends of the axial skeleton are involved, approximately half the lesions arising in the sacrum and/or coccyx, the others in the basioccipital and basisphenoid regions of the skull. A vertebral origin is found only in 15% of patients. Adjacent vertebrae may be involved. A fatal outcome results from a local extension, metastatic spread being unusual.

The usual clinical presentation is of a man between 40 and 70, the clinical symptoms and signs depending on the site of obstruction. Constipation is often a feature of those arising from the sacrum.

Radiological features. In the sacral area the tumour typically arises in the midline and involves the fourth or fifth sacral vertebrae (Fig. 6.32). The lesion is purely lytic, relatively well-defined, usually being oval or slightly lobulated. It may contain areas of calcification. The sacral margins may occasionally be sclerotic. The soft tissue structures within the pelvis are displaced anteriorly. Tumours arising at the basi-occipital or hypophyseal regions are accompanied by erosion and destruction of the dorsum sellae and clivus. Once again a lobulated or rounded area of bone destruction is associated with a large soft tissue mass displacing nasopharynx anteriorly and sometimes containing amorphous calcification. Here the differential diagnosis is from chondrosarcoma whereas in the sacrum the possibility of plasmacytoma should be considered.

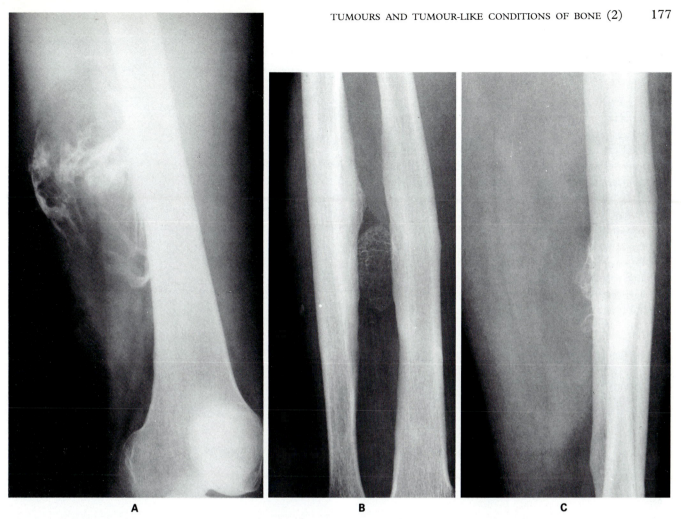

A   **B**   **C**

Fig. 6.31 Parosteal lipoma. Two examples are shown of parosteal lipomas arising in middle-aged patients. Both presented with a painless, rather firm mass, apparently attached to bone. **A**. A large lesion arising on the lateral aspect of the femur. Note the strands of ossification surrounding the radiolucent areas of fat. **B**. and **C**. A more discrete tumour arises from the interosseous membrane of the forearm. A fatty radiolucency is present, together with ossification in the soft tissues and some periosteal new bone formation.

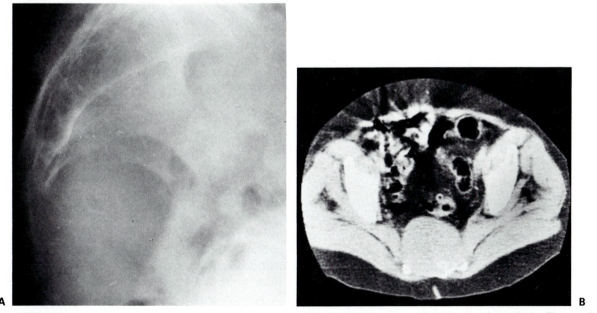

A   **B**

Fig. 6.32 Chordoma of the distal sacrum. **A**. A lateral film demonstrates a large soft-tissue mass displacing bowel anteriorly. The anterior cortex of the distal sacral vertebrae are ill defined and the coccyx is not seen. **B**. Computerized tomography demonstrates the typical well-defined soft tissue mass extending anteriorly from the sacrum. The anterior cortex of the sacrum has been destroyed. Chordomas usually exhibit an apparent disproportion between the size of the soft tissue mass and the extent of the bony involvement. L20, W200.

TUMOURS PRESUMED TO ARISE FROM OTHER TISSUE IN BONE: EPITHELIAL ORIGIN

IMPLANTATION DERMOID CYSTS

These rare lesions almost always follow a penetrating wound associated with a crush fracture, when it is assumed that epithelial cells are carried into the underlying bony structure. Typically they arise in distal phalanges of adolescents or young adults, the left middle finger being the single commonest site. The lesion grows slowly over many years.

Radiologically a well-defined translucency results, with slight expansion and sharply defined margins around which a minimal sclerotic reaction may be visible (Fig. 6.33). Subungual fibromas represent the only serious differential diagnostic possibility. A glomus tumour is almost invariably extraosseous.

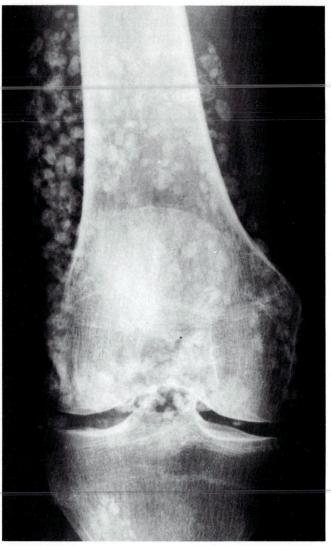

Fig. 6.34 Synovial chondromatosis. Hundreds of calcified lesions are shown in relation to the synovium, all of them approximately the same size. Nearly all were loose bodies.

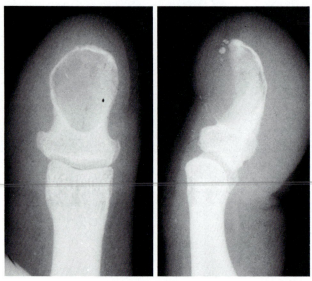

Fig. 6.33 Implantation dermoid cyst. A cystic lesion in the terminal phalanx of the thumb was found in an elderly woman many years after a penetrating injury. The sharp definition of its margins and the location of the lesion are characteristic.

TUMOURS RELATED TO JOINTS

1. SYNOVIAL CHONDROMATOSIS
(Osteochondromatosis)

This is a relatively unusual synovial disease, commonly regarded as a benign neoplasm, in which metaplastic cartilage formation occurs throughout the synovium. Typically young and middle-aged adults are affected, with a male preponderance and an affinity for large joints, in particular the knee. Minimal pain, swelling and limitation of movement are the usual presenting complaints. Cartilaginous lesions develop throughout the synovium later

becoming pedunculated and separating into the joint space. When large enough they undergo ossification. This condition undoubtedly progresses in phases, with episodes of intrasynovial disease and the shedding of loose bodies (Fig. 6.34).

In the early stages the only abnormality which may be detected on plain film is an apparent joint effusion. This may be delineated by CT, when a slight increase in density may be observed. Arthrography, however, demonstrates not only an irregular, nodular synovium (Fig. 6.35) but also cartilaginous loose bodies. Calcification and ossification of the cartilaginous masses result in numerous oval or rounded opacities, often of similar size, demonstrated on plain film. Serial examination may show these to be fairly constant in position. Scintigraphy using bone-seeking radiopharmaceutical often demonstrates an appreciable increase in activity localized particularly in

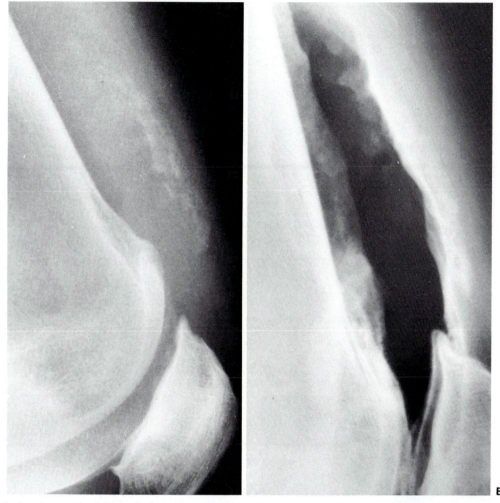

Fig. 6.35 Synovial chondromatosis. **A**. A preliminary film before knee arthrography demonstrates calcification in the thickened suprapatellar pouch. **B**. A localized view of the knee arthrogram demonstrates both nodular synovial thickening and intrasynovial calcification.

the larger masses, suggesting that active ossification and calcification are occurring. Eventually extensive capsular distension may result in marginal bony erosions occurring characteristically at the insertion of joint capsule, with clearly defined margins. Synovial chondromatosis also occurs in tendon sheaths and bursae. Chondrosarcoma is an extremely rare occurrence.

2. PIGMENTED VILLONODULAR SYNOVITIS
The aetiology of this disorder of synovium is not known. It is generally regarded as a benign neoplasm. The disease may be monoarticular or polyarticular, the latter being very rare. Adolescents and young adults are affected, usually complaining of local pain and swelling, occasionally with cystic masses related to a large joint, usually the knee or hip. Histologically, proliferation of villonodular masses of synovial tissue is associated with the deposition

of haemosiderin, a feature which may be detected by increased tissue attenuation on CT.

Radiologically, synovial thickening is usually evident, particularly with soft-tissue exposures. Features which suggest the diagnosis are sharply defined para-articular erosions with sclerotic margins, particularly if these lesions are present on both sides of the affected joint (Figs 6.36, 6.37). As in gout, integrity of the articular surfaces and preservation of the width of the joint space are maintained until relatively late in the disease. Disuse osteoporosis is not an initial feature. Calcification within the synovial mass is exceedingly rare, unlike malignant synovioma. Arthrographically, the thickening of the synovium is confirmed, usually being diffuse in larger joints, such as the knee, whereas in small joints, particularly metacarpo-phalangeal joints, the thickening is nodular (Fig. 6.38). The synovium of tendon sheaths and bursae may also be affected by this disease (Fig. 6.39).

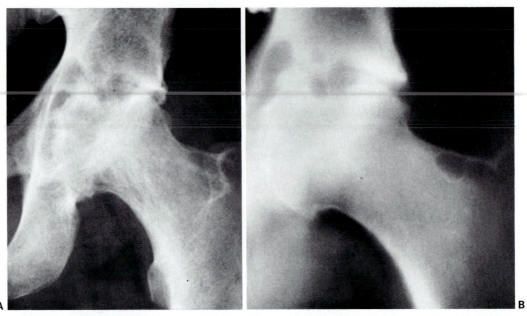

Fig. 6.36 Pigmented villonodular synovitis of the hip. **A.** Plain film illustrates sharply-defined radiolucent defects involving the acetabulum and the femoral head and neck. **B.** The sharply defined nature of the lesions confirmed on tomography. Note the sclerotic margins. This patient has relatively advanced disease and joint-space narrowing is present.

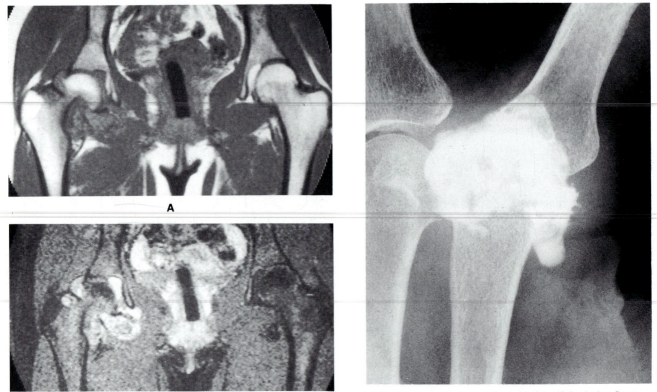

Fig. 6.37 Pigmented villonodular synovitis of the hip. Coronal T_1-weighted (**A**) and STIR sequence (**B**) demonstrate a lobulated synovial mass on the right with modestly high signal on the STIR sequence, though less so than the joint effusion associated with it. Note the replacement of the pulvina on the T_1-weighted sequence by tumour. A tampon is present in the vagina.

Fig. 6.38 Pigmented villonodular synovitis of the index finger metacarpophalangeal joint. An arthrogram confirms an enlarged joint space and thickened nodular synovium.

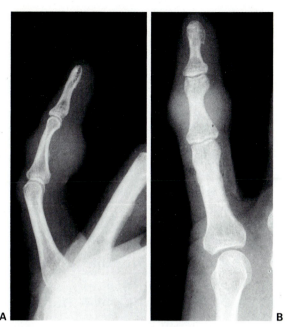

Fig. 6.39 A,B Pigmented villonodular synovitis of the flexor tendon sheath of the middle finger. A sharply circumscribed soft-tissue mass has caused slight pressure erosion of the middle phalanx.

3. SYNOVIOMA

This is a highly malignant tumour growing rapidly with early metastases to lymph nodes, unlike most other musculoskeletal tumours. Young adults are most commonly affected, the mean age being 35. The lesion arises in soft tissue adjacent to synovial structures of joints, tendon sheaths and bursae. 70% of cases involve the lower extremities, particularly around the knee. Clinically, a soft-tissue mass or ill-defined swelling is present in nearly three-quarters of patients, associated with local pain.

Radiologically, a soft-tissue mass is shown associated with a joint, about one patient in five demonstrating calcification of an amorphous nature. Ossification does not occur, unlike the later stages of synovial chondromatosis. About 10% of cases are associated with bone involvement, shown radiologically by irregular bone destruction, particularly at capsular attachments (Fig. 6.40).

This tumour may occasionally arise in the synovial lining of tendon sheaths, producing a similar soft-tissue mass. Secondary involvement of adjacent bone has been observed, particularly in the feet.

4. INTRAOSSEOUS GANGLION

This is a relatively uncommon lesion, representing ganglion material within a long tubular bone, the origin of which is unclear. Direct communication with a joint is demonstrated rarely. It may, on occasion, be shown to extend from an extraosseous lesion. Patients are between 30 and 60 years of age and two-thirds complain of local joint pain, often related to exercise. Most commonly the lesion occurs around the knee or ankle; hips and carpus are also common sites.

Radiologically, an oval or circular eccentric osteolytic lesion is shown, which is often expansile, with a thin

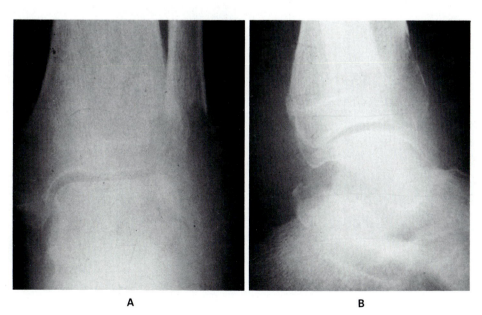

Fig. 6.40 Malignant synovioma of the ankle. Gross synovial thickening was present with hazy erosion of the capsular attachment. **A**. AP view. **B**. Lateral view.

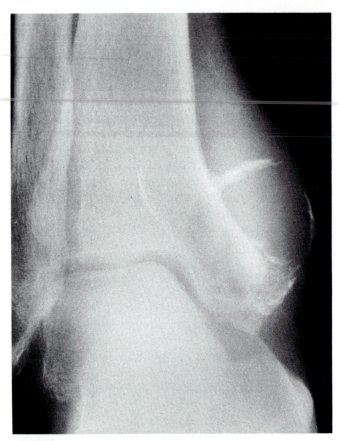

Fig. 6.41 Intraosseous ganglion. An oval, eccentric, osteolytic lesion arises from the medial malleolus with a thin sclerotic margin.

sclerotic rim. These may appear multilocular, varying between 1 and 5 cm in size (Fig. 6.41).

5. SUBARTICULAR ARTHRITIC CYST AND GEODE

Though not neoplasms, these space-occupying lesions may occasionally cause confusion. Described in detail elsewhere (Ch. 4), they most usually accompany rheumatoid disease, particularly with secondary degenerative change and osteoarthritis. The knee and hip are classic sites; the latter may present with a pathological fracture. The historical and radiological features of a pre-existing arthropathy should assist the diagnosis, together with the discrete sclerotic margins and close relationship with a joint (Fig. 6.42).

TUMOURS OF NO KNOWN ORIGIN

1. SOLITARY BONE CYST (*unicameral bone cyst*)

This entirely benign lesion is unlikely to be a true neoplasm, but is considered here since its diagnosis depends largely on radiological findings which can resemble those of known neoplastic conditions, and because of its predilection to recur after treatment.

Solitary bone cysts are always unilocular. The site of origin depends on the patient's age; prior to epiphyseal fusion the majority occur in the proximal humeri and

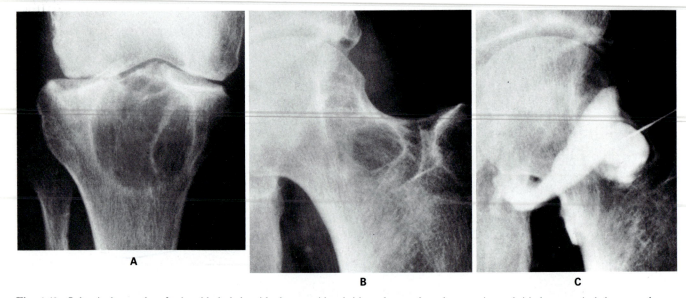

A

B

C

Fig. 6.42 Subarticular geodes. **A.** An elderly lady with rheumatoid arthritis and secondary degenerative arthritis has a typical, large geode immediately beneath the articular surface of the tibia. **B.** A younger man with rheumatoid disease has an oval, well-defined defect in the upper femoral neck. This too has a sclerotic margin. **C.** Aspiration of the defect yielded synovial fluid and injection of contrast medium confirmed, communication between the subarticular geode and the joint cavity.

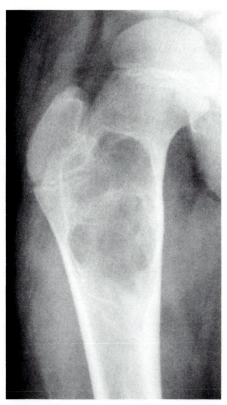

Fig. 6.43 Solitary bone cyst of the proximal femur showing expansion and thinning of the cortex, clearly defined endosteal margins but no calcification or periosteal new bone formation.

femora (Figs 6.43, 6.44) the former being the most usual site. Following skeletal maturation some lesions occur in such bones as the calcaneus (Fig. 6.45). Solitary bone cysts are commoner in males and develop during skeletal growth. Childhood and early adolescence is therefore the usual time for them to be discovered. More than half present due to a pathological fracture, a few may produce minor discomfort, others are found incidentally.

During the stage of skeletal development the lesion lies close to the metaphysis and is often situated in the midline, extending across the whole shaft. With further skeletal growth normal bone develops between the cyst and metaphysis so that the lesion is seen to be carried further the diaphysis. Hence those which develop early eventually lie in the middle of the shaft of a bone. The cyst contains clear liquid unless there has been contamination by bleeding following a fracture. It is lined by a thin layer of connective tissue.

Radiologically, an area of translucency in the metadiaphysis is characteristic. The overlying cortex is often thinned and slightly expanded with no periosteal reaction unless a fracture has occurred. The lesion may develop in relation to an apophysis, particularly the greater trochanter of the femur. In the earlier stages of growth, metaphysis cysts tend to have a continuous rounded, sharply-defined margin on the metaphyseal side but perhaps slightly less demarcation on the diaphyseal

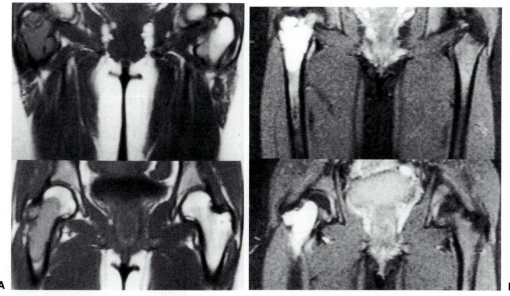

Fig. 6.44 A coronal T_1-weighted (**A**) and STIR sequence (**B**) with a typical liquid-containing lesion in the intertrochanteric region of the R. femur. The relatively classic characteristics of a liquid containing well-defined structure permit a confident diagnosis of a simple cyst.

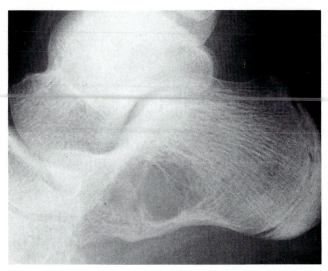

Fig. 6.45 Solitary bone cyst arising in a typical site in the os calcis. The margins in this bone tend to be less well defined.

side. Sclerotic reaction is usually present around the margin but may be quite discrete. A serpiginous margin may cause the cyst to appear multilocular. As normal bone grows in the metaphysis, subsequent examination demonstrates the apparent migration of the lesion along the shaft of the affected bone, with an increasing sclerotic reaction around its margins. On bone scanning no abnormality develops in the blood-pool phase, in contrast to aneurysmal bone cysts. The delayed image demonstrates increased activity only around the margins of the lesion, unlike fibrous dysplasia (Fig. 6.46). The only serious differential diagnostic possibility is a chondroma, but no calcification occurs in a simple bone cyst unless callus has formed from a fracture.

The prognosis depends partly on the patient's age. Before the age of 10 recurrences are frequent, whereas after that age primary healing usually occurs even after fractures. Because of the risk of pathological fracture the

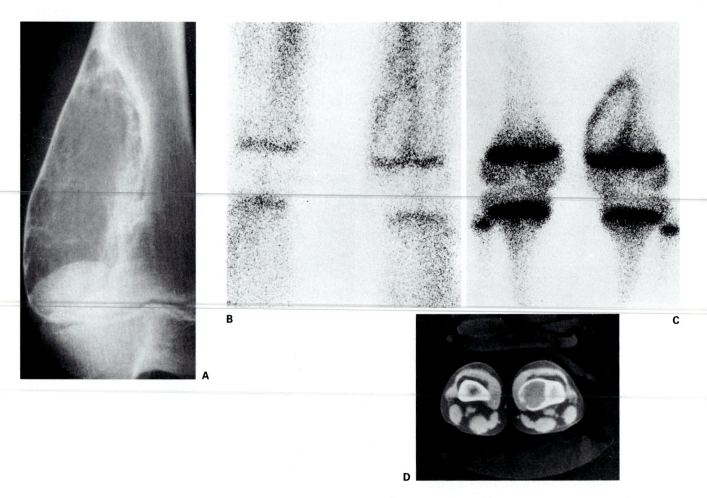

Fig. 6.46 Solitary bone cyst of the distal femur. The lesion is rather atypical (**A**) and plain-film diagnosis is not easy. However, it illustrates how further investigations can help in differential diagnosis. A bone scan, (**B**) in the blood-pool phase and (**C**) in the delayed phase, shows increased activity around the margin of the lesion corresponding to sclerosis on plain film. **D**. A CT scan demonstrates a soft-tissue density expansile lesion with no calcification. The differential diagnosis includes aneurysmal bone cyst, fibrous dysplasia (monostotic) and a chondroma. Aneurysmal bone cyst is vascular in the blood-pool phase of a bone scan, fibrous dysplasia markedly so on the delayed scan. Calcification may be expected on CT in a chondroma. L40, W400.

majority of patients are treated by curettage and packing with bone chips. Some lesions have been reported to regress satisfactorily after injection with steroids.

2. EWING'S SARCOMA: MALIGNANT ROUND-CELL TUMOURS

A group of highly malignant tumours involving bone is characterized histologically by numerous small round cells. Within this group are included Ewing's sarcoma, metastatic neuroblastoma, non-Hodgkin's lymphoma and undifferentiated tumours. Pathological distinction may be extremely difficult, even with the benefit of electron microscopy and histochemical techniques. Whilst it is clear that these entities show considerable overlap, Ewing's sarcoma is sufficiently distinctive to require definitive description.

Clinically, pain of several weeks' or months' duration is accompanied by localized tender swelling. The majority of patients are between 5 and 30 years of age. This rapidly progressive malignant tumour is characterized by pyrexia, anaemia and a raised ESR. These clinical symptoms and signs may closely simulate osteomyelitis but occur also in non-Hodgkin's lymphoma. It should be emphasized that the child with a Ewing's tumour is ill, in contrast to those with such benign lesions as eosinophilic granuloma which may cause similar radiological appearances. Histologically the malignant round cells typically contain glycogen granules. The lesion is most often found in a long bone, the diaphysis being more commonly affected than a meta-

physis. In about 40% of cases, however, the axial skeleton is involved, particularly the pelvis and ribs. Metastatic spread occurs early to lungs and to other bones where the radiological and histological findings are virtually identical. The time delay between the discovery of the primary lesion and the development of secondary deposits suggest that this tumour does indeed originate in bone, unlike some other malignant round cell tumours.

Radiologically the appearances are inconclusive. The lesion is essentially destructive, ill-defined and principally involves the medullary cavity. Cortical erosions and overlying periosteal reactions occur early; indeed a periosteal reaction may be the only sign of abnormality (Figs 6.47, 6.48). Although the onion-peel lamellar type of periosteal reaction is classically associated with this lesion it is observed only infrequently. Onion-peel periosteal reaction occurs in many other lesions, including osteosarcoma and infection. Elevation of periosteal new bone at the margins of cortical erosions (Codman triangles) may emphasize the shallow cortical erosions; known as 'saucerization' defects, they offer a highly suspicious diagnostic feature (Fig. 6.49). The tumour is highly vascular and grows rapidly. Angiographically, the extensive soft-tissue component and abnormal circulation is obvious (Fig. 6.50). The blood-pool phase of a bone scan also demonstrates increased vascularity, but, in the delayed phase, an increase in activity is evident only at the margins of the tumour with bone and in periosteal new bone. These modalities, CT and/or MRI, are necessary to delineate the soft-tissue extent of the tumour, which is often much greater than may be appreciated on plain films. A whole-body radio-

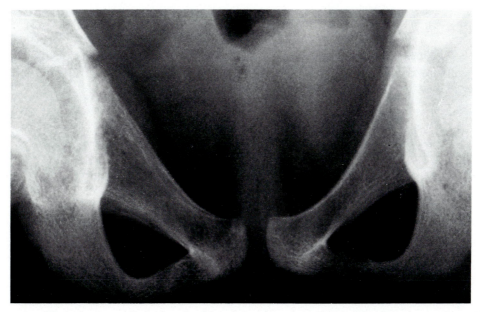

Fig. 6.47 Ewing's sarcoma. The only abnormal sign here is of lamellar periosteal new bone arising from the superior pubic ramus on the right.

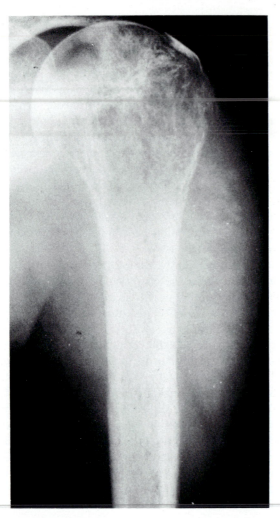

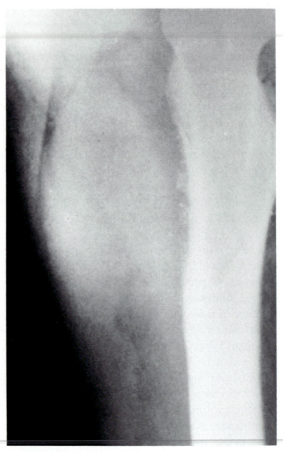

Fig. 6.48 Ewing's sarcoma. This tumour is much more advanced, with a well-defined soft-tissue mass, Codman's triangles, ossification and calcification in the soft tissues and ill-defined bony destruction. The radiological distinction from osteosarcoma is difficult.

Fig. 6.49 Ewing's sarcoma arising primarily in the soft tissues of the thigh. A well-marked erosion ('saucerization') defect has been caused with periosteal new bone formation.

nuclide bone scan is also of value in detecting recurrences and metastasis. The differential diagnosis may be difficult. Osteosarcoma may present almost identical radiological features and benign conditions, histiocytosis and aggressive osteomyelitis (particularly from *Staphylococcus*), require consideration.

REFERENCES AND SUGGESTIONS FOR FURTHER READING

See end of Chapter 7.

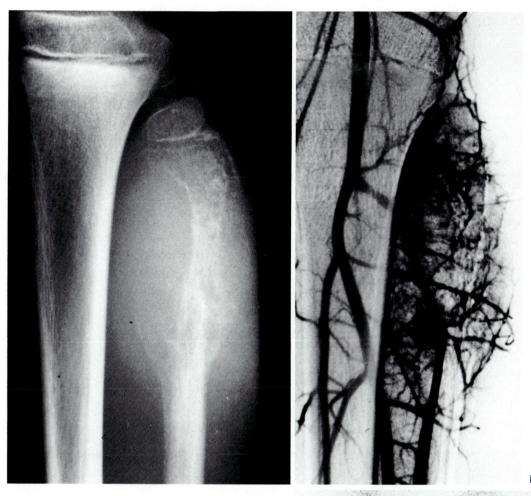

A

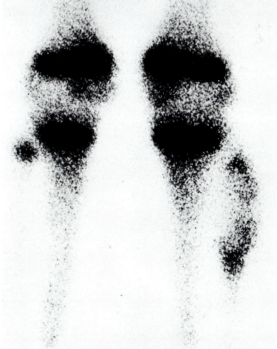

B

C

Fig. 6.50   Ewing's sarcoma of bone arising in the proximal fibula of an 8-year-old. **A**. An advanced tumour is shown on plain films, with Codman's triangles, a soft-tissue mass and ill-defined bone destruction. **B**. The subtraction print of femoral arteriogram demonstrates a very abnormal circulation with a large soft tissue mass. **C**. A bone scan, in the delayed phase, demonstrates increased activity where new bone formation is present on plain films. The lesion itself is photon-deficient. Osteosarcoma may present similar appearances.

CHAPTER 7

DISORDERS OF THE LYMPHORETICULAR SYSTEM AND OTHER HAEMOPOIETIC DISORDERS

Iain Watt

This important group of disorders is responsible for some of the most bizarre radiological abnormalities encountered in the skeleton and may be subdivided conveniently into diseases affecting:

1. the red blood cells
2. the white blood cells
3. the lymphoreticular system, and
4. the coagulation mechanism.

DISEASES PRIMARILY INVOLVING RED BLOOD CELLS

In the infant, red marrow extends throughout the medullary cavities of the whole skeleton. During the first few months of life red blood cells are also produced by the spleen and liver, this function being described as *extramedullary erythropoiesis*. As the physiological requirement for erythrocyte production diminishes progressively during the years of growth, a cessation of this function occurs in the liver and spleen and later by regression of the red marrow areas in the peripheral skeleton. By the age of 20 years red marrow is normally confined to the proximal ends of the femora and humeri and to the axial skeleton. Residual areas of fatty non-haematopoietic marrow in the appendicular skeleton, as well as the liver and spleen, may be reactivated should the need arise. Such a response occurs normally after a severe haemorrhage, but these episodes are insufficiently prolonged to cause radiological changes.

Chronic haemolytic anaemias, however, in which red blood cells suffer extensive destruction, are followed in many instances by such a degree of marrow hyperplasia that striking skeletal abnormalities result. The great majority of these diseases are congenital and hereditary in origin. The red blood cells are abnormal in shape, in fragility and in the type of haemoglobin which they contain. The clinical picture is that of any chronic anaemia. Dyspnoea, pallor, fatigue and weakness are often accompanied by jaundice due to erythrocyte destruction. If extramedullary haematopoiesis occurs, the liver and spleen may be enlarged, particularly the latter, especially when the anaemia is profound. Cardiac enlargement and failure may occur, many of the more severely affected patients dying before puberty.

Radiological changes in the skeleton, resulting from marrow hyperplasia, vary greatly with disease severity. In children, the changes are widespread and are usually demonstrated most easily in the extremities and the skull. To some degree, marrow hyperplasia causes destruction of many of the medullary trabeculae. This is followed by thinning and expansion and even perforation of the overlying cortex. In many patients this hyperplasia achieves its compensatory object, so that a state of erythrocytic balance is reached. The areas of bone destruction show features of repair, by formation of fibrous tissue and the development of reactive bone sclerosis. The latter thickens the remaining trabeculae and, in some, the endosteal aspect of the cortex, to produce an overall increase in bone density. As age advances, the peripheral bones, now in a state of balance, tend to revert to a normal appearance, but some residual increase of density may remain. Evidence of continued erythropoiesis to a greater degree than normal is then confined to the physiological red-marrow areas.

Extramedullary haematopoiesis, in addition to producing evidence of hepatosplenomegaly, may be revealed by the presence of sharply defined paravertebral soft tissue masses of haematopoietic tissue especially around the thoracic spine (Fig. 7.1).

THALASSAEMIA (*Cooley's anaemia*)

Described by Cooley in 1927, this condition, known also as *Mediterranean anaemia*, is by no means confined to Mediterranean countries or races. Geographical distribution extends eastwards in a broad band through Asia and West Africa. In such areas it is commonplace. It may be encountered anywhere in the world in individuals having a heredity originating from these areas.

The disease is due to abnormalities of the haemoglobin molecule, of which many have been established. Homo-

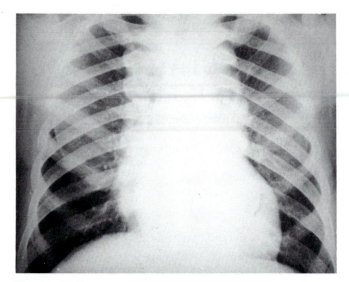

Fig. 7.1 Thalassaemia. Rounded soft-tissue masses due to extramedullary haematapoiesis are present adjacent to the thoracic spine.

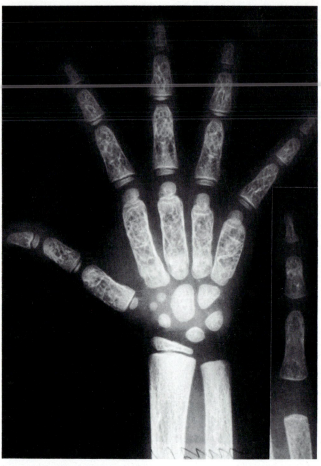

Fig. 7.2 Thalassaemia (boy aged 7). Gross marrow hyperplasia has expanded and thinned overlying cortical bone. Medullary trabeculae have been destroyed and the residual ones are coarsened. **Inset** — early changes of the same type in a finger of a child aged 4.

zygous subjects, who have inherited the trait from both parents, develop the more severe form of the disease, known clinically as *thalassaemia major*, whereas heterozygous subjects develop a minor form. Both may vary greatly in severity, so that distinction between them and other haematological variants is of relatively little radiological importance. Severe forms usually become manifest in the first two years of life. Although the majority of these patients die before puberty, some survive to early adult life. Those with less severe disease live correspondingly longer and minimal manifestations may be found only by examination of the blood of individuals who otherwise appear entirely normal. The important clinical features, in addition to those of other anaemias, are dwarfing, delay in development of secondary sexual characteristics, and either 'mongoloid' or 'rodent' facies due to expansion of the underlying facial bones as a consequence of erythroblastic hypertrophy.

Radiological changes. Hyperplasia of the marrow destroys many of the medullary trabeculae and expands and thins the overlying cortex. In children this is evident especially in the *hands*, when the shafts of the phalanges and metacarpals become biconvex instead of being biconcave (Fig. 7.2). The *feet* are affected in the same way. Similar abnormalities in the *ribs* (Fig. 7.3) and *long bones* (Fig. 7.4) may produce apparent failure of modelling with, for example, flask-shaped femora (Fig. 7.5). In the *skull* the diploic space is widened and gross thinning of the outer table may be followed by marked diploic thick-

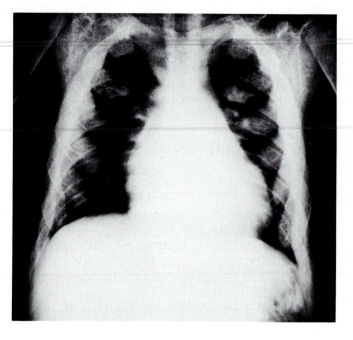

Fig. 7.3 Thalassaemia (boy aged 15). A chest film shows gross expansion of bone structures due to marrow hyperplasia. Note particularly involvement of the ribs and scapulae.

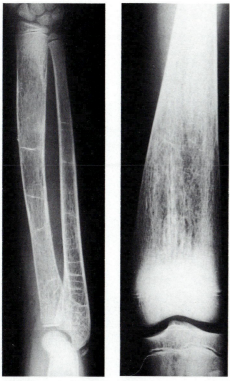

Fig. 7.4   Fig. 7.5

Fig. 7.4 Thalassaemia. Considerable bone expansion, cortical thinning and simplification of trabecular pattern is demonstrated in the forearm of a boy of 15.

Fig. 7.5 Thalassaemia. Considerable marrow expansion has produced a flask shape of the distal femur. The coarsened trabecular pattern and cortical thinning are obvious.

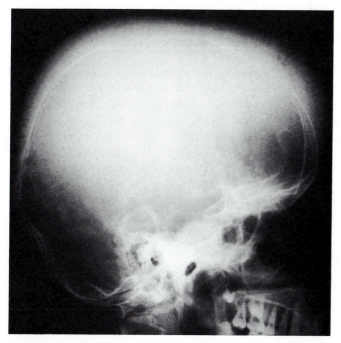

Fig. 7.6 Thalassaemia. Thickening of the outer table of the skull in the frontal area with perpendicular striation — the 'hairbrush sign'.

ening, starting in the frontal region, but usually exempting the occipital bone in which the marrow content is minimal (Fig. 7.6). The 'classical' appearance of the 'hairbrush' spicules is relatively uncommon. These changes appear considerably later than those in the short bones of the extremities. Development of the air spaces of the skull, especially the maxillary antra and the mastoids, is impaired as a result of hyperplasia of the marrow, accounting for the clinical manifestation of 'rodent' facies, with malocclusion. The *spine* shows only diffuse demineralization with the same generalized coarsened trabecular pattern as that observed in the appendicular skeleton. Vertebral collapse is uncommon.

Osseous abnormalities of this type may be observed also in a number of lesser forms of thalassaemia and its variants, including those associated with other abnormal haemoglobins and the sickle cell trait. In all these conditions, however, the changes tend to be very much less prominent than in thalassaemia major.

SICKLE CELL DISEASE

This chronic haemolytic anaemia is also congenital and hereditary in origin. The erythrocytes, when hypoxic, become abnormal in shape, being unusually long and slender. The abnormal haemoglobin which they contain has a reduced oxygen-carrying capacity. The disease occurs almost exclusively in black races, especially those in Central Africa or their descendants, who are homozygous for the sickling trait. This trait may be crossed with normal or abnormal haemoglobins, including thalassaemia. In these crossed types, the patient is less severely affected, both clinically and radiologically. Differentiation of the true homozygous state from the variants (of which combination with haemoglobin-C is the most common) is of some importance. The former group rarely survive after the age of 30, whereas the latter may have a normal lifespan. The former are characterized clinically by early onset of the severe anaemic picture, with frequent skeletal and abdominal crises. These acutely painful episodes, lasting for several days, are due essentially to infarction, attributed to vascular blockage by collections of erythrocytes which have undergone sickling in areas of capillary stasis with resultant hypoxia.

Infarcts may affect many systems. The fundamental skeletal abnormalities consist of hyperplasia of marrow with superimposition of areas of bone necrosis due to infarction and subsequent growth disparities. A further clinical complication is the development of infection within these infarcts, particularly in lesions developing in the long bones of children.

Radiological changes. The chronic haemolytic state is reflected by the development of characteristic and diagnostic radiological abnormalities, affecting primarily the erythropoietic skeleton, and also the soft tissues involved by extramedullary haematopoiesis. The frequency with which abnormalities are discovered increases with age. All variants of sickle-cell disease produce essentially similar radiological abnormalities.

1. *Marrow hyperplasia* is fundamental. In this disease, however, the effects on the skeleton, which are so prominent in thalassaemia major, occur in modified form, even in its worst clinical manifestations being less severe. A generalized osteoporotic appearance is evident throughout the haematopoietic areas of the skeleton, but even in infants and children it is recognized more easily in the axial than the peripheral skeleton. This feature is not diagnostic, but in a black child should arouse suspicion. Unlike severe thalassaemia, significant modelling abnormalities are uncommon so that the air spaces of the paranasal sinuses are rarely affected. The diploic space of the skull may be widened, with consequent bossing. If a state of erythrocytic balance is achieved, diffuse trabecular thickening is likely to develop.

Such an appearance may be shown incidentally in an asymptomatic adult sickle-cell trait carrier. In more advanced cases, a coarse medullary pattern is associated with enlarged vascular channels in bone, especially in proximal or middle phalanges.

2. *Endosteal apposition of bone.* Inward cortical thickening is separated occasionally by a thin zone of translucency, to result in the appearance in the long bones of 'a bone within a bone'. This sign may be observed in other conditions, including Gaucher's disease (see below). The medullary cavities, in severe cases, may ultimately be grossly narrowed and almost obliterated, so that a diffuse and generalized increase in bone density results. This does not occur in the axial skeleton, which is a persistent red marrow area, and this provides an important diagnostic feature, even in the absence of other signs.

3. *Infarction of bones* provides the diagnostic hallmark of this disease. Infarction of various tissues is considered to be the cause of the classical, clinical episodes of sickle-cell crises. Unlike thalassaemia, in which infarction is virtually unknown, this type of involvement of the skeleton is common. The consequent radiological abnormalities are comparable to those observed in other systemic disorders such as dysbaric osteonecrosis (caisson disease) and Gaucher's disease. Such infarcts are usually multiple and most commonly affect the *femoral* and *humeral* heads (Fig. 7.7), in particular the medullary bone. Medullary infarcts may be of two varieties, either with sharply defined margins or producing diffuse sclerosis. In their mildest form they may be recognized in an asymptomatic patient. The classical 'snowcap' sign refers to the subarticular area of increased density, particularly in a humeral head, which reflects the revascularization of an area of bone which has been necrotic (Fig. 7.8). At this phase of development bone scans are usually abnormal

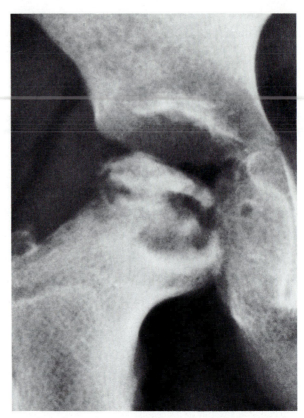

Fig. 7.7 Sickle cell disease. Infarction in the proximal femoral metaphysis has produced a large defect with avascular necrosis of the femoral head. These features are similar to those of Perthes' disease.

with increased activity. However, in acute infarction a photon deficiency is often present within 24 hours of the insult (Fig. 7.9). Repairing bone is brittle, however, and fractures easily — varying from 'osteochondritis dissecans' to complete collapse.

Femoral heads affected in *childhood* present an appearance exactly comparable to Perthes' disease (Fig. 7.7). In young black children the areas of predilection for infarctions are the small tubular bones of the hands and feet (Figs 7.10, 7.11), causing destructive changes accompanied by massive and painful soft-tissue swellings and periosteal reactions which may be florid and reflect associated infarction of cortical bone. These findings may indicate the correct diagnosis, but other causes of infantile periosteal reactions such as cortical hyperostosis of both the infantile or traumatic types, or possibly hypervitaminosis A, may require consideration. The formation of perpendicular bony spicules on the skull, uncommon even in thalassaemia, is distinctly unusual. More important is the possibility of superadded infection, discussed below.

Infarcts of vertebral bodies are another characteristic radiological stigma. Generalized depressions of the central portions of the vertebral plates are common, and may be demonstrated in an asymptomatic patient. The de-

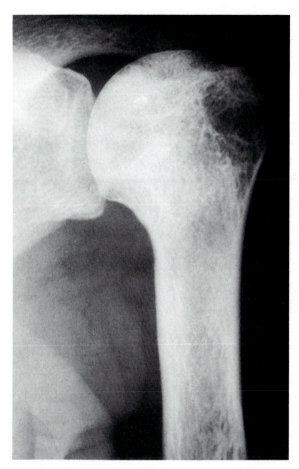

Fig. 7.8 Sickle cell disease. Endosteal bone deposition has resulted in diffuse sclerosis beneath the articular surface (the 'snow-cap' sign) due to medullary infarction. Note the lack of distinction between cortical and medullary bone in the upper humeral shaft, again due to endosteal deposition of bone.

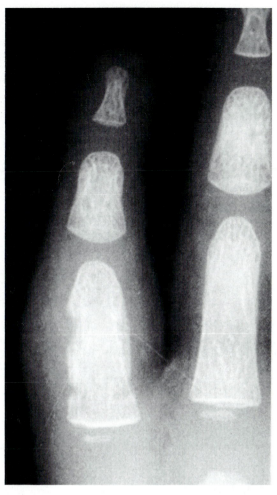

Fig. 7.10 Sickle cell disease. Soft-tissue swelling surrounds an expanded proximal phalanx. Medullary expansion is present with simplification of trabecular pattern and penetration of the cortex. The distinction between these changes and osteomyelitis is extremely difficult.

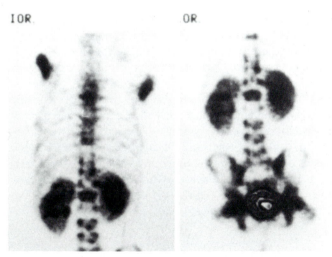

Fig. 7.9 Sickle cell disease. A bone scan performed 16 hours after the onset of severe pain in a boy with known sickle-cell disease. Acute infarction of L2 has resulted in a relative photon deficiency in this area. Previous infarctions, in varying phases of evolution, are shown as areas of increased activity (see particularly L1 and mid-thoracic vertebrae).

pressions are often concave and rounded, simulating an ordinary nucleus pulposus impression on a bone which is already porotic. Infarction may be diagnosed when the centre of the depression is flat and the sides slope obliquely (Fig. 7.12).

The diaphyses of the long bones, especially in the older child and the adolescent, are sites of predilection for infarction. Typically they involve the zones between the mid diaphysis and the metaphyses, the so-called 'intermediate fifths'. When the metaphysis is involved significant deformity may occur due to growth arrest. Central metaphyseal defects and lucencies are typical. These in turn may produce fragmentation and deformity of the epiphyses. They may also be the site of pathological fractures. Infarcts may be massive, causing bone destruction, sequestration, reactive sclerosis and even the formation of involucrum. The pattern may suggest acute pyogenic osteomyelitis.

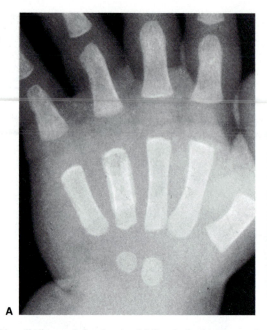
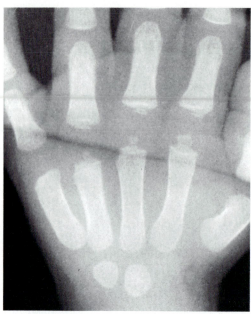

Fig. 7.11 Sickle-cell disease, infarction in childhood. **A**. At presentation, periosteal new bone formation surrounds the diaphysis of the fourth finger metacarpal. **B**. 10 months later resolution has occurred and growth has proceeded normally. The distinction between infarction and infection may be very difficult. In this case no specific treatment was given.

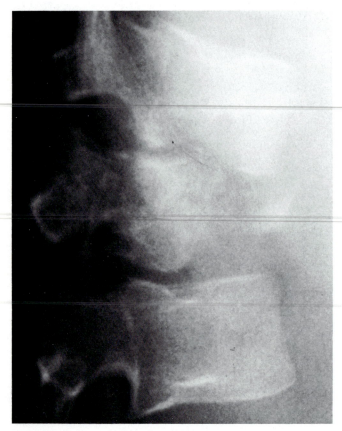

Fig. 7.12 Sickle cell disease. Flat depressions within the vertebral bodies with sloping sides typify metaphyseal infarct ('the vertebral step sign'). Frank destruction of the vertebral body with narrowing of the contiguous disc spaces is due to associated *salmonella* osteomyelitis.

4. *Superadded infection*. The areas of bone necrosis caused by infarction are especially susceptible to infection, classically by *salmonella* organisms of the paratyphoid B group. Differentiation between the pure infarct and those which have been infected in this way may be extremely difficult (Fig. 7.13) both radiologically and pathologically, since cultures are often sterile. Such lesions are liable to occur especially in the tubular bones of the hands and feet in infants and in the long bones and the spine of older children (Fig. 7.12). In the adult, septic arthritis may be superimposed on an adjacent infarct. With appropriate treatment, either by conservative antibiotic therapy or by active surgical measures, including sequestrectomy, healing usually takes place with remarkable rapidity.

5. *Soft-tissue involvement*, as in the other chronic haemolytic anaemias, and such disorders of the marrow as Gaucher's disease, is shown by hepatosplenomegaly caused by *extramedullary haematopoiesis*. Heterotopic masses of haematopoietic tissue may develop in the dorsal paravertebral areas. Release of iron pigments by accelerated destruction of erythrocytes may precipitate the formation of *biliary calculi*.

ERYTHROBLASTOSIS FETALIS
(haemolytic disease of the newborn)

Haemolytic anaemia occurring in the fetus and newborn results from immunological incompatibility between the blood of the mother and the fetus, most commonly due

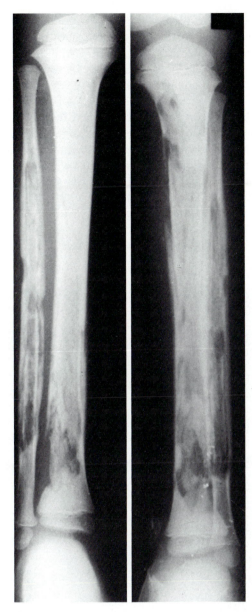

Fig. 7.13 Sickle-cell disease with salmonella osteomyelitis. (Nigerian boy aged 4). Extreme destructive changes in the long bones have been caused by infection superimposed upon infarction. Numerous sequestra are present. (Courtesy of Mr Geoffrey Walker.)

to Rh factor, although other haematological errors of this type are known. The severity of the affection of the infant may vary widely, from a mild anaemia to icterus neonatorum and fetal hydrops.

The Rh-positive erythrocytes of the fetus, crossing the placental barrier in a mother without Rh antigen, stimulate maternal formation of anti-Rh antibodies which traverse the placenta to enter the fetal circulation, there to haemolyse the fetal red blood cells. The danger of infants being affected by this incompatibility increases with the number of conceptions, but early recognition of

the disorder and the adoption of prophylactic measures has greatly reduced its incidence.

Radiological changes. The only skeletal abnormality is the development of transverse metaphyseal translucencies in the long bones. These translucencies are non-specific, since they may occur also with other severe maternal illnesses during pregnancy and also in congenital syphilis. With successful treatment the translucent areas ossify with residual growth lines. In the spine, such growth lines often cause 'ghost shadows' within the vertebral bodies. *Fetal hydrops* may be diagnosed sonographically (Ch. 44) by the detection of growth retardation, effusions and subcutaneous oedema. The fetus is displaced by enlargement of the placenta.

OTHER CHRONIC ANAEMIAS

The anaemia of infants suffering from **iron deficiency** may produce radiological changes in the skull due to marrow hyperplasia similar to those of the less severe congenital anaemias. An inadequate diet is the usual cause, but malabsorption or abnormal loss of iron may be important factors. The widening of the diploic space and the subsequent bossing of the skull vault are again characteristic, but the disease has never been reported to cause changes sufficiently severe to involve the long bones and facial bones.

Hereditary spherocytosis is an inherited defect in which the red blood cells are of an abnormal round shape. The anaemia which results may produce mild changes comparable to the other congenital anaemias. Removal of the spleen permits the bone structures to revert to a normal appearance.

Fanconi's syndrome of congenital aplastic anaemia with multiple congenital anomalies (not to be confused with the other syndrome described by the same author and concerned with osteomalacia and an abnormal renal tubular mechanism) is of interest in that the haematological changes are unlikely to appear before the age of 2 years. These consist of hypoplastic anaemia, marrow hypoplasia and skin pigmentation. The defect is inherited and congenital abnormalities of the skeleton are associated, e.g. deficient formation of the bones of the thumb, first metacarpal and radius; other abnormalities such as congenital dislocation of the hip and clubfoot also have been observed. These are evident long before the haematological abnormalities become apparent, and the latter are not responsible for any skeletal abnormalities. Some cases have terminated in leukaemia.

POLYCYTHAEMIA

This condition is due to overproduction of red cells. Although occasionally responsible for bone infarction, it produces no characteristic radiological changes in the skeleton. Transition to myeloid metaplasia is common. Pulmonary abnormalities in polycythaemia may occur in the form of increased reticulation or fine mottling.

DISEASES PRIMARILY INVOLVING WHITE BLOOD CELLS

LEUKAEMIA

Children are most commonly affected, almost invariably by an acute form. In adults the disease may also be acute, but it is more commonly chronic. Haematopoietic tissue is widely distributed throughout the skeleton of a child but is confined in the adult to the 'red marrow' areas of the axial skeleton and the proximal ends of the humeri and femora. Thus radiological changes in the bones are commonly in the younger age-groups. More than half the children affected show skeletal abnormalities, while in adults these are found in fewer than 10% of cases. While the diagnosis is usually confirmed by examination of the blood and sternal marrow, bone changes may precede the development of a grossly pathological blood picture, especially in the so-called *aleukaemic* type.

Differentiation between myeloid and lymphatic types of leukaemia cannot be made by radiological examination.

Radiological changes are observed mainly in children and consist of the following:

1. *Metaphyseal translucencies.* In children the most characteristic sign, occurring in 90% of cases, is the presence of bands of translucency running transversely across the metaphyses (Figs 7.14, 7.15). Such bands may be narrow and incomplete in the early stages of the disease, but in the course of a few weeks they may be found to traverse the metaphysis completely and be as much as 5 mm in width. The most rapidly growing areas — knees, wrists and ankles — are commonly affected first, but later the metaphyses of the shoulders, hips and vertebral bodies also may be involved. With treatment, remission may occur, and the bands of translucency resolve.

2. *Metaphyseal cortical erosions* on the medial side of the proximal ends of the humeral (Fig. 7.16A) and tibial shafts sometimes occur as an early feature. It is usually bilateral.

3. *Osteolytic lesions* develop in over half the cases.

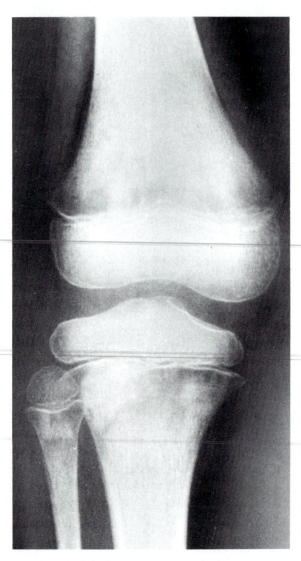

Fig. 7.15 Lymphatic leukaemia. Metaphyseal radiolucencies are present around the knee. Endosteal sclerosis is present adjacent to these lesions, obscuring the corticomedullary junction. Minor periosteal new bone formation is present in the upper tibia and fibula.

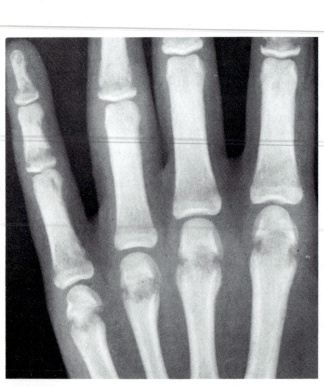

Fig. 7.14 Acute leukaemia. Extensive metaphyseal radiolucencies are present with adjacent periosteal new bone formation.

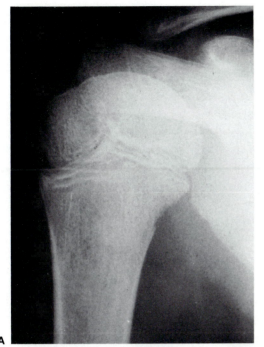

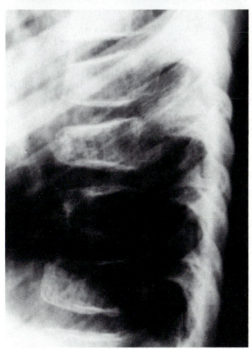

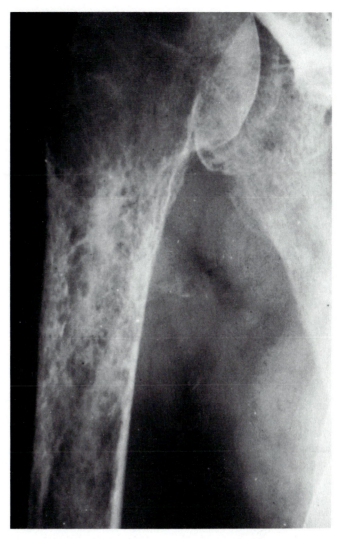

Fig. 7.16 Lymphatic leukaemia. **A**. Erosion of the medial side of the proximal metaphyses of both humeri were present in this 8-year-old. The disease was in an aleukaemic phase, not an uncommon finding even when skeletal changes are present. **B**. The same child complained of back pain. Multiple vertebral collapse is shown with the preservation of disc-space height. Overall bone density is reduced with a simplified trabecular pattern.

Fig. 7.17 Chronic lymphatic leukaemia — adult type. Diffuse medullary infiltration is shown in the humerus and scapula with cortical erosion.

(Fig. 7.17). When the vertebral bodies are involved, collapse often takes place before specific areas of rarefaction can be identified (Fig. 7.16B).

4. *Periosteal reactions* are usually associated with underlying lesions.

5. *Osteosclerosis* of the metaphysis is a rare but well-recognized primary manifestation. It may develop during treatment.

In *metastatic neuroblastoma* skeletal changes take place which may be indistinguishable from leukaemia. Separation of the sutures of the skull in the former condition is a helpful differentiating sign.

In *adults* skeletal lesions are rare. As has been stressed before, the deposits occur essentially in red marrow areas. Changes include porosis, translucent areas of leukaemic bone destruction (which tend to be oval with the long axis parallel to the shaft), and vertebral destruction and

Usually they are punctate and diffusely scattered, though solitary and larger lesions may occur. While any portion of the skeleton may be involved by such leukaemic deposits, they are commonest in the shafts of the long bones

collapse. Periosteal reactions are unusual. Occasionally, generalized osteosclerosis of the marrow area is evident. This is likely to be caused by trabecular thickening during periods of remission and may be patchy in type. In some instances, however, the leukaemic changes may be a secondary and terminal process in myeloid metaplasia.

MYELOID METAPLASIA
(myelofibrosis and myelosclerosis)

This syndrome is characterized by the triad of myelofibrosis, myeloid metaplasia and features in the peripheral blood film which simulate leukaemia. The relationship between myeloid metaplasia, myelosclerosis and other diseases including polycythaemia rubra vera and chronic myeloid leukaemia, is intimate. The typical patient is a middle-aged or elderly adult, the primary disorder being metaplasia of the marrow cells to fibrous tissue. The usual presenting complaints are fatigue and abdominal fullness due to hepatosplenomegaly. Obliteration of the haematopoietic tissue results in progressive anaemia, the appearance of immature red and white cells in the peripheral blood and compensatory splenomegaly. In the later stages of the disease, the fibrous tissue becomes converted to bone and endosteal cortical thickening develops. Polycythaemia may be followed by myeloid metaplasia and it appears probable that nearly half of the developed cases of myeloid metaplasia previously had some form of this blood disorder. Purine hypermetabolism may manifest itself as secondary gout.

Radiological changes. In the sclerotic stage of the disease increased density of the bones may be diffuse or patchy in nature. Areas of relative translucency due to fibrosis may persist. The increased density is due to new bone deposition on the trabeculae and also to the endosteal cortical thickening. Narrowing of the medullary space becomes clearly visible and resembles, in the long bones, the later stages of sickle-cell anaemia. Irregular periosteal reactions, particularly near the ends of long bones, may occur. These may be well organized and continuous with the cortex or separated from it by a zone of translucency. While the red marrow areas (particularly the pelvis) are especially subject to these pathological changes, the whole skeleton may be affected. Density of the skull is associated with obliteration of the diploic space, though some persistent areas of fibrosis may remain translucent. Splenomegaly is almost invariably evident (Fig. 7.18).

Differentiation must be made from other conditions causing a generalized increase of bone density. The congenital sclerosing dysplasias, including osteopetrosis, are likely to be encountered in adult life only as an incidental finding or in association with a pathological fracture. *Fluorosis* is likely to occur in an endemic area. *Mastocytosis* may cause some confusion, but the lesions are usually less diffuse and are accompanied by urticaria pig-

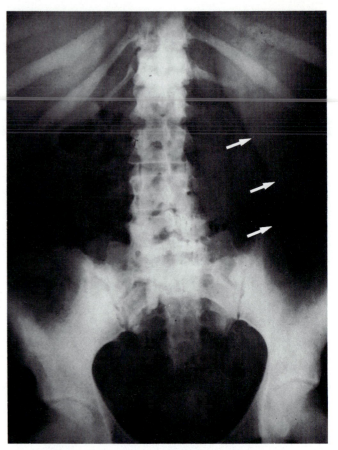

Fig. 7.18 Myeloid metaplasia (woman aged 63). All the bones are diffusely dense with lack of distinction between cortical and medullary bone. The spleen is grossly enlarged (arrows).

mentosa. Sclerosing and widespread *metastasis*, particularly prostatic, should never be forgotten.

DISORDERS OF THE LYMPHORETICULAR SYSTEM

Four main groups of disorder will be considered, divided for convenience as follows:

A. Lymphomas: including Hodgkin's and non-Hodgkin's lymphomas;
B. Plasma cell disease: plasmacytoma and multiple myeloma;
C. Histiocytosis;
D. Storage disorders: Gaucher's disease and Niemann-Pick disease.

THE LYMPHOMAS

The classification of the proliferative disorders of the lymphoreticular system is changing constantly and is based essentially upon histological features detected in lymph nodes. Consequently caution is necessary in extending such classifications to bone or bowel lymphoma. **Malignant lymphoma** is a generic term embracing all previously named tumours, including Hodgkin's disease, lymphadenoma, lymphosarcoma, reticulum-cell sarcoma and others.

Malignant lymphomas may be subdivided into two groups: Hodgkin's disease and a group of non-Hodgkin's lymphomas.

HODGKIN'S DISEASE

This defined tumour has an agreed classification on histological grounds, named after Rye. This comprises nodular sclerosing Hodgkin's disease, a complaint of young women involving intrathoracic lymph nodes, and three others: lymphocyte-dominant Hodgkin's disease, mixed Hodgkin's disease and lymphocyte-depleted Hodgkin's disease. The last three comprise a spectrum with, in order listed, worsening outlook. Bone involvement always implies a less favourable prognosis. It is a

feature of widespread disease and has been found at postmortem in more than half of cases. Skeletal lesions at presentation are far less common. Primary Hodgkin's disease of bone probably does not occur. There is no correlation between the variety of Hodgkin's disease and the nature of the individual bony lesions it produces.

The age of onset varies widely from childhood to old age but the diagnosis is most commonly made in young adults. The red marrow areas are the most frequent sites of presentation, the majority of lesions being found in the *spine*, *thoracic cage* and *pelvis*. Bone pain may precede, by several months, the development of these lesions and the importance of serial radiological examination either radiographic or scintigraphic must be stressed.

Radiological changes in the skeleton. The majority of early bone lesions are destructive and often large at the time they are first observed, either from direct involvement from affected soft tissues, particularly lymph nodes, or from infiltration of bone marrow. About a third are essentially osteolytic in type (Fig. 7.19). The majority are however of mixed type with patchy sclerosis and destruction (Fig. 7.20). Diffuse trabecular thickening causes sclerotic lesions in the remainder (Fig. 7.21). Such an appearance may develop in a few months, being preceded

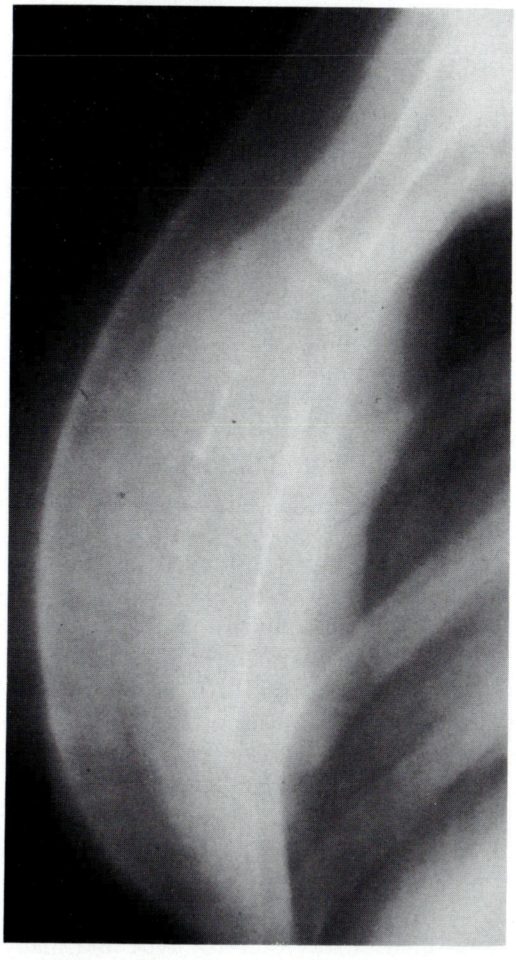

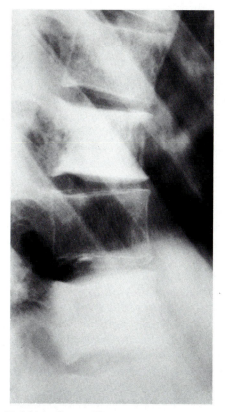

Fig. 7.19 Hodgkin's disease. An expanding, destructive lesion involves the body of the sternum, with anterior and posterior soft tissue masses. Bizarre changes in this bone should always arouse suspicion of a lymphoma.

Fig. 7.20 Hodgkin's disease. The common pattern of endosteal sclerosis and patchy bone destruction is shown in the vertebral body of T9 in an adult man. Similar changes are also present at T11. These features are virtually diagnostic.

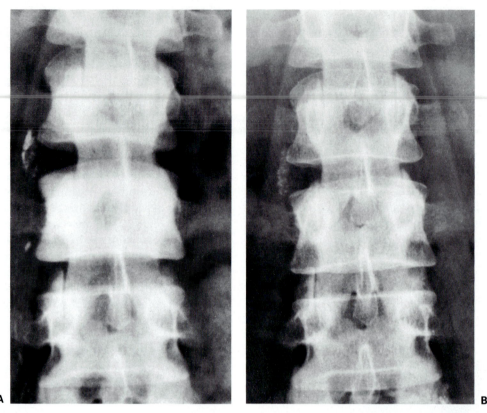

Fig. 7.21 Hodgkin's disease. **A.** Diffuse sclerosis is present in the bodies of L2 and L3 in a young woman at presentation with the disease. **B.** $2\frac{1}{2}$ years later, following treatment, the appearances have reverted to normal. (Lymphographic contrast medium is present in para-aortic nodes.)

by bone pain, and may well show no preliminary bone destruction. It may also follow treatment of a formerly osteolytic lesion. Conversely, some sclerotic lesions may be observed to become osteolytic or normal following treatment (Fig. 7.21). Whereas the osteolytic lesions may thin, displace and erode the overlying cortex and develop associated soft-tissue masses, the primary sclerotic lesion does not cause enlargement of the affected bone. Skeletal *scintigraphy* is a sensitive means of detecting the presence of bony lesions, particularly when sclerotic deposits have developed. The method is less reliable when purely lytic lesions are present. *MRI* is extremely sensitive (Fig. 7.22).

The *spine* is by far the most frequently involved area. A feature which is almost diagnostic is anterior erosion of a vertebral body (Fig. 7.23). This may or may not present reactive sclerosis in its margin and is attributed to involvement of adjacent paravertebral lymph nodes. Several vertebrae may be affected and the osteolytic lesions are likely to collapse. Soft-tissue masses will stimulate paravertebral abscesses. The sclerotic type shows a diffuse increase of density, possibly also with some anterior erosion but without increase in size of the affected body. A solitary dense vertebra, especially in young adults, is suggestive of this disease. In all these types the intervertebral discs are usually spared, aiding differentiation from an infection. Even in the rare cases where a disc space does become narrowed, preservation of density of the vertebral end-plates usually permits differentiation from an infective discitis where loss of this density is an early diagnostic sign. Lesions in the *ribs* may be found by themselves, sometimes being observed in a chest radiograph. They are usually osteolytic and expanding in type.

The *sternum* is also a not infrequent site for a lesion to appear, again usually osteolytic, but sometimes mixed in type with perpendicular spicules of new bone. Presternal and retrosternal soft-tissue swelling is not uncommon (Fig. 7.19). In the *pelvis*, mixed or sclerosing types tend to preponderate. The medial portions of the innominate bones are often dense. Osteolytic lesions, rather non-specific in appearance, are not uncommon in the ischia and change from either type to the mixed pattern may be observed in serial examinations. In the *long bones* the sites of predilection are the red marrow areas in the proximal portions of the femora and humeri. These are much more often of the osteolytic type and many small translucencies, oval in the long axis of the bone, may extend throughout the marrow cavity and may cause endosteal scalloping of the cortex. While such an appearance

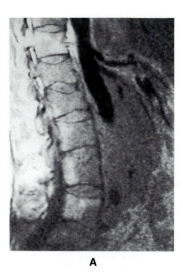
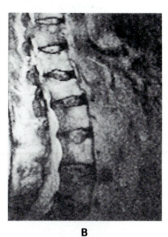
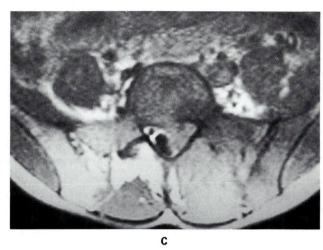

Fig. 7.22 Hodgkin's lymphoma. T_{18}-weighted (**A**) and STIR (**B**) sagittal images demonstrate extensive abnormality of the marrow of the lumbar spine. In addition a huge mass of lymph nodes is demonstrated anteriorly, wrapped around the abdominal aorta and displacing the superior mesenteric artery. An axial image (**C**) demonstrates not only body and left ala of the sacrum but also subcutaneous and intrathecal extension of tumour. The cauda equina is 'isplaced to the right.

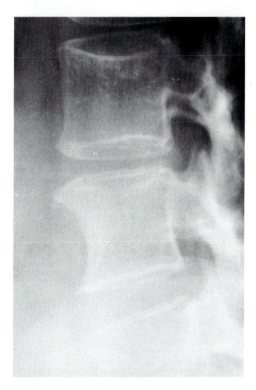

Fig. 7.23 Hodgkin's disease. A typical anterior scalloping of L4 is due to pressure erosion from enlarged lymph nodes. The cortex is preserved, as are the disc spaces.

is a feature of this disease, it may be observed also in *non-Hodgkin's lymphoma, leukaemia* and *Gaucher's disease.* Fusion of such areas may produce a honeycomb pattern, with coarse residual trabeculation, very like the medullary changes of Gaucher's disease. Organized periosteal reactions are not infrequent. Such a feature is rare in

Gaucher's disease. The skull, clavicles and scapulae are sometimes affected. Pathological fractures are uncommon. With sclerosing lesions in elderly individuals, confusion with *Paget's disease* may easily arise, but the characteristic enlargement of the affected bone in that disease will probably be absent. Differentiation, in all these lesions, must be made from *metastasis.* Intrathoracic disease may present with *hypertrophic osteoarthropathy.*

NON-HODGKIN'S LYMPHOMA

This forms a much more difficult spectrum of disease with no simple classification. That commonly used is based on lymph-node histology (Rappaport), though the application of such a classification to bone disease may not be reliable. Broadly speaking, non-Hodgkin's lymphoma in bone may be divided into three groups. The first, with larger cells histologically, essentially with a poor prognosis, was formerly called *reticulum cell sarcoma.* Another with multiple small round cells, and a much less aggressive nature, was called *lymphosarcoma.* This group merges into a spectrum with other small round-cell tumours including *Ewing's sarcoma* and *chronic lymphocytic leukaemia.* The third group is *Burkitt's lymphoma* (see below), which may be distinguished by nature of presentation and the age of patient.

It is difficult to assess how many patients actually present with primary skeletal non-Hodgkin's lymphoma; the proportion is probably less than one third, the majority of patients having diffuse disease at diagnosis. Experience suggests that reticulum cell sarcoma may present as a primary bone tumour, although in older patients particularly it can be multifocal and systemic. It is unlikely that lymphosarcoma ever presents primarily in the skeleton.

RETICULUM CELL SARCOMA

This condition represents about 3% of all apparent primary malignant tumours of bone. The presentation is of localized pain and swelling, often over a protracted period. The tumour may be asymptomatic, lesions presenting with pathological fracture. Males are affected twice as commonly as females. The majority are observed in the third and fourth decades although presentation during later years is not unusual. The lesions may be multifocal in the older age group. These tumours may be confused with other malignancies including osteosarcoma, metastasis and malignant round-cell tumours. Indeed differentiation between these tumours in a young adult may be extremely difficult, not only on clinical and radiological grounds, but also histologically.

The lesion may arise as an apparently *primary* tumour within bone marrow tending to remain confined to the skeleton, although it may spread to other bones and only at a later stage to lymph nodes and viscera. The latter structures, in contrast, may be involved first in the *extra-skeletal* form of reticulum cell sarcoma, which invades the skeleton only in its later stages.

In its primary form the condition is localized to a single bone with a marked predilection for the long bones. Nearly half the cases occur in the vicinity of the knee (Fig. 7.24) often with an associated synovial effusion. The proximal end of the humerus is another common site (Fig. 7.25) and about a third of cases are found in the flat bones of the axial skeleton. Spinal, rib and pelvic involvement tends to occur with the extraskeletal form, and in the older age group.

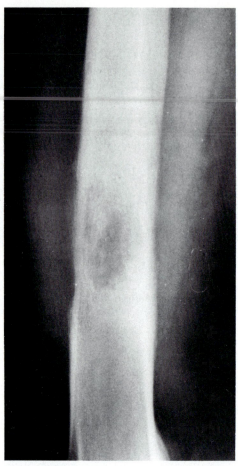

Fig. 7.24 Non-Hodgkin's lymphoma — reticulum cell sarcoma. A purely destructive lesion is present in the distal femur of a woman patient. The margins are ill-defined with cortical destruction. Periosteal new bone formation is present adjacent to this destruction. These appearances resemble metastasis and osteosarcoma.

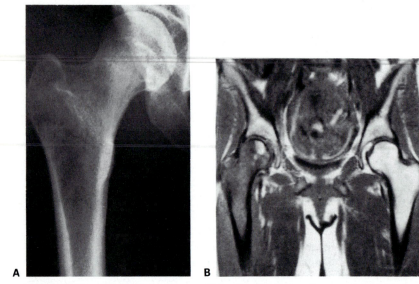
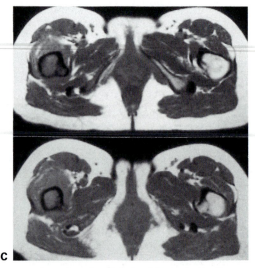

Fig. 7.25 Non-Hodgkin's lymphoma. Plain film (**A**) is virtually normal save for the slight suggestion of patchy ill-defined bone destruction. Subsequent T$_1$-weighted coronal (**B**) and axial (**C**) MR images demonstrate not only extensive marrow replacement but also a substantial enveloping soft-tissue mass. The degree and extent of tumour involvement of bone was virtually impossible to appreciate from film examinations.

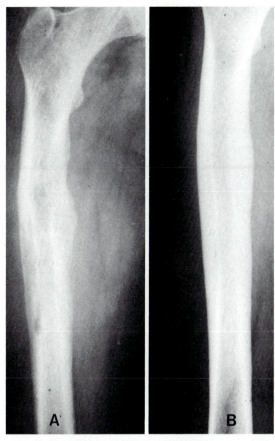

Fig. 7.26 Non-Hodgkin's lymphoma — reticulum cell sarcoma. Advanced changes are shown in the femoral shaft, with dramatic resolution 11 months later following local radiotherapy.

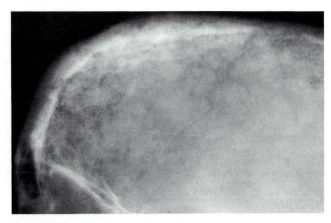

Fig. 7.27 Non-Hodgkin's lymphoma — reticulum cell sarcoma. Extensive patchy destruction of the cranium was present in this adult patient with generalized disease.

The tumour is extremely radiosensitive and radiotherapy alone or combined with amputation has resulted in many long survivals (Fig. 7.26). Even though a primary lesion may have regressed entirely with radiotherapy, generalized skeletal dissemination is likely to occur eventually.

Radiological changes. The earliest evidence of the tumour is diffuse medullary destruction of a patchy nature with very poorly defined margins (Fig. 7.25, 7.27). At this stage it may be impossible to differentiate the lesion radiologically from any other aggressive neoplasm. In particular, an *osteolytic metastasis* is likely to present the greatest difficulty. The lesion may resemble other primary malignant neoplasms stimulating little or no reactive bone formation such as *Ewing's tumour, fibrosarcoma* or *malignant fibrous histiocytoma*. Radiological confusion with osteomyelitis may also arise, particularly as overlying periosteal reaction is present in half the cases (Fig. 7.24). Indeed periosteal reaction may be present before medullary changes become evident. Scintigraphically the features are unremarkable. Usually increased activity is detected. Multifocal lesions may be found. Radiologically the area of destruction spreads widely through the marrow cavity and remains patchy in nature. Much of the adjacent cortex undergoes resorption with the development of well-defined soft-tissue swellings from soft-tissue tumour extension. Cortical thickening and reactive sclerosis are not prominent features, although they may occur exceptionally.

In the generalized form of the disease, lesions may be detected throughout the skeleton and each present the same characteristics as a solitary focus (Fig. 7.28). The patient is likely to be over the age of 40. The ultimate degree of osseous destruction may be extreme.

LYMPHOSARCOMA

This malignant tumour is rarer than Hodgkin's disease and mainly affects an older age group: patients in the fifth and sixth decades. Nonetheless a number of cases have been observed in children and in these a male sex preponderance has been found. A proportion of these patients develop frank lymphocytic leukaemia.

The incidence of bone lesions is of the order of 10–20%, although more are detected at post-mortem. Prognostically bone lesions imply a poor outcome. Primary skeletal involvement is probably extremely rare.

Radiological changes in the skeleton resemble very closely those of Hodgkin's disease; other lesions grow more rapidly and are almost always osteolytic in type. Areas of destruction, commonly in red marrow areas, may be large with diffuse and irregular margins, and with scalloping of the inner aspects of the cortex. They may be solitary or multiple and, because of their osteolytic nature, pathological fractures are common. The latter affect especially the femoral and humeral necks and may cause collapse of vertebral bodies. When the lesions are multiple they all tend to be of the same osteolytic type, unlike Hodgkin's disease when all the different types of bone change may be present. Erosion of the cortex is likely to be followed by the formation of large associated soft-

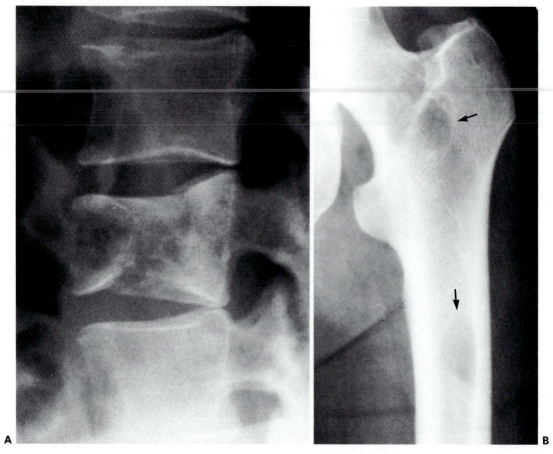

Fig. 7.28 A,B Non-Hodgkin's lymphoma — reticulum cell sarcoma. Multifocal disease was found at presentation in an elderly patient with low back pain. In addition to a pathological fracture of a lumbar vertebral body, ill-defined endosteal defects are present in the femoral shaft (arrows).

tissue masses with relatively little periosteal reaction. Such erosions usually take place through an area of cortex which has already been thinned and expanded by underlying pathological process, emphasizing the radiological similarity of the individual lesions to Ewing's sarcoma.

BURKITT'S TUMOUR

An exceptional and particularly aggressive form of lymphoma is common in African children and has been reported in other parts of the world. Large, destructive lesions develop especially in the mandible and maxilla (Fig. 7.29).

Radiologically these lesions are purely osteolytic and grow rapidly. The jaw lesions are characterized by the resorption of the lamina dura with multiple lytic foci which eventually coalesce with radiating spicules of bone. Spinal lesions are characterised by lytic, ill-defined destructive foci with paravertebral masses. In long bones the permeative lytic nature of the tumour, particularly with cortical erosions, may resemble a Ewing's sarcoma.

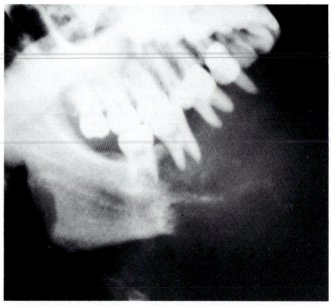

Fig. 7.29 Burkitt's tumour. A large destructive lesion in the mandible of this African child is typical of this form of lymphoma.

Foci develop in soft tissues, particularly the kidneys, ovaries and abdominal lymph nodes.

The disease is associated with a virus (Epstein-Barr) and is especially prevalent in endemic malarial areas. Regression can occur following the use of cytotoxic drugs.

MASTOCYTOSIS

The rare condition of urticaria pigmentosa is associated with enlargement of the liver, spleen and lymph nodes due to the proliferation of mast cells. The disease is relatively benign, but a few instances of leukaemic termination have been recorded. Bone changes are usually identified in early adult life.

Radiological changes. In probably a third of cases, generalized skeletal changes are present. These are diffuse or circumscribed areas of increased density, apparently due to thickening of the medullary trabeculae (Fig. 7.30). It may be difficult to identify the endosteal margin of the cortex. The absorption of some trabeculae and the thickening of others may cause the osseous structures to have a coarse pattern but the generalized increase in density usually pre-dominates. Any bone may be affected. At this stage it is possible to demonstrate only a few mast cells in the bone marrow. The appearance may closely resemble *myelosclerosis*, the *sclerosing types of leukaemia, chronic anaemias* and *osteopetrosis*. Occasionally the dense areas are sharply defined, of considerable size and localized to

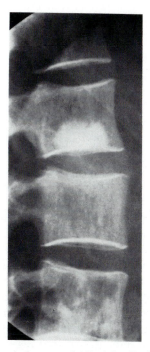

Fig. 7.30 Mastocytosis (man aged 34). A localized area of endosteal sclerosis is present in the body of L1. In addition, ill-defined thinning of trabeculae is demonstrated in L2 and patchier changes in the upper surface of L3.

a few areas. Particularly in young adults, differentiation from *Hodgkin's disease* must be made.

PLASMA CELL DISEASES

Plasma cells represent the end-product of B-lymphocyte maturation. Pathological proliferation produces either a local tumour (plasmacytoma) or disseminate disease (myelomatosis).

PLASMACYTOMA

This condition is unifocal, causing a localized destructive lesion in the skeleton, in a red marrow area. Many other descriptive terms, such as solitary myeloma, for this localized lesion have been used. Although for many years it may remain localized, and without health disturbance, ultimately it undergoes transition to generalized myelomatosis. A latent interval of 5–10 years is usual. Consequently the outlook is better than multiple myelomatosis. In comparison with the latter these lesions are uncommon. The exact incidence is difficult to assess since they are frequently asymptomatic. For example, a plasmacytoma in a rib may be noted incidentally on a routine examination of the chest.

When symptoms occur they are commonly those of bone pain, particularly backache. The vertebral bodies, especially in the thoracolumbar and lumbar regions, are the most common sites for these lesions and are likely to undergo partial collapse. The pelvis, especially the ilium, femur and humerus, are the next most commonly involved sites.

The vast majority of affected individuals are between 30 and 60 years of age so that this is almost entirely a disease of late middle age. The differential diagnosis always includes a solitary osteolytic metastasis.

Radiological changes. These lesions arise in areas of red marrow function. Bone expansion, which may be considerable with thinning of the overlying cortex, is common but, when a vertebral body is affected, collapse may precede such apparent expansions. The margins are usually well-defined and sharply demarcated and characteristically without a sclerotic reaction (Fig. 7.31). Coarse trabecular strands of increased density may give a network appearance in the area of destruction, and exceptionally the lesion may be entirely sclerotic. Large lesions in flat bones may assume a soap-bubble appearance (Fig. 7.32).

Differential diagnosis of these tumours may be difficult. In view of the age group concerned the most important is an osteolytic metastasis. In vertebrae, such metastases are likely to involve the pedicles more commonly. Metastatic disease apart, the development of a solitary osteolytic lesion in a vertebral body in a patient of the late middle age should always be considered as a plasmacytoma. Chordoma may produce similar features.

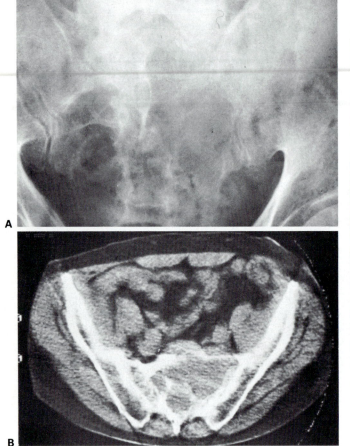

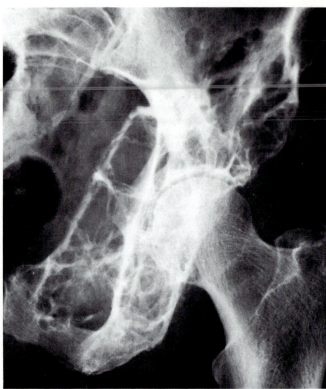

Fig. 7.32 Plasmacytoma of pelvis. This very extensive lesion was unaccompanied by any systemic abnormality. Bone expansion is associated with coarse trabeculation, producing a soap bubble appearance.

Fig. 7.31 Plasmacytoma of sacrum. **A**. An adult man exhibits a well-defined radiolucent defect involving the left sacral ala. **B**. CT scan demonstrated extensive destructive nature of the tumour, seen clearly to cross the mid line. Note the marked cortical thinning with absence of sclerosis or periosteal new bone formation.

Other differential diagnoses to be considered, especially with an expanding lytic focus in a rib, are *fibrous dysplasia*, a *'brown' tumour of hyperparathyroidism* and, particularly when the lesion is adjacent to an articular surface, a *giant-cell tumour*. Resemblance to a giant-cell tumour may be close; however, these lesions are found in early adult life and furthermore have a different distribution, commonly affecting the appendicular skeleton, whereas plasma-cytoma is more likely to be axial. Scintigraphy and CT afford no specific diagnostic features. Increased activity is observed on the blood-pool phase of a bone scan, while the delayed phase shows increased activity around the margins. CT confirms the extent of these tumours but does not afford tissue-specific information.

MULTIPLE MYELOMATOSIS

The disseminated or generalized form of plasma cell infiltration of bone marrow is known as multiple myelomatosis. This entity may be preceded by a solitary plasmacytoma or arise de novo.

It is much more common for the widespread form to present radiologically as a fully developed entity in the over-40 age group. Men are affected twice as often as women. Persistent bone pain or a pathological fracture are usually the first complaints.

Plasma cell proliferation causes elevation of the total serum proteins, due to the production of abnormal im-munoglobulins. Such proliferation eventually takes place at the expense of all other marrow functions so that a non-specific leucopenia and secondary anaemia develop. In about half of cases, presence of an abnormal urinary protein constituent, Bence-Jones proteose, may be demonstrated. Abnormal proteinuria causes cast formation in the renal tubules with impairment of renal function. Hyper-calcaemia, hypercalcuria and atypical amyloidosis occur, the last in about 10% of all cases. The hypercalcaemia and hypercalcuria are unassociated with an elevation of either the serum alkaline phosphatase or phosphate levels.

The pattern of bone destruction may vary from diffuse osteoporosis, through small and almost insignificant areas of translucency, to rounded or oval defects with sharply defined margins. The last, regarded as characteristic, develops relatively late. Frequently they coalesce to produce even larger areas of osteolysis.

Radiological changes. The two cardinal features are generalized reduction in bone density and localized areas of radiolucency in red marrow areas. The axial skeleton, therefore, is affected predominantly. Lesions may be observed also in the shafts of long bones and in the skull. In spite of positive bone-marrow aspiration, radiological features may be absent in as many as one third of cases, at least at initial presentation. This group of patients tend to develop generalized osteoporosis.

Since the detection of skeletal lesions is important in management, radiology plays a large part in assessing the extent of disease. Generally speaking a radiographic skeletal survey is superior to scintigraphic investigation using a bone-scanning agent, because the lesions are essentially osteolytic with no bone reaction. A bone scan is superior, however, in detecting lesions in the ribs because the associated fractures are demonstrated more easily. MRI may be unreliable in the detection of lesions.

Diffuse osteoporosis alone can cause suspicion of the disease in an elderly patient. Even though senile osteoporosis may be expected, the possibility of myelomatosis always merits consideration, particularly when symptomatic bone pain is present. The smaller areas of radiolucency are poorly demarcated and appear to be irregular accentuations of the generalized osteoporotic process (Fig. 7.33). The rounded and oval defects that develop are characterized by the sharp definition of their edges. Reactive marginal sclerosis is absent. Typically the cortex is eroded from within sharply defined margins (Fig. 7.34). Exceptionally, however, *sclerosing changes* have been reported. These have varied, some resembling focal lesions of prostatic metastases, some the spiculation of osteosarcoma and some a generalized diffuse increase in density. This very rare form of multiple mylomatosis occurs in probably 2% of cases, and is frequently accompanied by a peripheral neuropathy.

Treatment, as in other conditions, may alter these appearances and, during its course, it is common to observe some lesions resolving whilst others evolve.

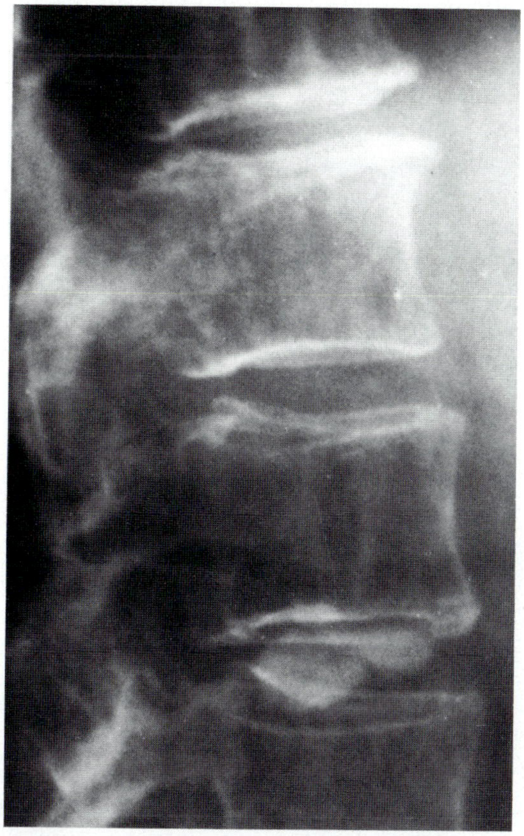

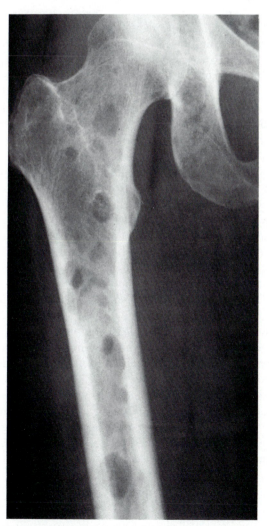

Fig. 7.33 Myelomatosis. Diffuse marrow involvement has resulted in an overall reduction in bone density similar to that seen in osteoporosis. However the rather patchy nature of radiolucencies should raise the possibility of myeloma.

Fig. 7.34 Typical localized lesions of myeloma are demonstrated in the upper femur of an adult woman. The sharply defined rounded defects with endosteal erosion of the cortex are characteristic.

The *distribution of lesions* is very widespread and destructive foci are commonly located in the long bones in addition to the axial skeleton. Involvement of the *skull* is variable. Diffuse and irregular translucencies with generalized osteoporosis are not uncommon. Such changes eventually become pronounced and extensive. The disease will not always be evident by the presence of the classical 'rain-drop' lesions, circular defects varying in diameter from a few millimetres to 2 or 3 cm. Indeed, the skull may be normal, even in the presence of many lesions elsewhere in the skeleton. Areas of osteolysis may be observed also in the *mandible*, a site only rarely affected by metastasis. Myelomatous lesions, may erode the cortex and extend into the adjacent soft tissues. The resulting soft-tissue masses are helpful in differentiating the advanced forms of the disease from the lesions of *metastatic carcinoma* which much less commonly produce extension into the soft tissues. The *spine* is often merely osteoporotic, but as the disease advances, multiple foci of destruction, almost invariably accompanied by some degree of collapse of the affected bodies, are likely to be present. With such collapse, paravertebral soft-tissue shadows are common. Differentiation from inflammatory lesions can be made, as the intervertebral disc spaces and the articular surfaces are not affected. The pedicles and posterior elements are involved less frequently and at a later stage than occurs with metastases. In the thorax a destructive rib lesion with a large associated soft-tissue mass is much more suggestive of myelomatosis than of a plasmacytoma. Diffuse involvement, however, is more usual, numerous cystic foci of characteristic appearance being visible. The *clavicles* and *scapulae* may also show these destructive changes.

The *long bones* are affected most commonly in the persistent red-marrow areas of the proximal ends of the humeri and femora. Lesions, however, are by no means found only in such areas and irregular or punched-out translucencies in the shafts of other bones may be the first radiological manifestation of disease. In some advanced cases lytic defects may be due also to *secondary amyloidosis*, which can complicate many chronic disorders, such as rheumatoid disease and long-standing infections.

Pathological fractures are very often the initiating factor in the diagnosis of the disease. These fractures heal remarkably quickly and soundly with massive callus and new bone formation. This response is somewhat surprising in view of the numerous cystic lesions and widespread osteoporosis which are likely to be present without any evidence of reactive sclerosis.

HISTIOCYTOSIS

The basic pathological abnormality in this group of diseases is a proliferation of histiocytic cells occurring particularly in the bone marrow, the spleen, the liver, the lymphatic glands and the lungs. In the more chronic forms these cells become swollen with lipid deposits, essentially cholesterol (though the blood cholesterol level remains normal) and they present the pathological appearances of 'foam cells'. Some of these become necrotic and are replaced by fibrous tissue.

Various forms of the condition have been regarded in the past as separate entities. These forms are outlined below but it must be emphasized that this subdivision is entirely arbitrary since histiocytosis essentially presents a spectrum of disease.

EOSINOPHILIC GRANULOMA

This is the most mild expression of histiocytosis. Pathological changes are predominantly bony, although occasionally pulmonary involvement may occur. Children, especially boys, between 3 and 12 years are most commonly affected, although these lesions may be observed in adolescents, young adults and exceptionally the middle-aged. Any bone may be affected. A quarter of cases occur in the skull. The skull, pelvis and femora between them account for nearly two thirds of all cases.

Clinically pain and swelling may be accompanied by mild fever. Histologically the eosinophilic infiltration is found around collections of histiocytes. In this relatively mild form necrosis and fibrosis are rare and the appearance of foam cells suggests a more serious variety.

Radiological changes. Translucent areas of bone destruction, with sharply defined margins and often of considerable size, are characteristic. The round or oval defects may have scalloped margins (Fig. 7.35). Although in the active phase they provoke no sclerotic margin, the healing phase, which usually develops by spontaneous regression, is marked by peripheral sclerosis round the lesion and slow reconstitution of the bony structure. This healing phase may be accelerated by biopsy, radiotherapy or steroid injection. True expansion is uncommon except

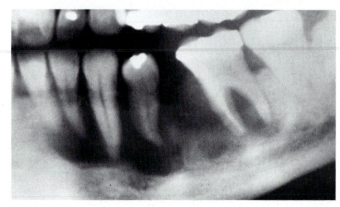

Fig. 7.35 Histiocytosis. A purely osteolytic lesion is present in the mandible, with well-defined, slightly scalloped margins. The lamina dura has been destroyed. The teeth seem to 'float in air'.

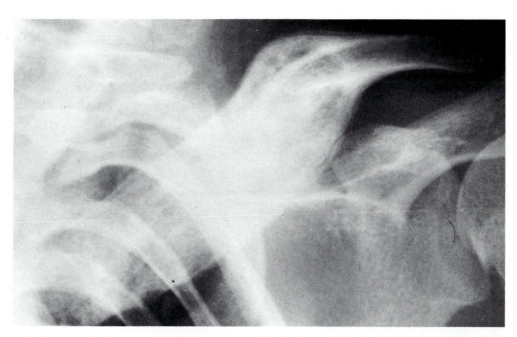

Fig. 7.36 Histiocytosis. Extensive involvement of a bone, here the clavicle, is often associated with layered periosteal new bone causing bony expansion. Ill-defined areas of resorption may be visualized in the lesion. This was the only abnormality found in a young girl over several years' follow-up.

in ribs and vertebral bodies. Apparent expansion may result from thickening of the overlying periosteum, especially if the cortex has been partially eroded (Fig. 7.36) or infarction has occurred. In approximately two-thirds of patients the lesions are *solitary*. Differential diagnosis of a solitary lesion of this type may be extremely difficult and is either from osteomyelitis or Ewing's tumour, which has a similar age incidence. Skeletal survey may disclose the presence of other asymptomatic lesions, facilitating the diagnosis. Multiple eosinophilic granulomas are usually found to be in different phases of evolution. As one lesion revolves another may appear in a different part of the skeleton. In the skull particularly, new lesions several centimetres in diameter may appear in as many weeks. Button sequestra may be observed. Skeletal scintigraphy is a sensitive means of detecting the lesions, particularly in the healing phase, and may be used in follow-up studies.

Solitary lesions in the spine may collapse, partially or completely, the latter presenting the classical appearance of *vertebra plana* (Fig. 7.37). The most commonly affected site is the thoracic spine. The lesions at one time were considered to represent an 'osteochondritis' and were named *Calvé's disease*. During the phase of collapse, the walls of the affected vertebral body tend to bulge laterally and paravertebral soft tissue shadows may be evident. The disc spaces on either side remain intact and may even be widened. As healing occurs, remarkably good reconstitution of these vertebral bodies may take place if sufficient years of growth remain. The vast ma-

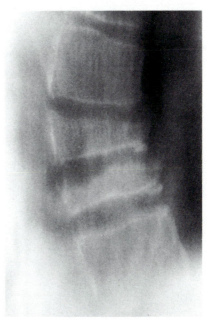

Fig. 7.37 Histiocytosis. Vertebral lesions in the thoracic spine are shown on a lateral tomogram. The bodies of T7 and 8 have collapsed with a slight increase in bone density. Note the relative preservation of the disc spaces.

jority of vertebra plana lesions, especially in a relatively healthy child, are caused by an eosinophil granuloma, and confirmatory biopsy is usually unnecessary. The differential diagnosis of collapse of a single vertebral body includes the relative rarities of Ewing's tumour, metastasis from a neuroblastoma, benign osteoblastoma or, most exceptionally, a bizarre and atypical tuberculous focus.

This benign form of histiocytosis occasionally affects long bones and initially has a predilection for the dia-

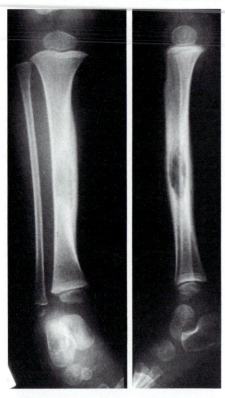

Fig. 7.38 Histiocytosis. A healing diaphyseal lesion exhibits periosteal new bone formation and minimal sclerosis around the margins of the radiolucency.

physis (Fig. 7.38). However, metaphyseal involvement may occur again causing confusion with a pyogenic infection. A rare entity, *chronic granulomatous (Landing-Shirkey) disease,* tends to cause skeletal lesions, including those in the metaphyses, which simulate closely the radiological appearance of multiple eosinophil granulomas. This condition is usually due to inherited and inadequate responses of leukocytes to infection.

HAND-SCHÜLLER-CHRISTIAN DISEASE

This is a more chronic form of the disease, with dissemination of lesions in the lungs, lymph nodes, liver and spleen, in addition to virtually constant and early involvement of the skeleton.

The early case reports drew attention to a syndrome consisting of skull defects, exophthalmos and diabetes in-

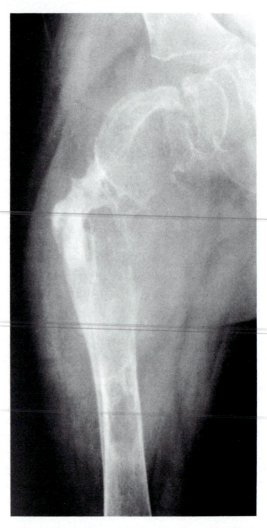

Fig. 7.40 Histiocytosis. Hand-Schüller-Christian type. Very extensive radiolucencies are present both in the metaphysis and diaphysis of this child's femur. A healed pathological fracture is present. Histiocytosis should always be considered in the differential diagnosis of bizarre bone lesions.

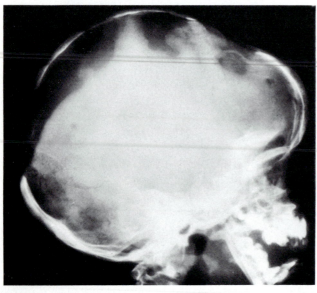

Fig. 7.39 Histiocytosis. Extensive skull involvement in a child with the Hand-Schüller-Christian type of lesion. The areas of destruction in the flat bones of the skull have a map-like configuration.

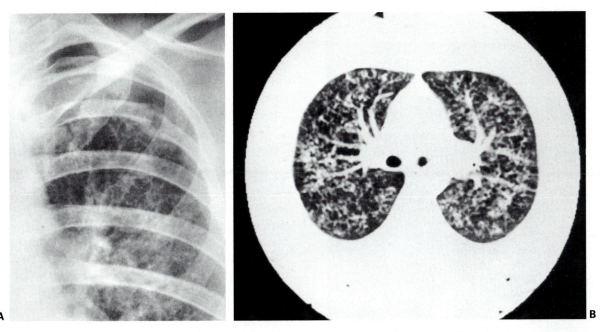

Fig. 7.41 Histiocytosis. Adult pulmonary involvement (man aged 20). **A**. A localized view from a chest X-ray demonstrates a coarse interstitial pulmonary fibrosis. Note also a pathological fracture of the left fourth rib due to a bony deposit. **B**. A CT scan demonstrates clearly peripheral interstitial pulmonary fibrosis with focal emphysema. (L 374, W 400.)

sipidus, the last two being associated with lesions round the orbit and the hypophysis respectively. Children below the age of 5 years are most frequently affected, though sporadic cases occur at later ages up to middle life. The course of the disease is chronic, often extending over 10 or more years. It is characterized by soreness of the mouth and loose teeth, due to deposits in the gums and jaws, and skin lesions. Abnormalities in the temporal bone are common, with an associated otitis media. The eventual prognosis is good, since spontaneous remission, possibly initiated or accelerated by radiotherapy, takes place in the majority of cases. Over 10%, however, terminate fatally.

Radiological changes. The bone defects are essentially the same as those of eosinophil granulomas. They are, however, very much more numerous and particularly affect the flat bones. In the skull they frequently coalesce to produce widespread irregular defects usually likened to a map and described as the 'geographical skull', both tables often suffering extensive osteolysis (Fig. 7.39). Lesions in the mandible and maxilla begin round the tooth roots, so that the teeth, which are never affected, remain dense and appear to 'float in air' (Fig. 7.35). Several vertebrae may be completely or partially collapsed and extensive lesions may develop in the scapulae, ribs and pelvis. Osteolytic pelvic lesions or vertebral collapse in a child are suggestive of this disease. Long bone involvement is less common (Fig. 7.40).

In a relatively early stage, sclerotic reaction round the sharply defined margins of these lesions will be absent. When healing does occur the lesions fill in by sclerosis

in the same way as eosinophil granulomas. New lesions may appear after the original ones have begun to heal, emphasizing again the wide spectrum of radiological change in histiocytosis.

The lungs show a fine nodular infiltration in the acute phase. With healing, these fibrose and persist as linear strands of increased density, but the presence of pulmonary changes in histiocytosis indicates a worse prognosis (Fig. 7.41).

LETTERER-SIWE DISEASE

This is an acute or sub-acute disseminated form of the disease, occurring very rarely in infants below the age of 2 years and presenting a much more severe clinical picture. It is characterized by a pyrexia, with a rash and mouth sores, bleeding gums, respiratory symptoms and failure to thrive. Particular involvement of the extraskeletal tissues occurs with enlargement of the liver, spleen and lymph nodes. The disease usually ends fatally, often in a few months and at the most in 2 years. In those cases with a rapidly fatal outcome, skeletal lesions are unlikely to be demonstrated radiologically, having insufficient time to develop. Nevertheless, histological change may be present in the bone marrow, with widespread masses of histiocytes and eosinophilic infiltration, comparable with the early histological picture of the benign eosinophil granuloma. Only in the rare cases that survive do fibrosis and cholesterol-containing foam cells become apparent.

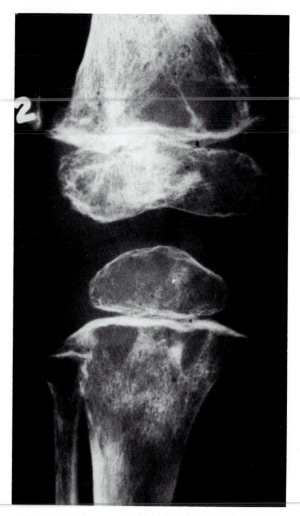

Fig. 7.42 Histiocytosis, Letterer-Siwe type. Massive destructive lesions are present throughout the skeleton, but affecting particularly the metadiaphyseal areas of the long bones. A similar appearance could be produced by metastases from a neuroblastoma or the advanced stages of leukaemia.

Radiological changes. Bone lesions, when they occur, are indistinguishable from those of Hand-Schüller-Christian disease, but tend to be even more widely spread, both in the flat bones and even more in the metadiaphyseal areas of the long bones (Fig. 7.42). They show no trace of the sclerotic reaction round their sharply-defined, punched-out margins. Diffuse pulmonary infiltration is common. This may closely resemble miliary tuberculosis and is a variety of honeycomb lung.

In summary, *histiocytosis* is a disease primarily of childhood, although exceptionally, its more benign manifestations may be observed in early adult life. The older the child, and the more the lesions are confined to the skeleton rather than other tissues, the better the prognosis. It must be appreciated that the benign eosinophil granuloma may deteriorate to a chronic, multifocal form of the spectrum, and rarely vice-versa.

STORAGE DISORDERS OF THE LYMPHORETICULAR SYSTEM

A number of conditions have been described in which the lymphoreticular system is the site of abnormal deposition of lipoproteins, usually as a result of inborn errors of metabolism. The commonest of these rare disorders are Gaucher's disease and Niemann-Pick disease.

GAUCHER'S DISEASE

Young Jewish females are particularly susceptible to this hereditary condition caused by deficiency of B-glucosidase. It is not confined to this ethnic group or sex. Although manifestations of the condition commonly become apparent in the later years of childhood and in early adult life, the disease may be so chronic, and of such insidious onset, that it may be recognized for the first time only in middle age or even later life. In infancy the rapidly fatal course of this systemic disease is characterized by gross neurological changes and pulmonary infiltration.

In the juvenile and young adult variety, the principal complaint is of weakness and fatigue with progressive dementia. On clinical examination splenic enlargement is detected in 95% of cases. Bone pain may be present, sometimes severe. In the chronic form of the disease characteristic and diagnostic bone changes may be expected. Histological examination reveals numerous large histiocytes within which an abnormal lipoprotein, *kerasin*, is present. These cells are disseminated throughout the marrow of the haematopoietic skeleton, in addition to the spleen and liver.

Radiological changes. Diffuse infiltration of the bone marrow causes widespread and irregular medullary radiolucency. When collections of the abnormal histiocytes occur destructive medullary lesions become visible and *abnormal modelling* of the long bones may be evident. Expansion of the distal ends of the femora begins with a loss of the normal concavity of the medial sides. Eventually this justifies the classical description of 'flask-shaped', on the analogy of the contour of the Erlenmeyer flask (Fig. 7.43). This feature is, however, not diagnostic of Gaucher's disease and may be seen in other conditions including haemolytic anaemias (thalassaemia), leukaemia, and osteopetrosis. Other bones, notably the tibia and humerus, may be similarly affected. *Destructive lesions* cause localized endosteal cortical erosions, with sharply-defined scalloped borders. As these lesions increase in size and coalesce, the areas of bone abnormality may become exceedingly widespread, both in the individual bone and in the skeleton as a whole. *Infarction* of bone is not uncommon (Fig. 7.44). The femoral and humeral heads, especially the former, are often involved in this way. In a child such infarction may simulate Perthes' disease. In an adult the destructive changes in the femoral

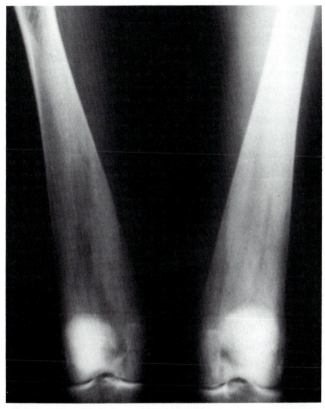

Fig. 7.43 Gaucher's disease (woman aged 20). Abnormal modelling of the distal ends of the femora has resulted in typical flask-shaped appearance. An osteolytic lesion with a coarse trabecular pattern is present in the right femur.

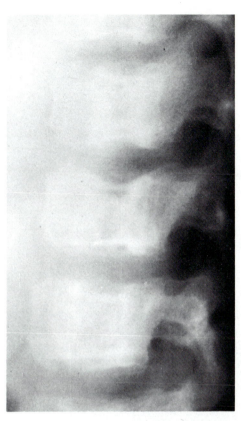

Fig. 7.44 Gaucher's disease. Infarctions in vertebral bodies have produced the 'bone within a bone' appearance throughout the lumbar spine in this child.

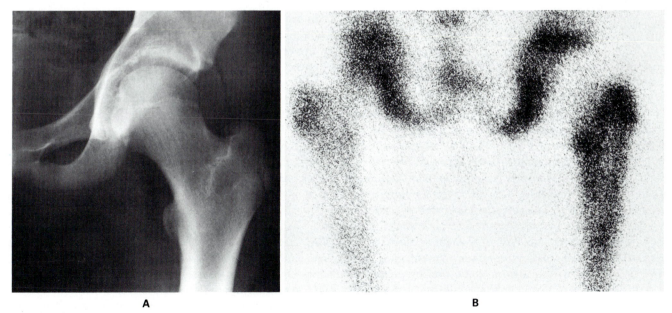

A   B

Fig. 7.45 Gaucher's disease — acute bone infarction. **A.** A radiograph of a 13-year-old girl, with known Gaucher's disease, presenting with acute hip pain of 12 hour's duration. Slight endosteal sclerosis is shown in the inferior pubic ramus and an area of ill-defined radiolucency in the intertrochanteric region. **B.** The delayed phase of a bone scan reveals the femoral head and neck to be markedly photon-deficient consistent with acute infarction. Abnormally increased activity is present also at site of previous disease.

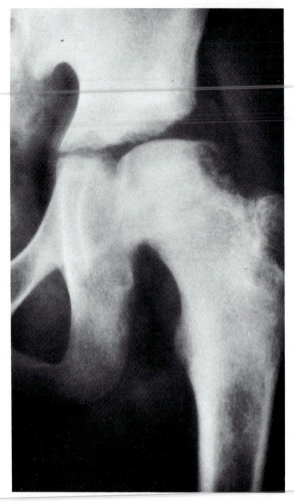

Fig. 7.46 Gaucher's disease. This adolescent has considerable deformity of the femoral head and acetabulum secondary to episodes of infarction. Evidence of degenerative arthritis is present already.

head that develop cannot be differentiated from avascular necrosis of other origin. Bone scintigraphy may be helpful in the assessment of acute bone pain in order to detect early infarction (Fig. 7.45). Subsequent disruption of articular surfaces promotes osteoarthritis (Fig. 7.46).

Pathological fractures may follow relatively minor trauma. While fractures may occur through any affected bone, compression of a vertebral body is the usual lesion. As in many other conditions, these compression fractures are most likely to be found in the lower dorsal or lumbar regions, the areas of greatest stress. Frank zones of osteolysis in the spine are rare in Gaucher's disease, but generalized osteoporosis is common. Pathological fractures also occur in the femoral neck causing coxa vara, and in sites where no concomitant radiological abnormality can be identified.

Usually bone trabeculae are destroyed, but the chronic form of the disease may be characterized by *sclerotic reaction* within the bone. A coarse network of dense medullary strands results which may give the appearance of a honeycomb. In addition, endosteal thickening may develop, as in the later stages of sickle cell disease and myelosclerosis, the appearances again being suggestive of 'a bone within a bone'. On the outer surface, diffuse periosteal reactions may develop, usually overlying an intact cortex.

As a result of these reactive changes in the later stages of the disease, the radiological picture may be confusing. It is particularly important for differentiation from *chronic osteomyelitis* to be made, as misguided surgical intervention has sometimes been followed by chronic and resistant infection with persistent discharging sinuses.

Unlike some of the other diseases in this group, notably the chronic haemolytic anaemias, the distribution of these lesions tends to be peripheral rather than central. The chronic form of the disease may cause characteristic changes in the first decade; the diffuse medullary osteoporosis and abnormality of modelling in the distal ends of the femora are likely to be the first radiological manifestations. The changes may be widespread and may resemble thalassaemia, except that the bones of the hands and feet are usually completely or relatively exempt.

In the adult, the long tubular bones are usually the site of lesions, destructive processes in the pelvis and thoracic cage being rarely evident. Nevertheless involvement of the axial skeleton does occur, as shown by the frequency of spinal osteoporosis and occasional vertebral collapse, which may be apparent even in the absence of other radiological evidence of this disease. No characteristic lesions are recognized in the skull, but diffuse osteoporosis has been reported. Frank cystic areas of destruction have been noted round the tooth roots in the mandible.

In the radiological assessment of any skeletal abnormality, appreciation of associated abnormalities of soft tissue is important. In this instance the combination of the changes described above, with a patient with an appropriate ethnic background and with *splenomegaly*, provides a strong diagnostic triad. Enlargement of the spleen, and often the liver, is almost constant in this disease. Pulmonary involvement is unusual, but an appearance suggestive of interstitial fibrosis may be observed, particularly in young children, even in the absence of skeletal involvement.

NIEMANN-PICK DISEASE

This rare disorder of the lymphoreticular system, of a type similar to Gaucher's disease, has, in its classic form, a predilection for Jewish girls under the age of 2 years. The abnormal lipoprotein in the 'foam cells' in this instance is *sphingomyelin*. Osseous changes, are less severe than in Gaucher's disease. Nevertheless, careful study may disclose generalized osteoporosis, minor coarsening of the trabeculae and minor modelling abnormalities.

Overt areas of osteolysis do occur, but are unusual and may resemble the lesions of histiocytosis. On the other hand interstitial pulmonary infiltration, causing a 'honeycomb' lung appearance and hepatosplenomegaly, are common in classic cases, for which the prognosis is grave. Other types of the condition have been recognized in older children.

DISORDERS OF THE COAGULATION MECHANISM

HAEMOPHILIA AND ITS VARIANTS

The normal process of blood coagulation depends on a number of factors. Many of these have been recognized and their individual deficiencies have led to descriptions of several disease entities within the haemophiliac group.

From the radiological aspect the most important of these disorders are classic **haemophilia**, due to deficiency of Factor VIII and the rarer **Christmas disease,** due to deficiency of Factor IX. These hereditary diseases primarily affect males, being X-linked, usually recessive disorders. The degree of affliction is related to the level of deficiency.

The bleeding tendency is usually observed during the first year of life and may affect any tissue system. Christmas disease is usually less severe. Bleeding is considered to result from trauma, possibly very slight, rather than being spontaneous. Bleeding into joints is characteristic. Such episodes commonly become more frequent during the later years of childhood and adolescence. Milder forms of the disease may cause formation of large, soft-tissue haematomas without significant joint involvement. This is true of **von Willebrand's disease**, which affects both sexes equally and is transmitted in an autosomal dominant manner. If, however, the Factor VIII level is low, bleeding into joints can occur in this condition.

Radiological changes in the skeleton are caused by bleeding into joints, within bony structures and beneath the periosteum. Frequent repetition of such episodes, particularly at an early age, increases their severity.

Intra-articular haemorrhage. In the early stages of the disease, the soft-tissue distension of a joint due to a haemarthrosis cannot be distinguished radiologically from a frank traumatic or inflammatory synovial effusion. Frequent repetition of haemorrhagic incidents results in synovial thickening and articular erosions. Initially these erosions tend to be marginal in distribution. At the same time the bony structures in the vicinity of an affected joint are likely to become porotic, partly through disuse, but even more through persistent hyperaemia associated with organization of the haemarthroses. This latter factor, as with hyperaemia of any other cause, commonly causes enlargement of the growing epiphyses (Fig. 7.47). Such epiphyses may also become abnormal in shape and often

fuse prematurely. Differentiation from a chronic inflammatory synovitis, particularly tuberculous, may present radiological difficulty. The trabecular pattern of the bone becomes coarse and often has a lattice appearance. Secondary degenerative changes develop prematurely (Fig. 7.48).

The knee is affected almost invariably, involvement being frequently bilateral. The intercondylar notch becomes wide and deep. The patella may develop an unusually rectangular shape and its proximal articular surface is a common site of an erosion.

The elbows and ankles also are affected commonly. A characteristic abnormality in the former joint is an enlarged and deformed radial head. The shoulders and wrists are less frequently involved. Bleeding into the hip is unusual, but when this does occur avascular necrosis of the femoral head causes an appearance comparable to Perthes' disease. Distended joint capsules, particularly those of the elbows, may become radiologically dense by deposition within them of haemosiderin (Fig. 7.49).

Intra-osseous haemorrhage. Juxta-articular cystic lesions may be observed in the later stages of the disease, with a peculiar predilection for the proximal humeral epiphyses and the olecranon processes. While many are comparable to the post-traumatic subarticular cysts of degenerative joint disease, the fact that some of these cysts are remote from the articular surfaces has led to the belief that they

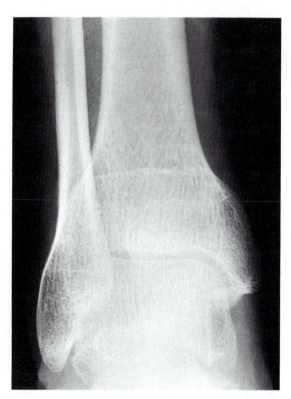

Fig. 7.47 Haemophilia. The former epiphyses are disproportionately large, presenting a 'squared' appearance. Hyaline cartilage thickness at the ankle joint is reduced.

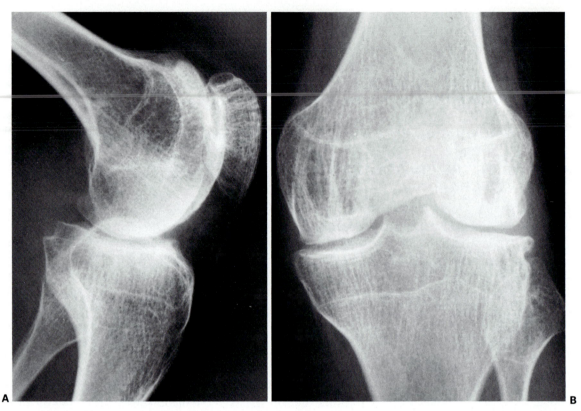

Fig. 7.48 A,B Haemophilia. Typical appearances in an adult patient subject to recurrent haemarthroses since childhood. As well as the enlarged, squared appearance of the former epiphyses, hyaline cartilage width is reduced, and osteophytes are present due to secondary osteoarthritis. Areas of radiolucency within medullary bone probably represent old intraosseous haemorrhages.

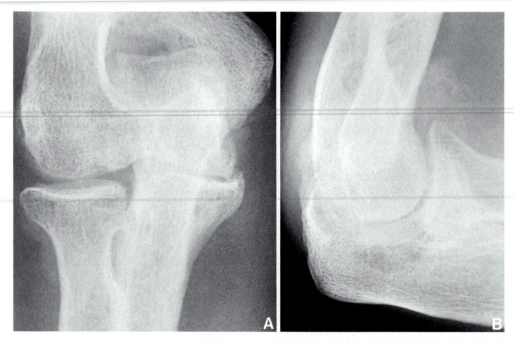

Fig. 7.49 A,B Haemophilia. Repeated intra-articular haemorrhages have caused overgrowth of the epiphyses, particularly the head of the radius. The joint capsule is distended and the synovium is amorphously dense due to the deposition of haemosiderin from recurrent haemarthroses. A subarticular cyst is present in the olecranon fossa, and degenerative changes, in the form of hyaline cartilage thinning and osteophyte formation, are present.

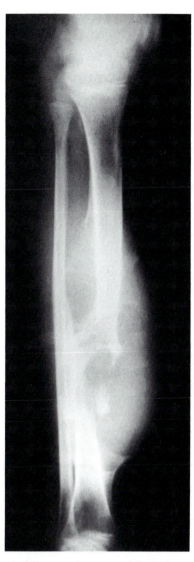

may be caused by haemorrhage within the bone itself.

Subperiosteal haemorrhage. Large osteolytic lesions known as *haemophiliac pseudotumours* occur in about 1 or 2% of severely affected patients. They have been observed especially in the iliac wings and in the shafts of the long bones of the lower limb, although other bones, including the calcaneus, have been involved (Fig. 7.50). These destructive lesions have been attributed to bleeding below the periosteum and often are accompanied by large swellings, sometimes relatively painless, of the soft tissues. Relation to a former traumatic incident may occasionally be established. Absorption of the underlying cortex and medulla with elevation of the periosteal margins results in an appearance which may be highly suggestive of a malignant bone tumour. Calcification is not uncommon within the space-occupying lesions. A diagnostic clue, however, may be provided by evidence in an adjacent joint of a haemophiliac arthropathy. Failure to appreciate the nature of this entity, nevertheless, has resulted in iatrogenic disasters by unnecessary amputation.

The diagnosis of haemophilia is likely to be made clinically, but the radiologist must be aware of its skeletal manifestations, including not only the typical arthropathies and bone cysts, but also and importantly the rare haemophiliac pseudotumours.

Fig. 7.50 Haemophiliac pseudotumour. A huge destructive lesion in the tibia, with relatively well-defined margins, is associated with some periosteal reaction. Although an initial impression may be of a malignant tumour changes of haemophilic arthropathy can be seen in the knee and ankle.

REFERENCES AND SUGGESTIONS FOR FURTHER READING (CHAPTERS 5–7)

Bullough, P. G., Vigorita, V. J. (1984) *Atlas of Orthopaedic Pathology.* Gower Medical, New York.

Dahlin, D. C., Krishnan, K. U. (1986) *Bone Tumors.* 4th edn. C. C. Thomas, Springfield.

Galasko, C. S. B., Isherwood, I. (Eds.) (1989) *Imaging Techniques in Orthopaedics.* Springer, Berlin.

Resnick, D., Niwayama, G. (1988) *Diagnosis of Bone and Joint Disorders.* 2nd edn. W. B. Saunders, Philadelphia.

Murray, R. O., Jacobson, H. G., Stoker D. (1989) *The Radiology of Skeletal Disorders.* 3rd edn. Churchill Livingstone, Edinburgh.

Wilner, D. (1982) *Radiology of Bone Tumors and Allied Disorders.* W. B. Saunders, Philadelphia.

Yaghmai, I. (1979) *Angiography of Bone and Soft Tissue Lesions.* Springer, Berlin.

CHAPTER 8

METABOLIC AND ENDOCRINE DISORDERS AFFECTING BONE

Jeremy W. R. Young

In general, metabolic bone disease affects the skeleton in one of two ways; there is either too much, or too little calcified bone. The latter change, which comprises the majority of metabolic bone disease, is due either to a decrease in the amount of bone formed, or to excessive resorption of bone. In turn this may be due to a variety of causes but most commonly to abnormalities of Vitamin D and calcium metabolism, which in turn arise from abnormality of diet or renal function, endocrine abnormalities (particularly of the parathyroid gland), drug therapy or poisoning.

For the most part metabolic processes involve the skeleton as a whole. The radiographic changes of metabolic bone diseases are therefore predominantly diffuse or at least multifocal, involving many areas of the skeleton, although on occasion, isolated lesions may be found, such as brown tumours in hyperparathyroidism. Another feature of metabolic bone disease is the tendency to involve specific locations, and to be symmetrical in the body, as seen in the 'Looser's zone's' of osteomalacia (see below). Radiographic evaluation of metabolic disease, and in particular the evaluation of changes in bone density, is difficult, as up to 40% of bone mass may be lost before it becomes apparent radiographically. Various techniques have been devised for the measurement of bone density. The more important ones are described below.

BONE DENSITY MEASUREMENTS

Radiogrammetry. This measures the cortical thickness of metacarpals and other tubular bones from standard radiographs (Fig. 8.1). It is particularly useful in serial studies, and comparison with a large normal population can be made. Although inexpensive and easy to perform, it does not reliably reflect bone mineral content.

Single photon absorption. This couples a monoenergetic photon source such as iodine-125 with a sodium iodide scintillation counter. The mineral content in the scan path is calculated from the difference in photon absorption between bone and soft tissue. The major criticism is that this measures mineral content in the appendicular skeleton, and that cortical bone measurements in the peripheries correlate poorly with dual photon absorptriometry in the spine.

Dual photon absorptiometry. As a photon source this uses gadolinium-153 which emits photons at two different energy levels. This allows scanning of the spine and femur, as it is independent of variation in soft tissue thickness. Because of the need to normalize the results due to different bone thickness, the technique cannot measure absolute bone mineral content, but is useful in quantitating mineral content changes. Nevertheless good correlation with CT mineral density evaluation has been obtained.

Neutron activation analysis. This technique uses high-energy neutrons to activate calcium-48 to calcium-49. The decay back to ^{48}Ca can then be measured with a gamma counter. As approximately 98% of body calcium is in the bones, this gives a reasonably accurate determination of total body calcium. With modifications, assessment of regional calcium can also be made. However, the technique is only available in a few specialized centres.

Quantitative computed tomography. CT is very effective for bone mineral content measurements, and has the advantage of being able to measure small volumes of bone, thus enabling measurement of both cortical and cancellous bone. In practice the mid-portion of a vertebral body is used. A mineral reference phantom such as potassium phosphate solution is needed for calibration. Either single- or dual-energy techniques may be used, although the accuracy of single-energy CT is variable and depends upon the amount of fat in the bone marrow.

Single-slice techniques are not suitable for bone mineral density readings in the femur, due to the complex trabecular architecture in this region. However this can be obtained by a complex multislice three-dimensional technique with sophisticated computer-generated histograms. At present CT analysis would appear to be the most reliable and adaptable technique for bone density measurements.

Other techniques. The above techniques are those

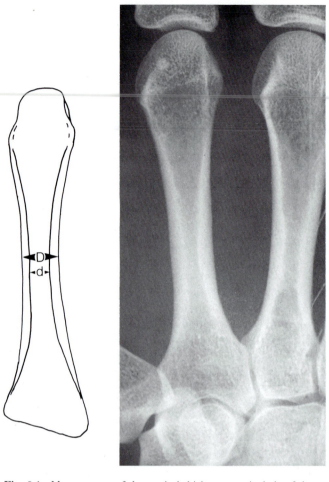

Fig. 8.1 Measurement of the cortical thickness, particularly of the right second metacarpal shaft, has been used widely in assessing bone mass. The measurement D – d = total thickness of cortical bone and is probably the most satisfactory of the simple indices that have been proposed. (Paterson, C. R. (1974) *Metabolic Disorders of Bone*. Blackwell, Oxford.)

most widely known and used at this time. Other techniques however are also in use or are being developed. **Dual Energy Projection Radiography** uses a CT scanner, with the patient scanned during longitudinal motion, multiple readings being obtained through the region of interest. Calibration with a multichamber phantom is again used, and a 'mineral equivalent' value is expressed in g/dl of potassium phosphate. The technique is again only available in specialized centres.

Magnetic Resonance Imaging has been suggested as another technique by virtue of the fact that T_1 and T_2 relaxation times for lumbar vertebral marrow have shown a decrease with increasing age, except for T_2 in women. This is explained by the replacement of active with fatty marrow. More rapid loss of bone mineral content in elderly women may explain the fact that T_1 and T_2 values are greater than in men of the same age. Calibration phantoms will have to be designed, however, to compensate for variations in signal sensitivity and magnetic field variations, if the technique is to become an accurate method for the determination of bone mineral content.

BIOCHEMISTRY

Biochemical findings in metabolic and endocrine disease of the bone are variable, but can be extremely helpful in making the diagnosis. They are summarized in Table 8.1.

CHANGES DUE TO VITAMIN D ABNORMALITIES

Vitamin D is derived either from the diet, or via the action of ultraviolet light on the skin. After hydroxylation of cholecalciferol in the liver, further hydroxylation occurs in the kidney to generate the active form of Vitamin D, 1,25,-dihydroxycholecalciferol (1,25 DHCC), which has several modes of action. In bone, homeostasis is maintained as 1,25 DMCC has two actions; mobilization of

Table 8.1 Laboratory changes in metabolic bone disease

	Serum Levels				Urine Levels	
	Calcium	Phosphorus	Alkaline phosphatase	Urea or creatinine	Calcium	Hydroxy proline
Osteoporosis	N	N	N	N	N	N or ↑
Hyperparathyroidism						
Primary	↑	↓	N or ↑	N or ↑	N or ↑	↑
Secondary	N or ↓	↑	↑	↑	↓	↑
'Tertiary'	↑	N or ↓	N or ↑	↑	N or ↑	N or ↑
Hypoparathyroidism	↓	↑	N	N	↓	N
Pseudohypoparathyroidism	↓	↑	N	N	↓	N
Hyperthyroidism	N or ↑	N	N	N	↑	↑
Rickets/osteomalacia						
Vitamin D deficiency	↓	↓	↑	N	↓	N
Vitamin D refractory	N	↓	↑	N or ↑	↓	N
Hypophosphatasia	N or ↑	N	↓	N	N or ↑	↓

N = normal   ↑ = elevated   ↓ = lowered

calcium and phosphorus, and promotion of mineralization and maturation. The former requires the presence of both 1,25 DMCC and parathormone. Also, 1,25 DMCC absorption of calcium and phosphorus is promoted in the intestines. In addition, it affects the kidney, both directly, on proximal renal tubular function, and indirectly, by stimulating production of relatively inert 24,25 dihydroxycholecalciferol, which has a negative feedback effect, limiting 1,25 DHCC production. Finally, there are receptors in other organs, particularly the pituitary, placenta and breast, which are thought to reflect the increased demand for calcium during growth, pregnancy and lactation.

RICKETS AND OSTEOMALACIA (VITAMIN D DEFICIENCY)

Rickets and osteomalacia are the same basic disorder, occurring in children and adults respectively. The pathological changes result from an interruption of development, and in particular, mineralization of the growth plate in the developing skeleton, or from lack of mineralization of osteoid in the mature skeleton. They occur as a result of a lack of the actions of Vitamin D which in turn may be due to dietary lack, lack of production by the body, failure of absorption, or defective metabolism. In practice, as the body can normally generate sufficient vitamin D when there is adequate ultraviolet light, nutritional deficiency only occurs when there is a dietary lack together with too little exposure to ultraviolet light. This is most commonly seen in black immigrants who make their homes in the colder and less sunny areas of Northern Europe. It may also occur in the neglected elderly, particularly in larger cities in the higher latitudes.

Malabsorption states, including Crohn's disease and scleroderma, can result in osteomalacia (see Table 8.2). Liver disease, whether ductal or hepatocellular, is also a cause of osteomalacia, although osteoporosis is also found histologically. The osteomalacia of liver disease is multifactorial, but appears largely due to malabsorption of Vitamin D, as bile salts are necessary for Vitamin D absorption in micelle form. In coeliac disease, the small bowel is less responsive to the action of vitamin D in calcium transport.

Table 8.2 Malabsorption states causing osteomalacia

Crohn's disease

Coeliac disease

Lymphoma

Amyloidosis

Small bowel fistula

Postoperative states (bowel resection)

Hepatobiliary disease

Drug therapy may produce osteomalacia, particularly long-term anticonvulsant therapy (phenytoin/dilantin). A similar effect has also been reported with *rifampicin*, and *glutethimide*.

Finally, many toxins have been found to cause osteomalacia by causing tubular damage and phosphate deficiency. These include *aluminium hydroxide, magnesium sulphate,* and *cadmium,* the latter being associated with alkaline battery manufacture, or the painful condition of '*itai-itai*' (ouch, ouch) reported in Japan in patients drinking cadmium-polluted water.

RICKETS

There are many causes of rickets in childhood. In general, however, the radiological features are similar, although varying in severity and location.

The skeletal effects are due to a lack of calcification of osteoid. Consequently the most obvious changes are at the *metaphysis,* where the most rapid growth is occurring. The initial abnormality is a loss of the normal 'zone of provisional calcification' adjacent to the metaphysis, although usually by the time radiographs are obtained, significant metaphyseal abnormality is seen. This begins as an indistinctness of the metaphyseal margin, progressing to a 'frayed' appearance with a widening of the growth plate, due to lack of calcification of metaphyseal bone (Fig. 8.2). Weight bearing and stress on the uncalcified bone give rise to splaying, and cupping of the metaphysis (Fig. 8.3).

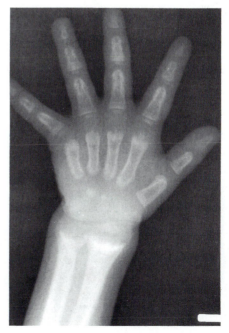

Fig. 8.2 Rickets. There is obvious 'fraying' of the metaphyseal margin, with a wide growth plate seen at the distal radius and metacarpals.

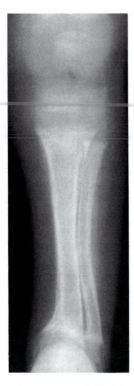

Fig. 8.3 Rickets. There is splaying of all of the visible metaphyses, with in addition, some characteristic S-shaped bowing of the bones of the lower leg.

A similar but less marked effect occurs in the subperiosteal layer, which may cause lack of distinctness of the cortical margin. Eventually a generalized reduction in bone density is seen, and in long-standing cases fractures may occur. Looser's zones are not seen as often as in osteomalacia (see below). In the epiphysis, there may be some haziness of the cortical margins.

With treatment, mineralization occurs, giving rise to a dense white line at the zone of provisional calcification adjacent to the metaphysis, but becoming contiguous with

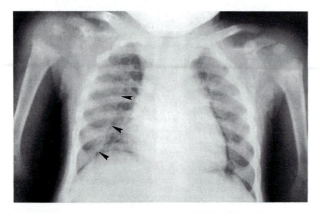

Fig. 8.4 Rickety rosary has occurred, with widening of the anterior ribs clearly demonstrated. The classic metaphyseal changes of rickets are also seen in the proximal humeri.

the metaphysis during the healing process. In cases of intermittent dietary vitamin deficiency, or inadequate treatment, the metaphysis will show patchy sclerosis.

In severe cases of rickets additional deformities of the bones occur, with bowing of the long bones (particularly of the lower limbs) (Fig. 8.3), thoracic kyphosis with a 'pigeon chest', enlargement of the anterior ribs, causing the 'ricketic rosary' (Fig. 8.4), and bossing of the skull.

Rickets may be seen in low-birthweight and premature infants, and may be severe, causing spontaneous fractures and respiratory difficulty. Affected infants are usually below 1000 g in weight, or less than 28 weeks' gestation.

VITAMIN-D-RESISTANT RICKETS (FAMILIAL HYPOPHOSPHATASIA)

This condition is usually inherited in a dominant sex-linked fashion. Affected women pass the disease on to half of their sons and daughters, whilst affected men pass the disease on to none of their sons and half of their daughters. The disease is similar to rickets in radiographic appearance, but it is refractory to vitamin D therapy, and growth retardation may be marked. The radiographic changes are variable from mild to severe, and may be similar to the metaphyseal dysplasia of the Schmid variety (see Ch. 1).

Acquired hypophosphataemia rickets

Rarely, hypophosphataemia has been seen in association with tumours of bone or soft tissues, frequently fibrous in origin. It has also been reported in association with *prostatic carcinoma*, and *oat cell carcinoma* of the lung and a similar condition has also been reported with other conditions, e.g. *neurofibromatosis, fibrous dysplasia*.

Vitamin-D-resistant rickets associated with renal tubular disorders

A variety of renal dysfunction syndromes produce rickets and osteomalacia. These include *hypercalcaemia, renal phosphate loss* and *secondary hypophosphataemia, amino aciduria* and *renal tubular acidosis*. In *renal tubular acidosis* affected patients demonstrate retarded growth and short stature. As well as the changes of osteomalacia, nephrocalcinosis and nephrolithiasis are seen (Fig. 8.5).

OSTEOMALACIA

This refers to the changes resulting from vitamin D deficiency in the mature skeleton. Bone pain is a frequent complaint. Serum alkaline phosphatase is elevated, and serum phosphorus is low. The hallmark of osteomalacia is the pseudofracture or 'Looser's zone'. This is a narrow zone of lucency, usually running perpendicular or nearly perpendicular to the bone cortex. Initially poorly defined, these zones become progressively more prominent, with

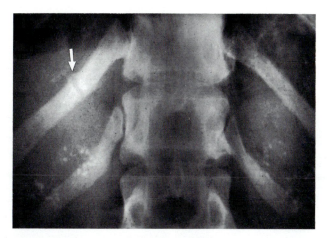

Fig. 8.5 Renal tubular acidosis. The combination of nephrocalcinosis and osteomalacia (Looser's zone — arrow) in the right 11th rib is characteristic, although symptomatic bone disease affects only a minority of patients. (Courtesy Dr. D. J. Stoker and Institute of Orthopaedics.)

sclerotic margins (Fig. 8.6). They are generally accepted as occurring at sites of stress as subclinical stress fractures that are repaired by unossified osteoid. They are frequently bilateral and symmetrical, and occur at regular sites (Fig. 8.7) such as the pubic rami, proximal femur (Fig. 8.8), scapula (Fig. 8.6), lower ribs, and ulna (Fig. 8.9). Osteopenia develops with 'pencilling-in' of the vertebral bodies, and loss of vertebral height in a characteristic 'codfish vertebra' pattern (Fig. 8.10).

Bowing of the long bones may occur. Compression wedge fractures of the vertebra are less common than

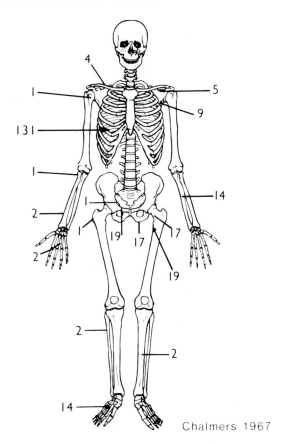

Chalmers 1967

Fig. 8.7 Looser's zones in osteomalacia. Sites of incidence in a group of middle-aged and elderly patients with dietetic osteomalacia. (Courtesy of Dr. D. J. Stoker and Institute of Orthopaedics.)

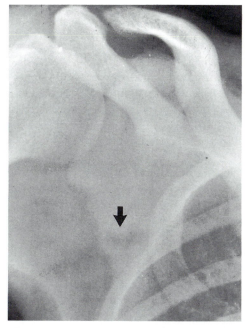

Fig. 8.6 Looser's zones. There is lucency with surrounding sclerosis in the lateral border of the scapula — a common site.

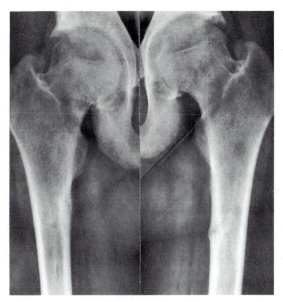

Fig. 8.8 Looser's zones. Symmetrical lucencies are seen involving the medial cortex of the proximal femur bilaterally — another characteristic site.

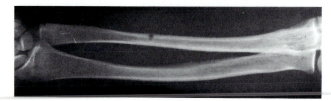

Fig. 8.9 Looser's zone. The characteristic lucency of the mid ulna is seen.

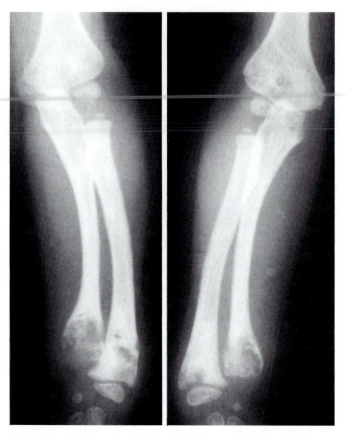

Fig. 8.11 Hypophosphatasia. In this child metaphyseal ossification is delayed in the ulnae whilst the distal radii contain islands of non-ossified tissue. (Courtesy of Dr. D. J. Stoker and Institute of Orthopaedics.)

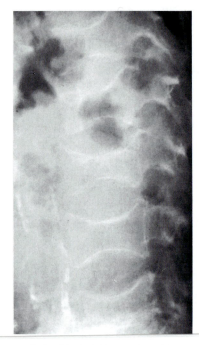

Fig. 8.10 Osteomalacia. Marked biconcavity of the vertebral bodies (codfish vertebrae). (Courtesy of Dr. D. J. Stoker and Institute of Orthopaedics.)

in osteoporosis. The histopathology of osteomalacia is characteristic, with excessive osteoid, and/or failure of ossification of new bone.

Hypophosphatasia

Inherited as an autosomal recessive trait, this rare disorder presents with a radiographic picture which varies from a mild to a very severe form of rickets, depending upon the age of onset, the neonatal variety being most severe, and generally lethal. There is a low serum alkaline phosphatase, and increased urinary phosphoethanolomine. In severe cases an exaggerated fraying of the metaphysis is seen, with uncalcified osteoid extending into the metaphysis (Fig. 8.11). Craniostenosis and nephrocalcinosis may occur, and deformities, particularly of the distal phalanges and tibia are seen.

Familial hyperphosphataemia

An extremely rare condition of autosomal recessive inher-

itance, this presents in early infancy. The radiographic appearance is similar to that of Paget's disease, but occurring in infancy, and demonstrating more symmetry; the conditions however are unrelated. The skull vault is thickened and the long bones are tubular, enlarged and bowed, but with cortical irregularity (Fig. 8.12). Serum alkaline phosphatase is elevated.

Fibrogenesis imperfecta ossium

This rare disorder presents with coarsening of the trabecular pattern of the bones, and in particular the ends of the long bones. Multiple fractures are seen. Serum alkaline phosphatase is elevated.

Axial osteomalacia

This rare condition is characterized by a coarsening of the bony trabeculae, similar to that seen in fibrogenesis imperfecta ossium, but only involving the vertebra, pelvis and ribs. Histologically osteomalacia is found, but serum alkaline phosphatase levels are normal.

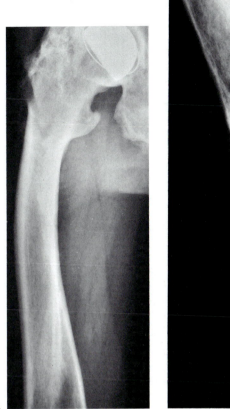
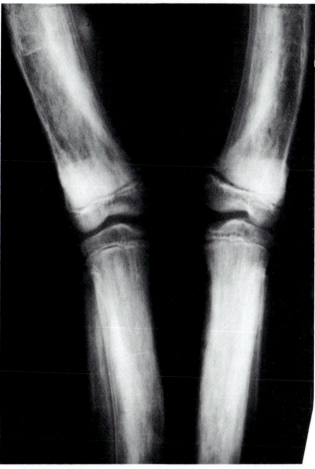

A   B

Fig. 8.12 Familial hyperphosphataemia. **A.** The femur is abnormal with some bowing, increased width, and prominent but irregular cortex, somewhat resembling Paget's disease (Courtesy of Dr C. S. Resnik). **B.** The radiological appearances in this child are diagnostic. The bones are widened with loss of differentiation of cortex and medulla. A coarse trabecular pattern and bowing are also evident. These features resemble those of Paget's disease. (Courtesy of Dr. D. J. Stoker and Institute of Orthopaedics.)

VITAMIN C DEFICIENCY

Vitamin C deficiency leads to a deficiency in the formation of bone matrix, as it is necessary for the formation of hydroxyproline, which is vital for collagen. About 90% of the matrix of mature bone is collagen, and hence a lack of collagen will have a severe effect on bone formation. In childhood, this gives rise to scurvy. The adult counterpart is osteoporosis.

Scurvy

Scurvy is rare before six months of age since the storage of vitamin C in the neonate is generally adequate. Children present with limb pain and irritability. Radiographically, four characteristic signs are seen. 1. The epiphysis is small, and sharply marginated by a sclerotic rim (Wimberger's sign) (Fig. 8.13). 2. The zone of provisional calcification at the growing metaphysis is dense, giving a white line (Frankel's line) (Fig. 8.13). 3. Beneath this is a lucent zone, due to lack of mineraliz-

ation of osteoid (Trumerfeld zone). 4. Finally, as this area is weakened, it is prone to fractures which manifest themselves at the cortical margin, giving rise to (Pelkan's) spurs.

In addition, due to capillary fragility, subperiosteal haemorrhages occur (Fig. 8.14), which may give rise to periosteal elevation, and subsequent new bone formation, particularly following treatment. This dense periosteal new bone should be differentiated from that found in battered infants.

Following treatment, dense bands of bone may be left, resembling growth arrest lines.

OSTEOPOROSIS

Osteoporosis is the most frequent metabolic bone disease, and is due to a decrease in bone mass. It is the result of many underlying causes (Table 8.3). In general, the loss of bone mass gives rise to increased incidence of fractures,

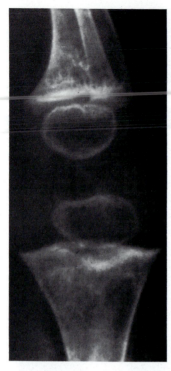

Fig. 8.13 Scurvy. The margins of the epiphyses are sclerotic (Wimberger's sign). There is a narrow epiphyseal plate, with increased density of the zone of provisional calcification (Frankel's line). The lucent zone beneath this is due to lack of mineralized osteoid (Trumerfeld zone).

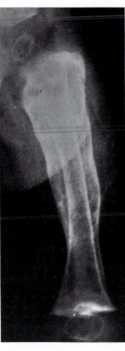

Fig. 8.14 Scurvy. Subperiosteal haemorrhage has elevated the periosteum. The healing stage shows marked periosteal new bone formation. (Courtesy of Dr. C. S. Resnik.)

Table 8.3 Causes of generalized osteoporosis

Age-related conditions (senile and postmenopausal states)

Deficiency states
  Malnutrition
  Calcium deficiency
  Scurvy

Drugs
  Steroids
  Heparin

Metabolic
  Hyperthyroidism
  Hyperparathyroidism
  Cushing's disease
  Acromegaly
  Pregnancy
  Diabetes mellitus
  Hypogonadism

Alcoholism

Chronic liver disease

Anaemias

Idiopathic

particularly in the femoral neck, spine (compression fractures), distal radius, and pubic symphysis.

In osteoporosis the microstructure of the bone is normal, but the quantity of bone is diminished. This eventually gives rise to a clear loss of bone density, radiographically best described as *osteopenia*. This radiographic appearance of generalized osteopenia however is not specific to osteoporosis and can be seen in a variety of conditions (Table 8.4).

Table 8.4 Major causes of diffuse osteopenia

Osteoporosis

Osteomalacia

Hyperparathyroidism

Neoplasia (particularly multiple myeloma)

In addition there are many conditions that can give rise to localized osteopenia (Table 8.5).

Table 8.5 Major causes of localized osteoporosis

Immobilization

Post-fracture

Sudeck's atrophy

Arthritis

Infection

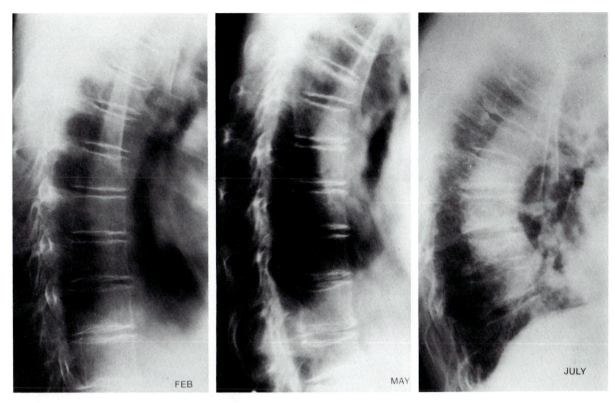

Fig. 8.15 Post-menopausal osteoporosis. Serial films in this patient show the progressive development of kyphosis as a result of anterior wedging of the thoracic vertebral bodies during the course of six months. (Courtesy of Dr. D. J. Stoker and Institute of Orthopaedics.)

In osteoporosis trabecular loss is most evident radiographically in the spine, where there is a loss of density, which may be appreciated as 'pencilling in' of the vertebra by the more radiographically dense end-plates (Fig. 8.15). Biconcave vertebral bodies (cod-fish vertebrae) may occur. In the femoral neck the osteopenia is manifested by an apparent increase in density of the residual trabecula (Fig. 8.16). Endosteal and intracortical resorption of bone is prominent, producing cortical thinning most evident in the appendicular skeleton.

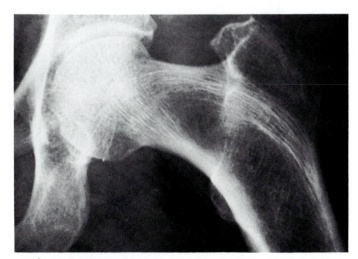

Fig. 8.16 Osteoporosis. In this patient, resorption of the secondary trabeculae has left the primary trabeculae to delineate the lines of stress within the femoral neck.

Postmenopausal and senile osteoporosis (involutional osteoporosis)

Postmenopausal osteoporosis occurs in women typically aged 50–65. There is a disproportionate loss of trabecular bone, giving rise to rapid bone loss, and a proportionate increase in fractures, particularly of the vertebrae and distal radius. In the vertebra, loss of height and anterior wedging occur, which may lead to a marked kyphotic deformity (Fig. 8.15). The changes of osteoporosis have been linked to reduced oestrogen levels, although additional factors such as skeletal size, level of activity, nutritional status and genetic determinants have been proposed. In general, once osteoporosis is established, oestrogen therapy does not affect the radiographic density of the bone. Blood chemistry is usually normal, although urinary hydroxyproline levels may be elevated in the acute stage.

Senile osteoporosis differs from postmenopausal osteoporosis in that there is proportionate loss of cortical and trabecular bone. Fractures occur most commonly in the

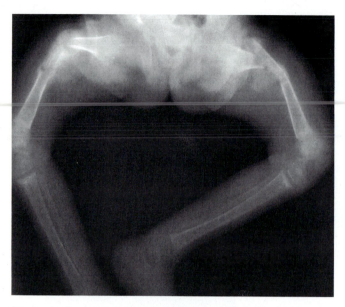

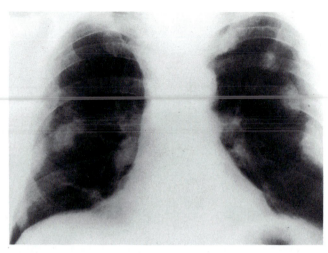

Fig. 8.18 Cushing's disease. Excessive callus formation is seen at multiple fracture sites in the ribs. The patient had functional adrenal carcinoma.

Fig. 8.17 Osteogenesis imperfecta. There is diffuse osteoporosis, with fractures of both femora. These are already showing marked callus formation.

femoral neck, proximal humerus, tibia and pelvis. There is no dramatic increase in bone loss in the post-menopausal stage, and patients tend to be older. The ratio of affected women to men is approximately 2:1. The aetiology is uncertain, but reduced intestinal absorption, diminished adrenal function and secondary hyperparathyroidism may play a role.

Idiopathic juvenile osteoporosis
This disorder is a rare self-limiting disease that affects both sexes and occurs typically before puberty. Patients present with bone pain, backache or limp related to fractures, characteristically of the metaphysis of the long bones with minimal trauma. Compressions of the vertebrae with kyphosis may result. The diagnosis is one of exclusion, particularly from leukaemia, lymphoma and hypercorticosteroid states. Another radiographic diagnostic consideration is *osteogenesis imperfecta*, as this also presents with diffuse osteoporosis, and multiple fractures (Fig. 8.17). Blood chemistry is normal.

Idiopathic male osteoporosis
A number of male patients present with generalized osteopenia before the age of 60. No definite predisposing factors have been found. Hypercalciuria and increased calcium absorption seem to be constant findings, and the condition may be an acquired defect in bone metabolism. Again, this is a diagnosis of exclusion.

ENDOCRINE-INDUCED OSTEOPOROSIS
Abnormality of function of the adrenal, pituitary and

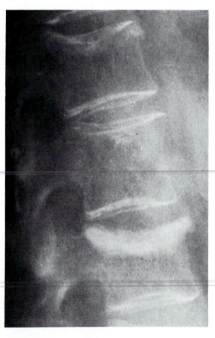

Fig. 8.19 Cushing's disease. Generalized reduction in bone density simulates post-menopausal osteoporosis in this patient. The compression fracture of the superior border of the body of L4 has characteristically produced dense callus. This feature is almost, but not entirely, pathognomonic of glucocorticosteroid excess. (Courtesy of Dr. D. J. Stoker and Institute of Orthopaedics.)

thyroid glands, hyperfunction of the parathyroids and hypofunction of the pancreas and gonads have all been linked with osteoporosis. As well as osteoporosis, other skeletal abnormalities are associated with particular endocrine disorders.

Steroid-induced osteoporosis (Cushing's disease)
Glucocortical excess may be related to therapy, but can

be due to a number of causes although it is usually secondary to Cushing's disease. Histological studies have revealed decreased bone formation and increased resorption. Biochemically there is a negative calcium balance and hypercalciuria. Exuberant callus formation at fractures is seen, particularly in long bones, ribs (Fig. 8.18) and vertebral bodies. In the latter case, a characteristic increased density of the end-plates occurs (Fig. 8.19). Avascular necrosis may occur, particularly of the femoral head. In children, growth may be retarded. Rib fractures may be multiple, painless and unsuspected.

Hypogonadism. In boys, this results in delayed closure of the epiphyseal plates. As a result, the patients have long limbs in relation to their trunks. A similar hypogonadal disorder in girls (Turner's syndrome), results in short stature, increased carrying angle at the elbow, a short fourth metacarpal and changes of Blount's disease at the knee. Congenital cardio-vascular anomalies also occur, most commonly coarctation of the aorta.

THE THYROID GLAND

Hyperthyroidism. In hyperthyroidism, a generalized osteoporosis may be seen. There is an increased metabolic ratio, with an increase in both bone formation and resorption. Increased cortical striations of the long bones are seen. *Thyroid acropachy* is a rare condition which usually follows therapy for previous hyperthyroidism or occurs in patients who have been on thyroid for many years. There is a characteristic periosteal thickening in the extremities and particularly in the hands (Fig. 8.20). It must be distinguished from hypertrophic osteoarthropathy, which is also found in the extremities (Figs 8.21, 8.22), but is usually exquisitely painful. Exophthalmus and pretibial myxoedema are frequently present. Rarely, hyperthyroidism appears in childhood, when accelerated skeletal maturation occurs.

Hypothyroidism. Although it is not associated with osteoporosis, it is appropriate to discuss this condition at this point. In children, skeletal maturation is delayed and growth is retarded. Epiphyses are late in appearing (Fig. 8.23) and fragmented, although when they do appear, the sequence is normal. This may cause an appearance in the hip that must be differentiated from Perthes' disease. Wormian bones are seen in the skull,

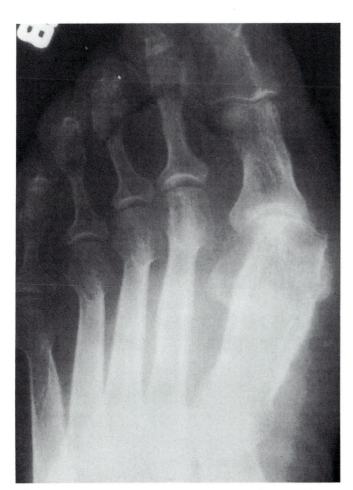

Fig. 8.20 Thyroid acropachy. A dense periosteal reaction is seen along the first metatarsal. Although this can occur in any of the digits, the first is a characteristic site.

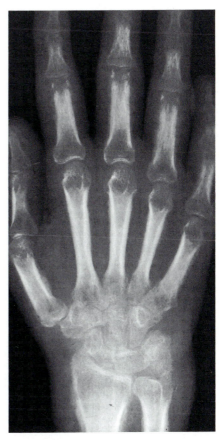

Fig. 8.21 Hypertrophic (pulmonary) osteoarthropathy. There is marked periosteal reaction along most of the visualized bones.

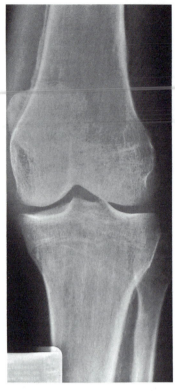

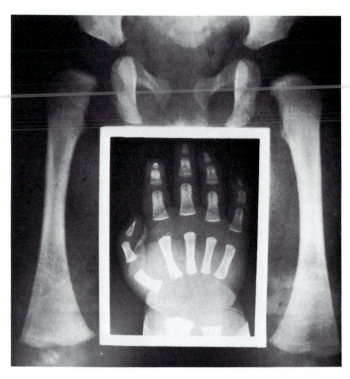

Fig. 8.22 Hypertrophic pulmonary osteoarthropathy of femur and tibia.

Fig. 8.23 Cretinism. Marked skeletal retardation was present in this 12-month-old child. Note that the carpal and proximal femoral centres have not yet appeared. (Courtesy of Dr. D. J. Stoker and Institute of Orthopaedics.)

and the sella is either small and bowl-shaped (young children), or of large rounded 'cherry sella' configuration (older children). The paranasal sinuses are underdeveloped. In the spine, bullet-shaped vertebral bodies are seen, especially at the thoracolumbar junction, where kyphosis may develop. All the long bones are short. In the pelvis the incidence of slipped capital femoral epiphysis is increased, and the pelvis itself is often narrow, with coxa vara deformities. In the adult the changes are exaggerated (Fig. 8.24).

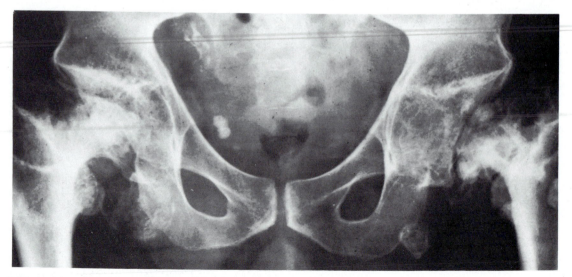

Fig. 8.24 Adult cretinism. This 39-year-old man received no therapy until four years before this film was obtained. Coxa vara is present, whilst the femoral heads are deformed and irregularly ossified in the absence of thyroid hormone during development. (Courtesy of Dr. D. J. Stoker and Institute of Orthopaedics.)

HYPERPITUITARISM (*acromegaly*)

It is questionable whether acromegaly is a cause for true osteoporosis. It will however be included in this section. Gigantism in the immature skeleton, and acromegaly in the adult, result from excessive growth hormone production by an eosinophilic adenoma. The radiographic features of acromegaly include enlarged mastoid air cells and sinuses, frontal bossing and prognathism (Fig. 8.25). Pituitary fossa enlargement may be seen on the plain film (Fig. 8.25), although CT or MRI are more helpful in evaluating for a pituitary adenoma (see Ch. 57). In the spine, enlargement of the vertebral bodies with posterior scalloping is seen (Fig. 8.26). The hands show characteristic enlargement of the bones and soft tissues with spade-like terminal tufts, or arrowhead distal phalanges

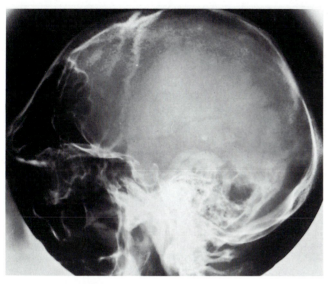

Fig. 8.25 Acromegaly. The frontal sinuses are markedly enlarged, and there is frontal bossing. A double floor with 'ballooning' is seen in the pituitary fossa.

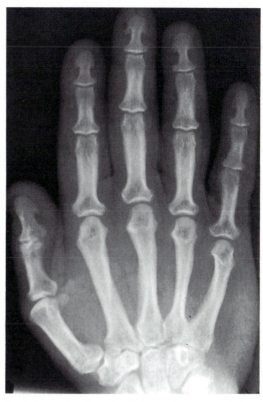

Fig. 8.27 Acromegaly. There is obvious enlargement of the soft tissues and phalanges with prominent joint spaces due to increased cartilage thickness. The distal phalanges show the characteristic 'arrowhead' configuration.

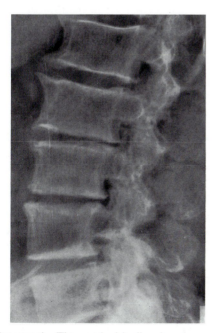

Fig. 8.26 Acromegaly. The vertebral bodies show bony overgrowth. Mild posterior scalloping is also seen at several levels. (Courtesy of Dr. C. S. Resnik.)

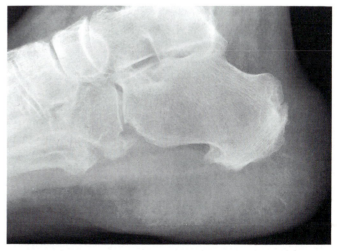

Fig. 8.28 Acromegaly. There is marked prominence of the soft tissues of the heel pad which measures approximately 35 mm.

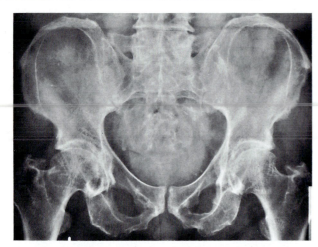

Fig. 8.29 Acromegaly. There is overgrowth of the bone in the iliac crests and irregular bony prominence of the sites of muscle attachments throughout the pelvis.

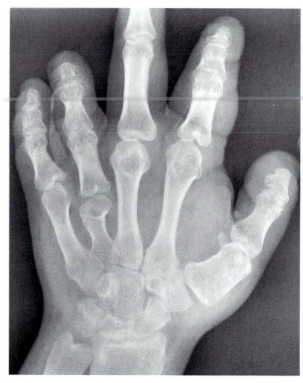

Fig. 8.30 Pseudohypoparathyroidism. A markedly short fourth metacarpal bone is seen. Although not specific for pseudohypoparathyroidism, this is a characteristic finding. (Courtesy of Dr. C. S. Resnik.)

(Fig. 8.27). Widening of the joint spaces due to overgrowth of articular cartilage may be seen (Fig. 8.27). The feet show evidence of increased thickness of the heel pads although this is no longer regarded as an infallible sign of acromegaly (Fig. 8.28). The long bones of the feet are elongated, although the feet usually remain slender. Prominence of muscle attachments, and premature or exaggerated degenerative change may be seen (Fig. 8.29). *Calcification* of the pinna of the ear occurs. Chondrocalcinosis has been reported as a rare variation, although crystal arthropathy has been suggested as the underlying cause by some authors.

THE PARATHYROID GLANDS

Hypoparathyroidism. Rarely, osteoporosis is seen in patients with hypoparathyroidism. The most common cause for hypoparathyroidism is parathyroid gland removal at thyroid surgery, or ^{131}I thyroid therapy. Rarely it can result from excessive therapeutic radiation, haemorrhage, infection, tumour deposition in the thyroid gland, or iron deposition in iron overload conditions. Idiopathic hypoparathyroidism, either autoimmune or familial, can occur without atrophy of the glands. It is associated with a variety of endocrine and immune deficiency states including *Addison's disease, ovarian dysgenesis, hypothyroidism* and *chronic mucocutaneous candidiasis*. Circulating antibodies to the parathyroid, thyroid and adrenal glands have been found. Calcium deposition in the basal ganglia occurs and osteosclerosis, particularly of the pelvis, inner table of the skull, proximal femur, and vertebral bodies can be seen, as well as abnormal tooth development. Serum calcium is low, and phosphate diuresis follows parathormone administration.

Pseudohypoparathyroidism. This is inherited in a dominant fashion and is characterized by hypocalcaemia and hyperphosphataemia which are unresponsive to parathormone. The parathyroid glands are normal, but there is 'end-organ' resistance to parathormone. This may be due to a defect in the adenyl-cyclase-cyclic AMP system in the renal tubules and bones. Basal ganglia calcification is more common than in idiopathic hypoparathyroidism. Short metacarpals are seen, particularly the fourth and fifth (Fig. 8.30). Abnormal dentition is also seen, with hypoplasia and cranial defects, and there may be calcification in the connective tissues of the skin, ligaments tendons and fascial planes. Coxa-vara, coxa-valga, cone-shaped epiphyses, and bowing of long bones are also reported. Secondary hyperparathyroidism is a feature of this disorder.

Pseudopseudohypoparathyroidism. This condition presents with the same clinical and radiographic appearances as pseudohypoparathyroidism, but with normal blood chemistry.

Hyperparathyroidism

This condition is divided into the primary, secondary and tertiary forms. In the **primary** form, increased hormone production occurs as a result of parathyroid adenomas (75%), hyperplasia or carcinoma. It occurs most commonly in middle-aged and elderly people, and is more common in women (2:1). *Symptoms* include weakness, lassitude, constipation, polydypsia, polyuria, peptic ulceration, renal calculi and psychiatric problems. *Radiographically*, bone resorption is seen, and although frank osteopenia is difficult to detect radiographically in early cases, bone mineral content measurements confirm bone mineral loss in approximately 50% of cases. More advanced cases demonstrate bone density loss, and sometimes a ground-glass appearance.

Subperiosteal erosion of bone, particularly along the radial aspect of the middle phalanx of the middle and index finger is virtually pathognomonic (Fig. 8.31), although fine-grain film or magnification views may be required to detect it. Other sites include the medial aspect of the proximal tibia (Fig. 8.32), femur and humerus, and the ribs. Loss of the lamina dura around the teeth occurs, although this is not specific for hyperparathyroidism.

Subchondral bone resorption is another common occurrence, being found at the distal, and sometimes proximal end of the clavicle (Fig. 8.33), symphysis pubis and sacroiliac joints. This may also occur at the vertebral end-plates, which may permit disc herniation (Schmorl's nodes).

Intracortical bone resorption is another feature of hyperparathyroidism, resulting from osteoclastic activity within the Haversian canals. This gives rise to small (2–5 mm) oval or cigar-shaped lucencies within the cortex (Fig. 8.34). This is a feature of rapid bone turnover, and is also seen in other conditions, such as *hyperthyroidism*,

osteomalacia and *acute (focal) osteoporosis* (Fig. 8.35). Loss of the corticomedullary junction may occur with a 'basket-work' appearance to the cortex. In the skull, a characteristic granular or mottled appearance may occur, giving rise to the so-called 'pepper-pot' or 'salt-and-pepper' (USA), skull (Fig. 8.36).

Subligamentous resorption occurs at sites of ligament or tendon insertions, and is seen in the ischial tuberosity, greater and lesser trochanters, inferior calcaneus and inferior surface of the distal clavicle (Fig. 8.33).

Brown tumours are locally destructive areas of intense osteoclastic activity. They present as a lytic lesion which may be expansive (Fig. 8.37), and may destroy the overlying cortex. Pathological fractures may occur (Fig. 8.38). The lesions are generally well defined, and may be multi-

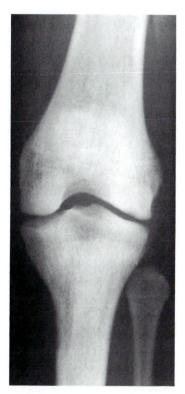

Fig. 8.32 Hyperparathyroidism. There is erosion of the medial side of the proximal tibia.

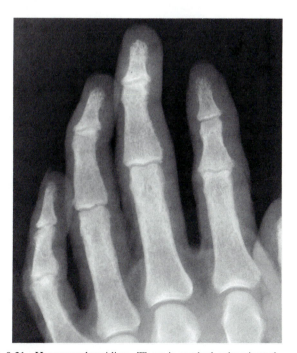

Fig. 8.31 Hyperparathyroidism. There is marked subperiosteal resorption of the radial aspect of many of the phalanges and erosion of the tufts. (Courtesy of Dr. D. J. Stoker and Institute of Orthopaedics.)

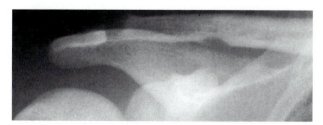

Fig. 8.33 Hyperparathyroidism. There is erosion of the distal end of the clavicle, as well as on the inferior surface at the site of the attachment of the coracoclavicular ligament.

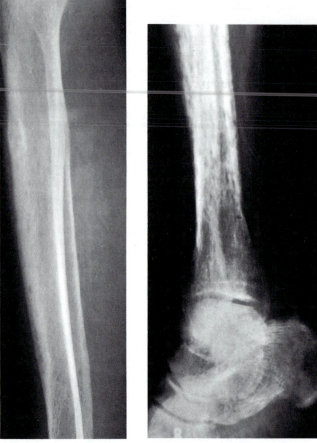

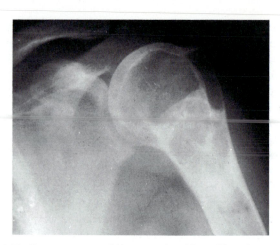

Fig. 8.37 Brown tumour of hyperparathyroidism. There is a well-defined, lytic, mildly expansive lesion of the proximal humerus.

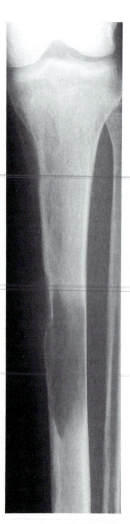

Fig. 8.34   *Fig. 8.35*

Fig. 8.34 Hyperparathyroidism. Intracortical bone resorption is seen, with multiple small oval lucencies within the cortical bone.

Fig. 8.35 Severe disuse osteoporosis. There is marked intracortical bone resorption, particularly evident in the tibia.

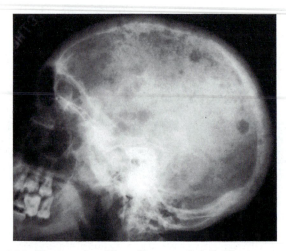

Fig. 8.36 Hyperparathyroidism. 'Pepper-pot' skull. There are multiple characteristic lucencies throughout the skull.

Fig. 8.38 Brown tumour of the mid tibia. The patient was found to have a parathyroid adenoma.

locular. Following treatment, they may resolve, but can persist for many years.

Rarely, an *erosive arthropathy* may also occur. This usually involves the hands, wrists and shoulders. It may simulate the appearance of rheumatoid arthritis, but subperiosteal resorption is usually a concurrent feature, and the distal interphalangeal joints are often involved, unlike rheumatoid arthritis.

Renal calculi have been reported in as many as 50% of patients. The majority are calcium oxalate, although a minority are uric acid stones. *Nephrocalcinosis* also occurs, but is less common.

Secondary hyperparathyroidism. Parathyroid hyperplasia involving all of the glands occurs in response to persistent hypocalcaemia. This can be seen in *rickets*, *osteomalacia* and *chronic renal failure*. The skeletal changes are similar to those of primary hyperparathyroidism, although brown tumours are less frequently seen. Nevertheless, as secondary hyperparathyroidism is so much more common than primary hyperparathyroidism, in practice brown tumours are more commonly seen as a result of the former. Calcification of arteries and soft tissues occurs, but is most common in the secondary hyperparathyroidism of renal osteodystrophy.

Renal osteodystrophy This is of particular interest as it combines the findings of osteomalacia, hyperparathyroidism and bone sclerosis.

As in hyperparathyroidism, the commonest finding is subperiosteal resorption, although in severe cases all features may be present. Calcification of arteries, articular cartilage and periarticular tissues also occurs. Osteomalacia is identified predominantly by the presence of Looser's zones. Osteosclerosis is seen in the skull, metaphyses of long bones, and adjacent to the vertebral body end plates, giving rise to the 'rugger-jersey spine' (Fig. 8.39).

In children, metaphyseal changes resembling rickets are seen, which together with cortical erosions can give rise to the so called 'rotting fence-post' appearance, particularly at the femoral neck (Fig. 8.40). Slipped capital epiphyses are also seen as a complication, most commonly involving the proximal femur.

A form of arthropathy has been associated with chronic renal failure, and is seen in patients on long term haemodialysis. This consists of changes resembling Charcot joints, but without the extensive bone debris. The most common sites are the shoulder and spine

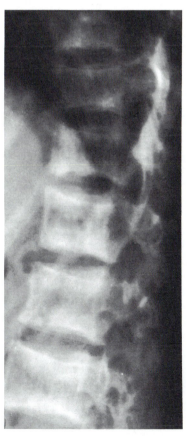

Fig. 8.39 Renal osteodystrophy. 'Rugger-jersey' spine. The typical end-plate sclerosis is seen, giving the characteristic alternating bands of sclerosis and lucency.

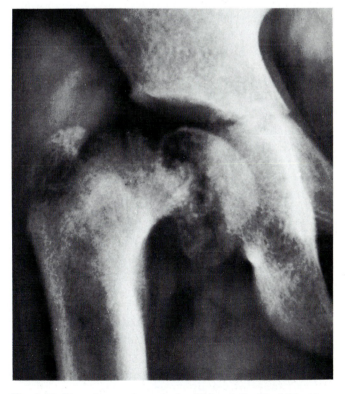

Fig. 8.40 Uraemic osteodystrophy in childhood. In this child with chronic renal failure, the combination of rickets and secondary hyperparathyroidism affects the skeleton. The femoral metaphysis is irregular and the capital epiphysis shows considerable displacement. The metaphyseal appearance has been likened to a rotting fence-post. (Courtesy of Dr. D. J. Stoker and Institute of Orthopaedics.)

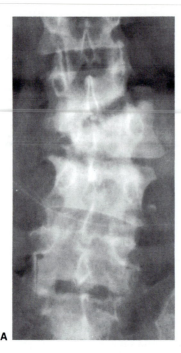

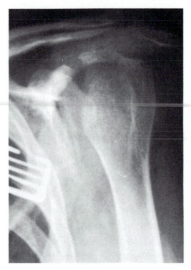

Fig. 8.41 Chronic renal failure: haemodialysis patient. **A**. There is an appearance resembling a Charcot spine, or even infection. **B**. A destructive arthropathy of the shoulder is also seen, without evidence of infection or neuropathy.

(Fig. 8.41). The aetiology is uncertain, although crystal deposition, and amyloid have been suggested.

Tertiary hyperparathyroidism. This term applies to cases in which secondary hyperparathyroidism gives rise to autonomous hyperparathyroidism. Treatment of the underlying disorder fails to control the hyperparathyroidism. Surgical removal of the autonomous parathyroid tissue is necessary.

DRUG- AND TOXIN-INDUCED OSTEOPOROSIS

Heparin, immunosuppressants, and *alcohol* have all been implicated in osteoporosis, as well as *corticosteroids*. The development of osteoporosis has been reported in patients who receive large doses of heparin (usually greater than 15,000 units per day), although the mechanism is uncertain. The activity of mast cells may be an important factor.

In alcoholics, the cause is not known, but it may well be, at least in part, dietary or due to concurrent osteomalacia, secondary to associated liver disease.

Pregnancy and related conditions

Rarely, osteoporosis may be observed during pregnancy, although the cause for this has not been determined.

Other causes of osteoporosis

Other causes of generalized osteoporosis included *multiple myeloma, glycogen storage diseases, marrow packing disorders* such as *Gaucher's disease, chronic liver disease, nutritional deficiency states*, and *chronic anaemias*. *Osteogenesis imperfecta* exhibits marked osteoporosis, Wormian bones,

and fractures which heal with marked callus formation (Fig. 8.17). Blue sclera and deafness are also found. *Homocystinuria* is another cause of osteoporosis.

Oxalosis

Primary hyperoxaluria is inherited as an autosomal recessive trait. The main feature is recurrent urinary calculi, progressing to renal failure. Calcium oxalate deposition in bone and soft tissues occurs in those who survive with dialysis (Fig. 8.42).

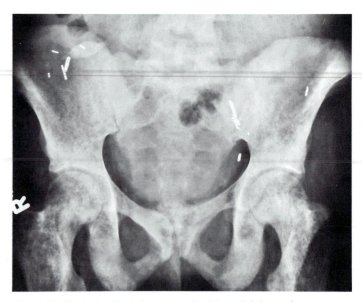

Fig. 8.42 Oxalosis. There is a generalized but slightly patchy increase in density of much of the visualized skeleton, due to calcium oxalate deposition.

Ochronosis (alkaptonuria)

This rare hereditary disorder of tyrosine metabolism is inherited as an autosomal recessive trait. Due to a lack of homogentisic acid oxalate, homogentisic acid accumulates in the tissues, particularly connective tissue. The radiographic features are mainly those of degenerative disease of the peripheral joints (Fig. 8.43) and calcification of spinal disc spaces, (Fig. 8.44). In the spine, advanced changes may lead to an appearance resembling ankylosing spondylitis. Although kyphoscoliosis may occur in the spine, in the major joints there may be considerable joint-space narrowing without marked osteophyte formation or sclerosis until the later stages.

Miscellaneous conditions

Wilson's disease (hepatolenticular degeneration) is a rare autosomal recessive disorder of copper metabolism that produces skeletal changes of osteomalacia, and a form of arthritis. Other metabolic disorders, such as *haemochromatosis* and *calcium pyrophosphate dihydrate deposition* disease also mainly produce joint disease. Haemochromatosis may also give rise to a generalized osteopenia.

Copper deficiency in infants is rare, but is reported in severely malnourished infants, and in infants on long-term parenteral nutrition. There is reduction in bone density, cortical thinning and metaphysical irregularity, with delayed maturation. However, unlike rickets, the zone of provisional calcification is preserved.

Homocystinuria. This is a rare disorder inherited in an autosomal recessive manner and due to a deficiency in the activity of the enzyme cystathiamine synthetase, which converts homocysteine to cystathionine and cys-

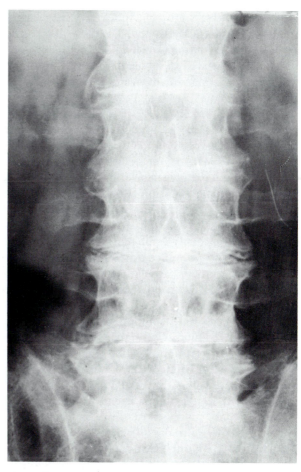

Fig. 8.44 Ochronosis. The intervertebral disc spaces are narrowed and calcified. Such widespread change is uncommon in uncomplicated degenerative spondylosis. (Courtesy of Dr. D. J. Stoker and Institute of Orthopaedics.)

teine. In one form of the disease (pyridoxine-resistant), changes in the skeleton include osteoporosis, arachnodactyly, epiphyseal enlargement, scoliosis, sternal deformity, and valgus deformity of the knees and hips. Being pyridoxine-resistant, this requires a low methionine diet. The other form of the disease is responsive to pyridoxine, and normal skeletal development follows.

LOCALIZED OSTEOPOROSIS

On occasion a localized osteoporosis may occur. The commonest cause for this is *disuse osteoporosis*, which may result from pain following trauma, severe vascular disease, infection or enforced immobilization. A rapid, aggressive-looking resorption of bone occurs, most marked in the cortical, and subarticular areas of the bones (Fig. 8.35).

Reflex sympathetic dystrophy syndrome (*Sudeck's atrophy*)

This is regarded as a distinct entity, including terms such

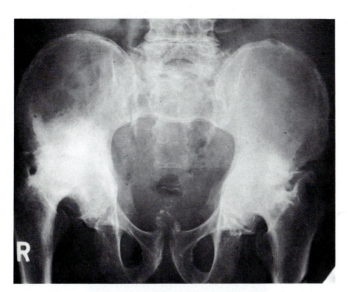

Fig. 8.43 Ochronosis. Gross narrowing of the joint spaces of both hips is associated with other evidence of severe degenerative disease. The intervertebral disc spaces are calcified and narrowed. (Courtesy of Dr. D. J. Stoker and Institute of Orthopaedics.)

as causalgia, Sudeck's atrophy, shoulder hand syndrome and reflex sympathetic dystrophy. The condition has been reported in association with prior trauma, surgery or infectious states, as well as vasculitis, calcific tendonitis, neoplasia, disc herniation, myocardial infarction, degenerative cervical spine disease and cardiovascular disorders. Symptoms usually include pain, swelling, stiffness, and weakness, but may be associated with hyperaesthesia, vasomotor changes and disability. It is thought to be related to abnormal neural reflexes. Endosteal bone resorption is the most prevalent form of demineralization in this condition, although subperiopheal resorption, periarticular porosis, intracortical resorption and subchondral erosions are also seen (see Fig. 9.23).

Idiopathic chondrolysis of the hip is a rare disorder of unknown aetiology. It affects predominantly adolescent girls and young women, particularly blacks, and gives rise to localized pain and marked osteoporosis. Early degenerative change results.

Transient (regional) osteoporosis. This is a rare condition of large joints where gross focal osteoporosis and pain occur. The femoral head is the commonest site. It occurs typically in young and middle-aged adults, and is more common in men. Interestingly, when it occurs in women, the left hip is almost exclusively affected, and the disease occurs in the third trimester of pregnancy. There is no history of trauma or infection. Some authors believe that it is a form of Sudeck's atrophy. Synovial biopsy may show mild chronic inflammation. Symptoms resolve spontaneously in 4–10 months.

Regional migratory osteoporosis. This condition is migratory in nature, and the hip is involved less frequently than other areas, such as the knee, ankle and foot. It is commoner in men than in women, and is most evident between 30 and 50. Clinically it is similar to transient osteoporosis of the hip, the involvement of each joint lasting approximately nine months. Recurrences in other bones may occur successively, or be separated by up to two years or more.

TOXIC EFFECTS ON THE SKELETON

Many toxins and poisons may affect the skeleton. Some common conditions are discussed below.

Hypervitaminosis A. *Overdosage of Vitamin A* may occur in children, but is rare in adults. It gives rise to hypercalcaemia, and an increase in periosteal new bone. Tender swellings of the limbs may occur. Radiographically, dense periosteal new bone is identified (Fig. 8.45), which, in contrast to infantile cortical hyperostosis, is not seen usually until after the first year of life. Withdrawal of Vitamin A supplements results in remodelling of the bone.

Lead poisoning occurs in children who ingest lead-containing paint or water from lead-containing pipes and

leads to lead deposition in the growing metaphyseal regions. This may cause modelling deformities and increased bone density, although most of this is due to reactive change (Fig. 8.46). Lead encephalopathy is a serious complication.

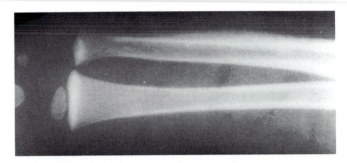

Fig. 8.45 Hypervitaminosis. There is increased cortical density, most marked in the ulna.

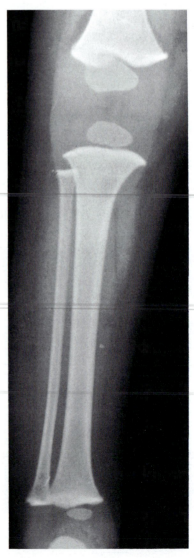

Fig. 8.46 Lead lines: metaphyseal bands of increased density.

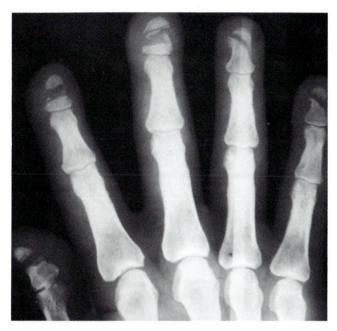

Fig. 8.47 Vinyl chloride poisoning. Inhalation or ingestion of vinyl chloride may produce this characteristic resorption of the central portions of the terminal phalanges. (Courtesy of Dr. D. J. Stoker and Institute of Orthopaedics.)

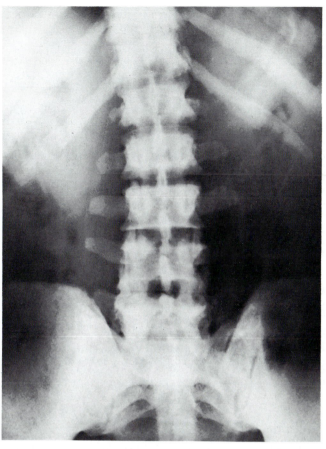

Fig. 8.48 Fluorosis. There is markedly increased density of all the visualized bones. (Courtesy of Dr. D. J. Stoker and Institute of Orthopaedics.)

Bismuth intoxication (often following treatment for syphilis in the past), causes a similar appearance.

Vinyl chloride poisoning found in workers in PVC manufacture causes Raynaud's phenomenon, and a characteristic form of acro-osteolysis (Fig. 8.47). Sacro-ileitis is also seen, and hemangiosarcoma of the liver has been reported.

Fluorosis, due to chronic fluoride poisoning, is endemic in some parts of the Middle and Far East, but may also occur in aluminium smelting industries, and from drinking wine when fluorine is used as a preservative. A generalized increased bone density is seen (Fig. 8.48), which is again due to osteoclastic response to the fluorine rather than to fluorine deposition *per se*.

Cortical thickening occurs, causing encroachment upon the medullary cavity, and ossification of ligamentous and musculotendinous attachments is seen. Endemic fluorosis is rare in children, unless there are exceptionally high levels of fluorine; it may be associated with crippling stiffness and pain.

REFERENCES AND SUGGESTIONS FOR FURTHER READING

General

Fogelman, I., Carr, D. (1980) A comparison of bone scanning and radiology in the evaluation of patients with metabolic bone disease. *Clinical Radiology*, **31**, 321–326.

Genant, H. K., et al (1980) Computed tomography of the musculoskeletal system. *Journal of Bone and Joint Surgery*, 62-A, 1088–1011.

Pitt, M. J. (1981) Ricketic and osteomalacia syndromes. *Radiologic Clinics of North America* **19**: 581–599.

Resnick, D. (ed) (1989) *Bone and Joint Imaging*. W. B. Saunders, Philadelphia.

Bone density

Dequeker, J., Johnston, C. C., Jr. (eds) (1982) *Non-invasive Bone Measurements: Methodological Problems*. I.R.L. Press, Oxford.

Genant, H. K., Cann, C. E. (1981) Vertebral mineral determination using quantitative computed tomography. In: DeLuca, H. F. (ed.) et al. *Osteoporosis: Recent Advances in Pathogenesis and Treatment*. University Park Press, Baltimore, pp. 37–47.

Genant H. K., Black J. E., Steigler, P. et al (1987) Quantitative computed tomography in assessment of osteoporosis. *Seminars in Nuclear Medicine* **17**, 316–323.

Singh, M., Riggs, B. L., Beabout, J. W., Jowsey, J. (1972) Femoral trabecular-pattern index for evaluation of spinal osteoporosis. *Annals of Internal Medicine*, 77, 63–67.

Endocrine disorders

Genant, H. K., Baron, J. M., Strauss, F. H., II, Paloyan, E., Jowsey, J. (1975) Osteosclerosis in primary hyperparathyroidism. *American Journal of Medicine* 59, 104–109.

Kho, K. M., Wright, A. D., Doyle, F. H. (1970) Heel pad thickness in acromegaly. *British Journal of Radiology*, 43, 119–125.

Meema, H. E., Schatz, D. L. (1970) Simple radiologic demonstration of cortical bone loss in thyrotoxicosis. *Radiology* 97, 9–15.

Osteomalacia and rickets

Callenbach, J. C., Shennan, M. B., Abramson, S. J., Hall, R. T. (1981) Etiologic factors in rickets of very low-birth-weight infants. *Journal of Pediatrics*, 98, 800–805.

Swischuk, L. E., Hayden, C. K., Jr. (1979) Rickets: A roentgenographic scheme for diagnosis. *Pediatric Radiology*, 8, 203–208.

Poisons and toxins

Betts, P. R., Watson, S. M., Astley, R. (1973) A suggested role of radiology in lead poisoning. *Annales de Radiologie* 16, 183–187

Caffey, J. (1951) Chronic poisoning due to excess of vitamin A. *American Journal of Roentgenology*, 65, 12–26.

Christie, D. V. (1980) The spectrum of radiographic bone changes in children with fluorosis. *Radiology*, 136, 85–90.

Grunebaum, M., Horodinceanu, C., Steinherz, R. (1980) The radiographic manifestations of bone changes in copper deficiency. *Pediatric Radiology*, 9, 101–104.

Harris, D. K., Adams, W. G. F. (1967) Acro-osteolysis occurring in polymerization of vinyl chloride. *British Medical Journal*, **iii**, 712–714.

Kilmar, S. P., Kemp Harper, R. A. (1963) Fluorosis in Aden. *British Journal of Radiology*, 36, 497–502.

Renal failure/haemodialysis

Elmstedt, E. (1981) Avascular bone necrosis in the renal transplant patient: A discriminant analysis of 144 cases. *Clinical Orthopaedics*, **158**, 149–454.

Goldman, A. B., Lane, J. M., Salvati, E. (1978) Slipped capital femoral epiphyses complicating renal osteodystrophy: A report of three cases. *Radiology*, **126**, 333–337.

Griffin, C. N. (1986) Severe erosive arthritis of large joints in chronic renal failure. *Skeletal Radiology*, **12**, 24–33.

Kaplan, P., Resnick, D., Murphey, M. et al (1986) Destructive noninfectious spondyloarthropathy in hemodialysis patients: A report of four cases. *Radiology*, **162**, 241–247.

Naidich, J. B., Massey, R. T., McHeffey-Atkinson, B. et al. (1988) Spondyloarthropathy from long-term hemodialysis. *Radiology*, **167**, 761–766.

Miscellaneous

Caffey, J. (1972) Familial hyperphosphatasaemia with ateliosis and hypermetabolism of growing membranous bone. *Bulletin of the Hospital for Joint Diseases*, **33**, 81–110.

Houang, M. T. D., Brenton, D. P., Renton, P., Shaw, D. G. (1978) Idiopathic juvenile osteoporosis. *Skeletal Radiology*, **3**, 17–23.

Kozlowski, K. et al. (1976) Hypophosphatasia. Review of 25 cases. *Pediatric Radiology*, **5**, 103–117.

Moule, N. J., Golding, J. S. R. (1976) Idiopathic chondrolysis of the hip. *Clinical Radiology*, **25**, 247–251.

Steinbach, H. L., Young, D. A. (1966) The roentgen appearances of pseudohypoparathyroidism and pseudo-pseudohypoparathyroidism. *American Journal of Roentgenology*, **97**, 49–66.

CHAPTER 9

SKELETAL TRAUMA: GENERAL CONSIDERATIONS

Jeremy W. R. Young

Skeletal trauma is one of the most important aspects of orthopaedic radiology, being by far the commonest problem presented to the musculoskeletal radiologist. Despite this fact however, trauma radiology continues to be the most neglected aspect of this subspecialty, particularly in teaching institutions. This may reflect an illogical approach to skeletal trauma historically, whereby fractures and dislocations were presented as a confusing list of unassociated injuries, often better known by eponyms. More recently there has been a trend towards classifying fractures by the force of injury causing them. This allows a more logical and thoughtful approach, and enhances understanding of fracture patterns, and associated injuries.

A fracture of a bone occurs when there is a break in the continuity of bone, which may be either complete or incomplete. When a loading force is applied to bone, it initially deforms elastically, i.e., as the load is removed the deformity of the bone is reversed, and the bone returns to normal. As the loading force is increased, the elasticity of the bone is overcome, and a plastic 'fracture' occurs, with the bone remaining deformed after cessation of the load. Finally, complete failure of the bone will occur, giving rise to a fracture. Repetitive loading of a bone at 'subfracture' levels may lead to the development of *stress* fracture (see below). Fractures are described in many different ways, as discussed below.

Terminology

The descriptive terms **open** or **closed** refer to whether the bone fragments communicate with the outside environment or not. If bone fragments penetrate the skin, the fracture is 'open' (Fig. 9.1). If the fracture remains covered with intact skin, it is called 'closed'. Although apparent on clinical inspection, various radiographic signs will suggest an open fracture (Table 9.1).

The nature of the fracture lines also describes the fracture. Generally a single fracture line follows one of three major types: transverse, oblique or spiral, although a combination of these is often present. In addition, if the injury produces more than one fracture line, the fracture is said

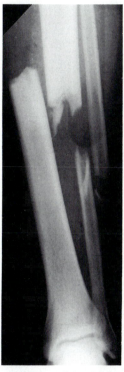

Fig. 9.1 A comminuted fracture of the tibia, with medial displacement and overriding of the distal fragment. Because of the proximity of the skin surface to the anteromedial aspect of the tibia, penetration of the skin is likely, and in fact, air is seen in the soft tissues, indicating that penetration has occurred. There is lateral angulation of the distal fragment. A segmental fibula fracture is noted.

Table 9.1 Radiographic signs of open fracture

Obvious protrusion of bone fragments beyond the soft tissue margins.

Absence of portions of the bone

Gross soft-tissue disruption extending to the bone surface

Subcutaneous gas

Foreign material within the fracture

to be *comminuted*. Comminuted fractures will often produce what is known as a 'butterfly' fragment (Fig. 9.2). A *segmental* fracture is one in which a segment of bone

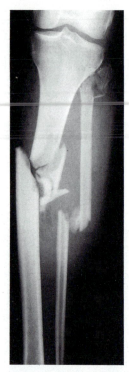

Fig. 9.2 A comminuted fracture of the tibia, with a triangular 'butterfly' fragment.

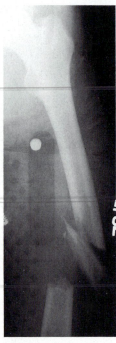

Fig. 9.3 Segmental fracture of the femur: by definition a comminuted fracture. In this case the isolated segment is clearly malaligned.

is isolated by fractures at each end (Fig. 9.3).

Fractures may also be termed 'incomplete' or 'complete'. *Incomplete* fractures occur most commonly in

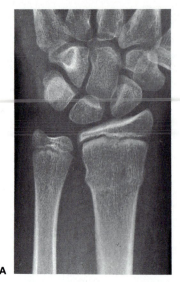
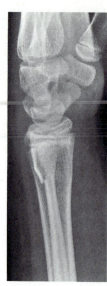

Fig. 9.4 A,B Torus fracture of the radius. The cortex is buckled on the dorsal surface. Apart from minor plastic deformity, the volar surface is intact.

children, when bone resilience is greater, and are of three types; *plastic fractures* occur when there is bending of the bone without cortical disruption, or acute angulation; a '*torus*' or buckle fracture is the term applied to a fracture of the cortex on the 'compressive' side of the bone with an intact cortex on the tension side (Fig. 9.4); *greenstick fracture* is the converse of the torus fracture, occurring only on the tension side.

Fractures should be evaluated for continuity and proximity of the fracture fragments.

Apposition refers to the position of the major fragments with respect to each other. Fragments which are not apposed are described as being *distracted* if the displacement is along the long axis of the bone, or *displaced* out of the long axis. In such cases, the fracture should be described according to the direction of displacement of the distal fragment relative to the proximal bone.

Alignment refers to the relationship along the axis of major fragments. Abnormality of alignment may be described in two ways. The most logical refers to the alignment of the distal fragment with respect to the proximal (Fig. 9.1). This has the additional advantage of following the same 'rules' as apply to displacement. The alternative method, commonly used by orthopaedic surgeons, is to describe the angulation as the direction of the apex of the angle at the fracture site.

'Varus' and 'valgus angulation' are terms that are commonly used, particularly by orthopaedic surgeons — they refer to the alignment of the distal fragment with respect to the midline of the body, with varus indicating angulation of the distal fragment towards the midline and valgus the reverse.

Impaction is the descriptive term for fractures in which the bone fragments are driven into each other.

Abnormality of *rotation* of the distal fragment is an important finding and should always be assessed. This requires visualization of both ends of the bone on the same radiograph, so that the orientation of the proximal and distal joints can be assessed.

Associated soft-tissue abnormalities

Although the majority of fractures are readily identified, on occasion they may be difficult or impossible to see on initial radiographs. Additional clues may be helpful in such cases.

For example, fractures around a joint may provide evidence of a joint effusion or haemarthrosis, providing the joint capsule remains intact. This can be particularly useful at the elbow, where elevation of the fat pads, either anterior or posterior, is good evidence of injury (Fig. 9.5). Lack of obvious bone injury should be regarded with caution, and delayed views after immobilization will often reveal a fracture.

A fat/fluid level (*lipohaemarthrosis*) within a joint, most commonly seen in the knee with the radiograph made with a horizontal beam, is also firm presumptive evidence of an intra-articular fracture, the fat being derived from the bone marrow (Fig. 9.6).

In the thoracic spine, a haemorrhage from a vertebral fracture can be seen as a localized paravertebral soft-tissue mass, giving an appearance similar to that seen in an abscess (Fig. 9.7).

Soft-tissue swelling in the retropharyngeal space has also been cited as being a reliable sign of cervical spine trauma, although more recently the value of this sign has been questioned.

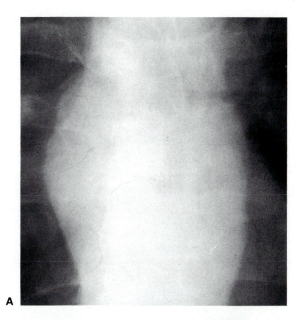

A

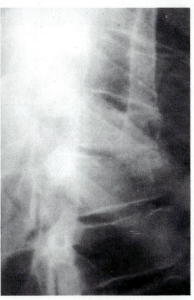

B

Fig. 9.7 A,B Compression fractures of the vertebral bodies of T7, T8 and T9 with large bilateral haematoma, which took many months to absorb, still being visible after the fracture had consolidated (Courtesy Dr. D. J. Stoker and Institute of Orthopaedics.)

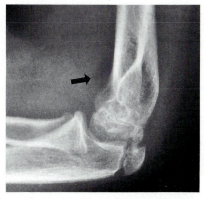

Fig. 9.5 Elbow effusion: elevation of the anterior fat pad (arrow). Although not pathognomonic for fracture, anterior fat pad elevation indicates significant effusion, and is frequently associated with a fracture. Careful inspection of the unfused radial head shows a minor cortical step-off of the metaphysis, indicating a fracture.

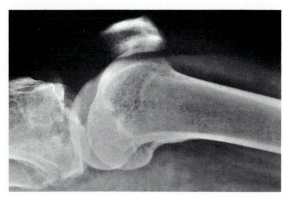

Fig. 9.6 A fat-fluid level (lipohaemarthrosis) is seen in the knee joint on this cross-table lateral view. This indicates intra-articular bone injury.

Fracture healing

After a fracture has occurred, the process of healing begins. Initially, a haematoma forms between the bone ends, occasionally causing periosteal elevation. Granulation tissue then forms between the fracture fragments, with immature osteoid (callus) laid down on the bone surface acting as an early bridge. This first becomes calcified, but eventually woven bone is laid down, leading to firm bone union.

The early stages of bone formation are not visible radiographically, but in a healthy person, new bone formation is visible within 4–6 weeks, with the healing process complete in 4–6 months for a single fracture in a large tubular bone. Delay in union however, may be evident by a delay in the appearance of new bone, and can occur from a variety of causes (see below).

EVALUATION OF SKELETAL TRAUMA

The vast majority of injuries can be adequately visualized by **plain radiographs**. On occasion however, other methods may be needed. **Tomography** has traditionally been used to assess fractures which are not visible, or poorly seen on plain radiographs. **Computed tomography** (CT) is vastly superior to tomography, with the additional advantage of imaging surrounding soft tissues. If CT is available, there are very limited indications for tomography, although this may be useful in cervical spine trauma (see Ch. 10), or in assessing the growth plate for early growth arrest following Salter/Harris fractures in children. In addition, tomography may be used to evaluate depression of bone fragments in tibial plateau fractures, or to determine the position of fragments in fractures of the tibial plafond, talus and calcaneus. In these cases however, it can be argued that CT provides information that is at least as good, if not better (Fig. 9.8) Tomography may also be helpful in suspected blowout fractures of the orbit (Fig. 9.9), as CT may miss fractures of the floor of the orbit, if only obtained in the axial plane. High-quality coronal CT however avoids this problem.

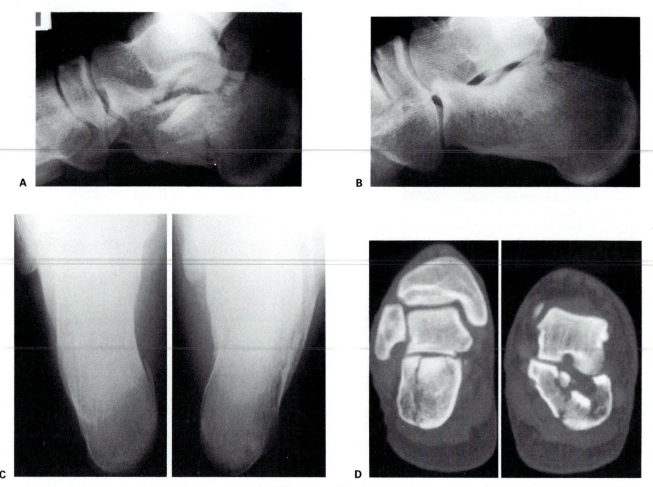

Fig. 9.8 There are comminuted fractures of both calcanea. The extent of the injury, and in particular of the articular involvement, is poorly displayed by the plain radiographs (**A,B,C**). **D.** CT images however demonstrate that there is an obvious disorganization of fragments at the articular surface on the left, and a mildly depressed segment on the right.

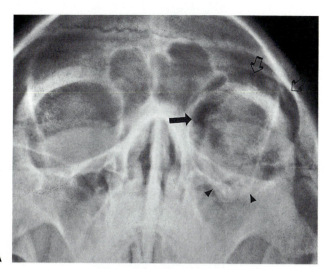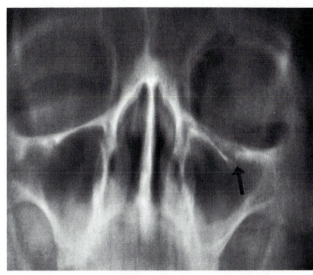

Fig. 9.9 A. Note orbital emphysema on the left, with air surrounding the eyeball (arrow), and beneath the eyelid (open arrows). This is highly suggestive of a blowout fracture. In this case there is irregularity of the inferior orbital rim (arrowheads), with an apparent soft-tissue density projecting into the maxillary sinus. **B.** Tomography confirms the fracture of the orbital floor (arrow).

Nuclear medicine can be helpful in detecting occult fractures, e.g. of the scaphoid or femoral neck, and stress fractures, although a positive scan may not be seen for 24 hours following injury, especially in older patients.

MRI is also gaining in popularity for its ability to distinguish between different pathologies. For example it is able to differentiate non-union from infected non-union by the increase in signal that is seen in areas of inflammation (Fig. 9.10). It is also superior to other techniques in evaluating joint injuries (see Ch. 4). The advantages of its ability to demonstrate soft tissue detail, its capability of multiplanar imaging, and its lack of ionizing radiation are responsible for the rapidly increasing use of MRI in musculoskeletal radiology.

COMPLICATIONS OF FRACTURE

In open fractures, there is an increased potential for *infection* at the fracture site. Closed fractures however are not as susceptible to this problem. Nevertheless there are potential problems in all fractures.

The tibia has long been singled out as a bone liable to *delayed union* or *non-union*. The reasons for this are obscure, but poor vascular supply and lack of immobilization have been cited. In practice it would appear that the reason for the high incidence of cases of delayed or non union may be due to the large number of 'high-energy' injuries seen in the tibia, particularly from pedestrian 'bumper' injuries, with a large amount of resulting necrosis of soft tissue and bone.

Delayed union. This may occur from many causes (Table 9.2).

Fig. 9.10 A. MRI scan demonstrates tissue of mixed signal intensity in the fracture gap of non-union of the distal femur (arrows) on T_1 images. **B.** Areas of increased signal intensity are shown on T_2 weighted images (dark arrows), indicating foci of infection.

Table 9.2 Causes of delayed union

Mechanical:	poor apposition
	inadequate stabilization
Pathological:	age — decreased osteoblastic activity
	dietary — vitamin deficiency (C and D)
	pathological fracture (underlying abnormality)
	infection

Non-union. This is the absence of bony union over a prolonged period (Table 9.3). The radiograph appearance is usually of a persistent fracture line, usually with sclerotic margins, and marked surrounding sclerosis (Fig. 9.11).

Table 9.3 Causes of non-union

1. Idiopathic (particularly tibia)
2. Poor stabilization
3. Infection
4. Pathological fracture
5. Massive initial trauma

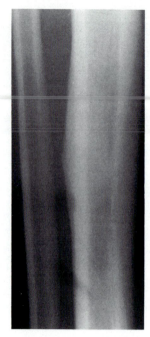

Fig. 9.13 Stress fracture: an area of increased sclerosis, with some dense periosteal new bone in the mid tibia.

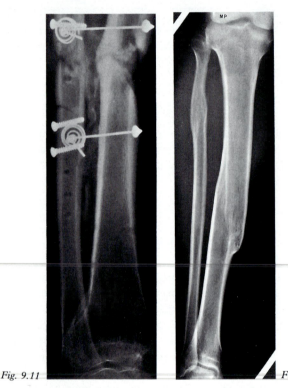

Fig. 9.11   Fig. 9.12

Fig. 9.11 Non-union of the tibia despite interosseous bone grafting, and surgical wiring: There is sclerosis around the fracture line, without firm evidence of bone bridging, one year after the fracture.

Fig. 9.12 Malunion of the tibial fracture, which has healed well, but shows lateral angulation of the distal fragment.

Malunion is the term given to a fracture which heals in an unsatisfactory anatomical position, either with excessive overlap of fragments, or unsatisfactory angulation or displacement of the distal fragment (Fig. 9.12).

SPECIAL TYPES OF TRAUMA

Stress (fatigue) fractures

These fractures result from chronic repetitive forces which by themselves are insufficient to cause fracture, but over the course of time lead to the classic changes of a stress fracture. They occur in many bones, and usually at characteristic sites, often as the result of athletic activity: for example the 'march' fracture of the second and third metatarsal head, the stress fracture of the mid and distal tibia and fibula in long-distance runners and ballet dancers, and fractures of the proximal fibula in paratroopers.

The earliest diagnosis can be made by *nuclear medicine* scanning, where activity will be seen before radiographic signs. When *radiographic signs* appear, they may take several forms, depending upon the stage of healing or the chronicity of the stress factors. A hairlike lucency may be seen traversing the bone, although this may not be apparent without tomography. New bone formation around the fracture may be the only sign, or may accompany the cortical fracture (Fig. 9.13). If the patient continues the activity, a form of chronic fracture will occur, with abundant sclerotic periosteal new bone and a persistent lucent fracture line, with surrounding sclerosis (Fig. 9.14).

A type of stress fracture is said to account for the pars interarticularis defects seen in spondylolisthesis (Fig. 9.15), whereby the continuance of the stress leads to a complete fracture, followed by non-union. Alternatively a congenital hypoplasia of the articular processes, or degenerative change within the posterior joints, may be the underlying cause. The defect in the pars interarticularis

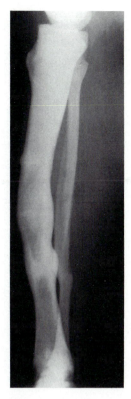

Fig. 9.14 Multiple stress fractures are seen, some with obvious horizontal lucencies running perpendicular to the bone cortex. The patient was a jogger who refused to give up jogging despite the pain!

is known as *spondylolysis*. When anterior displacement of the superior vertebral body on its neighbour is seen *spondylolisthesis*, is said to have occurred. Mild degrees of spondylolisthesis can occur when there is loss of articular cartilage at the posterior intervertebral joints as in degenerative disease. More severe spondylolisthesis results from pars interarticularis defects, and is graded according to severity: Grade I up to 25% displacement of the vertebral body: Grade II, up to 50%, Grade III, up to 75%, and Grade IV 100% displacement.

Avulsion fractures

These occur from avulsion of bone fragments at the site of ligamentous or tendinous attachments throughout the skeleton. Of note are abnormalities which have previously been classified as osteochondritis, but which represent avulsion fractures from chronic or repeated trauma. This includes *Osgood-Schlatter's* disease and *Sindig-Larsen* disease of the tibial tubercle and inferior patella respectively.

The diagnosis of Osgood-Schlatter's disease is made clinically, although it can be suggested radiographically when there is clear elevation of fragments of the tibial tubercle separated from the underlying bone (Fig. 9.16). Fragmentation alone without displacement does not constitute Osgood-Schlatter's disease, and merely represents multiple ossification centres.

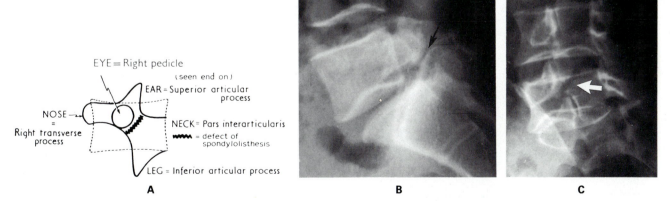

Fig. 9.15 A. Diagrammatic representation of an oblique view of a lumbar vertebra, presenting the "Scotty dog" appearance. The pars interarticularis defect corresponds to the dog's collar. **B,C.** Pars defect: oblique radiograph demonstrates the same appearances as in **A.** (Courtesy Dr. D. J. Stoker and Institute of Orthopaedics.)

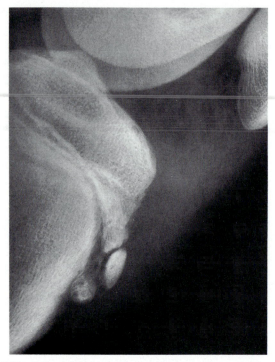

Fig. 9.16 Osgood-Schlatter's disease. Fragmentation may be seen and a portion of the tibial tubercle ossification centre is elevated.

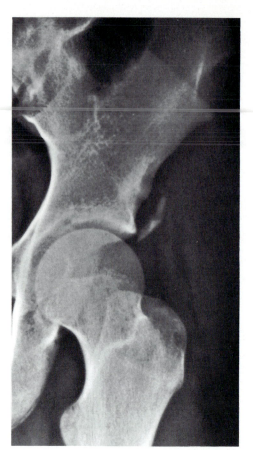

Fig. 9.18 Avulsion fracture of the anterior inferior iliac crest: This is the origin of the rectus femoris muscle.

Common avulsion injuries at the origin of muscle tendon insertions are seen at the inferior border of the ischium (hamstrings) (Fig. 9.17), anterior inferior iliac crest (rectus femoris), (Fig. 9.18) and lesser trochanter (iliopsoas) (see Table 9.4).

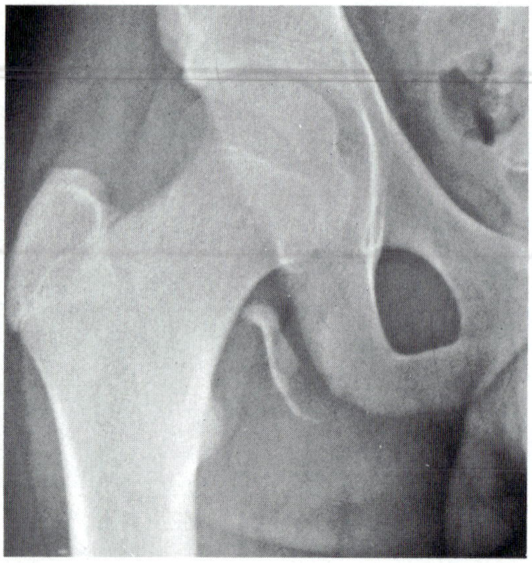

Table 9.4 Sites of avulsion fractures with muscle origin

Anterior superior iliac crest	Sartorius
Anterior inferior iliac crest	Rectus femoris
Ischial tuberosity	Hamstrings
Greater trochanter	Gluteals
Lesser trochanter	Iliopsoas
Posterior calcaneus	Achilles tendon
Olecranon process	Triceps
Superior patella	Quadriceps
Inferior patella (Sindig-Larsen)	Patella ligament
Tibial tuberosity (Osgood-Schlatter)	Patella ligament

Fig. 9.17 Note an avulsion of the inferior border of the ischium at the site of insertion of the hamstrings.

Pathological fractures

Pathological fractures are fractures through bone that has been weakened by an underlying disease. This does not necessarily mean an underlying malignancy, although the term 'pathological fracture' tends to suggest it. Pathological fractures occur through bone that is weakened by such conditions as osteoporosis or osteomalacia, bone tumours

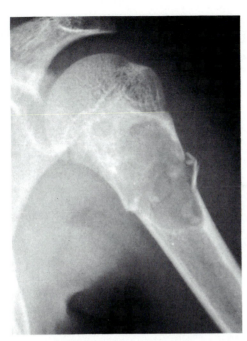

Fig. 9.19 Pathological fracture through a simple bone cyst of the proximal humerus.

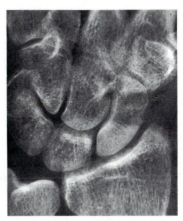

Fig. 9.20 Post-traumatic avascular necrosis of the proximal pole of the scaphoid. Although the fracture of the waist of the scaphoid has 'healed', avascular necrosis has occurred, with resulting sclerosis.

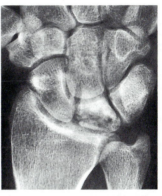

Fig. 9.21 Kienbock's disease: in fact, a form of traumatic avascular necrosis of the lunate.

(whether benign (Fig. 9.19) or malignant), or even tumour-like lesions of bone. In elderly patients of course, underlying malignancy should be considered, especially if the fracture occurs in a site other than those usually seen in osteoporosis such as the femoral neck, or in cases in which the severity of the injury is inappropriate to the fracture created.

Post-traumatic avascular necrosis

This occurs from a traumatic severance of the blood supply to the bone or a fragment thereof. There are several bones in the body in which this is likely to happen in areas when the blood supply is easily compromised. *Femoral neck* fractures may interrupt the vascular supply to the femoral head. In fractures of the wrist involving the *scaphoid*, the proximal pole is at risk as the vascular supply enters the bone more distally (Fig. 9.20). Similarly, *talar waist* fractures threaten the proximal fragment. Post-traumatic avascular necrosis may occur in part of a bone as described above, but may also involve the growing epiphysis such as the *head of the 2nd or 3rd metatarsal* (Frieberg's disease) or even the whole of a small bone, eg. *lunate* (Kienbock's disease) (Fig. 9.21). Frequently there is no clear history of predisposing fracture. However there is evidence that even conditions such as *Perthes' disease* may result from a traumatic effusion, which is also responsible for the widening of the joint space that may be seen in this condition. This radiographic abnormality may be seen in the 'irritable hip syndrome' of children, which may progress to frank necrosis of the femoral head. This has been attributed to interruption of the vascular flow, possibly on the venous side, by the formation of granulation tissue. A similar scenario has been suggested for *septic arthritis* (pus within the joint), and haemophilia (blood within the joint).

In avascular necrosis, the necrotic bone usually become denser than the surrounding bone (Fig. 9.20) which in turn may become more osteopenic due to disuse. Studies on the femoral heads removed following fracture in the process of hip prosthesis implantation show that this is due to revascularization, when a thin layer of calcifying osteoid is laid down on the necrotic trabecula. This feature may occur anytime from two months to two years following injury. Eventually collapse and fragmentation are likely to occur. MRI scan may be useful in the diagnosis.

Drillers' disease (vibration syndrome)

Drillers' disease is seen in workers with vibrating machinery, usually after five or more years of use. Degenerative cysts are found in the bone of the wrist,

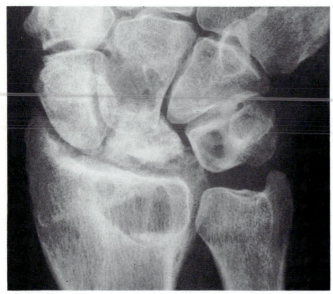

Fig. 9.22 Vibration syndrome. Fragmentation and flattening of the lunate due to avascular necrosis is typical of Kienbock's disease, accompanied by extensive cystic changes in the surrounding bones. These abnormalities occurred in a worker with compressed-air drills, who had been exposed to this repeated trauma for many years. (Courtesy Dr. D. J. Stoker and Institute of Orthopaedics.)

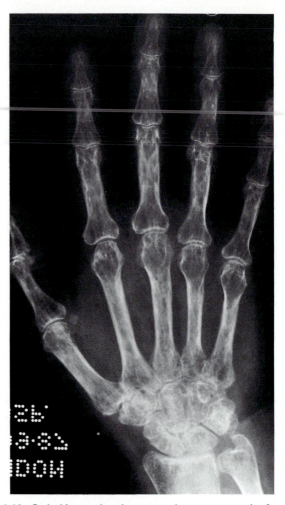

Fig. 9.23 Sudeck's atrophy: there was minor trauma to the forearm some weeks earlier. Note gross osteoporosis of the bones of the hand, wrist and forearm, most marked at the bone ends, but also causing cortical 'thinning' and resorption.

and occasionally hand (Fig. 9.22). They are however indistinguishable from the cysts also seen from heavy manual labour, and the exact aetiology is uncertain.

Sudeck's atrophy (*post-traumatic reflex dystrophy*)

This is a rare condition in which, following injury to a limb, intense pain and swelling occurs, resulting in severe disuse osteoporosis. Interestingly, the initial injury may be relatively minor; the effects however are dramatic (Fig. 9.23). An associated neurovascular reaction may be present.

Transient osteoporosis

This is a rare condition which usually affects the hip. Although this may represent a type of Sudeck's atrophy, a history of trauma is rare. Massive subarticular osteoporosis occurs, which is however self-limiting, with spontaneous resolution within 4–10 months.

Myositis ossificans (post-traumatic)

This usually occurs without overt underlying bone injury. The exact aetiology is uncertain, but it may be due to ossification of a haematoma or reactive periosteal elements which have been displaced into the soft tissues. The thigh is the commonest site. Hazy density in the soft tissues gives way to frank new bone formation, which may extend to the bone surface (Fig. 9.24). This may cause difficulty in distinguishing the lesion from parosteal osteosarcoma. Furthermore, unless adequate biopsy material is obtained, including the central and peripheral

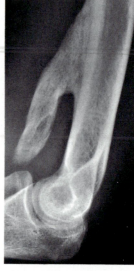

Fig. 9.24 Post-traumatic myositis ossificans. A well-defined bone density arises from the cortex of the distal humerus and extends into the soft tissues. There was a history of blunt trauma.

components of the lesion, histological differentiation may also be difficult.

A similar type of calcification or ossification may occur around joints following dislocation, and in cases of severe closed head injury (Fig. 9.25). Ligamentous avulsions or chronic ligamentous trauma may also result in calcification, such as calcification of the medial collateral ligament of the knee in cases of chronic subclinical trauma (Fig. 9.26) (**Pellegrini-Stieda lesion**).

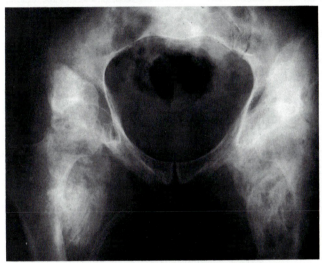

Fig. 9.25 Myositis ossificans associated with paraplegia. Very extensive soft-tissue ossification is visible round both hip joints. (Courtesy Dr. D. J. Stoker and Institute of Orthopaedics.)

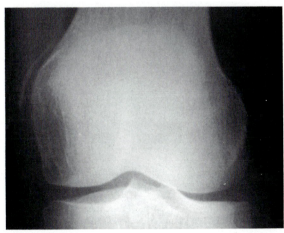

Fig. 9.26 Pellegrini-Stieda lesion. Post-traumatic calcification is shown in relation to the medial femoral condyle following a tear of the medial collateral ligament. (Courtesy Dr. D. J. Stoker and Institute of Orthopaedics.)

Compartment syndrome

Rarely, trauma to a limb will give rise to a potentially devastating situation whereby the tissue pressure within a closed 'compartment' causes progressive ischaemia and ultimately necrosis. The compartments of the limbs consist of areas surrounded by rigid osseous and fascial planes. Tissue oedema or haemorrhage may be the initiating factor and result from direct trauma and/or vascular interruption. The result of oedema within a closed compartment is to raise the tissue pressure, thereby further decreasing vascular perfusion. Prompt fasciotomy is required. *Volkmann's ischaemia* and contracture of the forearm, following fracture of the elbow, is probably a form of the compartment syndrome. Today the syndrome is most commonly seen in the leg as the result of road traffic accidents.

Arterial injury

Vascular trauma generally occurs as the result of penetrating injury, although it may be caused by sharp bone fragments from a fracture, either at the time of injury or during manipulation. The popliteal artery is commonly injured from fractures or dislocations around the knee. Brachial artery injury may also result from supracondylar fractures of the humerus or elbow dislocations, particularly in children. Branches of the internal iliac artery, especially the superior gluteal, pudendal, and vesical, are at risk in pelvic ring fractures (see below), and are responsible for the massive blood loss and associated high mortality rates (Fig. 9.27).

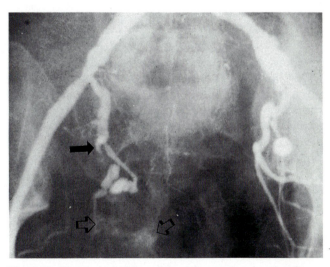

Fig. 9.27 Traumatic avulsion of the right superior gluteal artery (arrow) from pelvic trauma. Bleeding from branches of the internal iliac artery is also seen (open arrows). Marked diastasis of the right sacroiliac joint has occurred.

Joint injuries

Dislocations occur when there is a complete loss of normal articular contact between the bones comprising the joint (Fig. 9.28). *Subluxation* refers to a partial loss of articular contact. *Diastasis* refers to separation of fibrous joints, e.g.

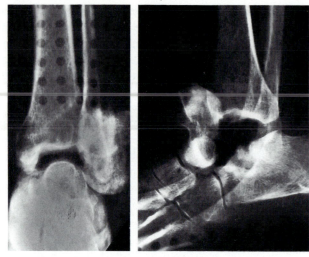

Fig. 9.28   Complete dislocation of the talus.

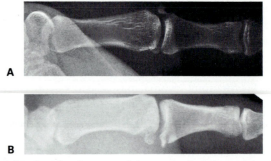

Fig. 9.30   Avulsion fractures of the proximal phalanx of the thumb. A. Fracture at the site of attachment of the radial collateral ligament. B. Fracture at the site of the attachment of the ulnar collateral ligament. In practice, the adductor of the thumb inserts in the same area, and may also be avulsed.

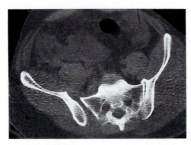

Fig. 9.29   CT image demonstrates complete diastasis of the right sacroiliac joint.

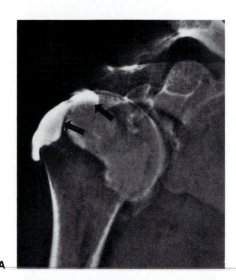

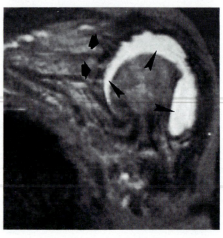

Fig. 9.31   Rotator cuff tear. A. Arthrography is performed by injecting contrast medium, with or without air, into the shoulder joint. Leakage of contrast into the subdeltoid bursa (arrows) indicates a rupture of the rotator cuff which normally separates the bursa from the joint. B. MRI demonstrates a large joint effusion, shown as high signal on this FLASH image. The effusion, which shows markedly increased signal intensity on this sequence, has tracked into the subdeltoid bursa (arrowheads), indicating rotator cuff rupture. In this case the subscapularis is seen to be retracted, with an irregular lateral margin (large arrows).

symphysis pubis; sacroiliac joint (Figs 9.27, 9.29).

Joint injuries may be difficult to diagnose radiographically, as they frequently comprise ligamentous injury without obvious bone involvement. In addition, subtle avulsion fractures adjacent to joints may be the only indicator of gross ligamentous injuries. These are most commonly encountered around the *ankle*, where avulsions of the medial and lateral malleoli indicate collateral ligament disruption. Other important areas are the base of the proximal phalanx of the *thumb* (Fig. 9.30), and corner avulsions of the *tibial plateau*. Plain radiographic signs of injury such as effusion or haemarthrosis may be helpful. Stress views of the involved joint have been advocated, but this may require the patient to be sedated as they may be extremely painful to obtain.

Assessment of joints

Arthrography has traditionally been used to assess joint abnormalities (Fig. 9.31A). Ultrasound has also been used, particularly to assess the shoulder joint for injuries to the rotator cuff (see below), and CT is also useful in the shoulder, especially when combined with arthrography, when injuries of the glenoid labrum may be seen.

Most recently however, magnetic resonance (MR) has made immense progress with its ability to define the soft tissues, ligaments and tendons. Although originally finding favour for its ability to diagnose meniscal tears in the knee (Fig. 9.32), more recent work suggests it can be useful for the shoulder (Fig. 9.31B), ankle and wrist, where ligamentous and tendinous abnormalities may be demonstrated (Fig. 9.33). In addition, it may be used to detect post-traumatic avascular necrosis (Fig. 9.34).

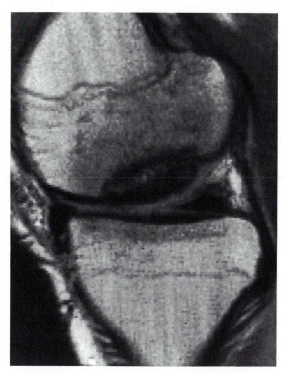

Fig. 9.34 Post-traumatic avascular necrosis of the femoral condyle. MRI demonstrates abnormal signal when compared to the surrounding bone. A focal defect is surrounded by a rim of low signal, indicating a non-viable osteochondral fragment. (Courtesy of Dr. David Nelson.)

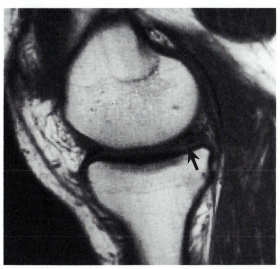

Fig. 9.32 Posterior horn tear of medial meniscus. MRI image (T₁) demonstrates a linear area of higher signal extending to the articular surface (arrow).

FRACTURES IN CHILDHOOD

Fractures in children differ from those in adults in several ways. They are often incomplete (torus or greenstick fractures) (Fig. 9.4), and 'plastic' fractures, without any cortical disruption, may occur. Children's bones have a greater capacity for remodelling than adult's bones, which allows for less exact corrective reduction, although rotational anomalies cannot be corrected by remodelling. Because of the hyperaemia associated with fracture healing, there may be increased growth in the affected limb. This helps to restore length when overlap of the main fragments occurs; but on occasion also can cause unwanted increased length in a limb.

Finally, because of the relatively weak epiphyseal plate, fractures through this region are common. Damage to the epiphyseal plate may result in partial or even complete growth arrest. The *Salter-Harris classification* of fractures of the epiphyseal plate is the one most commonly used (Figs 9.35, 9.36). Under this system, the potential for growth arrest increases with increasing type number, Types IV and V having the greatest potential for growth arrest (Fig. 9.37) However, it must be remembered that in a small child with uncalcified epiphysis, it may be difficult or impossible to accurately determine damage to the epiphyseal cartilage, and what may appear to be a

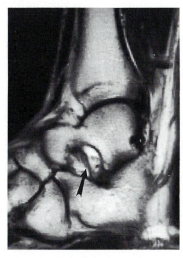

Fig. 9.33 MRI of the normal ankle. T₁ image, sagittal plane, showing the interosseous (talocalcaneal) ligament (arrow).

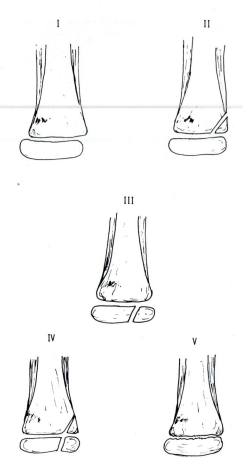

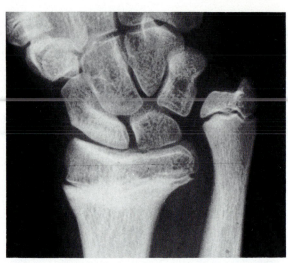

Fig. 9.37 Premature fusion of the distal radial epiphysis, following a fracture-separation seven years before, with relative overgrowth of the ulna.

Fig. 9.35 Salter-Harris classification. I — Injury through the epiphyseal plate only. II — Fracture through the epiphyseal plate and metaphysis. III — Fracture through the epiphyseal plate and epiphysis. IV — Fracture through the epiphyseal plate, metaphysis and epiphysis. V — Crush fracture of the epiphyseal plate.

simple Type I or II fracture may indeed represent a type IV or V injury, with the increased potential for growth arrest.

Growth arrest may take several forms, which have been classified by Bright. Type I and II growth arrests, which involve less than 25% of the area of the growth plate, can be treated by resection and implanting of inert material, but the more complex types may require radical resection and fusion with subsequent osteotomies or limb-lengthening procedures.

Slipped femoral capital epiphysis

This occurs in adolescent children and is probably related to trauma, which may be chronic. It represents a variety of Salter-Harris Type I fracture of the epiphyseal plate. It is most commonly seen in boys approaching puberty, particularly those who are overweight and sexually immature. The incidence in girls however is rising, possibly as a result of an increase in sporting and physical activity. It may be bilateral (30–40%).

The epiphysis is displaced from the metaphysis, usually in a posterior and slightly inferior direction reflecting an anterior and superior slip of the femoral neck with respect to the epiphysis. 'Frog's-leg' views as well as antero-posterior views may be needed to make the diagnosis and both hips should be examined because of the high incidence of bilateral involvement (Fig. 9.38).

Radiographic signs include blurring of the epiphyseal/metaphyseal junction due to superimposition; increased width of the epiphyseal plate; so-called elongation of the superior neck of the femur, whereby a line drawn along the superior neck fails to cut the epiphysis or cuts only a small portion (in normal patients this line usually cuts approximately one-fifth to one-fourth of the

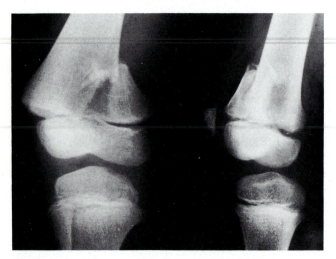

Fig. 9.36 Fracture-separation of the distal femoral epiphysis in an anteromedial direction, carrying with it a large fragment of the femoral metaphysis — the relatively common Salter-Harris Type II injury.

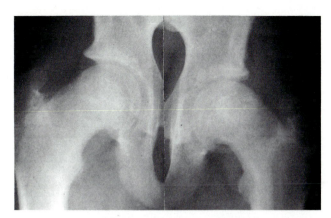

Fig. 9.38 Bilateral slipped capital femoral epiphyses. The diagnosis is more difficult when there is such symmetrical abnormality. There is however obvious blurring of the epiphyseal line, and elongation of the femoral neck. The femoral head does not project above the line of the femoral neck on either side.

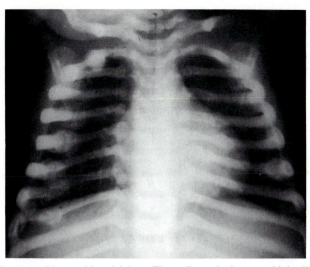

Fig. 9.40 Non-accidental injury. The radiograph shows multiple rib fractures at different stages of healing, probably the result of repeated compression injuries to the thorax. The child was admitted with a recent skull fracture. (Courtesy of Dr. D. J. Stoker and Institute of Orthopaedics.)

epiphysis); and loss of height of the epiphysis when compared to a normal contralateral hip. Careful follow-up of the contralateral hip is mandatory due to the high incidence of bilateral involvement.

A rare late complication of congenital slipped epiphysis is chondrolysis (Waldenstrom's disease), which ultimately causes joint-space narrowing and early degenerative arthritis.

The battered child
In 1946 Caffey described a syndrome of subdural haematoma, associated with multiple fractures of the long bones, often in various stages of repair. This is the condition known today as the *battered infant*. In addition, clinical inspection of such cases may demonstrate bruises, burns, evidence of malnutrition and signs of neglect. Inconsistencies in the history given by the parents or guardian are usual.

Radiographic findings include fractures in different stages of healing, periosteal reactions (Fig. 9.39) particularly in the bones of the distal forearm or leg, multiple growth recovery lines, and injuries to the skull and ribs (Fig. 9.40). Epiphyseal separations and metaphyseal in-

fractions are particularly common. Fractures in unusual sites (e.g. femoral shaft), and from apparently minor trauma, should also alert the physician to the possibility of non-accidental injury. Such findings warrant a complete skeletal survey and communication to the referring physician immediately, as many children subjected to battering die at a subsequent assault.

OTHER FORMS OF TRAUMA
Trauma may occur from a variety of other causes, including *ionizing radiation*, *frostbite* and rarely *electrical burns*, and *dysbaric osteonecrosis* (caisson disease).

Ionizing radiation may cause an area of osteonecrosis at the site of the insult, whether from radiation therapy or other causes, e.g. the mouth in radium dial workers in the past. The affected bone generally exhibits a patchy sclerosis, and may fracture spontaneously. Secondary malignant degeneration may occur, usually to osteosarcoma after a latent period of more than five years.

Frostbite may give rise to acro-osteolysis (Fig. 9.41), and in children, premature epiphyseal closure and growth arrest.

Caisson disease is found in deep-sea divers and tunnel workers, and is due to poor decompression giving rise to bubbles of nitrogen in the blood. These may block capillaries, causing avascular necrosis. Bone changes include areas of irregular bone density, usually in the long bones, and due to medullary infarction, and subarticular infarctions, particularly in the humeral and femoral heads (Fig. 9.42). A similar pattern of subarticular bone infarction is seen in a variety of other conditions. (Table 9.5).

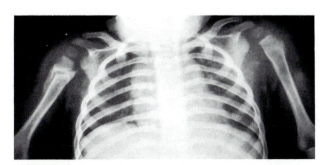

Fig. 9.39 Battered child. Healing fractures are seen in both proximal humeri.

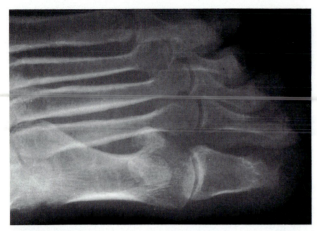

Fig. 9.41 Frostbite. Note acro-osteolysis of the toes, with almost complete resorption of the distal phalanges.

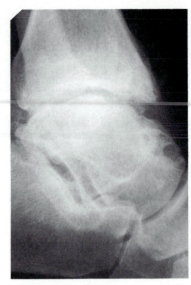

Fig. 9.43 Early Charcot joint, diabetic patient. Note irregularity of the talar dome, with increased density seen around the ankle joint.

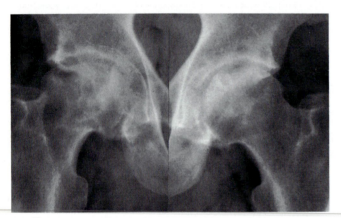

Fig. 9.42 Avascular necrosis of the hips. Note mixed sclerosis and lucency of the femoral heads, with collapse of the weight-bearing surface but maintenance of the joint spaces, indicating intact articular cartilage.

Table 9.5 Causes of subarticular bone infarction — avascular necrosis

Caisson disease

Sickle cell disease

Gaucher's disease

Pancreatitis

Chronic alcoholism (? pancreatitis)

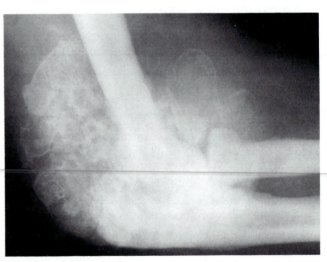

Fig. 9.44 Charcot joint: syringomyelia. The elbow joint shows marked irregularity, with abundant sclerosis, deformity and bone debris. On initial examination, the appearance resembles synovial osteochondromatosis. However the generalized sclerosis and joint destruction indicate the diagnosis.

CHRONIC TRAUMA TO THE JOINTS
(Neuropathic Arthropathy)

Brief mention will be made of this entity, although it is covered more fully in Chapter 10.

Repeated trauma to the joints in the absence of normal pain and proprioceptive sensation will give rise to a severe destructive arthropathy, first described by Charcot (Figs 9.43, 9.44, 9.45). Although seen originally in cases of neurosyphilis, there are a variety of causes (Table 9.6).

Most joints show evidence of *d*isorganization, increased bone *d*ensity, *d*ebris within the joint capsule, and bone *d*estruction, giving rise to *d*eformity — the so-called "5 Ds" (Fig. 9.44). On occasion however, a characteristic clear-cut destruction of the shaft of the bone is seen suggesting, at least superficially, a surgical procedure (Fig. 9.45).

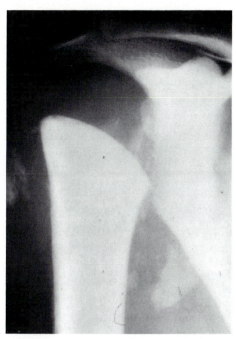

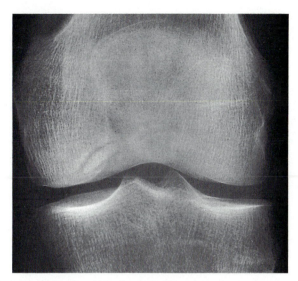

Fig. 9.46 Osteochondritis dissecans. Note defect in the femoral condyle, comprising a lucent ring with a more sclerotic centre.

Fig. 9.45 Charcot joint: syringomyelia. Same patient as in Fig. 9.44. There is the appearance of a surgical 'amputation' of the head of the humerus. Glenoid destruction, joint debris, and increased radiodensity of the bones indicate the true nature of the abnormality.

Table 9.6 Causes of Charcot joints

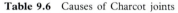

Diabetes (Fig. 9.43)

Neurosyphilis

Syringomyelia (Figs 9.44, 9.45)

Spina bifida

Leprosy

Congenital indifference to pain

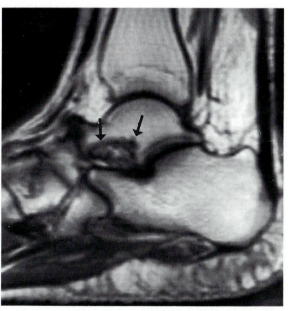

Fig. 9.47 Osteochondral fracture. Sagittal T$_1$ MRI of the ankle. There is a well defined area of abnormal signal in the inferior border of the talus at the insertion of the interosseous ligament (arrows). The ligament itself cannot be seen, indicating disruption (see Fig. 9.33).

OSTEOCHONDRITIS DISSECANS
(Osteochondral fractures)

Osteochondritis dissecans is really a misnomer, as the lesions clinically referred to as osteochondritis are usually the result of trauma, and indicate an osteochondral or chondral fracture occurring at an articular surface. After injury the detached portion of the bone may remain in situ, may be mildly displaced, or may become loose within the joint.

The most common site for osteochondritis dissecans is the distal femur. The medial condyle is involved in 85% of cases with the lesion classically on the lateral aspect of the medial femoral condyle (Fig. 9.46). Other forms of osteochondral fractures involve the weight-bearing sur-face of the joint, or the site of intra-articular ligamentous disruption (Fig. 9.47). Other sites of osteochondritis dissecans include the posterior patella and the talar dome.

Other forms of osteochondral fractures occur, with

direct trauma to the articular surface, as seen in the Hill-Sachs deformity of the femoral head, from anterior dislocations and the recently reported anterior femoral head defect following posterior dislocation of the hip.

REFERENCES AND FURTHER READING:

See end of Chapter 10.

CHAPTER 10

SKELETAL TRAUMA: REGIONAL

Jeremy W. R. Young

THE SKULL

The value of plain radiographic analysis of the skull continues to present a dilemma to physicians, and despite the large number of publications refuting the clinical value of plain radiographs, they continue to be widely requested. The logical approach would be that if there has been sufficient injury to necessitate examination, computed tomography should be performed, since whether a fracture is present or not, intracranial haemorrhage may occur (Fig. 10.1).

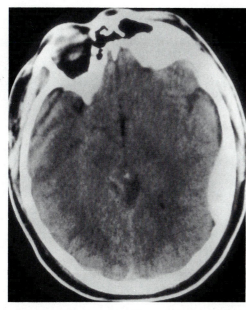

Fig. 10.1 Extradural haematoma: CT scan. A well-defined area of increased density is seen. The clear-cut convex inner margin is diagnostic of an extradural collection.

Basic skull radiography consists of a PA and a lateral view, although right and left lateral radiographs, submental-vertex view and Townes' view are also obtained in some centres. The majority of skull fractures are linear and on occasion these may cause a diagnostic problem, simulating or being simulated by vascular grooves

(see Ch. 53). In general, vascular grooves are less lucent and less sharply marginated, and are seen to branch and make curves rather than sharp angles.

Fractures which extend to the base of the skull may extend into the sphenoid sinus and an air–fluid level in the sphenoid sinus should always be sought on a cross-table lateral view. Similarly, fractures may extend into the frontal sinuses, causing air–fluid levels. *Otorrhoea* or *rhinorrhoea* may occur in basal skull fractures.

Fractures may occur in the temporal bones, and are generally of two varieties: longitudinal (along the axis of the temporal bone), or transverse. Both may cause damage to the auditory or facial nerve, but longitudinal fractures are more likely to cause injury to the tympanic membrane and ossicles.

Depressed fractures of the skull may be readily apparent clinically but can be missed. In general, however, they have a typical radiographic appearance of a crescent of dense bone, due to overlapping fragments (Fig. 10.2). Tangential views provide the conclusive diagnosis in these cases. Intracranial haemorrhage may be suggested by shift of the calcified pineal gland on the frontal views of the skull.

The advent of CT, however, and more recently magnetic resonance imaging (MRI) has revolutionized the radiological evaluation of head trauma. Fractures of the skull and facial bones, as well as intracranial haemorrhage, are readily seen.

THE FACIAL BONES

Usually the result of automobile accidents or assaults, facial bone injury generally involves one of four areas: mandible, zygomatic arch and orbit, nasal bones, or complex fractures of the Le Fort varieties (see below).

Radiographic examination of the facial bones will include lateral, PA (occipito-frontal) and Waters (occipito-mental) views. Although these provide moderately good information, overlying soft-tissue swelling can obscure detail considerably. Although additional views such as obliques may be helpful, CT has proved to be

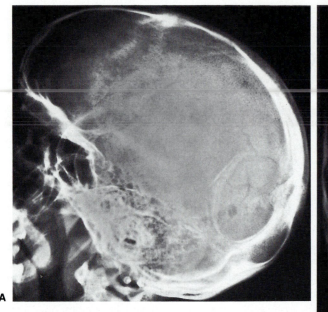

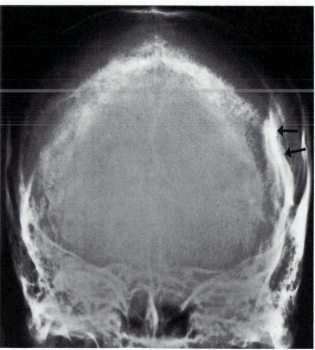

Fig. 10.2 Depressed skull fracture. **A**. A curvilinear density overlies the posterior parietal region on the lateral view. **B**. On the Townes view, the depressed nature of the defect can be appreciated (arrows).

vastly superior to the plain film in the evaluation of facial trauma. Most recently, three-dimensional images have provided exquisite detail, not available by any other technique (Figs 10.3 to 10.5).

The *mandible* is most commonly fractured at its weak spot, adjacent to the canine tooth (Fig. 10.5). However as it forms a 'ring' structure with the skull, there is a strong possibility of two fractures occurring, and this should always be excluded (Fig. 10.6).

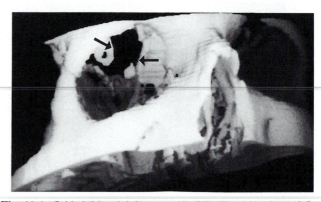

Fig. 10.4 Orbital 'blow-in' fracture: 3D-CT. There is a large defect in the medial and posterior orbital walls (arrows).

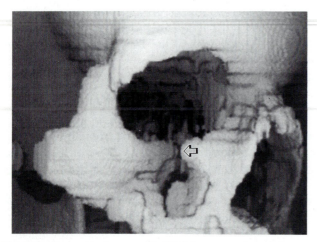

Fig. 10.3 Zygomatic fracture: 3D-CT. The zygomatic arch is obviously depressed on the right, with a comminuted fracture involving the interior orbital rim (arrow), and maxillozygomatic junction.

The *nasal bones* are best identified on the lateral view, although the frontal views or occlusal film will determine displacement of the nasal septum.

On plain radiographs, the *zygomatic arch* and *orbital rim* are best seen on the occipito-mental (Waters) view, although the submento-vertical and Townes' views are good for assessing the zygoma for depression. Fluid levels or opacification of the maxillary sinus are important hints of fractures extending into the sinus and may be the only sign of 'blow-out' fractures of the orbital floor. 'Blow out' fractures may also involve the ethmoid sinus walls, and air may penetrate the periorbital space, giving rise to orbital emphysema (see Ch. 9).

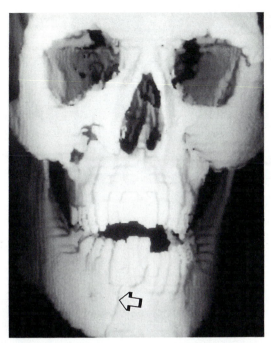

Fig. 10.5 Mandibular fracture (arrow): 3D-CT. Exquisite detail is provided by the 3D reconstruction.

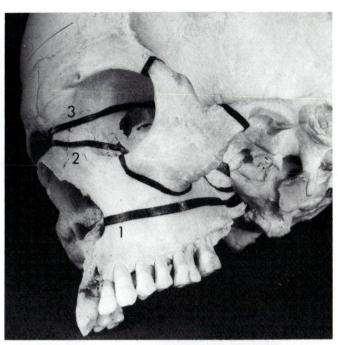

Fig. 10.7 Facial fracture lines. The lines of the common fractures are marked on the skull: 1. low transverse fracture; 2. pyramidal fracture; and 3. high transverse fracture. The numbers also relate to the Le Fort lines of weakness.

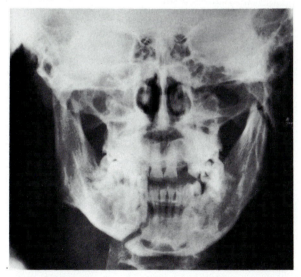

Fig. 10.6 Fractures of the mandible following direct injury. As with other bony rings, fractures in two places are common. Fractures involve the right canine region and the neck of the left condyle.

Le Fort defined lines of weakness within the facial bones, leading to the classification system based on the type of fracture pattern (Figs 10.7, 10.8). In practice, pure symmetrical Le Fort fractures of any one variety are rare, and a combination of the injuries usually occurs (Fig. 10.8).

THE SPINE

Spinal trauma is a common cause of disability, with approximately 150 000 persons suffering from spinal injury in the United States each year. It is predominantly an affliction of the young, with 80% occurring below the age of 40. Spinal injuries are common in multi-trauma patients, predominantly from motor vehicle accidents and from falls. Cervical spine injury occurs in over 20% of such cases.

Examination of the patient in the acute setting may be difficult due to combative or uncooperative behaviour, which may be the result either of head trauma or intoxication. Plain films are the primary method of evaluation and will detect abnormalities of alignment, as well as the majority of fractures. Additional methods of examination include tomography, computed tomography (CT) and magnetic resonance imaging (MRI). CT is able clearly to identify small bone fragments not seen on plain radiographs and has the advantage of better definition than tomography, as well as an ability to visualize the soft tissues. It also involves less radiation and may be quicker than tomography, and is only slightly more expensive. With the newer scanners, high-quality reconstruction in virtually any plane, and three-dimensional images may also be obtained (Fig. 10.9). However it must be remembered that despite the fact that CT is regarded by most authors as the 'gold standard' for examination of the spine, subtle undisplaced axially orientated fractures can

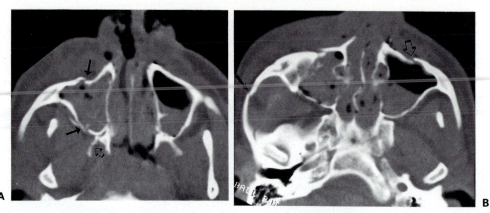

Fig. 10.8 CT of facial fracture. **A**. Fractures are identified through the anterior and lateral walls of the right maxillary sinus (arrows), and pterygoid plate (open arrow). There is complete opacification of the right antrum and nasal passage from haematoma, and a fluid level in the left antrum due to a maxillary fracture (not seen on this image). On another cut (**B**) the zygomatic arch fracture is also seen (arrow), and there is obvious depression of the zygoma. The left maxillary fracture is also seen (open arrow).

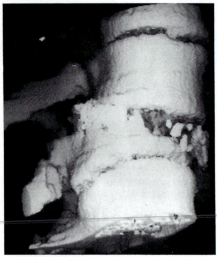

Fig. 10.9 3D CT of the spine. Note crush fracture of the body of LI, with anterior subluxation of T12 on L1.

be missed, and high-quality multidirectional tomography may prove superior in some cases.

MRI has yet to be fully evaluated in this field, but early results indicate that it may have a significant role. Advantages of MRI are its ability to visualize all of the soft tissues, including the substance of the spinal cord, where subtle injuries may be appreciated (Fig. 10.10). Disadvantages include its high cost, limited definition of small bony structures, and relatively poor resolution, although this is improving all the time.

CERVICAL SPINE

Normal radiographic anatomy. An understanding of the anatomy of the normal cervical spine is obligatory for correct evaluation. The anatomical features are identified in Figure 10.11. Alignment should be assessed along several anatomic lines as shown. These are: the anterior and posterior spinal lines, joining the anterior and posterior aspects of the vertebral bodies along the line of the longi-

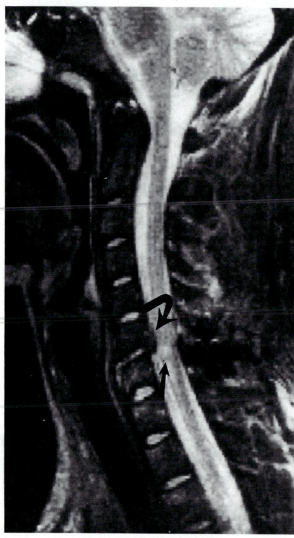

Fig. 10.10 MRI of the cervical spine: T_2-weighted image. There has been a fracture of C6, with mild posterior displacement of the dorsal fragment of the vertebral body (curved arrow). A focal area of high signal within the spinal cord at this level (straight arrow) indicates a focal cord injury.

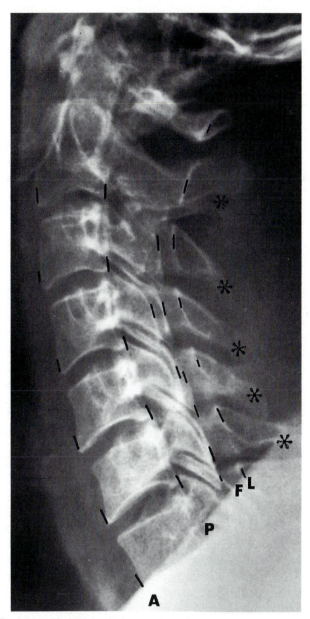

Fig. 10.11 Normal cervical spine. Five lines should be drawn in the mind. A and P are the anterior and posterior longitudinal lines respectively. These run along the margin of the anterior and posterior longitudinal ligament. L is the spinolaminar line, which runs between the anterior margin of the dorsal spines, outlining the posterior margin of the spinal canal. The asterisks represent the spinous line, along the posterior margin of the dorsal spines. F is the posterior pillar line, along the posterior margins of the articular pillars. N.B. Note divergence of the posterior pillar line in the upper and mid spine, due to mild positional rotation.

tudinal ligaments; the spinolaminar line, which joins the anterior margins of the junction of the lamina and spinous processes; and the spinous process line, joining the tips of the spinous processes. In addition, a fifth line should be drawn between the posterior margins of the articular pillars. This line defines the posterior aspect of the articular pillars and allows assessment of the laminar space between the posterior pillar and spinolaminar line. Abrupt

variation in this space has been shown to be an accurate method of determining rotational abnormality of a vertebral column, either with or without a fracture of the articular pillar (Fig. 10.12, 10.13). Prevertebral soft-tissue measurements have traditionally been regarded as being a valuable indicator of injury or normality. Recently however, Templeton et al (1987) have shown these to be of limited value, with the statistical likelihood of underlying injury occurring only at measurements above 7 mm at the C3 and C4 level, and a significant shift towards abnormality occurring only at measurements above 10 mm.

Radiographic evaluation. The condition of the patient will determine to a large extent the type and detail of the initial radiographic examination. The cross-table lateral view, with the patient supine, is the single most important radiographic examination and should be made as soon as the patient is stabilized. Evaluation of this film alone by an expert in the field will allow diagnosis of abnormality in the vast majority of cases. All seven vertebral bodies should be included on the radiographs. A normal cervical spine will demonstrate a gentle lordosis, but although lack of lordosis may be due to muscular spasm and indicate spinal injury, age, prior trauma, radiographic positioning, flexion of the spine, and the wearing of a hard collar (so commonly seen today) can all cause alteration in the natural lordosis.

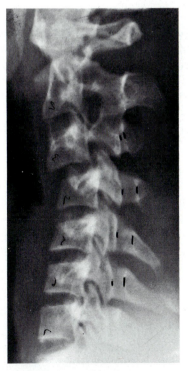

Fig. 10.12 Unilateral facet dislocation. There is an abrupt change in the laminar space (between the spinolaminar line and the posterior articular pillar line) at the C3-C4 level, indicating rotation. There is also a mild anterior subluxation of C3 on C4.

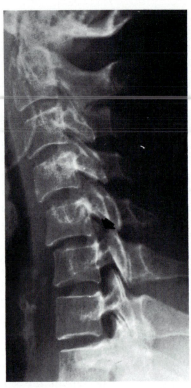

Fig. 10.13 Unilateral facet fracture/dislocation. There is a mild anterior subluxation of C5 on C6; also overlap of the posterior articular pillar lines at C6, but separation at C5, indicating rotation. The superior facet of C6 has been fractured, and rotated forwards with the anteriorly displaced inferior facet of C5 (arrow).

In the lateral radiograph of the resting cervical spine, as well as a normal lordosis, there should be no disruption of the anterior spinal line. In flexion, the mid and upper segments of the spine move forwards over the next inferior segment with concurrent sliding of each inferior articular facet over the superior facet of the level below, up to approximately 30% of the length of the articular surface. A unique phenomenon is seen in children up to the age of 8, approximately 25% of whom will demonstrate a 'pseudo-subluxation' at the C2/C3 level, attributed to laxity of the ligaments. This can be confirmed by examining the spinolaminar line, which will maintain a normal relationship in cases of pseudo-subluxation. In addition, in approximately 20% of patients in this age group, over half of the anterior arch of the atlas lies above the tip of the dens. This should not be misinterpreted as atlanto-axial dislocation. Furthermore, the space between the posterior surface of the anterior arch of C1 and the anterior surface of the dens may widen in flexion up to 6 mm in children, although it remains constant in adults.

Kyphosis, or a localized flexion angulation, may be mild or severe, and can occur as a result of narrowing of the vertebral bodies anteriorly, as in a wedge compression fracture. Alternatively, widening of the interspinous distance and/or interfacet joints posteriorly indicates posterior ligamentous disruption, as seen in hyperflexion sprains (Fig. 10.14) (see below). Both of these appearances indicate a hyperflexion force as the cause of injury, and they may occur together. Asymmetry of the disc space is also a useful sign, and may indicate ligamentous damage to the longitudinal ligament at the site of widening.

Additional plain radiographic examination of the patient with a spine injury may include an anterior posterior (AP) view, and an open-mouth AP odontoid view. The incidence of injury to C7 in cervical injuries has been reported at 30%, although this figure would appear to be on the high side. Tomography or CT may be needed to visualize this region fully. Oblique views are reported to be useful for defining the neural foramina, and may clarify a fracture of the articular pillars or a unilateral facet dislocation. 'Pillar views' of the cervical spine are also advocated by some authors. However, it can be argued that these additional views are superfluous; if an abnormality is not seen by routine plain film evaluation in a

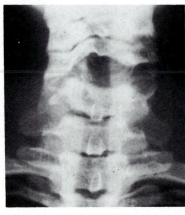
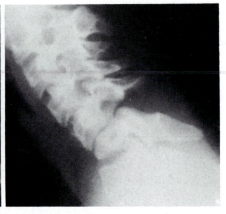

Fig. 10.14 Hyperflexion sprain/wedge compression fracture. There is a wedge compression fracture of C6 with marked widening of the interspinous distances of C5-6; also, widening of the facet joint at C5-6, with near 'perching' of the inferior facets of C5 on the superior facets of C6.

clinical setting suggestive of a fracture or dislocation, more definitive additional studies are mandatory in any case. These will include flexion/extension lateral radiographs, multidirectional tomography, CT, or MRI. These methods will provide additional information of abnormality, or confirm normality, and are indicated in the symptomatic patient, whether the oblique and pillar views demonstrate abnormality or not.

Classification. Most classification systems for cervical spine injury are based on the classic paper by Whitley and Forsythe (1960). These regard the forces acting on the spine as flexion, extension, rotation, compression, or a combination of the above. Each fracture force will be covered below.

Hyperflexion injuries

These include hyperflexion sprain, flexion compression fractures, flexion teardrop fractures and, if rotation also occurs, unilateral facet lock.

Hyperflexion sprain. These injuries usually involve anterior subluxation of a vertebral body, with respect to the vertebra located inferiorly. Flexion extension views are invaluable in cases in which injury is expected but not immediately visible, or when minor abnormality such as asymmetry of a disc space, or questionable 'fanning' of the spinous processes is seen. However they should *never* be obtained when there is clear radiographic evidence of bone displacement or ligamentous injury. Also, in the acute setting, muscular spasm may prohibit movement of the spine, thus invalidating the findings.

Hyperflexion sprain is associated with posterior ligamentous injury of the spine. Depending upon the severity, the ligaments will be involved in the following order: 1. *interspinous ligaments*, giving rise to widening of the interspinous distance: 2. the *ligamentum flavum* and *capsular ligaments*, which gives rise to more marked widening of the interspinous distance, and widening or subluxation of the facet joints; (Figs 10.14, 10.15); 3. the *posterior longitudinal ligaments*, allowing widening of the posterior disc space. In such cases, ultimately total subluxation of the facets may occur, giving rise to bilateral locked facets (Fig. 10.16). This is usually associated with anterior subluxation of 50% or more of the vertebral body above the injury, and will cause stripping or rupture of the *anterior longitudinal ligament*.

Flexion teardrop fracture. This occurs with flexion injuries when there is a compression fracture of the anterior aspect of the vertebral body inferior to the level of the injury (Fig. 10.17). This may also be associated with a posterior displacement of the posterior portion of the affected vertebral body, causing spinal cord compression.

Unilateral facet dislocation. When a rotational force is combined with hyperflexion, unilateral facet dislocation occurs. In such cases, the abnormal side rotates up and over the normal subjacent facet. The contralateral side acts as the fulcrum and is not involved in the injury. On the abnormal side, there is either 'locking' of the inferior

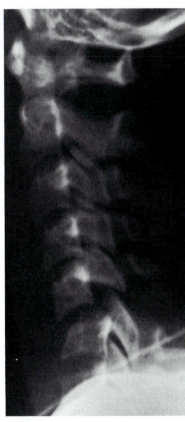

Fig. 10.15 Hyperflexion sprain. Note widening of the interspinous distance at C5/6, with additional widening of the facet joints, and superior subluxation of the facets of C4 on C5. The posterior intervertebral distance is also widened. This picture indicates severe ligamentous disruption.

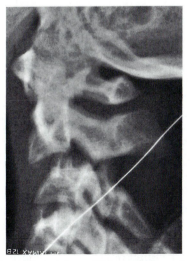

Fig. 10.16 Bilateral locked facet. C2 has leap-frogged over C3, and now lies with its inferior facets anterior to the superior articular facets of C3.

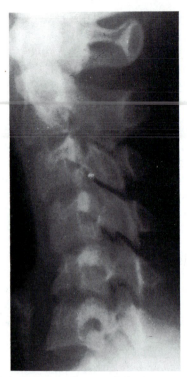

Fig. 10.17 Flexion teardrop fracture of C5. Note anterior compression of C5, with a fracture of the anterior inferior aspect. Some mild posterior displacement of the major dorsal fragment of the body of C5 is seen.

articulation of the facet of the rotated vertebra anterior to the superior articulation of the facet of the normally positioned lower vertebral body, or — as occurs in approximately 30% of cases — there is a fracture through one of the articular facets, usually the superior facet of the lower vertebral body. In general this fracture is horizontally orientated, indicating the rotational shearing nature of the force. Radiographically the vertebral body of the rotated vertebra is displaced anteriorly, varying in degree up to approximately 20% of the vertebral body. Change in the laminar/facet interspace is an accurate assessment of rotational anomaly (Fig. 10.12). An apparent shift of the spinous process may be identified on the frontal view, due to its being 'rotated' away from the midline.

Wedge fractures. These occur when there is wedging of the anterior aspect of the vertebra, without ligamentous injury or posterior displacement of fragments. This usually means less than 30% compression of the anterior vertebra, and is associated predominantly with axial loading, as well as hyperflexion.

Hyperextension injuries

In general, hyperextension injuries are associated with rupture of the anterior longitudinal ligament. This causes widening of the anterior disc space, and may cause prevertebral soft tissue swelling. It must be remembered, however, that positioning of the head in the neutral

position by a well-meaning passer-by, or the placement of a cervical collar at the scene of the accident, may largely restore any displacement, so that on initial inspection, the radiograph can appear grossly normal. Hyperextension tear-drop fractures may occur, usually at the anterior inferior aspect of the vertebral body involved, indicating the site of avulsion of the anterior longitudinal ligament. A further effect of hyperflexion, however, may be to cause an axial load on the posterior elements, giving rise to crush fractures of the articular pillars (Fig. 10.18) and narrowing of the interspinous distance. Fractures through the spinous process may also occur, due to axial compression. Facial injuries are often associated with these fractures.

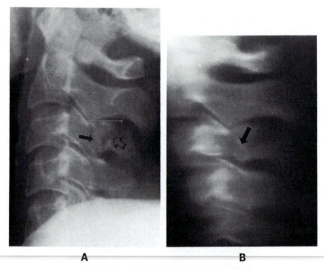

Fig. 10.18 Hyperextension fracture of the articular pillar of C3. **A.** There is obvious bone disruption of the posterior elements of C3, involving both the articular pillars, (closed arrow) and lamina (open arrow). **B.** Tomography demonstrates the crush fracture of the articular pillar, with posterior displacement of the postero-inferior fragment (arrow).

Hangman's fracture. This injury, misnamed because of a superficial resemblance to fractures seen in victims of hanging, occurs with hyperextension of the head, and therefore a form of axial loading on the posterior elements of the upper cervical spine caused by posterior rotation of the head in the sagittal plane (Fig. 10.19). The injurious force is in effect delivered by the occiput as it moves in an inferior and anterior direction, causing oblique fractures through the posterior arch of C2, which may extend into the body of C2. This fracture may be extremely unstable, although the spinal cord is usually spared due to the large AP diameter of the spinal canal at this level. The fracture may also extend into the vertebral canal, risking injury to the vertebral artery. A similar fracture pattern may occasionally be seen at lower levels in the spine.

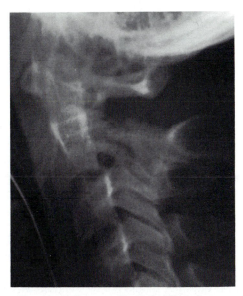

Fig. 10.19 Hangman's fracture. Classical oblique fractures through the pars interarticularis of C2 are associated with anterior subluxation of the body of C2.

Axial loading

Jefferson fracture: burst fracture of C1. In these injuries, axial loading causes compression of the lateral masses of C1 between C2 and the occipital condyles. Because of the anatomy of the region, this gives rise to lateral displacement of the masses of C1 (Fig. 10.20), thus disrupting the ring. This can be appreciated on the AP odontoid view, but usually gives rise to anterior displacement of the atlas relative to the odontoid process. Prevertebral soft-tissue swelling is usual.

Burst fracture. This is caused by axial loading and the vertebra is shattered, often in all directions. The importance of this injury lies in the possibility of posterior displacement of fragments into the spinal canal.

Miscellaneous

Spinous process fracture. This most commonly occurs at C7, and is often seen as an avulsion injury (clay shoveller's fracture). However, they may occur in direct trauma, or from compressive hyperextension (see

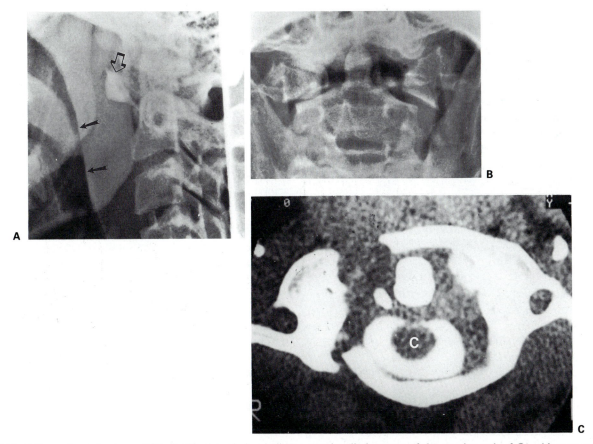

Fig. 10.20 Jefferson burst fracture of C1. **A.** The lateral view indicates anterior displacement of the anterior arch of C1 with respect to the odontoid process (open arrow). There is marked prevertebral soft-tissue swelling (closed arrows). **B.** The AP view demonstrates lateral displacement of the lateral masses of C2. **C.** Axial CT of Jefferson fracture of atlas. Contrast in sub-arachnoid space outlines cord.

above), or as the result of forced hyperflexion (Fig. 10.17).

Odontoid fractures. Fractures of the odontoid are divided into three types. In Type I, the fracture is through the upper aspect of the odontoid process. In Type II, the fracture occurs through the base of the odontoid (Fig. 10.21), and in Type III, the fracture extends into the body of C2 (Fig. 10.22). Non-united Type I fractures

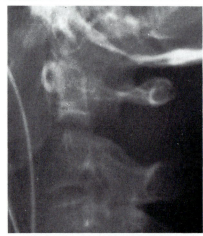

Fig. 10.21 Type II odontoid fracture. The fracture passes through the base of the odontoid process with slight separation, and anterior displacement of the odontoid process and ring of C1.

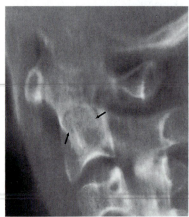

A

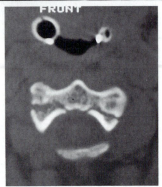

B

Fig. 10.22 Type III odontoid fracture. **A**. The lateral radiograph demonstrates interruption of the radiographic 'ring' of the body of C2 (arrows). **B**. CT demonstrates the nature of the fracture, through the body of C2.

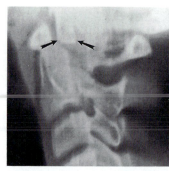

Fig. 10.23 Os odontoideum. The tip of the odontoid process is separated from the body, with smooth, well-corticated margins (arrows).

involving the superior aspect of the odontoid process are arguably the cause of the so-called os odontoideum (Fig. 10.23). Odontoid fractures may be best seen on the AP odontoid view, but should not be confused with artefacts from the posterior arch of the atlas (Mach effect) (Fig. 10.24), or overlying teeth. Type III fractures extending into the body of C2 may cause disruption of the cortical 'ring' of the lateral aspect of the body of C2, seen on the lateral view (Fig. 10.22). There may also be an anterior tilt of the dens and hence anterior displacement of C1 with respect to the ring of C2.

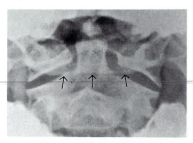

Fig. 10.24 Mach effect. An apparent fracture through the base of the odontoid process is due to the overlying posterior ring of C1 (arrows).

Rotational injuries. Pure rotational injuries are rare, but may give rise to rotational (rotatory) subluxation. This is a condition of a rotational anomaly, usually of C1 on C2, which in children may give rise to torticollis. Although the condition may be self-limiting, occasionally it persists. It is best appreciated on open-mouth odontoid views, in the AP and both oblique projections, although tomography may be needed for full evaluation (Fig. 10.25).

Additional rotational injuries are those associated with axial loading or hyperextension, both of which can give rise to unilateral facet dislocation (see above).

THORACOLUMBAR SPINE

Fractures in the thoracolumbar spine are generally the result of severe axial loading, as in falls from a height

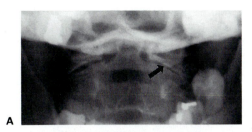

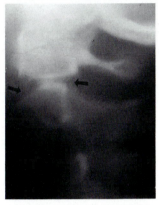

Fig. 10.25 Rotatory subluxation of C1 on C2. Despite a nearly perfect AP view (A), there is asymmetry of the C1/C2 articulation with narrowing of the left (arrow), which cannot be attributed to patient positioning. This suggests a rotation of C1 on C2, confirmed (B) by lateral tomograms, which indicate subluxation of the articular surfaces (arrowheads).

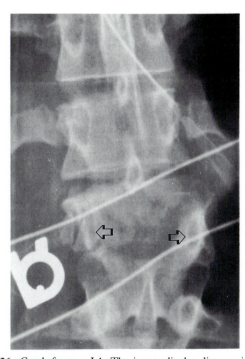

Fig. 10.26 Crush fracture L1. The interpedicular distance is widened, indicating lateral displacement of the pedicles, and hence 'bursting' of the ring formed by the vertebral body and posterior elements. Water-soluble contrast medium is present in the subarachnoid space.

(crush fractures) or acute flexion injuries, commonly seen in seat-belt injuries in car accidents (see below). Rotational forces however may play a role, particularly in the upper lumbar region. As in the cervical spine, ligamentous injury can usually be appreciated by subluxation, either anterior or lateral. Widening of the interpedicular distance or disc space, as well as paravertebral swelling in the thoracic region, are signs of injury which should be sought (Figs 10.26, 10.27).

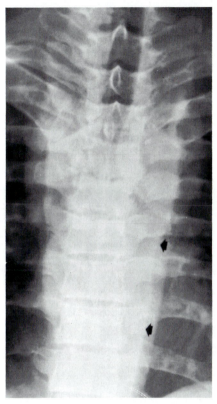

Fig. 10.27 Compression fracture: mild crush fracture of the body of T5, with a paraspinal soft-tissue 'mass' (arrows), due to haemorrhage.

Compression injuries cause 'burst fractures' or, when associated with flexion, wedge compression fractures, usually more marked at the anterior margin (Figs 10.28, 10.29). Lateral compression may also occur. Crush fractures are common in victims of falls, and are associated with fractures of the calcaneus, 'pilon' fractures of the tibial plafond, and vertical shear pelvic fractures (see below). These injuries therefore should warn of possible spinal trauma, particularly of the upper lumbar region. All forms of compression fracture require CT to evaluate for posterior displacement of fracture fragments, and impingement upon the spinal cord.

Seat belt injuries. These are caused by massive localized hyperflexion, typically the result of sudden

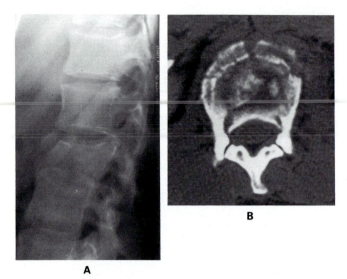

A

Fig. 10.28 Compression fracture of L2. **A**. Plain lateral radiograph indicates wedging of L2, with posterior bulging of the dorsal margin. **B**. CT scan demonstrates the extent of the impingement of the dorsal fragment upon the spinal canal.

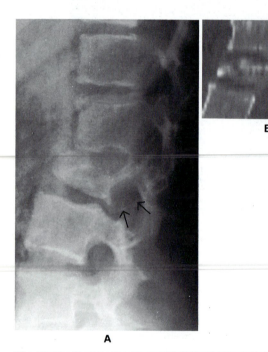

A

Fig. 10.29 Compression fracture L2. **A**. Again there is wedging and compression of L2, with evidence of body debris overlying the spinal canal (arrows). **B**. CT reconstruction indicates the position of the bone fragments and narrowing of the canal.

deceleration, in a car accident, when the occupant is restrained by a lap seat belt. In general there is very little, or no, anterior wedging of the vertebral body, suggesting a distracting hyperflexion force. The fractures are subdivided into three groups. Type I, the 'Chance fracture', extends horizontally from the spinous process into the vertebral body, passing through the articular pillars and

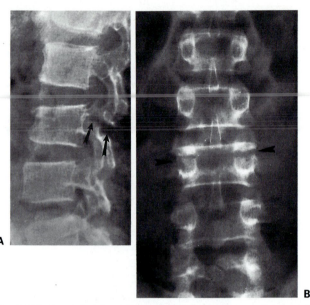

A   **B**

Fig. 10.30 Lap-belt injury: Smith fracture. **A**. There are horizontal fractures extending posteriorly from the dorsal surface of the vertebral body, through the pedicles (arrows). **B**. The AP view demonstrates the characteristic 'horizontal' defects in the pedicles (arrowheads).

pedicles; Type II, the Smith fracture, is similar, but does not involve the spinous process (Fig. 10.30); Type III involves one side only, due to a rotational component of the force responsible.

THE PELVIS AND HIP

Much confusion has arisen over pelvic fractures, due to a lack of a logical and meaningful classification system. Traditionally, pelvic fractures were classified by reference to historical descriptions of individual fractures, without any connection between them. These classifications included single fractures of the pelvis and thus were largely outdated by the work of Gertzbein and Chenoweth (1977) who demonstrated that there was always a second site of injury even in apparently single pelvic fractures. This is due to the fact that the pelvis is a bony ring, held together by ligamentous groups posteriorly and anteriorly. A search for a second site of injury should therefore always be made in fractures involving the pelvic ring.

The classification system of Young and Burgess (1987) developed from work by Pennal and Tile, which describes fractures relative to the force of injury, will be used in this text.

Lateral compression fractures. These are subdivided into three types, depending upon the severity of the injury, and progressive involvement of the posterior pelvis (Fig. 10.31). Pubic rami fractures are invariably present, and generally run 'horizontally', or in the coronal plane. Alternatively they may present as a 'buckle' fractures. A common association is a crush fracture of the

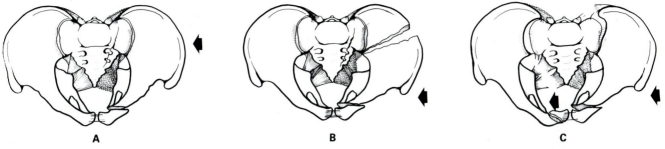

Fig. 10.31 Lateral compression pelvic fracture classification. **A**. Type I. Posteriorly positioned lateral force causes compression of the sacrum, and 'horizontal' or buckle fractures of the pubic rami. **B**. Type II. The force is delivered more anteriorly, causing inward rotation of the anterior pelvis around the anterior aspect of the sacroiliac joint. Either disruption of the posterior sacroiliac ligaments, or fracture of the iliac wing (shown here) results. **C**. Type III. The lateral force on one side is transmitted to the contralateral side, causing an externally directed force to 'open' the contralateral pelvis. Disruption of the major anterior ligamentous groups (anterior sacroiliac, sacrotuberous and sacrospinous) occurs. (Reproduced with permission of Urban and Schwartzenberg from Young and Burgess (1987).)

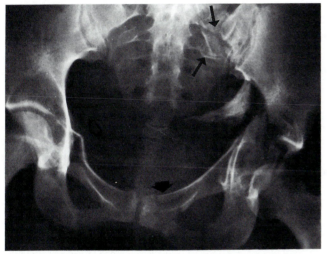

Fig. 10.32 Type I lateral compression fracture. A horizontal fracture of the left (closed arrow) and a buckle fracture of the right (open arrows) superior pubic ramus are seen. There is a crush fracture of the left sacrum (long arrows), and a fracture predominantly of the medial wall of the left acetabulum. (Reproduced with permission of Urban and Schwartzenberg from Young and Burgess (1987).)

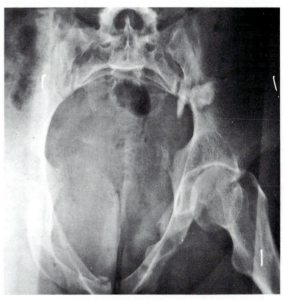

Fig. 10.33 Type II B lateral compression fracture. 'Horizontal' fracture of the right symphysis, and oblique fracture of the left iliac wing, arising from the sacroiliac joint. There is moderate medial displacement of the left anterior pelvis. (Reproduced with permission of Urban and Schwartzenberg from Young and Burgess (1987).)

sacrum (Fig. 10.32). Fracture of the medial wall of the acetabulum with or without central dislocation of the femoral head is also associated (Fig. 10.32). In Type I fractures, there is no ligamentous damage, and no posterior pelvic instability. However, with Type II injuries, there is medial displacement of the anterior pelvis on the side of injury, with either a fracture through the sacroiliac joint and iliac wing, or rupture of the posterior sacroiliac ligaments (Fig. 10.33). This allows some posterior instability. In Type III fractures, the lateral force on one side of the pelvis is transmitted through to the contralateral side, so that the force is directed outwards (Figs 10.31C and 10.34). This causes 'opening' of the pelvis on the contralateral side, with associated posterior ligamentous disruption.

Anterior posterior (AP) compression fracture. The damaging force in the AP (or PA) direction tends to cause 'opening' of the anterior pelvis (Fig. 10.35), with splaying of the symphysis pubis and/or fractures of the pubic rami, which however are in the vertical plane, in contrast to lateral compression fractures.

The more severe Types II and III fractures relate to increasing posterior ligamentous injury, and hence increasing instability (Figs 10.35, 10.36, 10.37). In Type II fractures, the anterior sacroiliac, sacrospinous and sacrotuberous ligaments are disrupted, allowing wide splaying of the anterior pelvis (Figs 10.35, 10.36). In Type III fractures, there is total disruption of the sacroiliac joint. (Fig. 10.37). Fractures of the anterior and

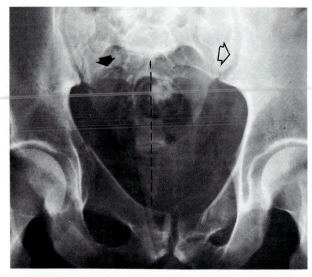

Fig. 10.34 Lateral compression Type III. There are crush fractures of the right sacrum (dark arrow) and left pubic rami. Note diastasis of the left sacroiliac joint (open arrow) and lateral displacement of the whole of the anterior pelvis to the left. Fractures of the right pubic rami are also seen.

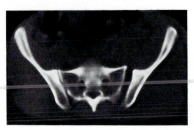

Fig. 10.37 Type III AP compression fracture. CT scan: complete diastasis of the left sacroiliac joint.

posterior acetabular pillars are common, and posterior hip dislocations are also associated, in contrast to lateral compression fractures, when the medial wall of the acetabulum is at risk (see above).

Vertical shear fractures. These commonly result from falls from a height. Fractures occur through the pubic rami and posterior pelvis, and are vertically oriented (Fig. 10.38). The large lateral hemipelvic fracture fragment containing the acetabulum is displaced superiorly.

Fractures of the posterior and superior acetabula are often associated with superior displacement of the femoral

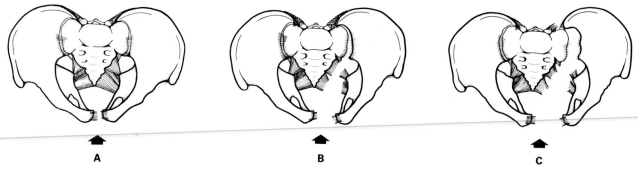

Fig. 10.35 Anteroposterior (AP) compression fracture classification **A**. Type I. Diastasis of the symphysis pubis only. **B**. Type II. Diastasis of the symphysis pubis, disruption of the sacrospinous and sacrotuberous ligaments, and anterior sacroiliac ligament. **C**. Type III. Total ligamentous disruption, including the posterior sacroiliac ligaments. (Reproduced with permission of Urban and Schwartzenberg from Young and Burgess (1987).)

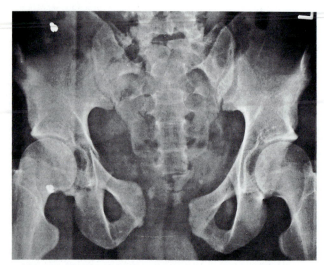

Fig. 10.36 Type II AP compression fracture. There is wide diastasis of the symphysis pubis and *anterior* left sacroiliac joint.

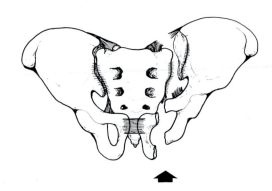

Fig. 10.38 Vertical shear fracture pattern. A superiorly directed force disrupts the left hemipelvis, with diastasis (or fracture) through the left sacroiliac region, and fractures of the pubic rami (or symphysis diastasis). The separated pelvic fragment containing the acetabulum is displaced superiorly. (Reproduced with permission of Urban and Schwartzenberg from Young and Burgess (1987).)

head. These injuries are associated with fractures of the lumbar vertebrae, and calcaneus.

Mixed fracture pattern. These arise from a combination vector of the forces causing injury, and give rise to a mixed pattern of fracture, the commonest being a mixed anterolateral pattern (Fig. 10.39), with signs of both AP and lateral compression.

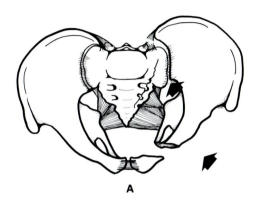

A

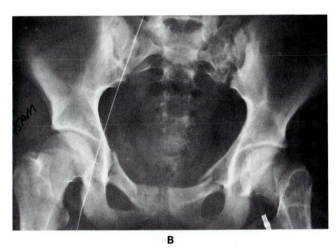

B

Fig. 10.39 Combined fracture pattern. **A**. AP and lateral compression. This type of injury gives fracture patterns of both AP and lateral compression, such as in **B**, where there are 'horizontal' fractures of the left pubic rami, indicating lateral compression, but disruption of the left sacroiliac joint, indicating AP compression.

Straddle fractures. It is questionable whether this term should be used at all, as it gives no useful indication as to the underlying mechanism of injury. Multiple fractures of the pubic rami can occur from lateral, anterior-posterior compression or vertical shear fractures and clues should be sought to the likely force vector, and to associated injuries (Fig. 10.40).

Isolated fractures. Isolated fractures of the sacrum, iliac crest, or inferior pubic ramus may occur, as these do not violate the integrity of the pelvic ring. Such sacral fractures are usually transverse and may be difficult to diagnose without a lateral view. Single fractures of a pubic ramus can be seen, resulting from a direct blow. However

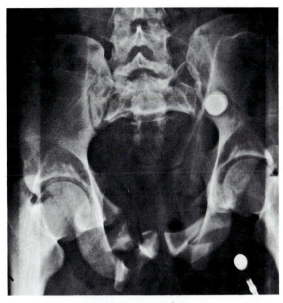

Fig. 10.40 The so-called 'straddle' fracture is not due to straddling, but, in this case, to AP compression. Diastasis of the left SIJ indicates a Type III AP compression fracture.

this is a rare occurrence, and additional injury to the pelvis should always be excluded.

Avulsion injuries. Avulsion injuries of the pelvis occur most commonly as the result of muscular exertion during sporting activities. The anterior superior iliac spine (sartorius), anterior inferior iliac spine (rectus femoris) and the ischial tuberosity (hamstrings) are the commonest sites.

Acetabular fractures. Acetabular fractures in general involve one or more of four regions: the posterior rim, the posterior pillar, the anterior pillar, or the quadrilateral plate. As expected, fractures of the posterior rim are usually caused by posterior dislocation of the femur (Fig. 10.41). These are commonly associated with cortical fractures of the anterior femoral head. Fractures of the posterior pillar may also be seen with posterior dislocations of the femur (Fig. 10.42), and, together with fractures of the anterior pillar, are common in AP com-

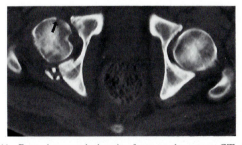

Fig. 10.41 Posterior acetabular rim fracture shown on CT. There has been a posterior hip dislocation. A characteristic defect described by Richardson et al (1990), is seen in the anterior femoral head (arrow): it is similar to the Hill-Sachs deformity of the humeral head in anterior humeral dislocations.

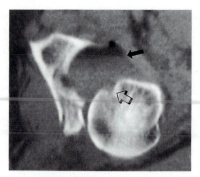

Fig. 10.42 Posterior acetabular pillar fracture. CT scan demonstrates an extensive fracture of the posterior acetabular pillar, again usually associated with posterior hip dislocation. A fat-fluid level is seen in the joint (arrow), with a small collection of air anteriorly, probably a 'vacuum' phenomenon. The cortical femoral head defect is again seen (open arrow).

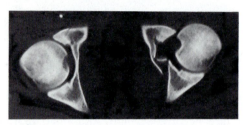

Fig. 10.43 Comminuted right acetabular fracture. CT indicates involvement of predominantly the quadrilateral plate, with disruption of the medial articular surface. A fracture through the anterior rim of the left acetabulum is also seen.

pression fractures of the pelvis. By contrast, fractures involving the quadrilateral plate are usually associated with lateral compression forces (Fig. 10.32). Undoubtedly CT provides the most detailed information about the fracture (Fig. 10.43), and there is a trend towards three-dimensional imaging of these fractures. The real advantage of conventional CT over plain radiography lies in its ability to detect small bone fragments within the joint space. Three-dimensional CT has been shown to miss small undisplaced fracture lines and intra-articular fragments, although it provides a dramatic representation of the overall fracture and orientation of fragments.

RIB FRACTURES

The lower ribs are commonly fractured, often from relatively minor trauma. Pneumothorax and haemothorax may be associated and should be excluded.

In contrast, fractures of the first and second rib are usually from major trauma, and serious associations including pneumothorax, haemopneumothorax, ruptured subclavian artery, pneumopericardium, and tracheobronchial fistula may be seen.

SHOULDER GIRDLE

THE CLAVICLE

Fractures of the clavicle involve the middle third in 80%, the outer third in 15%, and the medial third in 5% of cases. Over-riding of fragments and inferior displacement of the lateral fragment are common. Specific views however may be necessary to visualize the fracture. Fractures of the outer third are divided into two types, those in which disruption of the coracoclavicular ligaments does not occur (Type I), and those in which it does (Type II). Type II fractures are associated with greater displacement and a higher incidence of non-union.

THE SCAPULA

Fractures of the scapula are relatively rare, comprising only 1% of all fractures. They usually occur from major direct blows, and thus are commonly associated with other injuries, frequently of the ribs and clavicle. They may occur in any of the anatomical regions of the scapula, but are most common in the body (50–70%). Fractures of the glenoid rim occur in approximately 20% of shoulder dislocations. Isolated fractures of the spinous process are rare. Fractures of the coracoid process may occur from anterior humeral dislocations, or from avulsion injuries (coracoclavicular ligament, coracobrachialis), and may also be seen from shotgun or rifle recoils.

Dislocations. Dislocations around the shoulder are relatively common and usually involve the humeral head or acromioclavicular joint. The humerus is most commonly dislocated anteriorly (95%), or in practice, anteriorly, medially and inferiorly, coming to lie inferior to the coracoid process (Fig. 10.44). This may cause a cortical impaction both of the superior posterior aspect of the humerus (hatchet or Hill-Sachs deformity) (Fig.

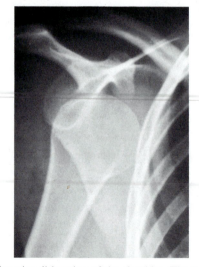

Fig. 10.44 Anterior dislocation of the shoulder. The humeral head lies medial and inferior to the glenoid in the subscapular fossa.

10.45), and inferior aspect of the glenoid, or may give rise to injury of the anterior portion of the glenoid labrum (*Bankart lesion*) (Fig. 10.46). Although more common

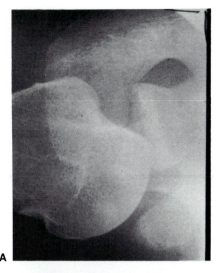

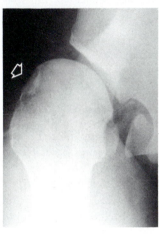

Fig. 10.45 Recurrent anterior dislocation of the shoulder. The characteristic defect is well shown in the axial projection (**A**). A large defect of this nature can even be visualized clearly in the AP projection, but it is rarely possible to identify small defects on a simple frontal projection; a film in 60° internal rotation or a Stryker view (**B**) is required.

after multiple or recurrent dislocations, the *Hill-Sachs* defect can occur after a single episode, and merely represents an osteochondral fracture. Anterior dislocations present no diagnostic difficulty.

Posterior dislocations however may be difficult to appreciate, although they should not be missed. In general, they can be appreciated on the AP view by persistent internal rotation of the humerus and asymmetry of the glenohumeral joint (Fig. 10.47). An axillary view may be impossible to obtain, but a transthoracic or 'swimmers' view or oblique (Y) view will confirm the diagnosis.

An unusual inferior dislocation (*Luxatio erecta*) is caused by severe hyperabduction of the arm, whereby the humeral head impinges upon the acromion, which in turn acts as a fulcrum and causes an inferior displacement of the humeral head with the arm 'locked' in abduction (Fig. 10.48).

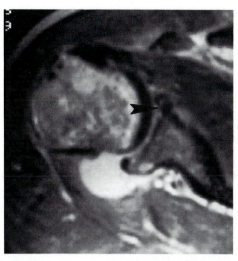

Fig. 10.46 Bankart lesion of the anterior glenoid labrum. MR image demonstrates disruption of the cartilaginous labrum (arrowhead).

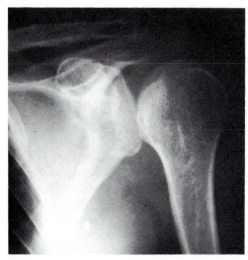

Fig. 10.47 Posterior dislocation of the shoulder. Note the circular appearance of the humeral head and the lack of parallelism between this and the glenoid fossa. The injury followed a severe electric shock causing muscle spasm, which had also precipitated compression fractures of the 5th and 6th thoracic vertebral bodies.

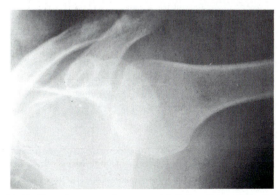

Fig. 10.48 Luxatio erecta. An unusual inferior dislocation of the humerus, which is 'locked' in abduction.

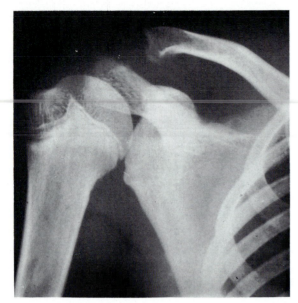

Fig. 10.49 Dislocation of the acromioclavicular joint following a fall on the point of the shoulder. The deformity is accentuated by examination in the erect position with weights being carried in both hands.

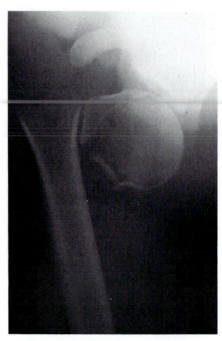

Fig. 10.50 Fracture of the surgical neck of the humerus: axial view. There is marked displacement of the distal humerus, with the comminuted fracture extending into the humeral head.

Acromioclavicular separation is usually the result of a fall on the outstretched arm or point of the shoulder. The importance of acromioclavicular dislocation lies in the trauma to the coracoclavicular ligament. This injury has been classified as sprain (Grade I), subluxation (Grade II), and dislocation (Grade III) (Fig. 10.49). Grade III injuries are in general obvious on plain radiography, with both acromioclavicular, and coracoclavicular separation. In Grade II injuries, stress views with weight bearing may be needed. In Grade I injuries, mild widening of the acromioclavicular space, but not the coracoclavicular space, may be seen on stress views.

Rotator cuff. This is the term applied to the conjoined tendons of the supraspinatus, infraspinatus, subscapularis and teres minor muscles. The rotator cuff passes between the humeral head and acromion before inserting into the greater tuberosity of the humerus. It separates the gleno-humeral joint from the subdeltoid bursa. Ruptures, either partial or complete, may be diagnosed by arthrography, although ultrasound and MRI are gaining popularity as diagnostic tools (see Fig. 9.31). Complete rotator cuff tears are commonly associated with narrowing of the acromiohumeral joint space.

THE UPPER LIMB

Humerus
Most injuries result from falls on the outstretched arm, particularly in elderly (osteopenic) women. Fractures of the surgical neck or greater tuberosity are the commonest injuries. Spiral and oblique fractures are common, usually with displacement or angulation of the distal fragment (Fig. 10.50), often requiring open fixation. Radial nerve injury occurs in up to 30% of cases.

Intra-articular fractures may be mild, as in the Hill-Sachs lesion, or severe, leading to fragmentation and intra-articular bone fragments. A 'drooping' shoulder may be seen, possibly as a result of capsular, muscular and neurological factors. Osteonecrosis has been reported in up to 50% of cases.

Supracondylar fractures are the commonest elbow injury in children (60%), resulting from a fall on the outstretched hand. No fracture line may be seen initially on the radiograph, but haemarthrosis with elevation of the anterior and/or posterior fat pads is highly suggestive. Volar displacement of the capitellum is also a helpful sign (Fig. 10.51). These fractures, with associated vascular damage, may be of importance in the development of **Volkmann's ischaemia** of the forearm. The second most common elbow fracture in children is that of the lateral epicondyle, although medial epicondylar fractures are also seen (Fig. 10.52).

Forearm fractures
Fractures of the bones of the forearm are extremely common, particularly of the radial head, olecranon process, distal radius and ulna. The forearm effectively acts as a ring structure and apparent single fractures may be associated with additional injury, either ligamentous or bony. This 'closed ring' concept explains double forearm frac-

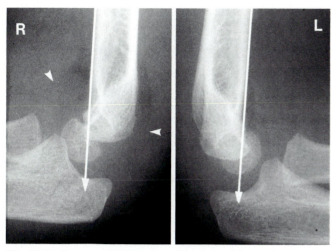

Fig. 10.51 Supracondylar fracture of humerus. The left humerus is normal; the line extending from the anterior cortex of the shaft passes through the middle third of the capitellum. A haemarthrosis of the right elbow joint displaces both fat pads and a similar line cuts the posterior third of the capitellum, indicating the anterior displacement of the fragment.

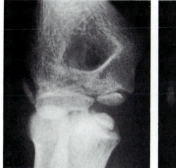
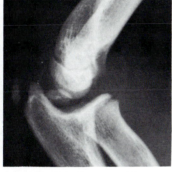

Fig. 10.52 Avulsion of medial epicondyle of the humerus. The centre for the lateral epicondyle has ossified in this child, therefore the medial epicondyle should also have appeared. It is not in its normal location but lies within the medial compartment of the elbow joint.

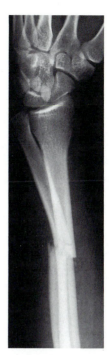

Fig. 10.53 Fractures through both forearm bones are seen.

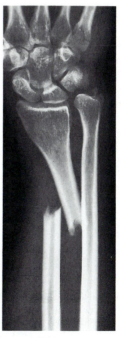

Fig. 10.54 Galeazzi fracture. Dislocation of the distal ulna accompanies the radial fracture.

tures (Fig. 10.53) i.e. *Galeazzi* fractures of the radius with distal ulnar dislocation (Fig. 10.54), and Monteggia fractures of the ulna with radial head dislocation (Fig. 10.55). It is therefore essential to examine the wrist and elbow carefully for additional injury in 'single bone' forearm fractures.

Fracture of the radial head is the commonest elbow injury in adults, usually occurring as a result of a fall on the outstretched arm. The fracture line may not be seen initially, but an elbow effusion is a good warning sign, warranting immobilization and repeat radiograph in 7–10 days.

Olecranon fractures result from falls onto the point of the elbow, or avulsions of the triceps insertions. They must be distinguished from the unfused ossification centre in children and young adults.

Injuries around the wrist. As mentioned above, injuries of the distal radioulnar joint are commonly associated with fractures of the radius and ulna, either alone or in combination. Injury to the wrist, and, in particular disruption of the triangular fibrocartilage complex

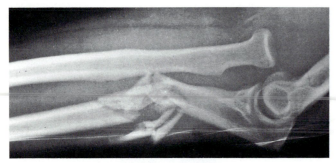

Fig. 10.55 Monteggia fracture/dislocation. There is a comminuted fracture of the ulna with dislocation of the radial head.

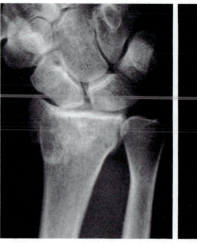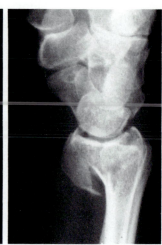

Fig. 10.57 Although commonly referred to as a *Smith's fracture*, the involvement of the articular surface indicates that this should more correctly be called a *reverse Barton's fracture*.

(TFCC) should be excluded in forearm fractures. TFCC disruptions may also be seen following a fall onto the outstretched hand. Arthrography is at present the method of choice in evaluating TFCC disruptions, although some authors suggest a role for MRI.

The distal forearm is one of the commonest sites of fracture in the entire body, and most fractures are associated with eponyms.

In **Colles'** fracture, the distal radius is fractured and angulated dorsally, giving rise clinically to the 'dinner-fork' deformity of the wrist (Fig. 10.56). The ulnar styloid is fractured in over 50% of cases, and there is almost invariably distal radioulnar dissociation.

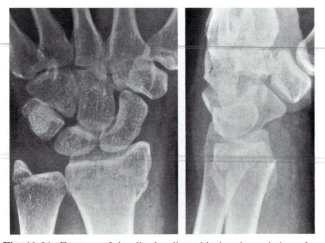

Fig. 10.56 Fracture of the distal radius with dorsal angulation of the distal fragment. Although frequently referred to as *Colles' fracture*, the extension of the fracture to the articular surface, seen on the AP view, indicates that this is a *Barton's fracture*.

Smith's fracture is the reverse of the Colles fracture, with volar angulation of the distal fragments of the radius (Fig. 10.57). In **Barton's** fracture, the fracture line extends through the dorsum of the distal radius to involve the articular surface. If the volar radial rim is involved this is a *reverse Barton's* fracture (Fig. 10.57).

FRACTURES OF THE CARPUS

The *scaphoid* bone is the most common carpal bone to be fractured. Once again, initial radiographic examination may be negative and a follow-up X-ray should be performed in 7–10 days after immobilization if there is a clinical suspicion (Fig. 10.58). Alternatively, a radio-nuclide bone scan may be helpful. Non-union and osteonecrosis of the proximal fragment are important complications, particularly in fractures of the proximal scaphoid, as the vascular supply enters in the middle of the bone. Dorsal avulsion fractures of the *triquetrum* are the second most common and may be appreciated best on the lateral view. The other carpal bones are only rarely injured, except for the *hamate*, the hook of which may be detached acutely by blows on the proximal palm of the hand, or by chronic trauma, such as from holding a tennis racquet or golf club.

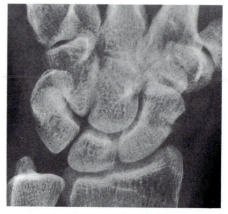

Fig. 10.58 Scaphoid fractures. There is a mild cortical irregularity of the radial side of the waist of the scaphoid. A faint fracture line extends through the waist.

Dislocation of the carpus

Dislocations of the carpus are complex, but are best appreciated by understanding two important concepts. 1. On the posteroanterior view, two major areas define the carpal relationship (Fig. 10.59): the proximal and distal carpal lines, following the proximal and distal margins of the scaphoid, lunate and triquetrum respectively. These lines should be roughly parallel, and the intercarpal joint spaces should be approximately equal. 2. On the lateral view of the normal wrist in its neutral position, a straight line can be drawn through the long axis of the radius, lunate and capitate (Fig. 10.60). This should intersect a line drawn along the long axis of the scaphoid at 30–60° (Fig. 10.61). A variation of the angle of any of these lines indicates *carpal instability*. Other patterns of instability are triquetrohamate instability (dissociation),

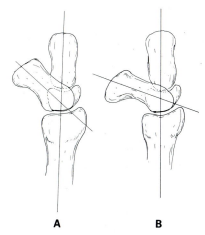

Fig. 10.61 **A**. In the normal wrist, the scaphoid long axis bisects the radial long axis at approximately 45° (30–60°). **B**. Rotatory subluxation: the long axis of the scaphoid is tilted in a volar direction.

and triquetrolunate dissociation, usually diagnosed by abnormal motion on fluoroscopy.

Examination of carpal trauma has led to the concept of two 'injury arcs' in the wrist (Fig. 10.62), enabling a sequence of injuries to be predicted. The sequence usually begins on the radial side with rotary subluxation of the scaphoid and scapholunate dissociation (see below). Stage II is the perilunate dislocation (see below), following failure of the radiocapitate ligament. In Stage III, injury to the radiotriquetral ligament and dorsal radiocarpal ligaments gives rise to triquetral malrotation and triquetrolunate dissociation, and in Stage IV injury there is disruption of the dorsal radiocarpal ligament, allowing complete dislocation of the lunate.

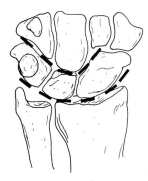

Fig. 10.59 Normal carpal relationship. The proximal and distal carpal lines define the normal carpal relationship on the PA projection.

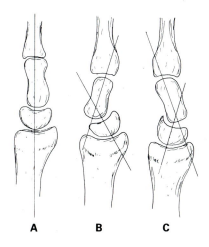

Fig. 10.60 **A**. Normal alignment of the wrist allows a continuous line to be drawn through the radius, lunate and capitate. **B**. Abnormal alignment: palmar flexion instability (volar intercalary segment carpal instability: VISI). The lunate is rotated towards the palmar surface of the wrist, with the capitate rotated towards the dorsal surface. **C**. Dorsiflexion instability (dorsal intercalary segment carpal instability: DISI) — the converse of B.

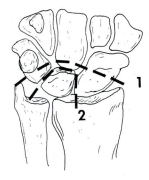

Fig. 10.62 Arcs of injury of the wrist. 1. The greater arc: pure injury of the greater arc gives rise to a transcaphoid, transcapitate, transhamate, and transtriquetral dislocation. 2. The lesser arc: injury here gives rise to lunate or perilunate dislocation.

In *lunate dislocation*, the normal anatomy of the proximal carpal row is lost, and the lunate is usually seen to overlap the capitate, hamate and triquetrum on the PA view, also taking on a triangular, rather than a rectangular

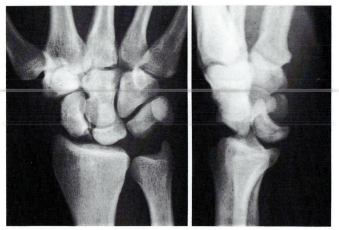

Fig. 10.63 In the anteroposterior projection the lunate bone appears to be triangular instead of quadrilateral in shape, and the lateral projection shows clearly that it is displaced forwards. The distal concavity no longer contains the base of the capitate. Because this appearance is perhaps intermediate between a lunate and a perilunate dislocation, it is better referred to as a dorsal midcarpal dislocation. A chip fracture of the proximal scaphoid is also present.

shape (Fig. 10.63). On the lateral projection, the lunate is seen overlying the volar aspect of the wrist, in an abnormal orientation.

In *perilunate (± transcaphoid fracture) dislocation*, the whole of the carpus (minus the proximal scaphoid pole in trans-scaphoid injuries), is dislocated posteriorly with respect to the lunate. This is usually evident of the PA view, but again is clear on the lateral projection (Fig. 10.64).

Scapholunate dissociation is identified by widening of the scapholunate joint, often exacerbated on clenching the fist (Terry-Thomas sign) (Fig. 10.65). This may be seen in rotational (rotary) dislocation of the scaphoid (Fig. 10.65).

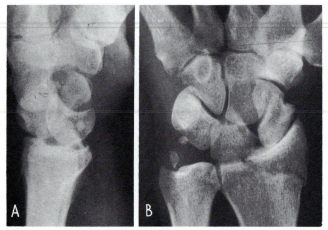

Fig. 10.64 A,B Perilunate dislocation of the carpus. With the exception of the lunate, the whole of the carpus has been dislocated dorsally in relation to the radius. Both the radial and ulnar styloid processes have been fractured. Note loss of articulation between lunate and adjacent carpal bones.

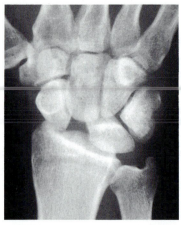

Fig. 10.65 Scapholunate dissociation: 'Terry-Thomas' or 'tooth gap' sign. There is wide separation of the scaphoid and lunate.

Arthrography is currently the method of choice for examining the intercarpal ligaments. Some authors advocate injection of all three wrist compartments, although careful examination with video fluoroscopy after injection of the radiocarpal joint will define the vast majority of injuries (Fig. 10.66). Although MRI has been proposed as a diagnostic tool for intercarpal ligament disruptions, results to date have not been convincing.

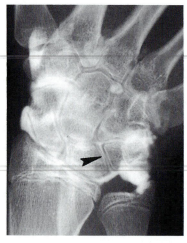

Fig. 10.66 Intercarpal ligament disruption: arthrogram. Injection of the radiocarpal joint has resulted in filling of the intercarpal joint as well. Contrast medium is seen passing between the lunate and triquetrum (arrowhead), indicating ligamentous disruption.

The hand

Hand injuries are common and usually present no diagnostic difficulty.

'Bennett's fracture' is a fracture dislocation of the base of the first metacarpal with involvement of the articular surface, usually associated with 'dislocation' of the major fragment (Fig. 10.67).

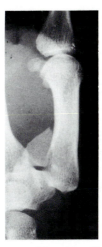

Fig. 10.67 Bennett's fracture-dislocation. The articular surface of the base of the first metacarpal is involved and the main portion of the bone is displaced proximally in relation to the trapezium.

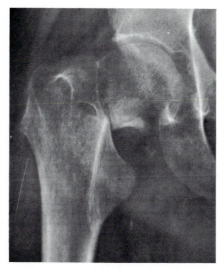

Fig. 10.69 A fracture of the femoral neck may be identified as a lucency interrupting the trabecular pattern, and the femur is externally rotated distal to the fracture.

Another important injury in the thumb is avulsion of the ulnar aspect of the base of the proximal phalanx, due to forced radial or posterior hyperextension. This injury is due to avulsion of either the ulnar collateral ligament or the adductor policis and creates instability and loss of forceful adduction if left untreated. Although named the 'mechanical bull' thumb, this is more common in skiing injuries, from falling into snow without releasing the ski pole. The 'boxer's' fracture of the fifth metacarpal is a common injury presenting in accident and emergency departments (Fig. 10.68).

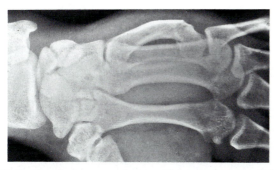

Fig. 10.68 Boxer's fracture: a fracture of the distal aspect of the 5th metacarpal, with volar angulation of the distal fragment.

THE LOWER LIMB

Fracture of the femoral neck and intertrochanteric fractures are common injuries following a fall, particularly in the elderly when osteoporosis is present (Fig. 10.69). Nevertheless, because of the age of many of the patients, underlying pathology such as metastasis should always be excluded. These fractures may be extremely difficult to define radiographically and radionuclide bone scan may be necessary. A faint ill-defined linear density across the

femoral neck, interruption of trabecular lines, and subtle cortical disruptions may be the only radiological signs.

Fractures of the femoral shaft are almost always a sign of significant trauma, often in multitrauma victims (Fig. 9.3). In trivial trauma, underlying pathology should always be suspected.

Fractures of the distal femur are frequently intra-articular and give rise to angulation of the distal fragments and disruption of the knee joint.

The knee and lower leg

Fractures around the knee include femoral fractures (see above), patellar fractures and tibial plateau fractures (Fig. 10.70). The only difficulty with patellar fractures may be in differentiating them from a bipartite patella when the fracture is single and involves the superior margins. This should be evident clinically and is usually clear radiographically although confusion may arise.

Fractures of the *tibial plateau* are obvious in general, but on occasion may not be evident as a fracture line. A cross-table lateral radiograph may demonstrate a fat/fluid level of lipohaemarthrosis in the suprapatellar bursa, indicating an intra-articular process (Fig. 9.6). Tomograms may be needed in tibial plateau fractures to determine any depression of fragments. CT is also gaining popularity as a method of evaluating their extent.

Injuries to the *menisci* traditionally have been examined by arthrography or arthroscopy. There is growing evidence however, that MRI may be the method of choice for the evaluation of knee abnormalities, especially with its additional advantage of superior visualization of the internal and external ligaments (Fig. 10.71) and surrounding soft tissues (Figs 10.72, 10.73).

Fractures of the shaft of the *tibia* are usually oblique

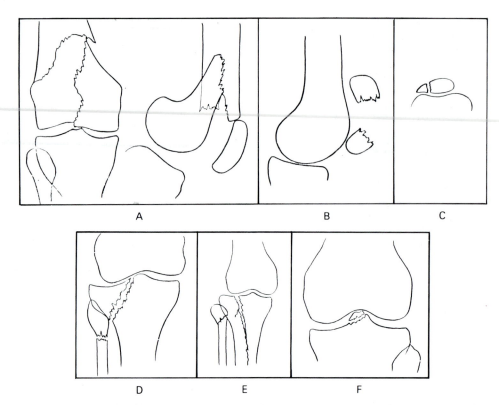

Fig. 10.70 Injuries of the knee and leg. **A**. *Supracondylar fracture of the femur* with extension to involve the articular surface. **B**. *Transverse fracture of the patella* with wide separation of fragments. **C**. *Vertical fracture of the patella* visible only in the axial projection. **D**. *Fracture of the lateral condyle of the tibia and neck of fibula*. This injury has resulted from forced abduction, with impact of the surface of the lateral femoral condyle upon the tibia. Involvement of the articular surface is minimal and this injury carries a good prognosis. **E**. *A more severe fracture of the lateral tibial condyle* with a crack running downwards into the tibial shaft. This has been caused by complete rupture of the internal lateral ligament and the cruciate ligaments, so that the lateral margin of the femur has impacted upon the surface of the lateral tibial condyle to produce the injury. The articular surface is involved. The neck of the fibula is also fractured. **F**. *Avulsion injury* to extrasynovial intercondylar region of tibia.

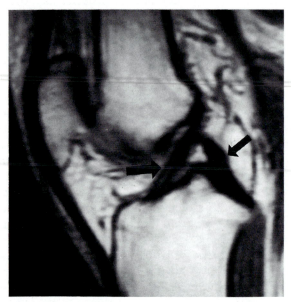

Fig. 10.71 MRI of the knee — T$_1$ sagittal image. Normal anatomy. The anterior (large arrow) and posterior (small arrow) cruciate ligaments are well seen.

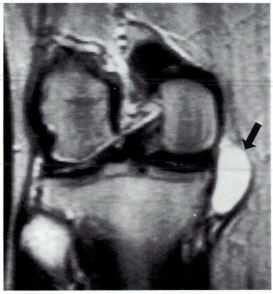

Fig. 10.72 Meniscal cyst: MRI (T$_2$). There is increased signal in a well-defined fluid collection (arrow) arising from the medial meniscus.

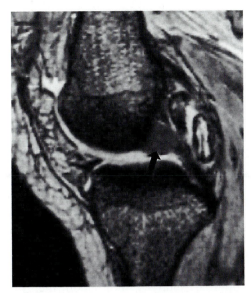

Fig. 10.73 Torn posterior cruciate ligament: MRI, gradient echo (FLASH) image. The anterior portion of the posterior cruciate ligament is abnormal, with loss of definition, and increased signal (arrow).

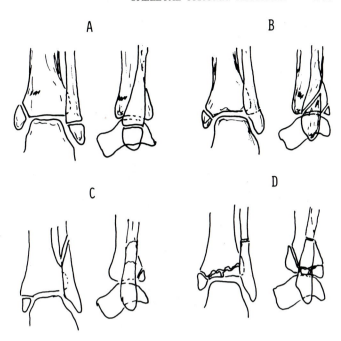

Fig. 10.74 Diagram of the major varieties of injuries of the ankle. **A**. Adduction/inversion injury of the ankle. The fracture on the tension side (lateral malleolus) is transverse. The medial malleolar fracture is oblique. **B**. Additional external rotation gives rise to an oblique or spiral fracture of the fibula ± fracture of the posterior aspect of the tibial plafond. **C**. Abduction (eversion) injury. The fracture on the tension side (medial malleolus) is transverse; with external rotation, fracture of the posterior aspect of the tibial plafond may occur, as shown. **D**. Forced dorsiflexion. Comminution of the tibial plafond is expected, particularly involving the anterior aspect.

or spiral, although transverse fractures also occur. There is invariably an associated fracture of the fibula, again indicating the association of double injuries with bony 'ring' structures. Complications of tibial fractures include a high incidence of open injuries and delayed union, usually the result of high-energy impact forces.

Stress fractures. These are found in those who inflict chronic stress on the leg (joggers, ballet dancers, etc). The proximal shaft is the commonest site, but they may occur at any site. Pain and with increased uptake on bone scan are the earliest signs. Periosteal reaction follows. Chronic stress fractures exhibit abundant surrounding sclerosis.

The ankle and foot

The most detailed (and complex) classification of *ankle fractures*, that of Lauge-Hansen, is based on classifying the injury according to the nature of the causative force, much as in the pelvis and spine. However, as well as using the parameters of external rotation, abduction, adduction, and dorsiflexion, the classification is complicated by whether the foot is in pronation or supination at the time of injury. A similar system regards ankle injuries as being the result of forced supination or pronation, and forced adduction or abduction with some variation being imparted by external (or rarely internal) rotation (Fig. 10.74) when injuries to the tibial plafond (usually posterior) may result. In practice, the injury patterns obtained using this less complicated system are the same as those described in the Lauge-Hansen classification.

Radiographically, symmetry of the ankle mortise should be sought, as asymmetry may be the only indication of

significant ligamentous injury. In addition, the nature of the injury to the malleoli (i.e. whether horizontal or oblique) will indicate the side from which the force of injury was derived, the horizontal fracture occurring on the side of injury, and the oblique fracture on the opposite side. If no fracture is present, stress views may be indicated, to evaluate for ligamentous damage. Again, however, MRI is gaining in popularity for evaluating the ankle, due to its ability to demonstrate ligamentous injury, particularly the internal ligaments, and injuries to the surrounding tendons (Fig. 10.75).

Talar fractures are generally avulsions or fractures through the waist, usually as a result of forced dorsiflexion. These are often associated with dislocations of the ankle or subtalar joint (Fig. 10.76). Avascular necrosis of the proximal fragment is a common complication. Talar dislocation may also result from forced plantar flexion injuries.

Calcaneal fractures are a frequent finding in falls from a height, and may be associated with fractures of the thoracolumbar spine. They are generally predominantly shearing fractures, but with a certain crushing component, due to the anatomy of the region: the talus, and hence the tibia, is offset medially in relation to the body

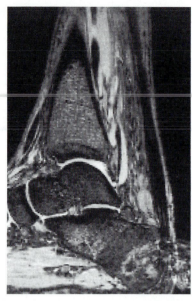

Fig. 10.75 MRI of the ankle: partial rupture of the Achilles tendon. There is widening of the tendon above its insertion, with areas of increased signal.

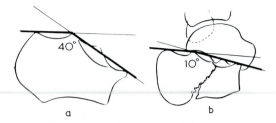

Fig. 10.77 Fracture of the calcaneus. The normal angle formed between the subtalar joint and the upper margin of the tuberosity of the calcaneus should be about 40°. Diminution of this angle should arouse suspicion of a fracture, but this may only be clearly shown in the axial projection. **A**. Normal Böhler's angle measurement. **B**. Increased angle with fracture of body of calcaneus.

Other notable fractures of the foot include *avulsion of the base of the fifth metatarsal* which must be distinguished from an unfused epiphysis. In addition, the 'Jones' fracture of the proximal diaphysis of the fifth metatarsal may proceed to non-union, or delayed union. The *Lisfranc fracture dislocation* of the tarsometatarsal junction is also an important injury, and although usually obvious (Fig. 10.78) is often overlooked when subtle. Malalignment of the second metatarsal and middle cuneiform on the frontal view is diagnostic in such cases. Failure to diagnose and treat this injury will give rise to significant long-term mid-foot problems.

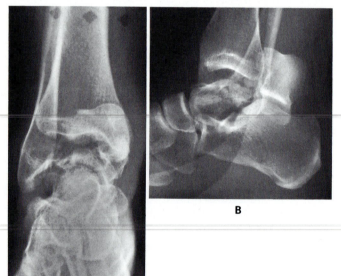

Fig. 10.76 A,B   Fracture dislocation of the talus. There is a fracture through the waist of the talus, with complete dislocation of the posterior fragment.

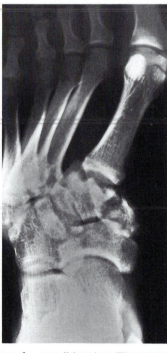

Fig. 10.78 Lisfranc fracture dislocation. There are fractures through the medial cuneiform, and bases of the second and third metatarsals, with lateral displacement of the 1st, 2nd, 3rd, and 4th metatarsals.

of the calcaneus. As such, the axial view of the talus may be helpful in the initial evaluation. Nevertheless, calcaneal fractures may be difficult to appreciate on plain radiographs. Flattening of Bohler's angle may be a helpful sign (Fig. 10.77). CT is particularly useful in the evaluation of calcaneal fractures (see Figs 9.8A, 9.8D).

REFERENCES AND SUGGESTIONS FOR FURTHER READING

Acheson, M. B., Livingston, R. R., Richardson M. I., et al (1987) High-resolution CT scanning in the evaluation of cervical spine fractures: comparison with plain film examinations. *American Journal of Roentgenology*, **148**, 1179–1185.

Amato, M., Totty, W. H., Gilula, L. A. (1984) Spondylosis of the lumbar spine: Demonstration of defects and laminal fragmentation. *Radiology*, **153**, 627–635.

Bloomberg, T. J., Nuttall, J., Stoker, D. J. (1978) Radiology in early slipped femoral capital epiphysis. *Clinical Radiology*, **29**, 657–667.

Bright, R. W. (1982). Partial growth arrest: Identification, classification, and result of treatment. *Orthopedic Transactions* **6**, 65–73.

Clanton, T. O., DeLee, J. C. (1982) Osteochondritis dissecans. History, pathophysiology and current treatment concepts. *Clinical Orthopedics*, **167**, 50–55.

Crowe, J. E., Swischuk, L. E. (1977) Acute bowing fractures of the forearm in children: A frequently missed injury. *American Journal of Roentgenology*, **128**, 981–986.

Daffner, R. H., Deeb, Z. L., Rothfus, W. E. (1986) Fingerprints of vertebral trauma — a unifying concept based on mechanisms. *Skeletal Radiology*, **15**, 518–525.

Daffner, R. H., Deeb, Z. L., Rothfus, W. E. (1987) Posterior vertebral body line: Importance in the detection of burst fracture. *American Journal of Roentgenology* **148**, 93–98.

Daffner, R. H., Riemer, B. L., Lupetin, A. R., Dash, N. (1986) Magnetic resonance imaging in acute tendon ruptures. *Skeletal Radiology*, **15**, 619–625.

Deutsch, A. L., Resnick, D., Mink, J. H. et al (1984) Computed tomography of the glenohumeral joint: Normal anatomy and clinical experience. *Radiology*, **153**, 603–608.

Dias, J. J., Stirling, A. J., Finlay, D. B. L., Gregg, P. J. (1987) Computerised axial tomography for tibial plateau fractures. *Journal of Bone and Joint Surgery*, **69B**, 84–89.

Fernbach, S. K., Wilkinson, R. H. (1984) Avulsion injuries of the pelvis and proximal femur. *American Journal of Roentgenology*, **137**, 581–586.

Fielding, J. W., Hawkins, R. J. (1977) Atlanto-axial rotatory fixation (Fixed rotatory subluxation of the atlanto-axial joint.) *Journal of Bone and Joint Surgery*, **59A**, 37–44.

Foster, S. C., Foster, R. R. (1976) Lisfranc's tarsometatarsal fracture-dislocation. *Radiology*, **120**, 79–85.

Gertzbein, S. D., Chenoweth, D. R. (1977) Occult injuries of the pelvic ring. *Clinical Orthopaedics*, **128**, 201–207.

Gilula, L. A., Weeks, P. M. (1978) Post-traumatic ligamentous instabilities of the wrist. *Radiology*, **129**, 641–647.

Goldberg, A. L., Rothfus, W. E., Deeb, Z. L. et al (1988) Impact of magnetic resonance on the diagnostic evaluation of acute cervicothoracic spinal trauma. *Skeletal Radiology*, **17**, 39–95.

Greaney, R. B., Gerber, F. H., Laughlin, R. I. et al (1983) Distribution and natural history of stress fractures in US marine recruits. *Radiology*, **146**, 339–346.

Harris, J. H., Jr., Harris, W. H. (1975) The Radiology of Emergency Medicine. Williams & Wilkins Co., Baltimore.

Hudson, T. M., Caragol, W. J., Kaye, J. J. (1976) Isolated rotatory subluxation of the carpal navicular. *American Journal of Roentgenology*, **126**, 601–605.

Judet, R., Judet, J., Letournel, E. (1964) Fracture of the acetabulum: Classification and surgical approaches for open reduction. *Journal of Bone and Joint Surgery*, **46A**, 1615–1631.

Keen, J. S., Goletz, T. H., Lilleas, T. et al (1984) Diagnosis of vertebral fractures. A comparison of conventional radiography, conventional tomography and computed axial tomography. *Journal of Bone and Joint Surgery*, **64A**, 586–594.

Lauge-Hansen, N. (1954) Fractures of the ankle: Genetic roentgenologic diagnosis of fractures of the ankle. *American Journal of Roentgenology*, **71**, 456–462.

McArdle, C. B., Crofford, M. J., Mirfakhraee, M. et al (1986) Surface coil MR of spinal trauma. Preliminary experience. *American Journal of Neuroradiology*, 7, 885–890.

Magid, D., Fishman, E. K. (1986) Computed tomography of acetabular fractures. *Seminars in Ultrasound, CT and MR*, 7, 351–357.

Milgram, J. W., Rogers, L. F., Miller, J. W. (1978) Osteochondral fractures: Mechanisms of injury and fate of fragments. *American Journal of Roentgenology*, **130**, 651–656.

Mirvis, S. E., Geisler, F. H., Jelnick, J. J., Joslyn, J. N., Gellad, F. (1988) Acute cervical spine trauma: Evaluation with 1.5 T MR imaging. *Radiology*, **166**, 807–816.

Mirvis, S. E., Young, J. W. R., Lim, C., Greenberg, J. (1986) Hangman's fracture: Radiologic assessment in 27 cases. *Radiology*, **163**, 713–717.

Mirvis, S. E. (1989). Applications of MRI and 3-D CT in emergency medicine. *Annals of Emergency Medicine*, **18**, 1315–1321.

Pavlov, H., Freiberger, R. H. (1978) Fractures and dislocations about the shoulder. *Seminars in Roentgenology*, **13**, 85–91.

Pennal, G. F., Tile, M., Waddell, J. P., Garside, M. (1980) Pelvic disruption: Assessment and classification. *Clinical Orthopaedics*, **151**, 12–23.

Reckling, F. W. (1982) Unstable fracture-dislocations of the forearm (Monteggia and Galeazzi lesions). *Journal of Bone and Joint Surgery*, **64A**, 857–863.

Resnick, D. (1989) (ed) Bone and Joint Imaging. W. B. Saunders, Philadelphia.

Resnick, C. S., Gelberman, R. H., Resnick, D. (1983) Transcaphoid, transcapitate, perilunate fracture dislocation (scaphocapitate syndrome). *Skeletal Radiology*, **9**, 192–197.

Richardson, P., Young, J. W. R., Porter, D. (1990) CT detection of cortical fracture of the femoral head associated with posterior inferior dislocation. *American Journal of Roentgenology*, **155**, 93–94.

Rogers, L. R. (1982) Radiology of Skeletal Trauma. Churchill Livingstone, Edinburgh.

Rosen, R. A., (1970) Transitory demineralization of the femoral head. *Radiology*, **94**, 509–514.

Ryan, M. D., Taylor, R. F. K. (1982) Odontoid fractures. *Journal of Bone and Joint Surgery*, **64B**, 416–421.

Salter, R. B., Harris, W. R. (1963) Injuries involving the epiphyseal plate. *Journal of Bone and Joint Surgery*, **45A**, 587–622.

Scott, W. J. R., Fishman, E. K., Magid, D. (1987) Acetabular fractures: Optimal imaging. *Radiology*, **165**, 537–539.

Templeton, P. A., Young, J. W. R., Mirvis, S. E., Buddemeyer, E. U. (1987) The value of retropharyngeal soft tissue measurement in trauma of the adult cervical spine. *Skeletal Radiology*, **16**, 98–104.

Thomason, M., Young, J. W. R. (1984) Os odontoideum. Case Report 261. *Skeletal Radiology*, **11**, 144–146.

Tile, M. (1986). Fractures of the Pelvis and Acetabulum. Williams and Wilkins, Baltimore.

Waddell, J. P., Johnston, D. W. C., Neidre, A. (1981) Fractures of the tibial plateau: A review of ninety-five patients and comparison of treatment methods. *Journal of Trauma*, **21**, 376–381.

Wang, S. C., Grattan-Smith, A. (1987) Thoracolumbar burst fractures: Two 'new' plain film signs with CT correlation. *Australasian Radiology*, **31**, 404–409.

Whitley, J. E. N., Forsythe, H. F. (1960) Classification of cervical spine injuries. *American Journal of Roentgenology*, **83**, 633–641.

Yeager, B. A., Dalinka, M. K: (1985) Radiology of trauma to the wrist: Dislocations, fracture dislocations, and instability patterns. *Skeletal Radiology*, **13**, 120.

Young, J. W. R., Burgess, A. R. (1987) Radiologic Management of Pelvic Ring Fractures, Urban-Schwartzenberg, Baltimore.

Young, J. W., Resnik, C. S., DeCandido, P., Mirvis, S. E. (1989) The laminar space in the diagnosis of rotational flexion injuries to the cervical spine. *American Journal of Radiology*, **152**, 103–107.

PART 2

THE RESPIRATORY SYSTEM

CHAPTER 11

THE NORMAL CHEST: METHODS OF INVESTIGATION AND DIFFERENTIAL DIAGNOSIS

Janet Murfitt

THE NORMAL CHEST: METHODS OF INVESTIGATION

1. Plain films:
   PA, lateral, AP, decubitus, supine, oblique; inspiratory–expiratory; lordotic, apical, penetrated, magnified
2. Tomography
3. CT scanning
4. Radionuclide studies
5. Needle biopsy
6. Ultrasound
7. Fluoroscopy
8. Bronchography
9. Pulmonary angiography
10. Bronchial arteriography
11. MRI
12. Digital radiography
13. Lymphangiography

The *plain chest film* is the most frequently requested radiological examination. Visualization of the lung fields is excellent because of the inherent contrast of the tissues of the thorax. A routine examination should include PA and lateral films. Comparison of the current film with old films is valuable and should always be undertaken if the old films are available. A current film is mandatory before proceeding to more complex investigations.

Simple tomography remains a useful investigation for determining that an abnormality suspected on a plain film is genuine and that it is intrapulmonary, although the high kVp film has reduced the need for tomography in these circumstances. In addition, it is still used in some centres to assess the peripheral lung mass and the abnormal hilum.

However *conventional CT* scanning, and *high-resolution CT scanning*, when available, are far superior for assessing chest wall lesions, the lung mass, the hilum and mediastinum, and for detecting pulmonary metastases and staging malignancy. High-resolution scanning is of proven value in the diagnosis of diffuse lung disease, particularly in the early stages when the chest radiograph is normal, and for follow-up. In many centres high-resolution scanning is used for the detection of bronchiectasis and surgery is undertaken without preoperative bronchography.

Radionuclide scanning is used as the first-line investigation of suspected pulmonary embolus in the majority of cases. A normal scan excludes the presence of an embolus. Large perfusion defects accompanied by smaller radiographic abnormalities or smaller ventilation defects indicate a high probability of pulmonary embolus.

However, *pulmonary angiography* remains the 'gold standard' for the diagnosis of pulmonary embolism. It is usually undertaken in patients with massive embolism when embolectomy or thrombolysis are contemplated.

Ultrasound is of use for investigating chest wall and pleural lesions and for localization of pleural fluid prior to a diagnostic tap or drainage. However, the acoustic mismatch between the chest wall and air-containing lung results in reflection of the ultrasound beam at the lung–pleura interface, so that the lung cannot be demonstrated.

Biopsy of pulmonary lesions using a fine needle for aspiration has a high diagnostic yield for malignancy, excluding lymphoma, with a low incidence of complications. A cutting needle is associated with a higher complication rate but is more helpful in the diagnosis of lymphoma and benign lung conditions.

The value of *MRI* for diagnosing pulmonary disease is still in the assessment stage. It appears to be helpful in the diagnosis of hilar masses and lymphadenopathy. The full potential of *Digital radiography* has not been determined up to now.

Diagnostic pneumothorax is an obsolete procedure which was once used to differentiate a pleural-based from a pulmonary lesion. The *barium swallow* has been supplanted by CT for assessing the nonoesophageal mediastinal mass, but may be indicated in the investigation of conditions which may be associated with pulmonary changes such as scleroderma, hiatus hernia and achalasia.

Chylous reflux with the formation of a chylothorax may be demonstrated by conventional *lymphangiography*.

THE PLAIN FILM

The PA view. By definition, the patient faces the film chin up, with the shoulders rotated forwards to displace the scapulae from the lung fields. Exposure is made on full inspiration for optimum visualization of the lung bases, centring at T5. The breasts should be compressed against the film to prevent them obscuring the lung bases.

There is no general consensus regarding the kilovoltage used for chest radiography although the high kVp technique is becoming widely used. High kVp, low kVp or intermediate kVp techniques are used with various film screen combinations, grids or air gap techniques.

Using a low kVp (60–80 kV) produces a high contrast film (Fig. 11.1). For large patients a grid reduces scatter. A film-focus distance (FFD) of 1.85 m (6') reduces magnification and produces a sharper image. With high kilovoltages (120–150 kVp) the contrast of the films is reduced (Fig. 11.2), with increased visualization of the hidden areas of the lung due to better penetration of overlying structures. The bones and pulmonary calcification are less well seen, although pulmonary markings are more clearly demonstrated. A grid or air gap is necessary to reduce scatter and improve contrast. An air gap of 15–25 cm between patient and film necessitates an increased FFD of 2.44 m (8') to reduce magnification.

An automatic exposure system and dedicated automatic chest unit are desirable in a busy department.

The lateral view. A high kVp or normal kVp technique may be used with or without a grid. For sharpness, the side of interest is nearest the film. With shoulders

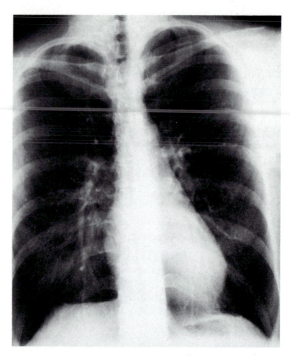

Fig. 11.2 Radiograph of same patient as in Fig. 11.1, taken at 140 kVp. Note the improved visualization of the main airways, vascular structures and the area behind the heart, including the spine.

parallel to the film the arms are elevated, or displaced back if the anterior mediastinum is of interest.

Lesions obscured on the PA view are often clearly demonstrated on the lateral view. Examples of this are anterior mediastinal masses, encysted pleural fluid (Fig. 11.4) and posterior basal consolidation. In contrast, clear-cut lesions on the PA view may be difficult to identify on the lateral film, both lung fields being superimposed (Fig. 11.3). This is particularly so with a large pleural effusion.

Other views. Additional plain films may assist with certain diagnostic problems. The hidden areas of the PA film, rib destruction, cavitation, calcification, an air bronchogram and the main airways may all be more clearly seen on a *penetrated film*. *Oblique views* demonstrate the retrocardiac area, the posterior costophrenic angles and the chest wall. In the *AP* position the ribs are projected over different areas of the lung from those in the PA view, and the posterior chest is well shown. Good visualization of the apices requires projection of the clavicles upwards, as in the *apical view* with the tube angled up 50–60°, or downwards, as in the *lordotic view* with the patient in a lordotic PA position. In this view a middle lobe collapse shows clearly as a well-defined triangular shadow.

A subpulmonary effusion is frequently difficult to distinguish from an elevated diaphragm or consolidation. In the *supine* and *decubitus* positions (Fig. 11.5), free fluid becomes displaced. On the supine projection this results

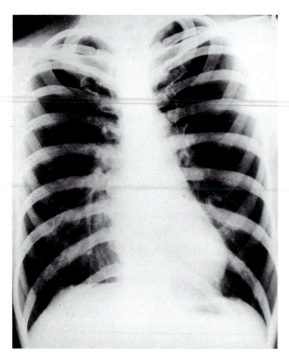

Fig. 11.1 Radiograph taken at 60 kVp.

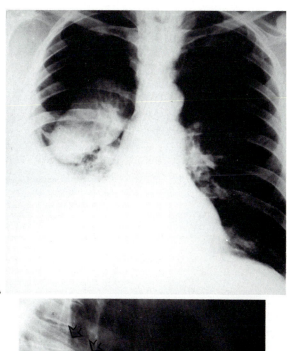

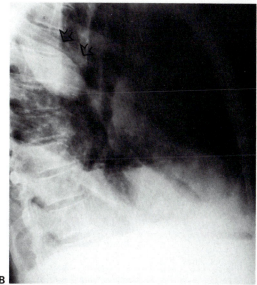

Fig. 11.4 Encysted pleural fluid. **A.** PA film. A large right pleural effusion and a large mass above. **B.** Lateral film. Loculated fluid is demonstrated high in the oblique fissure.

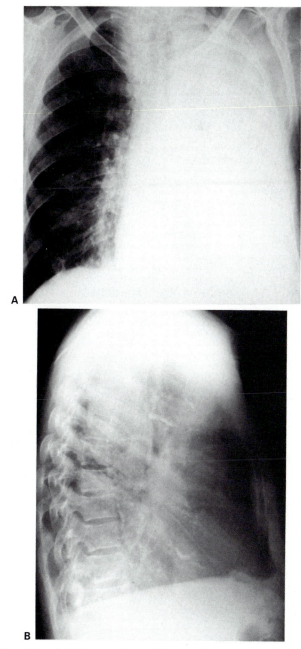

Fig. 11.3 **A.** Collapse and consolidation of the left lung. **B.** Lateral film. The appearances are less dramatic than on the PA film. Only the right hemidiaphragm is visible. The radiolucency of the lower vertebrae is decreased.

in the hemithorax becoming opaque with loss of the diaphragm outline, an apical cap, blunting of the costophrenic angle and decreased visibility of the pulmonary markings. On the PA view the apex of the effusion has a more lateral position than that of a normal diaphragm.

The decubitus film shows fluid levels particularly well. Small amounts of pleural fluid may be shown with the affected side dependent.

Paired *inspiratory* and *expiratory* films demonstrate air trapping and diaphragm movement. Small pneum-othoraces and interstitial shadowing may be more apparent on the expiratory film.

VIEWING THE PA FILM

Before a diagnosis can be made an abnormality, if present, must be identified. Knowledge of the normal appearance of a chest radiograph is essential. In addition the radiologist must develop a routine which ensures that all areas of the radiograph are scrutinized.

Some radiologists prefer initially to view the film without studying the clinical information. Comparison of the current film with old films is important and often extremely helpful. A suggested scheme is as follows, examining each point in turn.

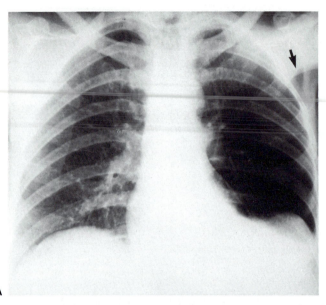
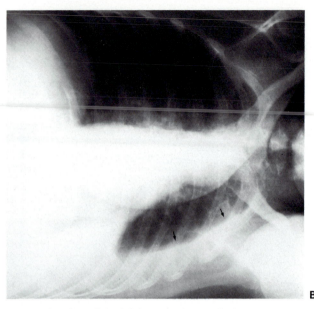

A   B

Fig. 11.5 Subpulmonary pleural fluid. **A.** Erect PA radiograph. There is apparent elevation of the left hemidiaphragm. Increased translucency of the left lung is due to a left mastectomy. Note the abnormal axillary fold (arrow). **B.** Left lateral decubitus film (with horizontal beam). Pleural fluid has moved to the most dependent part of the left lung (arrows).

1. Request form	Name, age, date, sex
	Clinical information
2. Technical	Centring, patient position
	Markers
3. Trachea	Position, outline
4. Heart and mediastinum	Size, shape, displacement
5. Diaphragms	Outline, shape
	Relative position
6. Pleura	Position of horizontal fissure
	Costophrenic, cardiophrenic angles
7. Lung fields	Local, generalized abnormality
	Comparison of the translucency and vascular markings of the lungs
8. Hidden areas	Apices, posterior sulcus
	Mediastinum, hila, bones
9. Hila	Density, position, shape
10. Below diaphragms	Gas shadows, calcification
11. Soft tissues	Mastectomy, gas, densities etc.
12. Bones	Destructive lesions etc

Technical

Centring. If the film is well centred the medial ends of the clavicles are equidistant from the vertebral spinous processes at the T4–5 level. Small degrees of rotation distort the mediastinal borders, and the lung nearest the film appears less translucent. Thoracic deformities, especially a scoliosis, negate the value of conventional centring. The orientation of the aortic arch, gastric bubble and heart should be determined to confirm normal situs and that the side markers are correct.

Penetration. The vertebral bodies and disc spaces should be just visible through the cardiac shadow. Underpenetration increases the likelihood of missing an abnormality overlain by another structure. Overpenetration results in loss of visibility of low-density lesions such as early tuberculous shadowing, although a bright light may reveal the abnormality.

Degree of inspiration. On full inspiration the anterior ends of the sixth ribs or posterior ends of the tenth are above the diaphragms, although the degree of inspiration achieved varies with the build of the patient. Pulmonary diseases such as SLE and fibrosing alveolitis are associated with reduced pulmonary compliance, which may result in reduced inflation with elevation of the diaphragms. On expiration the heart shadow is larger and there is basal shadowing due to crowding of the normal vascular markings.

The trachea

The trachea should be examined for narrowing, displacement and intraluminal lesions. It is midline in its upper part, then deviates slightly to the right around the aortic knuckle. On expiration, deviation to the right becomes more marked. In addition there is shortening on expiration, so that an endotracheal tube situated just above the carina on inspiration may occlude the main bronchus on expiration.

Calibre should be even and translucency of the tracheal air column decrease caudally. The right tracheal margin can be traced down to the right main bronchus. This border is the *right paratracheal stripe* and is seen in 60% of patients, normally measuring less than 5 mm. Widening of the stripe occurs with tracheal malignancy, mediastinal tumours, mediastinitis and pleural effusions.

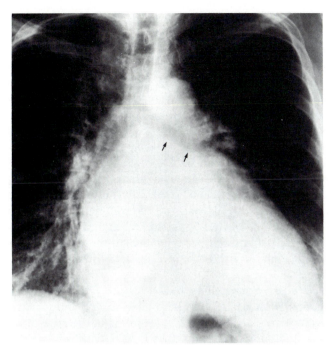

Fig. 11.6 Elevated left main bronchus (arrows) and widened carina. Patient with mitral valve disease and an enlarged left atrium.

The left paratracheal line is rarely visualized.

The *azygos vein* lies in the angle between the right main bronchus and trachea. Enlargement occurs in the supine position but also with portal hypertension, IVC and SVC obstruction, right heart failure and constrictive pericarditis. On the erect film it should be less than 10 mm in diameter. Its size decreases with the Valsalva manoeuvre and on inspiration.

Widening of the carina occurs on inspiration. The normal angle is 60–75°. Pathological causes of widening include an enlarged left atrium (Fig. 11.6) and enlarged carinal nodes.

The mediastinum and heart

The central dense shadow seen on the PA chest film comprises the mediastinum, heart, spine and sternum. With good centring two-thirds of the cardiac shadow lies to the left of midline and one-third to the right, although this is quite variable in normal subjects. The *transverse cardiac diameter* and the *cardiothoracic ratio* are assessed. Measurement in isolation is of less value than when previous figures are available. An increase in excess of 1.5 cm in the transverse cardiac diameter on serial films is significant. However the heart shadow is enlarged with a short FFD on expiration, in the supine and AP projections and when the diaphragms are elevated.

All borders of the heart and mediastinum are clearly defined except where the heart sits on the left hemidiaphragm. The right superior mediastinal shadow is formed by the SVC and innominate vessels; a dilated

aorta may contribute to this border. On the left side the superior mediastinal border is less sharp. It is formed by the subclavian artery above the aortic knuckle.

Various junction lines may be visualized. The *anterior junction line* is where the lungs meet anterior to the ascending aorta. It is only 1 mm thick. Overlying the tracheal translucency it runs downwards from below the suprasternal notch, slightly curving from right to left. The *posterior junction* line is where the lungs meet posteriorly behind the oesophagus and is a straight or curved line convex to the left, some 2 mm wide and extending from the lung apices to the aortic knuckle or below.

In young women the pulmonary trunk is frequently very prominent.

In babies and young children the normal *thymus* is a triangular sail-shaped structure with well-defined borders projecting from one or both sides of the mediastinum (Fig. 11.7). Both borders may be wavy in outline (the wave sign of Mulvey), from indentation by the costal cartilages. The right border is straighter than the left, which may be rounded. Thymic size decreases on inspiration and in response to stress and illness. The thymus is absent in di George's syndrome. Enlargement may occur following recovery from an illness. A large thymus is more commonly seen in boys.

Adjacent to the vertebral bodies run the *paraspinal lines* usually 1 or 2 mm wide. Enlargement occurs with osteophytes, a tortuous aorta, obesity, vertebral and adjacent soft-tissue masses, and a dilated azygos system.

A search should be made for abnormal densities, fluid levels, mediastinal emphysema and calcification. Spinal abnormalities may accompany mediastinal masses; for example, hemivertebrae are associated with neuroenteric cysts.

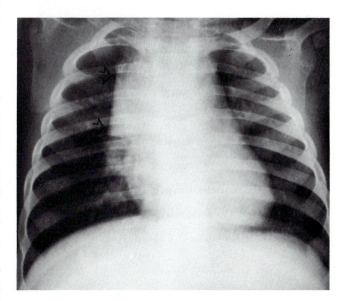

Fig. 11.7 Normal thymus in a child, projecting to the right of the mediastinum (arrows).

The diaphragm

In most patients the right hemidiaphragm is higher than the left. This is due to the heart depressing the left side and not to the liver pushing up the right hemidiaphragm; in dextrocardia with normal abdominal situs the right hemidiaphragm is the lowest. The hemidiaphragms may lie at the same level and in a small percentage of the population the left side is the higher; this is more likely to occur if the stomach or splenic flexure are distended with gas. A difference in height greater than 3 cm is considered significant.

On inspiration the domes of the diaphragms are at the level of the sixth rib anteriorly and at or below the tenth rib posteriorly. In the supine position the diaphragm is higher.

Both domes have gentle curves which steepen towards the posterior angles. The upper borders are clearly seen except on the left side, where the heart is in contact with the diaphragm, and in the cardiophrenic angles when there are prominent fat pads. Otherwise loss of outline indicates that the adjacent lung contains no air — for example, as a result of consolidation or of pleural disease.

Free intraperitoneal gas outlines the undersurface of the diaphragm and shows it to be normally 2–3 mm thick (Fig. 11.8).

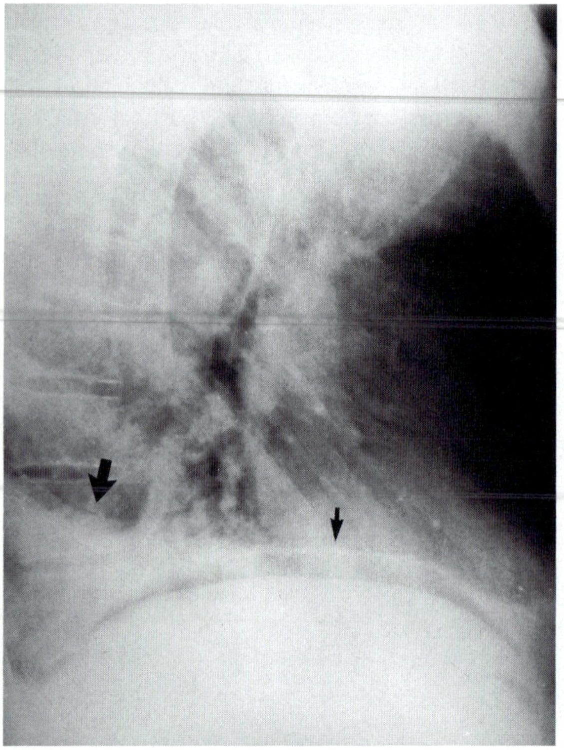

Congenital variations and other lesions of the diaphragm will be considered below.

The fissures

The main fissures. Visualization of the fissures occurs when the X-ray beam is tangential. On the PA film, the horizontal fissure is seen running from the hilum to the region of the sixth rib in the axillary line, and may be straight or have a slight downward curve. Occasionally it has a double appearance.

All fissures are clearly seen on the lateral film. The horizontal fissure runs anteriorly and often slightly downwards. Both oblique fissures commence posteriorly at the level of T4 or T5, passing through the hilum. The left is steeper and finishes 5 cm behind the anterior costophrenic angle, whereas the right ends just behind the angle.

Accessory fissures. The *azygos* fissure is shaped like a comma, with a triangular base peripherally, and is nearly always right-sided (Fig. 11.9). It forms in the apex of the lung and consists of paired folds of parietal and visceral pleura plus the azygos vein which has failed to migrate normally. Enlargement occurs in the supine position. At post-mortem the incidence is 1%, but radiologically it is 0.4%. When left-sided the fissure contains the hemiazygos vein.

The *superior accessory fissure* separates the apical from the basal segments of the lower lobes. It is commoner on the right side and has an incidence of 5%. On the PA film it resembles the horizontal fissure. The lateral film shows it running posteriorly from the hilum.

Fig. 11.8 Pneumoperitoneum after laparotomy. The thin right cupola (small arrow) is outlined by the adjacent aerated lung and the free abdominal gas. Posterior consolidation (large arrow) obscures the outline of the diaphragm posteriorly.

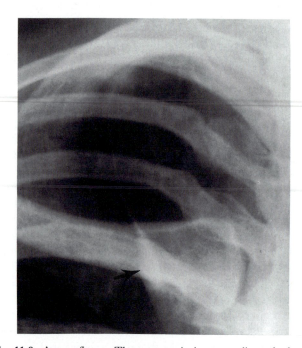

Fig. 11.9 Azygos fissure. The azygos vein is seen to lie at the lower end of the fissure (large arrow).

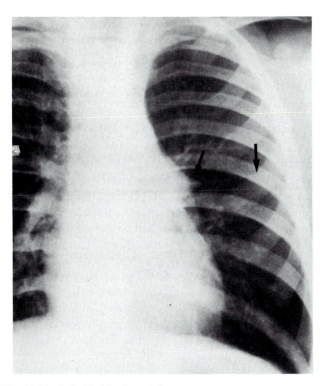

Fig. 11.10 Left-sided horizontal fissure.

The *inferior accessory fissure* appears as an oblique line running cranially from the cardiophrenic angle and separating the medial basal from the other basal segments. It is commoner on the right side and has an incidence of 5%.

The *left-sided horizontal fissure* (Fig. 11.10) separates the lingula from the other upper-lobe segments.

The angles. The normal costophrenic angles are acute and well defined, but become obliterated when the diaphragms are flat. Not infrequently the cardiophrenic angles contain low-density ill-defined shadows caused by fat pads.

The lung fields

By comparing the lung fields, areas of abnormal translucency or uneven distribution of lung markings are more easily detected. The size of the upper- and lower-zone vessels is assessed.

An abnormal shadow should be closely studied to ensure that it is not a combination shadow formed by superimposed normal structures such as vessels and costal cartilage. The extent and location of the shadow is determined and specific features such as calcification or cavitation noted. A general survey is made to look for further lesions and displacement of the normal landmarks.

The hidden areas

The apices. On the PA film the apices are partially obscured by ribs, costal cartilage, clavicles and soft tissues. Visualization is very limited on the lateral view.

Mediastinum and hila. Central lesions may be obscured by these structures or appear as a superimposed density. The abnormality is usually detectable on the lateral film.

Diaphragms. The posterior and lateral basal segments of the lower lobes and the posterior sulcus are partially obscured by the downward curve of the posterior diaphragm. Visualization is further diminished if the film is not taken on full inspiration.

Bones. Costal cartilage or bone may obscure a lung lesion. Determining whether a density is pulmonary or bony may be difficult; AP, expiratory and oblique films may be helpful before proceeding to tomography or CT.

The hilum

Normally the left hilum is 2.5 cm higher than the right. The hila should be of equal density and similar size, with concave lateral borders where the upper-lobe vessels meet the pulmonary arteries. However there is a wide range of normal appearances. Any shadow which is not obviously vascular must be regarded with a high index of suspicion and investigated further. Old films for comparison are helpful in this situation.

Of all the structures in the hilum, only the pulmonary arteries and upper lobe veins contribute significantly to the hilar shadows on the plain radiograph. Normal lymph nodes are not seen. Air can be identified within the proximal bronchi but normal bronchial walls are only seen end-on. The upper lobe bronchus may appear as a ring shadow adjacent to the upper outer hilum (Fig. 11.11) and is seen on the right side in 45% of cases and the left side in 50%. Normally there is less than 5 mm of soft tissue lateral to this bronchus. Thickening of the soft tissues suggests the presence of abnormal pathology such as malignancy.

The inferior pulmonary ligament is a double layer of pleura extending down from the lower margin of the inferior pulmonary vein in the hilum as a sheet which may or may not be attached to the diaphragm and which attaches the lower lobe to the mediastinum. It is rarely identified on a simple radiograph but is frequently seen at CT.

The pulmonary vessels. The left pulmonary artery lies above the left main bronchus before passing posteriorly, whereas on the right side the artery is anterior to the bronchus, resulting in the right hilum being the lower. Hilar size is very variable. The maximum diameter of the normal descending branch of the right pulmonary artery is 10–16 mm for males (9–15 mm for females).

The upper-lobe veins lie lateral to the arteries, which are separated from the mediastinum by approximately 1 cm of lung tissue. At the first intercostal space, the diameter of the normal vessels should not exceed 3 mm. The lower-lobe vessels are larger than those of the upper

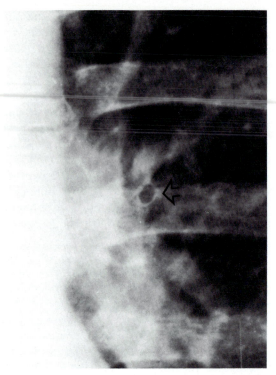

Fig. 11.11 Upper lobe bronchus seen end-on appears as a ring shadow.

lobes in the erect position, perfusion and aeration of the upper zones being reduced. In the supine position the vessels equalize. In the right paracardiac region the vessels are invariably prominent.

The peripheral lung markings are mainly vascular, veins and arteries having no distinguishing characteristics. There should be an even distribution throughout the lung fields.

Centrally the arteries and veins have different features. The arteries accompany the bronchi, lying posterosuperior, whereas veins do not follow the bronchi but drain via the interlobular septa, eventually forming superior and basal veins which converge on the left atrium. This confluence of veins may be seen as a rounded structure to the right of midline superimposed on the heart, sometimes simulating an enlarged left atrium. Pulmonary veins have fewer branches than arteries and are straighter, larger and less well-defined.

The bronchial vessels are normally not visualized. They arise from the ventral surface of the descending aorta at the T5–6 level. Their anatomy is variable. Usually there are two branches on the left and one on the right, which often shares a common origin with an intercostal artery. On entering the hila the bronchial arteries accompany the bronchi. The veins drain into the pulmonary veins and to a lesser extent the azygos system.

Enlarged bronchial arteries appear as multiple small nodules around the hilum and as short lines in the proximal lung fields and are seen with cyanotic heart disease. Focal enlargement may occur with a local pulmonary lesion. Occasionally, enlarged arteries indent the oesophagus.

Causes of enlarged bronchial arteries

1. General: cyanotic congenital heart disease, e.g. pulmonary atresia, severe Fallot's tetralogy
2. Local: bronchiectasis, bronchial carcinoma

The pulmonary segments and bronchi. The pulmonary segments (Figs 11.12, 11.13) are served by segmental bronchi and arteries, but unlike the lobes are not separated by pleura. Normal bronchi are not visualized in the peripheral lung fields.

The right main bronchus is shorter, steeper and wider than the left, bifurcating earlier. The upper lobe bronchus arises after 2.5 cm and is higher than the left, which arises after 5 cm. The bronchi divide between 6 and 20 times before becoming bronchioles. Terminal bronchioles are 0.2 mm wide. Each receives two or three respiratory bronchioles which connect with between 2 and 11 alveolar ducts. Each duct receives between 2 and 6 alveolar sacs which are connected to alveoli. The *acinus*, generally considered to be the functioning lung unit, is the portion of the lung arising from the terminal bronchiole (Fig. 11.14). When filled with fluid it is seen on a radiograph as a 5–6 mm-wide shadow, and this comprises the basic unit seen in acinar (alveolar) shadowing.

The primary lobule arises from the last respiratory bronchiole. The secondary lobule is between 1.0 and 2.5 cm in size and is the smallest discrete unit of lung tissue surrounded by connective tissue septa. When thickened, these septa become Kerley B lines (Fig. 11.15).

Other connections exist between the air spaces, allowing collateral air drift. The pores of Kohn, 3–13 μm in size, connect the alveoli. The canals of Lambert (30 μm) run between bronchioles and alveoli.

The lymphatics system. Lymphatics remove interstitial fluid and foreign particles. They run in the interlobular septa, connecting with subpleural lymphatics and draining via the deep lymphatics to the hilum. Normal lymphatics are not seen but thickening of the lymphatics and surrounding connective tissue produces Kerley lines, which may be transient or persistent. Thickened connective tissues are the main contributors to the substance of these lines (see Tables 11.1 and 11.2 below).

The lymph nodes. The intrapulmonary lymphatics drain directly to the bronchopulmonary nodes, and this group is the first to be involved by spread from a peripheral tumour. The node groups and their drainage are well described (Fig. 11.16). Extensive intercommunications exist between the groups but the pattern of nodal involvement can sometimes indicate the site of the

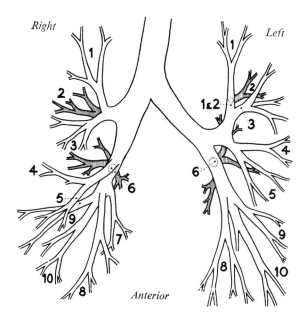

Fig. 11.12 Diagram illustrating the anatomy of the main bronchi and segmental divisions. Nomenclature approved by the Thoracic Society (reproduced by permission of the Editors of *Thorax*).

UPPER LOBE
1. Apical bronchus
2. Posterior bronchus
3. Anterior bronchus

Right	*Left*
MIDDLE LOBE	LINGULA
4. Lateral bronchus	4. Superior bronchus
5. Medial bronchus	5. Inferior bronchus

LOWER LOBE
6. Apical bronchus
7. Medial basal (cardiac)
8. Anterior basal bronchus   8. Anterior basal bronchus
9. Lateral basal bronchus   9. Lateral basal bronchus
10. Posterior basal bronchus   10. Posterior basal bronchus

primary tumour. Mediastinal nodes may be involved by tumours both above and below the diaphragm.

1. *The anterior mediastinal nodes* in the region of the aortic arch drain the thymus and right heart.
2. *The intrapulmonary nodes* lie along the main bronchi.
3. *The middle mediastinal nodes* drain the lungs, bronchi, left heart, lower trachea and visceral pleura. There are four groups:
   a. Bronchopulmonary (hilar) nodes which drain into groups (b) and (c). When enlarged they appear as lobulated hilar masses.
   b. Carinal nodes.
   c. Tracheobronchial nodes, which lie adjacent to the azygos vein on the right side and are near the recurrent laryngeal nerve on the left side.
   d. Paratracheal nodes are more numerous on the right side. There is significant cross-drainage from left to right.

4. *The posterior mediastinal nodes* drain the posterior diaphragm and lower oesophagus. They lie around the lower descending aorta and oesophagus.
5. *The parietal nodes* consist of anterior and posterior groups situated behind the sternum and posteriorly in the intercostal region, draining the soft tissues and parietal pleura.

Below the diaphragm

A pneumoperitoneum is often more obvious on an erect chest film, particularly a lateral, than an erect abdominal film. A search should be made for other abnormal gas shadows such as dilated bowel, abscesses, a displaced gastric bubble and intramural gas, as well as calcified lesions. Interposition of colon between liver and diaphragm, *Chilaiditi's syndrome* (Fig. 11.17), is a common and often transient finding, particularly in the aged, the obvious haustral pattern distinguishing it from free gas.

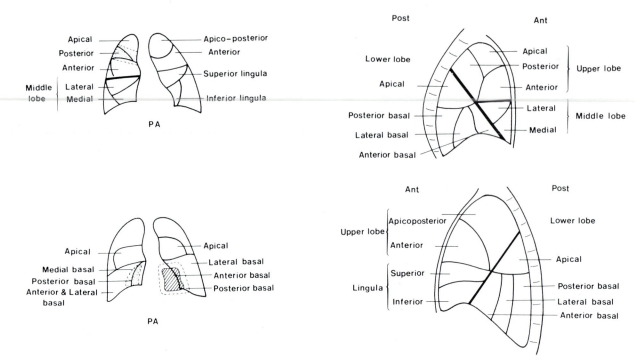

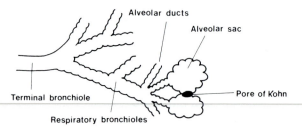

Fig. 11.13 Diagrams illustrating the approximate positions of the pulmonary segments as seen on the PA and lateral radiographs.

Fig. 11.14 A diagrammatic representation of the acinus.

Table 11.1 Kerley lines

A	lines	Thin non-branching lines radiating from the hilum, 2–6 cm long. Thickened deep interlobular septa.
B	lines	Transverse thin lines at the lung bases perpendicular to the pleura, 1–3 cm long. Thickened interlobular septa.
C	lines	A spider's-web appearance.

Subdiaphragmatic fat in the obese may be confused with free gas on a single film.

Soft tissues

A general survey of the soft tissues includes the chest wall, shoulders and lower neck.

It is important to confirm the presence or absence of breast shadows. The breasts may partially obscure the lung bases. Nipple shadows are variable in position and often asymmetrical; frequently only one shadow is seen.

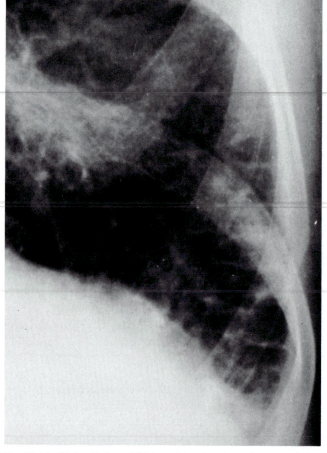

Fig. 11.15 Kerley B lines. Thickened interlobular septa in a patient with mitral valve disease.

Table 11.2 Causes of Kerley lines

Pulmonary oedema

Mitral valve disease

Pneumoconiosis

Lymphangitis carcinomatosa

Sarcoidosis

Idiopathic (in the elderly)

Fibrosing alveolitis

Alveolar cell carcinoma

Lymphoma

Lymphangiectasia

Lymphatic obstruction

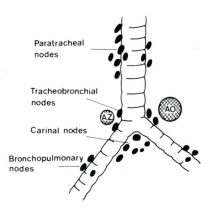

Fig. 11.16 The middle mediastinal nodes.

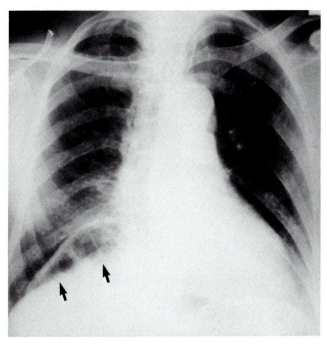

Fig. 11.17 Chilaiditi's syndrome. Interposition of colon between liver and diaphragm. Note the colonic haustral pattern.

Care is necessary to avoid misinterpretation as a neoplasm or vice versa. Nipple shadows are often well-defined laterally and may have a lucent halo. Repeat films with nipple markers are necessary if there is any doubt.

Skin folds are often seen running vertically, particularly in the old and babies. When overlying the lung fields they can be confused with a pneumothorax. However, a skin fold if followed usually extends outside the lung field.

The anterior axillary fold is a curvilinear shadow extending from the axilla onto the lung fields and frequently causing ill-defined shadowing which must be differentiated from consolidation.

At the apices the opacity of the sternocleidomastoid muscles curving down and slightly outwards may simulate a cavity or bulla. The floor of the supraclavicular fossa often resembles a fluid level. A deep sternoclavicular fossa, commonly present in the elderly, appears as a translucency overlying the trachea and simulating a gas-filled diverticulum.

Subpleural thickening seen peripherally is often due to subpleural fat or prominent intercostal muscles rather than pleural pathology.

Companion shadows are formed by the soft tissues adjacent to bony structures, are 2–3 mm thick and frequently seen running parallel to the upper borders of the clavicles and the inferior borders of the lower ribs.

Abnormalities of the soft tissues are discussed below.

The bones

All the bones should be surveyed. On occasions, identification of an abnormality in association with pulmonary pathology may help to narrow the differential diagnosis. Sometimes a normal bony structure appears to be a lung lesion and further films such as oblique, lateral, inspiratory and expiratory, or tomography, may be necessary.

The sternum. The ossification centres are very variable in number, shape, position and growth rate. Usually there are single centres in the manubrium and xiphoid, with three or four centres in the body. Parasternal ossicles, and in infants the ossification centres, may be confused with lung masses.

The clavicles. The rhomboid fossa is an irregular notch at the site of attachment of the costoclavicular ligament, with a well-corticated margin lying up to 3 cm from the medial end of the clavicle inferiorly, and it should not be mistaken for a destructive lesion. Superior companion shadows are usual. The medial epiphyses fuse late and may simulate lung nodules.

The scapulae. On the lateral film the inferior angle can simulate a lung mass. The spine of the scapula on the PA film casts a linear shadow which at first glance may seem to be pleural.

The ribs. Companion shadows are common on the upper ribs. Pathological rib notching, as seen with aortic coarctation, should not be confused with the normal notch on the inferior surface just lateral to the tubercle. The contours of the ribs are evaluated for destruction. However the inferior borders of the middle and lower ribs are usually indistinct.

The first costal cartilage calcifies early and is often very dense, partly obscuring the upper zone. Costal cartilage calcification is rare before the age of 20. Central homogenous or spotty calcification occurs in females whereas there is curvilinear edge calcification in males. On the lateral film the anterior end of the rib with its cartilage lying behind the sternum should not be confused with a mass.

The spine. Routine evaluation is made for bone and disc destruction and spinal deformity. A scoliosis often results in apparent mediastinal widening, and oblique films may be necessary to visualize both lung fields fully. The ends of the transverse processes on the PA film may look like a lung nodule.

In the neonate the vertebral bodies have a sandwich appearance due to large venous sinuses. Residual grooves may persist in the adult.

VIEWING THE LATERAL FILM

Routinely the left side is adjacent to the film to reduce

cardiac magnification, but if there is a specific lesion the side of interest is put adjacent to the film.

A routine similar to that used for the PA film should be employed. Important observations to make are (Fig. 11.18):

1. *The clear spaces.* There are two clear spaces and these correspond to the sites where the lungs meet behind the sternum and the heart. Loss of translucency of these areas indicates local pathology. Obliteration of the retrosternal space occurs with anterior mediastinal masses such as a thymoma (Fig. 11.19). Normally this space is less than 3 cm deep maximum; widening occurs with emphysema.

2. *Vertebral translucency.* The vertebral bodies become progressively more translucent caudally. Loss of this translucency may be the only sign of posterior basal consolidation.

3. *Diaphragm outline.* Both diaphragms are visible throughout their length except the left anteriorly where it merges with the heart. A small segment of the right hemidiaphragm is effaced by the IVC. The posterior costophrenic angles are acute and small amounts of pleural fluid may be detected by blunting of these angles (Fig. 11.20).

The fissures. The left greater fissure is steeper than the right and terminates 5 cm behind the anterior cardiophrenic angle. Loculated interlobar effusions are well shown and displacement or thickening of the fissures should be noted.

The trachea passes down in a slightly posterior direction to the D6–D7 level. It is partly overlapped by the

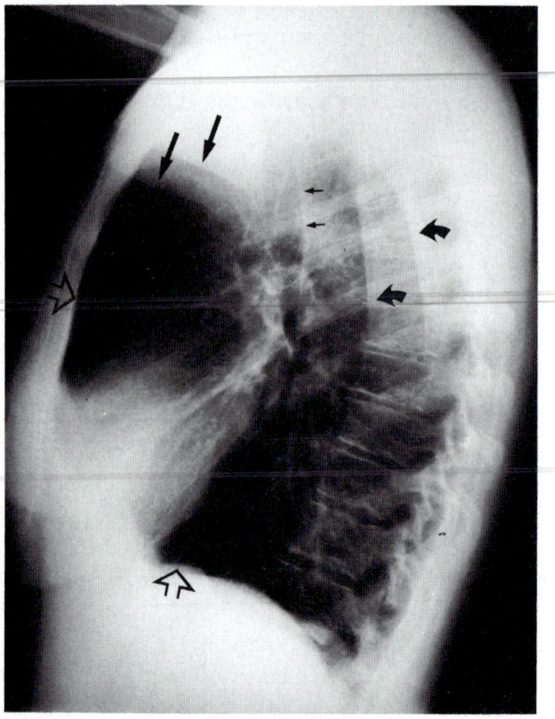

Fig. 11.18 Normal lateral film. Note the retrosternal and retrocardiac clear spaces (open arrows) and the increased translucency of the lower vertebrae. The axillary folds (large arrows) and scapulae (curved arrows) overlie the lung fields. The tracheal translucency is well seen (small arrows).

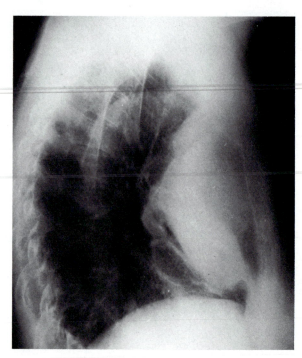

Fig. 11.19 Thymoma. Obliteration of the retrosternal space.

end-on may appear as a nodule overlying the trachea and above the aortic arch.

Shadowing seen in the region of the anterior cardio-phrenic angle is thought to be due to mediastinal fat and the interface between the two lungs.

The sternum should be studied carefully in known cases of malignancy or when there is a history of trauma.

INTERPRETATION OF THE ABNORMAL FILM
— HELPFUL RADIOLOGICAL SIGNS — DIFFERENTIAL DIAGNOSIS

THE SILHOUETTE SIGN

Described by Felson, the silhouette sign permits localiz-ation of a lesion on a film by studying the diaphragm and mediastinal outlines. These borders are seen because the adjacent alveoli are aerated. If this air is displaced, the borders are obliterated and the lesion can be localized. Conversely, if the border is retained and the abnormality is superimposed, the lesion must be lying either anterior or posterior. In 8–10% of people a short segment of the right heart border is obliterated by the fat pad or pul-monary vessels.

Obliteration of these borders may occur with pleural or mediastinal lesions as well as pulmonary pathology. The right middle lobe and lingula lie adjacent to the right and left cardiac borders; the apicoposterior segment of the left upper lobe lies adjacent to the aortic knuckle; the anterior segment of the right upper lobe and the middle lobe lie against the right aortic border. Pulmonary disease in these lobes and segments can obliterate the borders (Figs 11.21, 11.22, 11.23).

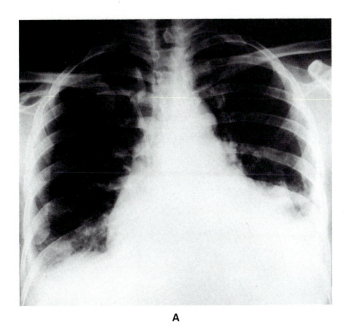

A

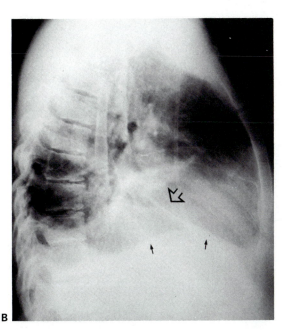

B

Fig. 11.20 A. PA film. A moderate-sized left pleural effusion and a small right effusion. **B.** Lateral film. There is loss of translucency of the lower vertebrae, thickening of the oblique fissure (open arrow) and absence of the left hemidiaphragm, with loss of the right hemidiaphragm posteriorly.

scapulae and axillary folds. Anterior to the carina lies the right pulmonary artery. The left pulmonary artery is posterior and superior and the veins are inferior. The venous confluence creates a bulge on the posterior cardiac border.

The normal posterior tracheal wall measures less than 5 mm. This measurement includes both tracheal and oesophageal walls plus pleura. Widening may occur with disease of all these structures. A branch of the aorta seen

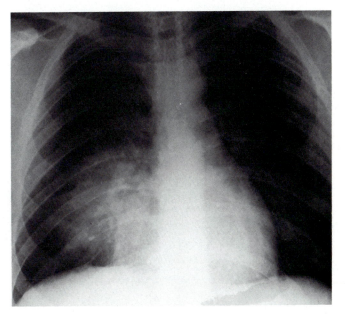

Fig. 11.21 Right middle lobe consolidation, demonstrating the silhouette sign with loss of outline of the right heart border.

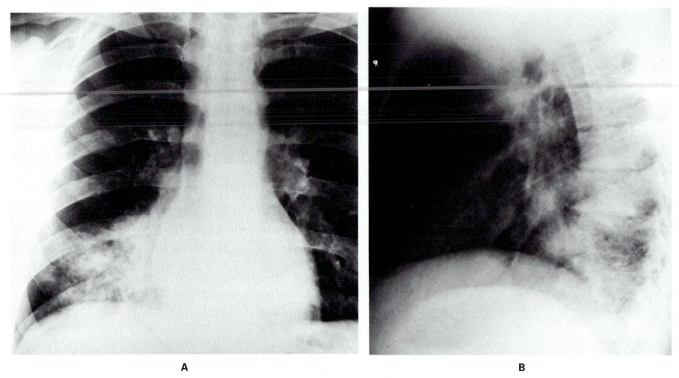

A   **B**

Fig. 11.22 Right lower lobe consolidation. **A.** Shadowing at the right base but the cardiac border remains visible. **B.** Lateral film. Consolidation in the posterior basal segment of the lower lobe with obliteration of the outline of the diaphragm posteriorly and loss of translucency of the lower vertebrae.

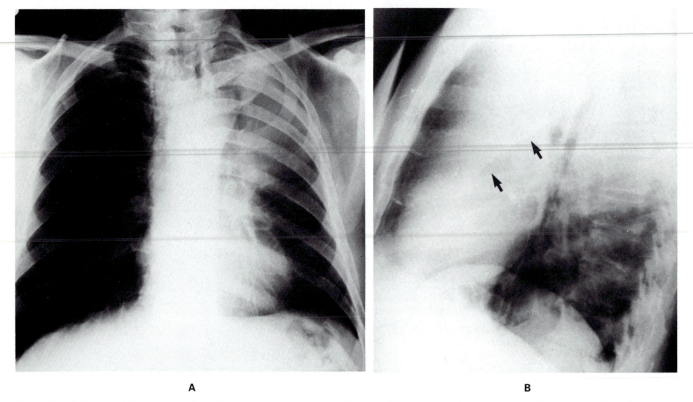

A   **B**

Fig. 11.23 Left upper lobe collapse. A carcinoma was present at the hilum. **A.** Shadowing in the upper zone with loss of outline of the upper cardiac border and aortic knuckle. There is tracheal deviation. **B.** Anterior displacement of the collapsed lobe and greater fissure.

Using the same principle, a well-defined mass seen above the clavicles is always posterior whereas an anterior mass, being in contact with soft tissues rather than aerated lung, is ill-defined. This is the *cervicothoracic sign*.

The *hilum overlay sign* helps distinguish a large heart from a mediastinal mass. With the latter the hilum is seen through the mass, whereas with the former the hilum is displaced so that only its lateral border is visible.

THE AIR BRONCHOGRAM
Originally described by Fleischner, and named by Felson, the air bronchogram is an important sign, showing that shadowing is intrapulmonary. The bronchus, if air and not fluid filled, becomes visible when air is displaced from the surrounding parenchyma. An air bronchogram is not seen within pleural fluid and rarely within a tumour, with the exception of alveolar cell carcinoma and, rarely, lymphoma. It may be seen in consolidation distal to a malignancy if the bronchus remains patent (Fig. 11.24). An air bronchogram is usually a feature of alveolar shadowing but is described accompanying interstitial diseases such as sarcoidosis (see Table 11.3).

ALVEOLAR (ACINAR) SHADOWING
The division of pulmonary shadowing into alveolar and interstitial is convenient but strictly incorrect; most dis-

Table 11.3 Causes of an air bronchogram

Common	Rare
Pneumonic consolidation	Lymphoma
Pulmonary oedema	Sarcoidosis
Hyaline membrane disease (Fig. 11.25)	Alveolar proteinosis
	Alveolar cell carcinoma
	Adult respiratory distress syndrome

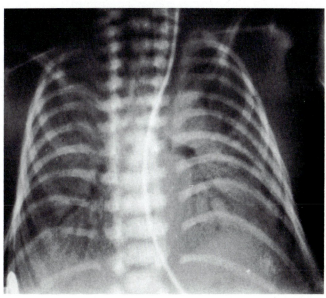

Fig. 11.25 Hyaline membrane disease. Extensive homogenous consolidation with a prominent air bronchogram.

ease processes are seen on histological examination to involve both the interstitium and acinus. A fluid-filled acinus forms a 4–8 mm shadow. These shadows rapidly coalesce into fluffy ill-defined round or irregular cotton-wool shadows, homogenous or patchy, but well defined adjacent to the fissures (Fig. 11.26). Vascular markings are usually obscured locally. The air bronchogram and silhouette sign are characteristic features. A ground-glass appearance or a generalized homogenous haze may be seen with a bat's wing or butterfly perihilar distribution (Fig. 11.27), sparing the peripheral lung fields, which remain translucent. This pattern is commonly due to cardiac failure and clears quickly with treatment. Other causes include pneumocystis infection, alveolar proteinosis and noncardiac causes of pulmonary oedema. Occasionally pulmonary oedema is unilateral or peripheral.

Infective processes are usually localized, and if generalized may well be due to an opportunistic infection. During resolution a mottled appearance can develop and this may give the impression that cavitation has occurred.

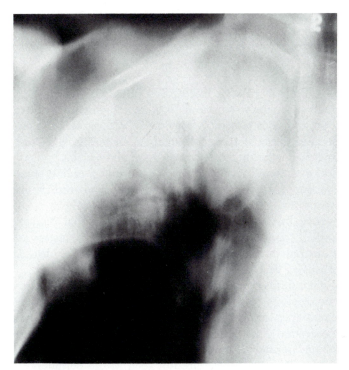

Fig. 11.24 Air bronchogram. An air bronchogram is clearly seen in the consolidated right upper lobe. A proximal carcinoma was present, although it is unusual for an air bronchogram to occur in the presence of a neoplasm.

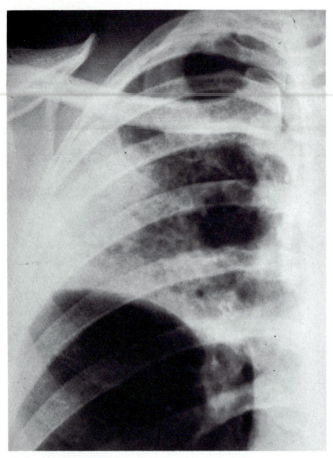

Fig. 11.26 Right upper lobe consolidation. Upper bowing of the horizontal fissure indicates some collapse. There is an acinar pattern with some confluence.

Table 11.4 Causes of alveolar shadowing

1. Pulmonary oedema		
	a. Cardiac	
	b. Non-cardiac	Fluid overload
		Hypoalbuminaemia
		Uraemia
		Shock lung
		Fat embolus
		Amniotic fluid embolus
		Drowning
		Hanging
		High altitude
		Blast injury
		Oxygen toxicity
		Aspiration (Mendelsohn's syndrome)
		Malaria
		Inhalation of noxious gases
		Heroin overdose
		Drugs (e.g. nitrofurantoin)
		Raised intracranial pressure
2. Infections		Localized
		Generalized, e.g. pneumocystis, parasites, fungi
3. Neonatal		Hyaline membrane disease
		Aspiration
4. Alveolar blood		Pulmonary haemorrhage, haematoma
		Goodpasture's syndrome
		Pulmonary infarction
5. Tumours		Alveolar cell carcinoma
		Lymphoma
		Leukaemia
6. Miscellaneous		Alveolar proteinosis
		Alveolar microlithiasis
		Radiation pneumonitis
		Sarcoidosis
		Eosinophilic lung
		Polyarteritis nodosa
		Mineral oil aspiration and ingestion
		Drugs

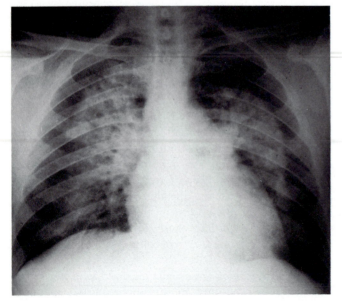

Fig. 11.27 Acute intra-alveolar pulmonary oedema with a bat's wing distribution.

THE DIFFUSE INTERSTITIAL PATTERN

'Diffuse interstitial pattern' is a radiological descriptive term and does not imply that the disease process is confined to the interstitium. In many cases both the alveolar cavity and the interstitial tissues are abnormal.

Correlation between the plain film radiographic changes and the severity of the clinical respiratory symptoms is often poor, the plain film sometimes being normal in the presence of extensive interstitial disease. Earlier changes can be detected with CT. A history of industrial dust exposure or bird-fancying, or of disease processes such as rheumatoid arthritis, is helpful.

The diffuse interstitial pattern (Fig. 11.28) is non-homogenous and includes various patterns including septal lines, miliary shadows, honeycomb shadowing and the ground glass pattern. Care is necessary to avoid mistaking normal vascular markings for early interstitial disease. Normal vessels are not seen in the periphery of the lung fields, and, unlike interstitial shadows, vessels taper and branch. Loss of volume may occur due to fibrosis but lobar collapse is not a feature.

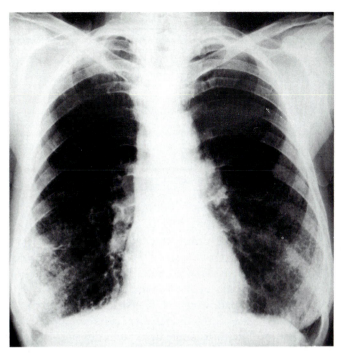

Fig. 11.28 Fibrosing alveolitis. Diffuse interstitial shadowing in the lower zones.

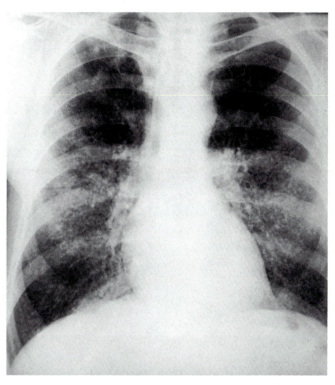

Fig. 11.30 Siderosis. Extensive dense miliary shadowing in an iron-foundry worker.

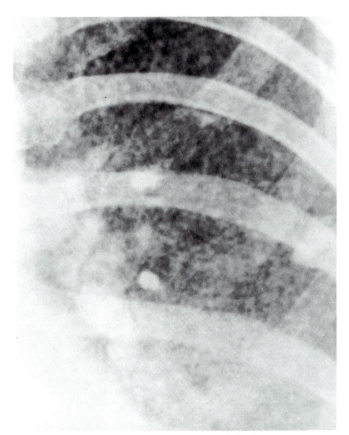

Fig. 11.29 Miliary tuberculosis. Widespread fine nodular shadowing without confluence.

The **miliary pattern** has widespread small discrete opacities of similar size up to 3 mm in diameter. This pattern is most often seen with tuberculosis (Fig. 11.29). Dense opacities occur with calcification and metallic dust disease (Fig. 11.30). **Ground glass** shadowing is a fine granular pattern which obscures the anatomical details and which may be seen with either an interstitial or an alveolar pattern (see Tables 11.5, 11.6 and 11.7).

HONEYCOMB SHADOWING

The parenchymal destruction which may occur with end-stage interstitial lung disease can result in the formation

Table 11.5 Causes of miliary shadowing

Soft-tissue density	High density	
Tuberculosis	Calcification:	Tuberculosis
Sarcoidosis		Histoplasmosis
Pneumoconiosis		Coccidioidomycosis
Hyaline membrane		Chickenpox
disease		
Histoplasmosis	Alveolar microlithiasis	
Metastases	Dust inhalation:	Tin
		Barium
		Beryllium
	Oil embolism (post-lymphangiography)	
	Ectopic bone (mitral valve disease)	
	Haemosiderosis	

Table 11.6 Causes of large nodular shadows

Malignancy	Metastases
	Alveolar cell carcinoma
	Lymphoma
	Primary
Tuberculosis	
Sarcoidosis	
Haemosiderosis	
Pulmonary infarcts, fat embolism	
Pulmonary sequestration	
Collagen disease	Wegener's granuloma
	Rheumatoid arthritis, etc.
Allergic lung disease	Drugs
	Extrinsic allergic alveolitis
Alveolar shadowing	Infections
	Pulmonary haemorrhage
	Pulmonary oedema
	Hyaline membrane disease
Artefacts	Skin nodules, e.g.
	neurofibromatosis
	Clothing
	Hair
Pleural	Tumours
	Loculated effusions

Table 11.7 Causes of diffuse interstitial shadowing

Infections	Bacterial: tuberculosis, mycoplasma, etc.
	Viral, fungal
	Protozoan: pneumocystis
	Parasites
Cardiac	Left heart failure
	Haemosiderosis
	Obstructed total anomolous pulmonary venous drainage
Neoplastic	Lymphangitis carcinomatosa
	Lymphoma
	Leukaemia
Collagen diseases	SLE, polyarteritis nodosa
	Scleroderma
	Rheumatoid arthritis
Drugs	Busulphan, methotrexate, bleomycin
Dust disease	
Honeycomb shadowing	
Miscellaneous	Fibrosing alveolitis
	Amyloidosis
	Oil embolism
	Extrinsic allergic alveolitis
	Chronic lipoid pneumonia
	Lymphoid interstitial pneumonia
	Desquamative interstitial pneumonia
	Gaucher's disease
	Tuberose sclerosis
	Pulmonary myomatosis
	Sarcoidosis
	Bronchiectasis
	Gaucher's disease
	Histiocytosis X
	Neurofibromatosis

Table 11.8 Causes of honeycomb shadowing

Common	Rare	Similar appearances
Histiocytosis X	Tuberous sclerosis	Bronchiectasis
Scleroderma	Amyloidosis	Cystic fibrosis
Rheumatoid lung	Gaucher's disease	
Fibrosing alveolitis	Neurofibromatosis	
Pneumoconiosis	Chronic lipoid pneumonia	
Sarcoidosis	Pulmonary lymphangiomyomatosis	
	Chronic lipoid pneumonia	

of cysts with walls 2–3 mm thick. When these cysts are 5–10 mm in diameter the term 'honeycomb shadowing' is used. This is associated with an increased risk of pneumothorax, often of the tension type.

Honeycomb shadowing is a particular feature of histiocytosis X. Frequently smaller cysts are found in fibrosing alveolitis, but larger cysts may develop.

THE SINGLE PULMONARY NODULE

Some 40% of solitary pulmonary nodules are malignant. A lateral film is often necessary to confirm that a lesion is intrapulmonary before investigating further. Typically an intrapulmonary mass forms an acute angle with the lung edge, whereas extrapleural and mediastinal masses form obtuse angles (Fig. 11.31).

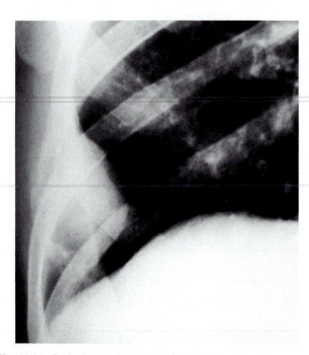

Fig. 11.31 Reticulum cell sarcoma of right lower rib with an extrapleural mass.

A nodule is assessed for its size, shape and outline and for the presence of calcification or cavitation. A search is made for associated abnormalities such as bone destruction, effusions, lobar collapse, septal lines and lymphadenopathy. If previous films are available it is possible to assess the doubling time, that is, the time taken for the volume of the mass to double. Usually malignant lesions have a doubling time of 1–6 months whereas benign lesions have a doubling time of over 18 months. Malignant lesions may grow spasmodically, however.

On occasions infective processes have a nodular appearance, which is usually ill-defined. Some change is seen with simple consolidation at follow-up after treatment.

Carcinomas are often upper-zone with irregular, spiculated or notched margins. Calcification favours a benign lesion, although a carcinoma may arise coincidentally at the site of an old calcified focus. Popcorn calcifications suggest a hamartoma. Calcified metastases are rare, the primary tumour being usually an osteogenic sarcoma or chondrosarcoma (Fig. 11.32).

Granulomas frequently calcify and are usually well defined and lobulated. Multiple lesions tend to be similar in size, whereas metastases are frequently of variable size but are well defined. Arteriovenous malformations characteristically have dilated feeding arteries and draining veins; they are multiple in 30% of cases. Rheumatoid nodules are invariably subpleural. Most bronchogenic cysts are intrapulmonary, arising in the lower zones.

A very large mass may be a primary tumour, a cannonball metastasis or a pleural fibroma.

Table 11.9 Causes of a solitary pulmonary nodule

Malignant tumour	Primary, secondary, lymphoma, plasmacytoma Alveolar cell carcinoma
Benign tumour	Hamartoma, adenoma
Granuloma	Tuberculosis, histoplasmosis, paraffinoma, sarcoidosis
Infection	Pneumonia, abscess, hydatid, amoebic, fungi, parasites
Pulmonary infarct	
Pulmonary haematoma	
Collagen diseases	Rheumatoid arthritis, Wegener's granulomatosis
Congenital	Bronchogenic cyst, sequestrated segment, congenital bronchial atresia
Impacted mucus	
Amyloid	
Intrapulmonary lymph node	
Pleural	Tumour (e.g., fibroma), loculated fluid
Nonpulmonary	Skin and chest wall lesions, artefacts

CAVITATING LESIONS AND CYSTS

A cavity is a lucency exceeding 1 cm in diameter surrounded by a complete wall which is 3 mm or more in thickness. Thinner walled cavities are cysts or bullae. Particular features of importance are the location of the cavity, its outline, wall thickness, a fluid level, contents of the cavity, satellite lesions and the appearance of the

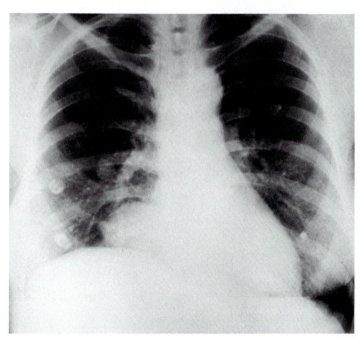

Fig. 11.32 Multiple calcified metastases from a chondrosarcoma of the right 10th rib.

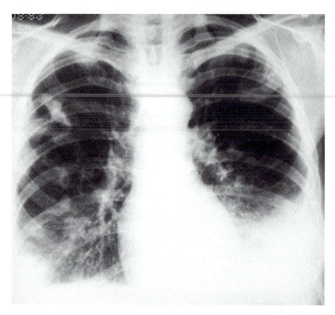

Fig. 11.33 Staphylococcal abscesses. Multiple cavitating abscesses in a young male heroin addict. Bilateral effusions also present.

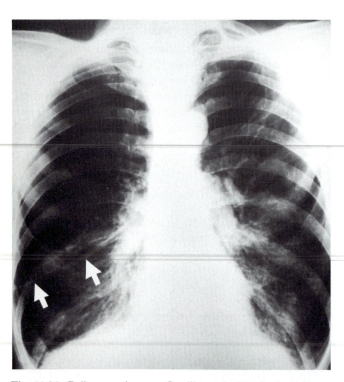

Fig. 11.34 Bullous emphysema. Curvilinear shadows in the right middle zone (arrows) with a lack of vascular markings in the upper zone due to the presence of bullae.

surrounding lung. CT or tomography often provide additional helpful information. Fluid is demonstrated only when using a horizontal beam.

Common cavitating processes are tuberculosis, staphylococcal infections (Fig. 11.33) and carcinoma. The tumour mass itself or the distal lung may cavitate.

The site. Tuberculous cavities are usually upper zone, in the posterior segments of the upper lobes or apical segments of the lower lobes. The site of lung abscesses following aspiration depends on the position of the patient at the time, but they are most often right-sided and lower zone. Traumatic lung cysts are often subpleural. Amoebic abscesses are nearly always at the right base, infection extending from the liver. Pulmonary infarcts are usually lower zone and sequestrated segments are left sided.

The wall of the cavity. *Thick walled* cavitating lesions include acute abscesses, most neoplasms (usually squamous-cell), lymphoma, most metastases, Wegener's granulomas and rheumatoid nodules. *Thin walled* lesions may be bullae (Fig. 11.34), pneumatoceles, cystic bronchiectasis, hydatid cysts, traumatic lung cysts, a carcinoma and chronic inactive tuberculous cavities. Pneumatoceles often develop in children after a staphylococcal pneumonia, and a rapid change in size is a feature.

Satellite lesions are a common feature of benign lesions, usually tuberculous.

Fluid levels and the meniscus sign. Fluid levels are common in primary tumours, and irregular masses of blood clot or necrotic tumour may be present. Fluid levels are uncommon in cavitating metastases and tuberculous cavities.

The meniscus sign is when an intracavitary body is surrounded by a crescent of air. It is commonly described with fungus balls such as an aspergilloma (Fig. 11.35).

Table 11.10 Cavitating pulmonary lesions

Infections	*Staphylococcus*
	Klebsiella
	Tuberculosis
	Histoplasmosis
	Amoebic
	Hydatid
	Paragonimiasis
	Fungal
	Abscess
Malignant tumours	Primary
	Secondary
	Lymphoma
Pulmonary infarct	
Pulmonary haematoma	
Pneumoconiosis	PMF
	Caplan's syndrome
Collagen diseases	Rheumatoid nodules
	Wegener's granulomatosis
Developmental	Sequestrated segment
	Bronchogenic cyst
	Congenital cystic adenomatoid malformation
Sarcoidosis	
Bullae, pneumatocele	
Traumatic lung cyst	

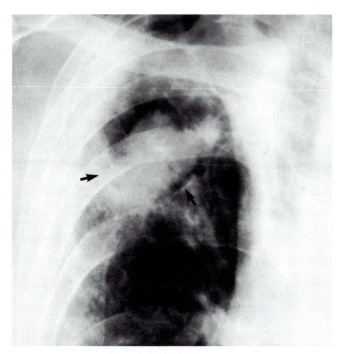

Fig. 11.35 Aspergillus mycetoma. A large mycetoma within an old tuberculous cavity in a fibrotic upper lobe. The mycetoma is surrounded by a halo of air.

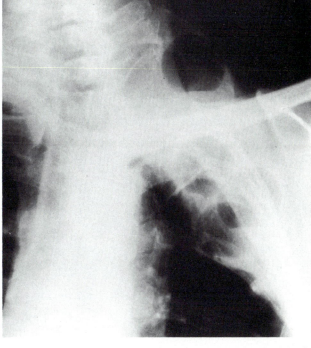

Fig. 11.36 Apical plombage. Hollow lucite spheres with fluid levels which have formed because of leakage of the walls of the spheres.

Table 11.11 Fluid levels on a chest radiograph

Intrapulmonary	
Hydropneumothorax:	Trauma Surgery, Bronchopleural fistula★
Oesophageal:	Pharyngeal pouch Diverticula Obstruction: tumour, achalasia Oesophagectomy: bowel interposition
Mediastinal:	Infections Oesophageal perforation: endoscopy, trauma
Pneumopericardium:	Diagnostic aspiration. Surgery Trauma
Chest wall:	Plombage with lucite balls (Fig. 11.36) Infections
Diaphragm:	Hernias, eventration, rupture

★ A bronchopleural fistula should be considered if a hydropneumothorax persists or enlarges after chest surgery.

The ball moves as the patient changes position.

Ruptured hydatid cysts have daughter cysts floating within the cavity, the *water-lily sign*. Other intracavitary lesions include inspissated pus, blood clot and caverno-liths. Blood clot occurs with cavitating neoplasms, tuberculosis and pulmonary infarcts.

CALCIFICATION

Calcification is most easily recognized on simple tomography and with low kVp films. In the elderly, calcification

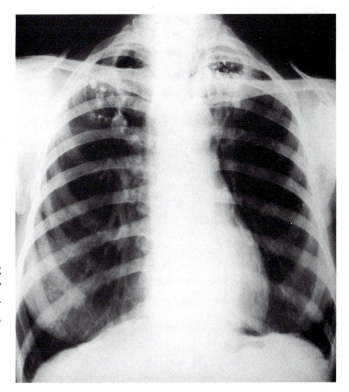

Fig. 11.37 Pulmonary tuberculosis. Numerous calcified foci in both upper zones with left upper lobe fibrosis.

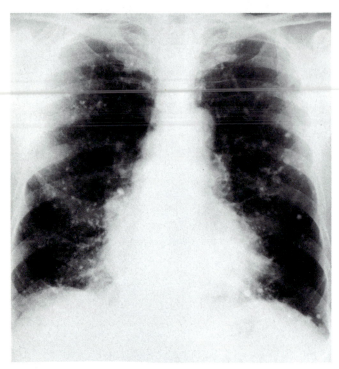

Fig. 11.38 Chickenpox. Widespread small calcified opacities following a previous chickenpox pneumonia.

of the tracheal and bronchial cartilage is common. Calcification of the bronchioles — osteopathia racemosa — is of no significance.

Tuberculosis is the commonest calcifying pulmonary process, with small scattered foci of various sizes, usually upper zone (Fig. 11.37). *Chicken-pox* foci are smaller (1–3 mm), regular-sized and widely distributed (Fig. 11.38). Characteristically the foci of *histoplasmosis* are surrounded by small halos.

Alveolar microlithiasis appears as tiny densities like sand grains in the mid and lower zones, due to calcium phosphate deposits in the alveoli. Punctate calcification may develop within the pulmonary nodules of *silicosis*. Popcorn calcification is often present in *hamartomas*. Occasionally *phleboliths* are present in arteriovenous malformations. Very rarely a fine rim of calcification forms in the wall of a *hydatid cyst*.

Pleural plaques may contain irregular areas of calcification.

Lymph-node calcification occurs in a number of conditions (Table 11.12). An eggshell pattern is characteristic of *sarcoidosis* and silicosis.

LINEAR AND BAND SHADOWS

There are many disease processes which may result in linear shadows within the lung fields. Causes which must be considered include the following:

Table 11.12 Calcification on the chest radiograph

Intrapulmonary	Granuloma infections	Tuberculosis Histoplasmosis Chickenpox Coccidioidomycosis Actinomycosis Hydatid cyst
	Chronic abscess	
	Tumours	Metastases (osteogenic/ chondrosarcoma) Cystadenocarcinoma Arteriovenous malformation Hamartoma, carcinoid
	Haematoma	
	Infarct	
	Mitral valve disease	
	Broncholith — tuberculosis	
	Alveolar microlithiasis	
	Idiopathic	
	Rare	Metabolic — hypercalcaemia Silicosis Sarcoidosis Rheumatoid arthritis Amyloid Osteopathia racemosa
Lymph nodes	Tuberculosis Histoplasmosis Sarcoidosis Silicosis Lymphoma after irradiation	
Pleural	Tuberculosis Asbestosis, talcosis Old haemothorax Empyema	
Mediastinal	Cardiac, vascular Tumours	
Pulmonary artery	Pulmonary hypertension Aneurysm Thrombus	
Chest wall	Costal cartilage Bone Breast	Tumours Fat necrosis
	Soft tissue	Parasites Tumours, etc.

Causes of linear bands

Pulmonary infarcts	Plate atelectasis
Sentinel lines	Kerley lines
Normal fissures and vessels	Thickened fissures
Pulmonary, pleural scars	Resolving infection
Bronchial wall thickening	Mucus-filled bronchi
Curvilinear shadows: bullae, pneumatoceles	
Artefacts	

Pulmonary infarcts are variable in appearance. Occasionally they form irregular thick wedge-shaped lines with the base adjacent to the pleura, but more usually they are nondescript areas of peripheral consolidation at the bases. Accompanying features are splinting of the diaphragm and a pleural reaction. Resolution tends to be slow, unlike infections, which often resolve quickly except in the elderly.

Plate atelectasis, described by Fleischner, is often seen postoperatively and is thought to be due to underventilation with obstruction of medium-sized bronchi. These lines are several centimetres long, 1–3 mm thick and run parallel to the diaphragms, extending to the pleural surface. Resolution is usually rapid.

Mucus-filled bronchi or bronchoceles are bronchi distended with mucus or pus beyond an obstructing lesion but with aeration of the distal lung from collateral air flow. Causes to consider include bronchopulmonary aspergillosis, malignancy, benign tumours and a congenital membrane. Typically the bronchus has a gloved-finger branching pattern. They are commonly found in the upper lobes.

Sentinel lines are thought to be mucus-filled bronchi and appear as coarse lines lying peripherally in contact with the pleura and curving upwards. They are often left-sided and associated with left lower lobe collapse. They may develop due to kinking of bronchi adjacent to the collapse.

Kerley B lines have been described above. Unilateral Kerley lines usually indicate lymphangitis carcinomatosa, but may be seen with early cardiac failure.

The normal and accessory *fissures* have been described. Thickening of the fissures is often seen accompanying cardiac failure. Bulging fissures indicate lobar expansion, which may occur with an acute abscess (Fig. 11.39), infections such as *Klebsiella*, *Pneumococcus* and *Staphylococcus*, tuberculosis and large tumours.

Old pleural and pulmonary scars are unchanged in appearance on serial films. Pulmonary scarring is a common end-result of infarction, appearing as a thin linear shadow often with pleural thickening and tenting of the diaphragm. Pleural scars extend to the pleural surface. Apical scarring is a common finding with healed tuberculosis, sarcoidosis and fungal disease (Fig. 11.40). **Curvilinear shadows** indicate the presence of bullae, pneumatoceles (Fig. 11.41) or cystic bronchiectasis.

Thickened bronchial walls cast thin parallel tramline shadows 1 mm thick, which when seen end-on appear as ring shadows. They are a common finding in bronchiectasis, recurrent asthma and bronchopulmonary aspergillosis.

APICAL SHADOWING

Apical pleural caps are present in 5% of the population. They are crescent-shaped, frequently irregular, and if

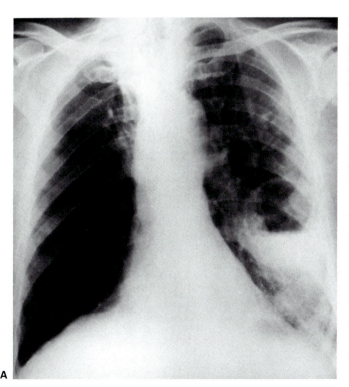
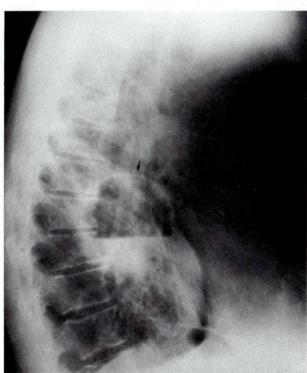

Fig. 11.39 A. A large lung abscess with a fluid level distal to a hilar carcinoma. There is an old right upper lobe collapse with compensatory emphysema. **B.** Note bulging of the oblique fissure adjacent to the abscess (arrows).

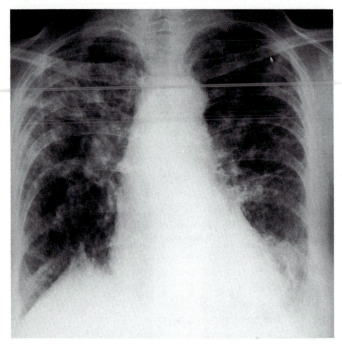

Fig. 11.40 Sarcoidosis. Fibrosis mainly affecting the upper zones with elevation of the hila and tenting of the right hemidiaphragm. A 55-year-old woman with a long history of sarcoidosis.

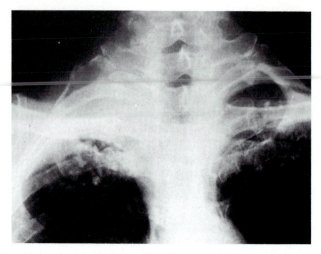

Fig. 11.42 Pancoast tumour. There is apical shadowing on the right side simulating pleural thickening. Note destruction of the first rib.

Table 11.13   Common causes of apical shadows

Pleural caps

Pleural fluid

Bullae

Pancoast tumour

Infections: tuberculosis

Pneumothorax

Soft tissue, e.g. companion shadows, hair (Fig. 11.43), sternocleidomastoid muscles

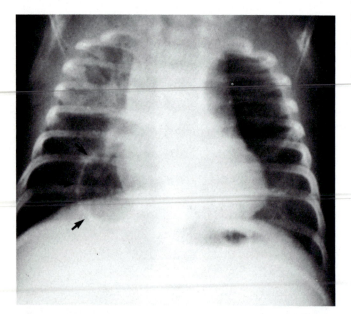

Fig. 11.41 Pneumatocele. Child with a staphylococcal pneumonia. Consolidation in the right upper lobe and a pneumatocele adjacent to the right heart border (arrows).

bilateral are usually asymmetrical. Their significance is uncertain but they may represent old pleural thickening. An apical cap should not be confused with a Pancoast tumour (Fig. 11.42) and adjacent rib destruction should be looked for.

The lung apex is a common site for tuberculosis and

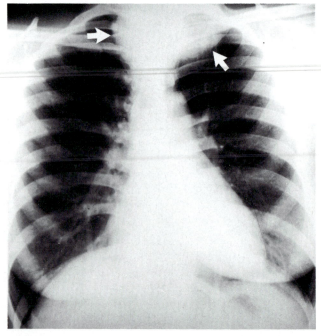

Fig. 11.43 A woman with her hair in a plait overlying the upper mediastinum and simulating mediastinal widening.

fungal diseases including histoplasmosis, coccidioido-mycosis, blastomycosis and aspergillosis. Assessment of active disease is difficult in the presence of fibrotic changes. Previous films for comparison are invaluable. Extrinsic shadows should be excluded (Fig. 11.43).

SIGNS OF LOSS OF VOLUME

With lobar or pulmonary collapse or fibrosis there is displacement or bowing of the pleural fissures (Fig. 11.44) with crowding of vascular markings within the collapse. Compensatory emphysema of the normal lung or lobes results in an increase in transradiancy with separation of the vascular markings. Mediastinal structures are displaced towards the affected side (Figs 11.44 and 11.45), and the ipsilateral hemidiaphragm may become elevated. Crowding of the ribs on the affected side is common in children. Lobar collapse displaces the hilum which changes shape. With major collapse there is herniation of the contralateral lung with displacement of the anterior mediastinal line.

HILAR ENLARGEMENT

The normal pulmonary hilum has a very variable appearance. It is difficult to detect minor degrees of pathological enlargement and to distinguish a prominent pulmonary artery from a small mass lesion, although branch vessels can often be traced back to an enlarged artery. A hilum should be assessed for its position, size

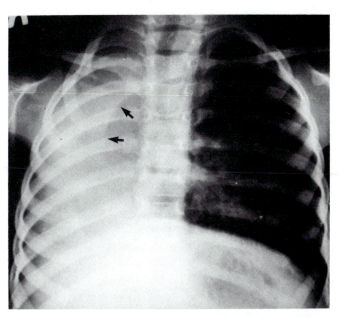

Fig. 11.45 Pulmonary agenesis. The right lung is absent. The heart and mediastinum are displaced to the right. Note herniation of the left lung across the midline (arrows). The rib spaces are narrowed on the right.

and density, with comparison between the two hila. Any possible abnormality can be assessed further with contrast-enhanced CT or simple tomography.

Enlarged lymph nodes appear as lobulated masses. The adjacent bronchi may be slightly narrowed. *Unilateral* en-

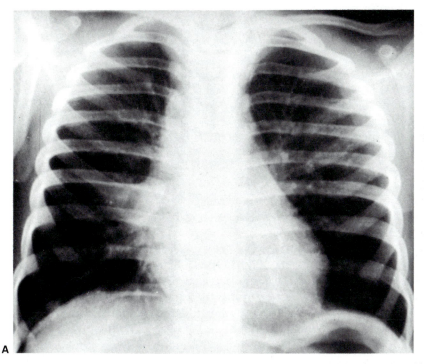
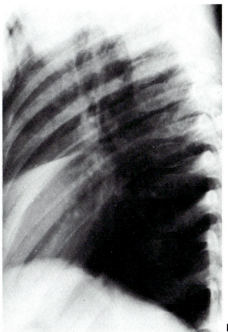

Fig. 11.44 Right middle lobe collapse. A. Loss of definition of the right heart border with adjacent shadowing. B. Lobar collapse with displacement of the fissures clearly shown.

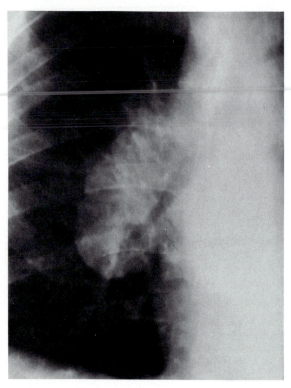

Fig. 11.46 A young man with Hodgkin's disease. An enlarged lobulated right hilum typical of glandular enlargement.

Table 11.14 Causes of hilar enlargement

Unilateral	Apparent	Rotation
		Scoliosis
		Small contralateral hilum.
	Lymph nodes	Tuberculosis
		Fungi
		Histoplasmosis
		Lymphoma
		Leukaemia
		Carcinoma
	Tumours	Benign
		Malignant
	Pulmonary artery	Aneurysm
		Embolus
		Poststenotic dilatation
	Superimposed anterior/posterior mass	
	Pericardial defect	
	Normal	Especially left
Bilateral	Expiratory film	
	Lymph nodes	Lymphoma
		Carcinoma
		Leukaemia
		Sarcoidosis
		Pneumoconiosis
		Glandular fever
		Whooping cough
		Tuberculosis
		Histoplasmosis
		Fungi
		Mycoplasma
	Pulmonary artery	Pulmonary hypertension
		Left heart failure
		Congenital heart disease

largement is seen with tuberculosis, whooping cough and malignancy. Nodes affected by lymphoma are often asymmetrically involved (Fig. 11.46). *Bilateral* involvement occurs with sarcoidosis, silicosis and leukaemia. Tuberculous lymphadenopathy without an identifiable peripheral pulmonary lesion is a common finding in the Asian population.

UNILATERAL HYPERTRANSLUCENCY

Comparison of the lung fields should reveal any local or general abnormality of transradiancy. Increased transradiancy may be accompanied by signs of obstructive or compensatory emphysema such as splaying of the ribs, separation of the vascular markings, mediastinal displacement and depression of the hemidiaphragm.

Rotation of the patient and scoliosis are the commonest causes of increased transradiancy. With rotation to the left, the left side becomes more radiolucent. Mastectomy is another important cause. An abnormal axillary fold is present after a radical mastectomy.

With conditions such as MacLeod's syndrome, congenital lobar emphysema and an inhaled foreign body, an expiratory film will demonstrate obstructive emphysema (Fig. 11.47). The mediastinum is displaced away from the affected side, with depression of the ipsilateral diaphragm. Congenital lobar emphysema usually affects the right upper or middle lobes. A small pulmonary artery

Table 11.15 Causes of a small hilum

Unilateral	Apparent: rotation, scoliosis
	Normal: especially the left side.
	Lobar collapse, lobectomy
	Hypoplastic pulmonary artery
	MacLeod's syndrome
	Unilateral pulmonary embolus
Bilateral	Cyanotic congenital heart disease
	Central pulmonary embolus

is a feature of MacLeod's syndrome and congenital hypoplasia or absence of the artery.

THE OPAQUE HEMITHORAX

All the causes described of unilateral hypertranslucency may be responsible for an apparent contralateral increase in density. Penetrated, lateral and high kVp films are usually helpful. Signs of collapse, fluid levels, mediastinal displacement and rib abnormalities are important findings. Pulmonary agenesis is associated with hypoplastic ribs and is invariably left-sided.

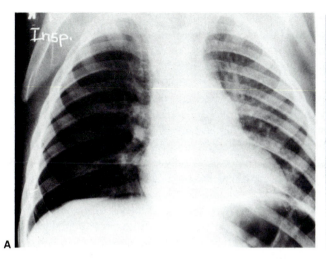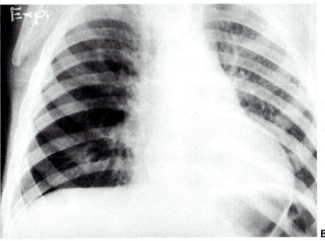

Fig. 11.47 Obstructive emphysema. This child inhaled a peanut. **A.** Inspiratory film shows a hypertransradiant right lung. **B.** Expiratory film. There is air trapping on the right side with further shift of the mediastinum to the left.

Table 11.16 Causes of unilateral hypertranslucency

Normal	Increased density in contralateral lung	E.g., pleural effusion, thickening Consolidation
Technical	Rotation Scoliosis	
Soft tissue	Mastectomy Congenital absence of pectoralis major Poliomyelitis	
Emphysema	Compensatory	Lobar collapse Lobectomy
	Obstructive	Foreign body Tumour MacLeod's syndrome Congenital lobar emphysema
	Bullous	
Vascular	Absent/hypoplastic pulmonary artery Obstructed pulmonary artery (e.g., by tumour or embolus) MacLeod's syndrome	
Pneumothorax		

Table 11.17 Causes of an opaque hemithorax

Technical	Rotation, scoliosis
Pleural	Hydrothorax, large effusion Thickening, mesothelioma
Surgical	Pneumonectomy, thoracoplasty
Congenital	Pulmonary agenesis
Mediastinal	Gross cardiomegaly, tumours
Pulmonary	Collapse, consolidation, fibrosis
Diaphragmatic hernias	

THE CHEST FILM OF THE ELDERLY PERSON

With age the thorax changes shape and the AP diameter increases. A kyphosis develops so that the chin overlies the lung apex. Very often only an AP film in the sitting position can be obtained, usually with a poor degree of inspiration so that the lung bases are poorly visualized.

Bone demineralization increases, with vertebral body compression and rib fractures being common. Bony margins become irregular. Costal cartilage and vascular calcification are prominent. Frequently there is calcification of the cartilagenous rings of the trachea and bronchi.

The major blood vessels become unfolded. On a lateral film the aorta is visualized throughout its length. Unfolding of the innominate and subclavian vessels results in widening of the upper mediastinum. Prominent hilar vessels accompany obstructive airways disease and the peripheral vessels become more obvious.

There may be changes due to old pathology with linear scars, pleural thickening, tenting of the diaphragm and calcified foci. Blunted costophrenic angles and flatter diaphragms are common findings in the elderly.

LIMITATIONS OF THE PLAIN CHEST FILM

Firstly the radiologist may fail to spot a lesion. Felson reported that 20–30% of significant information on a chest film may be overlooked by a trained radiologist.

Secondly, a disease process may fail to appear as a visible abnormality on a plain film. Examples include miliary shadowing, metastases and early interstitial disease. Such lesions are demonstrated earlier by CT. Inflamed bronchi are not easily seen and both bronchiectasis and obstructive airways disease may be associated with a normal chest film. Small pulmonary emboli without infarction can rarely be diagnosed without a radionuclide study.

Finally, the shadow patterns themselves are rarely specific to a single disease process. For example, consolidation due to infection or following infarction may have identical appearances.

OTHER METHODS OF INVESTIGATION

TOMOGRAPHY

Tomography is performed:

1. To improve visualization of a lesion
2. To localize a lesion and to confirm that it is intrapulmonary.
3. To evaluate the hilum and proximal airways.
4. To search for a suspected lesion e.g. metastases.
5. To evaluate the mediastinum and chest wall.

Technique. A recent chest film is mandatory. The examination should be closely supervised by the radiologist, with particular attention to the radiographic technique, ensuring that the area of interest is included on the films taken. Linear tomography is usually adequate, although more complex movements may be used. Cuts are made at 1 cm intervals routinely.

AP tomography supplemented with lateral tomography is satisfactory for peripheral lesions. The hilum is best visualized in the 55° posterior oblique position with the side of interest dependent (Fig. 11.48). On this view the bronchi are projected in profile. A penetrated view to show the carina is routinely obtained.

The peripheral mass. Features of diagnostic importance include calcification, cavitation, outline, bronchial narrowing and the presence of an air bronchogram (Fig. 11.49). Spiculation is a strong indicator of malignancy.

The hilum. Hilar tomograms are difficult to interpret. It is helpful to remember that normal-sized nodes are not usually seen, and that enlarged nodes are well defined. The vessels, unlike a mass lesion, branch and taper. If a mass is identified the adjacent bronchi should be assessed for narrowing or occlusion.

FLUOROSCOPY

Fluoroscopy is of value for assessing motion of the chest wall and diaphragm, and for demonstrating mediastinal shift in cases of air trapping. It is helpful in uncooperative children when the radiograph is nondiagnostic due to movement and poor inspiration.

Screening may be used to differentiate pulmonary from pleural lesions by rotating the patient and noting movement of the lesion with respect to the sternum and spine. Pulsation is often a misleading sign; it may be transmitted to a mass lying adjacent to a vascular structure. Masses of vascular origin change size with the Valsalva manoeuvre and with the position of the patient. Pulmonary lesions move with respiration whereas mediastinal lesions do not.

RADIONUCLIDE SCANNING

E. Rhys Davies

Radionuclide scanning of the lungs is of most value in the diagnosis of pulmonary embolism, a normal scan excluding the diagnosis. However the major drawback of this technique is its lack of specificity, so that interpretation on occasions must be guarded. A report should be made in the light of a current chest film and a ventilation scan.

The **main indications** for this examination are:

1. Diagnosis of pulmonary embolism
2. Evaluation of emphysema
3. To determine the extent of parenchymal disease, malignancy and infections associated with AIDS
4. Monitoring the effect of therapy.

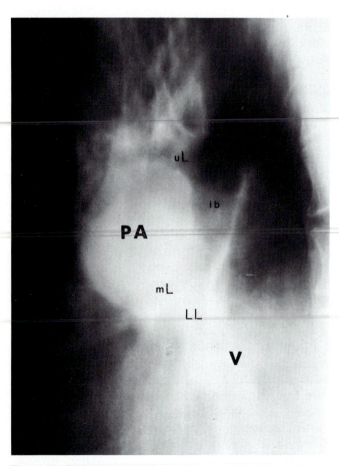

Fig. 11.48 Right posterior oblique (55°) tomogram of right hilum. PA = pulmonary artery, V = pulmonary vein, MB = main bronchus, uL = upper lobe bronchus, ib = intermediate bronchus, mL = middle lobe bronchus, LL = lower lobe bronchus.

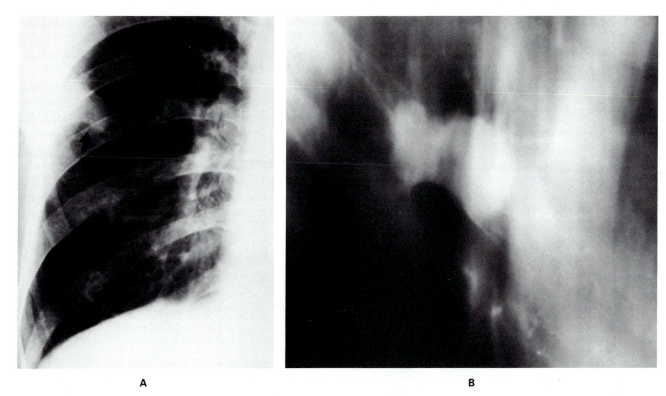

Fig. 11.49 Oat cell carcinoma. **A.** Peripheral mass adjacent to the ribs. **B.** Oblique tomogram shows an irregular mass with thin strands extending into the surrounding lung.

The following techniques are essentially complementary to each other and to a chest radiograph taken within 24 hours of scanning.

1. Ventilation studies

a. *Xenon-133*, with a principal photon energy of 80 keV and a half life of 5.7 days, is still used. The gas is delivered to the mouthpiece of a rebreathing system and after a single deep inspiration a 10-second image is recorded. This record shows the distribution of inspired air, with areas of low activity representing poor ventilation. Next, the mixture of air and ^{133}Xe is rebreathed for some minutes to reach equilibrium, after which rebreathing is discontinued and serial images are recorded during the 'washout' phase. Persistent activity denotes air trapping, e.g. in an emphysematous bulla.

b. *Krypton-81 m*, with a photon energy of 190 keV and a half-life of 13 seconds, is generated by the decay of cyclotron produced rubidium-81 (half-life 4.58 hours). Because of its short half-life, ^{81m}Kr is administered continuously during the investigation. Its distribution represents its rate of arrival and hence the ventilatory pattern. Naturally this pattern will be influenced by the posture of the patient as well as by disease.

^{133}Xe has the advantage of a relatively long shelf life so that it is readily available at all times, but its photon energy peak is relatively close to that of ^{99m}Tc which is used for perfusion studies. The labelled microspheres for the perfusion studies are fixed in the pulmonary capillaries and therefore the ventilation scan with krypton must precede the perfusion scan. This is an important disadvantage because it runs counter to the usual schemes of investigation. On the other hand, ^{81m}Kr can be separated satisfactorily from technetium, and despite the relative disadvantage of its cost and poor shelf life, it is favoured by most departments.

c. ^{99m}*Tc-labelled aerosols* have been developed in order to provide a relatively available ventilation technique. They have the disadvantage of disproportionate deposition of radioactivity in the larger air tubes.

It is essential to take *anterior*, *posterior* and *posterior-oblique views* in all instances. Other tangential views may be helpful in individual cases.

2. Perfusion studies

The principle of perfusion scanning is that particles greater than the size of the lung capillaries (80–100 μm) will be trapped during their first passage through the lungs. ^{99m}*Tc microspheres* of uniform size, about 40 μm, are the most satisfactory agents. These are cleared from the lungs over the next 12 hours or so, and then they are gradually broken down and metabolized in the liver. The patient rests for 5–10 minutes to achieve circulatory equilibrium; 40–80 MBq are injected intravenously during several resting respiratory cycles, in the supine position. This achieves good mixing, so that lung activity is proportional to its perfusion. The more dependent parts of the lung are slightly better perfused than the remainder, so that the anterior basal segments are less well perfused than the posterior. It is important to remember this when interpreting the scan, but if the same position is used always, this normal variation will be taken into account more easily.

Anterior, posterior and both posterior oblique views are carried out and, in a normal scan, activity is found over the whole thorax except the mediastinum. The size of the mediastinal defect is determined mainly by the size of the heart. This normal pattern is altered whenever the perfusion of a region of lung is diminished. This occurs when there is *mechanical obstruction of an artery* (Fig. 11.50), or *alveolar hypoxia* due to air trapping, *bronchial obstruction* (Fig. 11.51), *pneumonia* or redistribution of blood flow

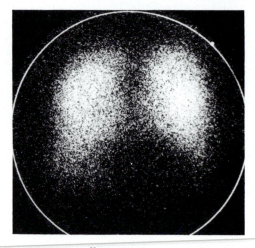

Fig. 11.52 Heart failure. ^{99m}TC-MAA scan, anterior view. The cardiac defect is large; activity over the upper lobes is greater than over the lower lobes because of redistribution of blood flow due to heart failure.

Fig. 11.50 A. Perfusion lung scan, ^{99m}Tc microspheres. There are several large defects in the right lung and a smaller defect in the left lung. **B.** Ventilation scan, ^{87m}Kr. There are no ventilation defects. These unmatched ventilation and perfusion scans are characteristic of pulmonary embolism.

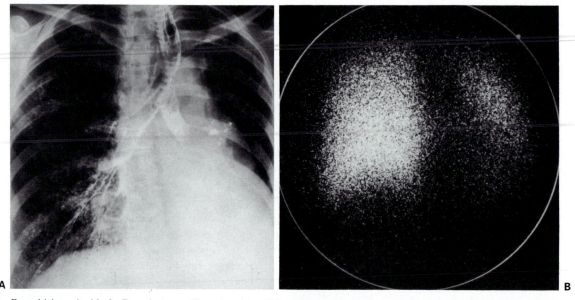

Fig. 11.51 Bronchial carcinoid. **A.** Bronchogram. There is a large filling defect in the left main bronchus and only a small amount of contrast medium has gone beyond it. The left lower lobe is collapsed. **B.** ^{99m}Tc-MAA scan, anterior projection. Right lung activity is even, there is some activity in left upper lobe, which is aerated, but none in left lower lobe, which is not aerated nor perfused.

as in *mitral stenosis with pulmonary hypertension* (Fig. 11.52). In normal lung, less than 1 in 1000 capillaries is occluded by microspheres and there is no haemodynamic upset. However, in severe pulmonary hypertension the capillary bed is already so reduced that a lung scan can be hazardous (especially if macro-aggregates are used, because they contain some particles up to 100 μm). Scanning is best avoided in these patients as it is unlikely to be useful.

3. Ventilation perfusion ratio (V/Q)

In normal scans the distribution of radioactivity is even and parallel in both ventilation and perfusion images. This pattern is disturbed in many diseases. Diminished ventilation leads reflexly to corresponding impaired perfusion, whereas the converse is not so, apart from exceptionally large or long-standing perfusion defects. Thus a bulla or collapsed segment will lead to impairment of activity in both scans, whereas embolus will lead to impaired perfusion and normal ventilation scans.

Pulmonary embolism

The investigation of suspected pulmonary embolism is probably the most widespread indication for lung scintigraphy. Uncertainties in clinical and plain radiographic diagnosis and the impossibility of using pulmonary angiography as the standard investigation have generated considerable demand for lung scintigraphy, with all its promise of being able to identify unperfused segments of lung. Alas, it is rarely possible to verify the diagnosis pathologically, and in the face of justifiable clinical anxiety over the consequences of overlooking pulmonary embolus, it is important to indicate clearly the degree of probability that a scan is positive or negative (Biello et al., 1979).

The characteristic appearance of a pulmonary embolus is a perfusion defect corresponding to an identifiable segment or lobe without a matching ventilation defect. If there is no radiographic abnormality or if the perfusion defects are substantially larger than radiographic abnormalities, or are multiple, there is a high probability of pulmonary embolism. At the other extreme, normal perfusion excludes pulmonary embolus, and focal matched defects with no corresponding radiographic abnormality, or a perfusion defect smaller than a radiographic abnormality, have a low probability for pulmonary embolism (less than 10%). Matched V/Q defects, with or without radiographic abnormalities, make up the most difficult diagnostic group. Usually the patients are known to have pre-existing lung disease such as pulmonary tuberculosis, fibrotic sarcoidosis, asthma or chronic bronchitis, all of which will produce abnormal scans of this kind. Occasionally in this group it will be necessary to give some consideration to pulmonary angiography, particularly if anti-coagulants are contra-indicated.

With meticulous technique and careful consideration of the clinical and radiological features, a firm opinion can be given in the vast majority of instances. In a small minority, resolution of the problem will remain difficult. It may be helpful to monitor the evolution of the signs by means of serial imaging and radiography.

Scintigraphy may underestimate the extent of embolic disease in two important situations. First, minute peripheral embolization following fragmentation of clot may be overlooked if the emboli are distributed evenly. Second, partial occlusion of both main pulmonary arteries by a saddle embolus may produce a symmetrical scan in the absence of total occlusion of the main pulmonary artery, or a recognizable peripheral defect. Disparities between arteriogram and scintigram are more apparent than real once it is appreciated that the presence of a patent small artery on the angiogram does not necessarily mean there is good flow through its capillary bed, which is the parameter being assessed by the scan. A normal four-view scan at the time of a suspected embolus is virtually certain evidence against embolization.

Individual arteries cannot be identified without arteriography and it is generally accepted this should be done when embolectomy is being considered on clinical grounds.

Scintigraphy may be repeated without hazard and serial scintigrams show improvement in perfusion within weeks or months of emboli. It is important sometimes to establish a baseline for future reference after an obvious embolus. Ventilation and perfusion studies are often useful both in the pre-operative assessment of patients with large bullae and in their assessment after lobectomy.

Other lesions that can cause localized perfusion defects include *lung tumours, pneumonia, exacerbation of chronic infection, tuberculosis, lung abscess, radiation pneumonitis, fibrosis*, and *under-ventilation associated with hypoplasia of pulmonary arteries*. The value of scintigraphy in assessing these lesions is limited and their importance is that they should not be confused with pulmonary embolus. This can be achieved by meticulous examination of a chest radiograph taken within 24 hours of the scans.

The investigation of pulmonary embolus is inseparable from the determination of its source. Ascending pedal *phlebography* is the traditional way of doing this and is still the best way of showing the precise location of the thrombus before operation. However, in any group of patients known to be at special risk, e.g. because of immobilization after operation, [131]I-*fibrinogen* given intravenously before operation will be incorporated into thrombi that are formed so that they can be detected by external counting. Usually the activity is measured at several points along both legs daily, and a rise of 30% between one of the counts and the adjacent counts is significant (Fig. 11.53). The method is much more reliable than clinical suspicion of deep vein thrombosis

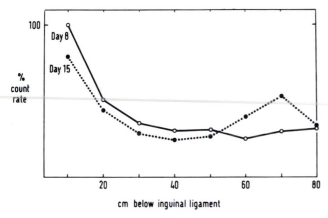

Fig. 11.53 Calf vein thrombosis. ^{131}I fibrinogen trace. On Day 8 the trace is normal, on Day 15 there is a significant rise of activity at 60 and 70 cm below the inguinal ligament, indicating thrombus formation in the calf.

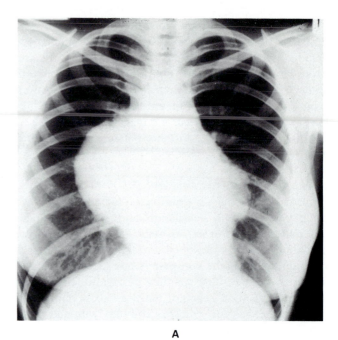

A

but loses its accuracy dramatically above the inguinal ligament.

The disadvantages of this technique are:

a. radiopharmaceutical is administered pre-operatively to *all* those at risk,
b. the test cannot be applied to the ilio-femoral venous segment where the clinically significant thrombi are likely to be,
c. fibrinogen uptake in arthritic knees may complicate the interpretation.

Alternatively, the radiopharmaceutical being given for a lung scan can be divided into two equal amounts that are injected synchronously into a dorsal pedal vein in each foot, with compression of superficial veins at the ankle. Rapid-sequence images of the limbs and abdomen can be taken to show the whole venous drainage including the inferior vena cava. Delayed transit, filling defects and asymmetric pattern are indications of abnormality and the technique has many obvious advantages. The lung scan is then done in the usual way.

Gallium scanning

^{67}*Ga citrate* is well known for being taken up in areas of inflammation, granulocyte activity, and in some tumours (Fig. 11.54). It has a physical half-life of 78 hours and several photon peaks, the most useful being at 240 keV. After intravenous injection, it is bound in vivo to transferrin and lactoferrin, and is excreted in the bile and urine. Because it is concentrated in lactating breasts and excreted in maternal milk, breast feeding should be discontinued temporarily if the investigation is unavoidable at this time. Images are usually taken at 6 hours but may be repeated up to 72 h if necessary.

The use of gallium citrate as an agent for detecting occult infection is usually directed extra-thoracically, though unsuspected thoracic infections can sometimes be

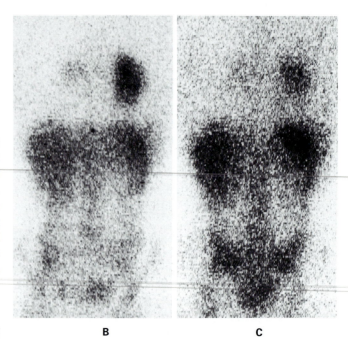

B   **C**

Fig. 11.54 Mediastinal lymphoma. **A.** PA chest radiograph. **B.** anterior and (**C**) posterior projections of ^{67}Ga citrate scan at 48 hours. There is high activity over the mediastinal abnormality. Note normal activity over lumbar spine, liver and spleen. The spleen is large but high activity is not in itself an indication that it is involved by lymphoma. Indeed the relatively low vascularity of splenic lymphoma may lead to lower activity than expected.

demonstrated. At one time, gallium^{-67} citrate scanning was advocated for staging carcinoma of the bronchus but it has now been superseded by high-resolution computed tomography.

The most practical use of ^{67}Ga scanning in lung disease is derived from the high affinity that granulomata have

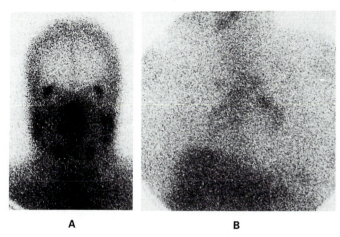

Fig. 11.55 Sarcoidosis. ⁶⁷Ga citrate scans of head (**A**) and chest (**B**), showing high activity in both hilar regions, the salivary glands, and more particularly the lacrimal glands.

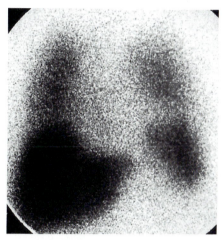

Fig. 11.56 ¹¹¹In leucocyte scan. There is normal activity in liver and spleen, and on each side of the heart there is pulmonary activity due to capillary trapping of damaged leucocytes.

for the compound. For example, the granulomata of sarcoidosis can lead to a typical uptake pattern in the hila, right paratracheal lymph nodes, and the parotid and nasolacrimal glands. Further, in sarcoidosis the scan may be used to assess the extent of extra-thoracic disease activity, and finally, to distinguish areas of active pulmonary disease from inactive fibrosis, a distinction that is not always possible from radiography (Goddard, 1988; Cooke, Davies & Goddard, 1989) (Fig. 11.55).

The role of ⁶⁷Ga citrate in detecting infection has been taken over to a large extent by ¹¹¹*In leucocyte* scanning. It is unusual to use the technique for pulmonary infections but it is important to recognise that abnormalities may be demonstrated in the lungs during leucocyte scanning. The labelling technique alters the properties of some of the white cells and makes them more liable to

sequestration in the lungs, thereby giving an innocent slight but diffuse activity on the scan. Careless injection technique may lead to overt clumping of cells. Finally, injection through central venous lines may lead to some disposition of white cells along the tube (Fig. 11.56).

CT OF THE LUNG
W. St C. Forbes and Ian Isherwood

Normal appearances

Anatomical considerations. The whole dynamic scale of tissue densities is present in each CT section of the thorax. Interrogation of the grey-scale image at a variety of window levels and widths is therefore necessary to witness the full range of anatomical structures.

The pulmonary vessels are clearly visible against the aerated lung at the appropriate window and can be traced to the periphery of the lung field. Secondary and frequently tertiary order bronchi can also be identified. The radial distribution of pulmonary arteries from the hila results in the differential 'sampling' of the vessels in transaxial sections. At the lung apices and bases, vessels pass obliquely through the thin sections whereas at central level a greater degree of arborization is encountered (Fig. 11.57). Apparent discontinuities in arborizing structures should not be interpreted as evidence of occlusive disease. Reference will always be made to sequential sections. There may be a relative paucity of pulmonary vasculature in either lung, denoting the position of the fissures.

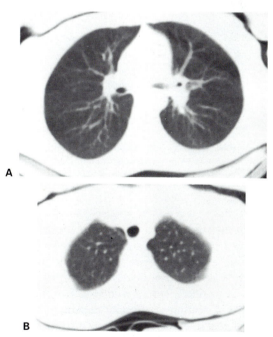

Fig. 11.57 Normal pulmonary vascularity. **A.** Hilar level (L –320, W400). **B.** Apical level (L –320, W400).

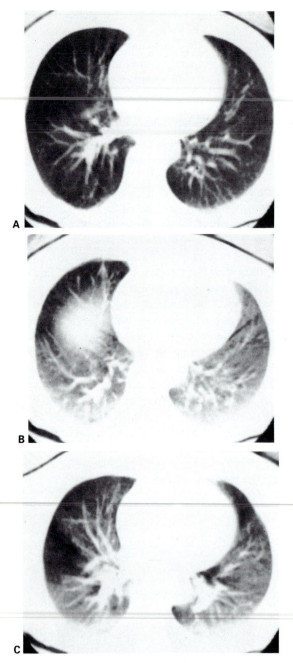

Fig. 11.58 Normal lungs. L −320, W400. **A.** Inspiration.
B. Expiration. Note intrusion of diaphragm dome into right lung
base section. **C.** Expiration at higher level demonstrating increase in
density in the dependent lung.

The dome of the diaphragm obtrudes into the basal
sections to a varying degree and may, as a result of the
partial volume effect, give rise to apparent increase in
density at the centre of the field.

Physiological considerations: respiratory phase. The density
of lung in a CT section is strongly dependent upon the
respiratory phase. In expiration there is a striking increase
in density, particularly in the dependent part of the lung.
Whilst the change is likely to be the result of inadequate

alveolar inflation, the effect of any related variations in
perfusion might also be considered (Fig. 11.58).

Suspended respiration in maximum inspiration is
necessary to obtain optimal scanning conditions. The
expiratory phase of respiration is not satisfactory for assessment of lung parenchyma.

Posture. The influence of gravity on pulmonary vessel
calibre is well demonstrated by CT. Dependent vessels
are notably larger whatever the position of the patient
(Fig. 11.59). In the supine position the gravity gradient
is from apex to base.

Posture also results in compression of the dependent
lung, most noticeable during expiration (Fig. 11.59). In
the lateral decubitus position the uppermost lung is in a
state of relative inspiratory apnoea, with diminution in
the vascular components.

Role of CT in diseases of the lung and pleura

Patterns of disease. Conventional radiological investigations usually reveal the anatomical distribution of lobar
or segmental disease. CT is of value in confirming such
disease and has a particular role in the identification of
segmental atelectasis (Fig. 11.60). The cross-sectional nature of the image makes it possible, for example, to
identify alveolar disease as predominantly in the outer
thirds of the lung fields (Fig. 11.61).

**Interstitial parenchymal disease: use of high-
resolution CT** (HRCT). Interstitial fibrosis may appear,
on conventional chest radiography, to affect the whole
lung field, but by CT it is observed to be predominantly
in the outer third (Fig. 11.61). The application of high-
resolution thin-section CT of the lungs using a bone
algorithm for reconstruction is used to detect interstitial
disease in the presence of a normal chest radiograph.

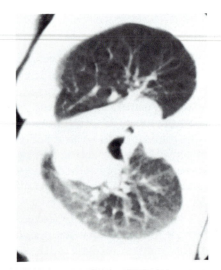

Fig. 11.59 Normal lung fields. Patient in right lateral decubitus
position. Note change in pulmonary vessels in dependent lung,
together with 'splinting' of upper lung in expiration. L −320, W400.

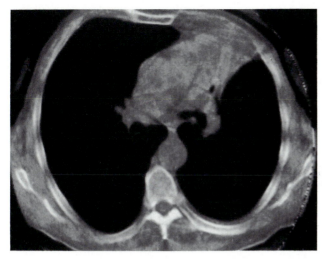

Fig. 11.60 Left upper lobe collapse. Note asymmetry of thoracic cavities. L + 20, W400.

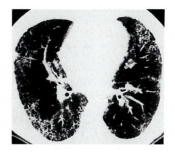

Fig. 11.62 Fibrosing alveolitis. 3-mm-interval sections. Subpleural 'honeycombing' with interlobular emphysema. Sawtooth interface.

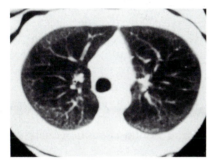

Fig. 11.61 Fibrosing alveolitis. Note increased alveolar density in outer third of the lung fields. L −325, W400.

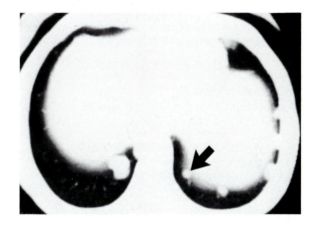

Fig. 11.63 Occult nodular metastases in posterior costophrenic sulci (arrow).

1–3 mm sections, using short scanning times, minimize movement artefact and overcome the partial volume effect of thicker sections. Targeting of images for maximal spatial resolution is required and each lung may be studied individually to examine a specific abnormality on a chest radiograph. In *fibrosing alveolitis* and *systemic sclerosis*, there is a subpleural crescent of increased attenuation posteriorly at the bases in early cases, progressing to peripheral 'honeycombing'. The pleural and mediastinal interfaces may become irregular with a saw-tooth appearance (Fig. 11.62). There is a good correlation between HRCT and histological findings from open biopsy. In *asbestosis* HRCT shows curvilinear subpleural lines, parenchymal bands, thickened inter- and intra-lobular lines, increased subpleural attenuation and honeycombing. HRCT has a positive predictive value of 100% in asbestosis with pleural thickening. It is a reliable and very accurate non-invasive method for assessing the presence and extent of *bronchiectasis*, eliminating the need for bronchography. Dilated bronchioles and *centri-lobular emphysema* can only be detected by HRCT. In *lymphangitis carcinomatosa*, HRCT can detect changes before they become evident on the chest radiograph. The interlobular septa become irregularly thickened and produce a reticular pattern. In *alveolar proteinosis*, the air-space opacification and thickening of the interlobular septae produce a characteristic 'crazy-paving' effect. HRCT may also be useful in demonstrating abnormalities in *sarcoidosis, histiocytosis X* and *drug-induced pneumonitis*, at an earlier stage than by other imaging techniques. An appropriate area or technique for biopsy can thus be accurately defined.

Pulmonary nodules. Computed tomography is a very sensitive technique for the identification of single, unsuspected nodules over 3 mm in diameter, but is relatively insensitive to the presence of smaller nodules. More nodules are detected by CT than by conventional chest radiology or even whole-lung tomography. Most metastatic disease of the lungs affects the outer third of the lung fields and the majority of metastases are subpleural (Fig. 11.63). Despite the improved sensitivity of CT, a proportion of nodules may still go undetected. In addition, there is a lack of specificity, particularly in those lesions less than 3 mm, with the result that many small nodules (up to 60%) are later found to be unrelated granulomata indistinguishable by CT from malignant metastatic disease. However there is still an incidence of false positive and false negative results in the assessment of pulmonary nodules. At present CT is the optimum means of detecting nodules in the lung parenchyma.

The principal role of CT in the evaluation of the pulmonary nodule is to confirm its solitary nature or detect other nodules not visible at simple X-ray, in determining the degree of malignancy and in contributing to staging procedures before treatment is instituted. The benign pathological character of a pulmonary nodule can be inferred primarily by the detection of calcium and the lack of growth over a two-year period. Other signs relating to marginal character and density are unreliable. Cavitation is detectable at an early stage, but may not necessarily indicate malignancy. Spread to hilum, pleura or chest wall, together with involvement of lymph nodes, is important pretreatment staging information (Fig. 11.64). Treatment planning together with monitoring of both single and multiple nodules after treatment, are most readily undertaken by CT.

High-resolution thin-section CT should not be used

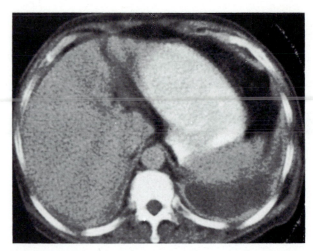

Fig. 11.65 Loculated left pleural effusion. L +30, W200.

for the detection of nodules because not all of the lung is examined using this technique.

Pleural disease. Differentiation between pulmonary and pleural disease may influence clinical management significantly, particularly in the identification of loculated pleural collections (Fig. 11.65). Identification of pleural and chest wall involvement in parenchymal disease is possible. Pleural plaques which may contain calcium and are often associated with asbestosis are visualized tangentially and can be seen to extend circumferentially (Fig. 11.66).

MRI IN CHEST DISEASES
Ian Isherwood and Jeremy P. R. Jenkins
The role of MRI and its relation to other imaging techniques in chest diseases has yet to be defined. The main advantages of MRI include a multiplanar facility and a high intrinsic soft-tissue contrast discrimination, allowing vascular structures and lesions in the mediastinal and hilar regions to be defined separately from other tissues without the need for contrast-medium administration. Disadvantages of MRI include respiratory and cardiac motion artefacts and an inability to visualize small branching pulmonary vessels and bronchi, and lung parenchyma. These structures, however, are better depicted on CT. The introduction of faster MR scan times, enabling images to be obtained within a single breath-hold, combined with a good signal-to-noise ratio (SNR), may alleviate some of these problems. At present, MRI is unable to provide the same anatomical detail and spatial resolution in the lung as high-resolution CT. The ease of performance and wider availability of CT makes it the procedure of choice in the assessment of most lesions in the thorax, including lung metastases. MRI can be useful in certain situations, e.g. in the separation of mediastinal masses from normal or abnormal vessels, the illustration of the craniocaudal extent of large lesions and

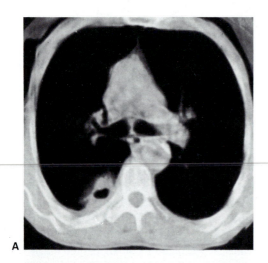

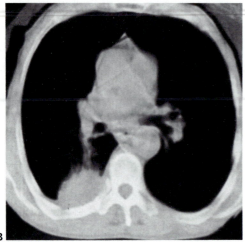

Fig. 11.64 A,B Bronchial carcinoma in right paravertebral gutter demonstrating cavitation and spread to hilum and chest wall. L –55, W400.

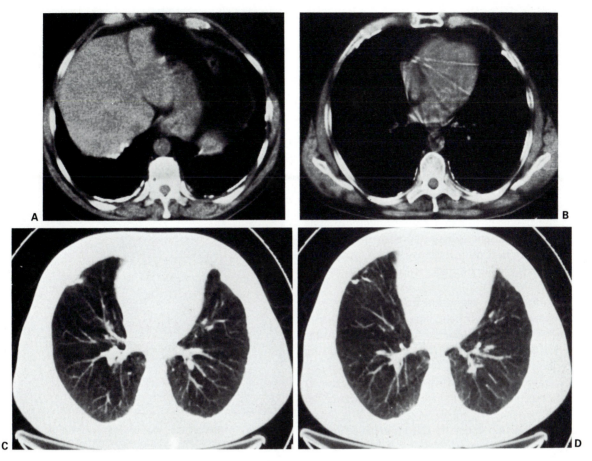

Fig. 11.66 Asbestosis. **A.** Diaphragmatic pleural calcification. **B.** Posterior pleural calcification. **C, D.** Anterior pleural calcification with early adjacent parenchymal fibrosis.

lesions at the lung apex, lung base and chest wall, and in the assessment of pathology affecting major vessels and the brachial plexus (see Ch. 12).

Anatomical detail of *lung parenchyma* is limited on MRI due to respiratory and cardiac motion artefacts, an intrinsically low SNR from the lung air-spaces, a poorer spatial resolution than conventional radiography and CT, and difficulty in precise localization of disease due to lack of normal anatomical landmarks. Normal lobar fissures and small peripheral pulmonary vessels and bronchi are not visualized, and alveolar and interstitial changes within the lung cannot be distinguished. MRI is unable to compete with thin-section high-resolution CT in the assessment or detection of small peripheral lung carcinomas, metastases, or calcifications. CT is the imaging method of choice in the detection and evaluation of lung nodules, including metastases.

Cystic lesions of the lung (e.g., bronchogenic cysts and bronchial atresia with mucocoele formation secondary to mucoid impaction) can be clearly demonstrated as areas of high signal on T_2-weighted images. Vascular lesions (e.g., scimitar syndrome and pulmonary A/V fistulae) may be missed on MRI due to lack of contrast from the low

signal or signal void from flowing blood within the vessel and the surrounding air space. This problem can be overcome by the use of phase-sensitive flow sequences, which provide increased signal from coherently flowing blood.

There is considerable overlap in the MRI characteristics of parenchymal consolidation, which may be due to a variety of causes. In the experimental situation it has been possible to separate cardiogenic from noncardiogenic pulmonary oedema although the clinical utility is unclear. MRI may be of value in assessing activity of interstitial lung disease by the demonstration of excess water in active pathology. Granulation tissue and compressed lung enhance markedly following intravenous administration of gadolinium-DTPA. Chronic inactive disease and tumour enhance, but to a lesser degree.

LUNG BIOPSY

Techniques:

1. Open biopsy is obtained at surgery and entails the risks of a thoracotomy and anaesthetic but an adequate specimen results. This technique is mostly used for diagnosing diffuse pulmonary disease.

2. Bronchoscopic biopsy can be used for central lesions. Brushings, washings and bacterial samples may be obtained. The success rate is high and the complication rate low.

3. Catheter biopsy is made with a French 7 or 8 catheter inserted via the cricothyroid membrane and screened into the relevant bronchus. Central masses can be biopsied.

4. Percutaneous biopsy. This may be performed with a fine needle for aspiration or with a cutting needle.

The procedure is contraindicated in patients on anticoagulants or with a bleeding diathesis, or if the mass is thought to be vascular. It is inadvisable in patients with bullae or in those who have had a pneumonectomy. The co-operation of the patient is essential and uncontrolled coughing a contraindication. Biopsy of a suspected hydatid cyst is inadvisable because of the theoretical risk of anaphylaxis.

The diagnostic yield of aspiration fine-needle biopsy is high for nonlymphomatous malignancy, in the region of 90%, but lower for benign lesions, around 85%. In addition there is a low complication rate. Large-bore cutting needles may be used for pleural-based or very peripheral lung lesions, having ascertained by CT that the lesion is avascular. There is a higher associated incidence of pneumothorax.

The site of the lesion must be determined. Biopsy is performed using biplanar screening or CT. The shortest route for the passage of the needle is determined, avoiding vascular structures. The puncture site is marked and anaesthetized before inserting the needle on suspended respiration. Ideally the biopsy is taken from the periphery of a mass, to avoid central necrotic tissue and to increase the likelihood of a positive biopsy. Some resistance is often experienced on entering the mass. Once its position is confirmed the biopsy is taken. With a fine needle, suction is applied with a syringe and several passes are made with the needle. Ideally a cytologist is at hand to prepare the slides.

Following the biopsy, films are taken to exclude a pneumothorax. The incidence of this is reported as some 15%, although only one-third of these require drainage.

Complications reported include:

1. Pneumothorax
2. Haemoptysis — incidence 5%, usually transient
3. Haemothorax
4. Empyema
5. Subcutaneous emphysema
6. Seeding of malignant cells along the needle track
7. Air embolism (very rare).

BRONCHOGRAPHY

Bronchography was once the definitive investigation for the diagnosis of bronchiectasis (Fig. 11.67) and for

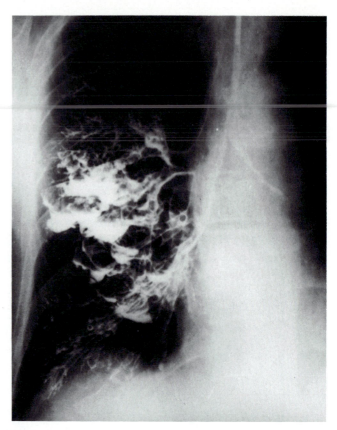

Fig. 11.67 Bronchogram. Patient with cystic bronchiectasis. The majority of the bronchi outlined with contrast medium are dilated.

assessing the extent of the disease. CT is now widely used, although its sensitivity is lower. Occasionally bronchography is used to investigate recurrent haemoptysis when all other investigations are negative, and for demonstrating bronchopleural fistulae and congenital lesions such as sequestration and agenesis. Rarely it is used to elucidate the nature of a lesion by assessing bronchial distortion and displacement.

Severe or partial impairment of pulmonary function, massive haemoptysis, recent pneumonia, active tuberculosis and a history of allergy are recognized contraindications. A limited examination is performed if pulmonary function is reduced.

The technique is well described elsewhere. Approaches include cricothyroid puncture, nasal or transoral drip, and tracheal intubation under local or general anaesthesia. Bronchography by inhalation of contrast medium is not widely performed. Physiotherapy before and after the procedure, and atropine to reduce the secretions, are essential. Films taken include AP, lateral, obliques and, if necessary, tomograms. Delayed films demonstrate distal filling.

All the bronchi should be surveyed for evidence of narrowing, occlusion, intraluminal filling defects and dilated mucosal glands, as seen with bronchitis and bronchiectasis.

ULTRASOUND

The acoustic mismatch between the chest wall and the adjacent aerated lung results in almost total reflection of the ultrasonic beam. Therefore ultrasound is used for assessing superficial pleural-based and chest-wall lesions only. It is helpful in the diagnosis and localization of pleural effusions and collections, for subphrenic collections, in differentiating fluid from a mass lesion, and for studying diaphragm movement.

A real time scanner with a 3.5 or 5.0 mHz transducer is preferred. On supine scanning the right diaphragm and surrounding areas are clearly seen through the liver (Fig. 11.68). However, on the left side visualization is hampered by intervening bowel. Filling the stomach with water to use as an acoustic window and scanning obliquely improve visualization. Scanning is performed in the supine or upright sitting position.

Pleural fluid appears as an anechoic area with a well-defined posterior wall in the posterior costophrenic angle (Fig. 11.69). Internal echoes may be due to blood or pus, septa indicating loculation and a thick wall suggesting an empyema.

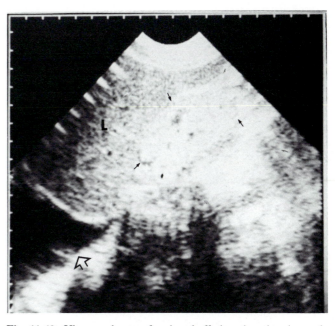

Fig. 11.69 Ultrasound scan of a pleural effusion. A patient in renal failure with acute glomerulonephritis. There is a moderate-sized effusion (open arrow) seen as a transonic area in the posterior sulcus above the diaphragm. Note the highly echogenic kidney (small arrows).

PULMONARY ANGIOGRAPHY

The main indications are:

1. Diagnosis of pulmonary embolism
2. Evaluation of pulmonary hypertension
3. Diagnosis of vascular lesions, e.g. pulmonary hypoplasia, arteriovenous malformations, pulmonary artery aneurysms.

In the majority of cases embolism is excluded by a normal radionuclide perfusion scan. However for a definitive diagnosis, particularly if surgery is anticipated, angiography is performed. In cases of pulmonary hypertension lower doses of contrast medium are used because of the increased risk of cardiogenic shock.

The right heart may be approached from the basilic vein after cutdown or via the femoral vein, provided femoral, iliac and IVC thrombus have been excluded by ascending phlebography in those cases of suspected embolism, to prevent dislodging a large clot. All procedures require ECG monitoring and pressure studies, including right heart and pulmonary wedge pressures. A fairly rapid injection of a large bolus of contrast medium (50–60 ml at 20–25 ml/s) is necessary with a rapid film sequence (Fig. 11.70). Improved arterial visualization is achieved with selective right and left artery injections, particularly if the peripheral vessels are of interest, but the main pulmonary artery only is injected if searching for a saddle embolus.

Magnification views help in the diagnosis of small peripheral emboli, as do occlusive balloons. DSA allows the use of smaller contrast volumes but disadvantages are the relatively poor resolution and artefacts due to chest motion affecting the quality of subtraction. DSA is

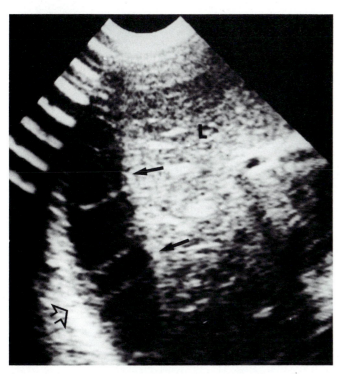

Fig. 11.68 Ultrasound scan of subphrenic abscess. There is a transonic area (arrows) between the liver (L) and diaphragm (open arrow). Strands crossing this area indicate loculation.

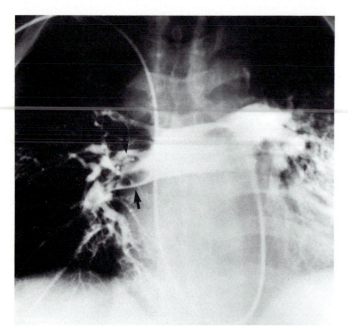

Fig. 11.70 Pulmonary angiogram. A 55-year-old man 4 days after a thoracotomy developed a DVT and pulmonary embolism. There are large thrombi (arrows) in the main arteries and peripheral perfusion is poor.

generally not considered to be satisfactory for demonstrating small peripheral emboli.

BRONCHIAL ARTERIOGRAPHY

Angiography followed by embolization of bronchial and intercostal branches is a recognized treatment for life-threatening or recurrent severe haemoptysis when surgery is contraindicated. Its value is limited in the investigation of pulmonary abnormalities, malignant and benign lesions often having similar vascular patterns.

The anatomy of the bronchial arteries varies greatly, the spinal branches often arising from the intercostal arteries or intercostal-bronchial trunks, in which case embolization should not be performed because of the risk of spinal cord infarction.

THE CHEST WALL

THE BONES

The sternum. *Developmental abnormalities* such as perforation, fissures and agenesis are rare. Several sternal abnormalities are associated with congenital heart disease and examples include sternal agenesis, premature obliteration of the ossification centres and pigeon chest, which are found with ventricular septal defects, and depressed sternum, associated with atrial septal defects and Marfan's syndrome. Delayed epiphyseal fusion is a feature of cretinism and double ossification centres are common in Down's syndrome.

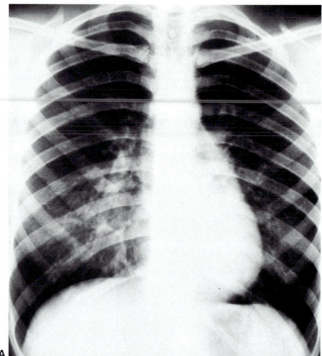

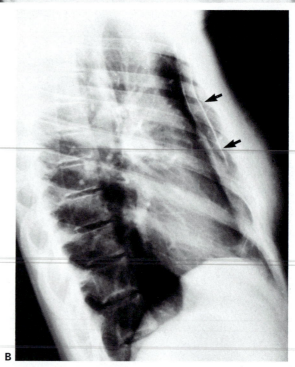

Fig. 11.71 Pectus excavatum (depressed sternum). **A.** Prominent shadowing adjacent to the right heart border. The heart is displaced to the left and has a straight left border. **B.** Note the posteriorly displaced sternum (arrows).

In the presence of a *depressed sternum* the anterior ribs are more vertical and the posterior ribs more horizontal than normal (Fig. 11.71), with displacement of the heart to the left. The heart appears enlarged, with a straight left border and indistinct right border with prominent lung markings and ill-defined shadowing in the right cardiophrenic angle. This should not be confused with consolidation. The lower thoracic spine is clearly seen through the heart.

Erosion of the sternum may occur with adjacent anterior mediastinal lymphadenopathy or tumours, aortic aneurysms and infective processes.

Primary *tumours* are rare and usually cartilagenous. The sternum may be the site of metastases, lymphoma and myeloma.

Sternal *fractures* are often seen with steering-wheel injury, an associated thoracic spine injury being common.

The ribs. *Rib notching* may affect the superior or inferior surface of the rib and be unilateral or bilateral.

Table 11.18 Causes of inferior rib notching

Unilateral	Blalock-Taussig operation	
	Subclavian artery occlusion	
	Aortic coarctation involving left subclavian artery or anomalous right subclavian artery.	
Bilateral	Aorta	Coarctation, occlusion, aortitis
	Subclavian	Takayashu disease, atheroma
	Pulmonary oligaemia	Fallot's tetralogy Pulmonary atresia, stenosis Truncus Type IV
	Venous	SVC, IVC obstruction
	Shunts	Intercostal-pulmonary fistula Pulmonary/intercostal arteriovenous fistula
	Others	Hyperparathyroidism Neurogenic Idiopathic

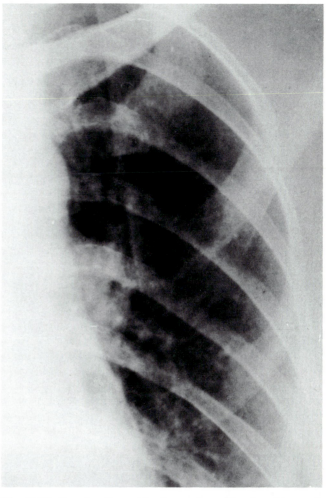

Fig. 11.72 Superior rib notching in a patient with a long history of paralysis following poliomyelitis.

Superior notching (Fig. 11.72) may be a normal finding in the elderly but has been recorded in patients with rheumatoid arthritis, SLE, hyperparathyroidism, Marfan's syndrome, neurofibromatosis and in polio victims.

Inferior notching (Fig. 11.73) develops as a result of hypertrophy of the intercostal vessels or with neurogenic tumours. Obstruction of the aorta results in reversed blood flow through the intercostal and internal mammary arteries. With coarctation the first and second intercostal arteries and ribs are not affected, the arteries arising proximally from the costocervical trunk. The lower ribs are not affected unless the lower abdominal aorta is affected. A preductal coarctation does not produce rib notching.

Congenital rib anomalies such as hypoplasia, bridging and bifid ribs are common. Hypoplastic first ribs, arising from D1, must be distinguished from cervical ribs (Fig. 11.74) which arise from C7, the transverse processes of which point caudally whereas the transverse processes of D1 are cranially inclined. Cervical ribs have an incidence of 1–2%.

With Down's syndrome there are often only 11 pairs of ribs.

An *intrathoracic rib* is uncommon. It appears as a ribbon-like shadow near to the spine, attached by one or both ends.

In *Tietze's syndrome* the anterior ends of the ribs are usually normal but are occasionally enlarged or look spotty.

At *surgery* a rib may have been removed (Fig. 11.75) or partially amputated. Periosteal stripping results in irregularity.

Soft-tissue masses such as a lipoma or neurofibroma may displace a rib and create a defect from pressure erosion.

Crowding of the ribs occurs with a scoliosis and major pulmonary collapse. It is an early sign of a mesothelioma. Hyperinflation results in the ribs having a horizontal lie.

Fractures are often difficult to spot on the high kVp film. There may be an accompanying extrapleural haematoma, a pneumothorax or surgical emphysema. Callus may simulate a lung mass. The sixth to ninth ribs

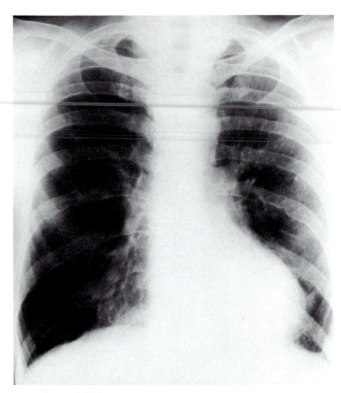

Fig. 11.73 Inferior rib notching. An elderly man who presented with hypertension. Coarctation of the aorta with rib notching most prominent in the 4th to 8th ribs.

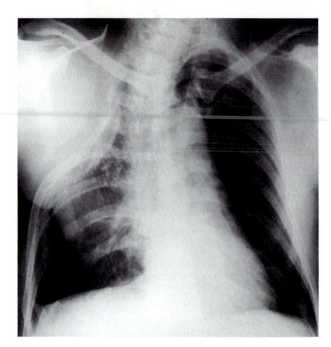

Fig. 11.75 Right thoracoplasty for tuberculosis. Removal of the upper ribs with collapse of the upper lobe.

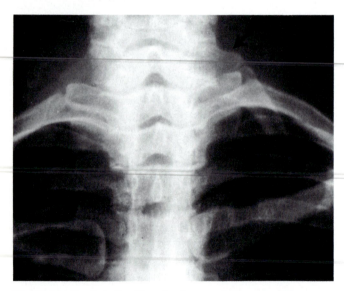

Fig. 11.74 Cervical ribs. Note the downward direction of the transverse process of C7 (arrow).

in the axillary line are the common sites for *cough fractures*. *Stress fractures* usually affect the first ribs. *Pathological fractures* occur due to a local rib lesion or to a generalized reduction in bone mass as found in senile osteoporosis, myeloma, Cushing's disease and other endocrine disorders, steroid therapy and diffuse met-

astases. Cushing's disease is associated with abundant callus formation.

The *Looser's zones* of osteomalacia represent areas of uncalcified osteoid and the resulting rib deformity creates a bell-shaped thorax.

Rib *sclerosis* occurs with generalized disorders such as osteopetrosis, myelofibrosis, fluorosis and metastases, or with localized lesions such as Paget's disease (Fig. 11.76), bony enlargement being characteristic. *Post-irradiation necrosis* results in non-united rib fractures, bony sclerosis or an abnormal trabecular pattern and soft-tissue calcification, and is often associated with a mastectomy.

Localized *rib expansion* occurs with fibrous dysplasia, Gaucher's disease and benign tumours such as eosinophilic granuloma, haemangioma, chondroma, the brown tumours of hyperparathyroidism and aneurysmal bone cyst. In Hurler's syndrome there is generalized expansion of the ribs sparing the proximal ends whereas in thalassaemia expansion is most marked proximally and the trabecular pattern is abnormal. Widening of the ribs is seen with rickets (Fig. 11.77) and scurvy.

Rib destruction due to an infection or tumour of the soft tissues, lung or pleura is usually accompanied by an extrapleural mass. Characteristically an actinomycosis infection is associated with a wavy periostitis of the ribs. Many malignant processes, including metastases, lymphoma and myeloma, commonly destroy the ribs.

The thoracic spine. A survey is made to check for abnormal curvature or alignment, bone and disc destruction, sclerosis, paravertebral soft-tissue masses and congenital lesions such as butterfly vertebrae. Scoliosis

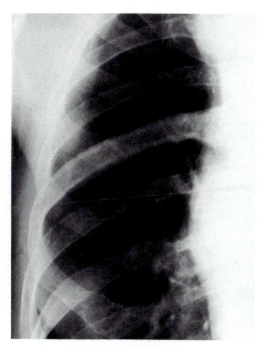

Fig. 11.76 Paget's disease. An enlarged 6th rib with a coarse trabecular pattern and of increased density.

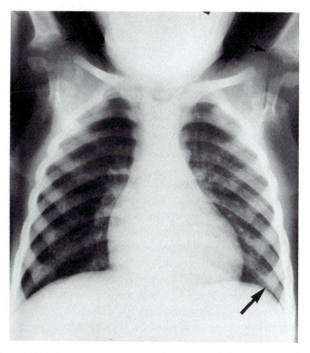

Fig. 11.77 Rickets. Enlargement and cupping of the anterior ends of the ribs. Note the metaphyseal changes in the humeri.

and Klippel-Feil syndrome are associated with an increased incidence of congenital heart disease. With a severe scoliosis, when the curve exceeds 60°, cardio-respiratory complications are common in adults.

With the *straight back syndrome* the normal kyphosis is reduced so that the sternum and spine are virtually paral-lel, resulting in compression of the mediastinum. On the PA film the heart appears characteristically enlarged, is displaced to the left and has a prominent left atrial appendage and aorta. On auscultation there is an ejection systolic murmur with accentuation on expiration.

Anterior erosion of the vertebral bodies sparing the disc spaces may occur with aneurysms of the descending aorta, vascular tumours, gross left atrial enlargement and neurofibromatosis, which may also cause posterior scalloping of the vertebral bodies and enlarged intervertebral foramina.

Destruction of a pedicle is typical of metastatic disease. A single dense vertebra, the *ivory vertebra*, is the classical appearance of lymphoma, but is also seen with other conditions such as Paget's disease and metastases. *Destruction of the disc* with adjacent bony involvement is characteristic of an infective process.

Disc calcification may be idiopathic or post-traumatic and occurs in ochronosis and ankylosing spondylitis.

SOFT TISSUES

Artefacts such as hair plaits and fasteners, buttons, clothing and jewellery overlying the lungs may simulate a lung lesion. Tracing the edges of a lesion will show whether it extends beyond the lung margins, in which case the lesion is nonpulmonary.

Skin lesions including naevi and lipomas may simulate lung tumours. Multiple nodules occur with neurofibromatosis. (Fig. 11.78) Pedunculated lesions have well defined edges, being surrounded by air, and lung markings should be visible through the lesion. It is most helpful to examine the patient.

The breast. Mastectomy is one of the commonest causes of a translucent hemithorax. With a simple mastectomy the axillary fold is normal, but following a radical mastectomy the normal downward curve of the axillary fold is replaced by a dense ascending line due to absence of pectoralis major (Fig. 11.79). Congenital absence of pectoralis major may also be found, sometimes associated with syndactyly and rib abnormalities (*Poland's syndrome*).

Surgical emphysema often accompanies a pneumothorax (Fig. 11.80) and pneumomediastinum. After surgery an increase in the amount of emphysema on serial films suggests the development of a broncho-pleural fistula.

Miscellaneous. Calcified nodes and parasites such as cysticercosis may overlie the lung fields. After lymphography, contrast medium may be seen in the thoracic duct in the left upper zone where the duct drains into the innominate vein, and there may be transient miliary shadowing in the lung fields due to oil emboli. Occasionally after Myodil (Pantopaque) myelography the residual Myodil tracked along the intercostal nerves and gave a bizarre appearance.

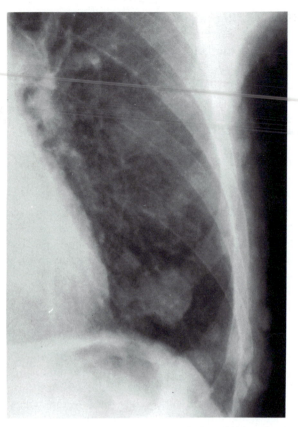

Fig. 11.78 Neurofibromatosis. Multiple soft-tissue lesions, those overlying the lung fields simulating intrapulmonary nodules.

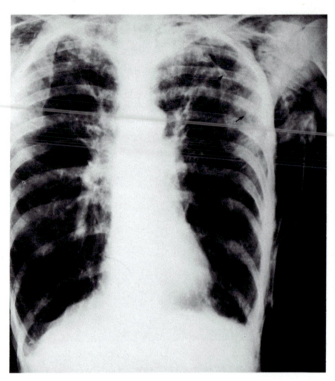

Fig. 11.80 Surgical emphysema following a small left pneumothorax (arrows) in a man with chronic obstructive airways disease.

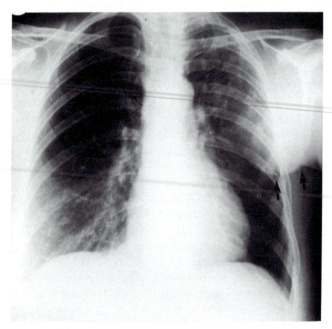

Fig. 11.79 Left mastectomy. Note the abnormal left axillary fold passing cranially (arrows). The left lung is hypertransradiant at its base. Note radiation necrosis of the upper ribs and soft-tissue calcification.

THE DIAPHRAGM

The normal appearances of the diaphragm have already been described.

Normal variants

1. *Scalloping* (Fig. 11.81). Short curves of diaphragm, convex upwards and mostly seen on the right side.

2. *Muscle slips* (Fig. 11.81) are most commonly seen in tall thin patients and in those with emphysema. They appear as small curved lines, concave upwards, and are more common on the right side.

3. *Diaphragm humps and dromedary diaphragm* (Fig. 11.81). These variants are probably mild forms of eventration. They arise anteriorly and are usually right-sided, containing liver. There is no diaphragm defect. On the PA film the hump appears as a shadow in the right cardiophrenic angle and must be distinguished from a fat pad, lipoma, pericardial cyst and Morgagni hernia. On the lateral film the hump overlies the cardiac shadow and should not be confused with middle-lobe consolidation. The dromedary diaphragm is a more severe form of diaphragm hump, appearing as a double contour on the PA view.

4. *Eventration* (Fig. 11.82). This is nearly always left-sided, the hemidiaphragm being considerably elevated with characteristically marked mediastinal displacement to the right, a feature rarely seen with paralysis of the

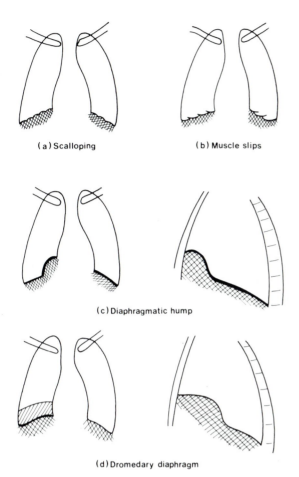

(a) Scalloping

(b) Muscle slips

(c) Diaphragmatic hump

(d) Dromedary diaphragm

Fig. 11.81 Diagrams to show the normal variants of the diaphragm.

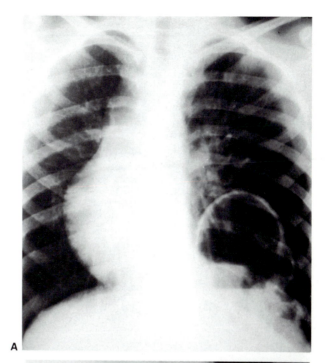

A

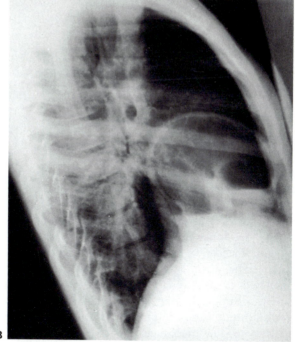

B

Fig. 11.82 Eventration. **A.** The left cupola is elevated and the heart displaced to the right. **B.** The lateral film shows the elevated left cupola with a distended stomach and a normal right cupola.

diaphragm. On fluoroscopy, movement is reduced, paradoxical or absent. The muscle is thin and weak. There may be an associated gastric volvulus, with rotation along its long axis resulting in the greater curve being uppermost. Eventration must be distinguished from absence and rupture of the diaphragm as well as paralysis.

5. *Accessory diaphragm.* This rare condition is asymptomatic and usually right-sided. The hemithorax is partitioned by an accessory diaphragm running parallel to the oblique fissure and resembling a thickened fissure. Its blood supply is often anomalous.

Diaphragm movement

Respiratory excursion is easily assessed at fluoroscopy. Normally the left side moves more than the right, with an excursion of between 3 and 6 cm. Paradoxical movement occurs when the pressure exerted by the abdomen exceeds that of the weak diaphragm so that movement is upwards on inspiration or sniffing. This may be seen with diaphragm paralysis, eventration and subdiaphragmatic infection. However, paradoxical movement is seen in a small number of normal subjects.

The elevated diaphragm

The causes are listed in Table 11.19.

Frequently no cause can be found to explain an elevated hemidiaphragm. The clinical history is important. It is essential to exclude an active lesion, particularly malignancy, by carefully assessing the lung fields, hila and mediastinum. Eventration is associated

Table 11.19 Causes of elevation of the diaphragm

Bilateral

1. Reduce pulmonary compliance	e.g. SLE, fibrosing alveolitis, lymphangitis carcinomatosa
2. Technical	Supine film, expiratory film, postoperative pain
3. Subdiaphragmatic	Ascites, obesity, pregnancy

Unilateral

1. Paralysis	Surgery and trauma Idiopathic Radiotherapy Neoplastic Diabetes mellitus Infections, TB glands, herpes zoster.
2. Congenital	Eventration and humps
3. Pulmonary	Pulmonary and lobar collapse Pulmonary hypoplasia Pneumonectomy Pulmonary embolism Basal pneumonia
4. Pleural	Thickening Pleurisy Subpulmonary effusion
5. Bony	Scoliosis Rib fractures
6. Subdiaphragmatic	Gas-distended viscus Subphrenic abscess Pancreatitis Abdominal mass Hepatomegaly Splenomegaly

Subphrenic abscess

These are often associated with recent surgery or sepsis. A subphrenic abscess is more common on the right side, where it is more easily diagnosed than on the left side. Ultrasound and CT are the investigations of choice, with percutaneous drainage if appropriate.

Plain film signs of a subphrenic abscess include:

1. Ipsilateral basal atelectasis and pleural effusion.
2. Elevated hemidiaphragm with paradoxical or decreased movement.
3. Abnormal gas shadow beneath the diaphragm due to infection with gas-forming organisms (Fig. 11.83). Horizontal beam films improve visualization of the abscess cavity.
4. Depression of the liver edge or gastric fundus.

The thickness of the diaphragm

The normal diaphragm is 2–3 mm thick. On the left side where the gastric bubble lies beneath the diaphragm, the stomach wall and diaphragm form a linear density 5–8 mm thick. Thickening may be a normal variant but occurs with tumours of the diaphragm, stomach and pleura, subpulmonary fluid, diaphragm humps, and abdominal lesions including a subphrenic abscess, hepatomegaly and splenomegaly.

Tumours of the diaphragm

Tumours of the diaphragm are rare. Benign lesions include lipomas, neurofibromas, fibromas and cysts.

with marked cardiac displacement. Pleural thickening is often accompanied by tenting of the diaphragm, with loss of definition and obliteration or blunting of the costophrenic angles and thickened fissures. Subpulmonary fluid may be difficult to distinguish from an elevated diaphragm. Typically it has a straighter upper border and will change shape with the position of the patient if it is not loculated. Loculated subpulmonary effusions are very difficult to distinguish from a high diaphragm on plain films. Ultrasound is the definitive diagnostic investigation.

Splinting of the diaphragm occurs with upper abdominal inflammatory processes, basal pneumonia and embolism.

Determining whether diaphragm elevation is due to paralysis or to an abdominal mass elevating it may be difficult. The position of the edge of the liver should be noted. If the liver edge is low then there is probably a mass within or between the liver and diaphragm, whereas a high diaphragm suggests paralysis as a cause. On the left side, the gastric bubble is assessed using the same principles.

A depressed diaphragm is seen with pulmonary hyperinflation and large pleural effusions.

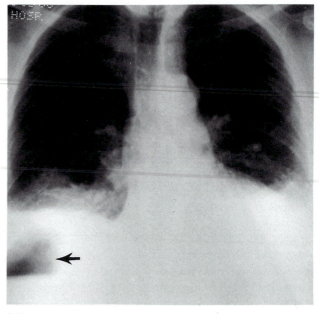

Fig. 11.83 Right subphrenic abscess following cholecystectomy. A large gas shadow with an air-fluid level is seen below the right hemidiaphragm. There are bilateral effusions with patchy shadowing at the right base.

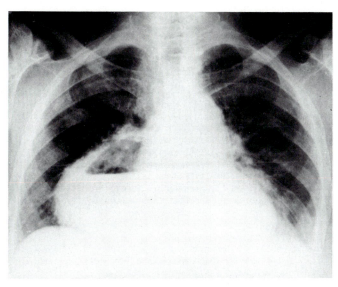

Fig. 11.84 Hiatus hernia. An elderly asymptomatic patient. A large fluid level superimposed on the cardiac shadow. A typical appearance of a hiatus hernia.

Pleural effusions are commonly present with sarcomas. Diaphragm tumours may appear as smooth or lobulated masses and need to be differentiated from lung and liver masses, hernias and diaphragm humps. CT is the most helpful investigation.

Hernias of the diaphragm. The classical appearance of a *hiatus hernia* with a fluid level superimposed on the cardiac shadow on the PA film is well known (Fig. 11.84). A *Bochdalek hernia* arises posterolaterally through the pleuroperitoneal canal and is usually congenital, presenting at birth as respiratory distress: 90% are left-sided. The hernia may contain omentum, fat, spleen, kidney or bowel. The ipsilateral lung is invariably hyploplastic.

Morgagni hernias are usually asymptomatic, presenting in adults as an incidental finding on a chest film. They are right-sided and anterior, appearing as an homogenous shadow in the cardiophrenic angle. The hernia contains fat or occasionally bowel.

Rupture of the diaphragm. This is usually the result of trauma but may be idiopathic or related to previous surgery. Presentation is commonly acute, but may be delayed, in which case bowel strangulation may occur. Some 90% of cases are left-sided. Herniation of the stomach with gastric obstruction is common and must be distinguished from a pneumothorax and eventration. The gastric walls rarely abut all the borders of the thoracic cage, but if there is a diagnostic problem, passage of a nasogastric tube or oral contrast medium should be helpful. Herniation of colon, spleen and kidney is less common. Appearances on the PA film may be normal if there is rupture without herniation, or the diaphragm may be elevated with an abnormal outline.

REFERENCES AND SUGGESTIONS FOR FURTHER READING

Alexander, G. (1966) Diaphragmatic movement and the diagnosis of diaphragmatic paralysis. *Clinical Radiology,* **17,** 79–83.

Bergin, C. J., Muller, N. L. (1985) CT in the diagnosis of interstitial lung disease. *American Journal of Roentgenology,* **145,** 505–510.

Boone, M. L., Swenson, B. E., Felson, B. (1964) Rib notching: Its many causes. *American Journal of Roentgenology,* **91,** 1075–1088.

Campbell, J. A. (1963) The diaphragm in roentgenology of the chest. *Radiologic Clinics of North America,* **1,** 394–410.

Favez, G., Willac, C., Heinzer, F. (1974) Posterior oblique tomography at an angle of 55 degrees in chest roentgenology. *American Journal of Roentgenology,* **120,** 907–915.

Felson, B. (1967) The roentgen diagnosis of disseminated pulmonary alveolar diseases. *Seminars in radiology,* **2,** 3–21.

Felson, B. (1973) *Chest Roentgenology.* W. B. Saunders, Philadelphia.

Felson, B. (1979) A new look at pattern recognition of diffuse pulmonary disease. *American Journal of Roentgenology,* **133,** 183–189.

Fleischner, F. G. (1941) Linear shadows in the lung. *American Journal of Roentgenology,* **46,** 610–618.

Freeman, L. M., Blaufox M. D. (1980) Radionuclide studies of the lung. *Seminars in Nuclear Medicine,* **10,** 198–310.

Fraser, R. G., Paré J. A. P. (1989–91) *Diagnosis of Diseases of the Chest.* Vol. 1 3rd edn. W. B. Saunders, Philadelphia.

Goralnik, C. H., O'Connell, D. M., El Yousef, S. J., Haage, J. R. (1988) CT-guided cutting-needle biopsies of selected chest lesions. *American Journal of Roentgenology,* **151,** 903–907.

Godwin, J. D., Tarver, R. D. (1985) Accessory fissures of the lung. *American Journal of Roentgenology,* **144,** 39–47.

Huston, J., Muhm, J. R. (1987) Solitary pulmonary opacities: Plain tomography. *Radiology,* **163,** 481–485.

Jereb, M. (1980) The usefulness of needle biopsy in chest lesions of different sizes and locations. *Radiology,* **134,** 13–15.

Keats, T. E. (1991) *An Atlas of Normal Roentgen Variants that may Simulate Disease.* 3rd edn. Year Book Medical Publishers, Chicago, pp. 427–500.

Kerr, I. H. (1984) Interstitial lung disease: The role of the radiologist. *Clinical Radiology,* **35,** 1–7.

Khouri, N. F., Stitik F. P., Erozan Y. S. et al (1985) Transthoracic needle aspiration biopsy of benign and malignant lung lesions. *American Journal of Roentgenology,* **144,** 281–288.

Lavender, J. P. (1982) Radioisotope lung scanning and the chest radiograph in pulmonary disease. In: Steiner, R. E., Lodge, E. (eds), *Recent Advances in Radiology 6.* Churchill Livingstone, Edinburgh.

McCleod, R. A., Brown, L. R., Miller, W. E., DeRemee, R. A. (1976) Evaluation of the pulmonary hila by tomography. *Radiologic clinics of North America,* **14,** 51–84.

Miller, W. E., Crowe, J. K., Muhm, J. R. (1976) The evaluation of pulmonary parenchymal abnormalities by tomography. *Radiologic Clinics of North America,* **14,** 85–104.

Milne, E. N. C. (1973) Correlation of physiologic findings with chest radiology. *Radiologic Clinics of North America,* **11,** 17–47.

Proto, A. V., Tocino, I. (1980) Radiographic manifestations of lobar collapse. *Seminars in Roentgenology,* **15,** 117–173.

Reed, J. C., Madewell, J. E. (1975) The air bronchogram in interstitial disease of the lungs. *Radiology,* **116,** 1–9.

Remy, J., Armand, A., Fardon, H. (1977) Treatment of haemoptysis by embolisation of bronchial arteries. *Radiology,* **122,** 33–37.

Ruskin, J. A., Gurney, J. W., Thorsen, M. K., Goodman L. R. (1987) Detection of pleural effusions on supine chest radiographs.

American Journal of Roentgenology, **148**, 681–683.

Sandler, M. S., Velchick, M. G., Alavi, A. (1988) Ventilation abnormalities associated with pulmonary embolism. *Clinics in Nuclear Medicine*, **13**, 450–458.

Savoca, C. J., Austin, J. H. M., Goldberg, H. I. (1977) The right paratracheal stripe. *Radiology*, **122**, 295–301.

Simon, G. (1975) The anterior view chest radiograph-criteria for normality derived from a basic analysis of the shadows. *Clinical Radiology*, **26**, 429–437.

Simon, G. (1978) *Principles of Chest X-ray Diagnosis*. 4th edn. Butterworths, London.

Simon, G., Bonnell, J., Kazantzis, G., Waller, R. E. (1969) Some radiological observations on the range of movement of the diaphragm. *Clinical Radiology*, **20**, 231–233.

Strickland, B. (1976) Sentinel lines — an unusual sign of lower lobe contraction. *Thorax*, **31**, 517–521.

Trapnell, D. (1973) The differential diagnosis of linear shadows in chest radiographs. *Radiologic Clinics of North America*, **11**, 77–92.

Vix, V. A., Klatte, E. C. (1970) The lateral chest radiograph in the diagnosis of hilar and mediastinal masses. *Radiology*, **96**, 307–316.

Radionuclides

Biello, D. R., Mattar, A. G., McKnight, R. G., Siegel, B. A. (1979) Ventilation perfusion studies in suspected pulmonary embolism.

American Journal of Roentgenology, **133**, 1033–1037.

Cooke, S. G., Davies, E. R., Goddard, P. R. (1989) Pulmonary uptake in gallium citrate scintigraphy — the 'negative heart' sign. *Postgraduate Medical Journal*, **65**, 885–891.

Goddard, P. R. (1988) Lung: pulmonary embolisms. In: Davies, E. R., Thomas, W. E. G. (eds.) *Nuclear Medicine: Applications to Surgery*. Castle House Publications, Tunbridge Wells, pp. 199–202.

Levenson, S. M., Warren, R. D., Richman, S. D., Johnson, G. S., Chabner, B. A. (1976) Abnormal pulmonary gallium accumulation in *P. carinii* pneumonia. *Radiology*, **119**, 395–398.

McIvor, J., Anderson, D. R., Britt, R. P. & Dovey P. (1975) Comparison of ^{125}I-labelled fibrinogen uptake and venography in the detection of recent deep vein thrombosis in the legs. *British Journal of Radiology*, **48**, 1013–1018.

Robinson, P. J. (1989) Lung scintigraphy: doubt and certainty in the diagnosis of pulmonary embolism. *Clinical Radiology*, **40**, 557–560.

M.R.I.

Hahn, D. (1988). Mediastinum and lung. In: Stark D. D., Bradley, W. G. (eds.) *Magnetic Resonance Imaging*. CV Mosby, St Louis, ch. 34, pp 804–860.

Webb, W. R. (1989). Magnetic resonance of the chest. *Current Opinion in Radiology*, **1**, 40–43.

CHAPTER 12

THE MEDIASTINUM

Roger H. S. Gregson

Mediastinal lesions are usually first demonstrated radiologically on a chest radiograph, which may show widening of the mediastinum, a soft-tissue mass or a pneumomediastinum. However the chest radiograph may appear normal in the presence of mediastinal disease, with computerized tomography (CT) subsequently revealing a small tumour or enlarged lymph nodes.

The frequency of different mediastinal mass lesions in a series of over 1000 surgical patients was:-

1. Neurogenic tumours	20%
2. Thymic tumours	20%
3. Benign cysts	20%
4. Lymph-node masses	15%
5. Teratodermoid tumours	10%
6. Thyroid tumours	5%
7. Mesenchymal tumours	5%
8. Miscellaneous masses	5%

Another large series of nearly 800 patients showed a completely different pattern of incidence of 65% for lymph-node masses, 10% for vascular abnormalities and 25% for all other mediastinal tumours. Most of these large series have a decided surgical bias and therefore exclude some mediastinal lesions such as hiatus hernia, aortic aneurysms and neoplastic or inflammatory causes of lymph-node enlargement. This makes them unhelpful to the radiologist when considering the possible differential diagnosis of the mediastinal abnormality on a chest radiograph. The commonest *radiographic* lesions are undoubtedly *lymph-node masses, vascular abnormalities* and *hiatus hernias* in adult patients and the normal *thymus gland* in infants and children. The typical sites for the common and rare mediastinal masses are shown in Figure 12.1 and Table 12.1.

ANATOMY

The mediastinum is situated between the lungs in the centre of the thorax and extends from the thoracic inlet above to the central tendon of the diaphragm below, with the sternum anteriorly, the thoracic spine posteriorly and the parietal pleura laterally.

The anatomical location of a mass lesion within the mediastinum affects its differential diagnosis, and therefore from a radiological point of view the mediastinum is best divided into three parts, which all extend from the root of the neck to the diaphragm. The *anterior* division lies in front of the anterior pericardium and trachea, the

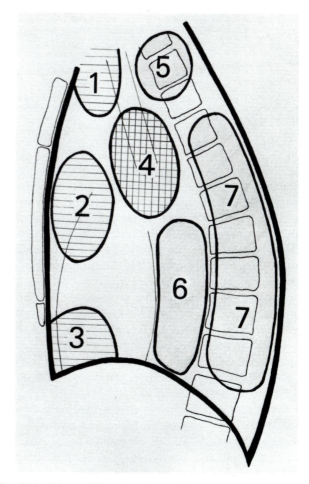

Fig. 12.1 Diagram illustrating the typical sites of the common and rare mediastinal masses listed in Table 12.1.

Table 12.1 The anatomical location of mediastinal masses

Position in mediastinum	Common lesions	Rare lesions
Anterior division	1. Tortuous innominate artery Lymph-node enlargement Retrosternal goitre Fat deposition	Aneurysm of innominate artery Parathyroid adenoma Lymphangioma
	2. Lymph-node enlargement Aneurysm of ascending aorta Thymoma Teratodermoid tumour	Sternal mass Lipoma Haemangioma
	3. Epicardial fat pad Diaphragmatic hump Pleuropericardial cyst	Morgagni hernia
Middle division	4. Lymph-node enlargement Aneurysm of aortic arch Enlarged pulmonary artery Dilatation of superior vena cava Bronchogenic cyst	Tracheal lesion Cardiac tumour
Posterior division	5. Neurogenic tumour Pharyngo-oesophageal pouch	
	6. Hiatus hernia Aneurysm of descending aorta Oesophageal dilatation Dilatation of azygos vein	Neuroenteric cyst Pancreatic pseudocyst Sequestrated lung segment
	7. Neurogenic tumour Paravertebral mass	Bochdalek hernia Extramedullary haemopoiesis

middle division within the pericardial cavity but including the trachea, and the *posterior* division lies behind the posterior pericardium and trachea. Some normal structures, such as the thoracic aorta and the mediastinal lymph nodes, are present in all these divisions and some very large mass lesions can involve adjacent divisions of the mediastinum. This makes the diagnosis of a mass lesion difficult, because its site of origin is obscure.

The anatomical structures that produce the outline of the mediastinum on a chest radiograph are discussed in Chapter 11. The way that the various mediastinal lines (such as the anterior and posterior junctional lines, the right paratracheal line, the azygo-oesophageal line and the right and left paraspinal lines) are produced on a chest radiograph becomes apparent at CT.

All the anatomical structures in the mediastinum are surrounded by fatty connective tissue and therefore the larger structures such as the ascending aorta, the innominate, carotid and subclavian arteries, the superior and inferior venae cavae, the brachiocephalic veins, the pulmonary arteries and veins, the trachea and main bronchi and the oesophagus are all well demonstrated by

CT in the normal adult patient. Their anatomy is illustrated diagrammatically at various critical levels through the mediastinum in Figure 12.2 and is further discussed below.

CT OF THE MEDIASTINUM
Ian Isherwood and W. St C. Forbes

Normal appearances

An understanding of the normal vascular structures of the mediastinum in cross-section is essential to permit an analysis of abnormal mediastinal masses. The ability of CT to identify small density differences in cross-section allows the demonstration of some structures not detectable by conventional techniques. Cardiac and vascular pulsation can, however, result in overlying artefacts and loss of marginal definition. CT angiography, i.e. high-dose intravenous contrast medium with first pass circulation studies, is of considerable value in the better definition of major vessels. An excess of fat in the mediastinum, e.g. in Cushing's syndrome, may allow identification of vascular structures without contrast enhancement.

The following normal features (Fig. 12.3) of the mediastinum are of particular importance:

Aortic arch (Fig. 12.3B). The ascending limb of the aortic arch lies anterior to the trachea and anterolateral to the superior vena cava. The descending limb is closely related to the oesophagus which may also contain air.

Right paratracheal stripe. The interface between the right upper lobe and the right lateral wall of the trachea is represented by the 'right paratracheal stripe' on a conventional chest radiograph.

Pulmonary arteries (Fig. 12.3C). The main pulmonary artery lies to the left, and anterior to the aortic root. The intrapericardial portion of the right pulmonary artery passes posterolaterally between the superior vena cava and the intermediate bronchus. CT offers a unique opportunity to make a direct measurement of the diameter of the vessel. The left pulmonary artery has a short intrapericardial course and passes posterolaterally anterior to the left main bronchus which may be displaced by it.

Pulmonary veins (Fig. 12.3D). The superior and inferior pulmonary veins draining into the left atrium on the posterior aspect of the heart lie caudal to the pulmonary arteries and anterior to the oesophagus.

Cardiac chambers (Fig. 12.3E). The approach to cardiac scanning is dealt with separately, but even a conventional CT scan of 2–10 seconds may permit some cardiac chambers to be identified, particularly the left atrium posteriorly and the ventricles at the diaphragmatic surface. The intraventricular septum is recognizable as a linear structure of fat density, passing obliquely from the left anteriorly towards the inferior vena cava posteriorly on the right side.

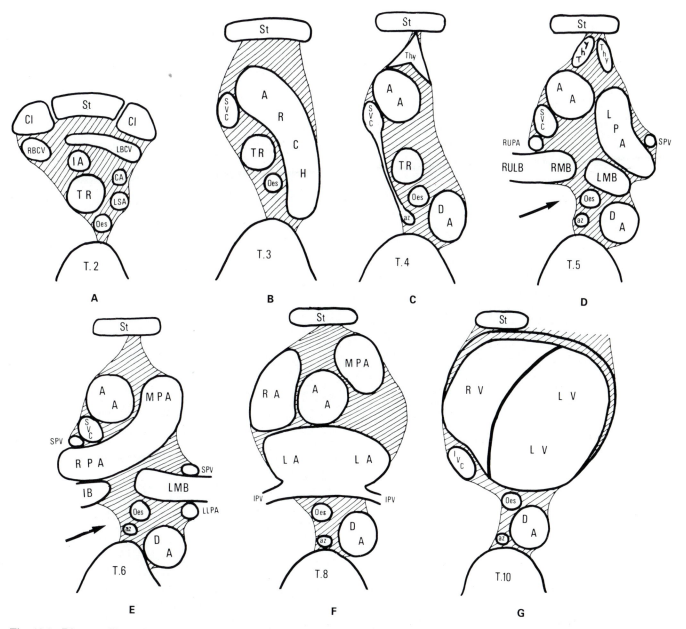

Fig. 12.2 Diagrams illustrating normal mediastinal anatomy at various levels through the thorax and features which can be identified by CT. **A.** Above the aortic arch through the sternoclavicular joints. **B.** Arch of aorta. **C.** Below the aortic arch through the aortopulmonary window. **D.** Left pulmonary artery. **E.** Main and right pulmonary arteries. **F.** Left and right atria. **G.** Left and right ventricles. Arch = arch of aorta; AA = ascending aorta; DA = descending aorta; IA = innominate artery; CA left common carotid artery; LSA = left subclavian artery; MPA = main pulmonary artery; RPA = right pulmonary artery; LPA = left pulmonary artery; RUPA = right upper lobe pulmonary artery; LLPA = left lower lobe pulmonary artery; SPV = superior pulmonary vein; IPV = inferior pulmonary vein; SVC = superior vena cava; IVC inferior vena cava; az. = azygos vein; RBCV and LBCV = right and left brachiocephalic or innominate veins; TR = trachea; RMB = right main bronchus; LMB = left main bronchus; IB = intermediate bronchus; RULB = right upper lobe bronchus; LV = left ventricle; RV = right ventricle; LA = left atrium; RA = right atrium; Oes = oesophagus; St = sternum; Cl = clavicle; Thy = thymus gland; → azygo-oesophageal recess (cf. Fig. 12.3).

Diaphragmatic crura. The diaphragmatic crura are clearly identified by CT as curvilinear structures of varying thickness demarcating the aortic hiatus. The right crus is longer and frequently thicker, particularly in males, than the left. The retrocrural space contains, in addition to the aorta, lymph nodes and the azygos vein. Localized thickening of the right crus should not be mistaken for lymph node enlargement.

Azygo-oesophageal recess (Figs 12.2D, 12.8B). The right lower lobe lies in intimate relationship with the posterior wall of the right main bronchus and the oesophagus and azygos vein medially. The azygo-oesophageal recess

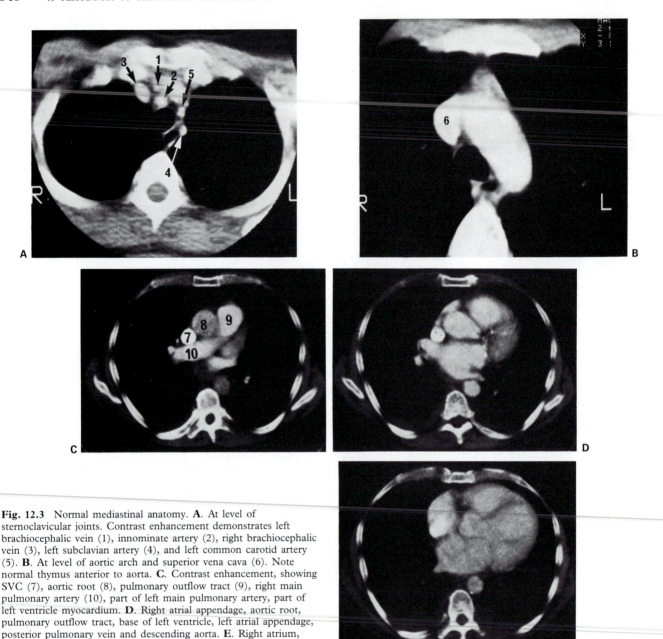

Fig. 12.3 Normal mediastinal anatomy. **A**. At level of sternoclavicular joints. Contrast enhancement demonstrates left brachiocephalic vein (1), innominate artery (2), right brachiocephalic vein (3), left subclavian artery (4), and left common carotid artery (5). **B**. At level of aortic arch and superior vena cava (6). Note normal thymus anterior to aorta. **C**. Contrast enhancement, showing SVC (7), aortic root (8), pulmonary outflow tract (9), right main pulmonary artery (10), part of left main pulmonary artery, part of left ventricle myocardium. **D**. Right atrial appendage, aortic root, pulmonary outflow tract, base of left ventricle, left atrial appendage, posterior pulmonary vein and descending aorta. **E**. Right atrium, right ventricle, intraventricular septum and left ventricle.

created in the mediastinum by the right lower lobe is known as the 'space of Holzknecht'. Enlargement of carinal nodes may be identified at an early stage by their intrusion into this easily recognized space.

Aortopulmonary window (Fig. 12.3C,D). The aorto-pulmonary window between the descending aorta and the left pulmonary artery is recognized on CT by the protrusion of a portion of left lower lobe into its posterior aspect. Hilar node enlargement or changes in pulmonary artery calibre can obliterate this recess at an early stage in its development.

Clinical applications

1. Evaluation of mediastinal mass. The location, size, contour and extent of mediastinal masses, whether neoplastic or vascular, are usually well demonstrated (Fig. 12.4). **CT** in the transverse plane frequently permits a clearer identification of abnormalities otherwise partially obscured in conventional radiographs, e.g. retrosternal or retrocrural areas. Whilst histological characterization is not possible, some information about the consistency of a mass can often be gained from variations in its attenuation characteristics. *Fat* and *calcification* are easily

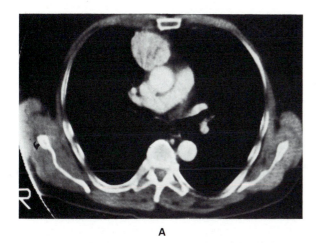

A

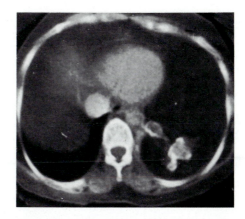

Fig. 12.5 Lipodermoid. Anterior mediastinal mass of fat density containing calcific deposits posteriorly. L0 W200.

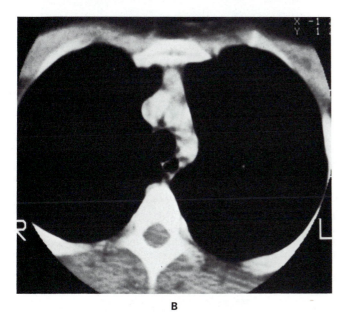

B

Fig. 12.4 Anterior mediastinal mass. Thymoma. **A.** Large tumour. **B.** Very small tumour.

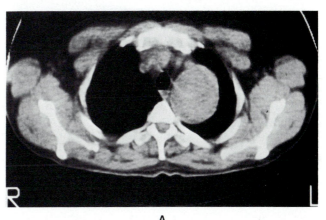

A

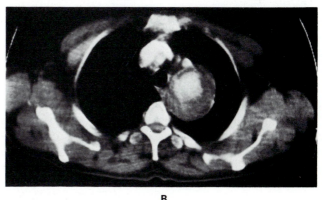

B

Fig. 12.6 Aortic aneurysm. **A.** Precontrast. Descending thoracic aortic aneurysm. **B.** Contrast demonstrates true lumen and surrounding thrombus.

detected and may permit a positive diagnosis of *lipoma* or *dermoid* (Fig. 12.5) to be established in situations where only a soft-tissue mass is visible by conventional techniques. Alteration in the shape of a mass resulting from a change in posture suggests it has a fluid content, and may also reveal a consistent relationship of the mass with an anatomical structure, e.g. *pericardial cyst*.

The high resolution of CT facilitates the visualization of the thymus. Small *thymic tumours* not visualized on a conventional chest radiograph are easily detected. The anatomical relationships of a larger mass can be precisely defined (Fig. 12.4).

CT angiography enables normal and ectatic vessels to be identified and the lumen of an aortic aneurysm to be differentiated from perivascular thrombus and the false lumen of a dissection (Fig. 12.6).

2. Evaluation of hilar mass. The hilum is frequently involved in mediastinal disease. A frequent problem on conventional radiography is the distinction of a true hilar mass from an enlarged vessel. CT demonstrates normal pulmonary vessels well and reveals, in transverse section,

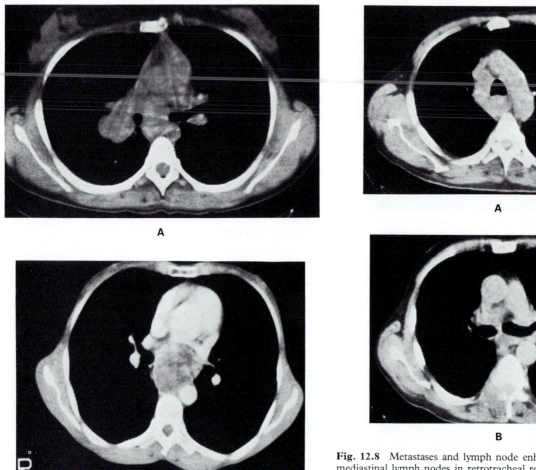

Fig. 12.7 Mediastinal lymph nodes. **A.** Enlarged hilar nodes. **B**. Posterior mediastinal nodes compressing the enhanced left atrium.

Fig. 12.8 Metastases and lymph node enhancement. **A.** Enlarged mediastinal lymph nodes in retrotracheal region. **B.** Same patient. Lymph node enlargement encroaching on the azygo-oesophageal recess. Note vertebral destruction.

enlarged mediastinal lymph nodes at an early stage, particularly those presenting in the *azygo-oesophageal* recess and the *aortopulmonary window* (Fig. 12.7).

3. Evaluation of paraspinal mass. It has been noted previously that an advantage of CT is its ability to demonstrate the dynamic range of tissue density. In the study of paraspinal disease, both soft tissue and bone can be studied together (Figs 12.8, 12.9).

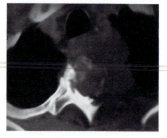

Fig. 12.9 Carcinoma of the bronchus. Transaxial sections showing destructive lesion of D2 and posterior ribs with associated paraspinal mass.

RADIOLOGICAL INVESTIGATION

Patients with mediastinal lesions may present with an asymptomatic abnormality discovered incidentally on a chest radiograph, or with clinical symptoms and signs suggestive of intrathoracic pathology. The clinical presentation may be quite unhelpful with symptoms such as *chest pain*, *cough* and *weight loss*, but more specific symptoms such as *dysphagia* or *stridor* are useful in localizing the mediastinal lesion to a particular anatomical site. Occasionally there is a very specific clinical problem, the best example of which is the patient who presents with *myasthenia gravis*. About 10–15% of patients with this autoimmune neurological condition turn out to have a thymoma on investigation.

There are various radiological methods of investigating

the mediastinum, but at present **CT** can still be regarded as the best single radiological investigation for evaluating a mediastinal abnormality demonstrated on a high-kV chest radiograph or for detecting occult mediastinal disease. Its uses include:-

1. The investigation of an obvious mediastinal mass;
2. The investigation of the widened mediastinum (e.g. fat deposition in an obese patient);
3. The investigation of the abnormal hilum;
4. The investigation of a suspected vascular abnormality (e.g. dissecting aortic aneurysm);
5. The staging of malignant disease (e.g. mediastinal lymph node involvement in a patient with a carcinoma of the bronchus);
6. The detection of mediastinal disease when the chest radiograph is normal (e.g. thymoma in a patient with myasthenia gravis).

The chest radiograph may be the only radiological investigation necessary to confirm the cause of a mediastinal mass lesion such as a hiatus hernia. CT can confirm the diagnosis of an aortic aneurysm, fat deposition or mediastinal haemorrhage and can detect a thymoma or enlarged mediastinal lymph nodes. It cannot however distinguish between reactive hyperplasia and inflammatory or neoplastic causes for the lymphadenopathy. CT has replaced conventional mediastinal tomography and limited the use of both barium studies and angiography. Even with CT a histological diagnosis cannot necessarily be made, as there are many mediastinal lesions which appear as masses of similar soft-tissue density, e.g. neurogenic tumours or bronchogenic cysts. The presence of calcification within the mass may not be diagnostic (e.g. a thyroid tumour or a thymoma) although the presence of fat usually is (e.g. a teratodermoid tumour).

Fine-needle aspiration biopsy of mediastinal masses can be used to produce a pathological diagnosis in about 80% of cases. This procedure is done under local anaesthetic with either fluoroscopic or CT-guided control, using a 19–21 gauge needle to produce both cytological and histological samples. Complications such as slight haemoptysis and minor pneumothorax occur in about 15% of patients, with a major pneumothorax in only 3%. This technique can be used instead of a diagnostic surgical procedure, but in about 20% of patients a specific pathological diagnosis cannot be made because of the limitations of cytology and histology on small samples of tissue, particularly in the diagnosis of lymphoma.

Investigations such as *radionuclide scanning*, *ultrasound*, *urography* and *myelography* are occasionally used to confirm the diagnosis of a mediastinal lesion. The role of *digital chest radiology* is still being evaluated.

In recent years *MRI* has become more widely available and is being increasingly used to investigate mediastinal lesions.

MRI OF THE MEDIASTINUM
Ian Isherwood and Jeremy P. R. Jenkins

MRI can stage certain mediastinal lesions more accurately than CT. The advantages of MRI include the differentiation of solid lesions from vessels, the direct visualization of the spinal canal and its neural contents, and the differentiation between chronic fibrosis (low signal) and recurrent lymphoma or tumour (intermediate signal). In children MRI may be the preferred technique, obviating the need for intravenous contrast enhancement, but in adults CT is more often used in conjunction with MRI. MRI is particularly indicated when the administration of intravenous contrast medium is contraindicated or when vascular opacification is suboptimal. Surgical clips can produce significant streak artefacts on CT, whereas on MRI only a localized signal void is produced. In the postoperative patient, where residual or recurrent tumour is suspected, distortion of the hilar and mediastinal anatomy can be more easily assessed on MRI because of its multiplanar capability and greater intrinsic soft-tissue and vascular contrast discrimination.

Anterior mediastinum

Mediastinal thyroid. This is the commonest mass lesion in the thoracic inlet. Sagittal and transverse T_1-weighted scans demonstrate its extent and relationship to adjacent major vessels. The thyroid gland gives a signal intensity slightly greater than muscle on T_1-weighted images and a much more intense signal on T_2-weighted scans. Thyroid masses have longer relaxation times than normal thyroid and thus are of lower and higher signal on T_1- and T_2-weighted images respectively. Measurement of relaxation times are unhelpful in separating this lesion from other tumours. Haemorrhage within cysts can be shown but calcification is better demonstrated by CT. The internal architecture of this tumour, including cystic and necrotic changes, can be shown on T_2-weighted scans but better assessed using intravenous gadolinium-DTPA.

Thymus. The *normal thymus* has a non-specific long T_1 and T_2 and appears of low signal, contrasting well with the high signal from surrounding fat on T_1-weighted scans but remaining isointense with fat on T_2-weighted images. The superior soft-tissue contrast resolution of MRI allowed the correct diagnosis to be made in a patient with an ectopic thymus in the posterior mediastinum because of its similarity in signal intensity characteristics to the normally positioned thymus. With increasing age, fat deposition within the normal thymus shortens its T_1 value, thereby reducing its contrast with adjacent fat.

The majority (90%) of *thymomas* are located in the anterior mediastinum and cannot be differentiated from other solid mediastinal tumours. Inhomogeneities in the tumour can occur due to cyst formation, necrosis or haemorrhage, and may be better delineated by the administration of gadolinium-DTPA. A disadvantage of gadolinium-DTPA enhancement in T_1-weighted images is the loss of contrast between fat and enhancing tumour. *Malignant thymomas* cannot be differentiated from benign tumours on signal intensity appearances or on relaxation time measurements, but can be recognized by evidence of invasion of adjacent structures.

Cystic mediastinal masses. MRI can demonstrate the cystic nature of lesions in the mediastinum when this is difficult to ascertain by other imaging techniques, including CT. *Simple cysts* typically have a very long T_1 and T_2, with a signal intensity similar to that of cerebrospinal fluid or urine. The actual signal intensity within the cyst does, however, depend upon its contents. It is important, therefore, to appreciate that the MRI appearance may be ambiguous and, in the presence of haemorrhage or an increase in the proteinaceous material within the cyst, may suggest a solid mass. A uniformly high signal intensity on T_1-weighted images, due to the presence of altered haemorrhage, is a typical feature of a benign cyst. In the assessment of *teratodermoids*, CT is superior to MRI because of its ability to detect calcification. Lipid is well shown by both techniques.

Middle mediastinum

Nodal disease. There is debate as to the relative merits of ECG-gated or rapid-acquisition non-gated T_1-weighted images in the demonstration of mediastinal and hilar nodes. Both techniques provide equivalent morphological detail and reduce cardiac and respiratory motion artefacts, but the rapid-acquisition non-gated scans are more heavily T_1-weighted, providing greater soft-tissue contrast between lymph nodes and fat. It is generally agreed that MRI is slightly superior to CT in the detection of lymph-node enlargement of the hilum but equivalent in the general assessment of enlarged nodes in the mediastinum. As hilar nodes are closely related to vessels, the superior contrast and multiplanar capability of MRI more than compensates for its slightly inferior spatial resolution. MRI can be of value in evaluating the *aortopulmonary window* and *subcarinal spaces* — areas that are difficult to delineate using the transverse plane of CT. MRI, however, has poorer spatial resolution and may not resolve small adjacent but separate nodes. *Calcification* within nodes, which may be useful as an estimate of benignity, is not easily detected. In patients with little mediastinal fat, small nodes can be difficult to define.

The diagnosis of nodal disease depends on the same *size* criteria as for CT. There is current debate as to the precise size criteria to be applied in different nodal areas, and also which dimension of the node (short or long axis) should be used for measurement. Generally, nodes greater than 10 mm are considered to be enlarged and involved by tumour. It should be recognized, however,

that not all enlarged nodes are tumorous and that metastases can occur in normal-sized nodes. It is not possible from measured relaxation time values or other MRI criteria to distinguish between tumour-involved nodes and reactive hyperplastic nodes. An in-vitro study of freshly removed lymph nodes from patients with lung cancer has shown significant ($p < 0.05$) differences in the mean T_1 values of tumorous (640 ms) and non-tumorous (566 ms) nodes. There was, however, too much overlap between the two groups for this to be of clinical relevance.

Although relaxation time values in themselves have limited value in the differentiation of pathology, the use of more sophisticated image analysis techniques, including texture analysis, may have great potential in detecting changes between tumour and non-tumour tissue which may not be demonstrable on visual inspection alone.

A new MRI lymphographic contrast agent, using an ultra-small (<10 nm diameter) superparamagnetic iron oxide preparation, has been developed, with early experimental results indicating a clinical potential for imaging the lymphatic system. Following intravenous administration the ultra-small iron oxide compound is able to bypass the mononuclear phagocytic system of the liver and spleen, cross capillary walls and achieve widespread tissue distribution, including lymph nodes and bone marrow. The particles accumulate in normal lymph nodes, reducing their signal intensity by a superparamagnetic effect. Malignant tissue is spared, and metastatic nodes, therefore, appear more intense than normal nodes. The use of such an agent could enable visualization of normal nodal anatomy and thus enhance the detection of nodal disease irrespective of size or anatomical distribution.

Lymphoma. MRI is not able to characterize tissue reliably. Most malignancies have a non-specific long T_1 and T_2, and their enhancement characteristics using gadolinium-DTPA are similar. Lymphoma usually has a homogeneous intermediate signal intensity on T_1-weighted images and appears isointense with fat on T_2-weighted scans. Nodular sclerosing Hodgkin's disease can appear heterogeneous, with low signal areas which are presumed to be due to a high fibrous content in this tumour type.

In the early post-treatment phase (8–12 weeks), responding lymphomas demonstrate heterogeneity in signal intensity, with a decrease in the T_2-weighted signal, associated with reduction in tumour size. Inactive residual masses assume a homogeneous low intensity signal pattern. Recurrent disease may be detected as an increase in signal intensity on the T_2-weighted images prior to evidence of a clinical relapse. Problems in interpretation, however, may result from intermixing of surrounding fat with an inactive mass. Post-radiation or reactive inflammatory changes may also simulate active disease. A low signal from *fibrosis* is a more reliable indicator of tissue type than a high signal intensity which is not specific for tumour. MRI, nevertheless, has a role in the assessment of response to treatment and in the detection of recurrent mediastinal disease.

Great vessels. Mediastinal disease can involve the mediastinal great vessels. Vascular abnormalities can be assessed with MRI without the need for the administration of intravenous contrast medium. The high intrinsic soft-tissue contrast, due to the low signal from flowing blood compared with the intermediate signal from the vessel wall and high signal from adjacent fat, gives MRI significant advantages over CT. Flow artefacts with signal within vessels during different phases of the cardiac cycle using conventional pulse sequences need to be recognized and correctly interpreted.

Aorta. Both acquired and congenital lesions of the thoracic aorta can be shown to advantage with MRI, which has significant advantages over CT and angiography, particularly in the evaluation of *aortic aneurysms*. The dimensions and extent of an aneurysm, the differentiation of a patent lumen from thrombus formation and the delineation of vessel wall from surrounding mediastinal fat can all be assessed. The use of multiplanar imaging allows the aortic valve and proximal origin of the great vessels to be demonstrated.

The origin and extent of *aortic dissection*, involvement of the arch and the dissecting flap can be well-shown on MRI (Fig. 12.10). The distinction between slow-flowing blood and thrombus may be difficult on conventional pulse sequences and does require a more flow-sensitive sequence (phase-sensitive or gradient-echo even-echo rephasing). The ability to measure blood flow velocity in vivo using flow-sensitive sequences enables a clear separation between the true and false lumens to be made, together with an assessment of the re-entry site in aortic dissection (see Ch. 25).

Mediastinal veins. Superior vena caval infiltration or obstruction secondary to thoracic tumour can be well

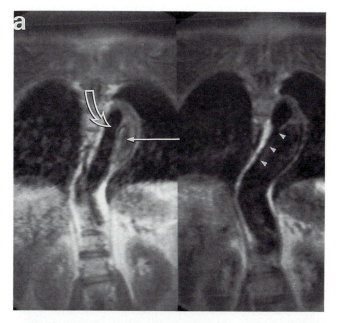

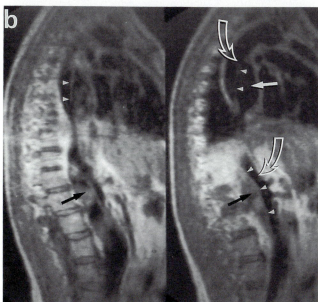

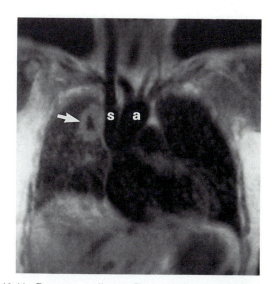

Fig. 12.10 Chronic aortic dissection on two contiguous (**a**) coronal and (**b**) sagittal ECG-gated spin echo (1100/26) images. The intimal flap (small arrowheads) with true (curved arrows) and false (short straight arrows) lumens are demonstrated. Note the signal from slow-flowing blood in the false lumen in the descending and abdominal aorta, with thrombus (long straight arrow) in (**a**).
(Fig. 12.10a reproduced with permission from: Mitchell et al (1988), *Clinical Radiology*, **39**, 458–461.)

Fig. 12.11 Recurrent malignant fibrous histiocytoma of the right lung (arrowed) following previous lobectomy on coronal T_1-weighted (spin echo 1100/26) image. The tumour is attached to and involves the lateral wall of the superior vena cava (s); a = aortic arch. (Reproduced with permission from: Jenkins, J. P. R., Isherwood, I. (1987). Magnetic resonance of the heart: a review. In: *Recent Advances in Cardiology 10*, D. J. Rowlands (Ed.), Churchill Livingstone, Edinburgh.)

shown on transverse and coronal T_1-weighted images (Fig. 12.11). The same flow void phenomenon is observed in veins as in arteries, but signals within veins due to slow flow can be difficult to interpret. The distinction between slow flow and thrombus may require the use of phase-sensitive or gradient-rephasing sequences. Gadolinium-DTPA can be useful in showing intraluminal tumour infiltration, which enhances compared with intraluminal thrombus (which shows no change in signal intensity). Gadolinium-DTPA can also enhance slow-flowing venous blood, producing an increase in intraluminal signal, but this is usually more pronounced than that from tumour enhancement.

Tracheal tumours. The reduced spatial resolution of MRI compared with CT accounts for the lower accuracy in the detection of 319 normal and 79 diseased bronchi confirmed bronchoscopically — 40% normal and 70% diseased bronchi were visualized on MRI and 98% for both groups on CT. MRI and CT are considered equivalent in the visualization of larger airways, but MRI has the possible advantage of imaging the whole trachea and major bronchi in a single oblique plane. CT is superior, however, to MRI in the detection of endotracheal and endobronchial lesions.

Posterior mediastinum

Neurogenic tumours. MRI is superior to CT in the detection and evaluation of neurogenic tumours within the posterior mediastinum (Figs 12.12, 12.13). This is due to the higher soft-tissue contrast discrimination, allowing direct visualization of the spine, spinal canal and cord (including nerve roots) without the need for intrathecal contrast medium, together with the multiplanar imaging facility. Calcification, which is common in neuroblastoma, is better shown by CT.

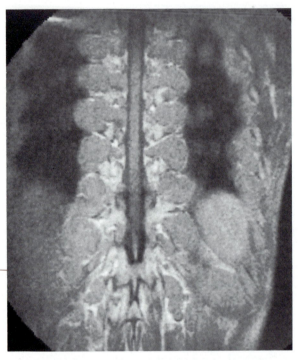

Fig. 12.12 Multiple paraspinal, intercostal and intra-abdominal neurofibromas, in a patient with neurofibromatosis, on a coronal T_1-weighted (spin echo 700/40) image through the thorax.

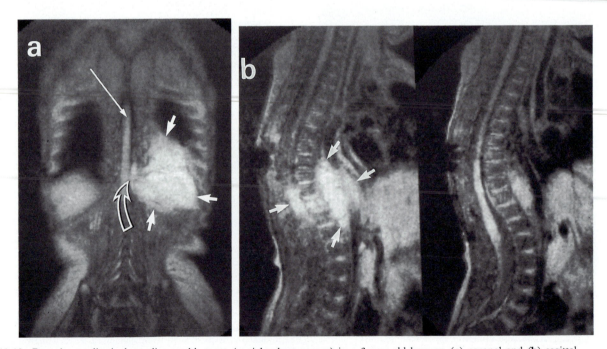

Fig. 12.13 Posterior mediastinal ganglioneuroblastoma (straight short arrows) in a 3-year-old boy, on (**a**) coronal and (**b**) sagittal T_1-weighted (partial saturation recovery 520/18) images. Note extension of tumour into the extradural space (curved arrow) displacing the spinal cord (straight long arrow).

Oesophageal lesions. Smooth muscle has similar values of relaxation time to skeletal muscle. There is therefore greater soft-tissue contrast between oesophageal tumour (high signal) and muscle (low signal) on T_2-weighted images. Conventional T_2-weighted images of the mediastinum are, however, prone to significant motion artefacts and have a much lower SNR than T_1-weighted images. On T_1-weighted images there is reduced tumour–to–muscle contrast. The use of MRI affords no advantages over CT in the assessment of oesophageal tumour, as MRI is unable to demonstrate small intraluminal and intramural tumours. Infiltration of the oesophageal wall cannot be detected, and difficulty does occur in separating tumour from intraluminal contents in stenotic lesions. Tumour enhancement may be achieved by the use of gadolinium-DTPA. Equivalent assessment of mediastinal infiltration can be demonstrated on both CT and MRI.

Extramedullary haematopoiesis. Extramedullary haematopoiesis has similar signal intensity characteristics to the spleen (long T_1/long T_2). The appearances are nonspecific and indistinguishable from other mediastinal tumours. Similar morphological criteria to those applied to CT can be used with MRI.

Diaphragmatic hernias. Coronal and sagittal plane imaging are particularly useful in delineating the diaphragm, which has a low signal (see Fig. 14.36). The relationship of intrathoracic masses to the diaphragm can be well visualized, as can the contents of the hernial sac, which determine the signal intensity.

Fibrosing mediastinitis. CT is superior to MRI in the detection of calcification invisible on chest radiographs, a feature which is important in suggesting the diagnosis of fibrosing mediastinitis. A low signal on both T_1- and T_2-weighted images, due to the presence of fibrosis, is very often sufficiently different from that from tumour to suggest the correct diagnosis.

ANTERIOR MEDIASTINAL MASSES

THYROID TUMOUR

Less than 5% of enlarged thyroid glands in the neck extend into the mediastinum to produce a retrosternal goitre. This can be due to non-toxic enlargement of the gland, thyrotoxicosis, carcinoma of the thyroid gland or Hashimoto's disease. An intrathoracic goitre also occasionally develops in a heterotopic thyroid gland in the anterior mediastinum.

A *retrosternal goitre* usually presents as a soft-tissue swelling that moves on swallowing in the root of the neck in a woman patient. The goitre is often asymptomatic, but can also produce dysphagia and stridor. Vocal cord paralysis or a superior vena caval compression syndrome indicate the development of malignancy.

A retrosternal goitre appears as an oval soft-tissue mass in the superior part of the anterior mediastinum, which extends down from the neck. The outline is well defined in the mediastinum but fades off into neck, due to its anterior location (a mass situated posteriorly in the thoracic inlet has a sharply defined upper and lower margin due to the posterior position of the lung apices). The soft-tissue mass more commonly projects to the right side of the mediastinum, with displacement and compression of the trachea to the left (Fig. 12.14). However, about 20% of thyroid goitres are retrotracheal, producing displacement of the oesophagus posteriorly and the trachea anteriorly (Fig. 12.15). The soft-tissue mass may also contain central nodular, linear or crescent patterns of calcification. This is of course not a diagnostic radiological sign, because calcification also occurs in thymic tumours, teratodermoid tumours, aneurysms and enlarged lymph nodes, as shown in Table 12.2. Rapid increase in the size of the mass indicates internal haemorrhage into a cyst. The diagnosis is confirmed by either *a radionuclide scan*, using either ^{99m}Tc sodium pertechnetate or ^{123}I sodium iodide, which shows an area of increased activity extending below the sternal notch, or *CT*, which shows a mass of mixed attenuation containing soft tissue, cysts and calcification, extending from one of the lower poles of the thyroid gland (Fig. 12.15). This has a higher attenuation level than soft tissue on an unenhanced scan, due to its iodine content.

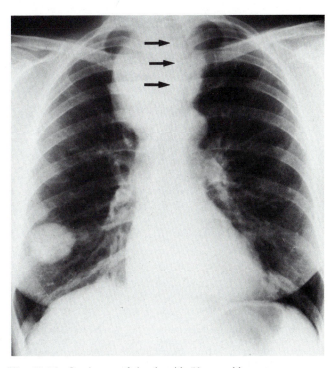

Fig. 12.14 Carcinoma of the thyroid. 53-year-old woman presenting with a painful goitre and dysphagia. PA film shows an oval mass in the superior part of the anterior mediastinum with displacement of the trachea (arrows) to the left and multiple pulmonary metastases.

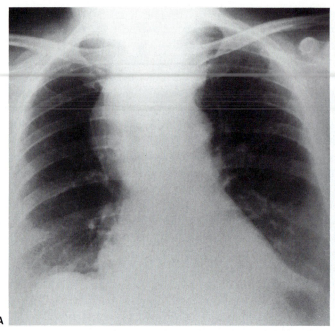

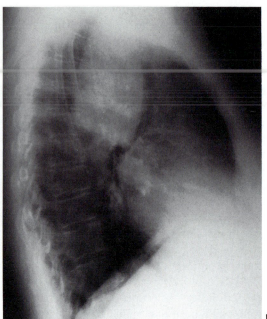

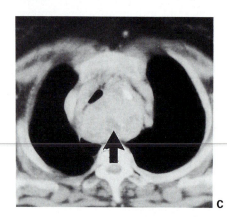

Fig. 12.15 Thyroid adenoma. 67-year-old woman presenting with a goitre. PA (**A**) and lateral films (**B**) show an oval mass in the superior part of the middle mediastinum with displacement of the trachea forwards and to the right. CT scan with contrast enhancement (L + 50, W500) (**C**) above the tracheal bifurcation shows a round mass of soft-tissue density (arrow), 8 cm in size, which contains calcification and cystic changes, in the middle mediastinum with compression of the trachea. Diagnosis confirmed by surgery.

Table 12.2 The causes of calcification in a mediastinal mass

Anterior mediastinum	Aneurysm of ascending aorta	
	Retrosternal goitre	
	Thymoma	
	Teratodermoid tumour	
	Lymphoma after radiothherapy	
	Haemangioma	
Middle mediastinum	Lymph-node enlargement:	Tuberculosis
		Histoplasmosis
		Lymphoma after radiotherapy
		Sarcoidosis
		Silicosis
		Amyloidosis
		Mucin-secreting adenocarcinoma
	Aneurysm of aortic arch	
	Bronchogenic cyst	
Posterior mediastinum	Aneurysm of descending aorta	Neuroblastoma
	Neurogenic tumour	Neurofibrosarcoma
	Neuroenteric cyst	Ganglioneuroma
	Abscess	
	Haematoma	
	Leiomyoma of oesophagus	

THYMIC TUMOUR

The normal thymus gland is the commonest cause of a mediastinal abnormality on a chest radiograph in infants. It produces a triangular soft-tissue mass, which projects to one side of the mediastinum — often the right. The normal thymus gland becomes more prominent on an expiratory or slightly rotated film, but may disappear radiologically in the presence of a severe neonatal infection, or after major surgery or the use of corticosteroids. The complete absence of the normal thymus gland occurs in immune deficiency disease involving the T-lymphocytes, such as Di George's syndrome.

The commonest of the thymic tumours in the mediastinum are the benign and malignant *thymoma*. Enlargement of the thymus can also be due to *hyperplasia* of the gland, *thymic cysts, thymolipomas, lymphoma, germ cell tumours* and *carcinoid tumours*. About 30% of thymomas are malignant.

A **thymoma** usually presents as an anterior mediastinal mass on a chest radiograph in an adult patient. The thymoma is often asymptomatic, but can also present with myasthenia gravis. About 10–15% of patients with myasthenia have a thymoma and about 10–15% of patients with a thymoma have myasthenia gravis. It is most important to assess the mediastinum by CT in all patients with myasthenia, because surgical removal of a thymoma, or occasionally even the gland, may reduce or abolish the effects of this autoimmune neurological condition. A thymoma can also present with red-cell aplasia or hypogammaglobinaemia. *Thymic hyperplasia* occurs in association with thyrotoxicosis, Addison's disease, acromegaly, systemic lupus erythematosus, rheumatoid arthritis and after stress atrophy. It is important to realize that enlargement of the thymus gland following chemotherapy for Hodgkin's disease or testicular tumours can be due to rebound thymic hyperplasia and not recurrent disease in isolation. *Thymic carcinoids* can present with Cushing's syndrome or hyperparathyroidism.

A thymoma appears as a round or oval soft-tissue mass, which projects to one side of the anterior mediastinum when large, but may be undetectable on the chest radiograph if small, indicating the need for CT (Figs 12.4, 12.16). The soft-tissue mass may also contain a peripheral rim or central nodules of calcification. A very

large soft-tissue mass with less radiographic density than expected for its size, and which alters in shape on respiration, is usually due to a *thymolipoma*. The presence of pleural metastases indicates a malignant thymoma, as these tumours tend to seed around the pleura (Fig. 12.17).

The diagnosis is confirmed by CT, which shows a mass of mixed attenuation containing soft tissue, calcification and cysts. Direct needle puncture of a thymoma with aspiration biopsy can be performed under CT or fluoroscopic guidance to confirm the diagnosis in patients with myasthenia gravis.

TERATODERMOID TUMOURS

The commonest of the **germ cell tumours** in the mediastinum are the *dermoid cyst* and the *benign* and *malignant teratoma*. This group of tumours also includes *choriocarcinomas*, *embryonal cell carcinomas*, *endodermal sinus tumours* and *seminomas*. These tumours are all thought to arise from primitive germ cell rests in the urogenital ridge. The dermoid cyst consists mainly of ectodermal tissues, whereas the solid teratoma usually contains tissues of ectodermal, mesodermal and endodermal origin. About 30% of teratodermoid tumours are malignant.

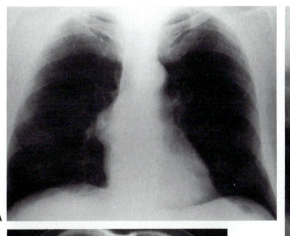

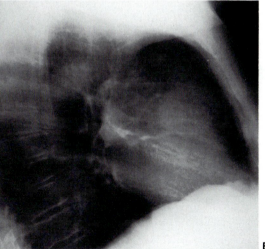

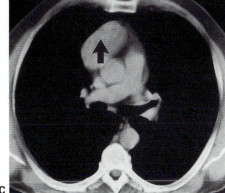

Fig. 12.16 Thymoma. 55-year-old man presenting with hypertension due to a phaeochromocytoma. PA (**A**) and lateral films (**B**) show a round mass in the anterior mediastinum overlying the right hilum. CT scan with contrast enhancement (L +50, W 500) (**C**) at the level of the tracheal bifurcation shows an oval mass of soft tissue density (arrow), 7 cm in size, in the anterior mediastinum. Diagnosis confirmed by surgery.

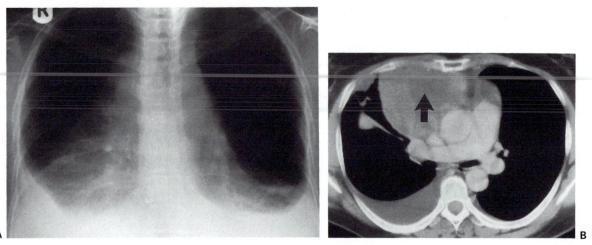

Fig. 12.17   Malignant thymoma. 43-year-old presenting with chest pain and dyspnoea. PA film (**A**) shows widening of the mediastinum on the right with bilateral pleural effusions. CT scan with enhancement (L +50, W 500) (**B**) at the level of the tracheal bifurcation shows an oval mass of mixed density (arrow), 9 cm in size, in the anterior mediastinum with a small pleural mass anteriorly on the right. Diagnosis confirmed by needle biopsy and surgery.

A teratodermoid tumour usually presents as an anterior mediastinal mass on a chest radiograph in a young adult patient. The tumour is often asymptomatic but can produce dyspnoea, cough and chest pain, and may become infected to form an abscess, which can rupture into the mediastinum, the pleural cavity or the bronchial tree. The striking diagnostic symptom of trichoptysis is rare.

A benign dermoid cyst appears as a round or oval soft-tissue mass, which usually projects to only one side of the anterior mediastinum. The outline is well defined, but becomes irregular in very large tumours due to peripheral atelectasis in the surrounding compressed lung (Fig. 12.18). The soft-tissue mass may also contain a peripheral rim or central nodules of calcification, a fat–fluid level or a rudimentary tooth, which is of course a diagnostic radiological sign. Rapid increase in the size of

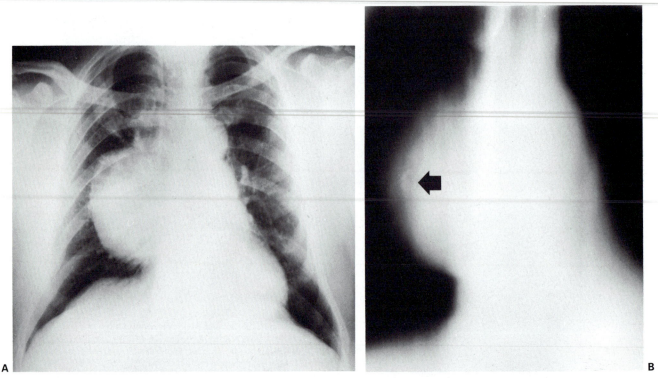

Fig. 12.18   Benign teratoma. 65-year-old man presenting with chest pain. PA film (**A**) and AP tomogram (**B**) show a large round mass which contains calcification (arrow) in the anterior mediastinum overlying the right hilum. Diagnosis confirmed by surgery.

the mass indicates either internal haemorrhage or the development of malignancy. An air–fluid level is present after rupture of an infected cyst into the bronchial tree. A malignant teratoma appears as a lobulated soft-tissue mass, which projects on both sides of the anterior mediastinum. The diagnosis is confirmed by CT, which shows a mass of mixed attenuation containing soft tissue, cyst fluid, fat, calcification or bone. Rarely, a teratodermoid tumour may occur in the posterior mediastinum.

FAT DEPOSITION

The excessive deposition of fat in the mediastinum usually presents as an incidental finding, with widening of the superior part of the mediastinum and large epicardial fat pads on a chest radiograph in an obese adult patient. This can also occur in patients with Cushing's syndrome, and in patients receiving long-term high-dose corticosteroid treatment. Steroids cause mobilization of body fat with its subsequent redistribution in the anterior mediastinum and cardiophrenic angles. This widening of the mediastinum can be difficult to differentiate from mediastinal haemorrhage, lymphadenopathy or a dissecting aortic aneurysm. The diagnosis is easily confirmed by CT, which shows an excessive amount of mediastinal fat (Fig. 12.19).

PLEUROPERICARDIAL CYST

A pleuropericardial cyst usually presents as an anterior (or middle) mediastinal mass on a chest radiograph in an asymptomatic adult patient. About 75% of pleuropericardial cysts occur in the right anterior cardiophrenic angle (Fig. 12.20). The cysts have thin walls lined by mesothelial cells and contain clear fluid (hence their name of 'spring-water' cysts). They appear as a round, oval or

triangular soft-tissue mass in the anterior or middle mediastinum and can alter in shape on respiration. The *differential diagnosis* of a soft tissue lesion in the right anterior cardiophrenic angle includes an epicardial fat pad, a partial eventration of the right hemidiaphragm, right middle lobe or pleural pathology, a Morgagni hernia and a right atrial or pericardial tumour.

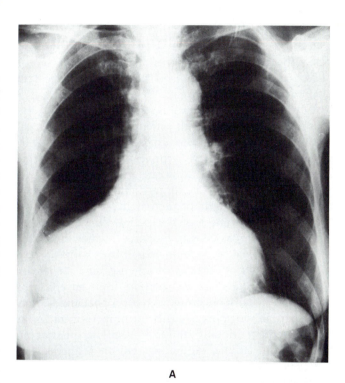

A

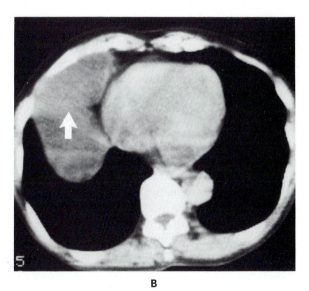

B

Fig. 12.20 Pleuropericardial cyst. 72-year-old woman presenting with dyspnoea. PA film (**A**) shows a large oval mass in the right cardiophrenic angle and CT scan (L +40, W 512) (**B**) below the tracheal bifurcation shows an oval mass (arrow) 10 cm in size, separate from the heart in the anterior and middle mediastinum. The density of the mass (average +9 HU) is typical of cyst fluid.

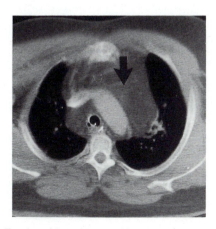

Fig. 12.19 Fat deposition. 40-year-old man presenting with chest pain after a road traffic accident and a widened mediastinum on a chest film. CT with contrast enhancement (L +50, W 750) above the tracheal bifurcation shows excess deposition of fat throughout the mediastinum, particularly anteriorly (arrow).

The diagnosis is confirmed by either *ultrasound*, which shows a transonic mass adjacent to the pericardium, or *CT*, which shows a thin-walled cyst containing fluid of low attenuation (0–20 HU) (Fig. 12.20). Direct needle puncture of a pleuropericardial cyst with aspiration of its fluid contents can be performed under CT or ultrasonic guidance.

MORGAGNI HERNIA

The foramen of Morgagni is a persistent developmental defect in the diaphragm anteriorly, between the septum transversum and the right and left costal origins of the diaphragm. A hernia through the foramen of Morgagni usually presents as an anterior mediastinal mass on a chest radiograph in an adult patient. The hernia is usually asymptomatic, but can produce retrosternal chest pain, epigastric discomfort and dyspnoea. Strangulation of the contents of the hernial sac is rare.

More than 90% of Morgagni hernias are situated in the right anterior cardiophrenic angle (Fig. 12.21), due to the protective effect of the pericardium on the left. The smaller hernias contain omentum, which appears as a round or oval soft-tissue mass, but with a lower radiographic density than would be expected for its size. This can be difficult to differentiate from an epicardial fat pad, a pleuropericardial cyst or right middle lobe pathology, although occasionally the properitoneal fat line can be seen continuing upwards from the anterior abdominal wall around the hernial sac on a lateral chest film. The larger hernias usually contain transverse colon, which appears as a soft-tissue mass containing either gas or an air–fluid level, but they can also contain liver, stomach or small intestine.

The diagnosis is confirmed by a barium meal and follow-through or a barium enema, which shows either upward tenting of the transverse colon towards the hernia or a loop of transverse colon above the diaphragm within the chest. The contents of the hernia are also easily confirmed by CT (Fig. 12.21).

PARATHYROID ADENOMA

An adenoma in an ectopic parathyroid gland in the chest usually presents with hypercalcaemia in an adult patient with hyperparathyroidism. It is a rare tumour, that occurs in the superior part of the anterior mediastinum, but due to its small size at presentation the mediastinum appears normal on a chest radiograph. It is also difficult to identify at CT. The diagnosis is confirmed by *a radionuclide scan*, using ^{201}Tl thallium chloride, with computerized subtraction of the thyroid image (using ^{99m}Tc sodium pertechnetate) to leave the parathyroid image, which shows an area of increased activity in the anterior mediastinum (Fig. 12.22).

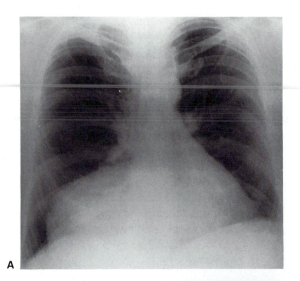

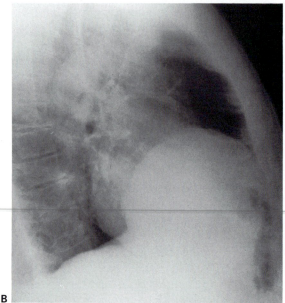

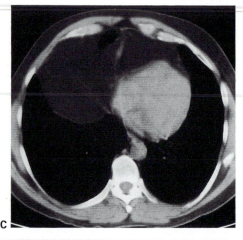

Fig. 12.21 Morgagni hernia. Asymptomatic 49-year-old man. PA (**A**) and lateral films (**B**) show a large round mass in the right cardiophrenic angle. CT scan (L +50, W 500) (**C**) below the tracheal bifurcation shows an oval mass of fat density, 18 cm in size, which contains transverse colon in the anterior mediastinum.

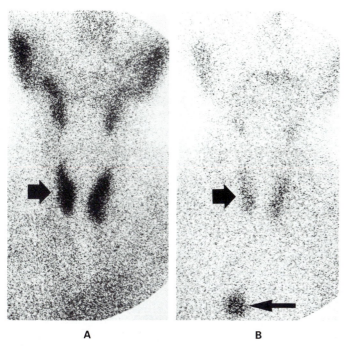

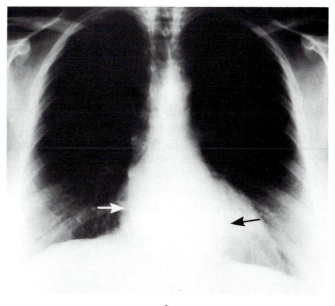

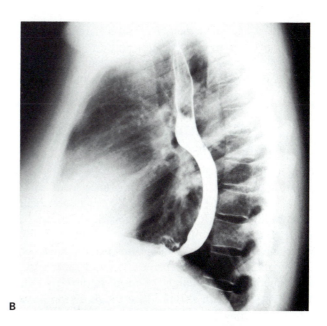

Fig. 12.22 Parathyroid adenoma. 64-year-old woman presenting with hyper-calcaemia. Radionuclide scans with ^{99m}Tc (**A**) and ^{201}Tl (**B**) show activity in the salivary glands and thyroid gland ($\rightarrow$) and in the parathyroid adenoma in the mediastinum ($\leftarrow$). The latter is shown only on the thallium scan, even without computerized subtraction of scan A from scan B.

LYMPHANGIOMA

A lymphangioma or cystic hygroma usually presents as a soft-tissue swelling that transilluminates in the root of the neck in children. It is a rare mesenchymal tumour that occurs in the superior part of the anterior mediastinum and it appears as an oval soft-tissue mass, which extends up into the neck and can alter in shape on respiration, but does not displace the trachea. An associated chylothorax may also occur. The diagnosis is confirmed by ultrasound or CT.

LIPOMA

A lipoma usually presents as an incidental mediastinal lesion on a chest radiograph in an asymptomatic adult patient. It is also a rare mesenchymal tumour, which occurs in the anterior (or posterior) mediastinum. It appears as a round or oval soft-tissue mass with a lower radiographic density than would be expected for its size, which can alter in shape on respiration (Fig. 12.23).

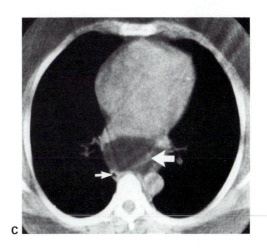

Fig. 12.23 Lipoma. Asymptomatic 42-year-old woman. PA film (**A**) and barium swallow (**B**) show an oval mass with less density than expected for its size, particularly in the lateral view, behind the heart. **C.** CT scan (L −150, W 800) below the tracheal bifurcation shows an oval mass of fat density ($\leftarrow$), 8 cm in size, in the posterior mediastinum, with displacement of the oesophagus ($\rightarrow$) to the right. (A and B courtesy of Dr P. Ho and C courtesy of Dr T. J. Bloomberg).

Malignant degeneration into a liposarcoma may also occur. The diagnosis is confirmed by CT, which shows a solid mass of tissue of fatty attenuation (−50 to −100 HU) (Fig. 12.23).

OTHER RARE ANTERIOR MEDIASTINAL MASSES

Apart from lymphangioma, lipoma and liposarcoma, other tumours of mesenchymal origin can also occur in the mediastinum and these include *fibroma*, *fibrosarcoma*, *haemangioma*, *haemangiopericytoma* and *haemangio-endothelioma*. About 50% of mesenchymal tumours are malignant.

The small benign tumours are usually asymptomatic, whereas the large benign tumours and the malignant tumours tend to produce symptoms such as retrosternal chest pain, back pain or dysphagia, depending upon their anatomical location. They appear as a round or oval soft-tissue mass in the anterior (or posterior) mediastinum or as widening of the mediastinum. The presence of phleboliths is of course diagnostic of a haemangioma.

A *plasmacytoma* of the sternum and an *osteochondroma* or a *chondrosarcoma* of a rib may also result in a tumour mass that involves the anterior mediastinum.

MIDDLE MEDIASTINAL MASSES

LYMPH NODE ENLARGEMENT

Lymph nodes occur in the anterior, middle and posterior mediastinum but are found predominantly in its middle division, where the paratracheal, tracheobronchial, bronchopulmonary (hilar) and subcarinal groups are situated (Fig 11.16).

Enlargement of lymph-node groups usually presents as a middle mediastinal mass on a chest radiograph in an adult patient. The enlarged lymph nodes are often asymptomatic, but can also produce cough, dyspnoea and weight loss or may be associated with generalized lymphadenopathy. There are many causes of enlargement of the mediastinal lymph-node groups and these include metastatic disease, lymphoma, leukaemia, sarcoidosis, tuberculosis, histoplasmosis and other infections and granulomas.

Metastatic disease can produce enlargement of any of the lymph-node groups within the mediastinum. The primary tumour is usually intrathoracic, such as a bronchial or oesophageal carcinoma, but may occasionally be extrathoracic in origin — breast carcinoma, renal carcinoma, adrenal tumours, testicular tumours and tumours of the pharynx and larynx. Associated pulmonary metastases or lymphangitis carcinomatosa are also frequently present. A bronchial carcinoma situated either peripherally or centrally in the lung metastasizes early to the mediastinal lymph nodes, producing either a unilateral hilar mass with an irregular outline (due to surrounding infiltration, atelectasis or consolidation), or widening of the superior part of the middle mediastinum due to superior vena caval compression syndrome. A bronchial carcinoma is the commonest primary tumour to metastasize to the mediastinal lymph nodes. A carcinoma of the breast may involve the lymph nodes of the internal mammary chain in the anterior mediastinum, and an oesophageal carcinoma may involve the posterior mediastinal lymph nodes. A renal carcinoma or an adrenal neuroblastoma can metastasize to the hilar lymph nodes, usually on the right, whereas a testicular teratoma or seminoma usually metastasizes to the paratracheal lymph nodes.

Hodgkin's disease, the **non-Hodgkin's lymphomas** (including Castleman's disease) and the lymphatic leukaemias usually involve the paratracheal and tracheo-bronchial lymph nodes, producing an asymmetrical bilateral widening of the superior part of the middle mediastinum. Involvement of the subcarinal lymph nodes splays the carina and unilateral or bilateral hilar masses can also occur. The lymphomas, particularly Hodgkin's disease, also frequently involve the anterior mediastinum, producing a lobulated soft-tissue mass due to indentation by the anterior ribs (Fig. 12.24). Parenchymal lung disease may also occur, and lymph node calcification occasionally develops in Hodgkin's disease after irradiation.

Radiotherapy to the mediastinum produces a reduction in the size of lymph-node masses in metastatic diseases

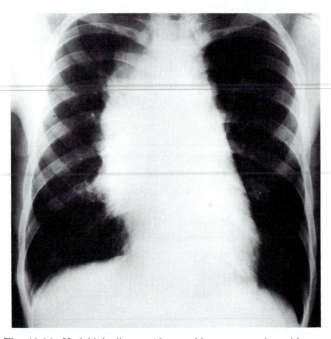

Fig. 12.24 Hodgkin's disease. 18-year-old man presenting with cervical lymphadenopathy. PA film shows asymmetrical lobulated widening of the mediastinum, due to involvement of the middle and anterior mediastinal lymph nodes, particularly on the right.

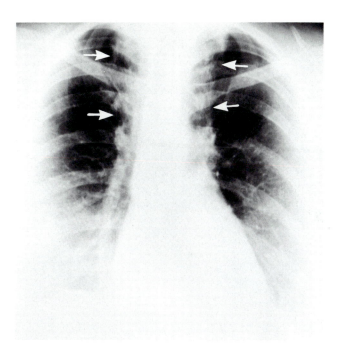

Fig. 12.25 Radiotherapy to the mediastinum. Asymptomatic 40-year-old woman with Hodgkin's disease in remission treated with mediastinal radiotherapy several years ago. PA film shows widening of the superior part of the mediastinum due to radiation fibrosis extending into the lungs (arrows).

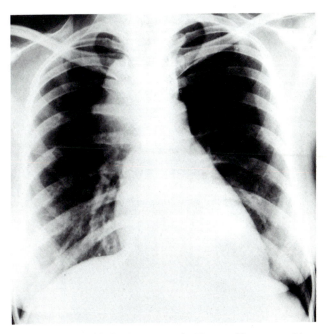

Fig. 12.26 Tuberculosis. Asymptomatic 29-year-old woman with chronic renal disease treated with immunosuppressive drugs. PA film shows a right paratracheal mass of enlarged lymph nodes in the middle mediastinum.

which respond to radiation, such as lymphoma and seminoma during treatment, but may also produce a *chronic mediastinitis* with *fibrosis* extending into the lungs. This is quite characteristic and appears as a straight line, widening the mediastinum on both sides and corresponding to the treatment field (Fig. 12.25). This mediastinal fibrosis may also develop at lower therapeutic doses in patients who are also receiving cytotoxic chemotherapy, particularly cyclophosphamide.

Sarcoidosis typically causes enlargement of the bronchopulmonary lymph nodes, producing bilateral lobulated hilar masses with well-defined outlines. Sarcoid granulomas also frequently involve the tracheobronchial, right paratracheal and left aortopulmonary lymph nodes. Parenchymal lung disease commonly develops, and peripheral calcification occasionally occurs in the lymph nodes.

Primary tuberculous infection of the lung in children or young adult patients produces an area of consolidation in one of the lobes, with a unilateral hilar mass and an associated pleural effusion. Calcification may develop in both the primary Ghon focus and the mediastinal lymph nodes as healing occurs. Tuberculosis can also produce a unilateral paratracheal mass of lymph nodes without obvious pulmonary or pleural involvement (Fig. 12.26). This type of infection occurs in the adult immigrant population and in patients who are immunosuppressed.

In the USA, **fungal infection** such as *histoplasmosis*, *coccidioidomycosis* and *blastomycosis* may produce enlargement of the hilar or paratracheal lymph nodes. Calcification may also develop in the lymph nodes in healing histoplasmosis. The only fungus in the UK which causes unilateral hilar lymphadenopathy is *actinomycosis* and this can be difficult to differentiate from a bronchial carcinoma.

There are many other inflammatory causes of unilateral or bilateral lymphadenopathy and these include *infectious mononucleosis* or glandular fever, *measles*, *whooping cough*, *mycoplasma* infection, *adenoviruses* and a *pyogenic lung abscess*. Peripheral calcification may occur in the hilar nodes in patients with *silicosis* and patients with *cystic fibrosis* may have enlarged hilar shadows due to enlarged lymph nodes or cor pulmonale.

The diagnosis of mediastinal lymph node enlargement is usually apparent on the chest radiographs, but can be confirmed by CT, which shows the lymph-node masses of soft-tissue attenuation distinct from the contrast-enhanced vascular structures (Fig. 12.27). Low-attenuation areas due to cyst formation or necrosis are occasionally seen in lymph nodes involved with Hodgkin's disease and metastatic testicular or squamous cell tumours, particularly after treatment with radiotherapy or chemotherapy.

AORTIC ANEURYSM

The thoracic aorta passes through all the anatomical divisions of the mediastinum and the great vessels arising

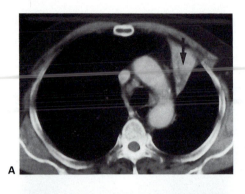

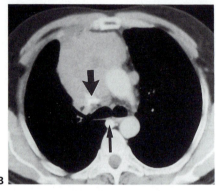

Fig. 12.27 A. Carcinoma of the bronchus. 67-year-old man presenting with haemoptysis and left upper lobe collapse seen on a chest film. CT scan with contrast enhancement (L +50, W 500) above the tracheal bifurcation shows the left upper lobe collapse (↓) and two lymph nodes (both less than 10 mm in diameter) found to be involved with tumour at mediastinoscopy. **B.** Non-Hodgkin's lymphoma. 56-year-old man presenting with superior vena caval compression syndrome and a widened mediastinum on a chest film. CT scan with contrast enhancement (L +50, W 500) at the level of the tracheal bifurcation shows a round mass of mixed soft-tissue density, 9 cm in size, in the anterior and middle mediastinum with compression of the superior vena cava (↓) and contrast medium filling the dilated azygos vein (↑). Diagnosis confirmed by surgical biopsy.

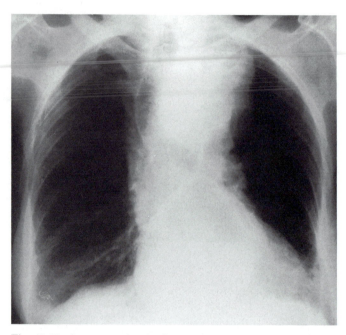

Fig. 12.28 Aneurysm of arch of aorta and hiatus hernia. 83-year-old woman presenting with dyspnoea and hypertension. PA film shows a large round mass, which has some calcification in its wall, in the middle mediastinum, with displacement of the trachea to the right, and another large round mass containing an air–fluid level behind the heart in the posterior mediastinum.

from it lie in the superior part of the mediastinum. Abnormalities of the aorta and great vessels usually present as a mediastinal mass or widening of the mediastinum on a chest radiograph in an elderly patient. An unfolded aorta or a tortuous innominate artery are usually asymptomatic but aortic aneurysms can produce chest pain, back pain, aortic incompetence, hoarseness and dysphagia. There are many causes of aneurysm of the thoracic aorta and these include atherosclerosis, hypertension, blunt chest trauma, syphilitic aortitis, a mycotic origin and congenital anomalies such as coarctation of the aorta, Marfan's syndrome and Ehlers-Danlos syndrome.

Aortic aneurysms produce either widening of the mediastinum or a round or oval soft tissue mass in any part of the mediastinum with a well-defined outline and sometimes a peripheral rim of calcification (Figs 12.28, 12.29). Curvilinear calcification in an ascending aortic aneurysm can be due to either syphilitic aortitis or atherosclerosis.

Displacement of the peripheral rim of calcification away from the wall of the aorta indicates a dissection. On fluoroscopy, aortic aneurysms appear as pulsatile masses, but this is not a diagnostic radiological sign because any mass lesion adjacent to the aorta transmits its pulsation. Aortic aneurysms may also involve adjacent bones, producing a pressure erosion defect of the sternum or anterior scalloping of one or two vertebral bodies.

The diagnosis can be confirmed by thoracic aortography or digital subtraction angiography but preferably by CT, which shows a dilated aorta containing a lumen of blood of high attenuation, due to contrast enhancement of the blood pool with water-soluble contrast medium (80–100 HU) and a layer of clot of lower attenuation on the wall of the aorta, which may contain calcification (Fig. 12.30) or by MRI (Fig. 12.10). The subintimal flap and false lumen of a *dissecting aortic aneurysm* can also be demonstrated by CT. Dissecting aortic aneurysms are now classified as Type A if they involve the ascending aorta (including the arch and descending aorta) and Type B if they only involve the descending aorta (see Ch. 25).

A *tortuous innominate artery* occurs in about 20% of elderly patients with hypertension and produces widening of the superior part of the mediastinum on the right without displacement of the trachea to the left. However, a true aneurysm of the innominate or subclavian arteries is a rare cause of a mass in the superior part of the mediastinum.

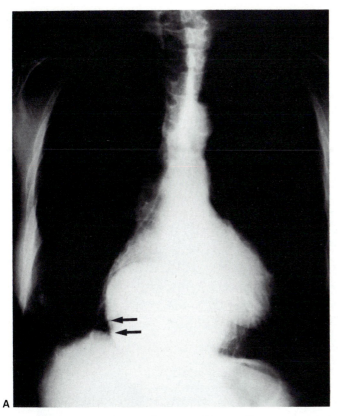
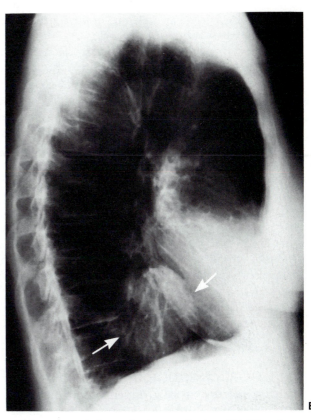

Fig. 12.29 Aneurysm of descending aorta. 59-year-old woman presenting with haematemesis from a benign gastric ulcer. (**A**) PA and (**B**) lateral films show a large round mass, which has some peripheral calcification in its wall (arrows), in the posterior mediastinum behind the heart. Diagnosis confirmed by ultrasound, using the liver as a window into the mediastinum.

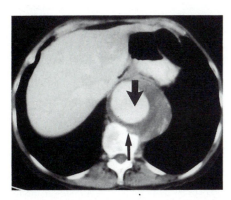

Fig. 12.30 Aneurysm of descending aorta. 45-year-old woman presenting with back pain. CT scan with contrast enhancement (L + 50, W 500) below the tracheal bifurcation shows an aneurysm of the descending aorta (↓), 8 cm in size, which contains thrombus, has calcification in its wall and is eroding the adjacent lower thoracic vertebral body (↑).

The common *tortuous aneurysmal descending thoracic aorta* produces widening of the mediastinum on the left, often at the level of the left hilum. The hilar vessels can be seen through this apparent hilar mass indicating that the descending thoracic aorta lies posterior to the hilum.

Dilatation of the main pulmonary artery can also produce an apparent left hilar mass, but in this case the main pulmonary artery lies anterior to the hilum. The causes of enlargement of the main pulmonary artery include primary or secondary pulmonary arterial hypertension, the poststenotic dilatation of pulmonary valve stenosis and a true pulmonary artery aneurysm.

Coarctation of the aorta, *kinking of the aorta* (pseudocoarctation) and *a right-sided aortic arch* can also produce an abnormal mediastinal configuration. The diagnosis of these other vascular abnormalities is confirmed by CT in some cases or by MRI.

DILATATION OF MEDIASTINAL VEINS

The superior vena cava lies in the middle mediastinum and the azygos vein lies in the posterior mediastinum. Dilatation of the veins in the mediastinum usually presents with cough, dyspnoea and swelling of the ankles in an adult patient.

Dilatation of the superior vena cava is produced by a raised central venous pressure, which occurs in congestive cardiac failure, tricuspid valve disease, constrictive pericarditis, a cardiomyopathy, a right atrial tumour, partial anomalous pulmonary venous drainage (to a right-sided superior vena cava) and a mediastinal tumour with a superior vena caval compression syndrome. A dilated superior vena cava produces widening of the superior part of the middle mediastinum on the right.

The causes of *dilatation of the azygos vein* include a raised central venous pressure, obstruction of the superior or inferior vena cava, portal hypertension and congenital azygos continuation of the inferior vena cava. A dilated azygos vein produces an oval soft-tissue mass in the right tracheobronchial angle. This can be difficult to differentiate from an enlarged azygos lymph node, although the azygos vein alters in size with a change in posture or during the Valsalva manoeuvre.

Total anomalous pulmonary venous drainage (to a right- or left-sided superior vena cava) or an *isolated left-sided superior vena cava* produce an abnormally wide mediastinal configuration, whereas complete transposition of the great vessels produces an unusually narrow mediastinal configuration. A left superior intercostal vein also produces an abnormal mediastinal configuration.

The diagnosis of these venous abnormalities is confirmed by venography but preferably by CT.

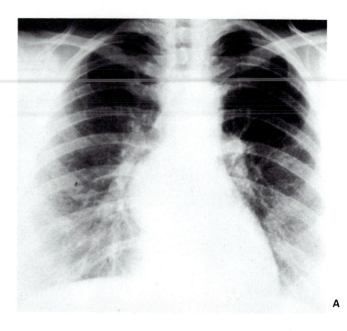

A

BRONCHOGENIC CYST

A bronchogenic cyst usually presents as a middle (or posterior) mediastinal mass on a chest radiograph in a child or young adult patient. The cyst is usually asymptomatic, but can also produce stridor in children and cough, dyspnoea and chest pain in adults. Infection with rupture into the bronchial tree is rare. The majority of bronchogenic cysts occur around the carina in the paratracheal, tracheobronchial or subcarinal regions. The cysts have thin walls lined by ciliated columnar epithelium of respiratory origin and contain mucoid material. They appear as a round or oval soft-tissue mass in the middle mediastinum, frequently on the right near the carina (Fig. 12.31), and can alter in shape on respiration. Rapid increase in the size of the mass indicates internal haemorrhage. An air–fluid level is present after rupture of an infected cyst into the bronchial tree.

The diagnosis is suggested by CT, which shows a mass containing fluid of either low attenuation (0–10 HU) or soft-tissue attenuation (10–50 HU) (Fig. 12.32), but is usually confirmed at surgery. A pericardial defect may occur in association with a bronchogenic cyst.

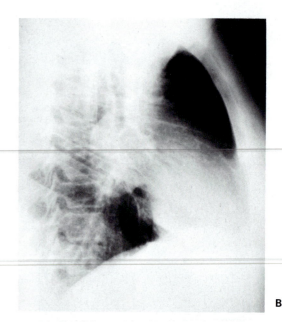

B

Fig. 12.31 Bronchogenic cyst. Asymptomatic 21-year-old woman. (**A**) PA and (**B**) lateral films show an oval mass in the middle mediastinum below the carina on the right. Diagnosis confirmed by surgery.

RARE MIDDLE MEDIASTINAL LESIONS

Tracheal tumours include *carcinoma*, *cylindroma* and *plasmacytoma* and usually present with stridor in an adult patient. They are rare tumours, which occur in the middle mediastinum. They appear as narrowing of the tracheal lumen by a small soft-tissue mass. The diagnosis is confirmed by conventional tomography or CT.

Tracheobronchomegaly or the Mounier-Kuhn syndrome,

and *tracheomalacia* may produce widening of the superior part of the mediastinum due to dilatation of the trachea.

POSTERIOR MEDIASTINAL MASSES

NEUROGENIC TUMOURS

The commonest of the neurogenic tumours in the mediastinum in adults are the *neurofibroma* and the *neurilemmoma* (or Schwannoma), which develop from

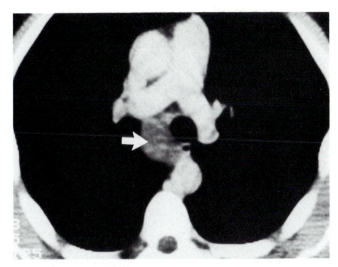

Fig. 12.32 Bronchogenic cyst. 25-year-old man presenting with cough. CT scan with contrast enhancement (L +40, W 512) at the level of the tracheal bifurcation shows a round mass (→), 3 cm in size, in the middle mediastinum. The density of the mass (average + 45HU) is typical of mucoid material.

the peripheral intercostal nerves; the *ganglioneuroma* and the *neuroblastoma*, which arise in the thoracic sympathetic ganglia, are the commonest of the neurogenic tumours in the mediastinum in children. This group of tumours also includes *neurofibrosarcomas*, *phaeochromocytomas* and *chemodactomas*, which occur in paraganglionic nerve tissue. About 30% of neurogenic tumours are malignant.

A neurogenic tumour usually presents as a posterior mediastinal mass on a chest radiograph in a child or young adult patient. The tumour is often asymptomatic but can produce back pain and may extend through an intervertebral foramen into the spinal canal (hence their name of 'dumb-bell' tumours) to produce a spinal cord compression syndrome. A neurofibroma or neurofibrosarcoma in the mediastinum may be part of the generalized *neurofibromatosis* of Von Recklinghausen's disease, but remember that a mediastinal mass in this neurocutaneous disease can also be caused by a *lateral thoracic meningocoele*.

A neurogenic tumour appears as a round or oval soft tissue mass with a well-defined outline in the paravertebral gutter, which usually projects to only one side of the posterior mediastinum (Fig. 12.33). A ganglioneuroma may appear as a rather elongated soft-tissue mass, in comparison to the more circular appearance of the neurofibroma, due to its extensive mediastinal origin. A neuroblastoma may contain central spicules or a peripheral rim of calcification. This can also occur in neurofibrosarcomas and ganglioneuromas. However, calcification is generally not a feature of the benign neurogenic tumours and does not occur in the mediastinal lymph-node metastases from an adrenal neuroblastoma.

Neurogenic tumours may also involve the posterior ribs or adjacent thoracic vertebrae. The benign tumours can produce splaying of several posterior ribs, a localized

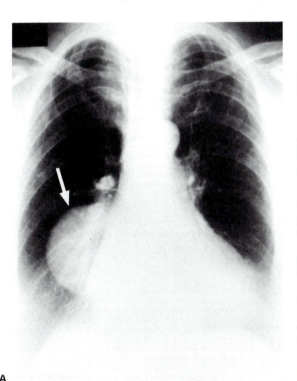
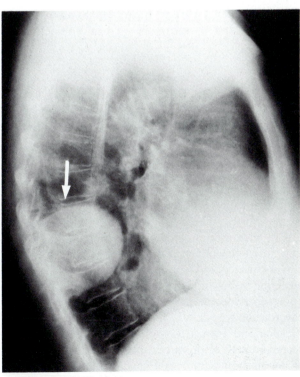

Fig. 12.33 Neurofibroma. Asymptomatic 57-year-old woman. (A) PA and (B) lateral films show a round mass in the posterior mediastinum behind the heart on the right. Lateral tomogram showed enlargement of the intervertebral foramen.

pressure erosion defect of one or two vertebral bodies, and of course rib notching. A bony destructive process indicates a malignant tumour. Enlargement of an intervertebral foramen is diagnostic of a dumb-bell neurogenic tumour, usually a neurofibroma. Rapid increase in the size of the mass or an associated pleural effusion indicates malignant degeneration.

The diagnosis is confirmed by CT, which shows a solid mass of soft-tissue attenuation which may contain calcification and involve the adjacent bones, or by MRI (Fig. 12.12). Intraspinal extension is easily demonstrated by computer-assisted myelography or MRI. Rarely a neurogenic tumour may occur in the anterior or middle mediastinum.

HIATUS HERNIA

A fixed or irreducible hiatus hernia is one of the commonest causes of a mediastinal mass and usually presents as a posterior mediastinal mass on a chest radiograph in an elderly patient. The hernia is often asymptomatic, but can produce dyspnoea, retrosternal chest pain and epigastric discomfort. Incarceration of the stomach is rare.

A hiatus hernia appears as a round soft-tissue mass containing an air–fluid level directly behind the heart, which lies to the left of the midline in the posterior mediastinum in about 70% of cases. The larger hernias can also contain liver, omentum and small intestine.

The diagnosis is easily confirmed by a penetrated PA film, a lateral film or a barium meal, which shows the stomach above the diaphragm within the chest (Fig. 11.84).

OESOPHAGEAL LESIONS

Lesions of the oesophagus usually present with dysphagia in an adult patient, but can also produce an aspiration pneumonitis, due to spilling over of the oesophageal contents into the trachea and main bronchi.

A *pharyngo-oesophageal pouch* or Zenker's diverticulum is produced by herniation of the pharyngo-oesophageal mucosa through Killihan's dehiscence, usually on the left, between the muscle fibres of the inferior constrictor muscle. The mediastinum appears normal on a chest radiograph when the pouch is small, but a large pouch appears as a round soft-tissue mass in the superior part of the posterior mediastinum, which contains an air–fluid level. The soft-tissue mass lies in the midline and displaces the trachea forwards.

A *carcinoma* and even a *leiomyoma* of the oesophagus may be large enough to produce a soft-tissue mass in the posterior mediastinum, and a large diverticulum of the lower oesophagus occasionally produces a soft tissue mass containing an air–fluid level behind the heart.

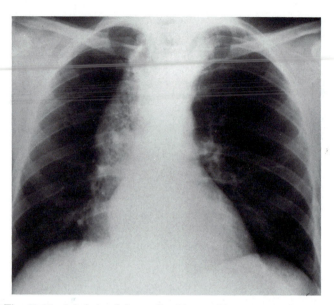

Fig. 12.34 Achalasia of the cardia. 31-year-old man presenting with dysphagia. PA film shows a dilated oesophagus containing food behind the heart on the right, with absence of air in the gastric fundus. Diagnosis confirmed by barium swallow.

There are several causes of a dilated or *mega-oesophagus*, and these include *achalasia* of the cardia, a *benign oesophageal stricture*, a *carcinoma* of the oesophagus, *presbyoesophagus*, *systemic sclerosis* and South American *trypanosomiasis* or *Chagas' disease*. The oesophagus dilates proximal to the long-standing obstruction or due to the degeneration of Auerbach's plexus in its wall. A mega-oesophagus produces widening of the posterior mediastinum behind the heart on the right, extending from the thoracic inlet to the diaphragm (Fig. 12.34). There is often an air–fluid level in the superior part of the posterior mediastinum, with the non-homogeneous mottled appearance of food particles mixed with air beneath it and no air in the fundus of the stomach. There may also be patchy pneumonic consolidation, bronchiectasis or even, occasionally, pulmonary fibrosis in both lower lobes, due to the recurrent aspiration pneumonitis.

The diagnosis of all oesophageal lesions is confirmed by a barium swallow, which can also be useful in the investigation of other posterior mediastinal masses. The dilated oesophagus is also easily confirmed by CT.

Oesophageal lesions are discussed in more detail in Chapter 28.

PARAVERTEBRAL LESIONS

Paravertebral lesions of the dorsal spine usually present with back pain in an adult patient. Apart from *neurogenic tumours*, which have been discussed above, the differential diagnosis of a paravertebral mass includes a traumatic wedge *compression fracture* of a vertebral body *with haematoma* formation, a pyogenic or tuberculous *paraspinal abscess, multiple myeloma, disseminated lymphoma, metastatic carcinoma with paraspinal extension* and *extramedullary haemopoiesis*, which will be discussed below.

They appear as an elongated or lobulated soft-tissue mass with a well-defined outline, which usually projects on both sides of the posterior mediastinum (Fig. 12.35). Paravertebral masses also usually involve the adjacent thoracic vertebrae or intervertebral disc spaces. This allows the radiologist to differentiate between the inflammatory lesions, which usually produce narrowing of the intervertebral disc space as well as bone destruction, and the neoplastic lesions, which only produce bone destruction.

The diagnosis is confirmed by a penetrated PA film, or CT (Fig. 12.35). Direct needle puncture of a paravertebral mass with aspiration biopsy can be performed under CT or fluoroscopic guidance to establish the exact diagnosis.

BOCHDALEK HERNIA

The foramen of Bochdalek is a persistent developmental defect in the diaphragm posteriorly, produced by a failure of the pleuroperitoneal canal membrane to fuse with the dorsal oesophageal mesentery medially and the body wall laterally. A hernia through the foramen of Bochdalek usually presents either with acute respiratory distress in the neonatal period or as a posterior mediastinal mass in an adult patient. The hernia is usually asymptomatic in an adult patient, but can produce abdominal discomfort. Strangulation of the herniating bowel is rare.

About 90% of Bochdalek hernias occur in the left hemidiaphragm, because of the protective effect of the liver on the right. The smaller hernias usually contain retroperitoneal fat, kidney or spleen, which appears as a soft-tissue mass in the posterior costophrenic angle. The smaller hernias can also contain the splenic flexure of the colon (Fig. 12.36).

The larger hernias contain jejunum, ileum and colon, which appears as multiple ring shadows in the hemithorax. The air-filled loops of bowel in the chest produce displacement of the heart and mediastinum into the contralateral hemithorax and a compressed hypoplastic lung in the ipsilateral hemithorax. The larger hernias can also contain liver.

The diagnosis is confirmed by a barium meal and follow-through, which shows loops of small intestine and colon within the hemithorax (Fig. 12.36). A radionuclide scan, ultrasound or intravenous urography can confirm the diagnosis by showing liver, spleen or kidney above the diaphragm. The contents of the hernia are also easily confirmed by CT. Thirteen pairs of ribs may occur in association with a Bochdalek hernia.

NEUROENTERIC CYSTS

The developmental anomalies produced by partial or complete persistence of the neuroenteric canal or its incomplete resorption include *gastrointestinal reduplications, enteric cysts, neuroenteric cysts, anterior meningocoeles* and *cysts of the cord.*

A neuroenteric cyst usually presents with respiratory distress or feeding difficulties in infants, whereas an anterior meningocoele is usually asymptomatic. An enteric cyst may produce chest pain in children or young adult patients if peptic ulceration occurs within it. Infection with rupture into the oesophagus is rare. These rare developmental cysts are closely related not only to the oesophagus, to which there may be fibrous attachments, but also to the thoracic spine, in which there may be congenital bony abnormalities such as block vertebra,

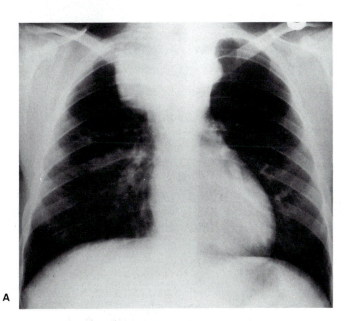

A

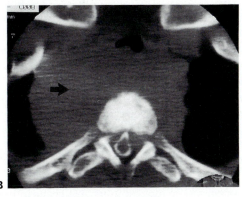

B

Fig. 12.35 Metastatic Ewing's sarcoma paravertebral mass. 22-year-old man presenting with spastic paraparesis. **A.** PA film shows an asymmetric paravertebral mass in the posterior mediastinum. **B.** CT scan after myelography (L +175, W 1400) shows an osteoblastic bone metastasis of the upper thoracic vertebral body of D2 with an associated paravertebral soft tissue mass (arrow), which is compressing the trachea and the spinal canal.

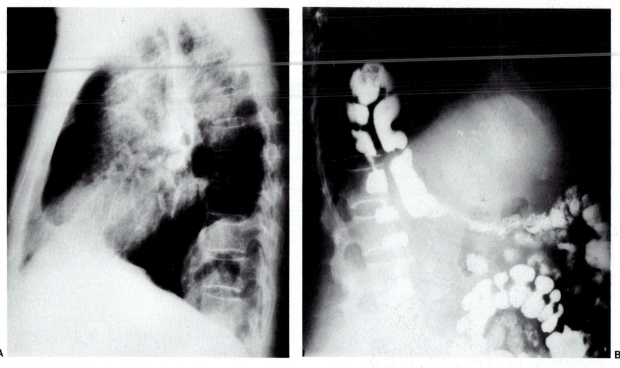

Fig. 12.36 Bochdalek hernia. Asymptomatic 65-year-old man. **A**. The lateral film shows an oval mass, which contains a loop of bowel, in the left posterior costophrenic angle. **B**. Barium meal and follow-through showed the splenic flexure of the colon within the hernia.

hemivertebra and butterfly vertebra (hence the split notochord syndrome). The cysts have thin walls lined by stratified squamous epithelium or ciliated columnar epithelium of both gastrointestinal and notochordal or neural origin and contain fluid material. They appear as a round or oval soft-tissue mass in the posterior mediastinum, frequently on the right. An air–fluid level is present after rupture of an infected cyst into the oesophagus.

The diagnosis of a meningocoele is confirmed by computer-assisted myelography, which shows the contrast medium entering the meningocoele in the prone position. The diagnosis of an enteric cyst is occasionally confirmed by a barium swallow, if the barium sulphate actually enters the cyst. The diagnosis of neuroenteric cysts may be suggested by CT, which shows a mass of soft-tissue attenuation, but is usually confirmed by surgery.

PANCREATIC PSEUDOCYST

A pseudocyst of the pancreas extending through the oesophageal or aortic hiatus into the chest usually presents with dyspnoea or dysphagia in an adult patient with acute pancreatitis. It is a rare abnormality which occurs in the posterior mediastinum and it appears as a round or oval soft-tissue mass behind the heart. A left basal pleural effusion or atelectasis in the lower lobes may also occur. The diagnosis is confirmed by CT, which shows a thin-walled cystic mass containing fluid of low attenuation (0–20 HU) extending from the abdomen into the chest through the aortic hiatus, behind the diaphragmatic crura.

EXTRAMEDULLARY HAEMOPOIESIS

Extramedullary haemopoiesis in the chest usually presents as an incidental mediastinal lesion on a chest radiograph in children or young adult patients with a chronic haemolytic anaemia, such as thalassaemia major. It is a rare abnormality which occurs in the posterior mediastinum and it appears as a lobulated paravertebral soft-tissue mass behind the heart. The diagnosis is confirmed by a penetrated PA film or CT. Extramedullary haemopoiesis may also occur in myelofibrosis.

OTHER RARE POSTERIOR MEDIASTINAL LESIONS

Apart from mesenchymal tumours, which have been discussed above, oesophageal varices and a cyst of the thoracic duct may produce a soft-tissue mass in the posterior mediastinum. An osteochondroma or a chondrosarcoma of a vertebra or rib may also result in a tumour mass that involves the posterior mediastinum.

OTHER MEDIASTINAL LESIONS

PNEUMOMEDIASTINUM

Air in the mediastinum usually presents as an incidental finding on a radiograph in an asymptomatic child or adult patient, but it may produce chest pain, which is made worse by breathing or swallowing. The air usually tracks upwards into the root of the neck to produce surgical emphysema. There are many causes of a *pneumomediastinum* and these include:

1. Perforation of the oesophagus following endoscopy, dilatation of a stricture or insertion of an Atkinson or Celestin tube, or after prolonged vomiting as in the Mallory-Weiss syndrome;
2. Rupture of the trachea or main bronchi following bronchoscopy or after blunt chest trauma;
3. After sternotomy;
4. Intermittent positive pressure ventilation, especially in neonates;
5. Asthma;
6. After prolonged coughing, as in whooping cough;
7. During pregnancy, especially at the time of childbirth;
8. Pneumoperitoneum due to any cause.

Air used to be deliberately introduced into the mediastinum during a diagnostic pneumomediastinum and it tracked into the mediastinum after diagnostic presacral pneumography, but today both these procedures are obsolete.

Air in the mediastinum appears as translucent streaks of gas outlining the blood vessels and other structures, with displacement of the parietal layer of the pleura laterally. A large volume of air tracks throughout the

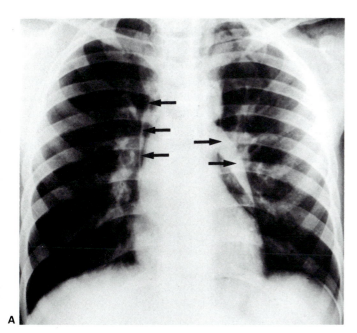

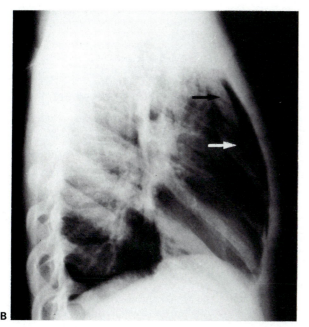

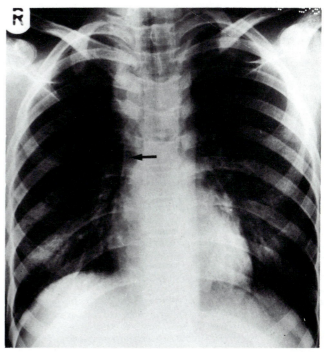

Fig. 12.37 Pneumomediastinum. 12-year-old boy with asthma. PA (**A**) and lateral (**B**) films show air in the mediastinum with displacement of the pleura (←) and demonstration of the thymus gland (→).

Fig. 12.38 Abscess. 15-year-old girl with a short history of pyrexia several days after a pharyngo-oesophageal tear produced by an explosion of a well-known fizzy drink into her mouth as she opened the bottle with her teeth. PA film shows a right paratracheal mass in the middle mediastinum and traces of the resolving mediastinal gas (arrow).

mediastinal tissue planes and up into the neck and so can easily be identified on a PA chest radiograph (Fig. 12.37), but a small volume of air behind the sternum or behind the heart can often only be seen on the lateral film.

The presence of chest pain and fever in a patient with a pneumomediastinum indicates *acute mediastinitis* and this is usually due to perforation of the pharynx, oesophagus or trachea. In addition to the streaks of gas, the mediastinum may be widened by the oedematous mediastinal tissues, which have a hazy outline, and there may be a small pleural effusion. An abscess occasionally develops from acute mediastinitis and appears as a round or oval soft-tissue mass (Fig. 12.38).

Chronic mediastinitis or *mediastinal fibrosis* usually presents with a superior vena caval compression syndrome. The commonest cause of chronic mediastinitis is radiotherapy (Fig. 12.25), but it may also be due to a chronic inflammatory condition such as tuberculosis or histoplasmosis. It can also occur in association with primary idiopathic retroperitoneal fibrosis, Riedel's thyroiditis and drug treatment with methysergide or prac-

tolol. The mediastinum is usually widened and there may be narrowing of the trachea. The diagnosis is confirmed by superior vena cavography or digital subtraction angiography, which shows either complete occlusions or stenoses in the mediastinal veins with retrograde filling of dilated veins such as the jugular, azygos and internal mammary veins (Fig. 26.26).

MEDIASTINAL HAEMORRHAGE

Mediastinal haemorrhage usually presents with widening of the mediastinum on a chest radiograph in a patient who has sustained either blunt or penetrating chest trauma. Mediastinal haemorrhage can also be due to a leaking aortic aneurysm, and can occur in association with bleeding disorders and after anticoagulant or thrombolytic therapy. The diagnosis is confirmed by CT, which is particularly important following trauma as it may also show a spinal fracture, pneumothorax, haemothorax or a false aneurysm. Arch aortography is however still essential in this situation.

REFERENCES AND SUGGESTIONS FOR FURTHER READING

Adler, O. B., Rosenberger, A., Peleg, H. (1983) Fine needle aspiration biopsy of mediastinal masses. *American Journal of Roentgenology*, **140**, 893–896.

Baron, R. L., Lee, J. K. T., Sagel, S. S., Peterson, R. R. (1982) Computed tomography of the normal thymus. *American Journal of Roentgenology*, **142**, 121–125.

Baron, R. L., Levitt, R. G., Sagel, S. S., Stanley, R. J. (1981) Computed tomography in the evaluation of mediastinal widening. *Radiology*, **138**, 107–113.

Cohen, A. M., Creviston, S., Li Puma, J. P., Lieberman, J., Haaga, J. R. Alfidi, R. J. (1983) Nuclear magnetic resonance imaging of the mediastinum and hili. *American Journal of Roentgenology*, **141**, 1163–1169.

Crowe, J. K., Brown, L. R., Muhm, J. R. (1978) Computed tomography of the mediastinum. *Radiology*, **128**, 75–87.

Day, D. L., Gedgaudas, E. (1984) The thymus. *Radiologic Clinics of North America*, **22**, 519–538.

Egan, T. J., Neiman, H. L., Herman, R. J., Malave, S. R., Sanders, J. H. (1980) Computed tomography in the diagnosis of aortic aneurysm dissection or traumatic injury. *Radiology*, **136**, 141–146.

Fon, G. T., Bein, M. E., Mancuso, A. A., Keesey, J. C., Lupetin, A. R., Wong, W. S. (1982) Computed tomography of the anterior mediastinum in myasthenia gravis. *Radiology*, **142**, 135–141.

Gamsu, G., Webb, W. R., Sheldon, P., et al (1983) Nuclear magnetic resonance imaging of the thorax. *Radiology*, **147**, 473–480.

Glazer, H. S. (1989) Differential diagnosis of mediastinal pathology. *CT Review*, **1**, 41–51.

Heitzman, E. R., Goldwin, R. L., Proto, A. V. (1977) Radiological analysis of the mediastinum utilizing computed tomography. *Radiologic Clinics of North America*, **15**, 309–329.

Husband, J. E. S. (1989) Thymic masses and hyperplasia. *CT Review*, **1**, 53–63.

Kirks, D. R., Korobkin, M. (1981) Computed tomography of the chest in infants and children: Techniques and mediastinal evaluation. *Radiologic Clinics of North America*, **19**, 409–419.

Lyons, H. A., Calvey, G. L., Sammons, B. P. (1959) The diagnosis and classification of mediastinal masses: A study of 782 cases. *Annals of Internal Medicine*, **51**, 897–932.

McLoud, T. C., Meyer, J. E. (1982) Mediastinal metastases. *Radiologic Clinics of North America*, **20**, 453–468.

Morrison, I. M. (1958) Tumours and cysts of the mediastinum. *Thorax*, **13**, 294–307.

Oudkerk, M., Overbosch E., Dee, P. (1983) CT recognition of acute aortic dissection. *American Journal of Roentgenology*, **141**, 671–676.

Pugatch, R. D., Faling, L. J., Robbins, A. H., Spira, R. (1980) CT diagnosis of benign mediastinal abnormalities. *American Journal of Roentgenology*, **134**, 685–694.

Siegal, M. J., Sagel, S. S., Reed, K. (1982) The value of computed tomography in the diagnosis and management of pediatric mediastinal abnormalities. *Radiology*, **142**, 149–155.

Von Schulthess, G. K., McMurdo, K., Tscholakoff, D., De Geer, G., Gamsu, G., Higgins, C. B. (1986) Mediastinal masses: MR imaging. *Radiology*, **158**, 289–296.

Westcott, J. L. (1981) Percutaneous needle aspiration of hilar and mediastinal masses. *Radiology*, **141**, 323–329.

Wychulis, A. R., Payne, W. S., Clagett, O. T., Woolner, L. B. (1971) Surgical treatment of mediastinal tumours: A 40-year experience. *Journal of Thoracic and Cardiovascular Surgery*, **62**, 379–392.

MRI

Mayr, B., Heywang, S. H., Ingrisch, H., Huber, R. M., Haussinger, K., Lissner, J. (1987) Comparison of CT with MR imaging of endobronchial tumors. *Journal of Computer Assisted Tomography*, **11**, 43–48.

Naidich, D. P., Rumancik, W. M., Ettenger, N. A., et al (1988) Congenital anomalies of the lungs in adults: MR diagnosis. *American Journal of Roentgenology*, **151**, 13–19.

Weissleder, R., Elizondo, G., Wittenberg, L. Lee A. S., Josephson, L., Brady, T. (1990) Ultrasmall superparamagnetic iron oxide; an intravenous contrast agent for assessing lymph nodes with MR imaging. *Radiology*, **175**, 494–498.

CHAPTER 13

THE PLEURA: COLLAPSE AND CONSOLIDATION

Michael B. Rubens

THE PLEURA

Basic anatomy. The pleura is a serous membrane which covers the surface of the lung, and lines the inner surface of the chest wall. The visceral pleura, over the lung, and the parietal pleura, over the chest wall, are continuous at the hilum, where a fold of pleura extends inferiorly to form the inferior pulmonary ligament. The two layers of pleura are closely applied to each other, being separated by a thin layer of lubricating pleural fluid. The parietal pleura and the visceral pleura over the periphery of the lung, are not normally visible radiographically. However, where the visceral pleura lines the interlobar fissures of the lung it is often visible, there being two layers of pleura outlined by aerated lung. The horizontal fissure of the right lung is often seen on a frontal chest film, and the oblique fissures will usually be seen on the lateral views. Some patients have one or more accessory fissures, the most common being the azygos fissure and the inferior accessory fissure of the right lower lobe. Occasionally anterior or posterior junction lines are seen in the frontal chest film, where the left and right lungs come into contact in the mediastinum.

Some physiological considerations. The normal anatomy of the lungs is maintained by a balance between different elastic forces of the chest wall and lungs. The lung has a natural tendency to collapse toward its hilum, and this is opposed by forces of similar magnitude in the chest wall tending to expand outwards. The visceral and parietal layers of pleura are thus kept in close apposition. If increased fluid or air collects in the pleural space, the effect of the outward forces on the underlying lung is diminished, and the lung tends to retract towards its hilum. Therefore, in an erect patient a small pleural effusion which has gravitated to the base of the lung causes retraction of the lower part of the lung, but has comparatively little effect at the apex. Conversely, a small pneumothorax will collect at the apex and have little effect at the lung base. Obviously large intrapleural collections will affect the entire lung. These basic patterns may be altered by the state of the underlying lung and the presence of pleural adhesions. Fibrotic, emphysematous or consolidated lung may not be able to retract and adhesions may prevent the usual distribution of air or fluid.

DISEASES OF THE PLEURA

Pleural fluid

Fluid which accumulates in the pleural space may be transudate, exudate, pus, blood or chyle: Radiographically these produce similar shadows and are therefore indistinguishable. However, there may be clinical data to point to the aetiology, or the chest film may show other abnormalities, such as evidence of heart failure or trauma, which indicate the cause. Sometimes the definitive diagnosis is only made after thoracentesis or pleural biopsy; not infrequently it remains obscure.

1. Transudates. Transudates contain less than 3 g/dl of protein, and are usually clear or faintly yellow, watery fluids. A pleural transudate may be called a hydrothorax. They are often bilateral. The commonest cause is *cardiac failure*, when the effusion usually accumulates first on the right, before becoming bilateral. Other causes are *hypoproteinaemia* (especially the nephrotic syndrome, hepatic cirrhosis and anaemia), *constrictive pericarditis*, *Meig's syndrome* and *myxoedema*

2. Exudates. Exudates contain in excess of 3 g/dl of protein, and vary from amber, slightly cloudy fluid, which often clots on standing, to frank pus. A purulent pleural effusion is termed an empyema. The commonest causes of pleural exudate are *bacterial pneumonia*, *pulmonary tuberculosis*, *carcinoma of the lung*, *metastatic malignancy* and *pulmonary infarction*. Less common causes are *subphrenic infection*, *connective-tissue disorders* (especially systemic lupus erythematosus and rheumatoid disease) and *non-bacterial* pneumonias. Unusual causes include *post-myocardial infarction syndrome, acute pancreatitis* and *primary neoplasia* of the pleura.

3. Haemothorax. Bleeding into the pleural space is almost always secondary to open or closed *trauma* to the chest. Rarely, it is due to *haemophilia.* The effusions associated with pulmonary infarction and carcinoma of the lung are frequently blood-stained but rarely pure blood.

4. Chylothorax. Chyle is a milky fluid high in neutral fat and fatty acids. Chylothorax may develop secondary to damage or obstruction of the thoracic lymphatic vessels. The commonest cause is chest *trauma,* usually surgical. Other causes include *carcinoma of the lung, lymphoma* and *filariasis. Lymphangiomyomatosis* is a rare cause.

Radiological appearances of pleural fluid

Free fluid. Pleural fluid casts a shadow of the density of water or soft tissue on the chest radiograph. In the absence of pleural adhesions, the position and morphology of this shadow will depend upon the amount of fluid, the state of the underlying lung and the position of the patient. The most dependent recess of the pleura is the posterior costophrenic angle. A *small effusion* will, therefore, tend to collect posteriorly and in most patients 1–2 dl of fluid are required to fill in this recess before fluid will be seen above the dome of the diaphragm on the frontal view (Fig. 13.1). Small effusions may thus be seen earlier on a lateral film than on a frontal film, but it is possible to identify effusions of only a few millilitres using decubitus views with a horizontal beam (Fig. 13.2),

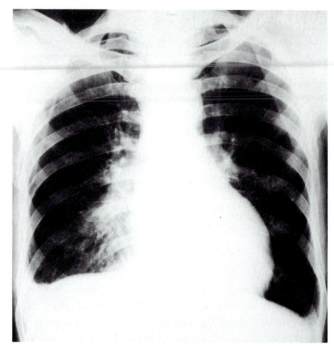

Fig. 13.1 Small bilateral pleural effusions. Man aged 58 with ischaemic heart disease. The left costophrenic angle is blunted by a small effusion. The right pleural effusion is larger, and fluid is beginning to extend up the chest wall.

ultrasound or CT (Fig. 13.23). As more fluid accumulates, the costophrenic angle on the frontal view fills in, and with increasing fluid a homogeneous opacity spreads upwards, obscuring the lung base. Typically this opacity has a fairly well-defined, concave upper edge, is higher

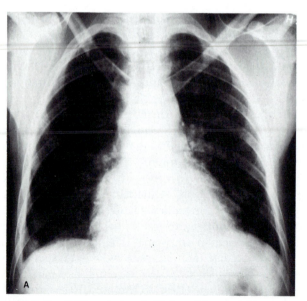

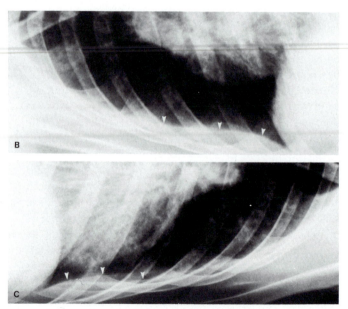

Fig. 13.2 Small bilateral pleural effusions. Man aged 34, renal transplant patient with cytomegalovirus pneumonia. The effusions probably relate to renal failure rather than the pneumonia. **A.** PA film shows subtle filling in of both costophrenic angles. **B,C.** Horizontal-beam right and left lateral decubitus films shown obvious free pleural effusions collecting along the dependent lateral costal margins (arrowheads).

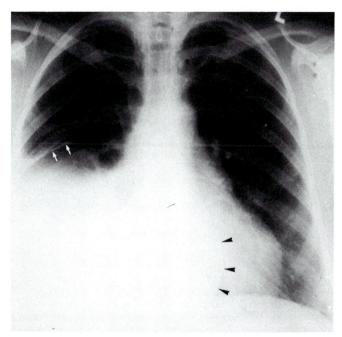

Fig. 13.3 Moderate-size pleural effusion in a woman of 56. Effusions of unknown aetiology. PA film demonstrates typical pleural opacity with concave upper border, slightly higher laterally, and obscuring the diaphragm and underlying lung. Fluid is extending into the fissure (arrows) and also into the azygo-oesophageal recess, producing a retrocardiac opacity (arrowheads).

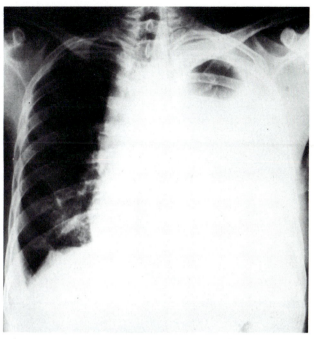

Fig. 13.4 Large pleural effusion. Man of 28 with well-differentiated lymphocytic lymphoma. PA film shows a large left pleural effusion extending over apex of lung and pushing the mediastinum to the right. A small right pleural effusion is also present, and right paratracheal shadowing represents lymphadenopathy.

laterally than medially and obscures the diaphragmatic shadow (Fig. 13.3). Frequently fluid will track into the pleural fissures. If the film is sufficiently penetrated, pulmonary vessels in the lung masked by the effusion will be seen. A *massive effusion* may cause complete radio-opacity of a hemithorax. The underlying lung will have retracted towards its hilum, and the space-occupying effect of the effusion will push the mediastinum towards the opposite side (Fig. 13.4). In the presence of a massive effusion, lack of displacement of the mediastinum suggests that the underlying lung is completely collapsed, and this is likely to be due to carcinoma of the bronchus. In the presence of pleural disease the ipsilateral hemidiaphragm is usually elevated. However, the weight of a large effusion may cause inversion of the diaphragm, and this sign is probably best demonstrated by ultrasound.

Atypical distribution of pleural fluid is quite common. *Lamellar effusions* are shallow collections between the chest wall and lung surface (Fig. 13.5), sometimes sparing the costophrenic angle. Occasionally quite large effusions accumulate between the diaphragm and undersurface of a lung, mimicking elevation of that hemidiaphragm. This is the so-called *subpulmonary pleural effusion*. The contour of the 'diaphragm' is altered, its apex being more lateral than usual, and there may be some blunting of the costophrenic angle or tracking of fluid into fissures (Fig. 13.6). On the left side increased

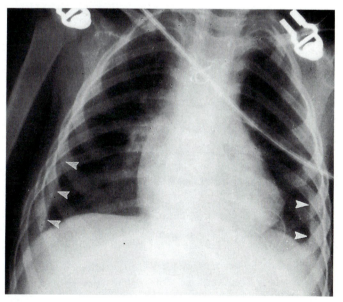

Fig. 13.5 Lamellar pleural effusions, post cardiac surgery. Erect AP film shows fluid filling both costophrenic angles and extending up the lateral chest wall (arrowheads).

distance between the gastric air-bubble and lung base may be apparent. A sub-pulmonary effusion in a free pleural space will move with changes of posture, as can be demonstrated by horizontal-beam lateral decubitus or supine films. A large right pleural effusion may collect in the

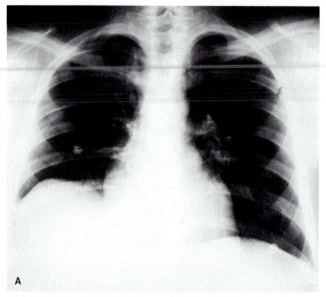

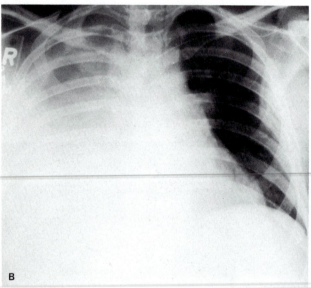

Fig. 13.6 Subpulmonary pleural effusion in a man of 21 with portal fibrosis. **A**. Erect PA film shows apparent elevation of right hemidiaphragm with apex more lateral than usual, and blunting of costophrenic angle. **B**. Supine film demonstrates shift of pleural fluid from below lung to collection posteriorly and laterally, veiling entire right lung.

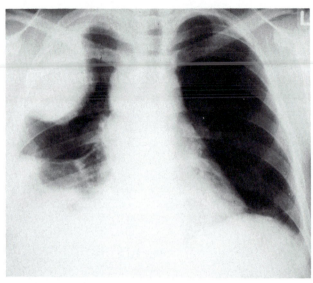

Fig. 13.7 Loculated pleural effusion in a man of 19 years with non-Hodgkin's lymphoma. Erect PA film shows well-circumscribed convex opacity adjacent to right upper costal margin and extending around apex of lung. Right paratracheal shadowing is partly due to lymph node enlargement, and partly due to loculated pleural fluid. Pleural fluid is also present at the right base extending into the horizontal fissure.

azygo-oesophageal recess and mimic a retrocardiac mass (Fig. 13.3). The reasons for atypical distribution of pleural fluid are often unclear, but it may be associated with abnormality of the underlying lung.

Loculated fluid. The pleural space may be partially obliterated by pleural disease, causing fusion of the parietal and visceral layers. Encapsulated and free pleural fluid can be distinguished by gravitational methods. Encapsulated fluid, however, may be difficult to differentiate from an extrapleural opacity, parenchymal lung disease or mediastinal mass, but there are some useful diagnostic points.

An encysted effusion is often associated with free pleural fluid or other pleural shadowing, and may extend into a fissure (Fig. 13.7). Loculated effusions tend to have comparatively little depth, but considerable width, rather like a biconvex lens. Their appearance, therefore, depends on whether they are viewed en face, in profile or obliquely. Fluoroscopy is often helpful in determining the best projection for radiographic demonstration. Extrapleural opacities tend to have a much sharper outline, with tapered, sometimes concave edges where they meet the chest wall. Parenchymal lesions may show an air bronchogram. The differentiation between pleural thickening or mass and loculated pleural fluid may be difficult on plain films, and CT and ultrasound are particularly useful in this context.

Fluid may become loculated in one or more of the interlobar fissures. This is an uncommon occurrence and is most often seen in heart failure. The appearances depend upon which fissure is affected and the quantity of fluid. Fluid collecting in the horizontal fissure produces a lenticular, oval or round shadow, with well-demarcated edges. Fluid extending into the adjacent parts of the fissure may make it appear thickened. In both frontal and lateral projections the shadow appears rounded. Loculated fluid in an oblique fissure may be poorly defined on a frontal radiograph, but a lateral film is usually diagnostic since the fissure is seen tangentially, and the typical lenticular configuration of the effusion is demonstrated (Fig. 13.8).

Loculated interlobar effusions can appear rounded on two views. Following treatment they may disappear rap-

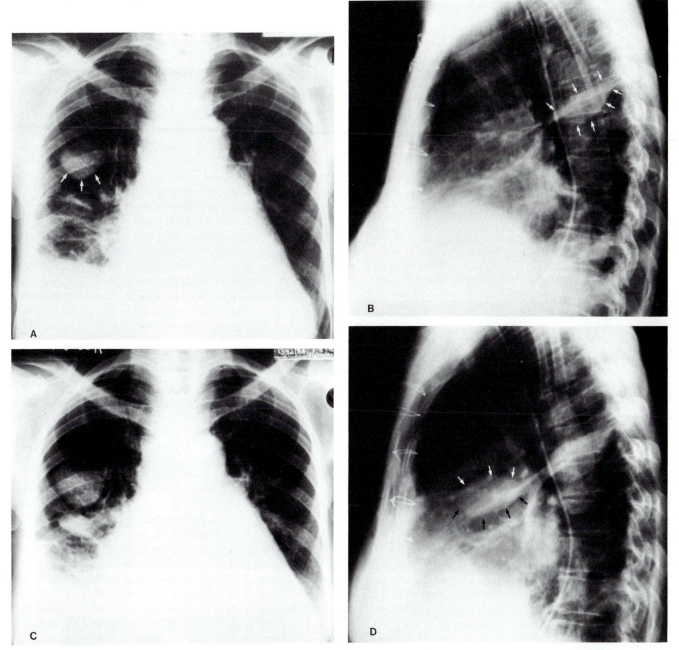

Fig. 13.8 Loculated interlobar pleural effusions in a woman of 60 after replacement of the aortic root. **A.** 19 days post-operatively a right mid-zone opacity appears (arrows), with a sharp lower margin and an indistinct upper margin. The right costophrenic angle has also filled in. **B.** Lateral projection demonstrates typical lenticular configuration of fluid loculated in the oblique fissure (arrows). **C.** Seven days later a second round opacity has appeared below the first. This opacity is well circumscribed. **D.** Lateral projection confirms that this is fluid loculated in the horizontal fissure (arrows).

idly, and are hence known as 'pseudo-' or 'vanishing' tumours. They may recur in subsequent episodes of heart failure.

Empyema may be suspected on a plain film by the spontaneous appearance of a fluid level in a pleural effusion, but is best diagnosed by CT or ultrasound (Figs 13.9, 13.10C). On CT an empyema usually has a lenticular shape and may compress the underlying lung.

Fluid, with or without gas, may be present in the pleura and both layers of the pleura may be thickened.

Ultrasound appearance of pleural fluid (Fig. 13.10)
Ultrasound is an excellent method for locating loculated pleural fluid prior to diagnostic or therapeutic aspiration. The fluid may be anechoic or contain particulate material. It is possible to visualize septations in loculated collections and also to identify pleural thickening and masses.

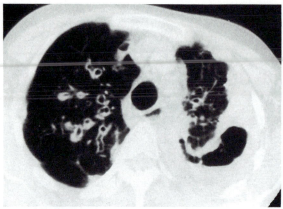

Fig. 13.9 Empyema complicating cystic fibrosis. CT shows fluid and gas collection in left pleural space posteriorly. The collection is surrounded by thickened pleura, and the underlying lung is compressed. There is bilateral bronchiectasis.

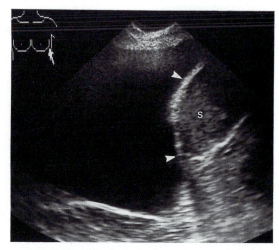

B

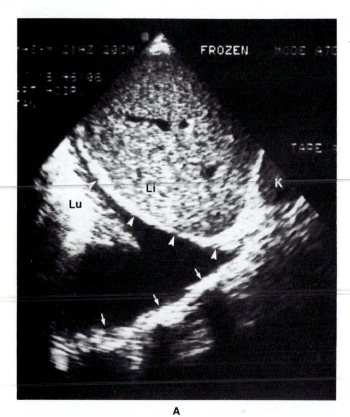

A

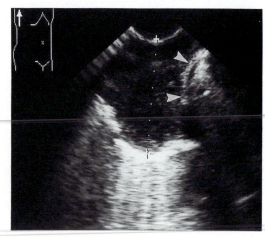

C

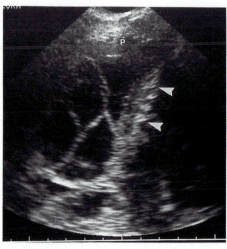

D

Fig. 13.10 **A**. Ultrasound of pleural effusion in a man of 47 with ischaemic heart disease. Liver scan performed for hepatomegaly; no evidence of pleural effusion clinically or on chest radiograph. Patient scanned supine. Sagittal section through liver (Li) and right kidney (K) demonstrates base of right lung (Lu) floating in echo-free effusion above diaphragm (arrowheads) and posterior chest wall (arrows). **B**. Large left pleural effusion due to carcinoma of bronchus. There is a large echo-free effusion above the left hemidiaphragm (arrowheads) and spleen(s). **C**. Empyema following right lower lobectomy. A poorly echogenic collection is seen above the diaphragm (arrowheads). **D**. Loculated pleural effusion due to tuberculosis. Ultrasound demonstrates thickening of the parietal pleura (P) and multiseptated fluid collection above the diaphragm (arrowheads).

Pneumothorax

Pneumothorax is the presence of air in the pleural cavity. Air enters this cavity through a defect in either the parietal or the visceral pleura. Such defects are the result of lung pathology, trauma or deliberate introduction of air, respectively giving rise to spontaneous, traumatic or artificial pneumothoraces. If pleural adhesions are present the pneumothorax may be localized, otherwise it is generalized. If air can move freely in and out of the pleural space during respiration it is an open pneumothorax, if no movement of air occurs it is closed, and if air enters the pleural space on inspiration, but does not leave on expiration, it is valvular. As intrapleural pressure increases in a valvular pneumothorax a tension pneumothorax develops.

Aetiology. *Spontaneous pneumothorax* is the commonest type, and typically occurs in young men, due to rupture of a congenital pleural bleb. Such blebs are usually in the lung apex and may be bilateral.

In older patients chronic bronchitis and emphysema are common factors. Rarer causes include bronchial asthma, rupture of a tension cyst in staphylococcal pneumonia, rupture of a subpleural tuberculous focus, rupture of a subpleural tension cyst in carcinoma of the bronchus, and rupture of a cavitating subpleural metastasis. Other associations include many of the causes of interstitial pulmonary fibrosis (cystic fibrosis, histiocytosis, tuberous sclerosis, sarcoidosis and some of the pneumoconioses).

Traumatic pneumothorax may be the result of a penetrating chest wound, closed chest trauma (particularly rupture of a bronchus in a road accident), rib fracture, pleural aspiration or biopsy, lung biopsy, bronchoscopy, oesophagoscopy, and positive-pressure ventilation. The pleura may also be violated during mediastinal surgery and nephrectomy.

Artificial pneumothorax as treatment for pulmonary tuberculosis is now of historical interest only, as is diagnostic pneumothorax.

Radiological appearances. A small pneumothorax in a free pleural space in an erect patient collects at the apex. The lung apex retracts towards the hilum and on a frontal chest film the sharp white line of the visceral pleura will be visible, separated from the chest wall by the radiolucent pleural space, which is devoid of lung markings (Fig. 13.11). The affected lung usually remains aerated: its perfusion is reduced in proportion to its ventilation and therefore its radiodensity remains normal. A small pneumothorax may easily go unseen and it may be necessary to examine the film with a bright light. An expiratory film will make a closed pneumothorax easier to see since on full expiration the lung volume is at its smallest, while the volume of pleural air is unchanged. A lateral decubitus film with the affected side uppermost is sometimes helpful, as the pleural air can be seen along the lateral chest wall. This view is particularly useful in

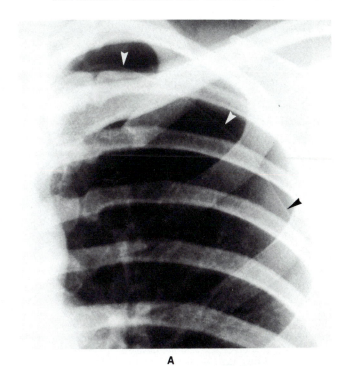

A

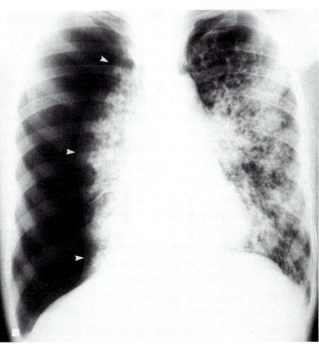

B

Fig. 13.11 Spontaneous pneumothoraces. **A.** Woman aged 22. PA film showing apical pneumothorax. The visceral pleura (arrowheads) separates aerated lung from the radiolucent pleural space. **B.** Adolescent boy of 16 with cystic fibrosis. PA film shows diffuse nodular and ring shadows in the lungs, left hilar enlargement and a large right pneumothorax (arrowheads).

infants, since small pneumothoraces are difficult to see in supine AP films, as the air tends to collect anteriorly and medially (Fig. 13.12).

A large pneumothorax may lead to complete relaxation

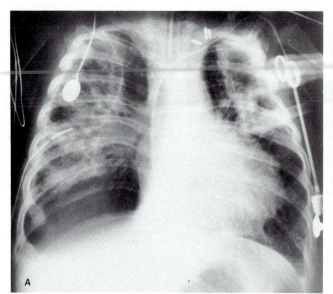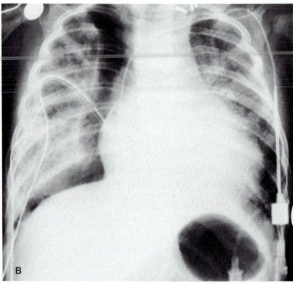

Fig. 13.12 Medial tension pneumothorax in a one-year-old-child on ventilator following closure of patent ductus arteriosus and resection of coarctation of aorta. **A**. Supine AP film demonstrates a right pneumothorax, the intrapleural air collecting anteriorly and medially, and the lung collapsing posteriorly and laterally. The pleural tube is situated laterally and is therefore not decompressing the pneumothorax. The right hemidiaphragm is depressed, and the mediastinum is displaced to the left, indicating a tension pneumothorax. **B**. Following insertion of another pleural tube more medially, the pneumothorax is smaller and the right hemidiaphragm and mediastinum have returned to their normal positions.

and retraction of the lung, with some mediastinal shift towards the normal side, which increases on expiration.

Tension pneumothorax (Figs 13.12, 13.13) may lead to massive displacement of the mediastinum, kinking of the great veins and acute cardiac and respiratory embarrassment. Radiologically the ipsilateral lung may be squashed against the mediastinum, or herniate across the midline, and the ipsilateral hemidiaphragm may be depressed. On fluoroscopy the mediastinal shift to the contralateral side is greatest in inspiration, an observation that distinguishes a tension pneumothorax from a large pneumothorax not under strain.

Complications of pneumothorax. Pleural adhesions may limit the distribution of a pneumothorax and result in a *loculated* or *encysted pneumothorax*. The usual appearance is an ovoid air collection adjacent to the chest wall, and it may be radiographically indistinguishable from a thin-walled subpleural pulmonary cavity, cyst or bulla. *Pleural adhesions* are occasionally seen as line shadows stretching between the two pleural layers, preventing relaxation of the underlying lung (Fig. 13.13). Rupture of an adhesion may produce a *haemopneumothorax*, or discharge of an underlying infected subpleural lesion, leading to a *pyopneumothorax*. Collapse or consolidation of a lobe or lung in association with a pneumothorax are important complications which may delay re-expansion of the lung.

Since the normal pleural space contains a small volume of fluid, blunting of the costophrenic angle by a short fluid level is commonly seen in a pneumothorax (Fig. 13.14). In a small pneumothorax this fluid level may be

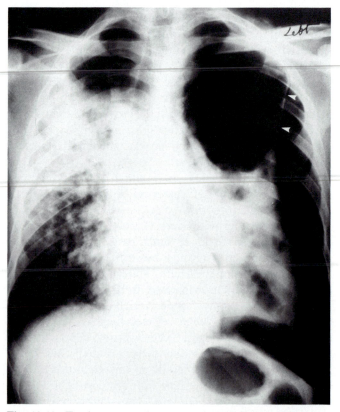

Fig. 13.13 Tension pneumothorax and pleural adhesion. Elderly man with spontaneous pneumothorax secondary to extensive cavitating pulmonary tuberculosis. The left lung is prevented from collapsing completely by the extensive consolidation, and by tethering of an adhesion (arrowheads). The mediastinum is displaced to the right.

the most obvious radiological sign. A larger fluid collection usually signifies a complication and represents exudate, pus or blood, depending on the aetiology of the pneumothorax.

The usual radiological appearance of a *hydropneumothorax* is that of a pneumothorax containing a horizontal fluid level which separates opaque fluid below from lucent air above. This demonstration requires a horizontal beam film (Fig. 13.15), so that if the patient is not fit enough

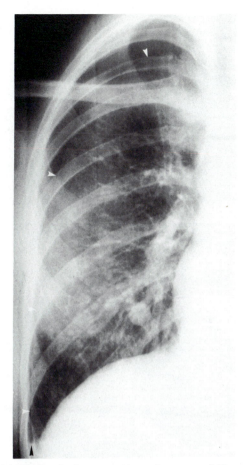

Fig. 13.14 Shallow hydropneumothorax in a man of 18 years. Spontaneous pneumothorax, probably due to rupture of subpleural cavitating metastatic osteogenic sarcoma. The primary tumour was in the right scapula, which has been removed, and pulmonary metastases are seen in the right lower zone. The visceral pleura is faintly seen (white arrowheads) and a short fluid level (black arrowhead) is present just above the right costophrenic angle.

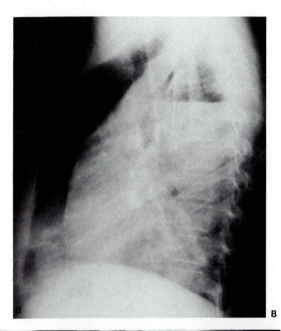

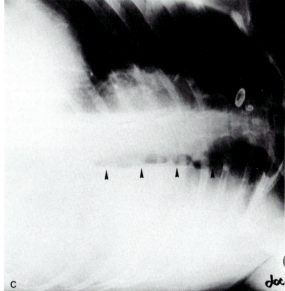

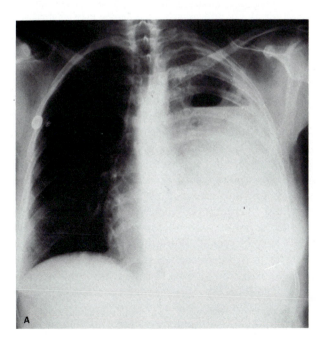

Fig. 13.15 Loculated pyo-pneumothorax in a woman of 45 following gunshot wound to chest. **A**. Erect PA film shows a fluid level in the left upper zone, and pleural thickening over the apex. **B**. Lateral film shows that the fluid level is situated posteriorly. The differential diagnosis lies between a pyo-pneumothorax and a lung abscess. **C**. Horizontal-beam left lateral decubitus film demonstrates a long fluid level (arrowheads) which can only be in the pleural cavity. Some smaller loculated collections are also seen.

for an upright film a lateral decubitus film or 'shoot-through' lateral film may be indicated.

If a pneumothorax becomes chronic, *thickening* of the visceral or parietal pleura may occur. The former may prevent re-expansion of the lung, and surgical decortication may be necessary if respiratory function is significantly impaired.

Bronchopleural fistula

Bronchopleural fistula is a communication between the airway and the pleural space. It is most frequently a complication of complete or partial *pneumonectomy*, and is discussed under 'Postoperative complications' in Chapter 18. Other causes include *carcinoma of the bronchus* and *ruptured lung abscess*. The radiological appearance is that of a hydro- or pyo-pneumothorax.

Pleural thickening

Blunting of a costophrenic angle is a frequent incidental finding on a chest X-ray. It is due to localized pleural thickening and usually results from a previous episode of pleuritis, although a previous history of chest disease is often lacking. In the asymptomatic patient and in the absence of other radiological abnormality it is of no other significance. It may mimic a small pleural effusion, and if a previous film is not available for comparison a lateral decubitus film or ultrasound scan will exclude free pleural fluid. Localized pleural thickening extending into the inferior end of an oblique fissure may produce so-called tenting of the diaphragm, and is of similar significance. This latter appearance may also result from basal intrapulmonary scarring, due to previous pulmonary infection or infarction.

Bilateral apical pleural thickening is also a fairly common finding. It is more frequent in elderly patients, and is not due to tuberculosis. Its aetiology is uncertain, but ischaemia is probably a factor. Such apical shadowing is usually symmetrical (Fig. 13.16). Asymmetric or *unilateral*

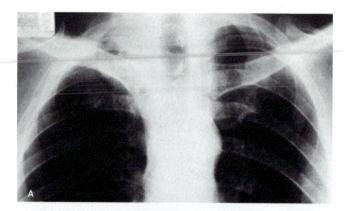

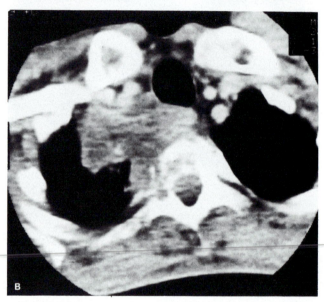

Fig. 13.17 Unilateral apical pleural thickening. Man aged 46 with pain in the right side of the neck and right arm. **A**. Dense pleural shadowing is present at the right apex. The left apex is clear. A dorsal spine film (not shown) demonstrated absence of the right pedicle of T3. **B**. CT demonstrates a right apical mass infiltrating the third thoracic vertebra. Histology: anaplastic carcinoma.

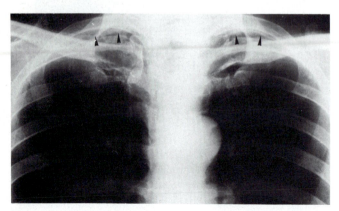

Fig. 13.16 Bilateral apical pleural thickening. An incidental finding in a 67-year-old man with ischaemic heart disease. The apical pleural shadowing (arrowheads) is symmetrical, although the edge is better seen on the left.

apical pleural thickening, however, may be of pathological significance, especially if associated with pain. If asymmetric, apical pleural shadowing may represent a *Pancoast tumour*, and it is important to visualize the adjacent ribs and spine (Fig. 13.17). Penetrated films and tomography may be indicated, since evidence of bone involvement will almost certainly indicate a carcinoma.

More *extensive unilateral pleural thickening* is usually the result of a previous thoracotomy or pleural effusion. Empyema and haemothorax are especially likely to resolve with *pleural fibrosis*. Chronic pneumothorax is a rarer cause. These causes of pleural fibrosis all involve the visceral layer and the thickened pleura may calcify. If the entire lung is surrounded by fibrotic pleura, this is termed a *fibrothorax*. The pleural peel may be a few centimetres thick, and may cause reduced ventilation of the surrounded lung and subsequent decrease in volume of that

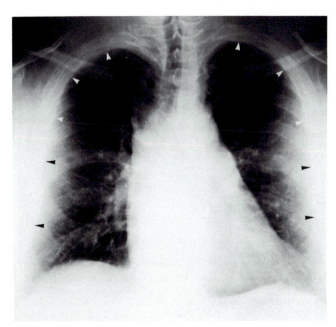

Fig. 13.18 Diffuse pleural thickening in a 60-year-old man with a history of asbestos exposure when working as a Post Office engineer and in gasworks. He was an asymptomatic tuberculosis contact. Both lungs are surrounded by pleural thickening (arrowheads).

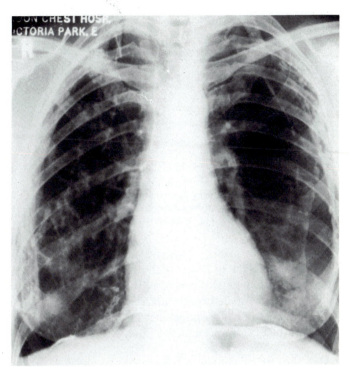

Fig. 13.19 Pleural calcification in a middle-aged woman with a history of recurrent episodes of pleurisy, presumed to be tuberculous. Extensive plaques of pleural calcification surround both lungs.

hemithorax. If the chest X-ray shows that the vascularity of the affected lung is decreased relative to the other lung, then significant ventilatory restriction is likely and surgical decortication may be necessary.

Bilateral pleural plaques are a common manifestation of asbestos exposure, and occasionally more diffuse pleural thickening is seen (Fig. 13.18).

Pleural calcification

Pleural calcification has the same causes as pleural thickening. Unilateral pleural calcification is, therefore, likely to be the result of previous empyema, haemothorax or pleurisy, and bilateral calcification occurs after asbestos exposure and in some other pneumonoconioses, or occasionally after bilateral effusions. As with the incidental finding of pleural thickening, pleural calcification may be discovered in a patient who is not aware of previous or current chest disease.

The calcification associated with previous pleurisy, empyema or haemothorax occurs in the visceral pleura, and associated pleural thickening is almost always present, and separates the calcium from the ribs. The calcium may be in a continuous sheet or in discrete plaques, usually producing dense, coarse, irregular shadows, often sharply demarcated laterally (Fig. 13.19). If a plaque is viewed en face it may cast a less well-defined shadow and mimic a pulmonary infiltrate. However, a lateral view will often demonstrate the calcified plaque over the anterior or posterior pleura but it may be necessary to fluoroscope the patient to obtain the best tangential projection for demonstration of the plaque.

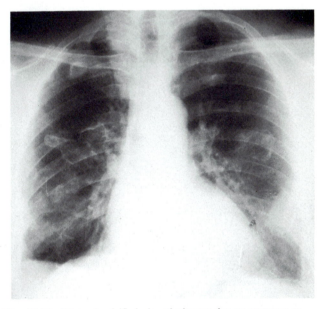

Fig. 13.20 Bilateral calcified pleural plaques due to exposure to asbestos. 48-year-old man with ischaemic heart disease — incidental finding. Pleural thickening is present in the periphery of both mid and lower zones, and calcified pleural plaques are seen en face in both lung fields.

The calcification associated with asbestos exposure is usually more delicate and bilateral (Fig. 13.20). It is frequently visible over the diaphragm (Fig. 13.21) and

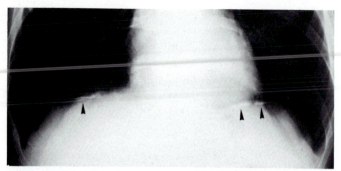

Fig. 13.21 Bilateral calcified pleural plaques due to exposure to asbestos in a 50-year-old man. Incidental finding in a tuberculosis contact. Pleural calcification is present over both domes of the diaphragm (arrowheads). The lungs appear normal.

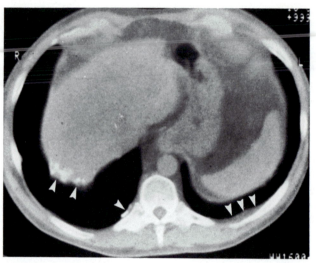

Fig. 13.23 CT demonstration of three pleural abnormalities not apparent on the PA chest film. 54-year-old man with a history of asbestos exposure. There is a small calcified pleural plaque in the right paraspinal gutter (single arrowhead); pleural calcification over the right hemidiaphragm (two arrowheads); and a small left pleural effusion (three arrowheads).

adjacent to the axillae. Tangential views show it to be situated immediately deep to the ribs, and it is in fact located in the parietal pleura (Fig. 13.22). The most sensitive method for demonstrating a pleural plaque is CT (Fig. 13.23), and ultrasound can be helpful in differentiating a plaque from loculated fluid.

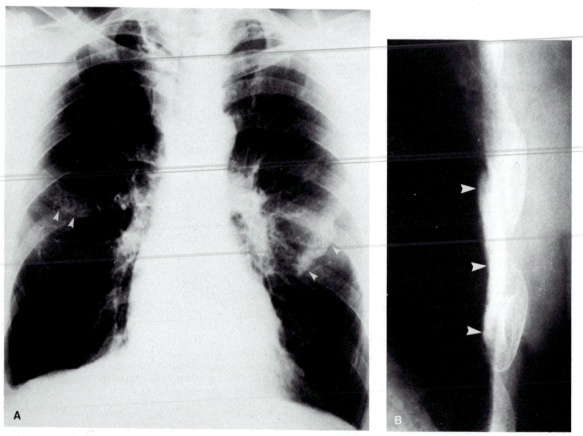

Fig. 13.22 Pleural calcification resulting from exposure to asbestos in a 51-year-old man with chronic obstructive airways disease. **A**. The lungs are hyperinflated. Calcified pleural plaques are present in both mid zones (arrowheads). **B**. An oblique film, aided by fluoroscopy, shows the left-sided plaque tangentially (arrowheads); it is situated in the parietal pleura, immediately deep to the ribs.

Pleural tumours

Primary neoplasms of the pleura are rare. Benign tumours of the pleura include local mesothelioma (or fibroma) and lipoma. The commonest malignant disease of the pleura is metastatic (Fig. 13.24), the most frequent primary tumours being of the bronchus and breast. Primary malignancy of the pleura (malignant mesothelioma) is usually associated with asbestos exposure.

Pleural fibromas usually present with finger clubbing and joint pains due to hypertrophic osteoarthropathy, but may be an incidental finding on a chest X-ray. The radiographic appearance is of a well-defined lobulated mass adjacent to the chest wall, mediastinum, diaphragm or a pleural fissure (Fig. 13.25). The mass may be small or occupy most of the hemithorax (Fig. 13.26). In the presence of osteoarthropathy, the diagnosis is almost certain, but if necessary, percutaneous needle biopsy is probably the investigation of choice.

Subpleural lipomas appear as well-defined rounded masses. They may change shape with respiration, being soft tumours, and if large enough may erode adjacent ribs. Since they comprise fat the CT appearance is diagnostic.

Malignant mesothelioma is usually due to prolonged exposure to asbestos dust, particularly crocidolite. The usual appearance is nodular pleural thickening around all or part of a lung (Fig. 13.27). A haemorrhagic pleural effusion may be present but the lung changes of asbestosis

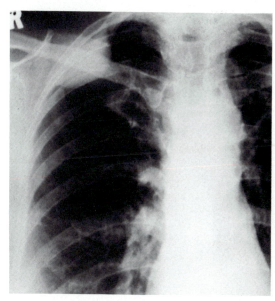

Fig. 13.25 Pleural fibroma or benign mesothelioma. Incidental finding in a 48-year-old woman with a past history of left apical tuberculosis. A sharply demarcated peripheral upper zone opacity is present, making an obtuse angle with the adjacent chest wall, and without other pleural abnormality. It was removed. Histology: benign fibrous mesothelioma.

may be absent. The effusion may obscure the pleural masses. Often the mediastinum is central, despite the presence of a large effusion, and this is thought to result from volume loss of the underlying lung secondary to

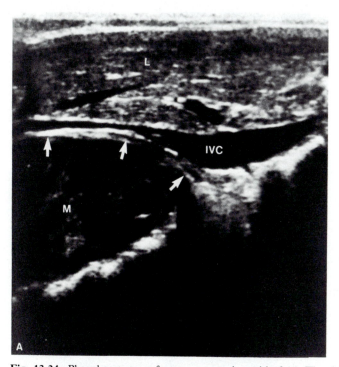

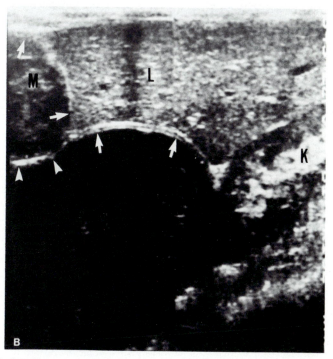

Fig. 13.24 Pleural metastases from a sarcoma in a girl of 14. The right hemithorax was opaque on the chest radiograph (not shown). **A**. Sagittal scan through the liver (L) and inferior vena cava (IVC). A pleural mass (M) with a few internal echoes lies adjacent to the diaphragm (arrows). **B**. Sagittal scan through liver and right kidney (K) demonstrates eversion of the diaphragm (arrows) by pleural fluid and a mass. An interface (arrowheads) is seen between the mass and pleural fluid. (Courtesy of Dr W. Lees.)

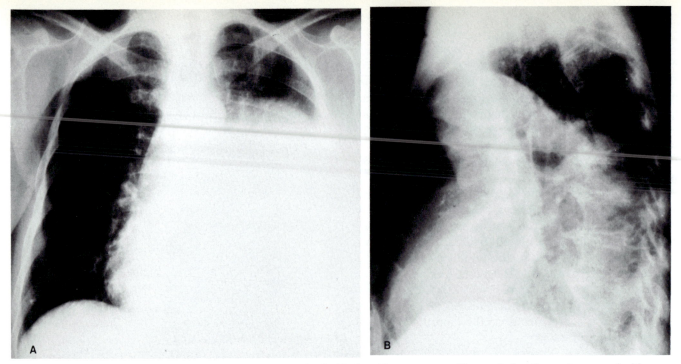

Fig. 13.26 Benign fibrous mesothelioma. 63-year-old woman who had had a right mastectomy 10 years before for carcinoma, and with a 30-year history of abnormal chest X-ray, left lung shadowing slowly increasing over the past 10 years. **A**. PA film shows opacity of left mid and lower zones. **B**. Lateral film shows a sharp upper border. A 2-kg mass, thought to be attached to the phrenic nerve by a narrow stalk, was removed surgically. The left lung completely re-expanded post-operatively. Histology: benign fibrous mesothelioma.

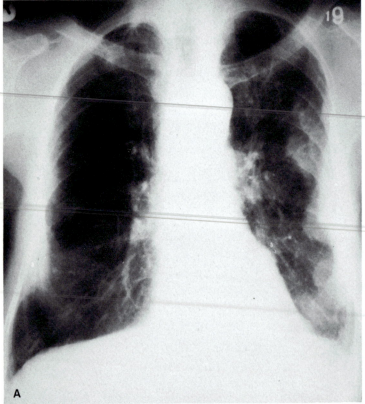

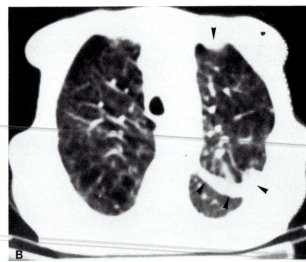

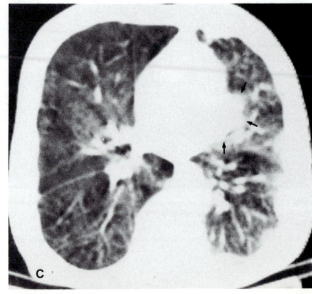

Fig. 13.27 Malignant mesothelioma. History of carcinoma of the colon 14 years previously. Presented with abnormal chest radiograph (**A**) which shows lobulated left pleural opacities. **B,C**. CT demonstrates reduced volume of left lung, peripheral pleural masses with extension into the oblique fissure (arrowheads), and masses adjacent to the left heart border (arrows), not seen on the chest radiograph. Percutaneous biopsy: malignant mesothelioma. (Courtesy of Dr B. Strickland.)

either ventilatory restriction by the surrounding tumour, or bronchial stenosis by tumour compression at the hilum. Rib involvement may occur with malignant mesothelioma, but the presence of a pleural mass and adjacent rib destruction is more likely to be due to metastatic bone tumour, or possibly a primary bone tumour.

The extent of malignant mesothelioma is best assessed by CT. CT may also help differentiate between malignant mesothelioma and benign pleural plaques. Nodular extension into fissures, pleural effusion and volume loss of the ipsilateral lung all suggest malignancy. A tissue diagnosis may be obtained by *percutaneous needle biopsy*.

THE LUNGS — COLLAPSE AND CONSOLIDATION

COLLAPSE

Partial or complete loss of volume of a lung is referred to as collapse or atelectasis. Current usage has made these terms synonymous, and they imply a diminished volume of air in the lung with associated reduction of lung volume. This contrasts with consolidation, in which a diminished volume of air in the lung is associated with normal lung volume. Fraser and Paré describe four different mechanisms which may cause pulmonary collapse.

Mechanisms of collapse

1. *Relaxation or passive collapse.* This is the mechanism whereby the lung tends to retract towards its hilum when air or increased fluid collects in the pleural space. It is discussed above under diseases of the pleura.

2. *Cicatrization collapse.* As discussed in the section on the pleura, normal lung expansion depends upon a balance between outward forces in the chest wall and opposite elastic forces in the lung. When the lung is abnormally stiff, this balance is disturbed, lung compliance is decreased and the volume of the affected lung is reduced. This occurs with pulmonary fibrosis.

3. *Adhesive collapse.* The surface tension of the alveoli is decreased by surfactant. If this mechanism is disturbed, as in the respiratory distress syndrome, collapse of alveoli occurs, although the central airways remain patent.

4. *Resorption collapse.* In acute bronchial obstruction the gases in the alveoli are steadily taken up by the blood in the pulmonary capillaries, and are not replenished, causing alveolar collapse. The degree of collapse may be modified by collateral air drift if the obstruction is distal to the main bronchus, and also by infection and accumulation of secretions. If the obstruction become chronic, subsequent resorption of intra-alveolar secretions and exudate may result in complete collapse. This is the usual mechanism of collapse seen in carcinoma of the bronchus.

Radiological signs of collapse

The radiographic appearance in pulmonary collapse depends upon the mechanism of collapse, the degree of collapse, the presence or absence of consolidation, and the pre-existing state of the pleura. Signs of collapse may be considered as direct or indirect. Indirect signs are the results of compensatory changes which occur in response to the volume loss.

Direct signs of collapse

1. *Displacement of interlobar fissures.* This is the most reliable sign, and the degree of displacement will depend on the extent of the collapse.

2. *Loss of aeration.* Increased density of a collapsed area of lung may not become apparent until collapse is almost complete. However, if the collapsed lung is adjacent to the mediastinum or diaphragm, obscuration of the adjacent structures may indicate loss of aeration.

3. *Vascular and bronchial signs.* If a lobe is partially collapsed crowding of its vessels may be visible; if an air bronchogram is visible, the bronchi may appear crowded.

Indirect signs of collapse

1. *Elevation of the hemidiaphragm.* This sign may be seen in lower lobe collapse, but is rare in collapse of the other lobes.

2. *Mediastinal displacement.* In upper lobe collapse the trachea is often displaced towards the affected side, and in lower lobe collapse the heart may be displaced.

3. *Hilar displacement.* The hilum may be elevated in upper lobe collapse, and depressed in lower lobe collapse.

4. *Compensatory hyperinflation.* The normal part of the lung may become hyperinflated, and it may appear hypertransradiant, with its vessels more widely spaced than in the corresponding area of the contralateral lung. If there is considerable collapse of a lung, compensatory hyperinflation of the contralateral lung may occur, with herniation across the midline.

Patterns of collapse

An air bronchogram is almost never seen in resorption collapse, but is usual in passive and adhesive collapse, and may be seen in cicatrization collapse if fibrosis is particularly dense.

Pre-existing lung disease such as fibrosis and pleural adhesions may alter the expected displacement of anatomic landmarks in lung collapse. There also tends to be a reciprocal relationship between the compensatory signs, e.g. in lower lobe collapse, if hemidiaphragmatic elevation is marked, hilar depression will be diminished.

Complete collapse of a lung

Complete collapse of a lung, in the absence of pneumothorax or large pleural effusion or extensive consolidation, causes opacification of the hemithorax, displacement of the mediastinum to the affected side and elevation of the diaphragm. Compensatory hyperinflation of the contralateral lung occurs, often with herniation across the midline (Fig. 13.28). Herniation most often occur in the retrosternal space, anterior to the ascending aorta, but may occur posterior to the heart or under the aortic arch.

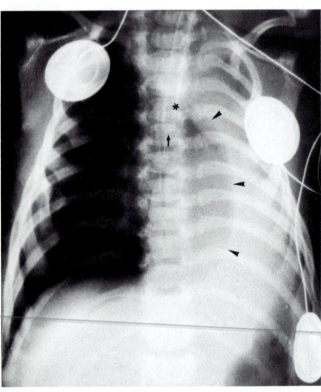

Fig. 13.28 Complete collapse of the left lung. A newborn child with complex cyanotic heart disease. The tip of the endotracheal tube (arrow) is beyond the carina (asterisk) and down the right bronchus, causing collapse of the left lung, and compensatory hyperinflation of the right lung, which has herniated across the midline (arrowheads).

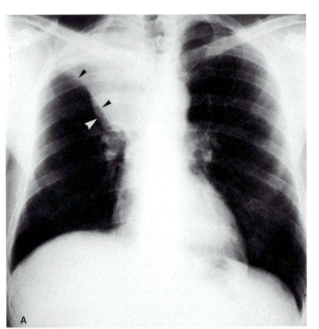

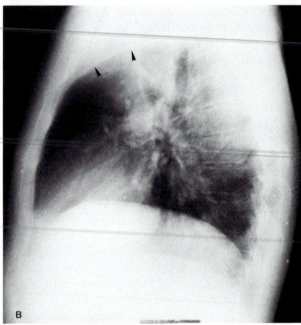

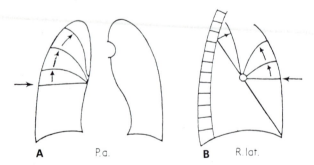

Fig. 13.29 Right upper lobe collapse. **A**. PA projection. Note how lesser fissure is drawn upwards, and often curved, towards the apex and mediastinum. **B**. Right lateral view. Lesser fissure also displaced upwards. Note some forward displacement of greater fissure above the hilum.

Fig. 13.30 Right upper lobe collapse. 54-year-old man with squamous carcinoma of right upper lobe. **A**. PA film shows a mass (white arrowhead) above the right hilum, and elevation of the horizontal fissure (black arrowheads). There is compensatory hyperinflation of the right lower lobe.
B. Lateral film shows anterior displacement of part of oblique fissure (arrowheads).

Lobar collapse

The following descriptions apply to collapse of individual lobes, uncomplicated by pre-existing pulmonary or pleural disease. The line drawings (Figs 13.29, 13.31, 13.33, 13.35, 13.38) represent the alteration in position of the fissures, as seen in the frontal and lateral projections, resulting from increasing degrees of collapse. Only the fissures are represented. The indirect signs of collapse are not indicated.

Right upper lobe collapse (Figs 13.29, 13.30). The normal horizontal fissure is usually at the level of the right fourth rib anteriorly. As the right upper lobe collapses, the horizontal fissure pivots about the hilum, its lateral end moving upwards and medially towards the superior mediastinum, and its anterior end moves upwards towards

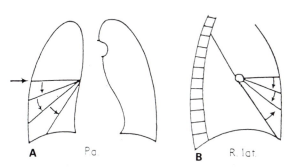

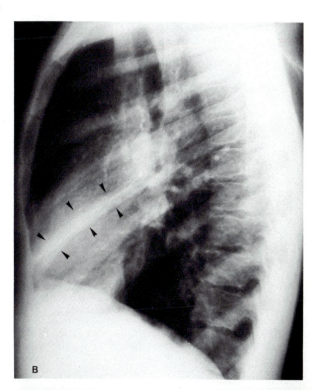

Fig. 13.31 Right middle lobe collapse. In both projections the lesser fissure is drawn downwards. In the PA view the fissure finally merges with the mediastinum and disappears. Note in the lateral view that the lower part of the greater fissure may be displaced forwards.

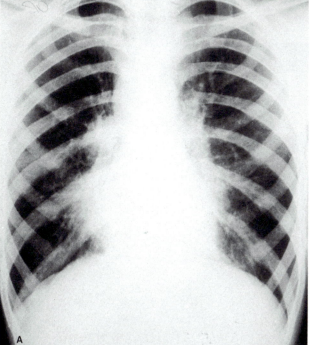

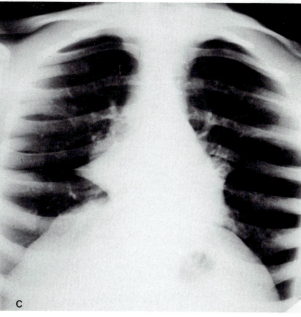

Fig. 13.32 Right middle lobe collapse. **A.** PA film shows obscuration of right heart border, indicating loss of aeration of part of right middle lobe. **B.** Lateral film shows complete collapse of right middle lobe (arrowheads) as a thin opacity between the displaced horizontal and oblique fissures. **C.** Lordotic film brings the collapsed wedge of tissue into profile — an elegant but unnecessary demonstration in this case.

the apex. The upper half of the oblique fissure moves anteriorly. The two fissures become concave superiorly. In severe collapse the lobe may be flattened against the superior mediastinum, and may obscure the upper pole of the hilum. The hilum is elevated, and its lower pole may be prominent. Deviation of the trachea to the right is usual, and compensatory hyperinflation of the right middle and lower lobes may be apparent.

Right middle lobe collapse (Figs 13.31, 13.32). In right middle lobe collapse the horizontal fissure and lower half

of the oblique fissure move towards one another. This can best be seen in the lateral projection. The horizontal fissure tends to be more mobile, and therefore usually shows greater displacement. Signs of right middle lobe collapse are often subtle on the frontal projection, since the horizontal fissure may not be visible, and increased opacity does not become apparent until collapse is almost complete. However, obscuration of the right heart border is often present, and may be the only clue in this projection. The *lordotic AP projection* brings the displaced fissure into the line of the X-ray beam, and may elegantly demonstrate right middle-lobe collapse. Since the volume of this lobe is relatively small, indirect signs of volume loss are rarely present.

Lower lobe collapse (Figs 13.33–13.36). The normal oblique fissures extend from the level of the fourth thoracic vertebra posteriorly to the diaphragm, close to the sternum, anteriorly. The position of these fissures on the lateral projection is the best index of lower lobe volumes. When a lower lobe collapses its oblique fissure moves posteriorly but maintains its normal slope. In addition to posterior movement, the collapsing lower lobe causes medial displacement of the oblique fissure, which may then become visible in places on the frontal projection.

Right lower lobe collapse causes depression of the horizontal fissure, which may be apparent on the frontal projection. Increased opacity of a collapsed lower lobe is usually visible on the frontal projection. A completely collapsed lower lobe may be so small that it flattens and

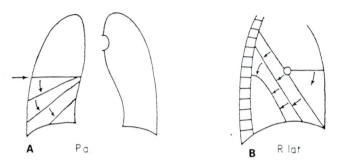

Fig. 13.33 Right lower lobe collapse. In the PA projection the greater fissure is not visible until the collapse is fairly complete. The lesser fissure is displaced downwards as in collapse of the middle lobe. The degree of displacement seen may be greater in collapse of the lower lobe than of the middle lobe, as the middle lobe tends to retract towards the hilum and the fissure may disappear. In the lateral view, the oblique fissure moves backwards, tending to retain its obliquity. The upper part of the oblique fissure may curve backwards and downwards, so becoming visible in the PA projection.

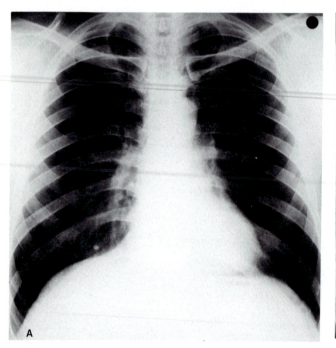
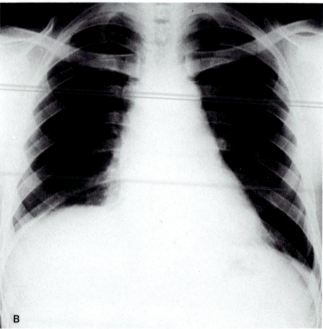

Fig. 13.34 Right lower lobe collapse. 49-year-old man with ischaemic heart disease. **A**. Normal preoperative film. **B**. Following coronary artery bypass surgery, the right lower lobe has collapsed with depression and medial rotation of the hilum, elevation of the right hemidiaphragm and hyperinflation of the right upper lobe.

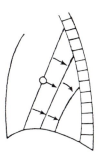

Fig. 13.35 Left lower lobe collapse. No fissure is visible in the PA projection. The lateral view shows that the greater fissure is displaced posteriorly as in collapse of the right lower lobe. The upper part of the fissure may also be drawn downwards as well as backwards.

merges with the mediastinum, producing a thin, wedge-shaped shadow. On the left this shadow may be obscured by the heart, and a penetrated view with a grid may be required for its visualization. If complete left lower lobe collapse is still in doubt, a right oblique film may demonstrate the wedge of tissue between spine and diaphragm. Mediastinal structures and parts of the diaphragm adjacent to the non-aerated lobe are obscured.

The hilum is usually depressed and rotated medially, and upper lobe hyperinflation is evident, but diaphragmatic elevation is not usual.

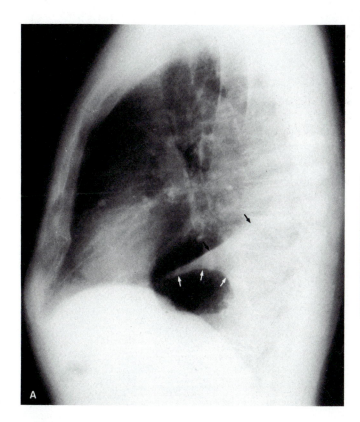

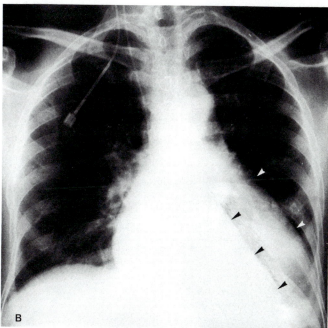

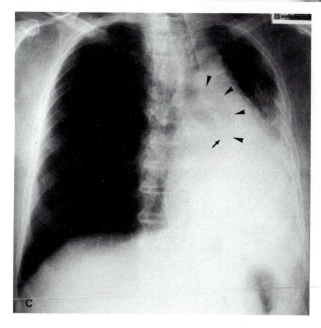

Fig. 13.36 Left lower lobe collapse. **A**. 66-year-old man with squamous-cell carcinoma of the left lower lobe. The oblique fissure is displaced posteriorly (black arrows). The left hemidiaphragm is obscured by the collapsed lobe, but the position of the stomach bubble (white arrows) indicates that the left hemidiaphragm is elevated. **B**. Postoperative film of patient with aortic valve replacement. The shadow of the collapsed left lower lobe (black arrowheads) is seen through the shadow of the heart (white arrowheads). **C**. 57-year-old man with oat-cell carcinoma occluding the left bronchus (arrow). The left lower lobe is collapsed, obscuring the left hemidiaphragm. The mediastinum is shifted to the left, and part of the hyperinflated right lung has herniated across the mid-line (arrowheads).

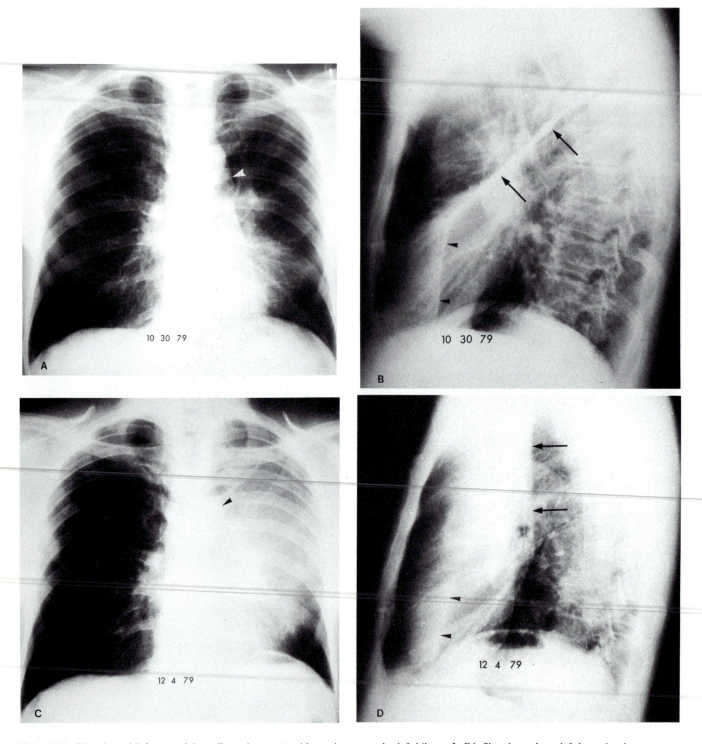

Fig. 13.37 Lingula and left upper lobe collapse in a man with carcinoma at the left hilum. **A**. PA film shows hazy left heart border, indicating loss of aeration of the lingula. A mass is present in the aorticopulmonary window (arrowhead). **B**. Lateral film shows collapse-consolidation of the lingula, with anterior displacement of the lower part of the oblique fissure (arrowheads). The upper part of the oblique fissure (arrows) is thickened, but in normal position. **C**. Five weeks later the left upper lobe has collapsed. A hazy opacity covers most of the left hemithorax. Vessels in the hyperinflated left lower lobe can just be seen through the haze, and the aortic knuckle is obscured (arrowhead). **D**. Lateral film shows that the oblique fissure is now displaced anteriorly (arrows).

Lingula collapse (Fig. 13.37). The lingula is often involved in collapse of the left upper lobe, but it may collapse individually, when the radiological features are similar to right middle lobe collapse. However, the absence of a horizontal fissure on the left makes anterior displacement of the lower half of the oblique fissure and increased opacity anterior to it important signs. On the frontal projection the left heart border becomes obscured.

Left upper lobe collapse (Figs 13.37–13.39). The pattern of upper lobe collapse is different in the two lungs. Left upper lobe collapse is apparent on the lateral projection as anterior displacement of the entire oblique fissure, which becomes oriented almost parallel to the anterior chest wall. With increasing collapse the upper lobe retracts posteriorly and loses contact with the anterior chest wall. The space between the collapsed lobe and the sternum becomes occupied by either hyperinflated left lower lobe or herniated right upper lobe. With complete collapse, the left upper lobe may lose contact with the chest wall and diaphragm and retract medially against the mediastinum. On a lateral film, therefore, left upper lobe collapse appears as an elongated opacity extending from the apex and reaching, or almost reaching, the diaphragm; it is anterior to the hilum and is bounded by displaced oblique fissure posteriorly, and by hyperinflated lower lobe anteriorly.

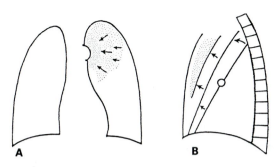

Fig. 13.38 Left upper lobe collapse. **A**. The greater fissure does not become visible in the PA projection. When the degree of collapse is fairly complete the lobe shows a uniform loss of translucency (this may be due to accompanying consolidation), which increases in density as the degree of collapse increases. Vessel markings seen through this opacity are those in the overexpanded lower lobe. **B**. In the lateral view, initially the fissure moves bodily forward, the lingula remaining in contact with the diaphragm. With increasing collapse the lingula retracts upwards, and the bulk of the upper lobe moves posteriorly, and becomes separated from the sternum by aerated lung. This is usually overexpanded lower lobe, though occasionally a portion of the right lung may herniate across the mid-line.

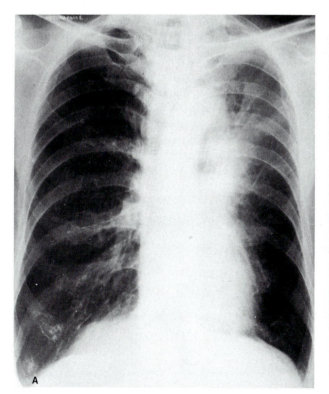 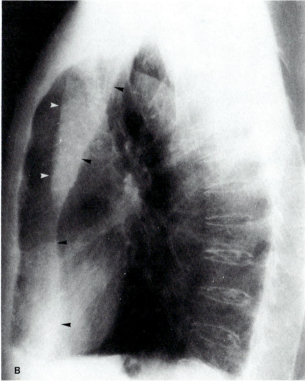

Fig. 13.39 Left upper lobe collapse due to squamous-cell carcinoma. **A**. PA film shows typical upper zone haze, through which are seen the elevated and enlarged left hilum, and vessels of the hyperinflated lower lobe. The contour of the aortic knuckle is indistinct, but the descending aorta is sharply outlined. **B**. Lateral film shows the collapsed left upper lobe between the anteriorly displaced oblique fissure (black arrows) and part of the hyperinflated lower lobe.

A collapsed left upper lobe does not produce a sharp outline on the frontal view. An ill-defined hazy opacity is present in the upper, mid and sometimes lower zones, the opacity being densest near the hilum. Pulmonary vessels in the hyperinflated lower lobe are usually visible through the haze. The aortic knuckle is usually obscured, unless the upper lobe has collapsed anterior to it, allowing it to be outlined by lower lobe. If the lingula is involved, the left heart border is obscured. The hilum is often elevated, and the trachea is often deviated to the left.

Rounded atelectasis (Fig. 13.40) is an unusual form of pulmonary collapse which may be misdiagnosed as a pulmonary mass. It appears on the plain film as a homogenous mass of up to 5 cm diameter, with ill-defined edges. It is always pleural-based and associated with pleural thickening. Vascular shadows may be seen to radiate from part of the opacity, resembling a comet's tail. The appearance is caused by peripheral lung tissue folding in on itself. It may be related to asbestos exposure, but is not of any other pathological significance.

CONSOLIDATION

Functionally the pulmonary airways can be divided into two groups. The proximal airways function purely as a conducting network; the airways distal to the terminal bronchioles are also conducting structures, but, more importantly, are the site of gaseous exchange. These terminal airways are termed acini, an acinus comprising respiratory bronchioles, alveolar ducts, alveolar sacs and alveoli arising from a terminal bronchiole. Consolidation implies replacement of air in one or more acini by fluid or solid material, but does not imply a particular pathology or aetiology. The smallest unit of consolidated lung is a single acinus, which casts a shadow approximately 7 mm in diameter. Communications between the terminal airways allow fluid to spread between adjacent acini, so that larger confluent areas of consolidation are generally visible and are frequently not confined to a single segment.

The commonest cause of consolidation is acute inflammatory exudate associated with pneumonia. Other causes include *cardiogenic pulmonary oedema, non-cardiogenic pulmonary oedema, haemorrhage* and *aspiration. Neoplasms* such as alveolar cell carcinoma and lymphoma can produce consolidation, and *alveolar proteinosis* is a rare cause. In an individual patient, consolidation may be due to more than one basic aetiology. For example, a patient with major head trauma may be particularly susceptible to infection, aspiration and non-cardiogenic pulmonary oedema.

When consolidation is associated with a patent conducting airway an *air bronchogram* (Fig. 13.41) is often visible. This sign is produced by the radiographic contrast between the column of air in the airway and the surrounding opaque acini. If consolidation is secondary to bronchial obstruction, however, the air in the conducting airway is resorbed and replaced by fluid, and the affected area is of uniform density.

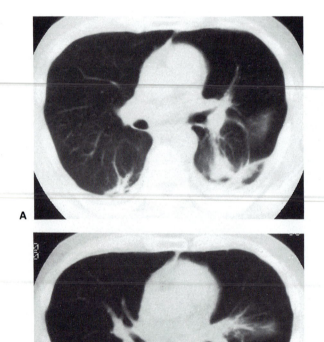

Fig. 13.40 A,B   Rounded atelectasis. Patient with history of asbestos exposure and left lung mass on chest radiograph. CT shows bilateral pleural-based masses with adjacent pleural thickening. Blood vessels are seen curving into the left-sided mass.

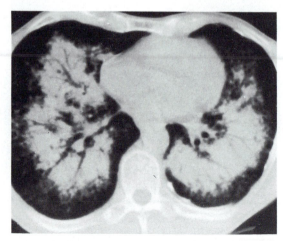

Fig. 13.41 Air bronchogram. CT shows patent, air-filled bronchi surrounded by widespread pulmonary consolidation.

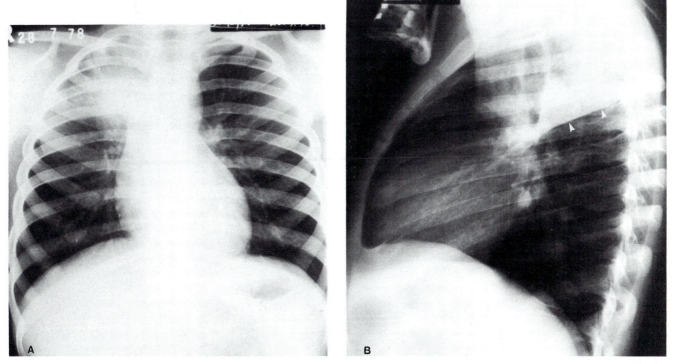

Fig. 13.42 Right upper lobe consolidation in a 6-year-old boy with aortic valve disease. **A.** Opacity in the right upper zone obscures the upper mediastinum. **B.** The lateral film shows consolidation anterior to the upper part of the oblique fissure (arrowheads), mostly in the posterior segment of the right upper lobe.

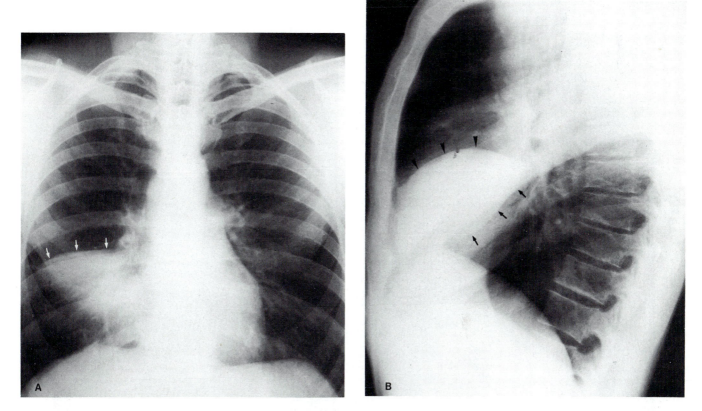

Fig. 13.43 Right middle lobe consolidation. 37-year-old man with squamous-cell carcinoma of the right middle lobe. **A.** PA film shows homogeneous opacity limited by horizontal fissure (arrows) and obscuring the right heart border. **B.** Lateral film shows consolidation bounded by horizontal fissure (arrowheads) and lower half of oblique fissure (arrows).

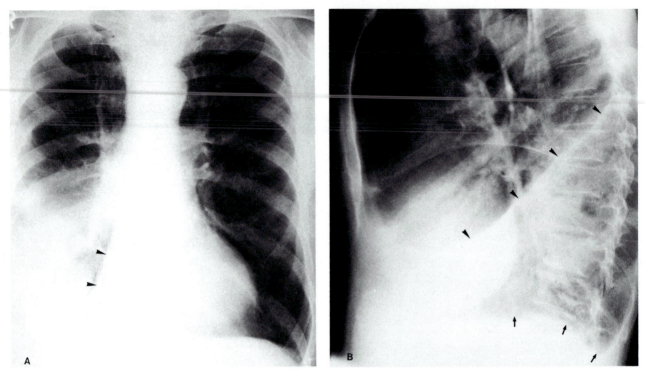

Fig. 13.44 Right lower lobe consolidation. *Aerobacter aerogenes* pneumonia in a chronic bronchitis. **A**. PA film shows right lower zone shadowing obscuring the diaphragm, but not the right heart border (arrowheads). **B**. Lateral film shows shadowing with air bronchogram, limited by oblique fissure anteriorly (arrowheads). The left hemidiaphragm is visible (arrows) but the right is obscured.

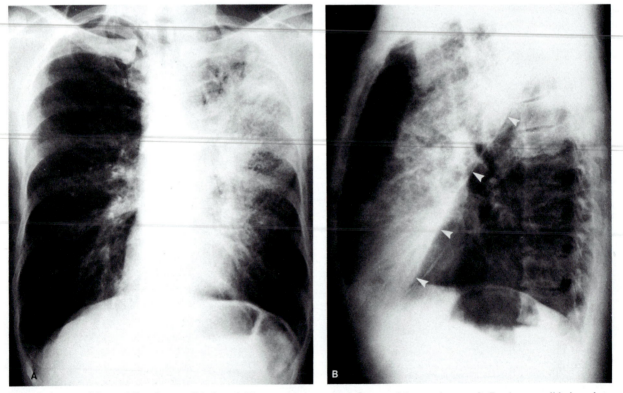

Fig. 13.45 Left upper lobe and lingula consolidation. A 70-year-old man with left upper lobe carcinoma. **A**. Patchy consolidation obscures the left heart border and aortic knuckle. **B**. The consolidation is bounded posteriorly by the oblique fissure (arrowheads).

The volume of purely consolidated lung is similar to that of the normal lung since air is replaced by a similar volume of fluid or solid. However, collapse and consolidation are often associated with one another. When consolidation is due to fluid, its distribution is influenced by gravity, so that in acute pneumonitis consolidation is often denser and more clearly demarcated inferiorly by a pleural surface, and is less dense and more indistinct superiorly.

Lobar consolidation

Consolidation of a complete lobe produces a homogenous opacity, possibly containing an air bronchogram, delineated by the chest wall, mediastinum or diaphragm and the appropriate interlobar fissure or fissures. Parts of the diaphragm and mediastinum adjacent to the non-aerated lung are obscured.

Right upper lobe consolidation (Fig. 13.42) is confined by the horizontal fissure inferiorly, and the upper half of the oblique fissure posteriorly, and may obscure the right upper mediastinum.

Right middle lobe consolidation (Fig. 13.43) is limited by the horizontal fissure above, and the lower half of the oblique fissure posteriorly, and may obscure the right heart border.

Lower lobe consolidation (Fig. 13.44) is limited by the oblique fissure anteriorly, and may obscure the diaphragm.

Left upper lobe and *lingula consolidation* (Fig. 13.45) are limited by the oblique fissure posteriorly. Lingula consolidation may obscure the left heart border, and consolidation of the upper lobe may obscure the aortic knuckle.

REFERENCES AND SUGGESTIONS FOR FURTHER READING

General

Felson, B. (1973) *Chest Roentgenology.* W. B. Saunders Co, Philadelphia.
Fraser, R. G., Paré, J. A. P. (1989–91) *Diagnosis of Diseases of the Chest*, 3rd edn. W. B. Saunders Co, Philadelphia.
Simon, G. (1978) *Principles of Chest X-ray Diagnosis*, 4th edn. Butterworths, London.

The pleura

Alexander, E., Clark, R. A., Colley, D. P., Mitchell, S. E. (1981) CT of malignant pleural mesothelioma. *American Journal of Roentgenology*, **137**, 287–291.
Albelda, S. M., Epstein, D. M., Gefter, W. B., Miller, W. T. (1982) Pleural thickening: Its significance and relationship to asbestos dust exposure. *American Review of Respiratory Disease*, **126**, 621–624.
Austin, J. H. M., Carsen, G. M. (1977) Radiologic diagnosis of pleural effusions. In: *Current Concepts in Radiology*, 3, 261–281. C. V. Mosby, St Louis.
Black, L. F. (1972) The pleural space and pleural fluid. *Mayo Clinic Proceedings*, **47**, 493–506.
Fleischner, F. G. (1963) Atypical arrangement of free pleural effusion. *Radiologic Clinics of North America*, **1**, 347–362.
Gaensler, E. A., Kaplan, A. J. (1971) Asbestos pleural effusion. *Annals of Internal Medicine*, **74**, 178–191.
Heller, R. M., Janower, M. E., Weber, A. L. (1970) The radiological manifestations of malignant pleural mesothelioma. *American Journal of Roentgenology*, **108**, 53–59.
Henschke, C. I., Davis, S. D., Romano, P. M., Yankelvitz, D. F. (1989) The pathogenesis, radiological evaluation and therapy of pleural effusions. *Radiologic Clinics of North America*, **27**, 1241–1255.
Hillerdal, G. (1983) Malignant mesothelioma 1982: Review of 4710 published cases. *British Journal of Diseases of the Chest*, **71**, 321–343.
Lipscomb, D. J., Flower, C. D. R., Hadfield, J. W. (1981) Ultrasound of the pleura: an assessment of its clinics value. *Clinical Radiology*, **32**, 289–290.
McLeod, T. C., Isler, R. J., Novelline, R. A., Putman, C. E., Simeone, J., Stark, P. (1981) The apical cap. *American Journal of Roentgenology*, **137**, 299–306.
Moskowitz, P. S., Griscom, N. T. (1976) The medial pneumothorax. *Radiology*, **120**, 143–147.

Rasch, B. N., Carsky, E. W., Lane, E. T., Callaghan, J. P. O., Heitzman, E. R. (1982) Pleural effusion: Explanation of some atypical appearances. *American Journal of Roentgenology*, **139**, 899–904.
Sargent, E. N., Gordonson, J., Jacobson, G., Birnbaum, W., Shaub, M. (1978) Bilateral pleural thickening: a manifestation of asbestos dust exposure. *American Journal of Roentgenology*, **131**, 579–585.
Stark, D. D., Federle, M. P., Goodman, P. C., Padrasky, A. E., Webb, W. R. (1983) Differentiating lung abscess and empyema: Radiography and computed tomography. *American Journal of Roentgenology*, **141**, 163–167.
Williford, M.E., Hidalgo, H., Putman, C. E., Korobkin, M., Ram, P. C. (1983) Computed tomography of pleural disease. *American Journal of Roentgenology*, **140**, 909–914.
Woodring, J. H. (1984) Recognition of pleural effusion on supine radiographs: How much fluid is required? *American Journal of Roentgenology*, **142**, 59–64.
Wright, F. W. (1976) Spontaneous pneumothorax and pulmonary malignant disease — a syndrome sometimes associated with cavitating tumours. *Clinical Radiology*, **27**, 211–222.

Collapse and consolidation

Krause, G. R., Lubert, M. (1958) Gross anatomico-spatial changes occurring in lobar collapse; a demonstration by means of three-dimensional plastic models. *American Journal of Roentgenology*, **79**, 258–268.
Proto, A. V., Tocino, I. (1980) Radiographic manifestations of lobar collapse. *Seminars in Roentgenology*, **15**, 117–173.
Robbins, L. L., Hale, C. H. (1945) The roentgen appearance of lobar and segmental collapse of the lung; preliminary report. *Radiology*, **44**, 107–114.
Robbins, L. L., Hale, C. H., Merrill, O. E. (1945) The roentgen appearance of lobar and segment collapse of the lung: technic of examination. *Radiology*, **44**, 471–476.
Robbins, L. L., Hale, C. H. (1945) The roentgen appearance of lobar and segmental collapse of the lung. III. Collapse of an entire lung or the major part thereof. IV. Collapse of the lower lobes. V. Collapse of the right middle lobe. VI. Collapse of the upper lobes. *Radiology*, **45**, 23–26, 120–127, 260–266, 347–355.
Schneider, H. J., Felson, B., Gonzalez, L. L. (1980) Rounded atelectasis. *American Journal of Roentgenology*, **134**, 225–232.

CHAPTER 14

TUMOURS OF THE LUNG

Ivan Hyde

PRIMARY MALIGNANT TUMOURS

CARCINOMA OF THE LUNG
(Bronchial or bronchogenic carcinoma)

There is an overwhelming preponderance of carcinoma compared to other malignant primary lung tumours. It is the cause of 35 000 deaths in England and Wales annually; it is the commonest cancer in men; in women it comes after breast, colon and skin cancer but its incidence is rising. Mortality rates are also still rising in the elderly but are falling in younger people because of lower cigarette consumption in that group. Cigarette smoking is responsible for the epidemic proportions of the disease but there are other known causes and predisposing factors. These are mostly to be found in industrial processes involving nickel, arsenic, asbestos, chromium and uranium. Its association with lung scars is higher than would be expected from chance and there is an increased incidence in sufferers from fibrosing alveolitis and systemic sclerosis. It is a disease of the over-50s and is rarely considered in the differential diagnosis of lung lesions in those under the age of 40 years. Nevertheless it has been found at all ages, including childhood.

Of 100 patients with carcinoma of the lung less than 10 will survive 5 years. Many will be inoperable when first seen. In general, operability is determined by absence of involvement of the mediastinum, but resection rates vary widely, depending on the surgeon's view of what is possible or achievable. Despite such differences, the 5-year survival rate in reported surgical series is remarkably constant at 25%. Moreover, the proportion of lobectomies to pneumonectomies does not influence the survival rate. These figures have remained unchanged over the last 30 years, the only improvement being in the operative mortality, from better peri-operative management. The conclusion to be drawn is that the dominant factor in survival lies in the nature of the disease process rather than in differences in timing or type of operation. Taking the group of peripheral carcinomas, 5-year survival following resection is related to tumour size, smaller lesions having a better prognosis. An exception to this rule is that those over 6 cm in diameter have more survivors than tumours one size below, indicating either that peripheral tumours may be large because they are fast-growing (and discovered earlier), or alternatively that they are slow-growing with consequently less tendency to metastasize. Amongst those surviving for 5 years there is a substantial mortality rate between 5 and 10 years.

Pathology. Carcinoma of the lung is divided pathologically into the following cell types with the approximate proportions of each shown:

Type	%
Squamous	50
Adenocarcinoma, including bronchioloalveolar cell	20
Small cell (oat cell)	20
Large cell	10

This does not mean that there is unanimity amongst pathologists concerning classification, merely that in the interests of comparable reporting the above is a satisfactory compromise. With rare exceptions carcinomas arise from some element of the bronchial mucosa or its metaplasia. All types are more frequent in cigarette smokers, the association being particularly strong with squamous and small-cell types, less strong in adenocarcinoma and weak in bronchioloalveolar carcinoma.

Small-cell carcinoma arises from the APUD system (amine precursor uptake decarboxylase) which secretes and stores 5-hydroxytryptamine and which is also the cell of origin of carcinoid tumours of the bronchus.

The distinctive feature of the *bronchioloalveolar carcinoma* is the manner of its spread over the inner surface of the terminal air spaces including alveoli, using the pulmonary architecture as a framework which initially remains intact. Primary adenocarcinomas of the alimentary tract metastasizing to the lung can produce an identical picture, so that a definition of this tumour includes a rider that no primary adenocarcinoma exists elsewhere.

It is probable that *squamous carcinoma* arises in an area of bronchial mucosal metaplasia, which would account for these tumours being predominantly central in position, where there is greatest exposure to inhaled irritants. The *adenocarcinoma*, unrelated to metaplasia, arises anywhere along the bronchial pathway and is usually peripheral because of the greater area at risk.

The majority of carcinomas arise peripherally in the lung, that is, distal to the division into segmental bronchi, but at presentation most will have spread centripetally. Those lesions which remain peripheral have a better prognosis. There is a poor correlation between cell type and prognosis, except for the general statement that prognosis is especially poor in small-cell and relatively more favourable in bronchioloalveolar carcinoma.

Investigations are directed to the establishment of a diagnosis, the determination of operability and the assessment of the patient's fitness for surgery. Once a suspicion of carcinoma has been raised the prime investigations are *sputum cytology* and *bronchoscopy*.

Tomography usually contributes little more than better definition of the lesion without answering the question: 'benign or malignant?' It is useful in settling doubts concerning such features as cavitation or calcification but its main function is to determine whether hilar and mediastinal nodes are involved.

CT scanning improves accuracy in the search for mediastinal involvement but it is not error-free and its precise place in pre-operative assessment is not yet fully evaluated. If it demonstrates normal hilar and mediastinal structures it is reliable, but if it reveals an abnormal mediastinum this does not necessarily imply inoperability, since enlarged nodes can be due to reactive changes. In that event recourse may then be had to *mediastinoscopy* but this too has limitations in the area which can be reached. If CT scanning is undertaken it is usual to include the adrenals, which are a common site of metastatic disease (Fig. 36.14).

Ventilation and perfusion *radionuclide scans* occasionally show unexpectedly large defects, and then there is likely to be extensive mediastinal involvement, but similar defects can result from pulmonary artery and vein occlusion. Large defects may also be found in the apparently normal lung, the first indication of serious chronic disease rendering pneumonectomy unduly hazardous.

Biopsy. An ideal biopsy is one obtained from a lesion visible at *bronchoscopy*; blind biopsy is disappointing. The fibreoptic bronchoscope has increased the area of accessible bronchial tree, but small peripheral lesions still constitute a problem, and it is here that *percutaneous needle biopsy* is invaluable. It is also useful for other lesions difficult of access by bronchoscopy. The determination of cell type is more reliable from bronchoscopic than from needle biopsy because of the larger specimen obtained. Nevertheless, for small-cell carcinoma both are reliable, and this is the most important discrimination because of the implications for treatment.

Radiological appearances. The diagnosis of carcinoma of lung starts in all but exceptional cases with an abnormality on a chest radiograph. If a previous series of chest radiographs happens to be available it is not uncommon to find in retrospect that a lesion had been missed months or even years before. This is not surprising when the opacity is very small and of low density, since only 25% of lung volume is unobstructed by the bony thorax. In a small number of cases the radiograph is still normal after the diagnosis has been established by bronchoscopy or other means.

The first indication of a central carcinoma may be a *hilar shadow* which is slightly more prominent or denser than normal (Fig. 14.1). A location within a bronchial lumen soon produces signs of obstruction — *atelectasis* or *hyperaeration*. Collapse of individual lobes or segments each have their distinctive radiographic signs but sometimes these are not obvious. A collapsed left lower lobe may be invisible on an underexposed PA radiograph but its presence may be inferred by the redistribution of the pulmonary vessels in the overexpanded upper lobe or by one or two curved basal 'sentinel' lines due to a drawing-down of bronchi by the loss of volume, the bronchi becoming visible from retained secretions. A collapsed upper lobe may paradoxically exist with a well-aerated lung apex, a circumstance often incorrectly ascribed to herniation of lung from the opposite side when it is more often due to the over-expanded apex of the lower lobe. This 'luftsichel' sign also explains why the outline of the

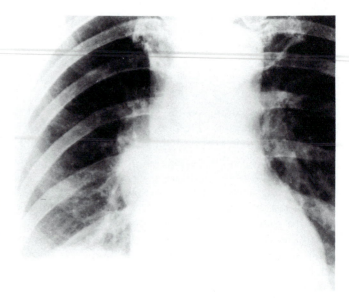

Fig. 14.1 Carcinoma of lung. Dense and enlarged right hilum.

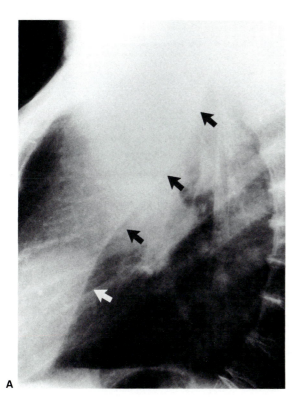
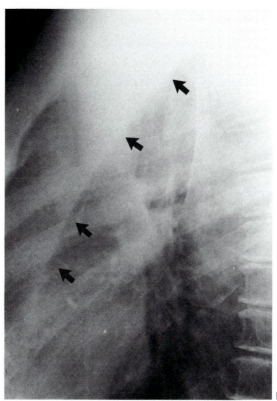

Fig. 14.2 A. The density of the collapsed left upper lobe covers the aortic arch and the latter was not visible on the PA chest radiograph. **B.** The arch is uncovered and was visible on the PA film.

aortic knuckle is sometimes unexpectedly preserved in collapse of the left upper lobe (Fig. 14.2). The presence of atelectasis should always initiate a search for evidence of a hilar mass.

The lung distal to a blocked lobar bronchus does not always collapse (Fig. 14.3); the air may be replaced by secretions or inflammatory exudate; microabscesses may form or lipid substances accumulate after release from chronic inflammatory cells. The result is a chronic fibrotic or lipoid pneumonia, hence the suspicion which attaches to a diagnosis of *unresolved pneumonia*. Air may return to an atelectatic lobe when mucosal oedema or infection subsides, so that re-expansion has to be interpreted with caution in determining aetiology. *Bronchography* is now rarely used but it can be useful in this situation as the appearances are always abnormal, bronchi even when patent showing irregularity, squeezing or pruning of side-branches.

Accumulation of secretions within bronchi distal to a blocked segmental bronchus may result in a mucocele which takes the form of an oval or branching opacity within aerated lung, the air reaching the segmental alveoli by collateral ventilation through the pores of Kohn (Fig. 14.4). Such collateral ventilation is inefficient, and the finger-like opacities are often the centre of a *focal hyper-inflation*. Regional hyperinflation can also result from a check valve bronchial obstruction.

Growth extends from the hilum along the connective tissue sheaths of bronchi and pulmonary vessels, its path revealed by dense streaks of opacity radiating from the hilar mass. As lymphatics become obstructed, the flow of lymph can be reversed, carrying tumour seedlings centrifugally. Lymphatic permeation of this nature results in fine linear shadows mingled with nodules of tumour. In an extreme case this leads to an appearance of *lymphangitis carcinomatosa* confined to one lung (Fig. 14.5).

An unusual form of carcinoma is one entirely confined within the mediastinum, some being genuine bronchial neoplasms. Radiographic signs may then be inconspicuous or even absent despite clinical signs of strangulation of mediastinal structures — great veins, pulmonary artery, oesophagus.

The majority of carcinomas arise at a *peripheral* site but by the time they are discovered many of them will have a band of growth extending into the hilum (Fig. 14.6). Initially they are roughly rounded in shape, growing as they do in compliant lung. A few retain this regular shape even when they achieve massive proportions but as a rule growth is attended by irregularity of outline, with extensions both proximally and distally.

Cavitation is not infrequent, particularly in squamous carcinoma, and there are a number of possible mechanisms — infection, infarction, discharge of secretions, dissection of air into the mass (Fig. 14.7). The

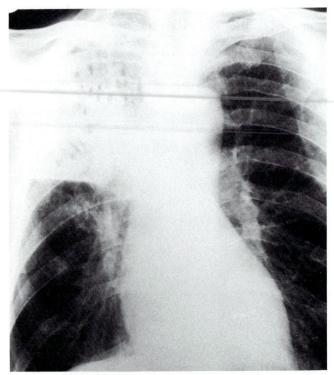

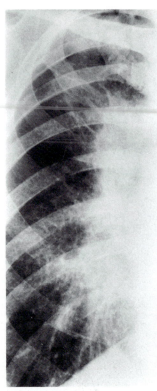

Fig. 14.3 Carcinoma of lung. Obstructive pneumonia of the right upper lobe containing translucent bronchi. There was bronchiectasis distal to the tumour.

Fig. 14.5 Centrifugal spread of carcinoma from the hilum into all lobes.

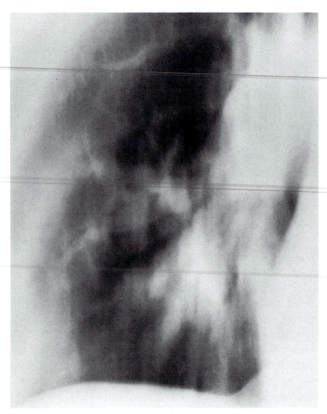

Fig. 14.4 Tomogram. Large dense right hilum; distended bronchi in middle and lower lobes. There was a tumour in the bronchus intermedius.

cavity may enlarge with the growth of the tumour, necrotic debris being shed into the lumen. A needle biopsy of such a lesion may yield a pus-like material which will not be diagnostic, and for this reason it is preferable to take biopsies from the growing edge rather than from the centre of a tumour. The cavities characteristically have thick irregular walls, a feature which is of use in the differential diagnosis of cavitating lung lesions. As a general rule the thicker the wall the greater the probability of malignancy. At one extreme a cavity with a uniform wall thickness of 1 mm is almost certain to be benign, and conversely, one with a wall thickness of 15 mm is almost certainly malignant.

Rupture of such a cavity is one cause of *pneumothorax*, a rare event in primary lung neoplasms but rather more frequent with certain pulmonary metastases. Carcinoma of the lung metastasizes widely but those sites commonly productive of symptoms or radiographic signs are mediastinum, bone and brain. *Metastasis to lung* is usually on the ipsilateral side, the opposite lung being relatively spared. Seedling deposits close to the pleura or pericardium are likely to stimulate the formation of an *effusion* which can be difficult to control.

A *paralysed diaphragm* due to tumour involvement of the phrenic nerve means that extension into the mediastinum has taken place and is inevitably a sign of inoperability. However, steps should be taken to try to

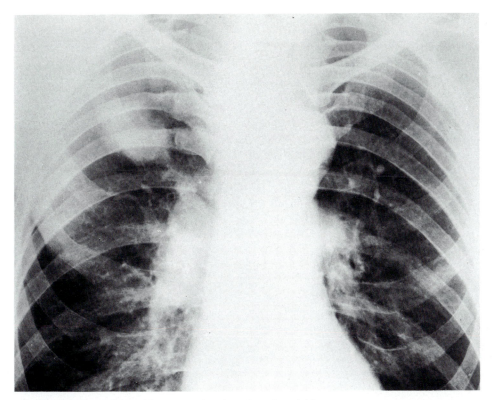

Fig. 14.6 Carcinoma in the right upper lobe with an extension into the enlarged hilum.

exclude paralysis from other causes and in this respect previous chest radiographs can be invaluable. A high diaphragm may be due to a localized weakness which does not have the same significance as total paralysis, and this is best assessed by fluoroscopic observation.

Hypertrophic pulmonary osteoarthropathy is most commonly caused by carcinoma of lung but it is not of itself a sign of inoperability.

The solitary lung lesion

A problem in differential diagnosis is presented by an apparently isolated single lesion. The questions that have to be answered are: 'is it a primary or secondary malignant lesion or is it benign?' There is no point in making a separate category of so-called coin lesions; the questions of management are the same irrespective of whether the lesions are strictly circular or not. In different series of such lesions the proportion of malignant primary tumours has varied between 36 and 52%. Several radiographic signs have been suggested as indicative of malignancy and conversely their absence as suggesting a benign nature.

The *character of the edge* — whether irregular, spiculated, notched; a halo of emphysema; a tail of one or two lines proceeding from the lesion to the pleura. All of these have been reported as more common in malignant lesions than in benign. Unfortunately none offer sufficient discrimination on which to base management of an individual case.

Two signs have more importance — the presence of *internal calcification* and *evidence of growth*. A carcinoma *may* arise in a calcified scar or it *may* engulf a calcification during growth but both are very rare phenomena. If it can be shown, if necessary with the aid of tomography, that there is genuine calcification within the lesion, then this is the most reliable sign of benignancy. CT may be helpful in this respect since it is more sensitive in detecting calcification.

Growth of a lesion over a period of time has to be interpreted with caution. Carcinomas usually grow rapidly and a definite change will be noted after a few weeks, but some carcinomas grow slowly, at much the same rate as benign lesions such as hamartomas or granulomas (Fig. 14.8). Nevertheless if a lesion is stable for two years that is reliable evidence that it is benign.

Regarding the management of these lesions, there is a strong body of opinion that they should always be removed unless they are calcified, or have been known to be stable for two years, or the patient cannot stand an operation. A more conservative approach involves biopsy, either percutaneously or by fibreoptic bronchoscopy, with excision if the biopsy shows anything other than a benign pathology. The case for biopsy is strengthened if the patient is under 35 years old or if operation carries an extra risk.

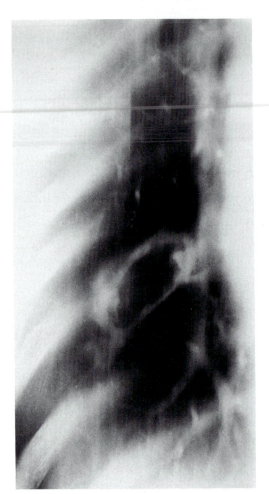

Fig. 14.7 Tomogram. Cavitating carcinoma. Irregular wall thickness.

Small-cell (oat-cell) carcinoma

These tumours are mostly centrally located, grow rapidly and disseminate early, particularly to the bone marrow and brain (Fig. 14.9). Surgery has little to offer except for those few cases where the lesion is a peripheral nodule, but even then it is not recommended if the tumour is visible at bronchoscopy. They are highly sensitive to combination chemotherapy, and the thrust of research at present is to determine what combination offers the best chance of remission (Fig. 14.10).

Approximately 30% of small-cell carcinomas secrete hormone-like substances which, if in sufficient quantity, result in corresponding endocrine and metabolic abnormalities. The substances produced are *parathormone*, *anti-diuretic hormone* and *cortico-trophin*, and the functional effects are, respectively, hypercalcaemia, fluid retention with hyponatraemia, Cushing's syndrome and gynaecomastia.

Other 'paramalignant' disorders seen are encephalopathy, myelopathy and myasthenia. In some instances it is difficult to differentiate these syndromes from the effects of metastases. Their manifestations may

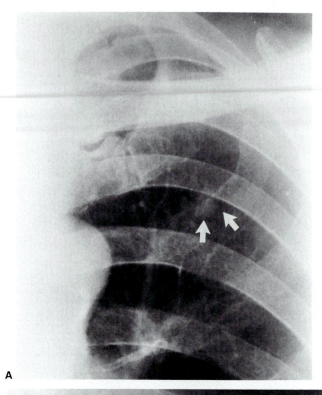

A

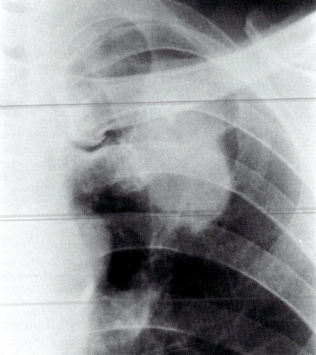

B

Fig. 14.8 Carcinoma growing slowly. No treatment. Between (A) and (B) there was an interval of $3\frac{1}{2}$ years.

appear in advance of any apparent lung neoplasm and they may remit with treatment of the primary. Other carcinoma cell types may have similar secretory properties, but less frequently than the small cell type.

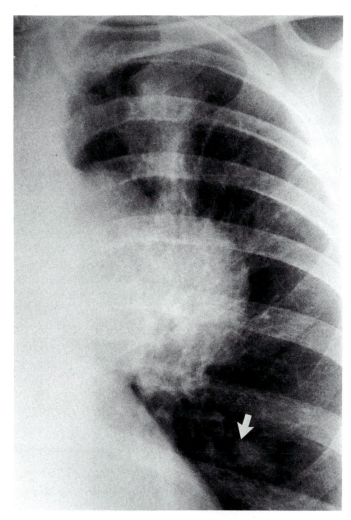

Fig. 14.9 Small-cell carcinoma at left apex with an extension to the large hilum. Secondary lung deposit inferior to the hilum (arrows).

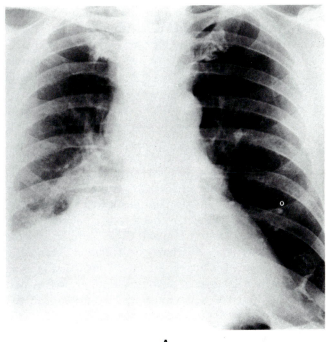

A

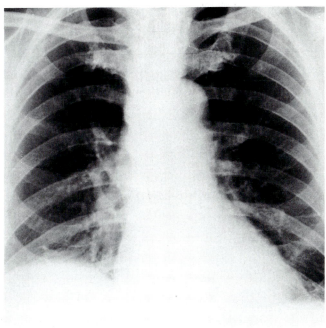

B

Fig. 14.10 A. Small-cell carcinoma. Remission with chemotherapy. Right lower lobe collapse; mediastinal adenopathy. **B.** 3 years later. No sign of disease.

Pancoast tumour

A carcinoma at the apex of the lung, whatever its histological type, has a propensity to invade the parietal pleura and soft tissues at the root of the neck. The term 'Pancoast tumour' refers to the syndrome of symptoms and signs so produced, which includes pain in the arm and paresis of sympathetic nerves on the same side. These tumours may be inconspicuous in the early stages, following as they do the line of the apical pleura, and be mistaken for postinflammatory pleural thickening so common at this site. Careful search should be made for evidence of rib erosion.

Bronchioloalveolar cell carcinoma

The tumour was so-called because of the doubt surrounding the identity of the cell line from which it arises, whether from bronchioles or alveoli. Many pathologists now believe that it can arise from a number of different cell types, including Type 2 pneumocytes, Clara cells (mucin secretors) and bronchiolar epithelium, or from a stem cell capable of differentiating into any of these cell lines. This places the tumour in the peripheral parts of the lung, from which it spreads into the alveolar spaces. It is not destructive of lung architecture which accounts for the relative preservation of regional lung perfusion.

By definition there must be no lesion in a major bronchus or an adenocarcinoma elsewhere in the body. The cells often secrete mucin and a profuse watery sputum is characteristic. Sputum cytology may reveal adenocarcinoma cells. It is not strongly related to cigarette smoking and its incidence is roughly equal in men and women. It tends to develop in damaged lungs and there may therefore be radiographic evidence of bronchiectasis, tuberculosis, rheumatoid pulmonary disease or systemic sclerosis.

It may be limited to a single, well-circumscribed, peripheral nodule, in which case surgical excision is likely to be curative because of the slow growth and late dissemination of this tumour. Another form of the disease is of multiple, ill-defined, variable sized nodules, either confined to one lung or bilateral. The nodules coalesce as they grow, and a lobar consolidation similar to pneumonia can result (Fig. 14.11). Consolidation is in part the result of airspace filling by tumour and in part by mucin. Surgery is not curative in the diffuse form, and eventual spread to the opposite lung is inevitable. *CT scanning* detects spread to the opposite lung earlier than the chest radiograph. Tumour growing alongside the bronchi makes them rigid but there is no obstruction. Atelectasis does not occur and air bronchograms are visible within the lung opacity. Bronchographic abnormalities consist of absence of normal changes of calibre during the respiratory cycle, a pruned-tree appearance from absence of filling of side branches and minor irregularities of the lumen. Septal lines and pleural effusion may be present. Cavitation is a rare event.

OTHER PRIMARY MALIGNANT TUMOURS OF LUNG

Most pathologists base their classification of these tumours on that proposed by the World Health Organization in 1967. Compared to carcinoma of lung, these tumours are relatively rare; they are not related to cigarette smoking and in general they occur in a younger age-group. Their slower rate of growth gives them a better prognosis than carcinoma. The symptoms, signs and radiographic appearances are largely determined by whether they arise within the air passages or lung.

CARCINOID

These tumours grow slowly and metastasize infrequently. Almost all arise within a major bronchus; a peripheral nodule is a rare exception. It grows through the bronchial wall and the intrabronchial tumour may be the tip of an iceberg, the greater portion being extrabronchial. The cell line is the APUD system of argentaffin cells, the same as the alimentary tract carcinoids. The age-group is younger than that for carcinoma and there is an equal incidence in men and women. The *carcinoid syndrome* from release

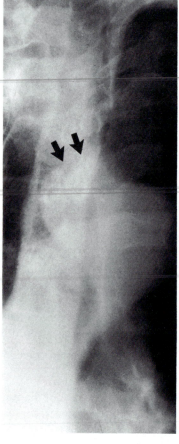

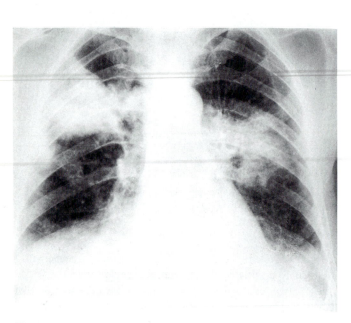

Fig. 14.11 Bronchioloalveolar carcinoma. Multiple consolidations. Small cavity lateral to the left hilum.

Fig. 14.12 Adenoid cystic carcinoma of trachea. There was severe stridor and a normal chest radiograph of lung fields.

of 5-hydroxytryptamine is rare, but when it occurs any endocardial fibrosis is located on the left side of the heart exposed to the drainage from the tumour. The radiographic signs are those of bronchial obstruction or a smoothly circumscribed mass.

ADENOID CYSTIC CARCINOMA (*cylindroma*)

This is a carcinoma of low-grade malignancy arising from the trachea, carina or main stem bronchi, locally invasive and spreading to regional hilar nodes but rarely metastasizing elsewhere (Fig. 14.12). It may extend outside or along the inside of the wall of the airway, the latter resulting in polypoid projections. Because of its site it commonly presents with obstructive symptoms, particularly stridor and 'asthma'.

This tumour, like others obstructing major airways, can give rise to alarming symptoms while the chest radiograph remains normal. Slowly growing tumours escape detection and the patient may be labelled as asthmatic. Any asthmatic whose symptoms and signs are in any way unusual should be regarded with suspicion, and any doubt settled by tomography of the major airways if necessary. These patients will usually have a characteristic flow/volume loop resulting from a test which plots rate of flow against lung volume; obstruction in a large airway limits the rate of flow through a large part of the expiratory phase, which is reflected in the flatter shape of the loop.

MUCOEPIDERMOID TUMOUR

Perhaps out of place here, this rare bronchial tumour has only exceptionally been reported as having malignant potential, although it is locally invasive. A small, entirely intrabronchial, sessile or polypoid tumour found at all ages, it consists of epidermoid elements and mucus-secreting acini. The same type of tumour is found in the salivary glands.

Bronchial adenoma is an old terminology for benign intrabronchial tumours. It is unsatisfactory on two counts; 90% of these tumours are carcinoids (which are of low-grade malignancy) and true adenomas are rare.

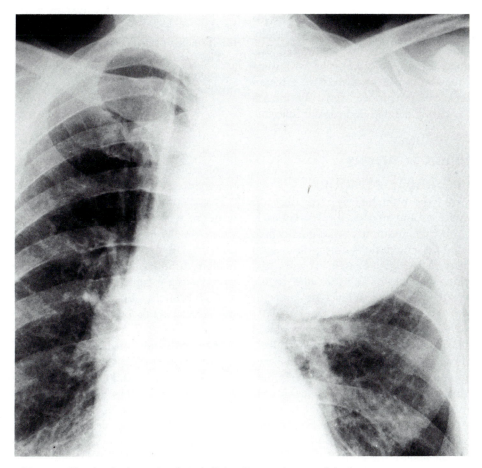

Fig. 14.13 Pulmonary blastoma. Despite the large size there is little effect on the rest of the lungs.

MIXED TUMOURS

Mixed tumours are those composed of two or more types of malignant cell. There are two lung tumours in this group:

1. Pulmonary blastoma. Embryonic connective tissue, muscle cells and columnar cell aggregations resembling fetal bronchioles make up this tumour. Because of its slow growth, peripheral site and absence of obstructive effects it may become a very large round mass before discovery (Fig. 14.13). Eventually metastasis to hilar nodes and elsewhere takes place.

2. Carcinosarcoma. The elements of this tumour are squamous carcinoma in a sarcomatous stroma. When found in the lungs it is usually a bronchial tumour, less often peripheral; it grows slowly and the prognosis after removal is relatively good.

PRIMARY SARCOMA OF LUNG

These are rare tumours outnumbered 500 to 1 by carcinomas. Leiomyo-, rhabdomyo- and fibrosarcoma are more frequent than any others and may arise from the tracheobronchial tree, lung or pleura. As a rule they affect a younger age-group than do carcinomas, and a number are found in children. The sex incidence is equal. Node involvement is unusual, and dissemination occurs late, so that prognosis after removal is relatively good, especially for fibrosarcoma. The tumour may be large when discovered; depending on the site of origin, pleural lesions are likely to signal their presence by a massive effusion and bronchial lesions by obstructive signs. Peripheral lesions typically have sharply defined and regular margins.

BENIGN TUMOURS

INTRABRONCHIAL TUMOURS

Tumours arising within the bronchial tree are likely to produce striking symptoms and signs at a relatively early stage, in contrast to benign pulmonary tumours which may remain undetected for long periods unless discovered incidentally on a chest radiograph. Cough, wheeze, and haemoptysis are common symptoms and the radiographic signs are those of atelectasis, bronchiectasis and air trapping.

The old term *bronchial adenoma* included carcinoid and adenoid cystic carcinoma, which are carcinomas of low-grade malignancy. True adenomas are rare and are either mucous gland adenomas (Fig. 14.14) or mucoepidermoids, the latter consisting of mixtures of mucous cells and squamous epithelium. *Papillomas* are warty tumours of the lining of the air passages and are predominantly lesions of childhood. They are frequently multiple, and in the condition of *papillomatosis* the entire bronchial tree may be stuffed with tumours which have a tendency to

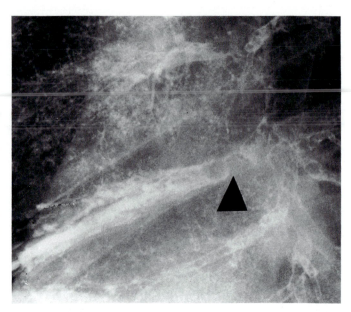

Fig. 14.14 Benign cystadenoma within the right middle lobe bronchus (large arrowhead). The lobe is collapsed (bronchogram).

cavitate. *Chondromas* arise from bronchial cartilage and protrude into the lumen, but, as in many endobronchial tumours, there may be a large extrabronchial extension. *Fibromas* and *lipomas* are usually endobronchial but can be found at other sites in lung, mediastinum or in relationship to the pleura.

The *granular cell myoblastoma* is a rare polypoid bronchial tumour which was thought to derive from muscle but it is now considered to have a neural origin.

PULMONARY TUMOURS

Hamartoma, *leiomyoma* and *neurofibroma* are other examples of benign tumours which can be endobronchial, but they are more often found as pulmonary nodules.

Benign pulmonary tumours are characteristically sharply defined, slow growing and smoothly rounded, except where they abut on a pleural surface which restrains their growth. Up to 10% of solitary pulmonary nodules are benign tumours. It may not be possible to determine whether these tumours arise from lung tissue, pleura or a small bronchus but this is not important radiologically, the critical factor being that they do not obstruct major air passages.

Hamartomas consist of mixtures of tissues normal to the organ in which they arise; in the case of the lung these are cartilage and epithelial elements. Most are under 1 cm in diameter and are found incidentally at postmortem. An average size of those found in life is about 3 cm. They grow very slowly but can reach a very large size. Those discovered are usually solitary and peripheral, with a sharply-defined but lobulated border. The density may be inhomogeneous because of fatty tissue. The cartilage

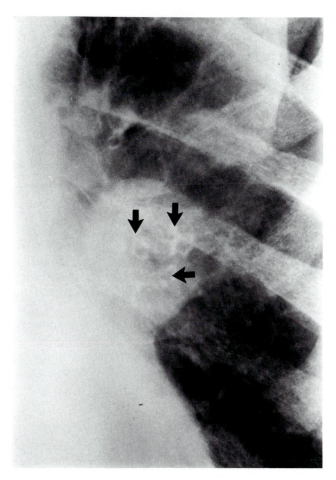

Fig. 14.15 Hamartoma. 'Popcorn' calcification is shown within the tumour (arrows).

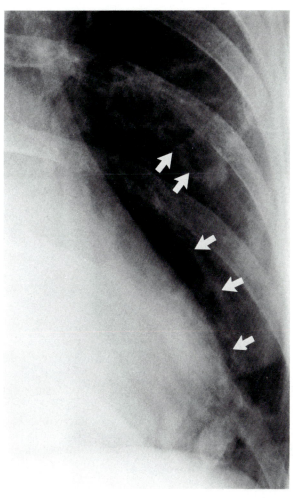

Fig. 14.16 Multiple pulmonary arteriovenous malformations. Enlarged feeding arteries (arrows).

element is a frequent source of calcification, seen radiographically as fine stippling, coarse irregular 'popcorn' granularity or linear streaks (Fig. 14.15).

Under the general term *angioma* are included lesions, arguably not true neoplasms and comprising blood-containing spaces. In the *capillary haemangioma* the spaces are of capillary size and these lesions are exemplified by the skin naevus. The spaces in the *cavernous haemangioma* are larger and their thin walls are lined by vascular endothelium. If there is a direct communication between the pulmonary artery and vein through the large spaces without the intervention of a capillary filter, the feeding artery and draining vein enlarge to accommodate what can be a considerable shunt. This is the *arteriovenous malformation or aneurysm* (Fig. 14.16). On a smaller scale the shunts are telangiectases, and both types are components of the Osler-Weber-Rendu disease (*hereditary haemorrhagic telangiectasis*).

The angiogram in arteriovenous malformation often reveals multiple lesions unsuspected on the plain radiograph, together with small areas of telangiectasia. Spontaneous rupture of an angioma sometimes takes place, resulting in a pulmonary haematoma. If the shunt through an arteriovenous malformation is sufficiently large there will be arterial desaturation and polycythaemia.

In *diffuse pulmonary telangiectasia* there are enormous numbers of small vessels producing nodularities and an exaggerated background of lung shadows which are readily confused with pulmonary fibrosis on the chest radiograph. The angiogram may show this intense hypervascularity but is sometimes normal. *Pulmonary haemangiomatosis* is an angiomatous infiltration within the walls of small arteries and veins, eventually causing their occlusion and resulting in pulmonary hypertension. In this condition death results from pulmonary hypertension, bleeding and respiratory failure. As the lung bases are affected in this disease it also mimics pulmonary fibrosis. The angiogram is similar to that of diffuse pulmonary telangiectasia except that there is prolonged retention of the contrast medium in the affected areas.

Neurofibromas are to be found wherever there are neural structures and therefore at any point throughout the bronchial tree. There is an association between

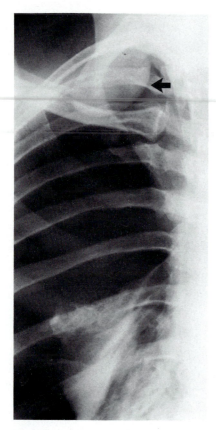

Fig. 14.17 Neurofibromatosis. Pneumothorax and an extrapleural neurofibroma (arrow).

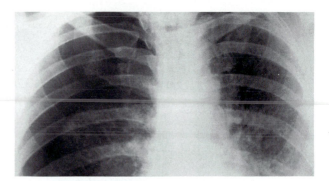

Fig. 14.18 Lymphangioleiomyomatosis. Right pneumothorax. Diffuse reticulonodulation in the lungs.

neurofibromatosis, diffuse pulmonary fibrosis and phaeochromocytoma. Pneumothorax occasionally complicates thoracic neurofibromatosis (Fig. 14.17).

TUMOUR-LIKE LESIONS

LYMPHANGIOMYOMATOSIS
(*Lymphangioleiomyomatosis*)
This is a rare and unusual disease of women of reproductive age, the major symptom being breathlessness, but the chest radiograph may be abnormal long before symptoms appear. Progressive respiratory insufficiency commonly leads to death within 10 years. Pathologically, there is a widespread infiltration of pleura, septa and alveolar walls by proliferating muscle and lymphatics. There are obstructive effects on lymphatics, veins and small airways. Radiographically, there is a fine reticulation, with miliary densities distributed widely and not sparing the lung bases, in contrast to eosinophil granuloma which it otherwise resembles closely (Fig. 14.18). Other features are: progressively enlarging lung volumes, small emphysematous cysts, pneumothorax, interstitial oedema, septal lines and chylous pleural effusions.

Lymphangiomyomatosis does not have a familial incidence, a point of differentiation from tuberous sclerosis which has the same pathological and radiological pulmonary manifestations.

Another disease of similar pathology is *metastasizing leiomyoma*, from uterine leiomyoma and consequently also confined to women. The pulmonary nodules in this condition are larger, over 1 cm in diameter, and the intervening lung is normal.

PULMONARY TUBEROUS SCLEROSIS
There is a characteristic triad of epilepsy, mental retardation and adenoma sebaceum diagnostic of this genetic disorder of mesodermal tissues. Mesodermal tumours of various kinds have been found in most organs and tissues of the body but the common sites are kidney, retina, brain and bone. The lungs are rarely affected, and then mostly in women. The disease may be limited to one organ, in which case epilepsy and mental retardation are unusual and symptoms are delayed until adult life.

Histologically there is a diffuse leiomyomatosis in alveolar walls, small airways and vessels, in places growing into small tumours budding into the lumen. This causes bronchial obstruction and distal destruction of alveolar walls. The radiographic counterpart of these changes is a diffuse reticulation or miliary pattern progressing to honeycombing. Pneumothorax is a common complication. The prognosis is poor once symptoms appear.

ROUND ATELECTASIS (*folded lung*)
The radiographic appearance of this lesion is of a pleural-based tumour-like mass almost always in the lower parts of the lungs. It has its origin in a sclerosing visceral pleuritis, which as it contracts rolls up a portion of the underlying lung in a spiral fashion. A radiological diagnosis is possible if pulmonary vessels and bronchi can be shown to curve towards the mass as though drawn into a vortex (Fig. 14.19). The same features are also shown on CT scanning.

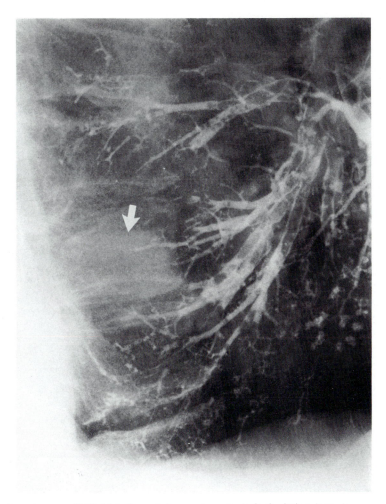

Fig. 14.19 Round atelectasis: bronchogram. Bronchi to lower lobe swept up towards the lesion (arrow).

PLASMA-CELL GRANULOMA

The histological components of this lesion are plasma cells and lymphocytes in a stroma of granulation tissue. It is now generally conceded that it is a post-inflammatory process occurring in all age groups and of equal sex distribution. When fat-laden mononuclear cells are present the terms *xanthogranuloma* or *fibroxanthoma* are sometimes applied. Usually a solitary well-circumscribed lesion, it can grow to great size but does not recur if removed. Calcification and cavitation are exceptional events. Other terms for this lesion are *histiocytoma* and *inflammatory pseudotumour*. It must not be confused with plasmocytoma, which is a true tumour.

SCLEROSING HAEMANGIOMA

Although this lesion has similarities to the plasma cell granuloma above, pathologists now believe that it is possible to differentiate them on histological grounds. Nevertheless there is still dispute about their origin, whether derived from vascular endothelium or Type 2 pneumocytes. In the latter case the vascular stroma is regarded as reactive rather than neoplastic. Despite these doubts the name is retained because it is the one by which it is most commonly known. It is a sharply circumscribed lesion predominantly affecting women under the age of 50, and it has a tendency to bleed, hence the frequent symptom of haemoptysis.

METASTATIC TUMOURS

Most pulmonary metastases have their origin in malignant tumours of the *genitourinary* and *gastrointestinal* systems, and when discovered unexpectedly a search is made for the primary site. The temptation to carry the search to absurd lengths has to be resisted. Histological examination of biopsy tissue narrows the possibilities, and then the question has to be asked whether a knowledge of the primary site will affect management of that particular case.

Haematogenous metastases are tumour emboli filtered by the pulmonary vasculature. Invasion of veins by the

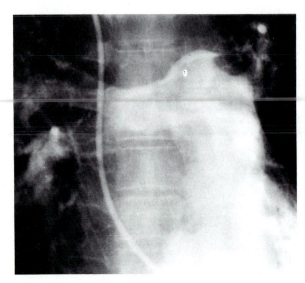

Fig. 14.20 Fibrosarcoma of pulmonary artery. Pulmonary angiogram. Large filling defects in pulmonary artery resembling emboli.

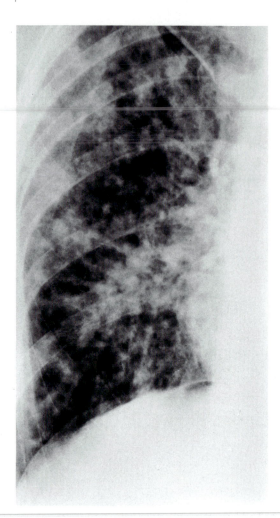

Fig. 14.22 Metastases with interstitial spread. The lung between nodules is abnormal. Origin unknown; the patient had both colon and breast carcinomas.

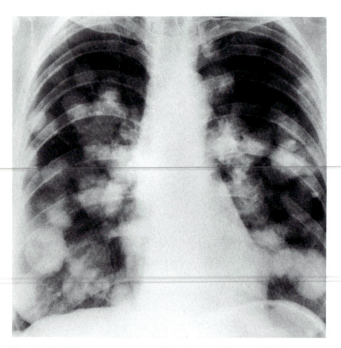

Fig. 14.21 Discrete metastases. Carcinoma of breast. The lung between lesions is normal.

primary tumour releases clumps of cells which pass via the cavae or vertebral venous plexus to the right heart and then to the pulmonary artery. The rare *sarcoma of the pulmonary artery* embolizes directly into the pulmonary artery (Fig. 14.20). Most of these tumour emboli are destroyed, but those that become established behave like primary neoplasms. The tumours may remain discrete and circumscribed (Fig. 14.21) or spread through the lymphatics of the broncho-vascular bundles to the hilum and mediastinum. In the latter case the lesions are irregular with intervening lung coarsened by lines and bands (Fig. 14.22). A miliary or snowstorm appearance indicates rapid growth (Fig. 14.23).

Lymphatic permeation can also take place directly from the primary, through the chest wall from breast or through the diaphragmatic crura from liver, adrenal or celiac nodes. The mediastinum and its nodes are the first in line with this type of spread (Fig. 14.24). Mediastinal and hilar node enlargement with clear lungs is a recognized pattern of metastatic spread from renal carcinoma.

The effects on pulmonary function bear little relation to the size of individual metastases but rather to their profusion. Showers of tumour emboli in the pulmonary capillaries can cause *pulmonary hypertension* even when the chest radiograph is normal. Tumour cells often stimulate a fibrotic reaction in lymphatics and capillaries, a feature found in *lymphangitis carcinomatosa* which is a mixture of miliary metastases, lymphatic permeation and interstitial

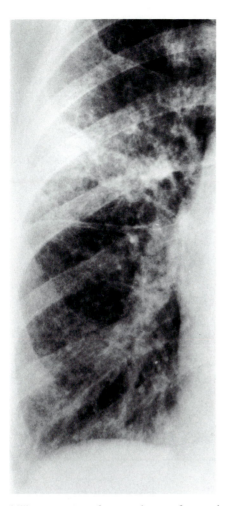

Fig. 14.23   Miliary metastases from carcinoma of stomach.

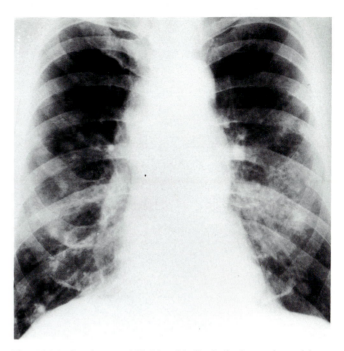

Fig. 14.24   Carcinoma of bladder. Mediastinal adenopathy and lung metastases.

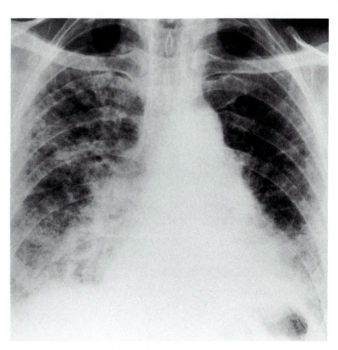

Fig. 14.25   Lymphangitis carcinomatosa.

fibrosis (Fig. 14.25). These patients are severely dyspnoeic. Massive *pleural effusion* can add to respiratory embarrassment and can be difficult to palliate. Metastases from carcinoma of thyroid may retain secretory function and can be detected by the increased uptake of ^{131}I even when the chest radiograph is normal.

At the extremes of growth rate there can be problems in the differentiation of metastases from other lesions. The sudden appearance of a profusion of lesions may seem altogether too rapid for the development of metastases and may suggest instead septicaemic abscesses (Fig. 14.26). At the other extreme is the solitary metastasis appearing many years after removal of a primary (Fig. 14.27). Multiple metastases from thyroid carcinoma can occasionally grow extremely slowly.

Calcification. Calcific densities within metastases result from a variety of pathological processes: bone formation (particularly seen in osteosarcoma), calcification in cartilage, dystrophic calcification, calcification in mucus (seen in papillary and mucinous adenocarcinoma) or following treatment.

Necrosis and cavitation is not a function of size and can occur in quite small metastases. Cavitation always carries a risk of *pneumothorax* (Fig. 14.28).

Trophoblastic tumours have variable malignant potential but all are liable to embolize to the lungs, where the benign varieties undergo absorption. Trophoblastic tissue is by its nature invasive, and the metastases have the same

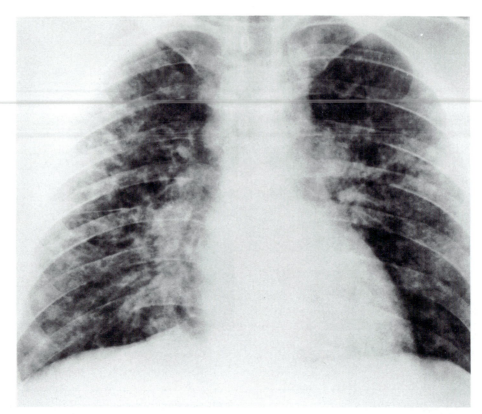

Fig. 14.26 Metastases from malignant melanoma. Chest radiograph was normal 12 days before this.

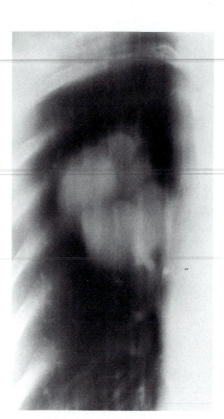

Fig. 14.27 Tomogram. Solitary fibrosarcoma metastasis. Fibrosarcoma removed from thigh 20 years before!

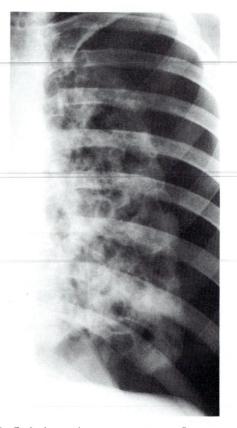

Fig. 14.28 Cavitating angiosarcoma metastases. Spontaneous pneumothorax.

characteristics. Their edge is poorly defined because they are surrounded by haemorrhage. An unusual complication sometimes follows removal of a molar pregnancy — the sudden onset of pulmonary oedema progressing into the adult respiratory distress syndrome with diffuse intravascular coagulation.

Occasionally an *endobronchial tumour* is biopsied and found to be a metastasis, usually from a primary in breast, colon or renal tract. Bronchial obstruction dominates the clinical and radiographic signs, a circumstance which is otherwise rare in metastatic disease.

MALIGNANT LYMPHOMA AND LEUKAEMIA

Proliferation of lymphocytes is a feature of malignant lymphoma and also of certain benign conditions. Distinction between them on histological grounds can be difficult, compounded by the fact that some of the benign disorders eventually become transformed into malignant lymphomas.

A number of conditions predispose to the development of malignant lymphoma. These include congenital immune deficiencies (Wiskott-Aldrich syndrome, ataxia telangiectasia), autoimmune diseases (rheumatoid, systemic lupus, myasthenia gravis), occupational exposure to benzene and other solvents, organ transplantation, Sjögren's syndrome and immunoblastic lymphadenopathy. There is also a slight excess in patients with sarcoidosis over the number expected from chance association. The drug *phenytoin* has an association with malignant lymphoma as well as with benign lymphoproliferative disorders. Most of the disorders which carry an increased risk have an abnormality of immune mechanisms, either immunosuppression, failure of immune surveillance or chronic subjection to antigenic stimulation. It is thought that there is a transformation by stages: first, a polyclonal proliferation of lymphocytes, followed by an escape of a malignant cell line.

Treatment of the malignant lymphomas is now highly effective, but radiotherapy and chemotherapy are not without risk and morbidity. Treatment therefore has to be tailored to the extent and site of the disease, hence the stress laid on diagnostic staging. The number and complexity of the imaging modes utilized in the staging process depends to some extent on the histological type. Centres dealing with the disease also vary in their requirements. Detailed histological classification is essential for the assessment of the efficacy of different treatment regimes under test, but it has few implications as far as radiological diagnosis is concerned.

Malignant lymphoma is divided into two groups — *Hodgkin's* and *non-Hodgkin's* — and each group is further subdivided, on histological criteria, into many varieties. Some confusion is created by the use of alternative names for the same histological type, e.g. lymphocytic lymphoma

and lymphosarcoma; histiocytic lymphoma and reticulum cell sarcoma.

Hodgkin's lymphoma is a nodal disease, starting in nodes and spreading from nodes. If it starts in the thorax the *mediastinal nodes* will almost invariably be enlarged, the hilar nodes less often. Although hilar node enlargement as the sole manifestation is unusual, it happens sufficiently often to limit the value of site as an infallible discriminant between lymphoma and sarcoidosis. The nodes are massive and merge with each other, presenting an undulating rather than a nodular margin. If *extension into the lung* takes place it does so along interlobular, perivascular and peribronchial lymphatic channels, forming deposits in the small *intrapulmonary nodes*. The latter are located at the sites of branching of the bronchovascular structures. In this way the disease can extend out to the pleura. Radiographically, the sharp outline of purely central nodal disease is then replaced by a shaggy edge from a mixture of linear streaks, bands and clusters of small nodules radiating into the lungs (Fig. 14.29). The

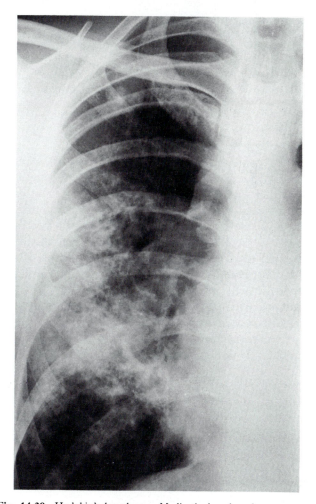

Fig. 14.29 Hodgkin's lymphoma. Mediastinal node enlargement. Mixed nodular and interstitial pulmonary spread into upper and middle lobes.

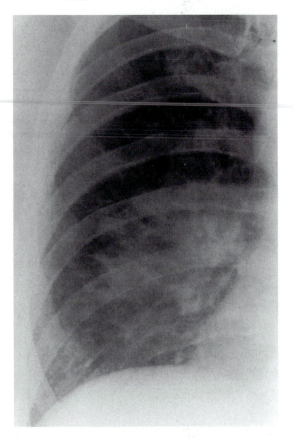

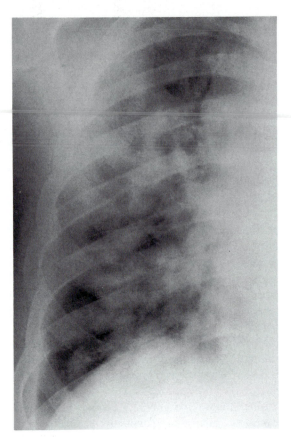

Fig. 14.30 Hodgkin's lymphoma. Right mediastinal and hilar node enlargement. Spreading consolidation in upper, middle and lower lobes. Nodules at the edge of the consolidation and distally.

Fig. 14.31 Hodgkin's lymphoma. Large, ill-defined nodules and a pleural effusion.

individual components of this shadowing may merge into a patchy haze of progressively diminishing density as it gets further out into the lung (Fig. 14.30). This pulmonary spread can take place rapidly over the course of a few days, causing confusion with oedema or infection. Dense coalescent *infiltrations* may result in segmental or lobar opacities, sometimes with air bronchograms. There may be *lung nodules*, either profuse and miliary, or larger — approximately 1 cm in diameter (Fig. 14.31).

Pulmonary lesions sometimes necrose with the formation of thick-walled *cavities*. An *effusion*, which may be chylous, may result from extension into the pleura and a careful search should then be made for evidence of rib erosion.

Hodgkin's disease beginning elsewhere in the body and spreading into the thorax differs from the pattern described above in that pulmonary lesions can develop without any obvious mediastinal or hilar node enlargement. This has been reported in up to 25% of cases, which contrasts with the exceptional rarity of primary pulmonary Hodgkin's disease. In other respects the radiographic signs are similar.

After successful treatment the chest radiograph may not return to normal. Nodes may *calcify*, *radiation pneumonitis*

appear or a residual mass of *pseudotumour* persist. To determine whether such a mass is due to pseudotumour or residual disease may require excision or biopsy. Pseudo-tumours consist of nonspecific inflammatory reactions or amyloid.

Radiation pneumonitis is strictly confined to the volume of lung irradiated, an important point in differential diagnosis. *Recall radiation pneumonitis* is a term applied to ill-defined opacities appearing in the radiation field but only after the withdrawal of steroid therapy. It has been described as occurring up to 6 years after radiotherapy and it responds to the reintroduction of steroids.

Non-Hodgkin's lymphoma. As far as the radiographic signs are concerned the differences between Hodgkin's and non-Hodgkin's lymphoma are quantitative rather than qualitative. The disease rarely starts in the thorax and it is usually at an advanced stage when it gets there. *Mediastinal* and *hilar node masses*, radiating *perihilar streaks with small pulmonary nodules* on the lymphatic pathways, *segmental* and *lobar opacities* are all features of the disease similar to those of Hodgkin's but *pulmonary lesions without nodal involvement* are more common (Fig. 14.32). A lobe solid with primary lymphocytic lymphoma is rare but not so exceptional as the equivalent in Hodgkin's

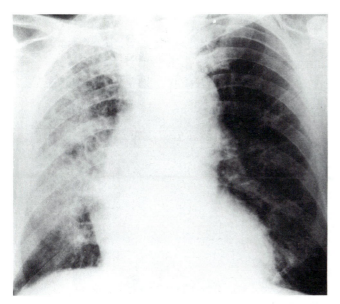

Fig. 14.32 Non-Hodgkin's lymphoma in Sjögren's syndrome. Mixed nodular and interstitial shadowing in right lung. Slow progression over 7 years. Minimal changes in left lung. No hilar or mediastinal adenopathy.

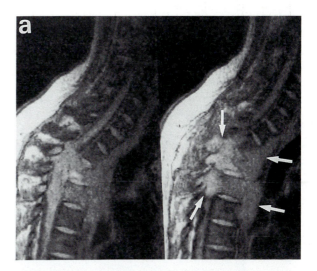

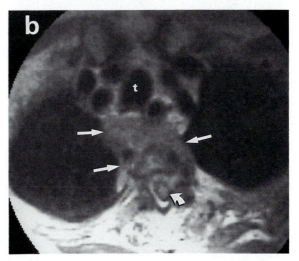

Fig. 14.34 Posterior mediastinal carcinoma (straight arrows) infiltrating two adjacent thoracic vertebral bodies with partial collapse and extradural extension, on T_1-weighted (**a**) sagittal (spin echo 740/40) and (**b**) transverse (partial saturation recovery 500/18) scans. Note low signal from dural sac (curved arrow); t = trachea.

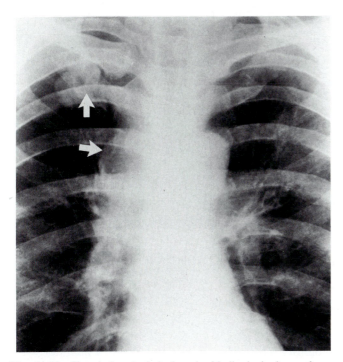

Fig. 14.33 Chronic lymphatic leukaemia. Mediastinal adenopathy. Deposit in right upper lobe (arrows).

disease. A *pleural plaque* or *effusion* is found in approximately 30% of patients.

Primary extranodal malignant lymphoma arises in lymphoid tissue related to mucosa (gut, salivary gland and bronchus). These mucosa-associated lymphocytes can pass through regional lymph nodes into the systemic circulation and spread to histologically related tissues. The lymphoma may remain localized for many years but when dissemination occurs it is characteristically into other mucosal sites. Some cases of *Sjögren's syndrome* are examples of this spread, from salivary gland to lung. It is now-believed that *pseudolymphoma*, *lymphomatoid granulomatosis* and *lymphocytic interstitial pneumonia* are also examples of extranodal mucosa-associated lymphoma.

Plasmacytoma or plasmacytic lymphoma are descriptive terms for the lesions of myelomatosis, and solitary tumours of this nature are identical to the disseminate form. Solitary tumours may present as pulmonary masses or obstructing endobronchial lesions.

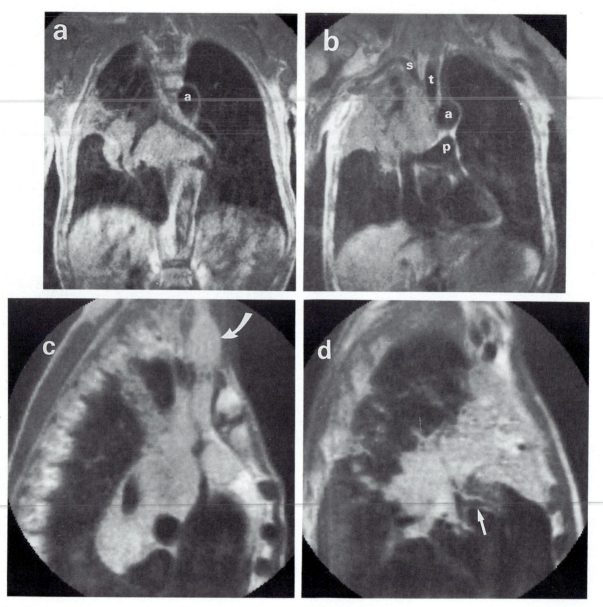

Fig. 14.35 Carcinoma of the lung with lymphadenopathy and distal collapse/consolidation on (**a, b**) coronal T$_1$-weighted (spin echo 560/26) (**c, d**) parasagittal intermediate-weighted (spin echo 1200/60) images. The collapse/consolidation in the anterior and posterior segments of the right upper lobe shows heterogeneity and higher signal than the more uniform intensity of the central tumour, but clear separation is difficult. Nodal disease in the neck (curved arrow) is demonstrated in (**c**). Straight arrow in **d** = middle lobe bronchus; a = aortic arch; p = left pulmonary artery; s = subclavian artery; t = trachea.

LEUKAEMIA

In almost all cases of leukaemia that come to postmortem there can be found microscopic infiltrations of leukaemic cells around bronchi and vessels and in alveolar walls. Macroscopic nodules from 1 mm to 2 cm in size may also be found. Nevertheless it is exceptional for these deposits to be visible on the chest radiograph; any abnormal opacity will almost certainly be the result of infection, infarction or haemorrhage. *Mediastinal* or *hilar node enlargement* is more frequent than pulmonary deposits (Fig. 14.33). Conversion of lymphoma to leukaemia is a

recognized complication, particularly with lymphoblastic lymphoma, and this conversion can sometimes be predicted if a mediastinal mass makes its appearance during the course of the disease. Leukaemia can also follow apparently successful treatment of lymphoma.

MRI IN TUMOURS OF THE LUNG
Ian Isherwood and Jeremy P. R. Jenkins

CT is an established technique in the staging of lung carcinoma, with MRI currently used in a problem-solving

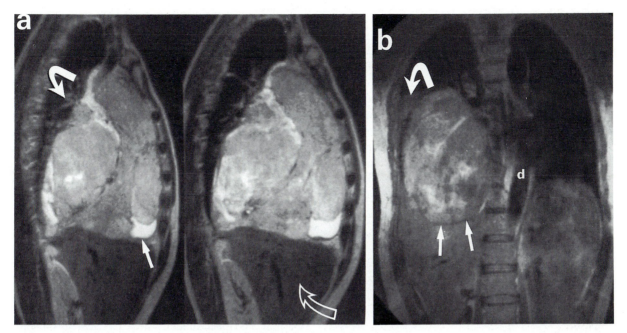

Fig. 14.36 Large pleural fibrosarcoma compressing lung (curved closed arrow) and displacing liver (curved open arrow) on (**a**) two contiguous sagittal T_2-weighted (spin echo 1660/80) and (**b**) coronal T_1-weighted (spin echo 560/26) images. The liver is not directly infiltrated and neither is the anterior chest wall. The diaphragm can be seen as a low-intensity line (straight arrows), most clearly beneath a small anterior pleural effusion in **a**. d = descending aorta. (Reproduced with permission from: Jenkins JPR (1990). Magnetic resonance imaging in oncology. In: R. J., Johnson, B. Eddleston, R. D., Hunter (Eds.) *Radiology in the Management of Cancer, Churchill Livingstone, Edinburgh.)*

role. Both CT and MRI are equally good at assessing tumour size. CT is more accurate in the demonstration of small nodules, except for those located close to hilar vessels, where MRI has advantage. MR images of the lungs have a low signal-to-noise ratio (SNR). Contrast between tumour and lung is essentially independent of pulse sequence, due to the inherently low proton density with aerated lung. Contrast and detail can be improved by enhancement of the mass with gadolinium-DTPA. A major disadvantage of MRI compared with CT is that peripheral pulmonary vessels and lobar fissures are not visualized, making it difficult to demonstrate the position of a lung mass with respect to a lobe or segment.

Superior sulcus tumours can be better visualized by MRI than by CT, due to improved anatomical display on coronal and sagittal plane images (Fig. 14.34). In a study of 31 patients with a superior sulcus tumour, the accuracy of MRI in the evaluation of tumour invasion of adjacent structures was 94%, compared with 63% by CT. T_1-weighted images showed the tumour as intermediate signal in contrast with the high signal from surrounding fat, enabling better delineation of chest wall invasion, adjacent vessels, brachial plexus and spinal structures.

In a small series of patients with proximal lung carcinoma and distal lobar collapse, evaluated by dynamic contrast-enhanced CT and MRI, CT was more successful than MRI in differentiating tumour mass from collapsed lung (Fig. 14.35). Dynamic contrast-enhanced CT was able to differentiate tumour from collapsed lung in eight of 10 patients, whereas MRI demonstrated signal intensity differences in only half those patients. It should be noted that in two patients in whom differentiation between tumour and collapsed lung was not achieved by contrast-enhanced CT, MRI showed separation, suggesting a possible complementary role for the techniques. T_2-weighted sequences were most useful in demonstrating a higher signal (longer T_2) from the collapsed lung than from the tumour. It is likely that the use of gadolinium-DTPA would improve the accuracy of MRI.

The *normal pleural space* cannot be resolved by MRI but adjacent *fat* is well shown. Early *chest wall invasion* by tumour is better demonstrated on MRI than CT. T_1-weighted images provide good morphological detail and contrast discrimination between tumour (intermediate signal) and fat (high signal). The presence of a high signal within chest wall muscle on T_2-weighted images suggests more extensive invasion. The changes however are non-specific. Similar increased signal intensity can occur with inflammatory disease. *Rib destruction* is not well shown on MRI. CT and MRI are unreliable in demonstrating mediastinal pleural infiltration, although the better contrast resolution of MRI has the greater potential. Microscopic invasion of the mediastinum by tumour without bulk change cannot be detected. Invasion can be assumed if interdigitation of tumour into the mediastinum, or chest wall, is present. Interruption of the normal low signal intensity line of the pericardium, which is less than 2 mm thick and best delineated on coronal and transverse ECG-gated T_1-weighted images, suggests *pericardial invasion*. Similarly, interruption of the low intensity line of the diaphragm adjacent to a mass, on sagittal and coronal images, suggests infiltration (Fig. 14.36).

Lymph node assessment is discussed elsewhere (Ch. 12). Vascular invasion by tumour is more clearly demonstrated by MRI than by CT whilst CT is more sensitive in the detection of pleural effusions. On MRI, effusions are more clearly shown on T_2- or proton-density-weighted images as a high signal, compared with a low signal on T_1-weighted scans. MRI is helpful in differentiating pleural from parenchymal disease and has the potential

to elucidate complex effusions. Lymphangitis carcinomatosa has the distinctive appearance of a hilar or mediastinal mass with peripherally dilated pulmonary lymphatics.

In the evaluation of distant metastases from carcinoma of the lung, MRI has the potential for characterizing some adrenal masses. On T_2-weighted images adrenal metastases have a high signal intensity (Fig. 36.15) whereas benign nonfunctioning adenomas give a low signal similar to surrounding liver. There is, however some overlap, which limits its clinical value. MRI is a more sensitive technique than CT in the detection of liver and CNS metastases.

REFERENCES AND SUGGESTIONS FOR FURTHER READING

Arnold, A. M., Williams, C. J. (1979) Small cell lung cancer: a curable disease? *British Journal of Diseases of the Chest*, **73**, 327–348.
Bragg, D. G., Colby, T. V., Ward, J. H. (1986) New concepts in the non-Hodgkin lymphomas: radiologic implications. *Radiology*, **159**, 291–304.
Castellino, R. A. (1986) Hodgkin disease: practical concepts for the diagnostic radiologist. *Radiology*, **159**, 305–310.
Cho, S. R., Henry, D. A., Beachley, M. C., Brooks, J. W. (1981) Round (helical) atelectasis. *British Journal of Radiology*, **54**, 643–650.
Corrin, B., Liebow, A. A., Friedman, P. J. (1975) Pulmonary lymphangiomyomatosis. *American Journal of Pathology*, **79**, 348–382.
Heath, D., Reid, R. (1985) Invasive pulmonary haemangiomatosis. *British Journal of Diseases of the Chest*, **79**, 284–294.
Herbert, A., Wright, D. H., Isaacson, P. G., Smith, J. L. (1984) Primary malignant lymphoma of the lung: histopathologic and immunologic evaluation of nine cases. *Human Pathology*, **15**, 415–422.
Lillington, G. A., Stevens, G. M. (1976) The solitary nodule. The other side of the coin. *Chest*, **70**, 322–323.
Ray, J. F., Lawton, B. R., Magnin, G. E., et al (1976) the coin lesion story: update 1976. *Chest*, **70**, 332–336.
Various authors (1977) Pulmonary neoplasms. *Seminars in Roentgenology*, **12**, 161–246.

MRI
Heelan, R. T., Demas, B. E., Caravelli, J. F. et al (1989) Superior sulcus tumours: CT and MR imaging. *Radiology*, **170**, 637–641.
Henschke, C. I., Davis, S. D., Romano, P. M., Yankelevitz, D. F. (1989) The pathogenesis, radiologic evaluation, and therapy of pleural effusions. *Radiologic Clinics of North America*, **27**, 1241–1255.
Libshitz, H. I. (1989) Imaging and staging of lung cancer. *Current Opinion in Radiology*, **1**, 21–24.
Naidich, D. P. (1990) CT/MR correlation in the evaluation of tracheobronchial neoplasia. *Radiologic Clinics of North America*, **28**, 555–571.
Templeton, P. A., Zerhouni, E. A. (1990) MR imaging in the management of thoracic malignancies. *Radiologic Clinics of North America*, **27**, 1099–1111.
Templeton, P. A., Caskey, C. I., Zerhouni, E. A. (1990) Current uses of CT and MR imaging in the staging of lung cancer. *Radiologic Clinics of North America*, **28**, 631–646.
Tobler, J., Levitt R. G., Glazer, H. S., Moran, J., Crouch, E., Evans, R. G. (1987) Differentiation of proximal bronchogenic carcinoma from postobstructive lobar collapse by magnetic resonance imaging: comparison with computed tomography. *Investigative Radiology*, **22**, 538–543.

CHAPTER 15

INFLAMMATORY DISEASES OF THE LUNG

Ivan Hyde

Terminology

The terminology used to describe inflammatory or any other disease of the lungs is designed to satisfy clinical and pathological criteria, and attempts to apply the same terms to radiographic appearances can lead to confusion. 'Infiltrate' or 'infiltration', often used to describe abnormal lung opacifications, means something quite different to a pathologist. Alternatively, radiographic shadows can be described in terms of their physical characteristics without any pathological overtones. Nevertheless it is difficult to avoid completely reference to such terms as 'atelectasis', 'consolidation' and 'interstitial'.

Three handicaps under which radiologists work are: 1. they deal with volumes compressed into two dimensions, with all the implications of superimposition; 2. terminology is imprecise and not uniform; 3. correlation between pathological and radiographic appearances is in many instances crude, particularly in the case of disseminate lung disease. Diagnosis based on purely radiographic appearances will almost always contain a large element of uncertainty, but this can be reduced by a search for ancillary clues which may be clinical, pathological, radiological or statistical.

Pneumonia is an inflammatory disease of lung, usually due to an infection by pathogenic organisms, and consolidation (the replacement of alveolar air by exudate) is assumed unless the term is qualified as in 'interstitial pneumonia'. It is seldom possible radiographically and without other evidence to differentiate inflammatory exudate from oedema fluid, blood or tumour.

Pneumonitis is a general term for any inflammatory reaction in the lung and consolidation is neither implied nor excluded. An inflammatory process that predominantly affects the alveolar wall is usually referred to as *alveolitis* in Great Britain or *interstitial pneumonitis (pneumonia)* in North America.

Bronchopneumonia is a multifocal bronchocentric infection based on the pulmonary lobule. The process spreads along the bronchial axis. Lesions are at first small but coalesce as they spread outwards. Their characteristic feature, both pathologically and radiographically, is inhomogeneity, in contrast to the homogeneity of lobar pneumonia.

Division of pneumonias into *primary* and *secondary* according to whether there is a precipitating cause is of limited help diagnostically.

ACUTE PNEUMONIA

A causative organism is only likely to be found in 50% of cases, usually because of prior treatment with antibiotics or an inability to provide a satisfactory sputum specimen. Of these organisms there will be a third each of bacterial, non-bacterial and viral. Of the bacterial causes the *pneumococcus (Streptococcus pneumoniae)* is most common, with much smaller numbers of *Staphylococcus aureus, Haemophilus influenzae, Klebsiella pneumoniae* and *Legionella pneumophila*.

Of the non-bacterial causes *Mycoplasma pneumoniae* is most common. In fact, it is the most common proven cause of primary pneumonia in Great Britain at the present time. Other non-bacterial causes found in small numbers are *Chlamydia psittaci* (psittacosis) and *Coxiella burnetti* (Q fever). The viruses are almost all *influenza* and *cold viruses*. Mixed infections are found in approximately 10% of cases.

Pneumococcal pneumonia is the archetype of classical lobar pneumonia (Fig. 15.1), with homogeneous lung opacification limited by fissures. Affected lobes retain normal volume and often show air bronchograms. The onset is so acute that opacification is often at its maximum on the initial radiograph. However, consolidation is not always obvious on the radiograph and its presence may be revealed more by the silhouette sign of boundary effacement than by pulmonary opacity.

The classic appearance is now the exception rather than the rule, largely because early antibiotic treatment aborts the progression. Consolidation may not spread uniformly throughout the lobe. From the initial focus of infection a tidal wave of inflammatory oedema spreads concentrically by all available routes, not only by the air passages but also through the substance of the lung via the pores

413

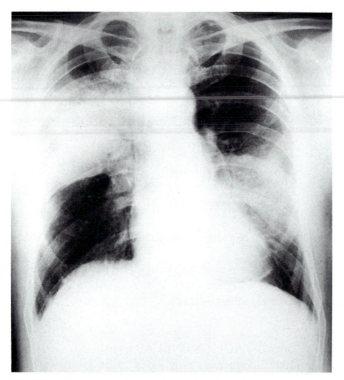

Fig. 15.1 Pneumococcal pneumonia. Lingula and right upper lobe consolidation with sparing of apex.

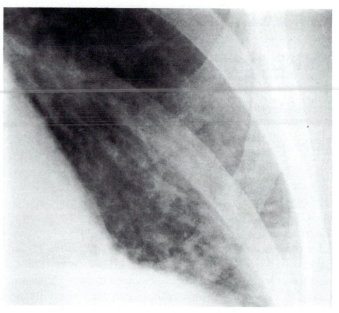

Fig. 15.2 Acute pneumonia. Oedema of interlobular septa.

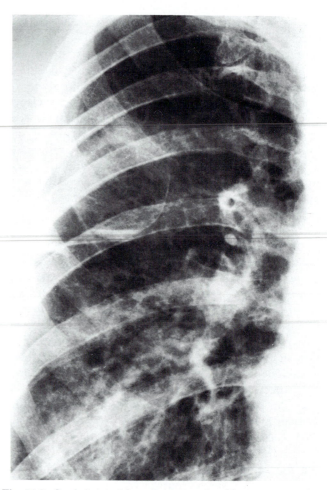

Fig. 15.3 Staphylococcal bronchopneumonia with a pneumatocele in the right upper lobe. The radiograph returned to normal.

of Kohn. The opacity may therefore not conform to segmental boundaries; it may produce rounded lesions with ill-defined margins. Kerley B lines may appear in the affected area from a temporary overloading of lymphatics and oedema of interlobular septa (Fig. 15.2). The distribution of the inflammatory exudate can be influenced to some degree by the effect of gravity until it becomes fixed by consolidation. Resolution is accompanied by diminution of the density of the opacity as air returns to the lobe. It is usually complete and lung architecture is restored to normal.

The complications of *empyema, lung abscess* or *delayed resolution* depend on such factors as host resistance and type of causative pathogen. If resolution is unduly delayed the exudate is invaded by fibroblasts and organization by fibrosis takes place.

There are no diagnostic features for particular pathogenic organisms but clues can sometimes be found in the radiographic pattern of pneumonia.

Staphylococcal pneumonia is usually a haematogenous dissemination and the lesions are therefore likely to be oval or round and multiple. However, this is not always the case, and the staphylococcus can be a secondary invader and then the lesions will be bronchopneumonic, irregular and patchy (Fig. 15.3). There is a strong tendency for colliquative necrosis to occur in the centre of staphylococcal consolidations (Fig. 15.4). As the consolidation around these *abscesses* recedes they are seen to have

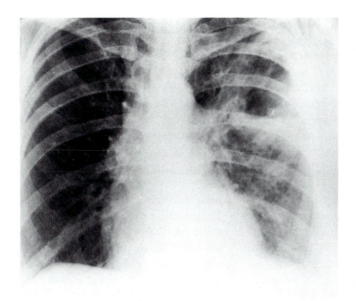

Fig. 15.4 Staphylococcal pneumonia of the left upper lobe with abscess formation. Influenzal illness one week before.

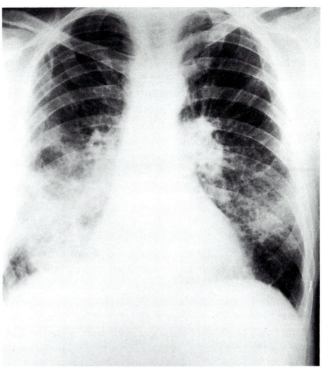

Fig. 15.5 Legionnaire's disease. Bilateral consolidations.

a thin wall. Resolution of the consolidation and resorption of the fluid contents leaves a *pneumatocele* with a wall of hair-line thickness. These may persist for months but eventually they disappear, usually leaving no trace. Empyema is another common complication of staphylococcal pneumonia — sometimes a result of injudicious needling of a lung abscess.

Legionnaires' disease. In 1976 an explosive epidemic of severe respiratory illness occurred at an American Legionnaires' convention in Philadelphia. It was a rapidly extending pneumonia complicated by shock, mental confusion, respiratory and renal failure, unresponsive to the usual antibiotics, with a case fatality of 16%. A previously unknown Gram-negative bacillus was eventually isolated and given the name *Legionella pneumophila*. The organism is ubiquitous in water, multiplying in water coolers, air-conditioners and showers, and infection takes place from inhalation of an aerosol mist.

It is prone to attack smokers and the debilitated. Radiographically there is spreading consolidation, and although it may be confined to one lobe initially it soon extends to others and to the opposite lung (Fig. 15.5). Another characteristic feature is the slow resolution over several weeks, but this is usually complete. Small *pleural effusions* are common; abscess and pneumatocele formation rare.

Friedländer (*Klebsiella*) pneumonia is typically a disease of elderly men. So voluminous is the inflammatory exudate that the affected lobe may be swollen and the fissures then bulge. Although this is regarded as a helpful sign it is in fact unusual, nor is it confined to Friedländer infections. The upper lobes are those most frequently involved, and, in common with other Gram-

negative pneumonias, there is a strong tendency to necrosis with the formation of multiple abscesses. If fibrosis takes place these cavities become permanent and, by virtue of their site, mimic tuberculosis. A septicaemic infection can occur in younger patients which is radiographically indistinguishable from many other overwhelming pulmonary infections or from pulmonary oedema (Fig. 15.6).

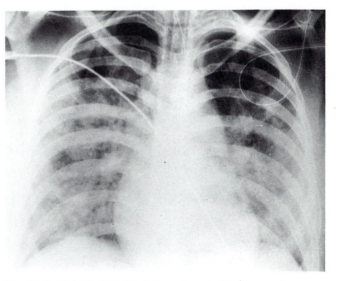

Fig. 15.6 *Klebsiella* (Friedländer) septicaemia. Diffuse, patchy, alveolar shadowing.

Haemophilus influenzae is a commensal of the upper respiratory tract, but since it is sometimes found in large numbers in the sputum in association with chronic lung diseases and treatment aimed at its eradication is often followed by clinical improvement, it is accorded a potentially pathogenic role. It is a secondary invader found in chronic bronchitis, cystic fibrosis and debilitated states. It is also found in influenza and other virus infections. Any pulmonary opacities found in *Haemophilus* infection are disseminate and bronchopneumonic; there are no characteristic radiographic appearances (Fig. 15.7).

Pseudomonas aeruginosa is an organism widely distributed in nature and of low pathogenicity. Most infections are either acquired in hospital or occur in immunocompromised patients. Pulmonary infections follow mechanical ventilation of the lungs, inhalation therapy or the use of aerosols. It is therefore an unwelcome visitor to ITUs where the incidence of its acquisition is directly proportional to the duration of mechanical ventilation and the use of broad-spectrum antibiotics. Pulmonary infection is a bronchopneumonia with a tendency to confluence and destruction of alveolar walls, resulting in microabscesses which progressively enlarge. An unusual manifestation consisting of large numbers of widespread small opacities suggests a septicaemic spread.

Melioidosis, a disease of tropical countries of the East, is caused by *Pseudomonas pseudomallei*. It may manifest years after the patient has left an endemic area. There are two pulmonary forms: 1. septicaemic disseminate necrotizing lesions; and 2. a chronic apical pneumonia which breaks down to form a thin-walled cavity.

Tularaemia. Discovered in Tulare, California, infection with the *Francisella tularensis* is endemic amongst small mammals and is spread by ticks. Humans acquire the infection either by inoculation or inhalation. Remarkably few organisms are required to cause illness. In the bacteraemic form there are small oval pulmonary lesions and hilar adenopathy. Inhalation infection causes one or more consolidations, also with hilar adenopathy. Untreated the consolidations cavitate and fibrose and then mimic tuberculosis.

LUNG ABSCESS

Gram-negative organisms have a particular propensity to cause pulmonary infections which break down with the formation of abscesses. Three circumstances favour their development: 1. aspiration of infected material; 2. infarction by septic material; and 3. infection by anaerobic organisms. The isolation of an organism from sputum does not necessarily mean that it is the sole cause, and a lack of response to treatment should lead one to suspect a mixed infection, particularly with anaerobic or microaerophilic organisms.

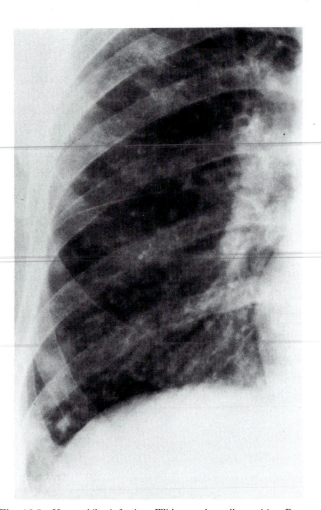

Fig. 15.7 *Haemophilus* infection. Widespread small opacities. Recent influenza.

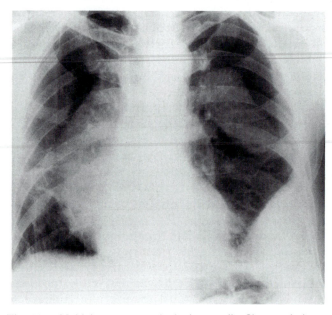

Fig. 15.8 Multiple empyemas. Aspirations sterile. Slow resolution. Probably anaerobic or microaerophilic infection.

Commonly multiple cavities form within an area of consolidation but they only become visible when the contents are discharged and air enters. *Gangrene of the lung* is a rapidly spreading necrosis, the separation of the slough first producing an air crescent between itself and viable lung before falling to the bottom of the cavity. The disease has a high mortality with or without surgical resection, and prognosis depends very much on finding an appropriate antibiotic.

Anaerobic and microaerophilic organisms can also be responsible for indolent pulmonary infections leading to bizarre empyemas clearing slowly over many months (Fig. 15.8).

ASPIRATION AND INHALATION

The effects of aspiration of particulate or liquid foreign material into the lungs are twofold: those due to mechanical bronchial obstruction and those due to the irritant properties of the aspirate. When the cough reflex is suppressed by stupor, alcohol or drugs, aspiration of food from the stomach during vomiting is likely to occur. The inflammatory response excited by vegetable matter is intense and commonly followed by secondary infection with commensals and anaerobic organisms. Aspiration of infected material from nasal and oral sepsis is a common cause of lung abscess. The radiological patterns are therefore those of atelectasis or suppurative bronchitis and pneumonia. Metallic or inorganic particles may excite little response, the mechanical effects of uncomplicated atelectasis or obstructive emphysema predominating, and they may remain undetected for long periods.

Aspiration of mineral oils results in **lipoid pneumonia** (Fig. 15.9). The prolonged use of liquid paraffin for constipation is the usual cause and a precipitating factor is chronic oesophageal obstruction. The oil floats to the top of any residue in the oesophagus, the optimum position for aspiration. The oil is almost inert and the reaction is indolent, granulomatous and fibrotic and any lung damage is permanent. Radiographically there are dense well-defined tumour-like masses or an extensive bilateral opacity spreading outwards from the hilar regions. Vegetable oils and animal fats such as milk induce a greater inflammatory response and the opacities are ill-defined and bronchopneumonic. Influenced by gravity, the lesions of aspiration and inhalation are found predominantly in the posterior parts of the lungs. Small aspirates are common in the aged from incompetence of the closing mechanism of the larynx. These recurrent aspirations produce coarse peribronchial thickening, small patches of pneumonia and eventually fibrosis and bronchiectasis.

Mendelson's syndrome is a chemical pneumonia caused by aspiration of acid gastric contents during anaesthesia. An intense bronchospasm is rapidly followed by a flood of oedema throughout the lungs, resulting in

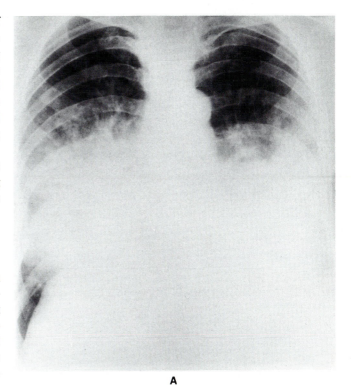

A

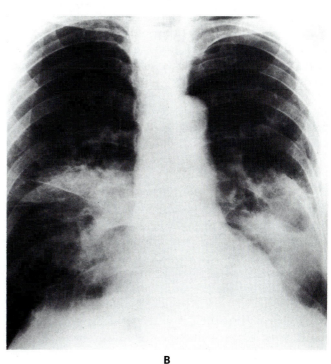

B

Fig. 15.9 A. Lipoid pneumonia. Aspiration of liquid paraffin. **B.** 8 years later. Significant clearance but massive residual fibrosis.

hypoxia and requiring high ventilation pressures. The radiographic appearance of massive pulmonary oedema taken together with the clinical presentation is pathognomonic (Fig. 15.10).

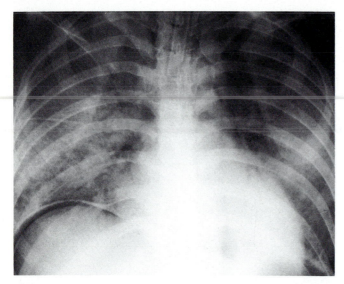

Fig. 15.10 Mendelson's syndrome. Postoperative aspiration of acid gastric contents.

In cases of *near drowning* the lungs show widespread, ill-defined alveolar opacities due to pulmonary oedema. The effects of salt water are less severe and of shorter duration than those due to hypotonic fresh water.

Inhalation of irritant gases (e.g. ammonia, chlorine, nitrogen dioxide) produces an acute focal or diffuse pulmonary oedema followed by functional derangements indicative of bronchiolar and alveolar damage. It is one cause of *bronchiolitis obliterans*. Widespread tubular bronchiectasis has been reported as a sequel to accidental smoke inhalation.

IMPAIRED DEFENCE MECHANISMS

There are a number of genetically determined abnormalities, the effects of which impair the defences of the lungs against infection. Acquired immunosuppression is dealt with at the end of this chapter.

Pulmonary cystic fibrosis. Patients are now surviving to adult life but the prognosis is poor. The susceptibility of the lungs to infection is related to the abnormal physicochemical properties of the bronchial mucus, making it more viscous and impairing mucociliary transport. Common infecting organisms are *Staphylococcus aureus*, *Pseudomonas aeruginosa*, *Haemophilus influenzae* and *Klebsiella*. Pneumothorax occurs in 20% of cases and is difficult to manage conservatively because 50% recur and prolonged tube drainage carries a high mortality. Surgical treatment is therefore undertaken more often than would otherwise be the case. Small haemoptyses are common and on rare occasions massive haemoptyses can be life-threatening. It is in such circumstances that control by bronchial artery embolization may need to be considered.

Primary immunodeficiency disorders. These are a diverse group of *abnormalities of immunoglobulins*. The deficiencies may be selective or total and the levels reduced or absent. Adult patients are survivors from the childhood affliction and the majority have an abnormal chest radiograph, the result of recurrent bronchopulmonary infections. Thoracic manifestations include atelectasis, bronchiectasis, thymoma and lymphocytic interstitial pneumonia. These patients are at increased risk of developing lymphoid neoplasms and carcinomas.

Chronic granulomatous disease. Only in rare instances do patients with this condition survive to adult life. Phagocytosis is normal but the polymorphs are incapable of destroying the ingested bacteria at a normal rate. Children suffer from recurrent pneumonias, but with increasing age these become less frequent. The lungs usually show bilateral interstitial fibrosis. Other thoracic complications are bronchiectasis and granulomatous mediastinitis.

Impaired neutrophil chemotaxis. Phagocytic cells are attracted to sites of bacterial infection by chemotactic substances released by the organisms or locally produced by the host. Activated complement is one such host substance. Instances have been found of impaired neutrophil chemotactic responses which have an adverse effect on the frequency and severity of infections. Abscesses and skin sepsis are the common manifestations and recurrent staphylococcal pneumonias are not infrequent.

Congenital dyskinetic ciliary syndromes. The 'immotile cilia syndrome' was the term originally applied to this group of conditions, but this is too restrictive, since it is now known that there can be abnormalities of synchrony as well as total immotility. It is a heterogeneous mixture of structural and functional abnormalities of cilia. It is now postulated that the beating of embryonic cilia determines organ situs and if the beat is abnormal the situs will be randomly allocated and 50% will have situs inversus. Sperm tails are also cilia, and males with the condition will be infertile. It also explains the curious combination of bronchiectasis, situs inversus and male infertility in *Kartagener's syndrome*.

The impairment of mucociliary clearance means that the lungs are more susceptable to bronchopulmonary infections, but this is only a serious problem if the infections are repeated and severe. The radiographic signs are those of bronchitis, tubular bronchiectasis, atelectasis and chronic obstructive airways disease.

Young's syndrome. This is a combination of obstructive azoospermia, sinusitis and chronic pulmonary infections. The latter begin in childhood and eventually most patients develop bronchiectasis. There is no structural abnormality of cilia but mucociliary transport is impaired. Spermatogenesis is normal, but the infertility of these men is due to a progressive obstruction of the epididymis by inspissated secretions.

UNRESOLVED PNEUMONIA

A pneumonic consolidation which stubbornly refuses to improve over a long period presents a problem in management. It is a circumstance where excision of the lesion may have to be considered if other diagnostic modalities have been inconclusive. Pathological examination of such lobes or lungs will usually reveal definitive or circumstantial evidence of aspiration. Proof of aspiration lies in the demonstration of identifiable particulate foreign material or extrinsic lipids. A suggestive histological pattern including foreign-body giant cells is circumstantial evidence of aspiration. Only a minority are post-infective. Isolated cases will be found to be rare examples of sarcoid reaction, lymphomatoid granulomatosis, chronic eosinophil pneumonia and other miscellaneous conditions.

A few cases in which all known causes have been excluded have responded favourably to steroids and there has been relapse, sometimes in another part of the lung, when they have been withdrawn. On continuous steroid treatment the lungs become virtually normal. To distinguish this group it has been called *cryptogenic organizing pneumonitis* or *bronchiolitis obliterans organizing pneumonia*.

ACTINOMYCOSIS AND NOCARDIOSIS

In the past these infections have been placed with the

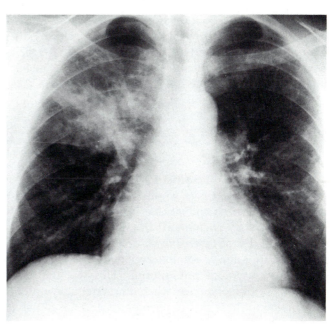

Fig. 15.12 Nocardiosis. Non-homogeneous consolidation.

mycoses but the organisms concerned are now regarded as branching bacteria.

Actinomycosis. The characteristic sulphur granules found in the exudate from actinomycotic lesions consist of clumps of *Actinomyces israeli*. It is a commensal in the mouth, and infection of the lung is by aspiration or direct extension from oesophagus, mediastinum or elsewhere. A chronic consolidation forms which as it progresses crosses pleural boundaries (Fig. 15.11). Perihilar consolidation fanning out into the lungs may closely simulate a carcinoma. When the pleura is reached a localized encysted abscess forms, which may erode a rib and break through onto the skin surface, leading to draining sinuses. An apical cavity simulating tuberculosis may form. An unusual form is that of an extensive bilateral patchy pneumonia.

Nocardiosis. *Nocardia asteroides* is a soil saprophyte of worldwide distribution and human infection is by inhalation. The lesions vary from a solitary nodule to a confluence of multiple areas of consolidation (Fig. 15.12). Nocardiosis is a suppurating bronchopneumonia and the consolidations can be notably dense. Multiple abscesses or a single thick-walled cavity may form. Hilar node enlargement and empyema are frequent accompaniments.

CHLAMYDIAE

The organisms responsible for the *psittacosis/lymphogranuloma-venereum/trachoma* group of diseases are now classified as *Chlamydiae*. They are obligate intracellular parasites but differ from viruses in having both RNA and DNA. *Psittacosis* is acquired from sick birds — parrots,

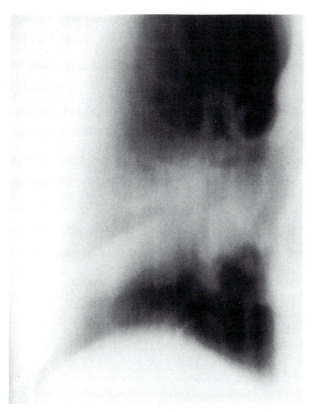

Fig. 15.11 Actinomycosis. AP tomogram. Dense consolidation in right middle lobe crossing the lesser fissure into the upper lobe. Removed surgically in the belief that it was a carcinoma.

budgerigars, domestic fowl. It presents as a lung consolidation of any size up to lobar, sometimes patchy rather than homogeneous, and a tendency to spread after diagnosis. A miliary pattern has also been described. The hilar nodes are often enlarged. Clearing of the lesions takes place slowly over several weeks.

Chlamydial pneumonias are now being seen more frequently than formerly.

MYCOPLASMA PNEUMONIA

Mycoplasma pneumoniae is an organism intermediate between the bacteria and viruses. It is the commonest isolate from primary pneumonias in Great Britain, accounting for 10–20% of cases, but in only a small proportion does it cause a major respiratory illness.

Primary atypical pneumonia. This was the name given to a respiratory illness where the systemic symptoms overshadowed those due to pneumonia and the course of the disease was less dramatic but more prolonged than that of typical pneumonia. Primary atypical pneumonia

is now known to have a number of causes, including adenovirus, psittacosis and Q fever, but the commonest cause is *Mycoplasma pneumoniae*.

The evolution of the pneumonia is slow so that it is possible to see a changing radiographic pattern. A fine reticulation first appears, representing interstitial inflammation, and this is followed by consolidation of the involved area as the alveoli become filled in with exudate (Fig. 15.13). On resolution the process is reversed. At its height there is usually a segmental or lobar consolidation but there are other possible patterns: 1. multiple irregular patches with ill-defined margins; 2. multiple well-defined small nodules; 3. rapid evolution into a fulminating fibrosing alveolitis; 4. massive bilateral bronchopneumonia with abscess formation. The last two are rare presentations. Hilar node enlargement is not uncommon but pleural effusions are rare. Resolution may take many weeks and abnormalities of pulmonary function may be detectable for up to four months.

Q FEVER

The 'Q' here refers to the question mark over the aetiology when first described and before it was traced to a *Rickettsia*, now re-classified as *Coxiella burnetti*. The reservoirs of infection are insects and mammals, most human disease in Great Britain being acquired from contact with farm animals or their products. Most patients will have an abnormal chest radiograph at presentation. A typical appearance is of a few roughly rounded, homogeneous consolidations in both lungs. The borders of the lesions are poorly defined except at pleural surfaces. They can be quite large consolidations, up to 10 cm in diameter. Alternatively the disease may present as a lobar consolidation. Linear streaks (*plate atelectases*) in association with the consolidations are also common. Nodes are not enlarged. During resolution, which takes one month on the average, the ill-defined borders become sharper as the lesions shrink and become more dense. Complications include endocarditis, meningoencephalitis and hepatitis.

ROCKY MOUNTAIN SPOTTED FEVER

The southern United States, as well as the Rocky Mountain regions, is the endemic area for this tick-born rickettsial disease. The lungs are involved as part of a bacteraemia. There is a vasculitis within the alveolar walls, with spill-over of haemorrhage and oedema into the alveolar spaces. Only a minority have a widespread interstitial radiographic pattern — in most there are variable numbers of alveolar opacities; an example of a predominantly interstitial histology but alveolar radiology. Pleural effusions are common. The major complication is secondary bacterial infection, which has been known to lead to adult respiratory distress syndrome. The disease has a 5% mortality (Fig. 15.33).

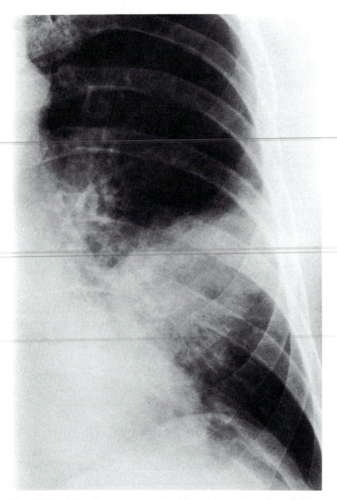

Fig. 15.13 *Mycoplasma* pneumonia. Linearities at the edge of the consolidation.

SCRUB TYPHUS

This rickettsial disease (*R. tsutsugamushi*), endemic in the countries of the Pacific basin, causes pulmonary abnormalities in approximately 10% of cases. The radiographic pattern is diverse and takes the form of interstitial, lobar or widespread pulmonary opacities. The latter presentation resembles adult respiratory distress syndrome both clinically and radiographically, but it clears rapidly with appropriate treatment.

VIRUS INFECTIONS

Characteristic features of virus pulmonary infections are described as widespread nodules, interstitial and peri-bronchovascular streaks radiating from the hila and mediastinal and hilar adenopathy. In contrast, bacterial infections are characterized by lobar or segmental consolidation, abscess formation and pleural effusion. In practice it is seldom possible to differentiate the two on radiographic grounds. Viral infections can present with every conceivable radiographic pattern.

The common cold

The common cold is an upper respiratory tract infection caused by many different varieties of virus — parainfluenza, rhino-, adeno-, or respiratory syncytial virus. Spread of the inflammatory process into the lower respiratory tract occurs in the predisposed — asthmatics, smokers, bronchitics — so that it is not surprising to find transient small pulmonary opacities should a chest radiograph be taken. Most pulmonary complications are the result of secondary bacterial invasion, analogous to the purulent sinusitis which so frequently starts from the common cold. There are however examples of virus pneumonia where the radiograph shows one or two patches of alveolar opacification with ill-defined borders (Fig. 15.14). The symptoms of these virus pneumonias are often atypical of other respiratory infections.

Influenza

It is the old and sufferers from chronic debilitating diseases who are most at risk of pulmonary disease during influenza infection. The influenza virus can cause pneumonia, but a more usual circumstance is a combination of viral and bacterial infection or bacterial secondary invasion in lung already made susceptible. Staphylococci, pneumococci and *Haemophilus* are common secondary invaders. A distinctive fulminating virus pneumonia is seen in epidemics of the disease. It is a rapidly extending bilateral and massive consolidation, indistinguishable from non-cardiac pulmonary oedema or adult respiratory distress syndrome (Fig. 15.15). Although prone to attack the debilitated, it also attacks young, previously healthy people and there is a high mortality. At postmortem an intense haemorrhagic oedema is found, involving all lung structures, as well as widespread necrosis of pulmonary epithelium.

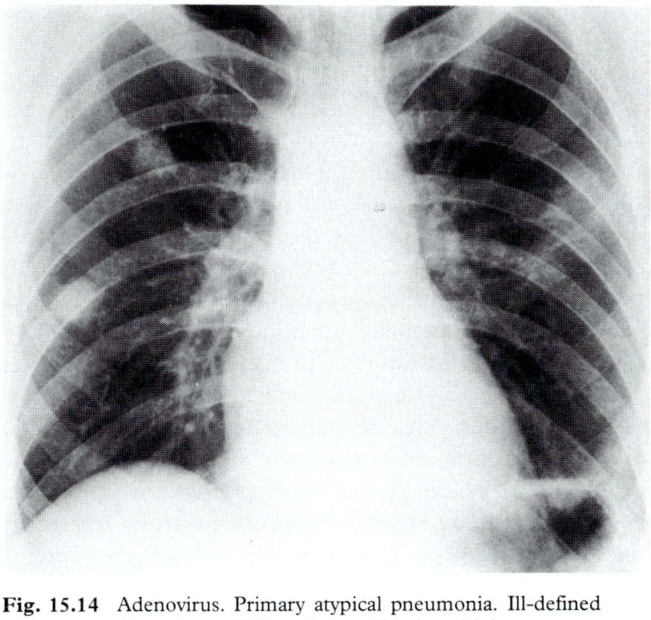

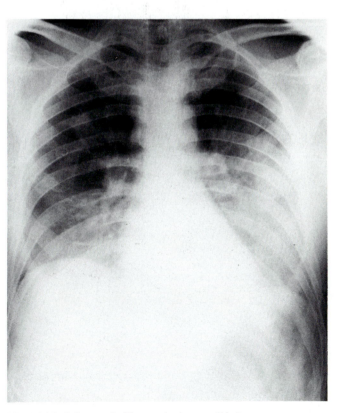

Fig. 15.14 Adenovirus. Primary atypical pneumonia. Ill-defined edges to small patches of bilateral consolidation. Major symptoms were myositis and dysphagia.

Fig. 15.15 Influenza A. Haemorrhagic consolidation at postmortem.

Varicella (chickenpox)

Septicaemic invasion of the lungs can occur in varicella. The patients are more likely to be adults than children and the exanthem particularly severe and haemorrhagic. The lungs are studded with nodules which can be very profuse and shifting. It is a rare complication but leaves its mark in later years by the presence of tiny calcified dots numbering from two or three up to dozens (Fig. 15.16). In Great Britain varicella is the commonest cause of these scars, but not all cases give a history of unusual respiratory disease during the original infection.

Measles giant-cell pneumonia

In addition to the common secondary respiratory infections associated with measles, there is a specific pulmonary viral infection characterized by multinucleate giant cells with cytoplasmic inclusions in the respiratory epithelium. Although a disease of childhood, it has been recorded in adults. The mediastinal and hilar nodes are commonly enlarged but other radiographic abnormalities are variable — streaky basal linearities, widespread reticulation or diffuse ill-defined opacities with a vague nodularity (Fig. 15.17). Remarkably swift resolution can take place, over the course of a few days.

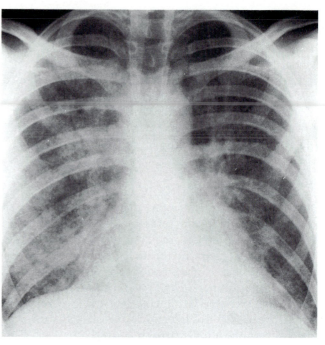

Fig. 15.17 Measles giant-cell pneumonia. Extensive ill-defined opacities with a suggestion of nodularity. Patient died. There was a possible T-cell deficiency.

Infectious mononucleosis

Less than 10% of cases have intrathoracic manifestations during the disease and node enlargement is most frequent. The lungs may show an isolated opacity or a reticulonodulation.

TUBERCULOSIS

Notifications of tuberculosis in Great Britain are of the order of 18 per 100 000 population annually. This rises to almost 400 per 100 000 amongst the immigrant population from the Indian sub-continent.

Epidemiologically the source of tuberculosis is a patient with open pulmonary tuberculosis. Infection from inoculation of the skin, from infected milk or from the handling of pathological specimens is rare where proper measures of control are exercised. Only those patients with sputum smears positive for tubercle bacilli are infectious, and after two weeks of adequate chemotherapy they can be regarded as non-infectious. Transmission is by droplet inhalation, and the dose of viable organisms received is critical. Children, the immunocompromised and some immigrant groups are particularly susceptible. All these factors are reflected in the recommendations current in Great Britain concerning isolation of patients, treatment of contacts and general control measures. A chest radiograph is part of these control measures, and follow-up of contacts for two years may be judged necessary.

The occupational risk of hospital personnel is, in

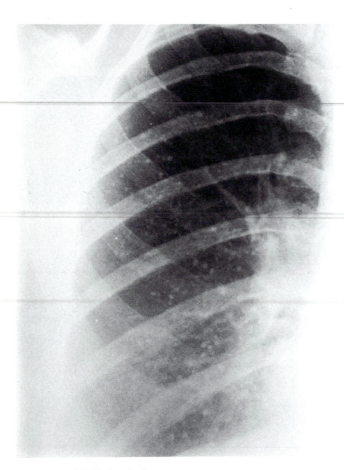

Fig. 15.16 Calcified varicella scars.

general, minimal and only a pre-employment chest radiograph is needed. Annual chest radiographs are not required. Those judged to be at higher risk should be offered an annual chest radiographic examination. Staff in any institution who will be in regular contact with children should have a chest radiograph as part of a pre-employment check, but routine periodic radiography is not necessary.

Tuberculosis is divided into primary and post-primary stages, separated by a latent interval which may stretch over decades.

PRIMARY PULMONARY TUBERCULOSIS

Organisms settle and multiply in an alveolus anywhere in the lungs, but most commonly in a subpleural site in the well-ventilated lower lobes. The initial pulmonary lesion is the *Ghon focus* and at an early stage there is spread along lymphatics, forming tubercles along the way, into the hilar nodes. The combination of Ghon focus, lymphatic infection and hilar node involvement is the *primary complex*. Bacilli are also carried centrifugally to the pleura where they may cause a lymphocytic serous *effusion*. Healing and progression proceed simultaneously, the balance between them determined by host resistance. A fibrous capsule walls off the lesion and calcium salts are deposited in the caseous material. From this point, if progression continues, there is little difference between lesions of primary and post-primary evolution. If the disease is not checked the caseous mass enlarges and is liquefied by enzymatic digestion. Expectoration of the contents of the *cavity* disperses infection to other parts of the lungs and if this is sudden and massive an acute, diffuse tuberculous bronchopneumonia results. A cavity breaking through to the pleura can result in *pneumothorax, effusion* or *caseous empyema*.

Miliary tuberculosis results from haematogenous dissemination after erosion of a vessel by a tuberculous lesion. It is usually an early primary event but is now being seen more often in patients with post-primary tuberculosis whose defences are waning.

Involved nodes may obstruct bronchi by external compression or by discharging caseous material into the lumen. *Epituberculosis* was a term used to describe a lobar opacity in primary tuberculosis resulting from a non-caseating inflammatory exudate and attributed to a hypersensitivity reaction. This concept seems to have been abandoned. Since most epituberculosis was to be found in the right middle lobe it was probably the result of bronchial obstruction by hilar nodes.

POST-PRIMARY PULMONARY TUBERCULOSIS

This follows the primary infection after a latent interval, however short or long, and could conceivably be either a reactivation or reinfection. It is now generally accepted that almost all post-primary tuberculosis is due to reinfection.

The lesions usually start in the subapical parts of the upper lobes or in the apical segment of the lower lobes as small areas of exudative inflammation. These extend, coalesce, caseate and cavitate. Typically there is a large cavity with several smaller satellite cavities, often bilateral but more advanced on one side. Cavity walls are lined by tuberculous granulation tissue and traversed by fibrotic remnants of bronchi and vessels. A vessel which has not been totally obliterated may dilate — a Rasmussen aneurysm.

Dispersion of infection from the cavities to other parts of the lungs takes place as in the primary form, and results in numerous small areas of caseous pneumonia, often in the lower lobes. Massive dispersal may lead to caseation of a whole lobe.

Adhesions usually limit pleural spread but sometimes the lung becomes encased in a thick coating of caseous material, fibrosis and hyaline connective tissue. Small cavities that heal leave radiating fibrotic strands puckering the lung. Large cavities become lined by columnar or squamous epithelium and are prone to secondary infection or fungal colonization.

NON-REACTIVE TUBERCULOSIS

This is a haematogenous dissemination in the immunosuppressed. Radiographically, it is miliary tuberculosis, but histologically it differs, in that the necrotic lesions are sharply demarcated from the surrounding lung, which shows little reaction. There is also an absence of giant-cell granulomas.

THE RADIOLOGY OF PULMONARY TUBERCULOSIS

Pulmonary tuberculosis has such a diversity of radiographic appearances that it is wise to include it in the differential diagnosis of virtually all pulmonary lesions.

Unusual though it is, tuberculosis can be confined to the lung bases. There is a characteristic sparing of the anterior parts of the lungs, a point of more importance in a negative rather than a positive sense. Lesions which are dominantly anterior, even though otherwise typical of tuberculosis, including cavitation, are likely to be of other aetiology.

A minimal apical lesion can easily be overlooked because of overlapping shadows of ribs and clavicle (Fig. 15.18). Comparison with the opposite side is then helpful, looking for asymmetries of density. The apical projection was designed to overcome this difficulty, but is rarely useful, and tomography is the best mode. The irregularity of outline and density of the lesion and the

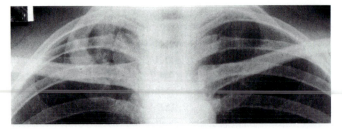

Fig. 15.18 Tuberculosis. Minimal apical lesion.

presence of small satellite shadows may give a spurious appearance of cavitation.

Until brought under control by natural healing or treatment, the lesions spread at an uneven rate, reparation and destruction proceeding simultaneously. Extensive areas of lung may become involved, irregularity and patchiness being the cardinal features, homogenous opacities unusual (Fig. 15.19).

Disease activity is monitored by periodic radiographs, the appearance of new lesions or the extension of old ones indicating continued activity whereas contraction indicates that the balance has been tilted in favour of healing. Once the radiographic signs have stabilized, any subsequent change in size or density must be regarded as suspicious of reactivation, fungal colonization or complication by neoplasm.

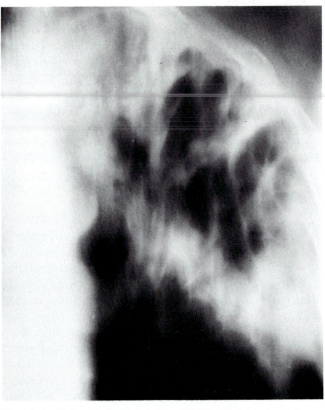

Fig. 15.20 Tuberculosis. Tomogram. Multiloculated cavity. A large part of the left upper lobe has been destroyed.

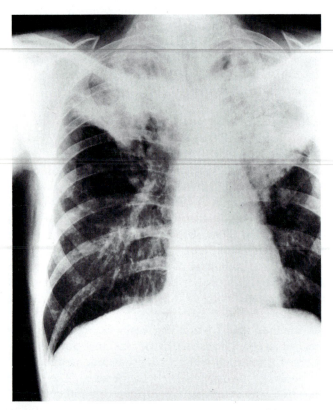

Fig. 15.19 Tuberculosis. Dense non-homogeneous opacities. Contracted right upper lobe. Small lesions in other areas.

Cavities may be thin- or thick-walled, central or eccentric, single or multiple (Fig. 15.20). Bullae are differentiated by their hair-line walls. Acute pneumonic lesions are especially liable to rapid breakdown into multiple round cavities. Tomography is necessary both to confirm cavitation and to display its structure.

All healed lesions leave fibrotic scars, very often containing calcifications. Since the upper lobes are predominantly involved, the effects of fibrotic contraction are seen in the drawing over of the trachea, elevation of hilar structures and bronchovascular distortions (Fig. 15.21). Air spaces in the fibrotic areas derive from bronchiectatic cavities and emphysematous bullae as well as true cavities. Atelectasis and bronchiectasis also result from endobronchial disease.

The large pleural effusion which may manifest early in primary tuberculosis is a reaction to subpleural tubercles. There are few bacilli in the fluid and resolution is uncomplicated. Large caseating lesions spreading into the pleura produce a more severe *pleuritis* which is commonly confined by adhesions. Whether localized or generalized, the result is a pleural space filled with tuberculous pus and caseous material which becomes grossly fibrotic. Complications which may arise from tuberculous empyema are *osteitis of rib*, chronically *discharging sinuses* to skin, *bronchopleural fistula* and *secondary infection*. These may

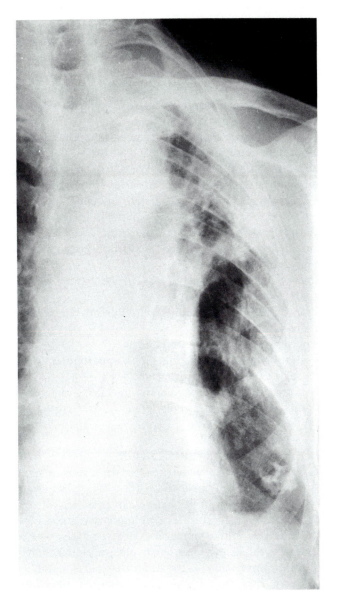

Fig. 15.21 Tuberculosis. Fibrotic shrinkage of upper lobe. Mediastinal and hilar displacement. Apex capped by thickened pleura.

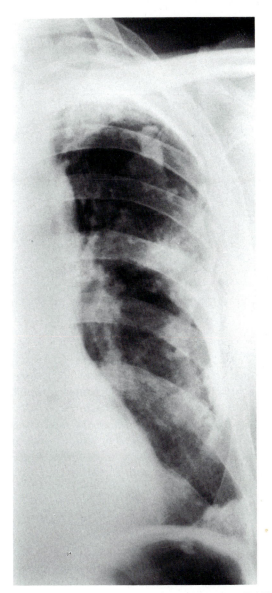

Fig. 15.22 Tuberculosis. Generalized pleural thickening. Calcified plaques on visceral pleura.

appear after years of apparently stable pleural disease. During healing the generalized empyema develops characteristic calcified plaques on the visceral pleura (Fig. 15.22). A cap of pleural thickening commonly accompanies apical disease.

Miliary tuberculosis may occur in the primary stage, when it is predominantly a disease of childhood, or in the post-primary stage, from waning of the body's defences brought about by steroids, immunosuppression, alcoholism or any debilitating disorder. Half the cases now presenting are over the age of 60 years. Radiographically there are enormous numbers of tiny opacities 1–2 mm in diameter, although superimposition may make it impossible to identify entirely discrete lesions. They are diffusely distributed throughout the lungs but there is

some latitude in the profusion, size and definition of the lesions (Fig. 15.23). The chest radiograph may be normal or it may only show the tuberculous lesion from which the dissemination arose. Healing of miliary tuberculosis often leaves a residue of a few small grains of calcification.

Disseminate lesions of larger size than miliary, and lesser profusion, are found if the defences are not totally submerged. This is the *acinar-nodose* pattern and the lesions are approximately 5 mm in diameter with indistinct margins. Localized dissemination also follows aspiration of infected material along bronchial pathways. A rare diffuse alveolar radiographic pattern of disease mimics pulmonary oedema.

A *tuberculoma* is a chronic, well-defined, rounded, granulomatous lesion which enters into the differential

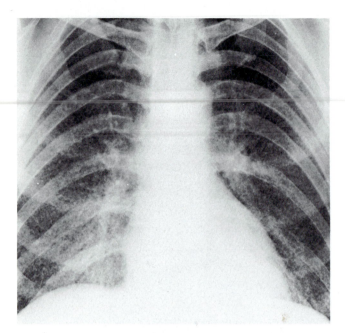

Fig. 15.23 Miliary tuberculosis. Enormous number of lesions. Sharp definition.

diagnosis of solitary or coin lesions. Internal calcification is then a valuable clue to its benignancy.

Considerable *enlargement of hilar and mediastinal nodes* may take place without any visible lesion in the lungs. If unilateral, this is likely to be confused with a malignant neoplasm and if bilateral, with sarcoidosis or lymphoma.

OTHER MYCOBACTERIAL PULMONARY INFECTIONS

There are a number of related bacilli with morphology and staining properties closely similar to those of the tubercle bacillus. Of these atypical mycobacteria, those most frequently the cause of human disease are *M. xenopi, M. kansasii* and *M. battei*. Their infectivity is low but their sensitivities to drugs differs from that of *M. tuberculosis*. In general they cause less fibrosis, are less prone to spread but more prone to cavitate than *M. tuberculosis* infections. A common pattern is of a cluster of small opacities grouped around a central lucency. The cavities are thin-walled. Pleural disease and node enlargement are rare. These differences are not however sufficient, in an individual case, to differentiate them from *M. tuberculosis* infections.

THE MYCOSES — PULMONARY FUNGAL DISEASES

Within the family of fungi, only a few cause invasive disease in humans. Outside this mainstream of fungal disease, a much larger number of fungi have been reported in isolated instances as causing disease.

Refinements of taxonomy are not of much importance in the clinical context, which is fortunate, because exact identification can be difficult even under ideal conditions. In human disease isolation is made difficult by problems in obtaining suitable pathological material, by diversity of cultural requirements and by cross-reactivity in skin testing and antibody production.

Something more than the presence of the fungus in the environment is required before it takes on a pathogenic role. Although the fungi of blastomycosis, cryptococcosis and histoplasmosis are present in Great Britain, these diseases very rarely occur as a native infection, such few cases as are found having been acquired in endemic areas, sometimes up to 20 years previously.

The following general statements are appropriate to fungal diseases:

Invasive disease is acquired by inhalation and the primary focus is in the lung;

Direct spread from animals to humans or between humans is rare;

The pathology is granulomatous;

Dissemination through the lungs is particularly likely to occur in the immunocompromised;

Systemic dissemination commonly affects the central nervous system and is usually lethal.

ASPERGILLOSIS

Aspergillus fumigatus is widespread in the atmosphere and it is inevitable that man inhales the spores from time to time. It is capable of multiplying in air passages when the conditions are favourable. The pulmonary manifestations are grouped into three categories: 1. *aspergilloma* — a ball of fungal hyphae growing in an old pulmonary cavity; 2. *invasive aspergillosis* — the fungus becomes a pathogen in its own right and invades pulmonary tissue causing necrosis; 3. *allergic bronchopulmonary aspergillosis* — asthmatics who develop transient pulmonary opacities. This is a useful classification but the boundaries of each are not rigid.

Aspergilloma. The fungus colonizes any chronic cavity or airspace except those in which tuberculosis is still active. The hyphae grow into a matted ball (a mycetoma) which lies free within the cavity. The radiographic feature is a crescent of air between the ball and the cavity wall, best shown by tomography (Fig. 15.24). Since most chronic cavities are in the upper lobes, this is where most aspergillomas will be found.

Air crescents are not always present, and the diagnosis of aspergilloma should be suspected in any chronic air space which becomes opacified. Other fungi are capable of forming mycetomas, and other pathologies can produce identical appearances: for example, haematoma, tumour, hydatid cyst. Rarely, a mycetoma disappears on the death of the fungus but it usually returns.

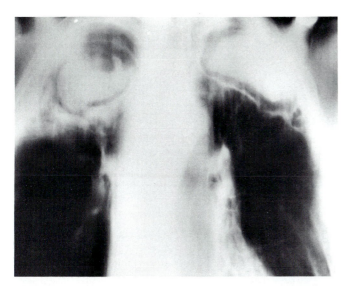

Fig. 15.24 Bilateral aspergillomas. Air crescents and fungal masses.

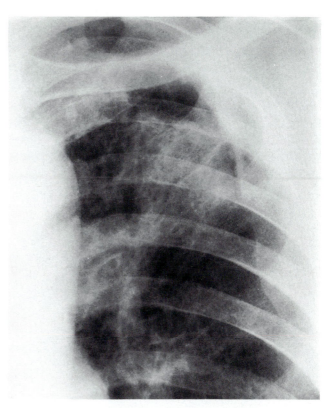

Fig. 15.25 Invasive aspergillosis. An old scarred tuberculous lesion reopacified. Irregular borders and a tail of opacity into the hilum.

Aspergilloma is an indolent condition but by no means always benign because of the tendency to bleed. Vascular granulation tissue forms in the wall of the cavity and sooner or later bleeding takes place. Small haemoptyses are frequent but occasionally a large haemoptysis can be life-threatening.

Medical treatment is unsatisfactory and surgery carries a high risk from the complications of bronchopleural fistula, pneumonia, empyema and further bleeding. In these circumstances control of bleeding by embolization of bronchial and intercostal arteries has to be considered. The effects are rarely permanent but it can be repeated.

Mycetomas are also sometimes found in allergic bronchopulmonary aspergillosis. They may also become invasive, spreading through the cavity wall into normal lung. Wider dissemination is only likely to occur in the immunocompromised host.

Invasive aspergillosis. In this form the aspergillus invades viable tissue and necrosis ensues. It is rarely primary, and predisposing factors are: chemotherapy, immunosuppression, or lung damage from other infections or radiotherapy. There is no characteristic radiographic pattern. It may take the form of a necrotizing bronchopneumonia with abscess formation, organizing lobar pneumonia, widespread lesions, even a miliary spread. It can mimic an aspergilloma, complete with air crescent, the differences being that it develops in apparently previously normal lung, the wall is thick and invaded by fungus and the core consists of fungus mixed with necrotic tissue (Fig. 15.25).

Allergic bronchopulmonary aspergillosis. The patient is usually an asthmatic subject who develops sensitivity to the aspergillus which has colonized the proximal bronchi. Local allergic reactions then take place, resulting in two types of pathological process: 1. transient pulmonary opacities; 2. bronchopulmonary damage. The transient pulmonary opacities are the same as those of other allergic reactions, an eosinophilic infiltration of alveolar walls and intra-alveolar exudate. The size varies from small nodules up to lobar dimensions. They are of low density and have ill-defined borders except at pleural boundaries (Fig. 15.26). A perihilar distribution of the opacity can simulate hilar adenopathy. Resolution is hastened by steroid therapy. Recurrences take place in the same or in different parts of the lungs.

The condition pursues an intermittent course over many years and the frequency of chronic changes increases with the number of acute episodes. Within areas previously the site of transient opacities, the bronchi dilate and contain plugs of tough, stringy mucus mixed with small numbers of the aspergillus. Mucoid impaction is a dilated bronchus packed tightly with this material. Because of their thickened walls, bronchi may be visible as tubes, rings or cavities or, if impacted, as bulbous 'glove finger' or branching opacities. Air may return to impacted bronchi if the material is coughed up. Plugging of central bronchi can lead to collapse of lobes or whole lungs. Continued damage and repair by fibrosis will lead to focal emphysema, permanent shrinkage and eventually end-stage upper lobe fibrosis. Thus, although pulmonary opacities are transient, in only a minority of cases does the chest radiograph become completely normal between

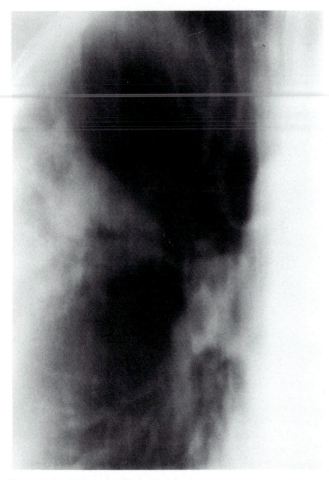

Fig. 15.26 Allergic bronchopulmonary aspergillosis. Tomogram. A wedge of opacity crossed by a patent bronchus.

acute episodes. A mycetoma may form, not always in the upper lobes.

Central bronchiectasis, in which normal bronchial calibre is resumed distal to the dilatation, is a highly characteristic feature and can be shown either by bronchography or narrow-section CT. However, the bronchiectasis may be of the non-specific tubular, cystic or varicose variety.

Other fungi and moulds can produce a picture so close to that of bronchopulmonary aspergillosis both clinically and radiologically that only skin testing and precipitin reactions will be able to differentiate between them.

HISTOPLASMOSIS

Lung infection by *Histoplasma capsulatum* is usually acquired by inhalation of soil dust contaminated by bird droppings. A tiny calcified dot may be the only indication that previous infection has taken place. When many of these are scattered throughout the lungs they closely resemble the scars of miliary tuberculosis or varicella

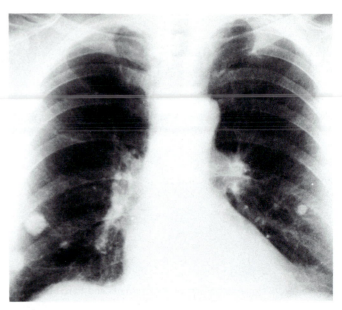

Fig. 15.27 Histoplasmosis. Nodules with calcification. Calcified right hilar nodes.

pneumonia except that they tend to be rather more variable in size (Fig. 15.27).

Progression of one or more of these foci leads to larger nodules. Hilar node enlargement is common and may be the only visible manifestation. Locally progressive disease may also take the form of a consolidation, acute or chronic, the latter associated with fibrosis and cavitation (Fig. 15.28). The presence of cavitation within an area

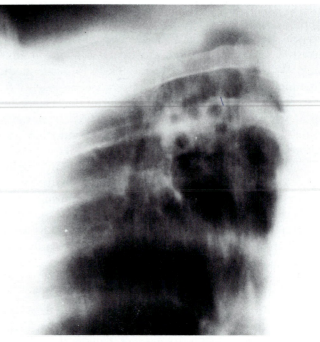

Fig. 15.28 Histoplasmosis. Tomogram. Chronic disease of the right apex. Multiple small cavities. Positive histoplasmin skin test. Confirmed by lobectomy.

of lung distorted by fibrosis is liable to be mistaken for tuberculosis. There is also a *miliary* form of diffuse lung dissemination.

An uncommon late manifestation of histoplasmosis is a *fibrosing mediastinitis* which can cause stenosis of cavae, oesophagus, trachea, bronchi or pulmonary artery. The chest radiograph will then show a widened mediastinum with large hilar shadows and opacities fanning out into the lungs. Kerley B lines may appear.

Systemic dissemination frequently gives rise to chronic ulceration of the upper air passages and destruction of the adrenal glands.

COCCIDIOIDOMYCOSIS

Some 60% of infections are asymptomatic and the commonest radiographic finding is a nodule which calcifies as it heals. Common presentations of symptomatic cases are segmental, lobar or patches of persistent consolidation together with enlarged hilar and mediastinal nodes. The adenopathy can be mistaken for sarcoidosis or lymphoma.

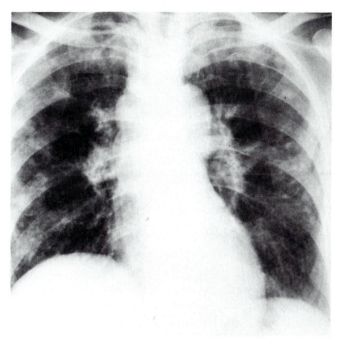

Fig. 15.30 Blastomycosis. Dissemination throughout the lungs. Multiple nodules some of which were cavitated. Mediastinal node enlargement.

Viable organisms persisting in healed lesions are a source of future reactivation.

Sequelae of chronic disease are fibrosis, calcification, cavitation, bronchiectasis and empyema. Cavities tend to be thin-walled but chronic apical fibrocavitary disease can be indistinguishable from tuberculosis. There is also a miliary form of coccidioidomycosis.

It is notable that most fungal infections have a form of disease which is indistinguishable radiographically from chronic tuberculosis.

BLASTOMYCOSIS

The asymptomatic nodule, chronic pneumonia, potential for re-activation and node enlargement are indistinguishable from other fungal infections (Fig. 15.29). Cavitation is less common but when it occurs it is similar to that in coccidioidomycosis. There is no great tendency to fibrosis and healed lesions leave only small scars. Dissemination throughout the lungs can have almost any radiographic pattern (Fig. 15.30).

CRYPTOCOCCOSIS (*torulosis*)

Cryptococcosis neoformans is a yeast form of fungus of world-wide distribution. The reservoir for human infection is probably pigeon droppings. Lung infection is usually benign, taking the form of one or more nodules of variable size. Growth of a nodule will form a mass

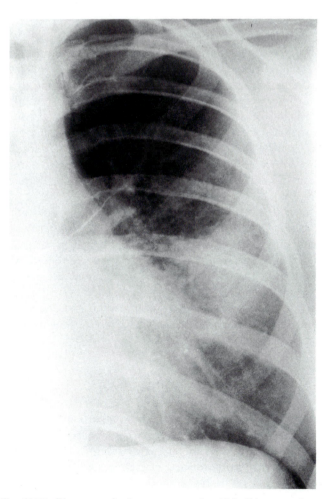

Fig. 15.29 Blastomycosis. Acute pneumonia which did not resolve. Fungus in sputum. Lingular consolidation. Resolved with treatment.

lesion (*toruloma*) simulating a carcinoma. Node enlargement and cavitation are rare.

CANDIDIASIS

Candida albicans is a normal mouth commensal which, when conditions are favourable, causes moniliasis (thrush), a superficial surface infection. It is rarely invasive but lung infection, when it occurs, is from haematogenous spread. The pulmonary lesion is a chronic pneumonia which breaks down with the formation of an abscess. A mycetoma may develop in the abscess, which is then indistinguishable from aspergilloma.

MUCORMYCOSIS

The *Mucorales* group of fungi are best known as causes of a spreading inflammation of the face and sinuses in diabetics or the immunosuppressed. Lung infection is a rapidly progressive, dense, cavitating bronchopneumonia.

WORMS AND OTHER PARASITIC INFECTIONS

There is a common pattern running through the pulmonary manifestations of many of these diseases and the condition of *tropical pulmonary eosinophilia* can be taken as illustrative.

The endemic areas of this disease are the tropical belts of all the continents. Diagnosis is based on the symptomatology, blood eosinophilia, an abnormal chest radiograph, antibodies to filarial antigens in the blood and the striking response to specific therapy with diethylcarbamazine. Although the parasites cannot be isolated from the lungs there can be no reasonable doubt of the filarial aetiology.

Pathologically there is an eosinophilic interstitial infiltration and intra-alveolar exudate, the usual signature of a pulmonary allergic response. Patients with the disease who travel to temperate zones may be misdiagnosed as asthmatics. If the asthma has unusual features such as recurrent fever, sweating, weight loss or a high ESR, suspicion should be aroused. Untreated the disease may persist for years, and can result in permanent lung damage with interstitial fibrosis.

The chest radiograph shows a subtle bilateral mid-zone haze which could readily be attributed to technical factors were it not for the accompanying loss of definition of pulmonary vessels and hila. Additionally there is a profusion of small, ill-defined, migrating nodules up to 5 mm in diameter scattered throughout the lungs, producing, in severe infestations, a 'snowstorm' picture. Larger areas of homogeneous consolidation appear transiently. There are also linear components, consisting of streaks radiating from the hila and peripheral reticulations.

PARASITIC WORMS

Ascaris, *Taenia*, *Ankylostoma* and *Strongyloides* are examples of parasitic worms which lodge in or traverse the lungs at some stage of their life cycles and in so doing give rise to one or two transient and migrating opacities as a result of an allergic response. Loeffler, who first described this condition, believed that his original cases were due to ascariasis. The term **Loeffler's syndrome** is now applied to almost any transient pulmonary opacities of a predominantly eosinophilic histology associated with a blood eosinophilia. The heavier the infestation the more profuse are the pulmonary lesions. *Strongyloides stercoralis* in particular is capable of causing widespread opacities and a serious pulmonary illness. Such *hyperinfection* can be activated by immunosuppression.

Worms or larvae which fail to complete their migration die and a chronic granulomatous nodule will be formed. If this is removed for histological examination it is easy to miss the remains of the worm within the granuloma.

Schistosomiasis. If the eggs lodge in pulmonary arteries of less than 100 μm the lesions they cause are small granulomas like miliary tuberculosis or sarcoidosis but if they lodge in arteries of larger size the irritation causes vascular necrosis and fibrotic occlusion. The latter results in pulmonary hypertension if sufficient vessels are occluded. A third type of reaction results in diffuse interstitial fibrosis.

Paragonimiasis. The *Paragonimus* worm is endemic in the tropics and infection is acquired from eating shellfish. The worm or eggs in the lungs excite a reaction consisting of a few alveolar opacities of up to 4 cm in diameter. One or more 'bubble' cavities appear within the opacities, and as the surrounding reaction subsides they are seen to have thin walls. Tuberculosis may be suspected, particularly as haemoptysis is a frequent symptom.

Armillifer armillatus. This is an arachnid infestation of birds, mammals and snakes endemic in Africa and South-East Asia. Humans are infected usually from eating snakes. The larvae migrate to the lungs where they encyst, die and calcify. The radiographic appearances are pathognomonic. There are numerous thin-walled cysts less than 1 cm in diameter in a subpleural position and containing the calcified bodies of the larvae. These appear as coils, targets and signet ring shapes.

HYDATID DISEASE

Dogs are the principal reservoir of the adult worm, *Echinococcus granulosus*, and most mammals serve as intermediate host for the larvae (echinococci). The hydatid is a parasitic echinococcal cyst consisting of three layers, an adventitia formed of compressed host tissue, a middle layer of friable ectocyst and an inner germinal layer from which is produced large numbers of scolices which are the heads of developing worms. Daughter cysts

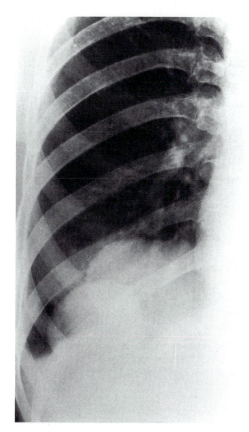

Fig. 15.31 Two hydatids. Small pleural effusion.

are formed if the viability is threatened but in the lung the cyst is unilocular (Fig. 15.31). Smoothly spherical and of homogeneous density, the cyst may grow to the size of a grapefruit. There is seldom significant reaction in the surrounding lung so that calcification is rare. Complications are those of rupture and infection.

Rupture may take place into the pleural cavity or into a bronchus. Communication with a bronchus leads to a detachment of the ectocyst from the adventitia and a crescent of air separates the two. Should the cyst itself rupture, the partial replacement of the fluid results in a fluid level.

Rupture of a *liver hydatid* into the right lung produces a characteristic combination of radiological signs. There is a basal opacity from lobar infection and atelectasis, and a pleural effusion. Bronchographically there is a local bronchiectasis and the bronchial fistula into the cavity may be shown. ^{99m}Tc-labelled iminodiacetic acid scanning shows a filling defect in the hepatic uptake followed by the appearance of the radionuclide in the cyst and its progress up the bronchial tree.

The leakage of hydatid fluid into the tissues is sometimes followed by a systemic reaction. Although these reactions are uncommon, when they occur the consequences can be serious.

TOXOPLASMOSIS

Epidemiological surveys have shown a high rate of subclinical infection. A protozoal disease, widespread amongst mammals and birds, human acquisition is from cats or from eating infected meat. One form of presentation is in the manner of a primary atypical pneumonia, with mild respiratory symptoms and mediastinal adenopathy or a pulmonary opacity.

ENTAMOEBA HISTOLYTICA

The *Entamoeba* is distributed worldwide but amoebiasis is a tropical or subtropical disease. The lungs can be involved by metastatic spread from the abdomen or by rupture of an hepatic amoebic abscess into the right lung base. In the latter case the radiographic signs are those of a lung abscess and bronchohepatic fistula.

IMMUNOSUPPRESSION AND PULMONARY INFECTION

Drugs are used to reduce antibody production in organ transplant recipients in order to prevent rejection, and in diseases where the immune response itself is damaging, as in systemic lupus. Impairment of immunological mechanisms is an unwanted side-effect of drugs used to kill malignant cells. Immunosuppression is therefore associated with administration of steroids, azathioprine and cytotoxics. The level of suppression is proportional to the intensity of the chemotherapy. Immunological impairment is also associated with other disease states, diabetes, alcoholism, exposure to ionizing radiations and the processes of ageing.

Not only is the risk of infection increased — the tissue response is altered, and potentially serious infections may give little clinical sign of their presence. For this reason periodic chest radiography is a reasonable precaution in those at risk.

The response to conventional pathogens may take a usual or an atypical form and this also applies with unusual pathogens. Certain organisms, notably *Pneumocystis carinii* and *Cytomegalovirus*, rarely if ever cause disease in the absence of immunosuppression. The organisms identified most often in these diseases are *Pneumocystis*, *Candida albicans*, *Mycobacterium tuberculosis*, *Aspergillus fumigatus* and the Herpes family of viruses.

There are many obstacles to accurate diagnosis. Infection has to be differentiated from the primary disease or a recrudescence, from the toxic effects of drugs and from graft rejection. Mixed infections are common and the isolation of an organism does not always mean that it is the principal agent. Similarly, seroconversion or the finding of high-antibody titres is not positive proof of causation. Isolation from sputum, blood, tracheal aspiration or bronchopulmonary lavage is too variable to be reliable.

Open lung biopsy is the optimum method for *Pneumocystis* but less reliable for other organisms. *Fibreoptic bronchoscopy and biopsy* are useful, particularly as they are less invasive. These last two methods are not without risk of pneumothorax or bleeding, and any clotting defect should be corrected beforehand. An advantage of biopsy is that it may differentiate infection from recurrence of tumour or other lesions. Unfortunately the biopsy may simply show nonspecific changes of organizing pneumonia, interstitial pneumonitis or haemorrhage. Even when determined efforts are made to reach a specific diagnosis using an extensive range of tests, success is elusive, and in about 40% of infections no pathogen will be found.

The *radiological signs* of these infections are nonspecific but the most characteristic feature is of *disseminate pulmonary lesions*, with only a few showing other patterns such as lobar consolidation or isolated nodules. *Abscesses* and cavitation are common and their presence amongst a diffuse alveolar or interstitial shadowing, especially if there are also focal nodules, is suspicious of a mixed infection. Enlarged nodes usually imply tumour rather than infection. In leukaemia pulmonary opacities imply infection since visible deposits rarely occur. Viral infections may be accompanied by a skin rash.

Bacterial infections. An existing tuberculous lesion can be reactivated and local or miliary spread ensue. Gram-negative bacteria characteristically cause micro-abscesses. Nocardia has less tendency to disseminate through the lungs and a local lesion progressing rapidly to cavitation is more characteristic.

Fungal infections. (Figs 15.32–15.34). *Candida albicans* infections may be bronchopneumonic, multinodular or

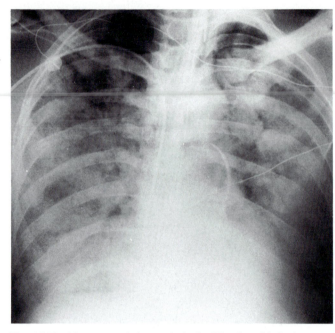

Fig. 15.33 Mucormycosis in an alcoholic. The fungal infection followed Rocky Mountain spotted fever. Mixed infection with Gram-negative organisms. Postmortem confirmation.

miliary. The latter may not be visible radiographically. The common pattern in fungal infections is disseminate nodules with abscesses, except for histoplasmosis, in which pulmonary dissemination is unusual. Aspergillus can produce focal lesions indistinguishable radiographically from an aspergilloma except that they occur in previously normal lungs (Fig. 15.25). It is an *invasive aspergillosis*.

Parasitic infection. In those who have lived in the tropics, fulminating *Entamoeba histolytica* or *Strongyloides*

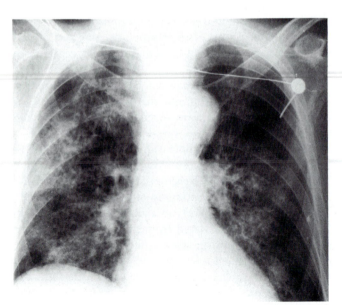

Fig. 15.32 *Candida albicans* bronchopneumonia. Mixed infection with Gram-negative organisms. Chronic alcoholic. Postmortem confirmation.

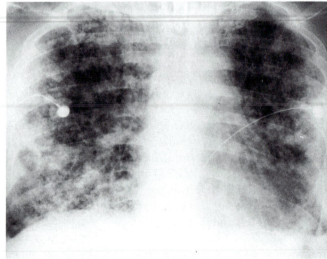

Fig. 15.34 Disseminated cryptococcosis. Mixed infection with Gram-negative organisms. On steroids for systemic lupus.

stercoralis pulmonary infections can occur. Strongyloides may be a focal nodular or a diffuse alveolar infection.

Viral infections. These are usually of the Herpes family, consisting of *Herpes simplex*, *varicella/zoster* and *Cytomegalovirus*.

Cytomegalovirus is usually acquired asymptomatically in normally immune-competent people, although occasionally there is an illness of infection similar to infectious mononucleosis. After primary infection the virus persists in latent form. In the immunocompromised host a reactivation of this latent infection may take place but this is not usually accompanied by clinical illness. It is a primary infection occurring in an immunocompromised host which is the cause of serious pulmonary and hepatic disease.

Diagnosis is made from the presence in cells obtained by biopsy or exfoliative cytology of characteristic 'owl eye' inclusions or from cell cultures. In the lungs it is found in pneumonic consolidations, in nodules, in widespread miliary lesions or in diffuse acinar perihilar opacities. Pathologically there is an interstitial infiltration and intra-alveolar exudate. The precise part which this virus plays in the pathogenesis of these lesions is uncertain because it is usually found in mixed infections.

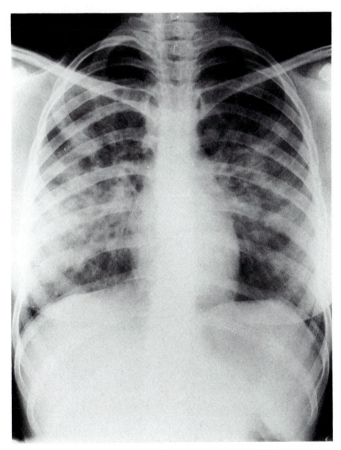

Fig. 15.35 *Pneumocystis carinii.* On cytotoxic drugs. Diffuse, patchy alveolar shadowing. Cleared on treatment.

Pneumocystis carinii **infection** (Fig. 15.35). This organism is worldwide in distribution but is only found in the lungs of humans and animals. Its natural habitat is not known. It is not decided whether it is protozoan or fungal but is usually classed as the former. It has not been cultured but it can be propagated in cultures of chick embryo lung cells. There is no positive evidence of transmission between humans or between animals and humans. The disease probably does not occur in otherwise healthy persons but asymptomatic infection is common, as revealed by the frequency of antibodies in the population. Immune deficiency is necessary for its expression. Untreated it is almost always fatal. The pathology is that of an acute fulminating pneumonia with interstitial infiltration and intra-alveolar exudate.

The earliest radiographic abnormality is a bilateral basal interstitial shadowing or perivascular cuffing, the latter leading to a loss of definition of hilar structures. As the opacity spreads peripherally it assumes an alveolar pattern similar to pulmonary oedema, generally homogeneous but within which there may be translucencies due to focal emphysema and air bronchograms. At a later stage many air cysts form, small at first but enlarging, some with fluid levels. Pneumothorax and pneumomediastinum are complications of the emphysema.

Open-lung biopsy or bronchoalveolar lavage are the most reliable diagnostic methods. Diagnosis from sputum, needle aspiration and fibreoptic biopsy is less reliable and antibody titres are unreliable. Since invasive methods are not without risk it is sometimes better to treat on suspicion without a confirmed diagnosis.

ACQUIRED IMMUNE DEFICIENCY SYNDROME (AIDS)

This syndrome is a highly lethal combination of opportunistic infections and certain rare malignancies in persons who have none of the usual reasons for being immunosuppressed. There is a progressive loss of cellular immunity, and humoral immunity is also impaired. An agent has now been identified, a human T-cell lymphotropic virus (HIV-1), which seems to be the pathogen, destroying helper T-lymphocytes. It is transmitted sexually and by infected blood. The population at most risk are promiscuous homosexuals, intravenous drug addicts and Africans. Haemophiliacs became infected through repeated exposure to blood products but screening tests and improvements in manufacture will substantially reduce or even eliminate this risk.

Some patients experience a transient illness during acute seroconversion shortly after exposure, characterized by general lymphadenopathy. Although radiographic abnormalities are rare at this stage, there may be patchy interstitial pulmonary opacities which resolve. Antibodies only become detectable 4–8 weeks after the first symptoms. The illness remits and there follows a latent interval which may last for many years before further manifestations appear.

Half of the patients with AIDS develop pulmonary infections, 85% of these being *Pneumocystis carinii pneumonia.* Cytomegalovirus, pyogenic bacteria and various mycobacteria account for substantial numbers. A small proportion is due to other viruses, fungi and protozoa. Regional and racial differences influence the relative frequency of the types of infection.

Pneumocystis carinii may be isolated from lungs which are radiographically normal, but when abnormalities appear they are as described in the previous section. However, atypical patterns arise — cavitating, nodular, honeycomb — but their presence should always be regarded as suspicious of mixed infections.

The chest radiograph in *Cytomegalovirus* infection is similar to that in the early stages of pneumocystis but lacks the later extensive consolidations. In *mycobacterial* infections the most frequent patterns are bilateral noncavitating consolidations, reticulonodulations or miliary. *Pyogenic* infections tend to conform to their usual pattern of segmental or lobar consolidation, and the patients are more acutely ill with high fever and purulent sputum.

Up to 25% of patients develop *Kaposi's sarcoma* or *lymphoma* and the characteristic features are hilar and mediastinal adenopathy, pleural effusion (especially if large) and nodules in the lungs. Kaposi's sarcoma, by the nature of its spread along lymphatics, will tend to produce peribronchial, septal or widespread linear opacities. Most patients will have evidence of the disease elsewhere, in skin or viscera.

Diagnostic clues with respect to the pulmonary complications of AIDS may be summarized:-

1. Hilar or mediastinal node enlargement or large pleural effusion — Kaposi's sarcoma or lymphoma.
2. Multiple bilateral nodular lung opacities — Kaposi's sarcoma or mycobacterial infection.
3. Massive consolidation simulating pulmonary oedema — *Pneumocystis carinii* pneumonia.
4. Unilateral lobar consolidation or abscess — pyogenic infection.

These are pointers, which, although useful, are frequently breached by anomalies and by the presence of mixed infections.

REFERENCES AND SUGGESTIONS FOR FURTHER READING

Berkman, Y. M. (1980) Aspiration and inhalation pneumonias. *Seminars in Roentgenology,* **15,** 73–84.

Bulmer, S. R., Lamb, D., McCormack, R. J. M., Walbaum, P. R. (1978) Aetiology of unresolved pneumonia. *Thorax,* **33,** 307–314.

Davison, A. G., Heard, B. E., McAllister, W. A. C., Turner-Warwick, M. E. H. (1983) Cryptogenic organizing pneumonitis. *Quarterly Journal of Medicine,* **52,** 382–394.

Janower, M. L., Weiss, E. B. (1980) Mycoplasmal, viral and rickettsial pneumonias. *Seminars in Roentgenology,* **15,** 25–34.

Jewkes, J., Kay, P. H., Paneth, M., Citron, K. M. (1983) Pulmonary aspergilloma: analysis and prognosis in relation to haemoptysis and survey of treatment. *Thorax,* **38,** 572–578.

Joint Tuberculosis Committee of the British Thoracic Society (1983) Control and prevention of tuberculosis: a code of practice. *British Medical Journal,* **287,** 1118–1121.

Malo, J. L., Pepys, J., Simon, G. (1977) Studies in chronic, allergic, bronchopulmonary aspergillosis. 2 — Radiological findings. *Thorax,* **32,** 262–268.

Murray, J. F., Garray, S. M., Hopewell, P. C., Mills, J., Snider, G. L., Stover, D. E. (1987) Pulmonary complications of the acquired immunodeficiency syndrome. *American Review of Respiratory Disease,* **135,** 504–509.

Scanlon, G. T., Unger, J. D. (1973) The radiology of bacterial and viral pneumonias. *Radiologic Clinics of North America,* **11,** 317–338.

Suster, B., Akerman, M., Orenstein, M., Wax, M. R. (1986) Pulmonary manifestations of AIDS: review of 108 episodes. *Radiology,* **161,** 87–93.

Tew, J., Calenoff, L., Berlin, B. S. (1977) Bacterial and non-bacterial pneumonia: accuracy of radiographic diagnosis. *Radiology,* **124,** 607–612.

White, R. J., Blainey, A. D., Harrison, K. J., Clarke, S. K. R. (1981) Causes of pneumonia presenting to a District General Hospital. *Thorax,* **36,** 566–570.

CHAPTER 16

CHRONIC BRONCHITIS AND EMPHYSEMA; PNEUMOCONIOSES

Michael B. Rubens

CHRONIC BRONCHITIS AND EMPHYSEMA

Chronic obstruction to bronchial airflow is an abnormality that unites the group of conditions termed chronic obstructive pulmonary disease or chronic obstructive airways disease. This group is the most common form of chronic lung disease and includes chronic bronchitis, pulmonary emphysema and asthma, which are discussed in this section. Other entities in this group (cystic fibrosis and bronchiectasis) are discussed elsewhere. (Chs 17, 19).

Definitions

Chronic bronchitis is defined in clinical terms as 'a chronic cough without demonstrable cause, with expectoration on most days during at least three consecutive months for more than two consecutive years'.

Emphysema is defined in morphological terms as 'an increase beyond the normal in the size of the air-spaces distal to the terminal bronchioles, with dilatation and destruction of their walls'.

Asthma is a clinical term referring to 'widespread narrowing of the bronchi, which is paroxysmal and reversible'.

Clinically and radiologically a patient may have manifestations of more than one kind of chronic obstructive airways disease. The clinical syndrome of asthma results from hyper-reactivity of the larger airways to a variety of stimuli, causing narrowing of the bronchi, wheezing and often dyspnoea.

Extrinsic or atopic asthma is usually associated with a history of allergy and raised plasma IgE. An important cause of extrinsic asthma is aspergillosis, and this is discussed in detail in Chapter 15. *Intrinsic* or non-atopic asthma may be precipitated by a variety of factors such as exercise, emotion and infection. In acute exacerbations of chronic bronchitis due to a chest infection, wheezing is a common feature.

The role of radiology in asthma is limited. Most asthmatics show a normal chest X-ray during remissions. During an asthmatic attack the chest X-ray may show signs of hyperinflation (Fig. 16.1), with depression of the diaphragm and expansion of the retrosternal air-space. Mediastinal emphysema may occur secondary to a rupture at terminal bronchiolar level or beyond, and occasionally this may lead to a pneumothorax. The peripheral pulmonary vessels appear normal, but if the central pulmonary arteries are enlarged, irreversible pulmonary arterial hypertension is probably present. The importance of radiology is to exclude complications such as a pulmonary infection, atelectasis due to mucus plugging or pneumothorax.

CHRONIC BRONCHITIS

The most consistent pathological finding in chronic bronchitis is hypertrophy of the mucus-secreting glands of the bronchi. Their secretions are more viscous than usual, leading to interference with the mucociliary transport mechanisms and plugging of the small airways.

Chronic bronchitics are almost always smokers, and are usually male. Other important aetiological factors are urban atmospheric pollution, a dusty work environment and low socio-economic group.

The role of radiology in chronic bronchitis is to detect and assess complications of the condition, and also to detect coincidental diseases. Pulmonary emphysema is a common complication which can be assessed radiographically, as can the development of cor pulmonale. The presenting symptoms of pulmonary tuberculosis and lung cancer can be masked by chronic bronchitis, and again the chest X-ray may help.

Radiological appearances. Approximately 50% of patients with chronic bronchitis have a normal chest X-ray. In patients with a plain film abnormality, the signs are due to emphysema, superimposed infection or possibly bronchiectasis.

An appearance which suggests chronic bronchitis is the so-called *'dirty chest'* (Fig. 16.2). There is generalized accentuation of the bronchovascular markings. Small, poorly-defined opacities may be seen anywhere in the lungs, but their perception can be extremely subjective. There is some correlation between the 'dirty chest' and

435

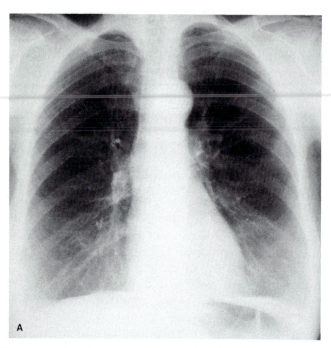
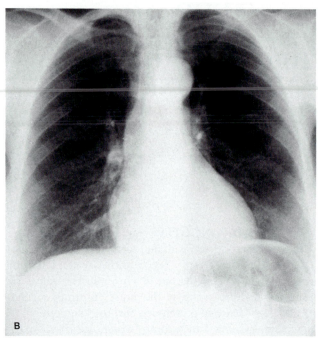

Fig. 16.1 Asthma in a woman of 64. **A**. During an asthmatic attack the lungs are hyperinflated, the diaphragm being depressed and flattened. **B**. During remission the chest radiograph is normal.

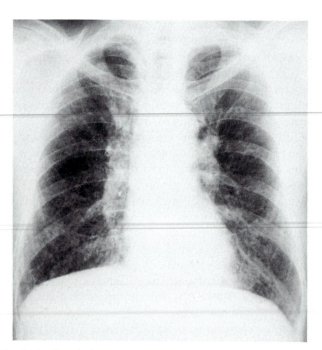

Fig. 16.2 Chronic bronchitis in a man of 62. Small poorly-defined opacities are present throughout both lungs, producing the 'dirty chest'. This contrasts with the clear lungs in Figure 16.1B.

Thin tram-line or tubular shadows may also be seen, suggesting bronchiectasis, but the precise nature of these shadows is uncertain. These opacities are usually related to the hila, and may be clearly demonstrated by tomography, but again are only suggestive and not diagnostic of chronic bronchitis.

If emphysema with air-trapping is present the lungs enlarge, the diaphragm becomes flattened and the retrosternal air-space increases. The number and size of the peripheral vessels decrease, and the central pulmonary arteries may enlarge. If cor pulmonale supervenes the heart enlarges.

EMPHYSEMA

As stated above, emphysema is defined in morphological terms as enlargement of the airways beyond the terminal bronchi, with dilatation and destruction of their walls. Classification of emphysema is also based, in part, on morphology, and a basic knowledge of lung structure is, therefore, pertinent. The trachea, bronchi and terminal bronchioles are strictly conducting airways. Beyond the terminal bronchioles, gas exchange takes place, so that respiratory bronchioles, alveolar ducts and alveolar sacs are both conducting and respiratory structures. The alveoli are purely respiratory in function. The secondary pulmonary lobule is a unit of lung structure supplied by between three and five terminal bronchioles; lung distal to a terminal bronchiole is called an acinus, and a secondary pulmonary lobule, therefore, comprises 3–5 acini.

the presence of perivascular and peribronchial oedema, chronic inflammation and fibrosis. If this pattern is particularly obvious, with fine linear shadows and hazy nodular opacities, the appearance may resemble interstitial fibrosis, lymphangitis carcinomatosis or bronchiectasis.

Types of emphysema and associated conditions

Involvement of the secondary pulmonary lobule by emphysema may be non-selective or selective.

1. *Pan-acinar emphysema* is a non-selective process characterized by destruction of all of the lung distal to the terminal bronchiole. It is sometimes termed pan-lobular emphysema. The lung may be involved locally or generally, but distribution throughout the lung is rarely uniform. It may be associated with centri-acinar emphysema, especially in chronic bronchitis, and is also seen in α-1-anti-trypsin deficiency.

2. *Centri-acinar emphysema* is a selective process characterized by destruction and dilatation of the respiratory bronchioles. The alveolar ducts, sacs and alveoli are spared until a late stage. It is sometimes called centrilobular emphysema. It is frequently found in association with chronic bronchitis.

3. *Paraseptal emphysema* involves the periphery of the secondary lobules, usually in the lung periphery, sometimes combined with pan- or centri-acinar emphysema, and occasionally causes bulla formation.

4. *Paracicatricial emphysema* refers to distension and destruction of terminal air-spaces adjacent to fibrotic lesions, and is most frequently seen as a result of tuberculosis.

5. *Obstructive emphysema* is strictly a misnomer, and the condition is better termed 'obstructive hyperinflation', since the distal airways are dilated but not necessarily destroyed. It is discussed here for the sake of completeness. It occurs when a larger bronchus is obstructed in such a way that air enters the lung on inspiration, but is trapped on expiration. Such one-way valve obstruction may be due to an inhaled foreign body (e.g. peanuts or teeth) or due to an endobronchial or peribronchial tumour. The lung beyond the obstruction becomes hyperinflated.

6. *Compensatory emphysema* is another process that is better regarded as hyperinflation. If part or all of a lung collapses, shrinks or is removed, the resulting space is occupied by displacement of the mediastinum or diaphragm, or usually, more significantly, by hyperinflation of the unaffected or remaining lung. This is discussed in the section on lobar collapse in Chapter 13.

7. A *bulla* is an emphysematous space with a diameter of more than 1 cm in the distended state, and its walls are made up of compressed surrounding lung or pleura, depending on its location.

Emphysema may be classified according to the presence or absence of air-trapping at respiratory bronchiole level. Pan-acinar, obstructive and congenital lobar emphysema are associated with air-trapping and usually cause symptoms. Centri-acinar, paraseptal and compensatory emphysema are not associated with air-trapping and are usually asymptomatic.

Radiological appearances

1. Pan-acinar emphysema

The radiographic features of pan-acinar emphysema are the results of destruction of lung tissue altering the vascular pattern, interference of ventilation decreasing lung perfusion, and air-trapping. The effects of pan-acinar emphysema are almost always apparent clinically by the time the radiographic manifestations occur, but a normal chest X-ray virtually excludes severe generalized emphysema.

The main radiographic signs are (Fig. 16.3):

a. Reduction of pulmonary vascularity peripherally.
b. Hyperinflation of the lungs.
c. Alteration of the cardiac shadow and central pulmonary arteries.

The vascular pattern in affected areas of lung is attenuated. Involvement of the lung may be localized or generalized, but if generalized is usually patchy. Involved areas have fewer vessels than normal, and those vessels that remain are small. Mild degrees of vascular attenuation are difficult to perceive, so it is worth comparing the size of vessels in different zones. If vessels are diminished in calibre and number in a particular zone, compared to another, that zone is likely to be emphysematous.

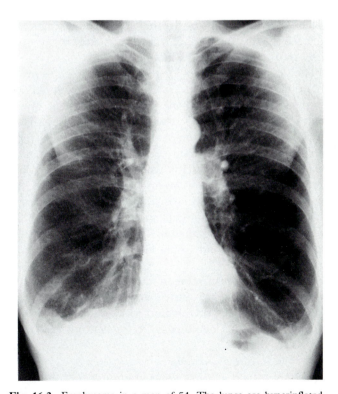

Fig. 16.3 Emphysema in a man of 54. The lungs are hyperinflated, the diaphragm being low and flat. The peripheral vascular pattern is attenuated in the right mid and left mid and lower zones. The central pulmonary arteries are enlarged, indicating pulmonary arterial hypertension. The heart is elongated.

Peripheral vascular attenuation is due to a number of factors. Perfusion of emphysematous lung is less than normal, and pulmonary blood flow is diverted to less affected areas of lung. Pulmonary vessels are displaced around emphysematous areas and bullae. Small arteries are obliterated by the primary emphysematous process, but these vessels are too small to be visualized radiographically, and this process, therefore, probably does not contribute to the oligaemic appearances, but may be a factor in increased radiolucency of affected areas.

Pan-acinar emphysema has a tendency to affect the lung bases, and may cause diversion of blood flow to the upper zones, which should not be mistaken for pulmonary venous hypertension. In α-1-anti-trypsin deficiency the changes of emphysema tend to be basal. Air-trapping causes hyperinflation of the lungs, and may lead to flattening of the diaphragm and increased anteroposterior diameter of the thorax. Flattening of the diaphragm is often best seen on the lateral projection, the level of the diaphragm often being as low as the 11th rib posteriorly. Some normal individuals can push their diaphragm as low on full inspiration, but on expiration the diaphragm will rise 5–10 cm, whereas in emphysema excursion of the diaphragm is usually less than 3 cm. In severe emphysema the diaphragm may actually be inverted.

The 'barrel chest' is caused by bowing of the sternum, and increased thoracic kyphosis. The retrosternal airspace may increase in depth, and extend inferiorly between the anterior surface of the heart and the sternum (Fig. 16.4).

The heart often appears long and narrow. This is probably due primarily to the low position of the diaphragm altering the projection of the heart. Enlargement of the central pulmonary arteries usually signifies pulmonary arterial hypertension (Fig. 16.3). If cor pulmonale develops, the heart may enlarge due to right ventricular dilatation. In patients with emphysema who develop left heart failure, the signs of hyperinflation may decrease, and the level of the diaphragm will rise. This is due to pulmonary oedema increasing the compliance of the lung and thus reducing the lung volume. In these patients the distribution of oedema fluid within emphysematous lung may be bizzare.

CT is more sensitive than the plain chest X-ray in detecting the presence and distribution of emphysema (Fig. 16.7). Vascular attenuation may be detected earlier, and bullae may be identified by CT when not visible on the chest X-ray.

2. Bullous disease of the lungs

Bullae are usually present in the lung in association with some form of emphysema, but occasionally bullae occur locally in otherwise normal lung (Fig. 16.5). They commonly occur in paraseptal emphysema, and in emphysema associated with scarring, but clinically the most important bullae are those due to pan-acinar emphysema, with or without chronic bronchitis.

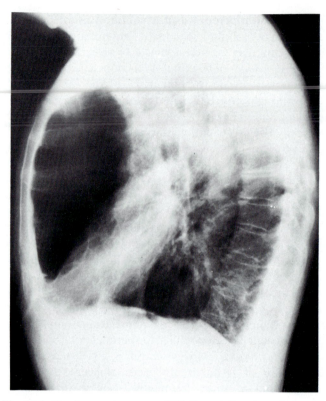

Fig. 16.4 Emphysema in a man of 52. Lateral film shows increased lung volume, which is producing a barrel chest. The retrosternal space is deeper than normal and extends more inferiorly than normal.

Bullae appear as round or oval translucencies varying in size from 1 cm in diameter to occupation of almost an entire hemithorax (Fig. 16.6). They may be single or multiple, and are usually peripheral. In asymptomatic patients and in those with pulmonary scarring, bullae tend to be apical, but in chronic obstructive airways disease bullae are found throughout the lungs (Fig. 16.7). Their walls may be visible as a smooth, curved, hair-line shadow. If the walls are not visible displacement of vessels around a radiolucent area may indicate a bullous area.

Bullae are usually air-filled but may become infected and filled with fluid. Associated inflammatory change may be present in the surrounding lung. A bulla will show a fluid level if it is partially fluid-filled, or will appear solid if completely fluid-filled (Fig. 16.8).

A giant bulla may be difficult to differentiate from a loculated pneumothorax, and tomography may be necessary to demonstrate the wall of the bulla or thin strands of lung tissue crossing it.

3. Emphysema with chronic bronchitis

Many patients with chronic obstructive airways disease have emphysema *and* chronic bronchitis. The chest X-ray may then show a combination of changes of hyperinflation, pulmonary arterial hypertension and increased bronchovascular markings of the so-called *'dirty chest'*.

At one end of the clinical spectrum is the *'pink puffer'* who, by major effort, ventilates sufficient alveoli to main-

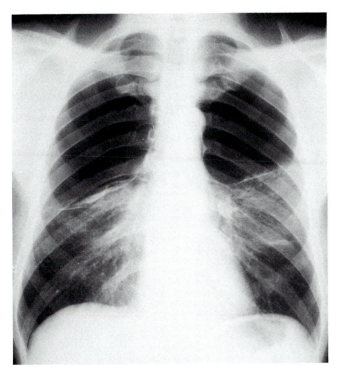

Fig. 16.5 Bilateral upper-zone bullae in a man of 35. 'Routine' chest X-ray — no history or symptoms of respiratory disease. Both upper zones are occupied by large bullae which are compressing the upper lobes. There is no evidence of generalized emphysema or air-trapping — the level and shape of the diaphragm are normal.

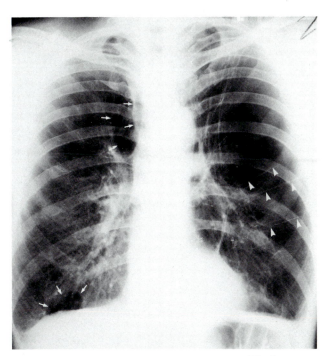

Fig. 16.6 Emphysema with bullae in a man of 61. The lungs are hyperinflated. A giant bulla occupies most of the left hemithorax, compressing the left lung. Strands of lung tissue (arrowheads) are seen crossing this bulla. Small bullae (arrows) are also present in the right lung.

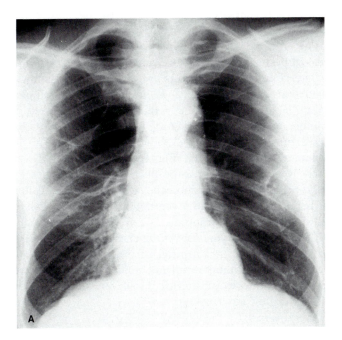

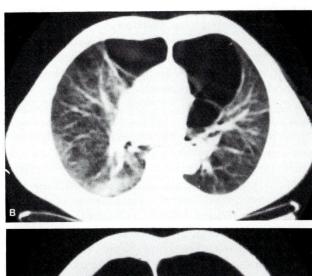

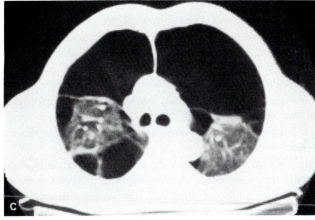

Fig. 16.7 Multiple bullae. **A**. The chest radiograph shows bullae in both upper zones, and in the periphery of the left mid and lower zones. **B, C**. CT scans demonstrate the bullae more clearly, making it easier to define their size, number and location more accurately. Comparison of expiratory and inspiratory scans makes it possible to differentiate between bullae that are ventilated and those with air-trapping. (Courtesy of Dr B. Strickland.)

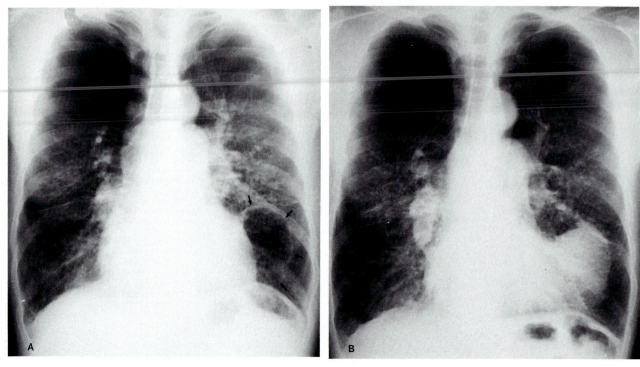

Fig. 16.8 Emphysema with infected bulla in a man of 48. **A.** The lungs are hyperinflated. The right upper zone is occupied by a large bulla, and another bulla is seen adjacent to the left heart border (arrows). The central pulmonary arteries are enlarged. **B.** Following a chest infection the left-sided bulla has filled with fluid and appears completely opaque.

tain normal blood gases; since there is no hypoxaemia, normal pulmonary artery pressure is preserved. Pink puffers tend to have predominantly pan-acinar emphysema, and the chest X-ray shows peripheral vascular attenuation and hyperinflation. This appearance may be termed the 'arterial deficiency' pattern.

At the other end of the clinical spectrum is the *'blue bloater'*, who chronically retains carbon dioxide due to poor alveolar ventilation. The respiratory centre becomes insensitive to the persistently raised concentration of arterial carbon dioxide, and chronic cyanosis occurs. Chronic hypoxaemia causes pulmonary arteriolar constriction, and in due course pulmonary arterial hypertension and cor pulmonale occur. Blue bloaters tend to have centri-acinar emphysema and less extensive pan-acinar emphysema. The chest X-ray shows increased bronchovascular markings, enlarged central pulmonary arteries and possibly cardiac enlargement. This appearance may be termed the 'increased markings' pattern of emphysema, and signs of hyperinflation are rarely severe. Most patients with chronic bronchitis and emphysema exhibit features between these extremes.

4. Unilateral or lobar emphysema (Macleod's or Swyer-James' syndrome)

This syndrome is characterized by a hypertransradiant hemithorax associated with air-trapping. It is probably the result of a childhood viral infection causing bronchiolitis and obliteration of the small airways; the involved distal

airways are ventilated by collateral air drift, and air-trapping leads to pan-acinar emphysema.

The affected lung is hypertransradiant, due to decreased perfusion, and may be smaller than normal. The ipsilateral pulmonary artery is present, but small, and the peripheral vascular pattern is attenuated. Air-trapping occurs in the affected lung, which tends to maintain its volume on expiration, resulting in displacement of the mediastinum to the normal side, and restriction of the ipsilateral hemidiaphragm (Fig. 16.9).

The syndrome may also be illustrated by radionuclide scanning, when a perfusion scan will show reduced flow to the affected lung, and a ventilation scan, using xenon, will demonstrate air-trapping.

The differential diagnosis of the chest X-ray appearance includes proximal interruption of the pulmonary artery, the hypogenetic lung syndrome and pulmonary artery obstruction due to embolism. However, none of these entities exhibit air-trapping.

5. Centri-acinar

This occurs principally in chronic bronchitis and uncomplicated coal-miners' pneumoconiosis. The radiological appearance is that of the primary condition. In later stages pan-acinar and bullous emphysema may become apparent.

6. Obstructive 'emphysema'

Obstructive hyperinflation may affect an entire lung, a lobe or a segment. The cause such as an inhaled foreign

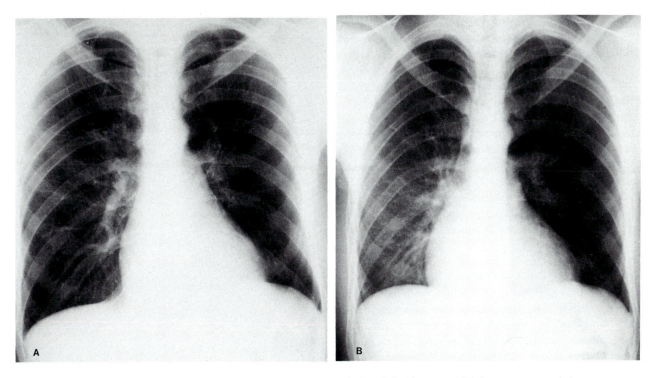

Fig. 16.9 Unilateral emphysema in a man of 30 with a history of repeated chest infections as a child, but no current respiratory symptoms. **A**. Inspiratory film shows normal right lung, and hypertransradiant left lung with small left pulmonary artery. **B**. Expiratory film demonstrates displacement of mediastinum to the right and restricted movement of the left hemidiaphragm, indicating air-trapping in the left lung.

body or tooth, or a central tumour, may be apparent on the chest X-ray. The vascular pattern of the affected part of the lung is attenuated, and this area may appear hypertransradiant. Fluoroscopy or an expiratory film will demonstrate air-trapping in the affected area with deviation of the mediastinum to the normal side, and restruction of the ipsilateral hemidiaphragm on expiration.

7. Compensatory 'emphysema'
The radiological signs resulting from collapse or removal of all or part of a lung are discussed in the section on lobar collapse (Ch. 13).

8. Congenital lobar emphysema
This is discussed in Chapter 19.

CRYPTOGENIC OBLITERATIVE BRONCHIOLITIS

This condition presents with dyspnoea, which may be progressive and severe. The clinical picture may suggest pulmonary thromboembolic disease, but the radiographic appearance is different. The chest X-ray shows symmetrical reduction of peripheral vascularity in the mid and lower zones, and evidence of mild hyperinflation of the lungs. *Bronchography* shows a characteristic appearance of non-filling of the side branches of the fifth and sixth generation bronchi, abrupt termination of bronchi, and either lack of normal tapering or generalized narrowing of bron-

chi. The cause is unknown, but there is an association with rheumatoid disease.

THE PNEUMOCONIOSES

Occupational disease of the chest may be due to inhalation of dusts or noxious fumes. Dusts may be inorganic or organic. In general, the organic dusts cause disease by hypersensitivity reactions, and they are considered in the section on extrinsic allergic alveolitis. Noxious gases usually produce an acute inflammatory reaction, often with pulmonary oedema, which may be fatal, or may be followed by resolution, with or without subsequent pulmonary fibrosis. The pneumoconioses considered in this section are diseases due to inhalation of *inorganic* dusts.

Dust particles larger than 5 μm in diameter are usually deposited onto the bronchial and bronchiolar walls and are coughed up, but smaller particles may reach the alveoli. Asbestos fibres are an exception, fibres longer than 30 μm sometimes penetrating the lung parenchyma.

The diagnosis of a pneumoconiosis depends upon a history of exposure to a dust, an abnormal chest X-ray and abnormal results of pulmonary function tests. Occasionally a lung biopsy is necessary. The history of exposure is not necessarily one of working with a dust, but may include living near a mine or factory.

The reaction of an individual to dust exposure depends

upon several factors, including the nature of the dust, the concentration of particles, the duration of exposure and the individual's susceptibility. Inorganic dusts are either active or inactive. The former are fibrogenic in the lung, and the latter are relatively inert. Frequently a patient will have been exposed to a combination of dusts. The important active dusts are silica and asbestos; coal dust is usually a combination of active and inactive components.

The ILO (International Labour Office) Classification of Radiographs of the Pneumoconioses has been devised to codify the changes in chest X-ray in a simple and reproducible manner. It is important in epidemiological and industrial medicine, and the interested reader is referred to the specialist publications at the end of this chapter.

SILICOSIS

Exposure to silica may occur in a variety of occupations, including granite, slate and sandstone quarrying, gold mining, sandblasting, foundry work, pottery and ceramics. Exposure usually lasts for several years before symptoms occur, unless the exposure is overwhelming. Silica causes a fibrotic reaction in the lung, which may progress after exposure has ceased, probably due to immunological processes. Silicosis predisposes to pulmonary tuberculosis.

Radiological appearance. Simple silicosis appears as multiple, nodular shadows of fairly uniform size, usually between 2 and 5 mm in diameter. The nodules have a fairly sharp outline, and are of uniform density (Fig. 16.10).

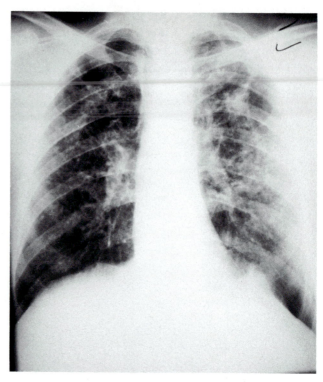

Fig. 16.11 Complicated silicosis in a maker of roofing felt, aged 63, exposed to silica sand and talc. In addition to widespread nodular opacities, densest in the mid and upper zones, confluent opacities are developing in the upper zones. Industrial talc is a mixture of silica and asbestos, and sputum examination revealed asbestos bodies. Lung biopsy showed mixed-dust pneumoconiosis.

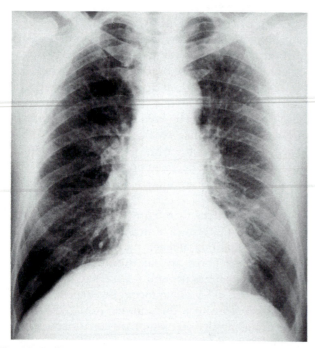

Fig. 16.10 Simple silicosis in a retired sandblaster aged 67. Multiple nodular opacities are present throughout both lungs, with relative sparing of the lower zones.

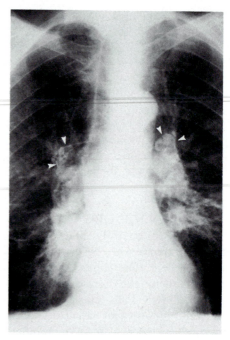

Fig. 16.12 Silicosis in a man of 69 with a history of exposure to a variety of dusts, including silica. Note bilateral hilar lymph node enlargement with 'egg-shell' calcification (arrowheads) typical of silicosis.

They appear initially in the mid and upper zones, but are later found in all zones, with relative sparing of the bases. The nodules rarely calcify. Reticular shadowing may occur at any stage, and septal lines may appear. Pleural changes are rare.

Complicated silicosis is characterized by confluence of nodules (Fig. 16.11) to form homogeneous, non-segmental areas of consolidation, usually in the upper lobes. These 'massive shadows' of fibrosis migrate towards the hila, leaving peripheral areas of emphysema. When complicated silicosis develops, the possibility of tuberculosis should be considered. Cavitation of a massive shadow is usually due to ischaemic necrosis or tuberculosis.

Hilar lymph node enlargement is common at any stage, and lymph node calcification may occur. Calcification may be diffuse throughout lymph nodes, or peripheral, giving an 'egg-shell' appearance (Fig. 16.12).

Extensive fibrosis may cause pulmonary arterial hypertension, and cor pulmonale may ensue.

In patients with rheumatoid disease, silicosis may be complicated by Caplan's syndrome, but, like massive fibrosis, this is commoner in coal worker's pneumoconiosis.

ASBESTOSIS

Asbestos exposure may occur in a variety of occupations. Asbestos mining and processing are obvious examples, but exposure may also occur in construction and demolition work, shipbuilding and manufacture of some textiles. Living near such workplaces also carries a risk of exposure. The duration of exposure may be very short, and the condition may become apparent only many years later.

The four types of asbestos that commonly cause disease are *chrysolite*, *crocidolite*, *amosite* and *anthophyllite*. Chrysolite (or white asbestos) is the commonest, and crocidolite (or blue asbestos) is the most pathogenic.

Fibrosis is probably the result of a number of mechanisms. Direct physical irritation is almost certainly a factor in the development of pleural plaques. Asbestos is a mixture of silicates, and release of silicilic acid may be locally irritant. Lastly, a toxic effect of asbestos on macrophages leads to the release of antigens and the subsequent production of auto-antibodies. This auto-immune response is probably the cause of the fibrosing alveolitis that is a common feature. Asbestos fibres may remain in the lung for years after exposure has ceased, and this may explain why the development of pulmonary fibrosis is sometimes delayed.

Inhaled fibres, sometimes longer than 30 μm, may reach the alveoli and penetrate the pleura and occasionally the diaphragm. The fibres gravitate to the lower lobes, so that changes are more severe in the lower zones, than in the mid and upper zones.

Symptoms of asbestosis are often not apparent until 20

or 30 years after exposure. Malignant disease is an important complication. *Lung cancer*, usually adenocarcinoma, is relatively common, especially when asbestos exposure is combined with cigarette smoking. Compared to the non-smoker without exposure to asbestos, asbestos alone increases the likelihood of lung cancer by a factor of 5, cigarette smoking alone by a factor of 10, and the combination of asbestos and cigarettes by a factor of 50! The combination of asbestos and cigarettes also predisposes to carcinomas of the oesophagus, larynx and oropharynx. *Mesothelioma of the pleura* is the other malignancy closely associated with asbestos exposure, and may develop after a latent period of 20 years. Other neoplasms associated with asbestos exposure are *carcinomas of the large bowel* and *renal tract* and *peritoneal mesothelioma*.

Radiological appearance

Asbestos exposure may produce changes in the lung parenchyma and in the pleura. Pleural changes, which include plaques, calcification, diffuse thickening and effusion, are seen on the chest X-ray more often than parenchymal changes.

Pleural plaques are usually bilateral, and most frequently are present peripherally in the mid zones, often adjacent to the ribs. They may be difficult to see unless viewed tangentially, so if they are suspected, fluoroscopy and oblique views are helpful (Fig. 16.13). They may also be demonstrated by ultrasound, and small plaques, especially

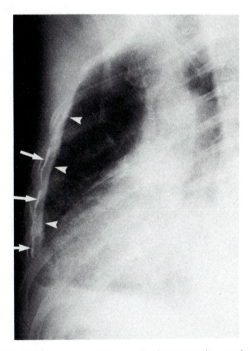

Fig. 16.13 Asbestos exposure in a retired construction worker. Oblique projection demonstrates extensive pleural thickening (arrowheads) and calcification (arrows) adjacent to the ribs.

close to the spine, may only be seen by CT. Plaques are common over the diaphragm but are difficult to see unless calcified. Occasionally it may be difficult to differentiate between plaques and companion shadows. The presence of bilateral pleural plaques is almost diagnostic of asbestos exposure.

Pleural plaques frequently calcify. Calcification is, therefore, most often seen in the periphery of the mid zones and over the diaphragm (Fig. 16.14). The calcium is situated in the parietal pleura, just deep to the ribs or diaphragm, usually forming linear shadows, occasionally with bizarre shapes. Again tangential views (Fig. 16.13) and CT may be helpful.

Diffuse pleural thickening is an unusual manifestation and small pleural effusions unrelated to malignant change occasionally occur. Mesothelioma is discussed in the section on the pleura.

Pulmonary fibrosis is usually present histologically by the time pleural calcification has developed, but may not be apparent on the chest X-ray. CT scanning is more sensitive than the chest X-ray in detecting early pulmonary fibrosis by demonstration of either nodular or linear shadows (Fig. 16.15). The earliest changes are frequently subpleural and may only be visible on high-resolution CT (Fig. 16.16).

The earliest sign of pulmonary fibrosis on the chest X-ray is a fine reticular pattern in the lower zones (Fig. 16.17). This becomes coarser, leading to loss of clarity of the diaphragmatic and cardiac outlines — the so-called 'shaggy heart'. At a later stage the whole lung may be involved, but the basal preponderance persists, and emphysematous bullae may develop.

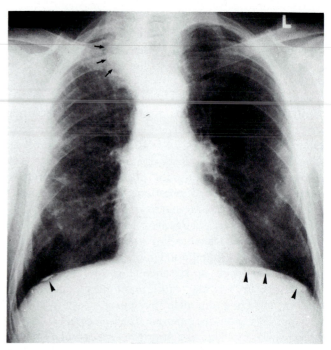

Fig. 16.14 Asbestos exposure in a man of 60. Pleural shadowing in the periphery of both mid zones is due to plaques. Pleural calcification is present along both domes of the diaphragm (arrowheads). The mass at the right apex is an adenocarcinoma (arrows).

COAL-WORKER'S PNEUMOCONIOSIS
Coal dust comprises mostly carbon, but it may contain small amounts of silica. Coal-workers are susceptible to coal-worker's *pneumoconiosis, silicosis, chronic bronchitis, emphysema* and *pulmonary tuberculosis.*

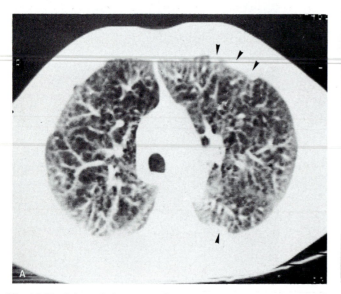
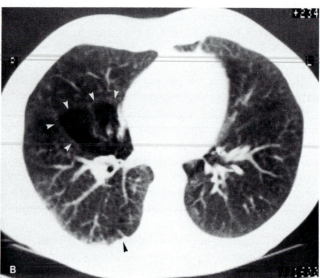

Fig. 16.15 Asbestosis in a man of 54 who had been a pipe lagger for 14 years. **A.** CT demonstrates pleural plaques (arrowheads) and diffuse reticular and nodular shadows. **B.** This section demonstrates further pleural plaques (black arrowhead) and bullae in the right lung (white arrowheads). The chest radiograph (not shown) demonstrated the pleural plaques but not the lung disease.

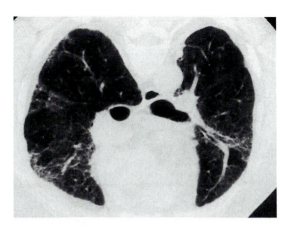

Fig. 16.16 Asbestosis shown in high-resolution CT with the patient prone. Bilateral subpleural reticular shadowing.

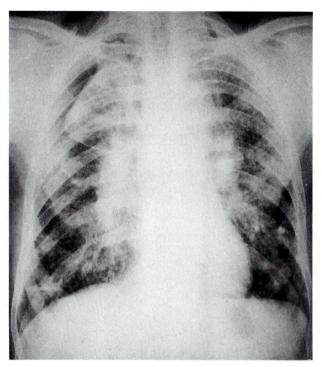

Fig. 16.18 Coal-worker's pneumoconiosis in a man of 59. Nodular opacities are present throughout both lungs, densest in the mid zones. A right apical pneumothorax is also present.

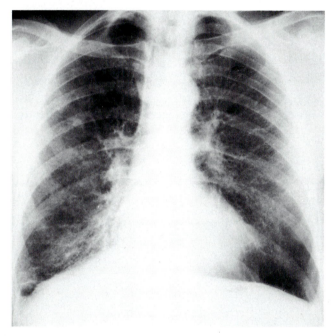

Fig. 16.17 Asbestosis in a man of 59 who had been exposed to asbestos for over 25 years. Fine reticulonodular shadowing is present in the mid and lower zones, best seen on the right side. Emphysematous bullae are present at the left base.

Coal dust is not fibrogenic, and deposits in the lung are surrounded by areas of focal dust emphysema. The corresponding radiographic appearance is 'simple' pneumoconiosis. 'Complicated' pneumoconiosis, characterized by *progressive massive fibrosis* (PMF), is the result of prolonged exposure, perhaps with a complicating factor such as silica exposure, infection, or an auto-immune process with the presence of rheumatoid factor, anti-nuclear factor or other auto-antibodies.

Radiological appearance

The earliest signs of simple pneumoconiosis on the chest X-ray are small, faint, indistinct nodular opacities, 1–5 mm in diameter. The nodules first appear in the mid zones, with subsequent involvement of the entire lung, although the mid zone preponderance persists (Fig. 16.18). The nodules are smaller and less well-defined than those of silicosis, and may rarely calcify. Coalescence of small nodules to form opacities of 1 cm diameter or more, or the appearance of new opacities of this size, signifies development of PMF (Fig. 16.19). These massive shadows are usually bilateral, and develop initially in the periphery of the upper and mid zones as round or oval shadows. They may become sausage-shaped and migrate towards the hila, leaving peripheral areas of emphysema and bullae. The massive shadows may develop scattered areas of calcification, and occasionally they cavitate, and may subsequently fill with fluid.

Simple coal-worker's pneumoconiosis does not usually progress if exposure to coal dust ceases, but PMF often does.

Caplan's syndrome may occur in patients with rheumatoid disease and coal-worker's pneumoconiosis. The appearance is of multiple, round, well-defined opacities, 1–5 cm in diameter, throughout the lungs, often developing rapidly, sometimes in successive crops (Fig. 16.20). These opacities represent necrobiotic nodules, and they may remain static, calcify or cavitate. The underlying changes of pneumoconiosis may not be obvious, and the appearance may then resemble pulmonary metastases.

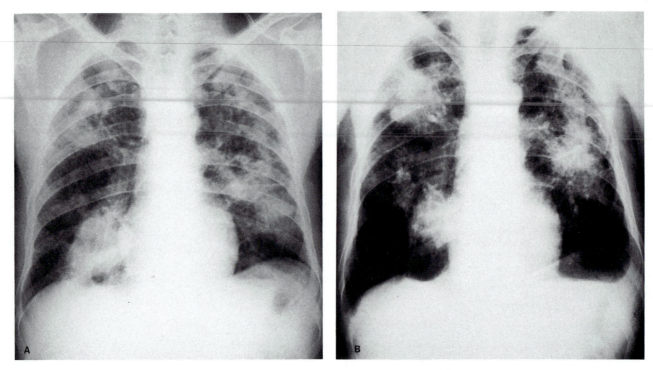

Fig. 16.19 Progressive massive fibrosis in a coalminer of 52. **A**. Nodular opacities are present throughout both lungs, and several areas of more confluent shadowing are present. **B**. Four years later, lower-zone masses have migrated centrally, leaving peripheral areas of emphysema. The upper lobe opacities have enlarged.

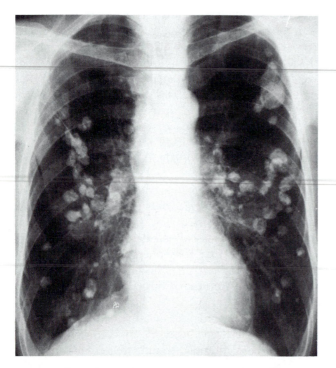

Fig. 16.20 Caplan's syndrome in a coalminer aged 54 with long-standing rheumatoid arthritis. Multiple rounded pulmonary opacities are present — some are partly calcified. The background changes of coal-worker's pneumoconiosis are minimal.

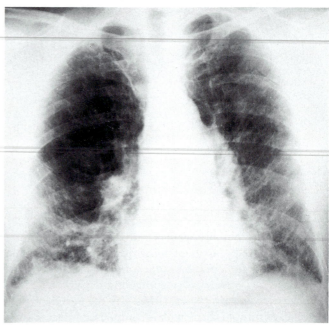

Fig. 16.21 Berylliosis. The patient had spent 35 years in the glass-blowing industry making neon lights. The chest radiograph shows diffuse reticular shadowing. The appearance is indistinguishable from end-stage sarcoidosis.

BERYLLIOSIS

Chronic beryllium poisoning may produce pulmonary manifestations that resemble a pneumoconiosis, but the changes are probably due to a specific antigen–antibody reaction. *Acute* berylliosis is a chemical pneumonitis and the radiological appearance is that of non-cardiogenic pulmonary oedema. *Chronic* berylliosis is a systemic disease characterized by widespread non-caseating granulomas, which in the lung produce appearances identical to sarcoidosis. There is widespread fine reticular and nodular shadowing, often with enlargement of the hila and mediastinal lymph nodes, and this may be followed by widespread fibrosis (Fig. 16.21).

PNEUMOCONIOSES DUE TO INACTIVE DUSTS

Inactive dusts do not cause fibrosis in the lungs, but may produce changes on the chest X-ray simply by accumulating in the lungs. Symptoms are usually absent.

Siderosis is due to prolonged exposure to iron oxide dust. Widespread reticulonodular shadowing occurs. When exposure ceases the shadowing may regress. In *silicosiderosis* fibrosis may occur, with a picture resembling that of silicosis.

Stannosis is caused by inhalation of tin oxide. Multiple, very small, very dense, discrete opacities of 0.5–1 mm diameter are distributed throughout the lungs. Particles may collect in the interlobular lymphatics and produce dense septal lines. The opacities are denser than calcium because of the high atomic number of tin.

Barytosis results from inhalation of particulate barium sulphate, causing very dense nodulation throughout the lungs. Following cessation of exposure the shadows regress.

REFERENCES AND SUGGESTIONS FOR FURTHER READING

Chronic obstructive airways disease

A report of the conclusions of a CIBA Guest Symposium: Terminology, definitions and classification of chronic pulmonary emphysema and related conditions (1959). *Thorax*, **14**, 286–299.

Anderson, A. E. Jr., Foraker, A. G. (1973) Centrilobular emphysema and panlobular emphysema: two different diseases. *Thorax*, **28**, 547–550.

Breatnach, E., Kerr, I. H. (1982) The radiology of cryptogenic obliterative bronchiolitis. *Clinical Radiology*, **33**, 657–661.

Carr, D. H., Pride, N. B. (1984) Computed tomography in pre-operative assessment of bullous emphysema. *Clinical Radiology*, **35**, 43–45.

Fletcher, C. M., Pride, N. B. (1984) Editorial: Definitions of emphysema, chronic bronchitis, asthma and air flow obstruction: 25 years on from the CIBA Symposium. *Thorax*, **39**, 81–85.

Goddard, P. R., Nicholson, E. M., Laszlo, G., Watt, I. (1982) Computed tomography in pulmonary emphysema. *Clinical Radiology*, **33**, 379–387.

MacLeod, W. M. (1954) Abnormal transradiancy of one lung. *Thorax*, **9**. 147–153.

Morgan, M. D. L., Strickland, B. (1984) Computed tomography in the assessment of bullous lung disease. *British Journal of Diseases of the Chest*, **78**, 10–25.

Patheram, I. S., Kerr, I. H., Collins, J. V. (1981) Value of chest radiographs in severe acute asthma. *Clinical Radiology*, **32**, 281–282.

Reid, L. (1967) *The Pathology of Emphysema*. Lloyd-Luke, London.

Simon, G. (1964) Radiology and emphysema. *Clinical Radiology*, **15**, 293–306.

Swyer, P. R., James, G. C. W. (1953) A case of unilateral emphysema. *Thorax*, **8**, 133–136.

Thurlbeck, W. M., Simon, G. (1978) Radiographic appearance of the chest in emphysema. *American Journal of Roentgenology*, **130**, 429–440.

Tomashefski, J. F. (1977) Definition, differentiation and classification of COPD. *Postgraduate Medicine*, **62**, 88–97.

The pneumoconioses

Becklace, M. R. (1976) Asbestos related diseases of the lung and other organs. Their epidemiology and implications for clinical practice. *American Review of Respiratory Disease*, **114**, 187–227.

Caplan, A. (1962) Correlation of radiological category with lung pathology in coal-workers' pneumoconiosis. *British Journal of Industrial Medicine*, **19**, 171–179.

Cunningham, C. D. B., Hugh, A. E. (1973) Pneumoconiosis in women. *Clinical Radiology*, **24**, 491–493.

Doig, A. T. (1976) Barytosis: a benign pneumoconiosis. *Thorax*, **31**, 30–39.

Epler, G. R., McLoud, T. C., Gaensler, E. A. (1982) Prevalence and incidence of benign asbestos pleural effusion in a working population. *Journal of the American Medical Association*, **247**, 617.

Greening, R. R., Helsep, J. H. (1967) The roentgenology of silicosis. *Seminars in Roentgenology*, **2**, 265–275.

Hardy, H. L. (1967) Current concepts of occupational lung disease of interest to the radiologist. *Seminars in Roentgenology*, **2**, 225–234.

Heitzman, E. R. (1973) *The Lung: Radiologic–Pathologic Correlations*. The pneumoconioses. C. V. Mosby, St. Louis, pp. 241–258.

ILO/UC International Classification of Pneumoconioses (1979) (ILO Occupational Safety and Health Series) International Labour Office, Geneva.

Katz, D., Kreel, L. (1979) Computed tomography in pulmonary asbestosis. *Clinical Radiology*, **30**, 207–213.

Parkes, W. R. (1982) *Occupational Lung Disorders*. 2nd edn. Butterworths, London.

Pendergrass, E. P. (1958) Silicosis and a few of the other pneumoconioses: observations on certain aspects of the problem with emphasis on the role of the radiologist. The Caldwell Lecture 1957. *American Journal of Roentgenology*, **80**, 1–41.

Rabinowitz, J. G., Efremidis, S. C., Cohen, B. et al. (1982) A comparative study of mesothelioma and asbestosis using computed tomography and conventional chest radiography. *Radiology*, **144**, 453–460.

Sander, O. A. (1976) The nonfibrogenic (benign) pneumoconioses. *Seminars in Roentgenology*, **2**, 312.

Sargent, E. N., Gordonson, J. S., Jacobson, G. (1977) Pleural plaques: a signpost of asbestos dust inhalation. *Seminars in Roentgenology*, **12**, 287–297.

Staples, C. A., Gamsu, G., Ray, C. S. et al. (1989) High resolution computed tomography and lung function in asbestos exposed workers with normal chest radiographs. *American Review of Respiratory Diseases*, **139**, 1502–1508.

CHAPTER 17

MISCELLANEOUS LUNG CONDITIONS

Ivan Hyde

SARCOIDOSIS

Sarcoidosis is a multisystem disease sometimes preceded acutely by erythema nodosum or arthropathy. Although worldwide in distribution there are *racial differences* in incidence, natural history and radiographic patterns. These differences are most obvious between the black and white races but there are also smaller variations within each group. The incidence in black people is 12 times that of white and the male/female ratio is 1:2 compared to 1:1 in white races. The influence of *genetic factors* is also apparent in the occasional clustering of familial cases, the fact that it is more prevalent in monozygotic than in dizygotic twins, and the fact that cases with the histocompatibility antigen HLA-B8 have less chance of developing progressive fibrosis. Genetic factors therefore can influence the natural history of the disease through the *immune response* which determines the outcome.

The immune response in the lungs is distinct from the systemic immune response. The latter includes a reduction in circulating lymphocytes and in T-cell proportions, an increase in gamma-globulin and anergy to tuberculin skin testing. In contrast, in the lungs there are increased proportions of lymphocytes and T-cells. The effects of the disease on function are those of impaired ventilation and alveolar gas diffusion.

There is no specific test for sarcoidosis, and the diagnosis is based on a combination of symptoms, signs, histological appearances and radiographic abnormalities. Histologically epithelioid granulomas are found which do not caseate whatever size they reach. The granulomas are found in the nodes, alveolar walls and bronchial submucosa. Healing is by fibrosis which is progressive as long as the disease is active. The end result therefore may vary from a normal chest radiograph up to a severe fibrotic lung disease. The histology is characteristic but not pathognomonic since it can be found in association with other lung diseases, particularly industrial berylliosis. Caution has to be exercised in the interpretation of biopsy material showing a sarcoid reaction, as it may not be representative of the whole. The *Kveim test* is an intradermal inoculation of an extract of sarcoid tissue, and if the re-

sulting skin reaction has sarcoid histology the test result is positive. Although useful, errors can result from the use of a weak antigen or misinterpretation of the histology of the granuloma.

A test which would predict those cases of active pulmonary sarcoid likely to respond to steroids would be valuable. Gallium-67 uptake by the lungs, blood levels of angiotensin-converting enzyme and measurements of the cellularity of bronchoalveolar lavage fluid have all been assessed as markers of activity but have not been universally accepted. Radiographic changes too do not correlate well with the inter-related triad of disease activity, functional abnormality and steroid responsiveness.

Radiological appearances. The radiographic abnormalities progress through three stages:

1. enlarged nodes only;
2. enlarged nodes with pulmonary lesions;
3. pulmonary lesions only.

The first stage is one of bilateral hilar node enlargement (Figs 17.1, 17.2), and so characteristic is this pattern that the diagnosis is often regarded as established without recourse to biopsy. An accompanying enlargement of right paratracheal nodes is not uncommon but the diagnosis must be regarded as suspect if the nodes are solely paratracheal, if the anterior mediastinal nodes are enlarged or if the hilar involvement is unilateral. The latter may be more apparent than real and tomography may reveal contralateral nodes not appreciated on the chest radiograph. The nodes rarely calcify and do so only when there is associated pulmonary disease. Sarcoidosis is one of the causes of *eggshell calcification* of nodes.

Even in Stage 1 a peripheral lung biopsy through the fibre-optic bronchoscope will show sarcoid granulomas, but these are fewer in number and have less fibrosis than in overt pulmonary disease. Resolution of the node enlargement is the rule and recurrence is rare. There is a small group of cases in which nodes persist for many years but even after such a long interval progression to pulmonary involvement can still occur. Progression to Stage 2 occurs in between one half and two-thirds of

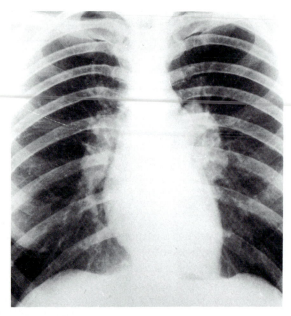

Fig. 17.1 Sarcoidosis. Bilateral hilar node enlargement.

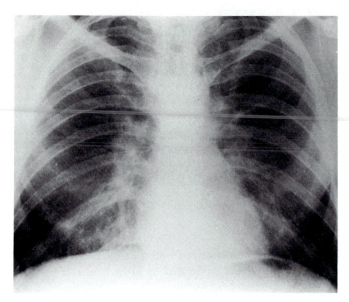

Fig. 17.3 Sarcoidosis. Right hilar adenopathy and micronodulation giving a fine granular appearance.

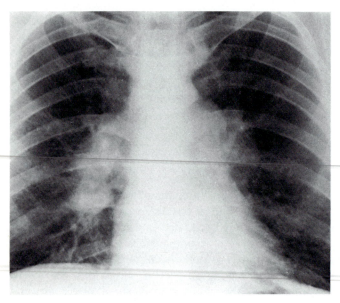

Fig. 17.2 Sarcoidosis. Hilar and tracheobronchial node enlargement. On the right the adenopathy extends to the segmental level of bronchial division.

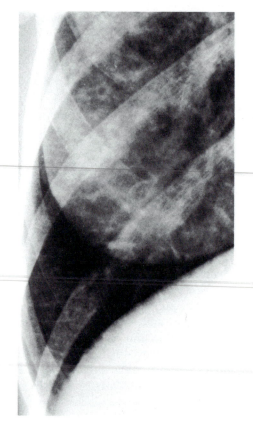

Fig. 17.4 Sarcoidosis. Basal septal lines. Reticulonodulation.

cases. If lung disease is present on the initial chest radiograph, 15–30% will develop progressive pulmonary fibrosis.

In Stages 2 and 3 the pulmonary ('parenchymal') disease takes several forms, all bilateral and widespread. Lobar localization is an exceptional presentation and this ultimately disseminates.

a. *Small nodules*: a profuse but not uniform scattering of enormous numbers of 2–3 mm lesions fittingly described as miliary. They appear most profuse in the thicker lower parts of the lungs (Fig. 17.3). The overall

effect may be a fine granularity, or the discrete opacities may fuse into a hazy loss of translucency in which the vessels become obscured.

b. *Reticulation*: a network of fine lines or linearities radiating from the hila. There may be a few Kerley B lines from lymphatic seedlings (Fig. 17.4). The latter are not due to the effects of nodal obstruction causing lymphatic congestion and they always imply pulmonary disease.

c. *Reticulonodular*: pure examples of nodular and reticular forms are less common than mixtures of the two (Fig. 17.5).

d. *Large nodules*: these are of the order of 1 cm in diameter and the edges may be well or poorly defined (Fig. 17.6). They may coalesce into larger opacities of segmental or lobar size, and lesions such as these are prone to rapid change, either of deterioration or improvement. Ill-defined large nodules and conglomerate opacities are often described as acinar, since air bronchograms may be visible within them, but this is an artificial division: they encroach on, rather than grow within, the alveolar spaces. Discrete nodules of 2–3 cm size are very rarely seen in Great Britain but are found in the United States, usually in black people. Cavitation within these lesions is sometimes seen.

The pulmonary disease may regress and the chest radiograph revert to normal but it is capable of reactivation in the same areas as the original disease. Infection superimposed on sarcoid disease will add its own contri-

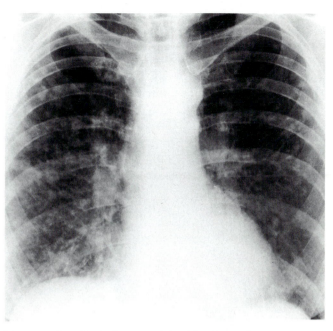

Fig. 17.6 Sarcoidosis. Larger nodules. No adenopathy.

bution to the overall radiographic appearances and it is one cause of cavitation.

e. *Fibrosis*: the fibrotic sequelae can vary between a few inconspicuous linear scars and widespread interstitial fibrosis which may resemble fibrosing alveolitis. Like fibrosing alveolitis it can also lead to honeycombing — clusters of thin-walled air cysts 1 cm in diameter. Condensation and contraction of the fibrous tissue result in distortion of the pulmonary architecture, elevation of the hila, the formation of bullae and bronchiectasis (Fig. 17.7). This end-stage fibrotic disease is often predominantly apical in distribution despite the diffuse nature of the original sarcoid lesions. Bullae have thinner walls than true cavities but it is not always possible to differentiate between them (Fig. 17.8).

Despite the fact that bronchial biopsy commonly reveals submucosal granulomas, bronchial stenosis is an unusual complication. When it occurs it is due to fibrotic strictures, and not to compression by node masses or to an intraluminal granulomatous mass. It follows that stenosis is not always relieved by the resolution of hilar adenopathy.

It will usually be detected first on bronchoscopy but it requires bronchography to reveal the true extent and multiplicity of the stenoses. Atelectasis and bronchiectasis may follow the bronchial obstruction. There is a notable absence of significant pleural involvement in sarcoid pulmonary disease but pneumothorax can result from rupture of a bulla.

Necrotizing sarcoid granulomatosis is a pathological curiosity dissimilar in almost all respects from classical sarcoidosis. Discussion centres around whether it is a nec-

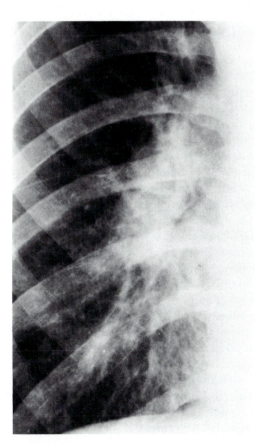

Fig. 17.5 Sarcoidosis. Hilar adenopathy and lines radiating from the hilum. Reticulonodulation.

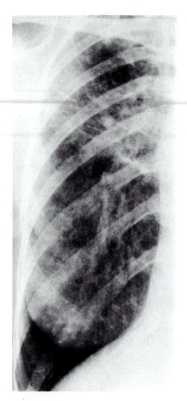

Fig. 17.7 Sarcoidosis (same case as Fig. 7.4). Coarse reticulation. Elevation of the hilum by fibrotic contraction.

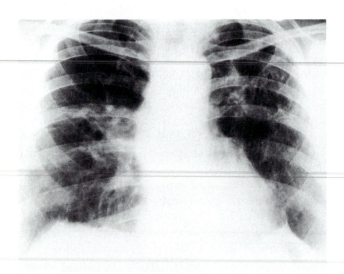

Fig. 17.8 Sarcoidosis. End-stage fibrotic disease. Apical bullae. Fibrotic contraction elevating left hilum.

rotizing angiitis with sarcoid reaction or sarcoidosis with necrosis of the granulomas and angiitis. It occupies a position between sarcoidosis and Wegener's granulomatosis. There is no other evidence of sarcoidosis, such as lymphadenopathy or extrapulmonary lesions. The granulomas coalesce, necrose and occlude the lumens of bronchi and vessels. Lung architecture is destroyed. Lung

distal to bronchial occlusion undergoes lipid consolidation. Although a miliary radiographic pattern has been reported, the lesions are more often *solitary masses* or *large nodules* with a localized or unilateral distribution.

FIBROSING ALVEOLITIS

A widespread fibrosis involving the alveolar walls is variously called diffuse pulmonary fibrosis, diffuse interstitial fibrosis, Hamman-Rich disease or fibrosing alveolitis. As there is also a concomitant or preceding chronic inflammatory cellular infiltration, the terms 'interstitial pneumonia' or 'pneumonitis' are also used.

There are a number of causes of alveolar injury which result in an exudation or cellular infiltration, which then shows a strong tendency to progressive fibrosis. Included amongst the known causes are the inhalation of certain *industrial dusts, drugs, infections, radiation injury* and *oxygen toxicity*. In the end stages, with severely fibrotic lungs and distorted bronchoalveolar architecture, it may not be possible to trace the signs of the initiating injurious agent. In Great Britain the preferred terminology for this group of conditions is 'fibrosing alveolitis' and if the cause is not known it is designated *cryptogenic*.

Cryptogenic fibrosing alveolitis

Although the cause is not known — and indeed there are likely to be many causes — the distinctive combination of symptoms, functional abnormalities, clinical signs, histology and radiographic appearances almost raise it to the status of a disease entity. The history is one of progressive exertional dyspnoea and cough with scanty sputum, finger clubbing, widespread crepitations, restricted ventilation and impaired gas exchange but little if any airways obstruction.

Histologically two patterns are recognized, one in which the cellular infiltration and fibrosis is limited to the alveolar walls, the other in which the alveolar spaces are also filled with mononuclear cells desquamated from the walls. They are labelled respectively *mural* (or usual interstitial pneumonitis — UIP) and *desquamative* (desquamative interstitial pneumonitis — DIP). Other distinguishing features are the variability of the histology, with more intense fibrosis in the mural type, whereas the desquamative has uniform histology, with less fibrosis, and is more responsive to steroid therapy, which gives it a better prognosis. An area of dispute is whether the two types represent the two ends of a scale or are of different pathogenesis.

Progressive fibrosis leads to contraction of lung substance and destruction of architecture. Dilatation of bronchioles accounts for honeycombing. Typically there is predominant involvement of the basal parts of the lungs with a tendency to spread upwards as the disease progresses. An overgrowth of smooth muscle in the alveolar walls and interstitial tissues may be striking, but is a nonspecific feature of a number of fibrotic and chronic inflammatory conditions.

The course of the disease varies from a devastating progression with death in a few weeks to an indolent process spanning many years. Death is usually due to respiratory or cardiac failure. Desquamative histology has a better prognosis, but it can hardly be called benign, with a reported mortality of 27% and a mean survival time of 12 years. Carcinoma of the lung of all histological types, including the bronchioloalveolar cell, complicates the disease process in about 10% of cases.

There is no doubt that immune mechanisms play a decisive role. In over 50% of cases rheumatoid-factor, nuclear, mitochondrial or smooth-muscle antibodies are found in the blood and immune complexes in the blood and lungs. Immune complexes formed from antigen/antibody combination are deposited in alveolar walls and capillaries, where they set in train a sequence of reactions which are locally damaging. They are found most often with a cellular histology, diminishing or disappearing in the predominantly fibrotic disease.

Diseases having an association with cryptogenic fibrosing alveolitis are generally those with an *autoimmune* pathogenesis: the connective tissue disorders rheumatoid arthritis, systemic lupus, systemic sclerosis, dermatomyositis/polymyositis being the most frequent. Other associates are Sjögren's disease, Hashimoto's thyroiditis, autoimmune haemolytic anaemia and idiopathic thrombocytopenic purpura. Cases with neurofibromatosis and an occasional familial incidence point to a possible genetic predisposition. The mural and desquamative forms do not differ in the variety of disease associates.

Radiological appearances. Characteristically the radiographic signs are basal in distribution. In the early stages the chest radiograph may be normal, but some apparently normal films when reviewed later will be seen to have a subtle shadowing, not surprisingly misinterpreted at the time as underexposure or breast shadows.

Computed tomography shows abnormalities at an earlier stage than chest radiography. The minimal change is a triangle of ground-glass haze at the bases, more easily appreciated on the right side where it fills the cardiophrenic angle. Although bilateral, it may be unequal on the two sides. The haze partially obscures pulmonary vessels and it is neither distinctly alveolar nor interstitial. With progression the changes spread upwards and out into the costophrenic angles.

Three other types of opacity may then be added to the basic pattern:

1. ill-defined and patchy;
2. small (2 mm) discrete miliary (Fig. 17.9);
3. profuse, small but of irregular outline.

The latter is a reticulation and the small shadows are superimposition of intersecting lines (Fig. 17.10).

It might be expected that a desquamative histology

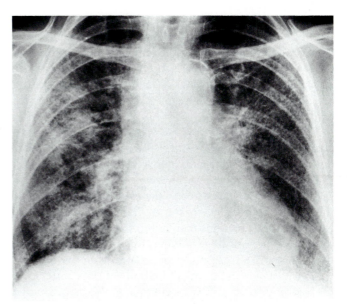

Fig. 17.9 Cryptogenic fibrosing alveolitis. Miliary opacities and a little reticulation. The apices are spared.

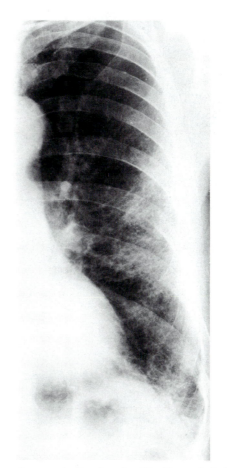

Fig. 17.10 Cryptogenic fibrosing alveolitis. Fine reticulation, predominantly peripheral and sparing the apices.

would have an alveolar pattern. It has been suggested that the ill-defined patchy opacities are the radiographic counterpart of desquamative histology, and miliary nodules that of the mural. However true this may be in isolated cases, it is generally agreed that radiographic appearances are not a reliable discriminator of histological type in the early stages.

The subtle and fine early radiographic opacities become coarser with progression of the fibrosis. Thicker lines and denser opacities appear as the lungs shrink. Since it is the gas-exchanging parts which are the site of the disease, the condensation and hence the dense opacities are in the surface 'cortex' of the lungs. This is more apparent in tomographic sections than in the chest radiograph. The densities represent large volumes of condensed lung. The diaphragms rise from underexpansion of the bases.

Honeycombing is a manifestation of late interstitial fibrosis (Fig. 17.11). It is exceptional in the desquamative type. Hilar and mediastinal node enlargement and pleural effusions are rare. Cor pulmonale, pulmonary embolism and infections are complications which contribute to the radiographic signs. Although bronchography is not required for primary diagnosis, the appearances are char-

acteristic should it be performed for other reasons. The bronchi fill right out to the pleural surface, another reflection of the condensation of alveolar spaces.

EXTRINSIC ALLERGIC ALVEOLITIS
(*hypersensitivity pneumonitis*)

Inhaled particles less than 10 μm in diameter are capable of reaching the alveoli, where their potential for causing damage to the gas-exchanging parts of the lungs is considerable. If the particles are antigenic and the lung previously sensitized, a hypersensitivity reaction ensues. Antibodies are meant to neutralize potentially harmful foreign material, but sometimes the combination of antigen and antibody is itself damaging and constitutes a disease process. Extrinsic allergic alveolitis is a syndrome caused by the inhalation of dusts containing certain organisms or proteins. In *farmer's lung* the offending organism is usually *Micropolyspora faeni* from damp mouldy hay. Pigeon breeders inhale dust from the desiccated droppings containing bird serum protein or from the feathers. *Mushroom growers* are affected by fungal spores from the compost used. *Air-conditioning systems* may circulate fungal spores and amoebae. A similar reaction in the lungs may be induced by *drugs*, in this case blood-borne, the most common examples being nitrofurantoin and salazopyrine.

Precipitating antibodies directed specifically against the antigen are found in the serum of patients but their presence only implies exposure, not necessarily disease. Some 40% of pigeon breeders have precipitins but few suffer from the disease. However the presence of precipitins to extracts of budgerigar excreta in those exposed is stronger evidence in favour of disease. The immunological reactions are predominantly Type III, that is, free-circulating antigen and antibody combine in the presence of complement to form complexes which are deposited in the alveolar walls. Activation of complement sets in train a sequence of reactions liberating a variety of damaging substances. The time-scale of the reaction is intermediate, which corresponds well with the clinical presentation. Type IV reactions also play a part, and here the antibody is produced and transported by lymphocytes which then aggregate at the site where the reaction takes place. The *granuloma*, a characteristic feature of Type IV reactions, is the fundamental histological lesion of extrinsic allergic alveolitis.

Acute symptoms characteristically begin some 6 hours after exposure. The patient experiences an influenza-like illness of malaise, headache, fever, cough and dyspnoea. If the dose of antigen is small and frequently repeated, acute symptoms may be absent, and the presentation is then one of an insidiously progressive dyspnoea. This is a common mode of presentation of disease from budgerigars. Monday-morning fever occurs in office workers in

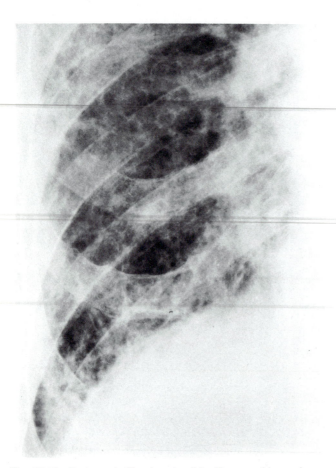

Fig. 17.11 Cryptogenic fibrosing alveolitis. Honeycombing and conglomerate fibrosis.

an air-conditioned environment and is traceable to contamination of humidifiers.

On auscultation there are usually inspiratory crepitations but finger clubbing is rare. Lung function tests show restricted ventilation and impaired gas transfer but little airways obstruction. The best test is a bronchial challenge by the inhalation of the allergen to reproduce the symptoms and functional abnormalities. It is now rarely used, but it was instrumental initially in establishing the pathogenesis of the disease.

Treatment is by removal from exposure or, if that is not possible, reduction of contact to a minimum. Steroids are of doubtful value. In only 50–60% of patients does the lung function return to normal and some continue to deteriorate after elimination of exposure.

The pathological lesions are *alveolar wall granulomas*, aggregates of normal constituent cells of granulation tissue — histiocytes, lymphocytes, fibroblasts, giant cells. They are widely but patchily distributed throughout the lungs, some areas being normal. After repeated attacks the acute changes give place to alveolar wall and peribronchial *fibrosis*, the granulomas then disappearing. Intra-alveolar exudate is not striking in biopsy specimens but radiographic signs of transient alveolar opacification occur in acute attacks. Bronchiolitis obliterans is common and found in 40% of specimens from farmer's lung. The pathology is similar whatever the aetiology, but occasionally it is possible to identify a specific characteristic such as the fungus which causes maple bark stripper's disease, or vegetable fibres in bagassosis (in cane-sugar workers). In the late stages there are extensive areas of dense fibrosis, representing large volumes of contracted lung in which alveolar architecture can no longer be recognized. *Honeycombing*, or larger air spaces arising from dilatation of small airways or from destruction of alveolar walls, then appears. These chronic changes are almost always in the upper parts of the lungs and are predominantly subpleural.

Radiological appearances. The chest radiograph may be initially normal, but as in cryptogenic fibrosing alveolitis, early changes may escape detection unless a high index of suspicion is cultivated. The minimal change consists of a widespread small nodulation, the individual nodules being 2 mm in diameter and having ill-defined edges, in contrast to the sharp definition of lesions of similar size in miliary tuberculosis (Fig. 17.12). Although widespread, they may be more profuse in certain areas, and typically the costophrenic angles are clear. All other radiographic changes are superimposed on this basic pattern. Patchy, ill-defined transient shadows described as 'clouding', 'mottling' or 'haze' are found in the early stages and probably represent alveolar filling during acute exacerbations. Septal lines are not uncommon (Fig. 17.13). The chronic stage is marked by the appearance of large dense opacities due to contraction and conden-

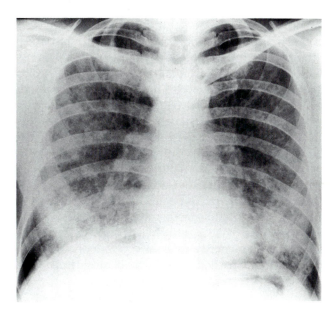

Fig. 17.12   Farmer's lung. Patchy alveolar opacification superimposed on a miliary nodulation. The costophrenic angles are clear.

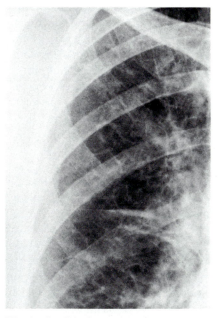

Fig. 17.13   Allergic alveolitis due to monoamine oxidase inhibitor drug. The interstitial shadowing was generalized throughout both lungs. Complete resolution within 7 days.

sation, almost always in the upper parts of the lungs. Cystic air spaces are due to bullae, bronchiectatic cavities and bronchiolar dilatations. A band of density which may be seen along the lateral chest wall, and graphically described as a 'white wall', is a condensation of subpleural alveolar spaces. Notably absent are pleural effusion, node enlargement and calcification. The sequence of radiographic changes from a diffuse abnormality to a progressive upper lobe fibrosis is highly characteristic.

Upper lobe fibrosis is a common end-stage of a number of disparate diseases, including extrinsic allergic alveolitis, cryptogenic fibrosing alveolitis, tuberculosis, bronchopulmonary aspergillosis, ankylosing spondylitis and many others. At this stage the natural history is the only means of differentiating between them.

PULMONARY EOSINOPHILIC CONDITIONS

Pulmonary eosinophilia is defined as the presence of transient radiographic opacities which contain eosinophils together with a blood eosinophilia. However, it is useful to consider pulmonary eosinophilia with a broader group of allied conditions, some of which fall outside the simple definition.

In this broader group the brunt of the changes may fall on the peripheral pulmonary tissues or on the bronchial tree. The pulmonary element is an eosinophilic exudate and an alveolar-wall granulomatous infiltration, either focal or diffuse. There is a tendency for recurrent acute attacks to lead to fibrosis.

The bronchial element consists of mucosal oedema and infiltration by eosinophils, and the functional effects are more impressive than the radiological. There is smooth-muscle spasm, reversible airways obstruction and the secretion of tenacious mucus. The sputum is eosinophilic and contains plugs or casts of the bronchi. There are secondary effects from infection and obstructive collapse, namely bronchiectasis and peribronchial fibrosis.

ASTHMA

Asthma is a state of bronchial hyper-reactivity. Stimuli ineffective in normal people produce bronchial constriction in asthmatics.

Extrinsic asthma is believed to follow inhalation of particles commonly found in the environment such as pollens, house dust and animal danders, to which the patient is allergic. The immunological response is Type I, characterized by an immediate weal on skin testing with allergens, histamine release from mast cells and attraction of eosinophils to sites of antigen/antibody reaction. The onset is in childhood and there are usually other allergic hypersensitivities such as hay fever and eczema. Patients have positive skin tests to a number of common allergens. These are all features of atopy.

Intrinsic asthma has a later onset and these patients are not atopic, the usual skin tests being negative. The onset sometimes follows a respiratory infection.

The state of heightened bronchial reactivity is also reflected in the fact that asthma may sometimes be provoked or made worse by exercise or respiratory infections. Eosinophilia in the blood is intermittent.

Radiological appearances. The chest radiograph in uncomplicated asthma is unremarkable and usually normal. During attacks the lungs are overexpanded and in severe chronic asthma this may persist. Signs of over-expansion are low diaphragms and a lung height greater than combined lung width, a reversal of normal. Bronchial wall and peribronchial thickening show as parallel lines, and once this feature makes its appearance it is often permanent.

Lobar or segmental collapse results from a combination of bronchial mucosal swelling and mucous plugging, and rapid re-expansion is the rule. Patchy, ill-defined opacities, sometimes widespread, appear transiently, but in the absence of histological verification it is not known how often these are due to eosinophilic consolidation or how often to collapse. Septal lines are sometimes seen. Rupture of alveoli results in pulmonary interstitial emphysema, mediastinal emphysema and pneumothorax.

The inter-relationship of asthma, pulmonary eosinophilia and aspergillosis is dealt with elsewhere (Ch. 15). Pulmonary eosinophilia can occur in *drug hypersensitivity* (aspirin, nitrofurantoin), after exposure to *industrial chemicals* (epoxy resins), during *parasitic infections* (Ch. 15) or the cause may be unknown.

CHRONIC EOSINOPHIL PNEUMONIA

Also known as *prolonged pulmonary eosinophilia*, the diagnosis of this unusual condition rarely presents a problem because of the highly characteristic constellation of symptoms and radiographic signs together with the blood eosinophilia, which may however be intermittent. Symptoms are often severe with fever, drenching sweats, loss of weight, dyspnoea and cough. Only one-third of patients have a history of asthma or other atopic conditions. It has been reported in identical twins. There is ventilatory restriction and impaired gas exchange with little, if any, airways obstruction.

Pathologically there is an alveolar exudate of eosinophils and macrophages but only mild alveolar wall infiltration. Ulcerative bronchiolitis obliterans is found in one-third of cases. A number of patients with this disease will have eosinophil infiltrations in other organs, with potentially serious consequences in those with myocardial involvement.

Radiological appearances. The radiographic signs have been described as pulmonary oedema in reverse, that is, ill-defined, non-segmental alveolar opacities in the peripheral parts of the lungs. This is the most distinctive pattern, but central opacities are also found. They are unevenly distributed and the densities are not homogeneous. Their subpleural position may mimic a loculated effusion, but true effusions are rare. Another distinctive and almost diagnostic sign is a vertical band of shadowing roughly parallel to the chest wall but separated from it

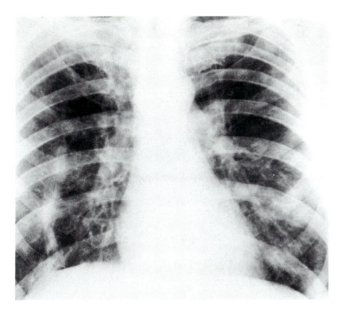

Fig. 17.14 Chronic eosinophil pneumonia. Alveolar opacities distributed peripherally. The vertical band in the right lung is characteristic.

and apparently bearing no relationship to pleura, fissures or hilum (Fig. 17.14). It is a band of subpleural alveolar opacification, for which there are two possible explanations: 1. the band is *en face* and not tangential to the X-ray beam; 2. a wide border of opaque lung clears from the periphery, leaving a translucent strip between the pleura and lung still affected. It is seen most often in the stages of resolution and may recur in exacerbations of the disease.

Treatment with steroids is rapidly effective, and total radiographic clearing may take no more than two or three days. Fibrotic scars are few and inconspicuous. Pulmonary function returns to normal with radiographic clearing. Relapse of symptoms and radiographic signs frequently follows reduction or withdrawal of steroids and the opacities may return in precisely the same sites, with or without the addition of fresh lesions elsewhere. They respond to the reinstitution of steroids in full doses. Recurrent disease has been reported over a period of 26 years.

EOSINOPHIL GRANULOMA

Eosinophil granuloma is a disease of unknown aetiology, conventionally grouped with Hand-Schüller-Christian and Letterer-Siwe's diseases as Histiocytosis-X disease. The pathology of eosinophil granuloma and Hand-Schüller-Christian disease is the same, the difference lying in the multi-organ distribution of the latter, especially in the cranium. Eosinophil granuloma of the lungs may or may not be associated with bone or soft-tissue lesions. Isolated lung disease is found in five times as many men as women, and generally pursues a benign course which

remits either spontaneously or as a result of treatment. There is no association with atopy or allergy and there is no blood eosinophilia.

There is a diffuse infiltration of alveolar walls with histiocytic granulomas, unusual in the numbers of eosinophils which they contain. The presence of Langerhans cells with granules is regarded as specific. The lesions are eventually replaced by fibrous tissue. Polypoid granulomatous lesions are also found in the bronchi.

Radiological appearances. The chest radiograph shows a fine, diffuse reticulation and sharply defined nodules, usually 2–3 mm in size but occasionally as large as 5–7 mm. The nodules may be predominantly basal or apical, but typically the costophrenic recesses are spared. As the lesions mature the nodules recede and the reticulation becomes more pronounced (Fig. 17.15). An alveolar haze resembling pulmonary oedema may be seen as a transient exudative phenomenon. Honeycombing and bulla formation result from the fibrosis, and the hair-line walls of these air spaces are particularly clearly seen because there are no dense fibrotic masses and the lungs are consequently well expanded. Bullous cysts may become very large. Pneumothorax occurs at some

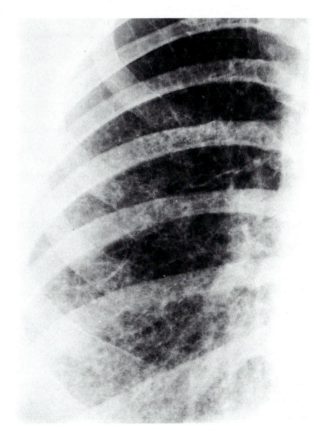

Fig. 17.15 Eosinophil granuloma. Reticulonodulation. The nodulation is receding. Honeycombing and commencement of bulla formation.

time in 25% of cases. Node enlargement and pleural effusions are rare.

PULMONARY HAEMORRHAGE AND HAEMOSIDEROSIS

Under this heading will be considered those states where there is multifocal bleeding at acinar level, that is, distal to the terminal bronchioles, but excluding those with a known bleeding state such as leukaemia, anticoagulation or diffuse intravascular coagulation. Haemoptysis is a common symptom but its severity does not match the large volumes of blood lost into the lungs, since most of it is beyond the mucociliary clearing processes. Bleeding is severe enough to cause anaemia, even at times requiring blood transfusion. Macrophages with engulfed red cells and haemosiderin fill the alveolar spaces and infiltrate the walls. These macrophages in sputum or bronchoalveolar lavage fluid are a diagnostic feature. After repeated attacks of bleeding, interstitial fibrosis is initiated but this is not sufficiently extensive to cause gross scarring or destruction of lung architecture.

Pulmonary haemosiderosis may conveniently be classified into 5 types:

1. Idiopathic;
2. Associated with renal disease;
3. Due to drugs (penicillamine) or industrial chemicals (hydrocarbon fumes);
4. Part of a widespread vasculitis (Wegener's granulomatosis);
5. Miscellaneous.

Idiopathic pulmonary haemosiderosis is predominantly a disease of childhood, in which there are repeated episodes of haemorrhage, sometimes accompanied by constitutional upset. The lungs return to normal between attacks but if these are frequently repeated permanent fibrotic changes eventually follow. The disease may remit spontaneously. The kidneys are not involved.

Pulmonary haemosiderosis with renal disease. Three subgroups can be identified on the basis of the renal histology:

  a. anti-glomerular basement membrane (GBM) antibody disease;
  b. immune complex renal disease;
  c. glomerulonephritis without either of the above.

The name *Goodpasture syndrome* should be reserved for those cases with GBM antibody. Immunofluorescence microscopy shows a linear deposit of the immunoglobulin on the glomerular capillaries, sometimes with similar deposits on the alveolar capillaries. In contrast, *immune complex renal disease* has lumpy or granular glomerular deposits. Damage to basement membranes by these deposits allows leakage to take place.

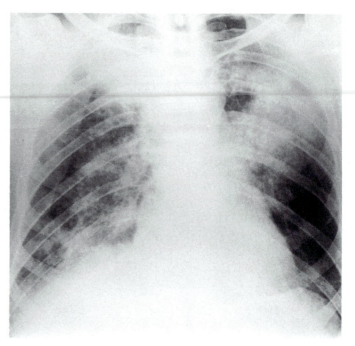

Fig. 17.16 Pulmonary haemorrhage. Goodpasture syndrome. Large alveolar opacities.

Infection, fluid overload, smoking and inhalation of toxic fumes are factors which are known to precipitate episodes of bleeding. Pulmonary function tests often indicate airways obstruction and there may be an increased uptake of *inhaled radioactive CO* by the leaked blood. The latter test is useful in differentiating haemorrhage from oedema and infection. Treatment regimes include steroids, immunosuppression and plasmaphoresis, and these are more effective in Goodpasture syndrome than in the other types.

Miscellaneous conditions. Included in this group of pulmonary haemosiderosis are cases of heart disease which chronically elevate left atrial pressure, notably mitral stenosis. The radiographic features in the lungs are distinctive, consisting of a permanent miliary stippling due to the focal nature of the bleeding.

With the exception of cardiogenic haemosiderosis noted above, the radiographic appearances of the other types are indistinguishable. Typically there are fleeting, migratory opacities with ill-defined margins, individually like pulmonary oedema (Fig. 17.16). At the edges of large confluent opacities, ill-defined nodules of acinar size (6 mm) may be seen. An air bronchogram is occasionally visible within the opacities. These are characteristics of an alveolar filling process or consolidation. In severe cases both lungs can be almost totally opacified, but conversely, the chest radiograph may be normal in an acute attack — the decisive factor is the volume of blood lost. As the opacities resolve, reticulation may become evident transiently, but a permanent reticular pattern is indicative of the evolution of interstitial fibrosis. Fibrosis only occurs after repeated episodes; usually resolution is rapid and complete. Differentiation from pulmonary infection can be difficult, especially as infection is one of the precipitating factors of haemorrhage, but clues to its presence are opacities which reach the apices or costophrenic angles, opacities limited by interlobar fissures, and loss of mediastinal silhouettes. The presence of septal lines indicates fluid overload.

GRANULOMATOSIS WITH ANGIITIS AND LYMPHOPROLIFERATIVE DISORDERS

Wegener's granulomatosis, lymphomatoid granulomatosis and bronchocentric granulomatosis are conditions in which pulmonary angiitis is a central pathological component. These overlap with certain lymphoproliferative disorders which in turn merge with the lymphomas. Indeed, it has been suggested that some of the diseases in this group, particularly lymphomatoid granulomatosis, lymphoid interstitial pneumonia and pseudolymphoma, are in reality unusual forms of lymphoma.

WEGENER'S GRANULOMATOSIS

The essential component of Wegener's granulomatosis is a necrotizing vasculitis, the lungs being involved as part of a widespread disease. A focal glomerulonephritis is part of the classical disease and is the most important determinant of prognosis. By *limited Wegener's granulomatosis* is meant a disease predominantly but not exclusively intrathoracic, and in this form renal lesions, when present, are focal and granulomatous, not glomerulonephritic.

Symptoms referable to the upper air passages are almost always present at some time in the course of the disease: nasal obstruction, purulent discharge, sinusitis, chronic ulceration — even in some cases, necrosis of nasal cartilage and bone. Cough, haemoptysis and pleurisy are usually accompanied by constitutional symptoms of malaise, weakness and fever. Rheumatoid and antinuclear factors are commonly found in the blood. Untreated, the disease has a poor prognosis with an average survival of five months, but steroids and cyclophosphamide have transformed the outlook.

Lesions occur in any part of the respiratory tract and take the form of inflammatory necrosis in the walls of small arteries and veins leading to occlusion of the lumen. Granulation tissue containing lymphocytes, polymorphs and giant cells represents a reparative process, but this also undergoes necrosis. The necrotic granulation tissue forms rubbery pulmonary masses which have a propensity to cavitate. Sometimes there is a profusion of miliary lesions. Ulceration of bronchial mucosa can result in airway narrowing and lobar collapse.

Patients with Wegener's granulomatosis form auto-antibodies against cytoplasmic components of their neutrophil polymorphs. This is the basis of the *anti-cytoplasmic antibody (ACPA) test* which is highly sensitive in the active disease but the titres fall as activity diminishes. It is not specific for Wegener's granulomatosis, positive tests being found in other cases of necrotizing or crescentic glomerulonephritis.

Radiological appearances. Single or multiple, well-defined, round or oval pulmonary masses 1–5 cm in diameter are typical radiographic presentations (Fig. 17.17). A lobar consolidation results if the lesions extend up to the pleural fissures. Cavitating lesions may have thick or thin walls, depending on how much of the necrotic material is expectorated. Multiple cavities can closely mimic tuberculosis.

A variation is a diffuse disease where the area of involved lung is still aerated but contains vaguely reticular or irregular nodular opacities.

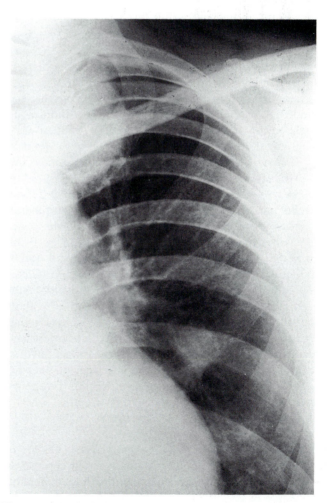

Fig. 17.17 Limited Wegener's granulomatosis. Circumscribed mass at left apex; small lesion in lingula. The large mass contained pus-like material.

Reactive hilar or mediastinal node enlargement can be mistaken for carcinoma, especially if associated with a wedge of pulmonary consolidation or a lobe collapsed from endobronchial disease.

The lesions are not static: new ones appear at the same time as others are resolving and leaving linear scars. Relapse may occur in previously affected areas. Other frequent radiographic signs are small pleural effusions and paranasal sinus opacification. Occasional complications are pneumothorax and subglottic stenosis. Calcification is notably absent from the lesions.

Non-healing granuloma, although of similar pathology, is a separate condition characterized by gross destruction of the facial structures and responding poorly to treatment which would normally be effective in Wegener's granulomatosis. The lungs and kidneys are not involved.

LYMPHOMATOID GRANULOMATOSIS

This is a lymphoproliferative disorder with angiitis, pathologically intermediate between Wegener's granulomatosis and lymphoma. Men are affected twice as frequently as women. The pulmonary disease has no distinctive clinical features but the combination with neurological symptoms and maculopapular skin lesions is suggestive of the diagnosis. Involvement of the central nervous system or peripheral nerves is found in up to one third of cases.

There are destructive lesions centred on vessels surrounded by lymphoid infiltrations and granulation tissue. Neighbouring bronchioles suffer damage to their walls and obliteration of the lumen. Almost half of the patients have lesions with the same histology in the kidneys and other organs.

Bilateral pulmonary consolidations with ill-defined margins are the early signs. They have a predominantly peripheral distribution, sparing the apices. As the opacities evolve they become more discrete and resemble metastases. They can change rapidly, waxing and waning simultaneously in different areas. There is cavitation in 30%. In a few cases the pattern is diffuse reticulonodular or interstitial. Only a minority resolve, with or without residual scarring, and in general the disease has a high mortality from pulmonary insufficiency, haemorrhage, secondary infection or central nervous system involvement. Hilar and mediastinal node enlargement does not occur except in the event of overt evolution to lymphoma, which happens in approximately 10% of cases.

BRONCHOCENTRIC GRANULOMATOSIS

This is a necrotizing granulomatous reaction centred on bronchi and bronchioles. Patchily distributed shallow ulcerations of the mucosa are followed by penetration of the wall, leading to destruction of cartilage in the larger bronchi. Bronchial walls are thickened and the lumen filled with masses of cheesy necrotic material. The process spreads outwards into lung tissue where the histology becomes that of an obstructive lipid pneumonia and an interstitial fibrosis. Pulmonary arteries and veins are involved incidentally by incorporation in the spreading inflammation, their lumens undergoing obliteration. There is no extrapulmonary involvement.

The disease has an equal sex incidence and the symptoms are those of chronic or recurrent pneumonia with airways obstruction. It is thought to be due to hypersensitivity to the aspergillus. Some sufferers are asthmatics, and the impacting bronchial material is then eosinophilic, otherwise it is polymorphonuclear. Steroid therapy is usually effective.

Radiological appearances. Typical radiographic presentations are a mass, a lobar consolidation or atelectasis. The opacities are frequently bilateral and migratory, with the lung apex a favourite site. Less frequent presentations are small nodules or diffuse reticulonodulation. Reactive hilar node enlargement has been reported but is unusual.

LYMPHOID INTERSTITIAL PNEUMONIA
(*pneumonitis*)

Areas of lung are diffusely infiltrated with mature lymphocytes within alveolar walls and in the interstitium. There is no node involvement. In places the infiltrate may form larger, round aggregates. It is a disease of slow evolution, with a variable outcome: resolution, interstitial fibrosis or malignant lymphoma; and it carries a 50% mortality. Frequently there is a disorder of immune globulins, indicated by its association with Sjögren's syndrome, Hashimoto's thyroiditis or amyloidosis and by the presence of rheumatoid and antinuclear factors. It has also been found in late-onset graft-versus-host disease following allogenic bone marrow transplantation.

Radiological appearances. Radiographic reticulation is the counterpart of the interstitial histology, usually bilateral and basal, proceeding to honeycombing in cases which fibrose. Added to this are coarse confluent shadows with air bronchograms suggestive of alveolar filling. This is an example of an interstitial process which, when sufficiently extensive, obliterates lung architecture and takes on the characteristics of an alveolar consolidation. There is no node or pleural involvement.

IMMUNOBLASTIC LYMPHADENOPATHY

As a cause of generalized lymphadenopathy this lies between a hyperimmune state and neoplasia. Within the enlarged nodes there is a proliferation of several types of cell but predominantly of lymphocytes, and including immunoblasts containing immunoglobulins. There is also a proliferation of small blood vessels, which accounts for its alternative name, angioimmunoblastic lymphadenopathy.

Other features of the disorder are hepatosplenomegaly, haemolytic anaemia, polyclonal hypergammaglobulinaemia, maculopapular skin rashes and cutaneous anergy.

Radiological appearances. In the thorax the hilar and paratracheal nodes are enlarged, sometimes recurrently during the course of the disease. Pulmonary involvement is usually the result of infection and takes the form of coarse basal reticulation, sometimes with an alveolar or nodular component. However, cases have been reported in which the pulmonary lesions had the same histology as the nodes. Spontaneous remission takes place in one-third, but the disease is fatal in the other two-thirds, from infection or renal and hepatic failure. A minority evolve into a malignant lymphoma.

SJÖGREN'S SYNDROME

Sjögren's syndrome is defined as dry mouth and dry eyes due to reduced exocrine gland secretions *plus* one of a number of connective tissue disorders. If the latter is missing it is called the *sicca syndrome* or *primary Sjögren's syndrome*. Women are more often affected than men. The salivary, lachrymal and mucous glands of the mouth, nose, eyelids, pharynx, bronchial tree and stomach may all be the site of the pathological changes which consists of a massive lymphoid infiltration with eventual atrophy of the gland acini. There are minor salivary glands in the lip and this is the easiest site for diagnostic biopsy. Although sarcoidosis may involve the salivary glands, with the same functional effects, it is by convention excluded from the definition of Sjögren's and sicca syndromes.

The frequency of pulmonary abnormalities has varied between 10 and 30% in different series. There are several pathogenic pathways.

1. *Infection*: reduced secretion with an increased viscosity lowers the resistance of the air passages to infection. Recurrent pulmonary infections are common events and can lead to bronchiectasis.

2. *Direct pulmonary infiltration*: infiltrations of lymphocytes and plasma cells surround and obstruct small airways.

3. *As a manifestation of associated diseases*: by definition Sjögren's syndrome is associated with a connective tissue disorder, which is usually rheumatoid arthritis or, less often, systemic lupus, systemic sclerosis, polyarteritis nodosa and polymyositis. Fibrosing alveolitis, lymphoid interstitial pneumonia, pseudolymphoma and malignant lymphoma also have associations with Sjögren's and sicca syndromes.

4. There is evidence pointing to a pathogenic role for *immune complex deposition* in alveolar capillaries.

The sicca and pulmonary components have a predictable symptomatology but there may also be complaint of

dysphagia or Raynaud's phenomenon; a few patients have renal tubular acidosis or primary biliary cirrhosis; there is a tendency to develop allergies to drugs. Hypergammaglobulinaemia is present in 50% of cases and there is a high incidence of organ-specific and non-organ-specific antibodies.

Sialographic abnormalities, although nonspecific, offer some diagnostic support, since they are found in 50% of cases, which is a much higher incidence than is found in the associated diseases uncomplicated by Sjögren's or sicca syndromes.

Radiological appearances. It is not surprising that such a heterogeneous condition has no characteristic radiographic pattern (Fig. 17.18). Infection and bronchial obstruction account for basal atelectasis, pulmonary consolidations, pleural effusion and bronchiectasis. The lymphocytic infiltrations and associated disease pathologies take a variety of forms — fine diffuse interstitial, coarse reticulonodular, diffuse alveolar; in cases with lymphocytic lymphoma, multiple discrete nodules and hilar node enlargement may be found.

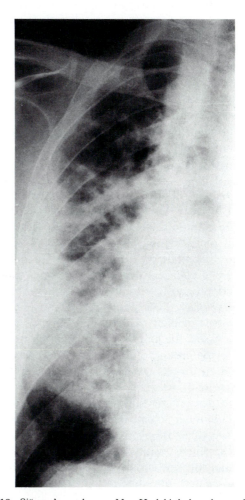

Fig. 17.18 Sjögren's syndrome. Non-Hodgkin's lymphoma. Dense conglomerate opacities mainly subpleural; coarse reticulation.

PSEUDOLYMPHOMA

Ambiguity surrounds the nature of this lymphoproliferative disorder; should it be placed with the post-inflammatory processes or the benign neoplasms? or indeed has it any separate existance apart from the lymphomas? On the face of it the issue seems simple enough. Considering only intrathoracic lesions, pseudolymphoma is a sharply demarcated massive infiltration of the lung by well-differentiated lymphocytes and other inflammatory cells. Growth can be extremely slow, nodes are not involved and there is no extrathoracic spread. Bronchial walls may be invaded but the epithelium is not breached. At the periphery of the mass the infiltration is interstitial, and such areas are indistinguishable from lymphoid interstitial pneumonia. A number progress to malignant lymphoma, which poses the question whether the condition is a pre-malignant phase or is malignant from the beginning. Lymphocytic lymphoma is monoclonal, whereas pseudolymphoma should be polyclonal, a separation which can be made on the basis of whether the cells stain for one or more light chains. Many pseudolymphomas have had to be reclassified on the basis of this test. The drug *phenytoin* has been responsible for some cases of pseudolymphoma, and in these the lymph nodes may be enlarged.

Radiological appearances. On the chest radiograph the lesions either appear as round isolated opacities or as consolidations of segmental or lobar size abutting on pleural surfaces. Both types are likely to show air bronchograms. The round lesions are usually 1–4 cm in diameter, single or multiple, with borders which shade off into surrounding lung.

CONNECTIVE TISSUE (COLLAGEN) DISEASES

The feature common to this group of diseases is inflammation of joints, serosa, blood vessels and connective tissue. The inflammation is followed by fibrosis and the laying-down of collagen. Any tissue or organ may be involved, and prognosis depends on the severity in vital organs, particularly kidney, central nervous system and lung. By virtue of their rich supply of blood vessels and connective tissue, the lungs are a frequent target. Criteria for entry to the group are not strict but, conventionally, rheumatoid arthritis, systemic lupus erythematosus (SLE), systemic sclerosis (SS), polyarteritis nodosa (PAN) and dermatomyositis/polymyositis (PMS) are regarded as founder members, with Henoch-Schönlein purpura, Goodpasture syndrome, Behçet's disease and others occupying a position on the periphery.

By rearranging the clinical signs various subdivisions have been created, the justification being an attempt to predict subsequent behaviour. *CREST syndrome* is a sub-set of SS characterized by cutaneous calcinosis, Raynaud's phenomenon, oesophageal abnormalities, sclerodactyly and telangiectasis. *Mixed connective tissue disease* consists of combined features of SLE, SS and PMS. The term 'overlap syndrome' was usually applied to cases occupying the middle ground between classic PAN and allergic angiitis, but it has been extended to include almost any combination so that it now lacks a precise definition.

POLYARTERITIS NODOSA

The classic form of polyarteritis nodosa affects medium-sized muscular arteries in any part of the body. There is inflammation in and around the vessel, followed by necrosis of the wall, which is thereby weakened and gives way, forming small aneurysms, the 'nodosa' of the title. Vessels are also occluded by the process. It is predominantly a male disease, in the ratio 3:1. Immunological mechanisms are involved and there is immune complex deposition in vessel walls, the antigen unidentified except in those cases due to drug hypersensitivity or to the hepatitis B antigen. The protean symptomatology reflects the widespread distribution of the lesions, affecting gut, skin, kidney, heart, central nervous system, joints and muscle. Visceral angiography shows aneurysms or other arterial abnormalities in over 60% of cases and is frequently of more diagnostic value than blind tissue biopsy.

Radiological appearances. Abnormalities in the lungs are unusual but nodules, segmental opacities, atelectases, small pleural effusions and diffuse interstitial fibrosis may be found. Opacities are usually transient, except for those caused by diffuse fibrosis.

The rare disease of **relapsing polychondritis** has similarities to polyarteritis nodosa and the two conditions are sometimes found together. There is inflammation, necrosis and fibrosis of cartilage and other tissues with a high glycosaminoglycan content, which includes the aorta. The destruction of the cartilage of the bronchial tree produces collapsible airways and ultimately fibrotic strictures. The lungs are exposed to the risk of infection because of defective clearance.

Allergic granulomatosis and angiitis (*Churg-Strauss disease*) is at one end of a scale with classical polyarteritis at the other, the middle ground being occupied by the *overlap syndrome* with features common to both. Like classical PAN, allergic granulomatosis and angiitis is a generalized necrotizing vasculitis but with certain differences. The lungs are always involved; it occurs in patients with an allergic diathesis, usually asthma; there is a blood eosinophilia; the pathology is granulomatous; and eosinophils figure more prominently in the infiltrations. The differences are therefore mostly one of degree rather than of kind. It is to be suspected in asthmatics with a multisystem disorder and affects the same organs as classical

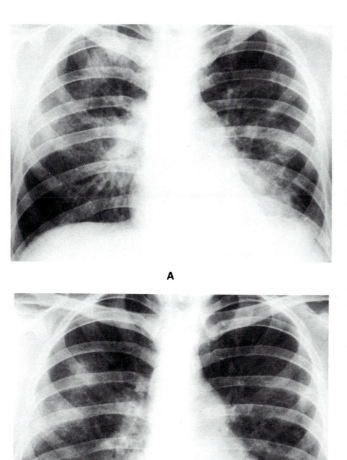

Fig. 17.19 A. Henoch-Schönlein purpura. Non-segmental, migratory, alveolar opacities in all lobes. **B**. 3 weeks later. Some lesions resolving; fresh ones have appeared at right base and right mid-zone.

PAN. The pericardium and myocardium are often affected.

Lung opacities are alveolar consolidations, sometimes massive, or a diffuse coarse reticulation, and typically they wax and wane. Infarcts following pulmonary arteritis account for some of the opacities. Sometimes the presentation is acute, suggesting a precipitating insult, and this *hypersensitivity vasculitis* can be induced by drugs, serum sickness or infection. Henoch-Schönlein purpura is a vasculitis of this type. These transient lung opacities are nodular, diffuse or patchy (Fig. 17.19 A, B).

SYSTEMIC LUPUS ERYTHEMATOSUS
Notable features of SLE are its female preponderance (F:M ratio 9:1), a butterfly facial rash, arthralgias, Raynaud's phenomenon, renal glomerulitis and nervous system involvement. The LE cell test has now been replaced by tests for *anti-nuclear antibody*, positive in 90% of cases but not an absolute requirement for diagnosis. Few patients have pulmonary symptoms or gross radiographic signs even though a majority have abnormal function tests of restrictive type. The presenting symptom may be dyspnoea without apparent cause. So-called 'shrinking lung' is the most typical feature, where the diaphragms are raised and move sluggishly. The loss of lung volume is not explained by pleural disease or pulmonary fibrosis and this can be confirmed by CT. It is probably an effect of chest wall and diaphragm weakness. Pathologically, the alveoli have a predominantly mononuclear infiltration and hyaline membranes. Interstitial fibrosis is not a major feature and evidence of it on the chest radiograph is rarely found. Patchy pulmonary opacities are caused by pulmonary oedema, infarction or secondary infection. Infective and infarctive lesions may cavitate. There is an entity of lupus pneumonitis which responds to steroids. Vascular thrombosis in the lungs and elsewhere is related to the presence of lupus anticoagulant, an antibody to certain clotting factors in the blood, which paradoxically increases coagulability in vivo. It is not specific to SLE and is found in other connective tissue diseases.

SYSTEMIC SCLEROSIS
The pathological abnormalities in the lungs in systemic sclerosis consist of proliferative endothelial obliteration of small arteries and an interstitial and peribronchial fibrosis. The consequences are inequalities of ventilation and perfusion, air-trapping, emphysema and pulmonary hypertension. Similar pathological changes in the diaphragm and intercostal muscles add to the respiratory dysfunction. In fact only a minority have lung disease. Radiographic changes therefore are usually inconspicuous and they are absent in the sub-set with CREST symptomatology (calcinosis, Raynaud's, oesophagus, sclerodactyly, telangiectasia). In the 'overlap' cases most have lung disease.

Systemic sclerosis carries an increased risk of carcinoma of the lung, particularly bronchioloalveolar cell, and at a younger age. Sjögren's syndrome also occurs with all types.

Radiological appearances. In those patients with an abnormal chest radiograph the typical pattern is a fibrosing alveolitis, reticular or reticulonodular opacities spreading upwards from the bases (Fig. 17.20). Honeycombing may develop. Small pleural effusions are not uncommon and occasional findings are pneumatoceles, pneumothorax, egg-shell calcification in the hilar nodes and evidence of pulmonary hypertension. Oesophageal

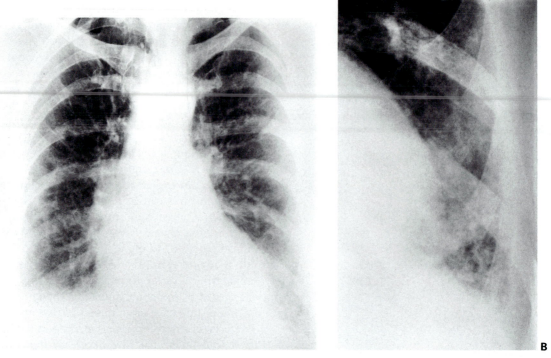

A

B

Fig. 17.20 **A**. Systemic sclerosis. Fibrosing alveolitis spreading upwards from the bases. **B**. Close-up. Coarse reticulation.

dysfunction can lead to aspiration pneumonitis but this is neither frequent nor important.

MIXED CONNECTIVE TISSUE DISEASE

This has features common to systemic lupus, systemic sclerosis and polymyositis, prominent amongst them being Raynaud's phenomenon, arthritis, muscle weakness and lymphadenopathy. It responds to steroids and pursues a relatively benign course due to the absence of severe renal disease. Its immunological characteristic is a high titre of antibody to ribonuclear protein, which is absent, or in low titre, in other connective tissue diseases. The chest radiograph is abnormal in most cases, with fibrosing alveolitis at the bases, small lung volumes and upper-lobe shrinkage. A notable characteristic is a deforming erosive arthritis and acro-osteolysis.

DERMATOMYOSITIS AND POLYMYOSITIS

Lung involvement is unusual in these conditions, but when present it takes the form of a basal fibrosing alveolitis. This can progress rapidly but more often it evolves slowly, with emphysema complicating the later stages.

BEHÇET'S DISEASE

The features of this disease of unknown aetiology are ulcerations in the mouth, eye and genitalia with arthritis

of large joints, thrombophlebitis and inflammatory lesions of the gut. It is found most often in the Middle East and is almost exclusively a disease of men. In association with these symptoms, the finding of multiple aneurysms and occlusions of pulmonary artery branches is pathognomonic. Obstruction of the cavae may also be found.

RHEUMATOID ARTHRITIS

The incidence of pleuropulmonary diseases directly related to rheumatoid arthritis and not just a chance association is low, no more than a few per cent. However, looked at from the other direction, the incidence of rheumatoid arthritis in fibrosing alveolitis is much higher than this. Intrathoracic manifestations of rheumatoid disease comprise pleural effusions, fibrosing alveolitis, rheumatoid necrobiotic nodules, angiitis and bronchiolitis obliterans. Occasionally these antedate overt joint disease.

Pleural effusions are usually straw-coloured exudates of moderate volume with a tendency to chronicity. The rare cholesterol effusion may remain unchanged over many years. Men are often more affected than women. Resorption of the exudate often leaves a fibrotic obliteration of the pleural space.

Cryptogenic fibrosing alveolitis and its relationship to rheumatoid disease has already been discussed but it has to be remembered that treatment with gold and penicillamine are potential causes of diffuse fibrosis (Fig. 17.21).

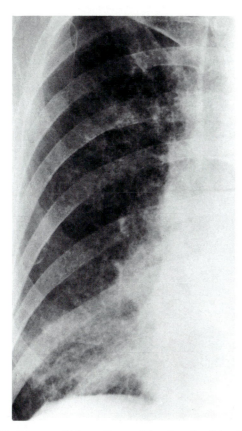

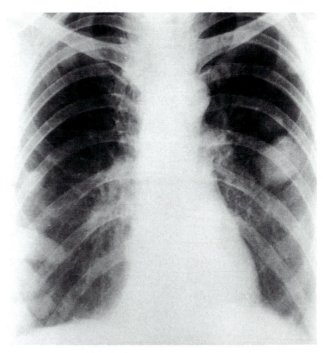

Fig. 17.22 Rheumatoid nodules. Seven can be seen. They later cavitated.

Fig. 17.21 Rheumatoid lung disease. Fibrosing alveolitis; also a mass at right hilum. At postmortem pulmonary arteritis was found; the mass was found to be necrotic. The patient had received gold treatment, but this bore no temporal relationship to the respiratory disease.

Rheumatoid lung nodules and subcutaneous nodules have the same histology, a necrotic centre surrounded by histiocytes, lymphocytes and fibroblasts. The nodules are round and well defined but with borders that are slightly irregular. The average diameter is 2–4 cm but an occasional one reaches large size. They occur in any part of the lungs and may be single or multiple but are never profuse (Fig. 17.22).

Cavitation is common and is a result of evacuation of the necrotic material (Fig. 17.23). The cavities may periodically fill and empty, they may become infected or rupture into the pleura, in which case there will be a pneumothorax or bronchopleural fistula. Some nodules resolve, leaving a scar, but in general they are indolent. Large cavities have been known to close after treatment with azathioprine.

In *Caplan's syndrome* there are numerous round opacities up to 5 cm in diameter, resembling metastases. It occurs against a background of simple pneumoconiosis, the two diseases modifying each other in this distinctive fashion. The solid fibrotic lesions eventually become hyalinized and may calcify. It was first described in coal-

miners but it is also found in asbestosis, silicosis and other industrial pneumoconioses (see Ch. 16).

Pulmonary angiitis is commonly found on histological examination of the lungs from rheumatoid patients, but this does not give rise to any recognizable radiographic pattern. Isolated case reports have described acute necrotizing angiitis in association with consolidative pulmonary opacities.

Obliterative bronchiolitis is a potential cause of respiratory failure, with a normal chest radiograph. It has been found in association with obstructive pneumonia and probably accounts for some large apical cavitating lesions.

Progressive upper-lobe fibrosis with bullous cystic changes indistinguishable from those found in ankylosing spondylitis has also been reported.

ANKYLOSING SPONDYLITIS AND PROGRESSIVE APICAL FIBROSIS

About 2% of long-standing ankylosing spondylitics develop progressive apical fibrosis. It begins as patchy opacities in the upper lobes, with an apical cap of pleural thickening. It may be unilateral at first, but always spreads to the opposite side. The opacities enlarge, and bullous air cysts appear within them, at which time there may be a complaint of haemoptysis. Like all chronic cavities, they are susceptible to fungal colonization. Bronchi in the affected area are distorted and bronchiectatic. Pathologically, the early changes are those of a patchy

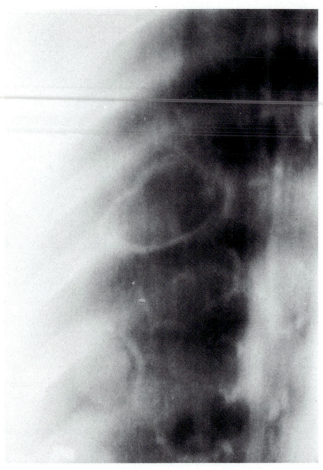

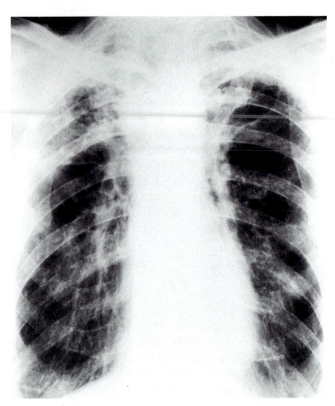

Fig. 17.24 Idiopathic progressive apical fibrosis. Nine years previously the chest radiograph was normal. The same pattern is found in many other diseases.

Fig. 17.23 Cavitating rheumatoid nodules. Tomogram. One cavity contains a central round opacity and an air crescent (compare with a mycetoma).

pneumonia, with infiltration by chronic inflammatory cells and fibroblasts. There is progression to an extensive fibrosis and hyalinization, destroying lung architecture.

Contracting fibrobullous disease of this nature is not distinguishable from that caused by tuberculosis, sarcoidosis, extrinsic allergic alveolitis, pneumoconiosis, post-radiation and rheumatoid arthritis. There is also a group of idiopathic cases to which none of these causes apply (Fig. 17.24).

PULMONARY ALVEOLAR PROTEINOSIS

When this disease was first described in 1958 the pathology was characterized as 'filling of the alveoli by a PAS-positive proteinaceous material rich in lipid' which still defines the essential elements of the process. Macroscopically, the lung is not uniformly affected but studded with nodules from a few millimetres up to 2 cm or more in diameter. The most plausible theory of causation is that it is a response to a variety of irritants, including

dusts, and that for some unknown reason there is impairment of clearance of the material so formed. This material is probably mainly formed from surfactant ingested by macrophages, which then disintegrate within alveoli. Leakage of serum into alveoli also plays a part. There is a striking absence of reaction within alveolar walls unless there are complications. Men are affected three times as often as women and no age is exempt. The disease is worldwide.

Radiological appearances. Radiologically the commonest pattern is one likened to pulmonary oedema with a bilateral, fine, diffuse, radiating perihilar shadowing. However, the nonuniformity of the pathology may be reflected in a superimposition of patchiness, taking the form either of a granularity or nodularity, seen within the general opacity or at its edges (Fig. 17.25). The granularity can be confused with sarcoidosis or miliary tuberculosis but the background opacity is finer than in these diseases. The irregular coarse linearities characteristic of fibrosis, or the mediastinal distortions of chronic tuberculosis, are not found unless there are infective complications, but small honeycomb cysts representing distended terminal air spaces may be found at the edges of lesions and are probably the source of the occasional *pneumothorax*.

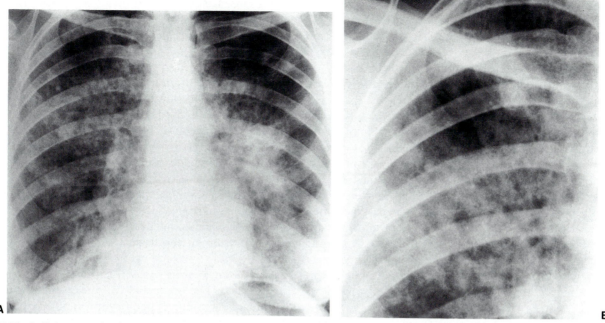

Fig. 17.25 A. Pulmonary alveolar proteinosis. Central alveolar patchy densities and vague nodulation. **B.** Close-up. Ill-defined alveolar opacities; air bronchogram visible.

Enlargement of hilar nodes, pleural effusions and cavitation only occur with complications. There are variations to the basic 'butterfly' distribution; the opacities can be solely or predominantly unilateral or may be confined to one lung segment.

The disease may remain static over many years or it may progress. A minority of cases resolve spontaneously, sometimes completely, others leaving a residue of fibrosis. Recurrence after spontaneous resolution is uncommon but is now seen frequently after treatment by broncho-alveolar lavage.

Diagnosis is confirmed by *biopsy* or by the finding of the proteinaceous material in the *sputum* or *lavage fluid*. Macrophages with lamellar inclusions of lipid in the lavage fluid are also diagnostic. *Bronchoalveolar lavage* is not only diagnostic but therapeutic. Each lung in turn is filled with saline which is then repeatedly exchanged, up to a total of 40 l or more. The return is at first opalescent but becomes progressively clearer. Functional improvement is immediate but radiographic clearing may be delayed and then incomplete. The procedure can be repeated as necessary.

The disease causes dyspnoea as a result of impaired gas transfer, and previously carried a high mortality rate from respiratory or cardiac failure, but lavage has improved the prognosis. There is an increased risk of infection, not only from the usual respiratory pathogens but also from *Nocardia, Aspergillus, Cryptococcus* and other opportunistic organisms, in these circumstances likely to be disseminate. The disease is occasionally found associated with leukaemia, Hodgkin's disease and immunoglobulin deficiencies.

AMYLOIDOSIS

Amyloid is a proteinaceous substance with specific chemical and staining properties. Amyloidosis is a group of conditions in which amyloid in unusually large amounts is deposited in connective tissue, around parenchymal tissue cells and in the walls of blood vessels. The conditions are grouped into *primary* and *secondary* categories according to whether there is a prior precipitating cause. Secondary amyloidosis may arise as a complication of *chronic infection* such as tuberculosis, osteomyelitis, bronchiectasis or leprosy but in Western countries infection now assumes less importance and the most common causes are *rheumatoid disease* and *neoplasia*. Chemical analysis and histological staining can differentiate between primary and secondary amyloid, but there is a borderland represented by myeloma in which secondary amyloidosis has a chemically primary amyloid. Secondary amyloid is derived from serum (*AA amyloid*) and primary amyloid (and myeloma amyloid) from immunoglobulin light chains (*AL amyloid*).

Both primary and secondary amyloidosis can occur in localized and generalized forms. Once generalized amyloidosis is established, it tends to be progressive and has a poor prognosis when vital organs become involved. In 75% of cases of the generalized disease there are amyloid deposits in the mucosa of rectal biopsy specimens. Secondary amyloid does not invoke an inflammatory response in the lungs, whereas primary amyloid does so. For this reason secondary amyloidosis in the lungs seldom causes symptoms, and the chest radiograph is normal unless the initiating cause is intrapulmonary.

Further subdivision of primary pulmonary amyloidosis is based on the site involved:

Tracheobronchial. This may take the form of a solitary endobronchial tumour mass or polyp, or it may grow down the trachea and into the bronchi in the form of nodular submucosal plaques. Radiologically, the predictable effects are those of obstruction, namely atelectasis, distal bronchiectasis and infection. On bronchography there is a nodularity of the wall of the air passages and multiple strictures (Fig. 17.26). The tumour masses may have to be removed piecemeal but they recur. Amyloid material is sometimes found in relationship to bronchial neoplasms, so that caution is required in the interpretation of a biopsy appearance as it may not be typical of the whole lesion.

Tracheopathia osteoplastica is a condition of cartilaginous masses lining most of the trachea and major bronchi. The masses contain amyloid deposits, calcific bodies and ossifications. It is thought to be an end-stage of tracheobronchial amyloidosis.

Pulmonary parenchymal amyloidosis. There are two varieties: *nodular* and *alveolar septal*. In the nodular variety the lesions are discrete and either solitary or multiple, sometimes in large numbers. In size they vary from one to several centimetres in diameter and they grow slowly. Approximately one-third cavitate or calcify, the latter resembling a fine stippling, best appreciated on tomography. Calcification of this nature in a solitary lesion is strong evidence of amyloidosis. The second variety, alveolar septal or interstitial amyloidosis, is a diffuse deposition of amyloid within alveolar walls, lobular septa and in the walls of pulmonary arterioles. Radiographically, there may be a diffuse reticulation or reticulonodulation, a honeycomb pattern or an appearance which mimics pulmonary oedema.

Nodal. Amyloidosis may be confined to nodes (Fig. 17.27). The frequency of mediastinal and hilar node enlargement differs significantly in different reported series. It can be massive, and the nodes frequently contain a coarse speckled or egg shell *calcification.*

Combinations of these varieties are sometimes found in the same patient. In all types the pleura is usually spared. *Cardiac amyloid* is a cause of pericardial effusion, impaired myocardial contractility and conduction defects, all leading to heart failure. As the pulmonary oedema of heart failure recedes, an underlying reticulonodular pattern may be revealed. The combination of increasing dyspnoea with reticulonodular shadowing in a patient

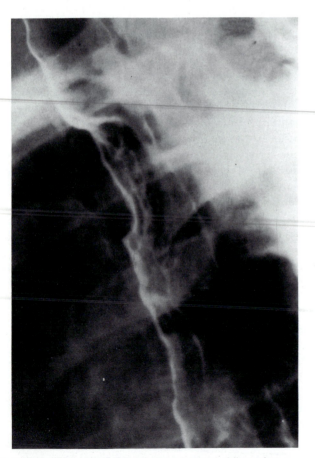

Fig. 17.26 Tracheal amyloidosis. Bronchogram; oblique view. Nodular filling defects in the lumen.

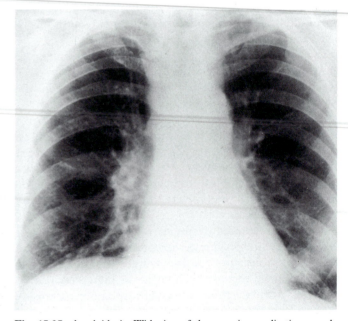

Fig. 17.27 Amyloidosis. Widening of the superior mediastinum and right hilar enlargement from adenopathy. Patient had lymphoplasmacytic lymphoma, but this was not present in the mediastinal nodes, which showed amyloidosis only.

with cardiac dysfunction without obvious cause is very suggestive of myocardial amyloidosis and alveolar septal amyloidosis.

BRONCHIAL ABNORMALITIES
Bronchial abnormalities which are a part of specific diseases are considered in their respective sections.

CHRONIC BRONCHITIS
The excessive mucous secretion which is the hallmark of *chronic bronchitis* impairs the defences of the bronchial tree against infection. Sooner or later the symptoms of recurrent bronchial infection are added to those of hypersecretion, and as the intervals between infections shorten, the patient may have sputum which is almost continually purulent. Damage to the bronchial tree is then manifested in changes in the bronchogram — patchy non-filling of some bronchi because of retained secretions; contrast medium filling the dilated ducts of mucous glands in the epithelium of major bronchi; the epithelium is thrown into concertina folds; the even bronchial tapering is replaced by minor dilatations and narrowings; small airways dilate into small cavities. There is no sharp cut-off point between these changes and those of minor tubular bronchiectasis, the difference is simply one of degree.

Although chronic bronchitis and chronic airways obstruction are often found together, their relationship is not a simple one of cause and effect; they are independent variables.

BRONCHIECTASIS
The incidence and severity of bronchiectasis has been changed substantially by improved medical management of pulmonary infections and by a reduction in the incidence of measles and whooping cough, which, with their frequent complications of secondary infection, were potent initiators of bronchiectasis. The bronchial tree was permanently subjected to aspiration from pools of chronic suppuration, so that surgical resection of the worst areas was no guarantee that spread to other parts would be prevented. Antibiotics have transformed the outlook so that those now most at risk are those who, by virtue of structural or functional abnormalities, are incapable of clearing the lungs of infection. Examples of such abnormalities are *cystic fibrosis of the pancreas*, *agammaglobulinaemia* and *deficient mucociliary clearance*. In parallel with the fall in the number of surgical resections there has been a fall in the number of bronchograms performed. Diagnosis and treatment can be based on symptoms, clinical signs and non-invasive radiography, so that it is no longer crucial to know the precise distribution of the bronchiectasis.

Radiological appearances. On a chest radiograph the only pathognomonic sign of bronchiectasis is a dilated, air-filled bronchus. Bronchial-wall or peribronchial thickening has to be present before these tubes become visible (Fig. 17.28). Cavities which fill and empty, branching band shadows, grossly scarred areas of persistent collapse, are all signs suggestive but not pathognomonic of bronchiectasis. In progressive upper lobe fibrosis such as is found in tuberculosis, sarcoidosis or extrinsic allergic alveolitis, the bronchi are distorted and usually dilated. Cavities in these areas are frequently bronchiectatic in origin.

Nevertheless there are circumstances when bronchography can be useful. The diagnosis may be uncertain and the chest radiograph unhelpful. The chest radiograph is sometimes normal even in the presence of extensive cystic bronchiectasis. In such cases CT is the preferred examination and often also in those in whom surgical resection is to be performed for localized bronchiectasis. The latter will be patients with resistant infection or haemoptysis and in these bronchography still has a place.

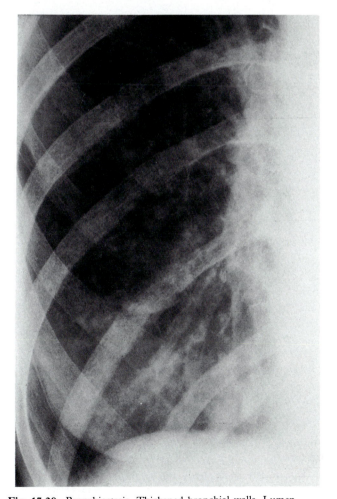

Fig. 17.28 Bronchiectasis. Thickened bronchial walls. Lumen dilated in places.

Tubular (or *cylindrical*) and *saccular* (or *cystic*) are descriptive terms applied to the morphology of bronchiectasis, referring respectively to dilatation along the bronchial axis or to peripheral expansions indicating the site of maximum damage to the airways. The side-branches of the bronchial axis are spaced at first at intervals of over 1 cm, but as the peripheral parts are reached the intervals reduce to 2–3 mm. The 'mm branching pattern' identifies any changes beyond as being at the bronchiolar level. Most cases of bronchiectasis however, are of mixed type but with one predominating.

A common pattern is of irregularly dilated tubes with clubbed terminations crowded together in shrunken lung (Fig. 17.29). Additional signs of chronic bronchitis are usually to be found in the large central bronchi. Saccules may remain small or enlarge to 2–3 cm in diameter, and it is the larger which fill with greatest difficulty during bronchography. They may fill with contrast medium after coughing or after a delay of some hours (Fig. 17.30).

Allergic bronchopulmonary aspergillosis may have a unique pattern of proximal bronchiectasis, with normal-calibre bronchi beyond the dilatation, but the common tubular bronchiectasis is more often found. Generalized bronchiectasis may be found in *α-1-anti-trypsin deficiency* which contrasts with the predominantly basal emphysema which is characteristic of this condition. Bronchiectasis in *cystic fibrosis* appears first in the upper lobes before spreading widely. However, bronchography is seldom required in these conditions.

BRONCHIOLITIS

Bronchiolitis is predominantly an acute infective disease of children, often of viral aetiology.

Bronchiolitis obliterans has a wider spread of age incidence and aetiology. It may be caused by, or follow, viral infections or inhalation of toxic fumes; it is found in association with the lung lesions of rheumatoid arthritis, connective tissue diseases, chronic eosinophil pneumonia, bronchocentric granulomatosis and allergic angiitis with granulomatosis; it is present in 25% of cases of farmer's lung; there is an association with bronchitis, emphysema and smoking; it is found in chronic graft-versus-host disease after organ or allogenic bone marrow transplantation.

Plugs of granulation tissue are found within the lumen of small airways, causing their destruction and obliter-

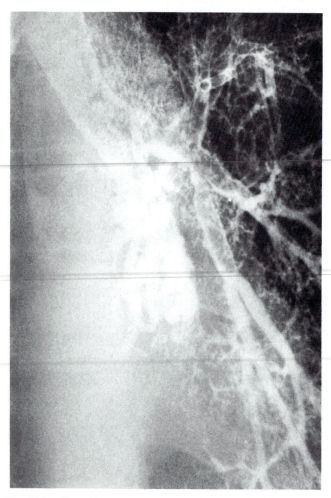

Fig. 17.29 Bronchiectasis. Diminutive left lower lobe, probably from infection in infancy which arrested further growth. Dilated mucous gland ducts visible on the lingula bronchus – chronic bronchitis.

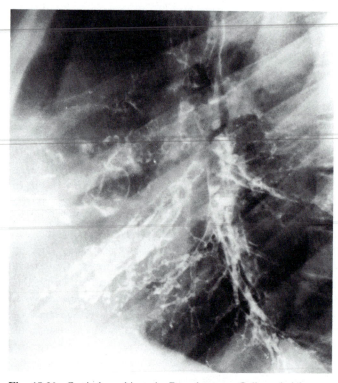

Fig. 17.30 Cystic bronchiectasis. Bronchogram. Collapsed right middle lobe, tubular (cylindrical) bronchiectasis and saccules filling with difficulty.

ation by scarring. The distribution of these changes is characteristically patchy. If the granulation tissue extends distally into the alveoli it is called *bronchiolitis obliterans organizing pneumonia*. The majority of cases respond to steroid therapy.

After excluding those cases having known precipitating factors such as described above, there remains a small number with severe, chronic irreversible obstruction of small airways for which the term *cryptogenic obliterative bronchiolitis* has been proposed. These patients are almost all women with severe dyspnoea, sometimes dating from a respiratory infection. Half of the patients have rheumatoid arthritis but no overt evidence of rheumatoid lung disease.

Radiological appearances. In pure *bronchiolitis obliterans* the chest radiograph is usually normal or shows no more than hyperinflation, but some show a nodular pattern. Bronchographic abnormalities are more impressive, with the contrast medium stopping well short of the periphery and a sparsity of side branches. These are the changes found in *unilateral lung transradiance*. There are matched, non-segmental ventilation/perfusion defects on lung scanning, with slow wash-in and slow wash-out. Bronchiolitis obliterans organizing pneumonia has a variety of radiographic patterns — a diffuse, ground-glass alveolar opacity, multiple nodular opacities with air bronchograms or reticulonodulation.

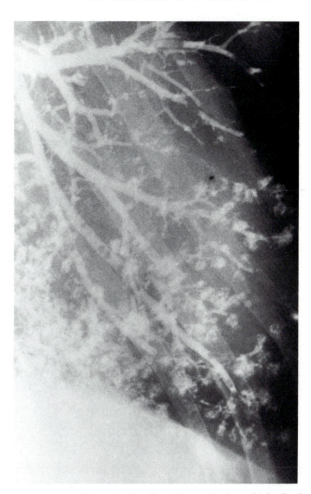

Fig. 17.31 Bronchiolectasis. Small cavities at the bronchiolar level; some have a crenated outline, 'mimosa' pattern.

BRONCHIOLECTASIS

Small peripheral saccular dilatations of the terminal and respiratory bronchioles are identified bronchographically at the level of the millimetre branching pattern (Fig. 17.31). The acinus — that is, the group of alveoli distal to the terminal bronchiole — may be incorporated in the saccules, which measure approximately 1 cm in diameter. Symptoms of chronic bronchitis and bronchiectasis are related to the numbers of such saccules. Bronchiolectasis has been found postmortem in patients who have had intermittent positive pressure ventilation with positive end-expiratory pressures. Patients treated identically who survived had no recognizable sequelae, from which it is assumed that the condition is potentially reversible.

BRONCHOCOELE

Accumulation of mucus, pus or caseous material within distended bronchi distal to a segmental bronchus but without collapse is known as bronchocoele, bronchial mucocoele or blocked bronchiectasis. An obstructing membrane found in some cases has been interpreted as indicating a congenital origin but obstruction from any cause, including bronchial carcinoma, is capable of producing an identical appearance (Fig. 17.32). It is relatively rare in bronchial carcinoma because of insufficient time available for its evolution before being overtaken by atelectatic changes from continued growth of the neoplasm. The characteristic appearance is a collection of oval or finger-like branching, homogeneous opacities along the axis of the bronchial tree, usually in an upper lobe. The low density makes it difficult to define on the plain radiograph but it is clearly seen on tomography. The 'cyst' does not fill on bronchography, the obstruction producing a sharp cut-off in the contrast column. Aeration of the segment of lung distal to the bronchocoele is maintained by collateral air flow from adjacent segments through the pores of Kohn. For reasons which are not clear, this collateral flow is largely one-way and the segment is hyperinflated. With increasing distension the bronchocoele assumes a round shape and it can then be mistaken for a bronchogenic cyst, even to the extent of the histology, since it is lined by respiratory epithelium.

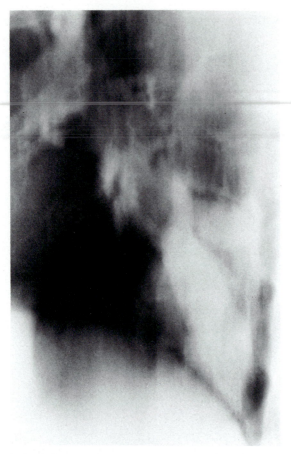

Fig. 17.32 Bronchocoele due to squamous carcinoma of bronchus. Lateral tomogram. Wide, branched bronchus. Inspissated gelatinous material was found distal to the obstructing carcinoma.

those that remain are usually referred to eponymously as either *Macleod's* or *Swyer-James syndrome*. The vessels in the affected lung are reduced in number and calibre, a fact adequately demonstrated by *whole-lung tomography* without the need for angiography. The small vessel size includes the hilum, a point of differentiation from emphysema in which these vessels are normal or enlarged (Fig. 17.33). Since the normal lung takes a larger proportion of the cardiac output, its vascularity is increased.

Bronchography usually shows bronchi slightly narrower than normal, with minor calibre irregularities, but, more importantly, the contrast medium stops well short of the periphery. This is because inspiration does not affect the aspiration of the contrast medium peripherally. The lung is aerated but poorly ventilated, with only a small change in volume between inspiration and expiration. As a consequence the mediastinum moves towards the impaired side during inspiration, and diaphragmatic excursion is reduced.

The condition is the end result of *bronchiolitis obliterans* in infancy. It has been observed to follow adenovirus and respiratory syncytial virus bronchiolitis, but it is the site of the damage rather than the type of infection which is critical. Lung development is incomplete at birth, and proliferation of newly formed alveoli continues for several years. Stunting of this growth is the cause of unilateral transradiance; the alveoli are fewer in number but larger in size. Functionally, there is airways obstruction and de-

BRONCHIAL MUCOID IMPACTION

Bronchial mucoid impaction has superficial similarities to bronchocoele but the aetiology and treatment of the two conditions are quite different. In the former, bronchial obstruction is caused by impaction of thick, tenacious plugs of mucus, often containing a fungal mycelium. The bronchus may be dilated and may or may not fill on bronchography, depending on the tightness of the impaction. If the plugs are coughed up, the obstruction is relieved. A branching opacity may be visible on the radiograph but is rarely as wide as a bronchocoele. The conditions in which it is commonly found are asthma, allergic bronchopulmonary aspergillosis and cystic fibrosis of the pancreas.

UNILATERAL LUNG TRANSRADIANCE

If the transradiance of one lung is greater than that of the opposite side it is usually due to one of the following: 1. technical radiographic factors; 2. abnormalities of the thoracic cage; 3. pulmonary embolism; 4. compensatory or obstructive emphysema. If these causes are excluded,

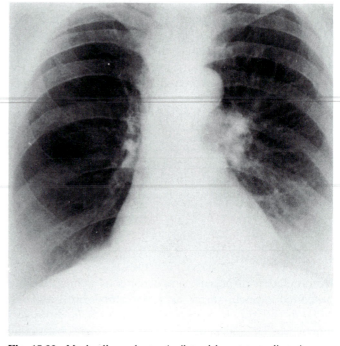

Fig. 17.33 Macleod's syndrome (unilateral lung transradiance). Small right hilum and reduced vessel calibre in right lung.

fective gas exchange. Although classically described as affecting one lung, it may in fact be segmental or lobar or even widespread in both lungs. In the latter case the distribution is patchy, enough undamaged lung remaining to support life. Symptoms are mild, rarely more than a tendency to recurrent respiratory infections and mild dyspnoea, despite the poor regional function.

TRACHEOBRONCHOMEGALY
(*Mounier-Kuhn abnormality*)

The trachea may be as wide as the vertebral bodies and of uneven contour, with bulging of the mucosa between the cartilage rings (Fig. 17.34). The dilatation may proceed no further than the main bronchi, or it may be associated with a generalized bronchiectasis. The hypothesis that it results from a defect of connective tissue receives some support from its occasional association with

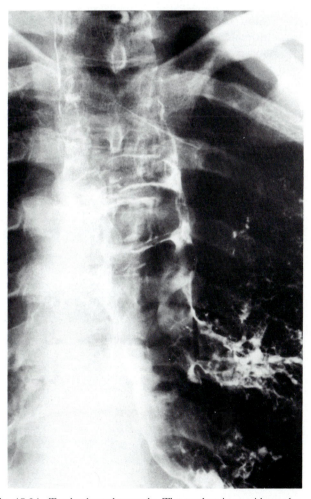

Fig. 17.34 Tracheobronchomegaly. The trachea is as wide as the vertebral bodies. The major bronchi are also wide; there was minor peripheral bronchiectasis in the lower lobes. The patient had recurrent chest infections.

Ehlers-Danlos syndrome, a generalized connective tissue disorder.

ADULT RESPIRATORY DISTRESS SYNDROME

This condition is an *acute respiratory failure from pulmonary oedema, non-cardiac in origin* which is precipitated by a variety of insults, most of which involve some form of *trauma* or *sepsis*.

The list of causes is long and includes such unexpected items as miliary tuberculosis, mountain sickness, burns and major haemorrhage.

Running through these diverse situations there is a common thread of symptoms, physiological disturbances, pathological events and radiographic abnormalities. Following the primary insult, there is a period of shock from which the patient recovers or is resuscitated. There follows a latent interval of hours or days before respiratory distress supervenes. The patient becomes dyspnoeic, tachypnoeic, cyanosed and hypoxic. The respiratory distress is refractory and mechanical ventilation is instituted. Improvement may then follow, or else a deterioration, requiring progressively higher ventilation pressures and oxygen concentrations. The mortality rate is approximately 40% and results from multiorgan failure, irreversible fibrotic lung disease or superadded lung infection.

This chain of events is initiated by damage to alveolar and capillary cells, which allows leakage of proteinaceous oedema fluid into the alveolar walls and air spaces. The damage can result from the release or activation of many injurious substances, including catecholamines, serotonin, vasoactive peptides and complement. The condition is further aggravated by ischaemia, overhydration, oxygen toxicity and consumption coagulopathy. With the latter, the clotting factors may be reduced to a level at which spontaneous bleeding is likely to occur.

Initially the histology is one of *haemorrhagic oedema*, followed within the first week by hyperplasia of Type 2 pneumocytes and the formation of hyaline membranes. Type 2 pneumocytes are the repair cells of the alveoli, and anything which delays or interrupts the repair process causes a *fibroblastic proliferation*. There is a rapid increase in lung collagen and within a few weeks the lungs are irreversibly fibrotic and the architecture destroyed.

Radiological appearances. When the symptoms of respiratory distress first arise, the chest radiograph is usually normal and this paradox will suggest massive pulmonary embolism. A few show evidence of interstitial oedema with Kerley B lines and perivascular cuffing but this is unusual. At 12 hours a pattern of bilateral patchy alveolar opacities appears. This will suggest pulmonary oedema unrelated to heart failure because the heart size is normal. Moreover there is no pleural effusion or pulmonary vessel engorgement. Thereafter there is a rapid

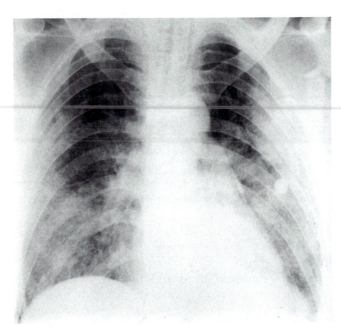

Fig. 17.35 Adult respiratory distress syndrome. Fat embolism from multiple skeletal trauma. Diffuse alveolar opacities.

and massive extension of the opacities, which are unaffected by diuretics.

After the first week *complications* make their appearance. Infection by Gram-negative organisms is common and will be suggested by the presence of multiple abscess cavities and pleural effusion. Interstitial pulmonary emphysema, pneumomediastinum and pneumothorax are usually complications of mechanical ventilation. Interstitial emphysema, producing as it does blebs of air within the pulmonary opacities, may give a spurious appearance of improvement. Segmental pulmonary angiography through an occluding balloon catheter has been performed in the ITU using a single film technique, and the results may have prognostic significance. Those showing pruning of pulmonary artery side branches, occlusions, filling defects or early pulmonary venous filling have a poor prognosis, as these changes are largely irreversible.

Examples of the adult respiratory distress syndrome may have their own individual features, relating to the nature of the initiating cause, as in 'pump' lung after cardiopulmonary by-pass, paraquat poisoning, toxic inhalations and fat embolism (Fig. 17.35).

OXYGEN TOXICITY
Exposure to concentrations of oxygen above 50% for more than three days is followed by signs of pulmonary damage. There is increased permeability of the capillary endothelium and alveolar epithelium, allowing leakage of proteinaceous fluid into the alveolar walls and air spaces. If exposure continues, fibroblastic proliferation and per-

manent interstitial fibrosis follow. Radiographically, the lesions are initially ill-defined alveolar opacities, changing in the proliferative stage to coarse, linear and reticular formations.

STAPHYLOCOCCAL TOXIC SHOCK SYNDROME
This is a clearly defined syndrome caused by *Staphylococcus aureus* of certain phage types. It came into prominence when reports appeared of it affecting menstruating women using a superabsorbent type of vaginal tampon which provided an ideal environment for the growth of the organism. An exotoxin is produced, and it is this which, when absorbed, causes the disease; no organisms are to be found in the blood or tissues remote from the primary site of infection. Abscesses and postoperative wound infection can also be the site of infection.

The illness has an acute onset with major systemic symptoms. Cardinal features are *hypotension*, *oliguria* and an *erythematous rash* which desquamates in the recovery stages. *Thrombocytopenia* is common and occasionally diffuse intravascular coagulation occurs. Pulmonary involvement is not invariable, but when it occurs it is indistinguishable from the adult respiratory distress syndrome due to other causes (Fig. 17.36).

THE LUNGS IN CHRONIC RENAL FAILURE
Microscopic calcification undetected during life is often found at postmortem in the lungs of patients who have

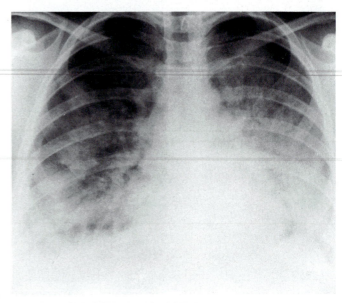

Fig. 17.36 Staphylococcal toxic shock. Extensive alveolar opacification. *Staphylococcus aureus* phage type 3C–55 isolated from a vaginal tampon.

had long-term haemodialysis. It is found in the lumen and walls of alveoli, in bronchi and vessels. If sufficiently profuse, it may appear on the chest radiograph as a fine diffuse micronodulation or as 'pulmonary oedema', but only rarely is it identifiable as discrete foci of calcification. It might be suspected if the 'pulmonary oedema' is unusually dense or fails to respond to appropriate treatment. Such patients will usually also have fibrotic changes in the alveolar walls.

PULMONARY ALVEOLAR MICROLITHIASIS

Innumerable fine calculi like grains of sand form within alveoli, but with surprisingly little change in other lung structures until late in the disease. There is an even distribution throughout the lungs, but the shadowing is denser at the bases where the lung is thicker. The outlines of heart and vessels are obscured and the lungs may seem to be encased in a cortical shell of calcification. The only condition likely to be confused with microlithiasis is *stannosis*. Genetic factors are involved and reduced mucociliary clearance has been reported but otherwise little is known of its aetiology.

IDIOPATHIC PULMONARY OSSIFICATION

This rare condition has also been described under a variety of other names, including ossifying pneumonitis, bony metaplasia of lung and arboriform pulmonary ossification. In its usual form the delicate branching or

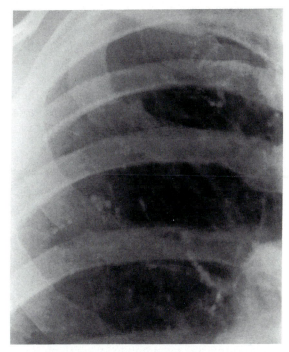

Fig. 17.38 Bronchial 'gravel'. Chains of small stones. Patient had severe respiratory infection 30 years before.

lace-like pattern of dystrophic bone formation in the lower parts of the lungs is sufficiently distinctive to suggest the diagnosis (Fig. 17.37). The cause is unknown and there are no symptoms attributable to the condition.

Another unusual calcification in the lungs takes the form of groups of tiny grains arranged in branching chains (Fig. 17.38). They clearly lie within the lumen of small airways. Patients with this 'bronchial gravel' may give a history of severe bronchopneumonia in the past.

THE ADVERSE EFFECTS OF DRUGS ON THE LUNGS

The two types of reaction to be considered here are those which can occur in all individuals and those in which idiosyncrasy or hypersensitivity are a pre-condition. Therapy with the drugs producing the first type of reaction is only justifiable in extreme circumstances, since almost by definition there is a narrow margin between therapeutic and toxic dose, and the research effort is directed to defining that margin or finding an effective but less toxic substitute. Most of the members of this group will therefore be used in tumour chemotherapy or immunosuppression. In the second group the reaction is unexpected, albeit well-recognized, and is frequently, though not always correctly, ascribed to allergy.

No list of drug reactions is ever complete. However thoroughly new drugs are tested in clinical trials, their introduction into widespread use will uncover unexpected reactions, hence the need for systems of surveillance.

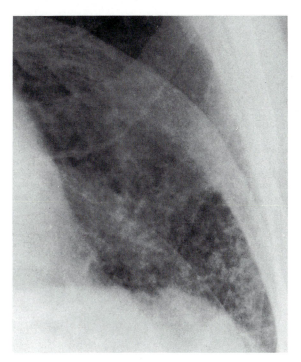

Fig. 17.37 Idiopathic pulmonary ossification. Close-up of left lung base. Fine stippled calcification.

The lungs, with their large capillary bed, are especially vulnerable to blood-borne injurious agents. Drugs may initiate, precipitate or potentiate asthma, common ones in this respect being *antibiotics, contrast media, aspirin* and *beta-adrenoceptor blockers.*

The gas-exchanging parts of the lungs may be damaged by a direct toxic action or by processes suggestive of immunological mechanisms. In either case *fibrosis* is liable to occur following an acute inflammatory oedema, or develop insidiously. *Nitrofurantoin* is a drug which provides a model of a hypersensitivity reaction. The onset is acute, with pulmonary oedema, either alveolar or interstitial, and there are septal lines and pleural effusions. Eosinophilia is often present. With continued use a fibrosing alveolitis occasionally develops. Drugs with a similar exudative response include *aspirin, thiazide diuretics, sulphonamides, amiodarone, methotrexate* and *monoamine oxidase inhibitors* (Fig. 17.13).

Immunological mechanisms are also thought to be involved in lupus-like reactions caused by drugs such as *penicillin, procainamide* and *isoniazide.* The pulmonary signs are a nonspecific pneumonitis, pleural effusions and pleural fibrosis.

Cytotoxic drugs such as *bleomycin, busulphan, cyclophosphamide* and *chlorambucil* are directly damaging to the lung, eliciting an intra-alveolar exudation followed by fibrous thickening of the alveolar walls. During their administration there is no interval of time after which the lungs can be considered safe from attack, but after withdrawal the risk of reactions declines rapidly, except in the case of cyclophosphamide where the risk can persist for months. *Radiotherapy* to the thorax potentiates the pulmonary toxicity of these drugs. Bleomycin and busulphan reactions are dose-dependent. Busulphan occasionally causes pulmonary calcification or ossification. The radiographic signs are widespread reticular or reticulonodular opacities. An acute stage with patchy alveolar opacities is sometimes observed. The differentiation of drug reactions from recurrence or progression of the disease for which they are being given, and also from opportunistic infection, is clearly important, and the contribution of radiology is useful but limited.

Few drug reactions feature hilar or mediastinal node enlargement, a useful point in differential diagnosis. The exception is *phenytoin* where the histology can be confused with lymphoma.

Penicillamine is unusual in the variety of its possible reactions. It can cause pulmonary eosinophilia, miliary shadows, pulmonary haemorrhage and fibrosing alveolitis.

In any diffuse lung disease the possibility that it may be due to drugs requires consideration and the appropriate enquiries should be made.

REFERENCES AND SUGGESTIONS FOR FURTHER READING

Breatnach, E., Kerr, I. H. (1982) The radiology of cryptogenic obliterative bronchiolitis. *Clinical Radiology*, **33**, 657–661.

Fairfax, A. J., Haslam, P. L., Pavia, D. et al (1981) Pulmonary disorders associated with Sjögren's syndrome. *Quarterly Journal of Medicine*, **50**, 279–295.

Davies, D., Crowther, J. S., MacFarlane, A (1975) Idiopathic progressive pulmonary fibrosis. *Thorax*, **30**, 316–325.

Gaensler, E. A., Carrington, C. B. (1977) Peripheral opacities in chronic eosinophilic pneumonia: the photographic negative of pulmonary edema. *American Journal of Roentgenology*, **128**, 1–13.

Himmelfarb, E., Wells, S., Rabinowitz, J. G. (1972) The radiologic spectrum of cardiopulmonary amyloidosis. *Chest*, **72**, 327–332.

Hunninghake, G. W., Fauci, A. S. (1979) Pulmonary involvement in the collagen vascular diseases. *American Review of Respiratory Disease*, **119**, 471–503.

Julsrud, P. R., Brown, L. R., Li, C-Y., Rosenow, E. C., Crowe, J. K. (1978) Pulmonary processes of mature-appearing lymphocytes: pseudolymphoma, well-differentiated lymphocytic lymphoma and lymphocytic interstitial pneumonitis. *Radiology*, **127**, 289–296.

Liebow, A. A. (1973) Pulmonary angiitis and granulomatosis.

American Review of Respiratory Disease, **108**, 1–18.

MacFarlane, J. D., Dieppe, P. A., Rigden, B. G., Clark, T. J. H. (1978) Pulmonary and pleural lesions in rheumatoid disease. *British Journal of Diseases of the Chest*, **72**, 288–300.

McLoud, T. C., Epler, G. R., Colby, T. V., Gaensler, E. A., Carrington, C. B. (1986) Bronchiolitis obliterans. *Radiology*, **159**, 1–8.

Scadding, J. G. (1974) Diffuse pulmonary alveolar fibrosis. *Thorax*, **29**, 271–281.

Talner, L. B., Gmelich, J. T., Liebow, A. A., Greenspan, R. H. (1970) The syndrome of bronchial mucocele and regional hyperinflation of the lung. *American Journal of Roentgenology*, **110**, 675–686.

Turner-Warwick, M. (1974) A perspective view on widespread pulmonary fibrosis. *British Medical Journal*, **ii**, 371–376.

Turner-Warwick, M., Dewar, A. (1982) Pulmonary haemorrhage and pulmonary haemosiderosis. *Clinical Radiology*, **33**, 361–370.

Williams, D. M., Krick, J. A., Remington, J. S. (1976) Pulmonary infection in the compromised host. *American Review of Respiratory Disease*, **114**, 359–394.

CHAPTER 18

CHEST TRAUMA; THE POST-OPERATIVE CHEST; INTENSIVE CARE; RADIATION CHEST TRAUMA

Michael B. Rubens

The thorax may be affected by direct trauma, or as a result of trauma elsewhere in the body. Direct trauma may be the result of penetrating or non-penetrating injury. The usual causes of penetrating injury are shooting, stabbing and shrapnel wounds.

Thoracic surgery is a special category of penetrating trauma. Non-penetrating injuries may be caused by falls, blows or blasts. Car accidents resulting in deceleration injuries are increasing in frequency. Trauma to other areas of the body may have thoracic complications. For example, bone fractures may cause fat emboli, and pulmonary complications following abdominal surgery are common.

Radiological techniques. The severely injured patient, the postoperative patient and the patient in the intensive care ward are true tests of the radiographer's skill. In no areas of radiography are good-quality films more necessary, and in no other group of patients are good-quality films more difficult to produce.

The injured patient is usually brought to the X-ray department, where, if possible, an erect PA film should be taken. A *high-kV technique* is desirable in order to see mediastinal detail, but if this is not possible a penetrated grid radiograph should be taken. A lateral film may be useful. If the patient is severely injured it is necessary to make do with supine films. In the acute stage multiple views for rib fractures are not indicated, since it is complications of the fractures that really matter, whether or not fractures are seen.

Ultrasound is an excellent method for examining the pleura, diaphragm and sub-phrenic areas. *Aortography* and *CT* may be indicated when vascular injuries are suspected.

The postoperative patient and the patient in the intensive care ward will usually be examined with mobile X-ray equipment. An erect AP film, with the patient sitting up, is preferable, but a supine film at end-inspiration is better than a film taken with the patient slouched and at end-expiration. The highest kV and mA possible and high-speed screens will minimize motion blurring. Horizontal-beam lateral decubitus films are often useful to assess pleural fluid, pneumothoraces and fluid levels.

The films of intensive care ward patients need to be examined with full clinical information, since many of the pathological processes to which these patients are susceptible produce similar radiographic manifestations. Serial films need to be evaluated for general trends, as day-to-day changes may not be apparent, and special attention needs to be given to monitoring and life-support devices.

INJURIES TO THE THORACIC CAGE

Rib fractures are common, and may be single, multiple, unilateral or bilateral. Healed rib fractures are a fairly frequent incidental finding on the chest X-ray. Acute rib fractures are often difficult to see if there is no displacement, and their presence may only be inferred by surrounding haematoma producing an extrapleural

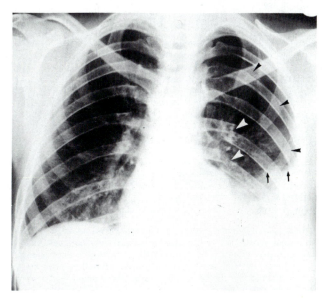

Fig. 18.1 Rib fractures and haemopneumothorax in a woman injured in a car accident. The left 7th and 8th ribs are fractured (white arrowheads). A pneumothorax (black arrowheads) is present, and a fluid level (arrows) is seen in the pleural space.

opacity. In cases of chest trauma, the chest X-ray is more important in detecting a complication of rib fracture than the fracture itself. However, fracture of the first three ribs is often associated with major intrathoracic injury, and fracture of the lower three ribs may be associated with important hepatic, splenic or renal injury.

Complications of rib fracture include a flail segment, pneumothorax, haemothorax and subcutaneous emphysema. A *flail segment* is usually apparent clinically, the affected part of the chest wall being sucked in during inspiration, possibly compromising the underlying lung. The chest X-ray will show several adjacent ribs to be fractured in two places, or bilateral rib fractures.

The fractured ends of ribs may penetrate underlying pleura and lung and cause a *pneumothorax, haemothorax, haemopneumothorax* (Fig. 18.1) or *intrapulmonary haemorrhage*. Air may also escape into the chest wall and cause *subcutaneous emphysema* (Fig. 18.2).

Stress fractures of the first and second ribs are sometimes an incidental finding on the chest X-ray. *Cough fractures* usually affect the sixth to ninth ribs in the posterior axillary line, but may not be visible until callus has formed.

Fractures of the sternum usually require a lateral film or tomography for visualization.

Fractures of the thoracic spine may be associated with a paraspinal shadow which represents haematoma.

Fractures of the clavicle may be associated with injury of the subclavian vessels or brachial plexus, and posterior dislocation of the clavicle at the sternoclavicular joint may cause injury to the trachea, oesophagus, great vessels or nerves of the superior mediastinum.

Herniation of lung tissue is usually associated with obvious rib fractures, but may only be apparent on tangential views in full inspiration.

INJURIES TO THE DIAPHRAGM

Laceration of the diaphragm may result from penetrating or non-penetrating trauma to the chest or abdomen. The left hemidiaphragm is involved more often than the right. The typical plain film appearance is of obscuration of the affected hemidiaphragm and increased shadowing in the ipsilateral hemithorax due to herniation of stomach, omentum, bowel or solid viscera (Fig. 18.3), although such herniation may be delayed. *Ultrasound* may demonstrate diaphragmatic laceration and free fluid in both the pleura and peritoneum. *Barium studies* may be useful to confirm herniation of stomach or bowel into the chest.

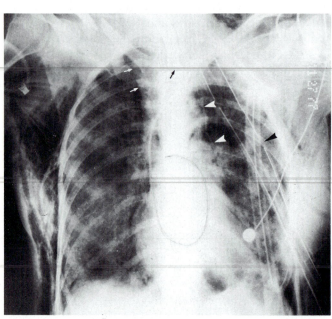

Fig. 18.2 Massive chest trauma in a women involved in a car crash. Gross subcutaneous emphysema extends over the chest wall, outlining muscle planes. The right clavicle is fractured. Several ribs were fractured, but not seen on this film. Mediastinal emphysema separates pleura from the descending aorta (white arrowheads). A mediastinal haematoma is present (white arrows). Widespread lung contusion is obscured by the subcutaneous emphysema. Note tracheostomy tube (black arrow), left pleural tubes, with side-hole indicated (black arrowhead), Swan-Ganz catheter and ECG lead.

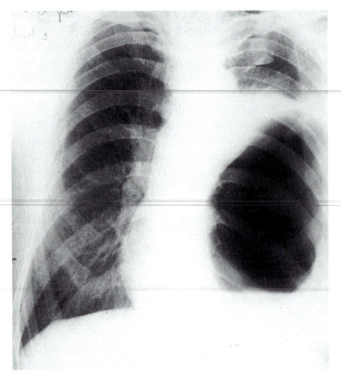

Fig. 18.3 Rupture of diaphragm in a man of 58 who fell from a building 13 years before, breaking ankles and injuring chest, and now presented with persistent vomiting. The chest radiograph demonstrates distended stomach in the left hemithorax, confirmed by barium swallow. Thoracotomy revealed stomach herniating into left pleural cavity through a 5-cm rent in the left hemidiaphragm.

INJURIES TO THE PLEURA

Pneumothorax, as mentioned above, may be a complication of rib fracture, and is then usually associated with a haemothorax (Fig. 18.1). If no ribs are fractured, pneumothorax is secondary to a pneumomediastinum or a penetrating chest injury (Fig. 18.4). Pneumothorax due to a penetrating injury is liable to develop increased pressure, resulting in a tension pneumothorax, which may require emergency decompression.

Haemothorax may also occur with or without rib fractures (Fig. 18.5), and is due to laceration of intercostal or pleural vessels. If a pneumothorax is also present a fluid level will be seen on a horizontal-beam film (Fig. 18.1).

Pleural effusion may also result from trauma. Open injuries to the pleura are prone to infection and development of an empyema.

INJURIES TO THE LUNG

Pulmonary contusion is due to haemorrhagic exudation into the alveoli and interstitial spaces and appears as patchy, non-segmental consolidation (Figs 18.5, 18.7). Shadowing appears within the first few hours of penetrating or non-penetrating trauma, and usually shows improvement within two days, and clearing within 3–4 days (Fig. 18.6). When contusion due to a bullet wound clears, a longitudinal haematoma in the bullet track may become visible (Fig. 18.4).

Pulmonary lacerations as a result of non-penetrating trauma may appear as round thin-walled cystic spaces. When the injury is acute, the laceration may be obscured by pulmonary contusion, but as the surrounding consolidation resolves, laceration will become evident. If the laceration is filled with blood it appears as a homogeneous round opacity, and if partly filled with blood it may show a fluid level. Such pulmonary haematomas or blood cysts gradually decrease in size, but may take a few months to resolve completely. Pulmonary haematomas are often multiple (Fig. 18.7).

Torsion of a lung is a rare result of severe thoracic trauma, usually to a child. The lung twists about the hilum through 180°. If unrelieved the lung may become gangrenous and appear opaque on the chest X-ray.

Atelectasis and **compensatory hyperinflation** after a chest injury may be due to aspiration of blood or mucus into the bronchi. Atelectasis may also occur secondary to decreased respiratory movement.

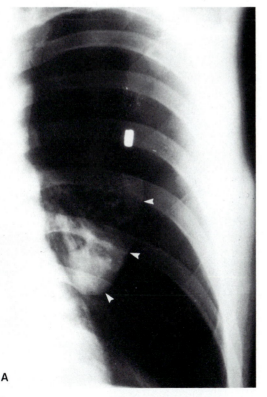
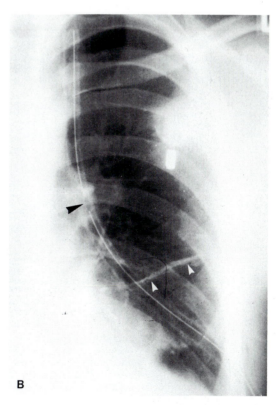

A   B

Fig. 18.4 Penetrating chest injury — man with bullet wound. **A.** Large pneumothorax (arrowheads), and bullet in chest wall. **B.** Following insertion of pleural tube (black arrowhead), the lung re-expands, revealing haematoma in bullet track. Band shadow in lower zone (white arrowheads) represents subsegmental atelectasis.

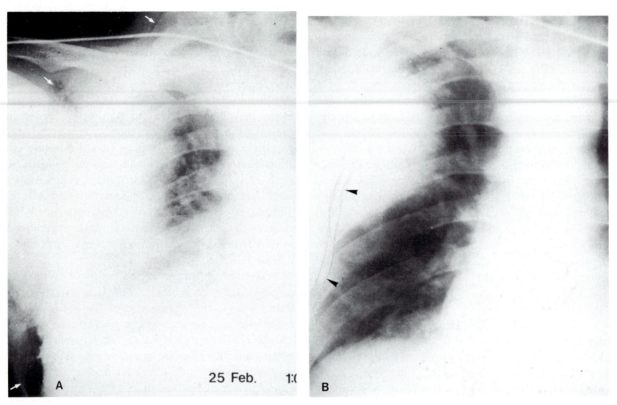

25 Feb.   1:

Fig. 18.5 Pulmonary contusion and haemothorax in a man with a gunshot injury. **A.** Subcutaneous emphysema is present over the chest wall (arrows), and dense shadowing extends over most of the hemithorax. **B.** Following the insertion of a pleural drain (arrowheads) the lower half of the shadowing, due to blood in the pleural space, has gone. The remaining opacity is pulmonary contusion. A few bullet fragments are visible above the contusion.

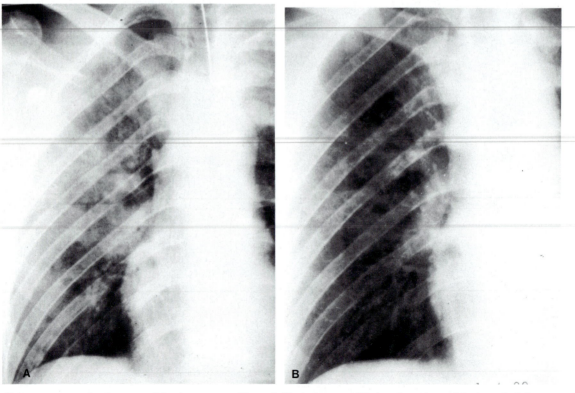

Fig. 18.6 Pulmonary contusion in a man following a car accident. **A.** Extensive consolidation throughout right lung. Left lung was clear. No rib fractures. **B.** Four days later the shadowing has resolved.

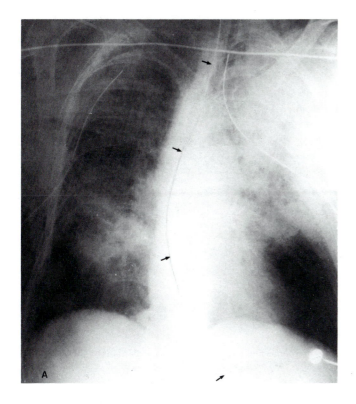

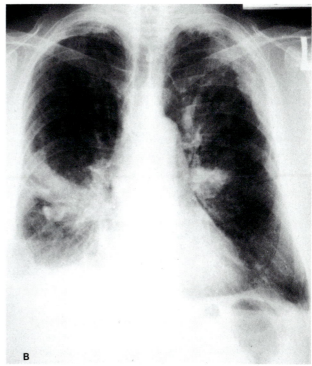

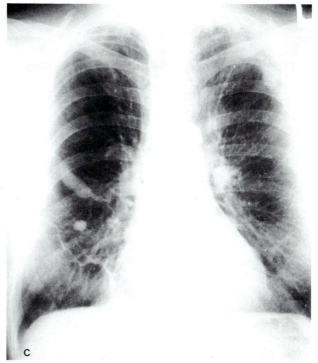

Pulmonary oedema as a manifestation of the adult respiratory distress syndrome may occur after major trauma.

Fat embolism is a rare complication of multiple fractures, due to fat globules from the bone marrow entering the systemic veins and embolizing to the lungs. Poorly-defined nodular opacities appear throughout both lungs. The opacities resolve within a few days. The diagnosis is confirmed if fat globules are present in the sputum or urine.

INJURIES TO THE TRACHEA AND BRONCHI

Laceration or **rupture** of a major airway is an uncommon result of severe chest trauma, usually in a car crash. Fracture of the first three ribs is often present, and mediastinal emphysema and pneumothorax are common (Fig. 18.8). The injury is usually in the trachea just above the carina, or in a main bronchus just distal to the carina. If the bronchial sheath is preserved there may be no immediate signs or symptoms, but tracheostenosis or bronchiectasis may occur later. Tomography may be helpful in diagnosis, but bronchoscopy is the best diagnostic method in the acute stage.

INJURIES TO THE MEDIASTINUM

Pneumomediastinum or mediastinal emphysema are terms that describe the presence of air between the tissue planes of the mediastinum. Air may reach here as a result

Fig. 18.7 Pulmonary contusion and haematoma in a youth of 18 trampled on by a bull. **A.** Extensive consolidation is present throughout both lungs, particularly in the left upper zone. Subcutaneous emphysema is seen over the right hemithorax. Bilateral pleural tubes and a nasogastric tube (arrows) are present. **B.** Six days later the contusion has resolved and multiple pulmonary haematomas and some extrapleural haematomas have become visible. **C.** One month later the haematomas are smaller.

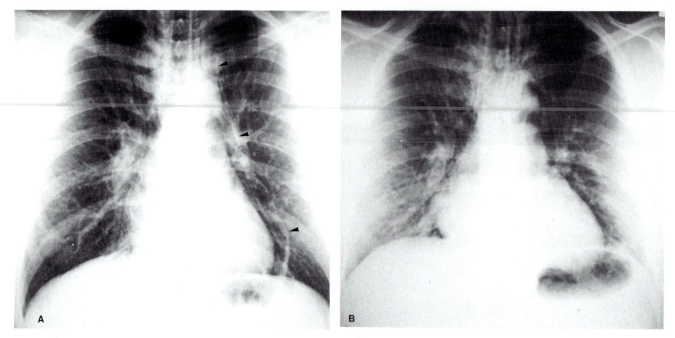

Fig. 18.8 Ruptured trachea in a man suffering a deceleration injury with dysnpoea and chest pain. **A.** Pneumomediastinum with linear lucencies in the mediastinum and displacement of mediastinal pleura (arrowheads). **B.** One hour later, following a bout of coughing, a left pneumothorax has developed. Bronchoscopy revealed a ruptured trachea.

of interstitial pulmonary emphysema, perforation of the oesophagus, trachea or a bronchus, or from a penetrating chest injury. *Interstitial pulmonary emphysema* is a result of alveolar wall rupture due to high intra-alveolar pressure, and may occur during violent coughing, asthmatic attacks or severe crush injuries, or be due to positive pressure ventilation. Air dissects centrally along the perivascular sheath to reach the mediastinum. Rarely, air may dissect into the mediastinum from a pneumo-peritoneum. A pneumomediastinum may extend beyond the thoracic inlet into the neck, and over the chest wall. Pneumothorax is a common complication of pneumo- mediastinum, but the converse never occurs.

Pneumomediastinum usually produces vertical translucent streaks in the mediastinum. This represents gas separating, and outlining the soft-tissue planes and structures of the mediastinum. Gas shadows may extend up into the neck (Fig. 18.9), or dissect extrapleurally over the diaphragam, or extend into the soft-tissue planes of the chest wall, causing subcutaneous emphysema (Figs 18.9, 18.10). The mediastinal pleura may be displaced laterally, and become visible as a linear soft-tissue shadow parallel to the mediastinum (Figs 18.2, 18.8–10). If mediastinal air collects beneath the pericardium the central part of the diaphragm may be visible, producing the 'continuous diaphragm' sign (Fig. 18.10).

Sometimes it may be difficult to differentiate between pneumopericardium and pneumomediastinum. In pneumo-pericardium gas does not extend beyond the aortic root

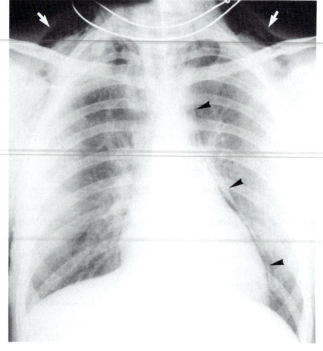

Fig. 18.9 Pneumomediastinum in a man after a car crash. Note linear lucencies in the mediastinum extending into the neck, and subcutaneous emphysema over the supraclavicular fossae (arrows). The mediastinal pleura is outlined by air and displaced laterally (arrowheads).

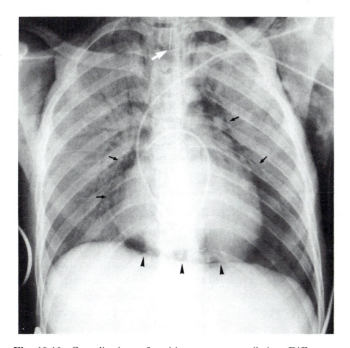

Fig. 18.10 Complications of positive pressure ventilation. Diffuse consolidation in a boy aged 15 following presumed viral pneumonia. Note endotracheal tube (white arrow) and Swan-Ganz catheter, both well positioned. Pneumomediastinum is indicated by linear lucencies in the mediastinum, lateral displacement of the mediastinal pleura (black arrows) and infrapericardial air, producing the 'continuous diaphragm' sign (arrowheads). There is extensive bilateral subcutaneous emphysema.

or much beyond the main pulmonary artery (Fig. 18.14). In pneumomediastinum, gas often outlines the aortic knuckle and extends into the neck. In pneumopericardium a fluid level is often seen on horizontal-beam films, and the distribution of air may alter with changes in the patient's position. The patient's position has little or no effect on a pneumomediastinum. Pneumomediastinum is relatively more common in neonates and infants, and may displace the thymus or resemble a lung cyst.

Mediastinal haemorrhage may result from penetrating or non-penetrating trauma, and be due to venous or arterial bleeding. Many cases are probably unrecognized, as clinical and radiographic signs are absent. Important causes include car accidents, aortic rupture and dissection, and introduction of central venous catheters. There is usually bilateral mediastinal widening (Fig. 18.11), but a localized haematoma may occur (Figs 18.2, 18.19).

Aortic rupture is usually the result of a car accident. Most non-fatal aortic tears occur at the aortic isthmus — the site of the ligamentum arteriosum. Only 10–20% of patients survive the acute episode, but a small number may develop a chronic aneurysm at the site of the tear. The commonest acute radiographic signs are widening of the superior mediastinum, and obscuration of the aortic knuckle (Fig. 18.11). Other radiographic signs include deviation of the left main bronchus anteriorly, inferiorly

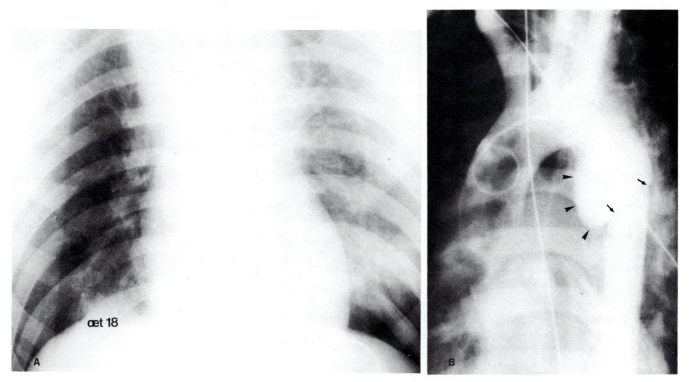

Fig. 18.11 Mediastinal haemorrhage in a youth of 18 after a car crash. **A.** Chest radiograph shows bilateral widening of the superior mediastinum. The aorta is obscured. **B.** Arch aortogram demonstrates an aneurysm of the aortic isthmus (arrowheads) with intimal tear (arrows).

and to the right, and rightward displacement of the trachea, a nasogastric tube or the right parasternal line. A left apical extrapleural cap or a left haemothorax may be visible. Aortography is the definitive investigation, but CT or MRI may be diagnostic.

Cardiac injury may result from penetrating or blunt trauma. Penetrating injuries are usually rapidly fatal but may cause tamponade, ventricular aneurysm or septal defects. Blunt trauma may cause myocardial contusion and infarction.

Oesophageal rupture is usually the result of instrumentation or surgery, but occasionally occurs in penetrating trauma, and is rarely spontaneous due to sudden increase of intraoesophageal pressure (Boerhaave's syndrome). Clinically there is acute mediastinitis, and radiographically there are signs of pneumomediastinum, with or without a pneumothorax or hydropneumothorax, which is usually left-sided. The diagnosis should be confirmed by a swallow using water-soluble contrast medium or barium. The former is safer, and the latter radiographically superior, but carries a theoretical risk of granuloma formation in the mediastinum.

Chylothorax due to damage to the thoracic duct may become apparent hours or days after trauma. Thoracic surgery is the commonest cause.

THE POSTOPERATIVE CHEST

Intrathoracic surgery is performed most frequently for resection of all or part of a lung, or for cardiac disease. This section will discuss the usual acute changes apparent radiographically following such surgery, followed by a description of complications and late changes, and finally a description of thoracic complications of nonthoracic surgery.

THORACOTOMY

Lung resections are usually performed posterolaterally through the fourth or fifth intercostal space. Part of a rib may be resected or the ribs may simply be spread apart. Rib fractures sometimes occur, but often the surgical route is not obvious on the chest X-ray, or is marked only by some narrowing of the intercostal space, or some overlying soft-tissue swelling and subcutaneous emphysema.

Following *pneumonectomy* it is important for the remaining lung to be fully ventilated, and for the mediastinum to remain close to the midline. Excessive mediastinal shift may compromise respiration and venous return to the heart. On the initial postoperative film the trachea should be close to the midline, the remaining lung should appear normal or slightly plethoric, and the pneumonectomy space usually contains a small amount of fluid. A drainage tube may or may not be present in the

space. Over the next several days the pneumonectomy space begins to obliterate by gradual shift of the mediastinum to that side, and accumulation of fluid. The space is usually half-filled within about a week, and completely opacifies over the next 2–3 months (Fig. 18.12). If the mediastinum moves towards the remaining lung, this may indicate too rapid accumulation of fluid in the pneumonectomy space, or atelectasis in the remaining lung. A sudden shift may indicate a bronchopleural fistula (Fig. 18.13).

Following *lobectomy* the remaining lung should expand to fill the space of the resected lobe. Immediately postoperatively, pleural drains are present, preventing accumulation of pleural fluid, and the mediastinum may be shifted to the side of the operation. With hyperinflation of the remaining lung the mediastinum returns to its normal position. When the drains are removed a small pleural effusion commonly occurs, but usually resolves within a few days, perhaps leaving residual pleural thickening.

With *segmental* or *subsegmental lung resections* a cut surface of the lung is oversewn, and air leaks are fairly common, sometimes causing persistent pneumothorax, which may require prolonged drainage. Wire sutures or staples may be visible at the site of a bronchial stump or lesser lung resection.

Complications of thoracotomy

Postoperative spaces may persist following lobectomy and segmental or subsegmental resections. They are air spaces that correspond to the excised lung. Fluid may collect in them, but they usually resolve after a few weeks or months. If they persist and are associated with constitutional symptoms, increasing fluid and pleural thickening, an empyema or bronchopleural fistula should be suspected.

Empyema complicating pneumonectomy, or rarely lobectomy, usually occurs a few weeks after surgery, although it may occur months or years later. Rapid accumulation of fluid may push the mediastinum to the normal side. If a fistula develops between the pneumonectomy space and a bronchus or the skin, the air-fluid level in the space will suddenly drop (Fig. 18.13). Increasing gas in the pneumonectomy space may also indicate infection by a gas-forming organism.

Bronchopleural fistula is a communication between the bronchial tree (or lung tissue) and the pleural space. The commonest cause is a complication of lung surgery, but it may be the result of rupture of a lung abscess, erosion by a lung cancer or penetrating trauma. Bronchopleural fistula complicating complete or partial lung resection may occur early, when it is due to faulty closure of the bronchus, but it more commonly occurs late due to infection or recurrent tumour of the bronchial stump. The usual radiographic appearance is the sudden appearance of, or increase, in the amount of air in the pleural space, with a corresponding decrease in the

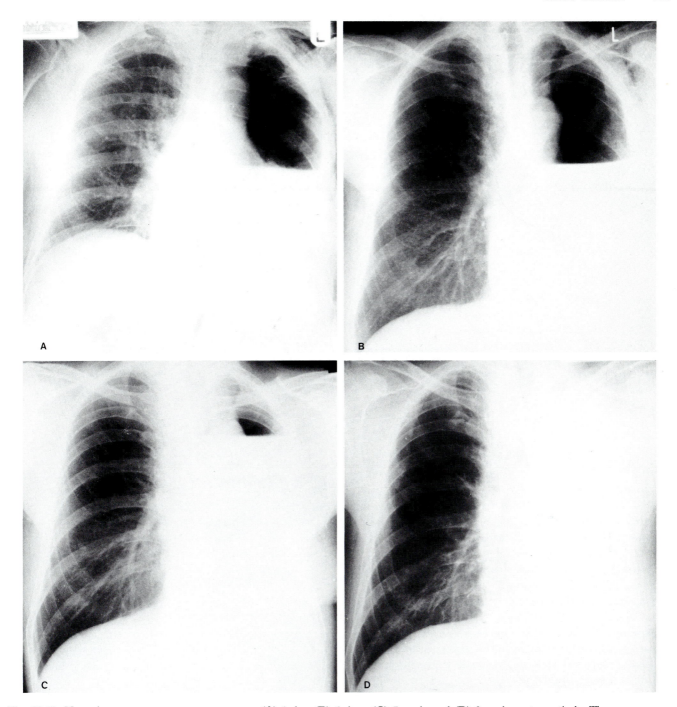

Fig. 18.12 Normal postpneumonectomy appearance. (**A**) 1 day, (**B**) 6 days, (**C**) 5 weeks and (**D**) 8 weeks postoperatively. The pneumonectomy space is gradually obliterated by the rising fluid level and mediastinal shift.

amount of fluid in the space. A fluid level is almost always present (Fig. 18.13). If fluid enters the airways and is aspirated into the remaining lung, widespread consolidation may be seen on the chest X-ray. Sinography of the pleural space or bronchography may demonstrate the fistula.

Pleural fluid is usually seen on the chest X-ray following thoracic surgery. If the amount is excessive it

may be due to bleeding or chylothorax.

Diaphragmatic elevation may indicate phrenic nerve damage and is best assessed by fluoroscopy or ultrasound.

Other pulmonary complications of thoracic surgery include *atelectasis*, *aspiration pneumonia*, *pulmonary embolism* and *pulmonary oedema*, both cardiogenic and noncardiogenic. These may also complicate nonthoracic surgery and are discussed below.

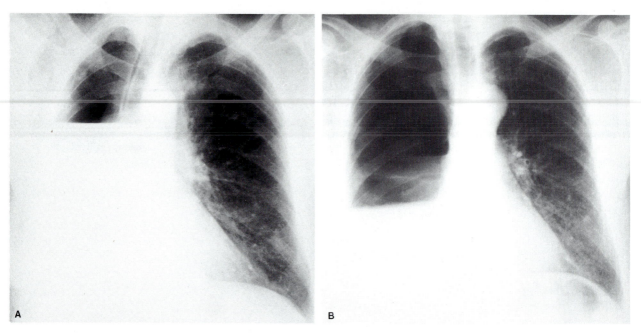

Fig. 18.13 Bronchopleural fistula. **A**. 13 days after right pneumonectomy the space is filling with fluid and the mediastinum is deviated to the right. **B**. Two days later, after coughing up a large amount of fluid, the fluid level has dropped and the mediastinum has returned to the midline. Bronchoscopy confirmed a right bronchopleural fistula.

CARDIAC SURGERY

Most cardiac operations are performed through a *sternotomy* incision, and wire sternal sutures are often seen on the postoperative films (Figs 18.24, 18.25). Mitral valvotomy is now rarely performed via a *thoracotomy* incision, but this route is still used for surgery of coarctation of the aorta, patent ductus arteriosus, Blalock-Taussig shunts and pulmonary artery banding.

Following cardiac surgery, some widening of the cardiovascular silhouette is usual, and represents bleeding and oedema. Marked widening of the mediastinum suggests significant *haemorrhage*, but the necessity for re-exploration is based upon the overall clinical situation. Some air commonly remains in the pericardium following cardiac surgery, so that the signs of *pneumopericardium* may be present (Fig. 18.14).

Pulmonary opacities are very common following open-heart surgery, and left basal shadowing is almost invariable, representing atelectasis. This shadowing usually resolves over a week or two. Small *pleural effusions* are also common in the immediate postoperative period.

Pneumoperitoneum is sometimes seen, due to involvement of the peritoneum by the sternotomy incision. It is of no pathological significance.

Violation of left or right pleural space may lead to a *pneumothorax*. Damage to a major lymphatic vessel may lead to a *chylothorax* or a more localized collection — a *chyloma*. Phrenic nerve damage may cause paresis or paralysis of a hemidiaphragm.

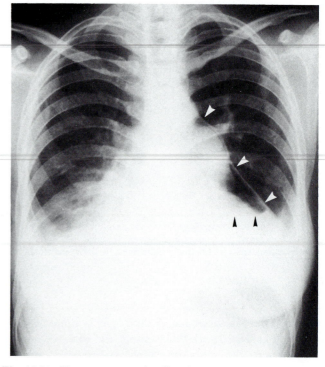

Fig. 18.14 Haemopneumopericardium in a woman two days after closure of atrial septal defect. The pericardium is outlined by air (white arrowheads) which does not extend as high as the aortic arch. A fluid level (black arrowheads) is present in the pericardium, and there are bilateral pleural effusions.

Surgical clips or other metallic markers are sometimes used to mark the ends of coronary artery bypass grafts. *Prosthetic heart valves* are usually visible radiographically, but they may be difficult to see on an underpenetrated film. Their assessment fluoroscopically, angiographically or ultrasonographically is outside the scope of this chapter.

Sternal dehiscence may be apparent radiographically by a linear lucency appearing in the sternum and alteration in position of the sternal sutures on consecutive films. The diagnosis is usually made clinically and may be associated with osteomyelitis. A first or second rib may be fractured when the sternum is spread apart. The importance of this observation is that it may explain chest pain in the postoperative period.

The *post-pericardotomy* syndrome is probably an auto-immune phenomenon, usually occurring in the month after surgery. It presents with fever, pleurisy and pericarditis. Pleural effusions may be visible and the cardiac silhouette may enlarge. Ultrasound will demonstrate pericardial fluid. Patchy consolidation may occur in the lung bases.

LATE APPEARANCES AFTER CHEST SURGERY
Following thoracotomy, the appearance of the chest X-ray may return to normal, or evidence of surgery may persist. Resected ribs or healed rib fractures are usually obvious (Fig. 18.15). There may be irregular regeneration of a rib related to disturbed periosteum. A rib space may be narrowed where a thoracotomy wound has been closed (Fig. 18.15). Rib notching may result from a Blalock-Taussig shunt between subclavian and pulmonary arteries. Pleural thickening often remains after a thoracotomy.

Rearrangement of the remaining lung occurs after lobectomy, so that the anatomy of the fissures may be altered. Following oesophageal surgery, stomach or loops of bowel may produce unusual soft-tissue opacities or fluid levels, if they have been brought up into the chest.

Surgery is now rarely performed for pulmonary tuberculosis, but many patients who have had such surgery are still alive. The object of surgery was to reduce aeration of the infected lung, usually an upper lobe. *Thoracoplasty* involved removal of the posterior parts of usually three or more ribs so that the underlying lung collapsed (Fig. 18.16). Occasionally, thoracoplasty was combined with pneumonectomy for the treatment of chronic tuberculous empyema. An alternative approach was *plombage*, which was the extrapleural insertion of some inert material to collapse the underlying lung. Solid or hollow lucite balls (Fig. 18.17) were commonly used. Other substances included crumpled cellophane packs and paraffin (Fig. 18.18).

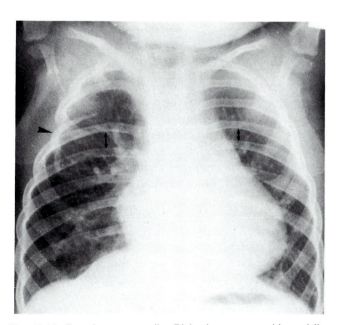

Fig. 18.15 Post-thoracotomy ribs. Right thoracotomy with partially excised regenerating right fourth rib (arrowhead) after repair of tracheo-oesophageal fistula. Left thoracotomy, indicated by narrowed fifth intercostal space, for pulmonary artery banding for multiple ventricular septal defects.

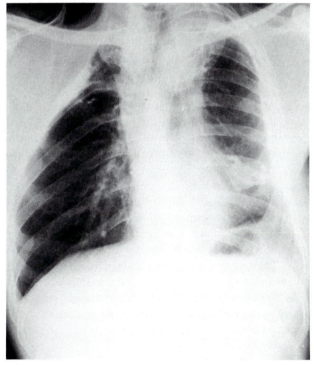

Fig. 18.16 Thoracoplasty. The first five right ribs have been removed. Left upper lobe fibrosis, bilateral apical calcification and extensive left pleural calcification are due to tuberculosis.

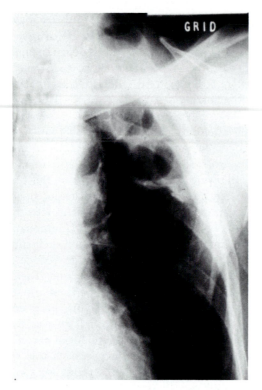

Fig. 18.17 Plombage. Several hollow balls have been inserted extrapleurally at the left apex. The balls are slightly permeable, and the shallow fluid levels do not indicate a complication.

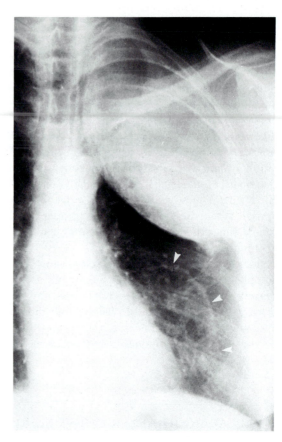

Fig. 18.18 Oleothorax. Plombage has been performed by instilling paraffin extrapleurally through a thoracotomy with excision of the fifth rib. A thin rim of calcification has developed in the extrapleural collection. Some paraffin has tracked inferiorly behind the lung and produced a calcified pleural plaque which is seen en face (arrowhead).

THORACIC COMPLICATIONS OF GENERAL SURGERY

Atelectasis is the commonest pulmonary complication of thoracic or abdominal surgery. Predisposing factors are a long anaesthetic, obesity, chronic lung disease and smoking. It is a result of retained secretions and poor ventilation. Postoperatively it is painful to breath deeply or cough. The chest X-ray usually shows elevation of the diaphragm, due to a poor inspiration. Linear, sometimes curved, opacities are frequently present in the lower zones, and probably represent a combination of sub-segmental volume loss and consolidation (Fig. 18.4B). These shadows usually appear about 24 hours postoperatively and resolve within two or three days.

Pleural effusions are common immediately following abdominal surgery and usually resolve within two weeks. They may be associated with pulmonary infarction. Effusions due to subphrenic infection usually occur later.

Pneumothorax complicating extrathoracic surgery is usually a complication of positive pressure ventilation or central venous line insertion. It may complicate nephrectomy.

Aspiration pneumonitis during anaesthesia is common, but fortunately is usually insignificant. When significant, patchy consolidation appears within a few hours, usually basally or around the hila. Clearing occurs within a few days, unless there is superinfection.

Pulmonary oedema in the post-operative period may be cardiogenic or noncardiogenic. The latter includes fluid overload and the adult respiratory distress syndrome.

Pneumonia may complicate postoperative atelectasis and aspiration pneumonitis. Postoperative pneumonias, therefore, tend to be associated with bilateral basal shadowing.

Subphrenic abscess usually produces elevation of the hemidiaphragm, pleural effusion and basal atelectasis. Loculated gas may be seen below the diaphragm, and fluoroscopy may show splinting of the diaphragm. Subphrenic abscess can be demonstrated by CT or ultrasound.

Pulmonary embolism may produce pulmonary shadowing, pleural effusion or elevation of the diaphragm. However, a normal chest X-ray does not exclude pulmonary embolism, and the investigation of choice is a perfusion lung scan.

THE PATIENT IN INTENSIVE CARE

Patients are admitted to an intensive care ward postoperatively, following major trauma or following circulatory or respiratory failure. A number of monitoring and life-support devices may be used in their care. Radiology plays an important part in the management of these devices.

Central venous pressure (CVP) catheters are used to monitor right atrial pressure. The end of a CVP line needs to be intrathoracic and is ideally in the superior vena cava (Fig. 18.22B). CVP lines may be introduced via an antecubital, subclavian or jugular vein. Subclavian venous puncture carries a risk of pneumothorax and mediastinal haematoma (Fig. 18.19). Rarely, perforation of the subclavian vein leads to fluid collecting in the mediastinum or pleura (Fig. 18.20). All catheters have a potential risk of coiling and knotting, or fracture leading to embolism.

Swan-Ganz catheters are used to measure pulmonary artery and pulmonary wedge pressures. The latter is an index of left atrial pressure. Swan-Ganz catheters are usually introduced via an antecubital or jugular vein. An inflatable balloon at the catheter tip guides it through the right heart. Ideally the end of the catheter should be maintained 5–8 cm (2–3 in) beyond the bifurcation of the main pulmonary artery in either the right or left pulmo-

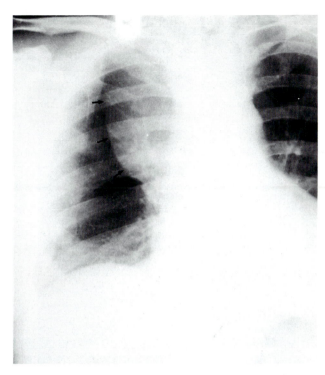

Fig. 18.19 Mediastinal haematoma. Following unsuccessfully attempted placement of a central venous line via the right subclavian vein, a large extrapleural haematoma (arrows) is present.

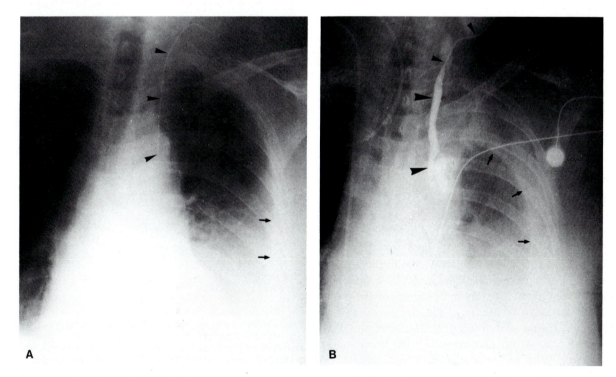

Fig. 18.20 Perforation of innominate vein. **A.** A central venous catheter (arrowheads) has been introduced via the left jugular vein. Its tip points inferiorly, rather than to the right along the axis of the innominate vein. A pleural effusion (arrows) is present. **B.** Next day the effusion is larger. Injection of contrast medium into the catheter (larger arrowheads) demonstrates extravasation and communication with the pleural effusion.

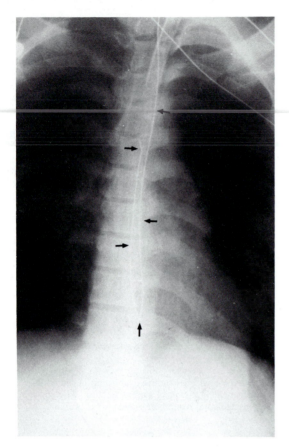

Fig. 18.21 Nasogastric tube coiled in oesophagus. The tube does not reach the stomach, but has folded back on itself (arrows).

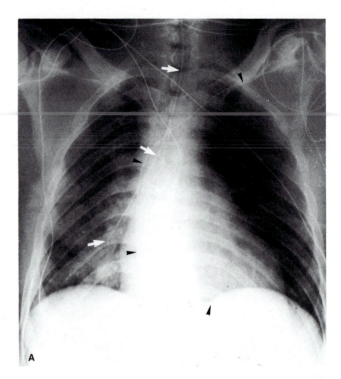

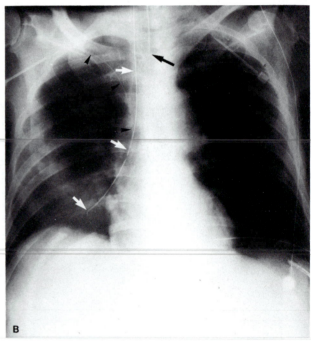

nary artery (Fig. 18.10). When the pulmonary wedge pressure is measured the balloon is inflated, and the flow of blood carries the catheter tip peripherally, to a wedged position. After the measurement has been made the balloon is deflated and the catheter returns to a central position, otherwise there is a risk of pulmonary infarction. The inflation balloon is radiolucent. The balloon should normally be kept deflated to minimize the risk of thrombus formation.

Nasogastric tubes may not reach the stomach or may coil in the oesophagus (Fig. 18.21) or occasionally are inserted into the trachea and into the right bronchus (Fig. 18.22).

Endotracheal tubes are used for access to the airways for ventilation and management of secretions, and also to protect the airway. The chest X-ray is important in assessing the position of the tip of the endotracheal tube relative to the carina. Extension and flexion of the neck may make the tip of an endotracheal tube move by as much as 5 cm. With the neck in neutral position the tip of the tube should ideally be about 5–6 cm above the carina. A tube that is inserted too far usually passes into the right bronchus (Fig. 18.23), with the risk of collapse

Fig. 18.22 Nasogastric tubes in right bronchus. **A.** The nasogastric tube (arrows) passes down the trachea and into the right bronchus. The patient had been 'fed' via the tube, causing patchy consolidation in the right lung. A temporary pacing electrode (arrowheads) is present. **B.** This patient, with chronic renal failure, developed peritonitis following peritoneal dialysis. Drains are present in the abdomen. A nasogastric tube (white arrows) has been passed beyond an endotracheal tube (black arrow) and into the right bronchus! Two venous lines are present; the right-sided catheter (arrowheads) is well placed for central venous pressure measurements.

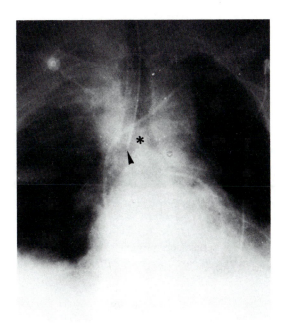

Fig. 18.23 Endotracheal tube too low. The tip of the endotracheal tube (arrowhead) is beyond the carina (asterisk) and in the right bronchus. A well-positioned Swan-Ganz catheter is present.

of the left lung. If the inflated cuff of the tube dilates the trachea, there is a risk of ischaemic damage to the tracheal mucosa. A late complication of an overinflated cuff is tracheostenosis.

Tracheostomy tubes are usually inserted for long-

term ventilatory support. The tube tip should be situated centrally in the airway at the level of T3 (Fig. 18.2). Acute complications of tracheostomy include pneumothorax, pneumomediastinum and subcutaneous emphysema. Long-term complications include tracheal ulceration, stenosis and perforation.

Positive pressure ventilation may be complicated by interstitial emphysema, pneumomediastinum, pneumothorax and subcutaneous emphysema (Fig. 18.10).

Pleural tubes are used to treat pleural effusions and pneumothoraces. If the patient is being nursed supine, the tip of the tube should be placed anteriorly and superiorly for a pneumothorax, and posteriorly and inferiorly for an effusion. A radio-opaque line usually runs along pleural tubes, and is interrupted where there are side holes. It is important to check that all the side holes are within the thorax (Figs 18.2, 18.4). Tracks may remain on the chest X-ray following removal of chest tubes, causing tubular or ring shadows.

Mediastinal drains are usually present following sternotomy. Apart from their position, they look like pleural tubes.

Intra-aortic balloon pumps are used in patients with cardiogenic shock, often following cardiac surgery. The pump comprises a catheter, the end of which is surrounded by an elongated, inflatable balloon. It is inserted via a femoral artery and is positioned in the descending thoracic aorta. The pattern of inflation and deflation of the balloon is designed to increase coronary perfusion

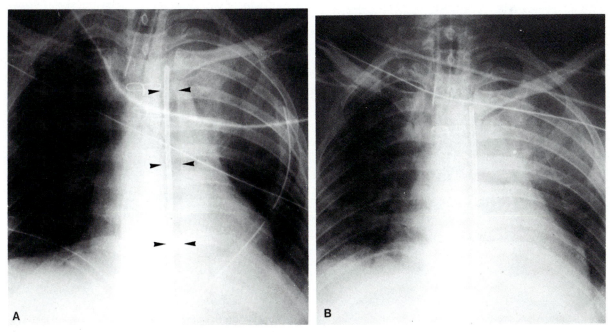

Fig. 18.24 Intra-aortic balloon pump. Post-coronary artery bypass surgery. **A**. Bilateral pleural and mediastinal drains and endotracheal tube are present. The pump is well sited, and its balloon is seen to be inflated (arrowheads). **B**. The drains have been removed. When this radiograph was exposed the balloon was deflated.

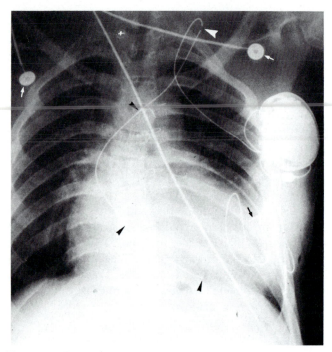

Fig. 18.25 Fractured pacing wire. Patient with surgically repaired complete atrioventricular canal. A permanent transvenous pacing system is present; the power unit is in the left axilla; the electrode (arrowheads) reaches the right ventricle by traversing the innominate vein, superior vena cava and right atrium. The electrode is fractured (white arrowhead). Note disconnected epicardial electrodes (black arrow) and ECG electrodes (white arrows).

during diastole, and to reduce the left ventricular afterload. The ideal position of the catheter tip is just distal to the origin of the left subclavian artery (Fig. 18.24). If the catheter tip is advanced too far it may occlude the left subclavian artery, and if it is too distal the balloon may occlude branches of the abdominal aorta.

Pacemakers may be permanent or temporary. Temporary epicardial wires are sometimes inserted during cardiac surgery, and may be seen as thin, almost hair-like metallic opacities overlying the heart. Temporary pacing electrodes are usually inserted transvenously via a subclavian or jugular vein (Fig. 18.22A). If a patient is not pacing properly, a chest X-ray may reveal that the position of the electrode tip is unstable, or a fracture in the wire may be seen (Fig. 18.25). A full discussion of the radiology of pacemakers is outside the scope of this chapter.

RADIATION INJURY OF THE LUNG

Radiation injury of the lung usually results from treatment of a pulmonary or mediastinal neoplasm by radiotherapy. It may also be a complication of the treatment of breast cancer. The changes seen on the chest X-ray are often remarkably geometric, and correspond to the shape of the treatment portal.

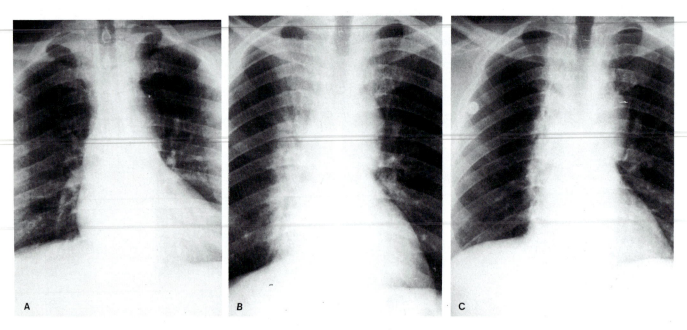

Fig. 18.26 Radiation pneumonitis in a man of 45 with diffuse histiocytic lymphoma who developed upper thoracic spinal cord compression. **A.** After surgical decompression the lungs are clear and the patient commenced radiotherapy to the spine. **B.** Ten weeks later there is paraspinal consolidation with air bronchograms. **C.** 14 weeks after treatment paraspinal pulmonary fibrosis has developed. The changes correspond to the shape of the treatment portal.

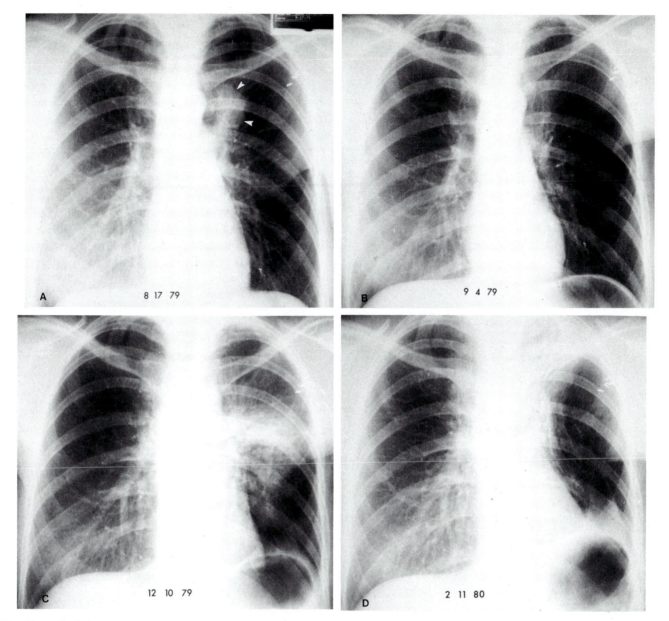

Fig. 18.27 Radiation pneumonitis in a woman of 32 one year after a left mastectomy for carcinoma. Surgical clips overlie the left axilla. **A**. Medial left upper zone opacity (arrowheads) is caused by metastasis to left internal mammary lymph nodes. **B**. 18 days later, following radiotherapy, the left upper mass has gone. **C**. 16 weeks after treatment there is extensive consolidation in the left mid and upper zones. **D**. Five months after treatment there is gross left upper lobe fibrosis, the mediastinum has shifted to the left and the left hemidiaphragm is elevated. The patient remained asymptomatic throughout this time.

The earliest pathological changes in the lung are alveolar and bronchiolar desquamation and accumulation of exudate in the alveoli. This is followed by organization and fibrosis.

The affect of radiation on the lung depends upon several factors. Healthy lung tissue is more resistant to damage than diseased lung. Previous radiotherapy and associated chemotherapy increase the likelihood of fibrosis. The total dose, the time over which it is given and the volume of lung irradiated are other factors. Radiographic changes are rare at a dose rate of 20 Gy (2000 rad) over 2–3 weeks, but are usual with doses of 60 Gy (6000 rad) or more over 5–6 weeks.

The radiological changes correspond to the pathology. The acute or exudative phase is not usually evident until a month or more after treatment, and may take up to six months to appear.

Consolidation, usually with some volume loss, occurs. It

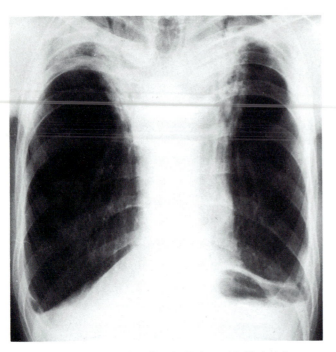

Fig. 18.28 Massive radiation fibrosis. Patient with Hodgkin's disease treated with mediastinal irradiation and chemotherapy (MOPP — Bleo). Note gross bilateral upper lobe fibrosis with extensive air bronchogram.

is not segmental or lobar, but corresponds to the shape of the radiation portal. An air bronchogram may be visible. The patient is usually asymptomatic, but may have a pyrexia or cough. *Fibrosis* then occurs, and is usually complete by 9–12 months (Fig. 18.26). Fibrosis, if extensive and severe enough, may cause displacement of fissures, the hila or mediastinum, and compensatory hyperinflation of the less affected lung (Fig. 18.27). Very dense fibrosis may produce an air bronchogram (Fig. 18.28).

A pleural effusion as a result of irradiation is rare, and is more likely to be due to the malignant disease being treated. Pericardial effusion may occur as a late complication of irradiation. Necrosis of ribs or a clavicle may be seen on the chest X-ray following radiotherapy.

The diagnosis of radiation pneumonitis and fibrosis is usually easy, based on the history and characteristic shape, but occasionally apical fibrosis following treatment of breast cancer may resemble tuberculosis.

REFERENCES AND SUGGESTIONS FOR FURTHER READING

Trauma
Ball, T., McCrory, R., Smith, J. O., Clements, J. L., Jr. (1982) Traumatic diaphragmatic hernia: errors in diagnosis. *American Journal of Roentgenology*, **138**, 633–637.
Cochlin, D. L., Shaw, M. R. P. (1978) Traumatic lung cysts following minor blunt chest trauma. *Clinical Radiology*, **29**, 151–154.
Fishbone, G., Robbins, D. I., Osborn, D. J., Grnja, V. (1973) Trauma to the thoracic aorta and great vessels. *Radiologic Clinics of North America*, **11**, 543–554.
Harvey-Smith, W., Bush, W., Northrop, C. (1980) Traumatic bronchial rupture. *American Journal of Roentgenology*, **134**, 1189–1193.
Parkin, G. J. S. (1973) The radiology of perforated oesophagus. *Clinical Radiology*, **24**, 324–332.
Reynolds, J., Davis, J. T. (1966) Injuries of the chest wall, pleura, pericardium, lungs, bronchi and oesophagus. *Radiologic Clinics of North America*, **4**, 383.
Sefczek, D. M., Sefczek, R. J., Deeb, S. L. (1983) Radiographic signs of acute traumatic rupture of the thoracic aorta. *American Journal of Roentgenology*, **141**, 1259–1262.
Williams, J. R., Stembridge, V. A. (1964) Pulmonary contusion secondary to non-penetrating chest trauma. *American Journal of Roentgenology*, **91**, 284–290.
Wiot, J. F. (1975) The radiologic manifestations of blunt chest trauma. *Journal of the American Medical Association*, **231**, 500.

The postoperative chest
Carter, A. R., Sostman, H. D., Curtis, A. M., Swett, H. A. (1983) Thoracic alterations after cardiac surgery. *American Journal of Roentgenology*, **140**, 475–481.
Goodman, L. R. (1980) Postoperative chest radiograph: I. Alterations after abdominal surgery. *American Journal of Roentgenology*, **134**, 533–541.
Goodman, L. R. (1980) Postoperative chest radiograph: II. Alterations after major intrathoracic surgery. *American Journal of Roentgenology*, **134**, 803–813.
Goodman, L. R., Putman, C. E. (1983) *Intensive Care Radiology: Imaging of the Critically Ill.* 2nd edn. W. B. Saunders, Philadelphia.
Melamed, M., Hipona, F. A., Reynes, C. J., Barker, W. L., Pardes, S. (1977) *The Adult Postoperative Chest.* Charles, C. Thomas, Springfield, IL.
Shipley, R. T. (1988) The chest radiograph after extrathoracic surgery. *Seminars in Roentgenology*, **23**, 49–60.
Spirn, P. W., Gross, G. W., Wechsler, R. J., Steiner, R. M. (1988) Radiology of the chest after thoracic surgery. *Seminars in Roentgenology*, **23**, 9–31.
Thorsen, M. K., Goodman, L. R. (1988) Extracardiac complications of cardiac surgery. *Seminars in Roentgenology*, **23**, 32–48.
Wechsler, R. J., Steiner, R. M., Kinori, I. (1988) Monitoring the monitors: the radiology of thoracic catheter, wires and tubes. *Seminars in Roentgenology*, **23**, 61–84.

Radiation injury of the lung
Boushy, S. F., Belgason, A. H., Borth, L. B. (1970) The effect of radiation on the lung and bronchial tree. *American Journal of Roentgenology*, **108**, 284–292.
Freedman, G. S., Lofgren, S. B., Kilgerman, M. M. (1974) Radiation-induced changes in pulmonary perfusion. *Radiology*, **112**, 435–437.
Gross, N. J. (1977) Pulmonary effects of radiation therapy. *Annals of Internal Medicine*, **86**, 81–92.
Libshitz, H. I., Southard, M. E. (1974) Complications of radiation therapy: the thorax. *Seminars in Roentgenology*, **9**, 41–49.
Polansky, S. M., Ravin, C. E., Prosnitz, L. R. (1980) Lung changes after breast irradiation. *American Journal of Roentgenology*, **139**, 101–105.

CHAPTER 19

THE CHEST IN CHILDREN

Donald Shaw

TECHNIQUES

Plain radiographs remain the basis for evaluation of the chest in childhood. In the neonate, satisfactory films can be obtained in incubators using modern mobile X-ray apparatus. The baby lies on the cassette and the film is exposed. Although automatic triggering of the exposure can be made using variations of temperature at the nostril and of electrical impedance across the chest in the differing phases of respiration, an experienced radiographer will usually be able to judge the end of inspiration. An adequate inspiration will be with the right hemidiaphragm at the level of the eighth rib posteriorly. Films in expiration frequently show a sharp kink in the trachea to the right and varying degrees of opacification of the lung fields, with apparent enlargement of the heart. Films should be well collimated and the baby positioned as straight as possible and lordotic films avoided, especially if the heart size is of particular interest. As much monitoring equipment as possible should be removed. Magnification radiography in the neonate allows better evaluation of the lung granularity in hyaline membrane disease, but the construction of most incubators makes this technique difficult and its vogue has passed.

Children over five years can usually cooperate sufficiently to stand for a PA film like adults. Below this age some form of chest stand is needed in which an assistant, preferably the mother, can hold the child in front of a cassette with a suspended protective lead apron behind which she stands. With proper collimation, the dose to the mother is small and her position allows the child to be held straighter than from a position to the side. The difference between a PA and an AP projection in the small child is usually negligible. High kilovoltage techniques with added filtration and the use of a grid allow evaluation of the trachea and major bronchi, which is important in stridor, in investigating mediastinal masses and to assess isomerism in congenital heart disease.

Fluoroscopy. Limitation of radiation exposure is vital in childhood, but quick fluoroscopic examination of the chest can frequently prove extremely useful, in particular, in the evaluation of differing lung radiolucencies in suspected foreign-body aspiration. With obstructive emphysema, the effected lung will show little volume change in respiration and the mediastinum will swing contralaterally in expiration. Prior to the advent of computed tomography, fluoroscopy had been advocated for the detection of dubious lung metastases.

A *barium swallow* is a useful adjunct to the evaluation of paediatric lung disease, especially when there is stridor, or mediastinal masses or vascular anomalies are suspected.

Tomography. Conventional tomography generally gives poor results in children, usually because the time of traversing the arc is a relatively long time for the child to be still. The indication was typically to detect metastases, especially in Wilm's tumour or osteosarcoma. *Computed tomography*, which is superior for this despite the larger radiation dose, has also been used to evaluate mediastinal masses. If such a mass is posterior and adjacent to the vertebral column, intrathecal water-soluble contrast medium before CT scanning has been advocated, but intraspinal extension can usually be detected without this.

Angiography. Angiography is infrequently used in extracardiac chest pathology. It provides valuable information, however, in arteriovenous malformation and pulmonary sequestrations. *Digital vascular imaging* has proved a less invasive technique in such cases. *Embolization of bronchial arteries* has been used in bronchiectatic severe haemorrhage.

Radionuclide scanning. Perfusion studies with technetium-99 m macroaggregates are well established in adults, but in children, combination with a ventilation scan using krypton-81m is a more useful technique in investigating the small lung, differing radiolucency and suspected bronchiectasis.

Ultrasound. Ultrasound has a relatively small role. It can be particularly useful in detecting the correct site for aspiration of pleural or pericardial effusions, and may show whether a mass close to the chest wall is solid or cystic.

MRI. Experience in the use of this method is increas-

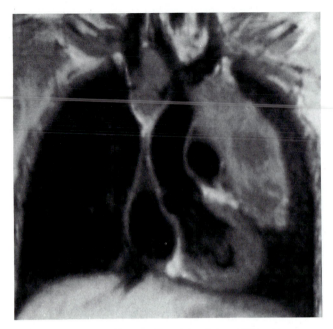

Fig. 19.1 Coronal MRI scan (T$_1$-weighted) in a child with a mediastinal mass. Note how the heart and great vessels are readily differentiated by low signal due to blood flow from the glandular masses due to Hodgkin's disease.

ing. The advantages of an inherently higher contrast resolution are partly offset by image degradation, particularly due to respiratory movement. The longer scanning times often associated with a noisy environment may require the child to have a general anaesthetic or at least to be heavily sedated. Evaluation of mediastinal structures, however (Fig. 19.1), has proved successful, particularly in cases of tumour, aberrant pulmonary vessels and extrinsic compressive lesions of the airways. Extension into and involvement of the spinal canal and spinal cord is also well assessed (Fig. 12.13). MRI has proved particularly useful in the differentiation of physiologically prominent thymic shadows from shadows caused by a pathological process such as lymphoma. As elsewhere in the body, MRI is of value in the evaluation of musculoskeletal lesions, particularly rib and shoulder girdle tumours.

As yet, parenchymal lesions cannot be investigated with as good a resolution as can be achieved by CT, the preferable technique for evaluation and enumeration of pulmonary metastases and detection of calcified lesions.

SPECIFIC FEATURES OF THE CHEST RADIOGRAPH IN CHILDREN

The thymus. The normal thymus is a frequent cause of widening of the superior mediastinum during the first years of life. The lateral margin often shows an undulation — the thymic wave — which corresponds to the indentations of the ribs on the inner surface of the thoracic cage. Particularly on the right, the thymus may have a triangular 'sail-like' configuration. The thymus may involute in times of stress, and a decrease in size can be induced by steroids. At times, the differentiation of physiological thymus from pathology in the anterior mediastinum can be difficult. Ultrasound examination will usually differentiate cystic lesions from the homogeneous normal thymic tissue. Occasionally the normal thymus can act as a significant space-occupying lesion in the superior mediastinum and in such cases differentiation may be helped by computed tomography or MRI.

The cardiothoracic ratio. In toddlers, the cardiothoracic ratio can at times exceed 50% and care should be exercised in overdiagnosis of cardiomegaly.

Kink of the trachea to the right. This is a frequent feature of a chest film taken in less than full inspiration. This is a physiological buckling and does not represent a mass lesion.

The soft tissues may be prominent in children, and the anterior axillary fold crossing the chest wall can at times mimic a pneumothorax. Similarly, skin folds can at times cast confusing shadows. Plaits of hair over the upper chest can mimic pulmonary infiltrations.

Pleural effusions. Whereas in adults an early sign of pleural effusion is blunting of the costophrenic angles, in childhood it is more common to see separation of the lung from the chest wall with reasonable preservation of the clarity of the costophrenic angles, and accentuation of the lung fissures.

THE SMALL LUNG

Discovery of a small lung on a radiograph can be elucidated by ventilation and perfusion radionuclide lung

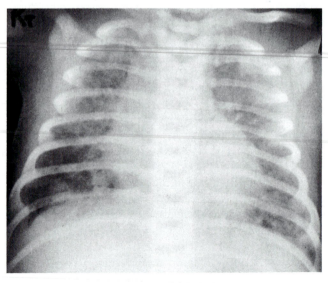

Fig. 19.2 Wet lung, or transient tachypnoea of the newborn. Patchy parenchymal shadowing on the first day of life.

scans using krypton-81 and technetium-99 m macro-aggregates. The complete absence of V–Q in one lung in the presence of an ipsilateral opaque hemithorax, with mediastinal shift to the affected side, is highly suggestive of a diagnosis of pulmonary aplasia or of extreme pulmonary hypoplasia.

The complete absence of perfusion in a small lung, with a decreased ventilation, is typical of congenital absence of the pulmonary artery. Both perfusion and ventilation are shown to be decreased in the presence of a small hemithorax, as may be seen in *MacLeod's syndrome*, with postinfective maldevelopment, with aplasias of single lobes and with pulmonary hypoplasia. A segmental perfusion defect in a fully ventilated lung is associated with pulmonary sequestration.

RESPIRATORY DISTRESS IN THE NEWBORN

Transient tachypnoea of the newborn, or wet lung disease (Fig. 19.2)
The amount of fluid in the newborn lung varies, but typically is quickly cleared after birth. Some babies, however, show a transient respiratory distress due to excess lung fluid. Predisposing conditions include prematurity, a diabetic mother and Caesarian section. The radiographs show diffuse parenchymal patchy shadowing with perihilar streakiness. The prognosis in this condition is good and there is usually progressive clearing, complete within two or three days.

Hyaline membrane disease (Fig. 19.3)
In this condition a deficiency of the pulmonary surfactant leads to alveolar collapse. Conditions which predispose to this include prematurity, Caesarean section and perinatal asphyxia. In mild hyaline membrane disease, the radiological appearances consist of a mild granularity through out the lung fields. As the condition becomes more severe, an air bronchogram becomes apparent. In the most severe cases the lungs are virtually opaque, with loss of differentiation of the cardiac and thymic and diaphragmatic contours. Uncomplicated hyaline membrane disease is a symmetrical condition.

Bronchopulmonary dysplasia (Fig. 19.4)
Severe hyaline membrane disease is typically treated by artificial ventilation of the lungs. If ventilation needs to be prolonged (especially if high pressures and high inspiratory oxygen tensions are required), damage can occur to the lungs. The hyaline membrane present in the alveoli becomes organized and fibrous tissue develops within the lungs. As a consequence, areas of the lungs collapse, with compensatory emphysema developing in residual aerated alveoli. This leads to a coarse reticulation and at times to variable amounts of segmental collapse, and occasionally to considerable areas of localized

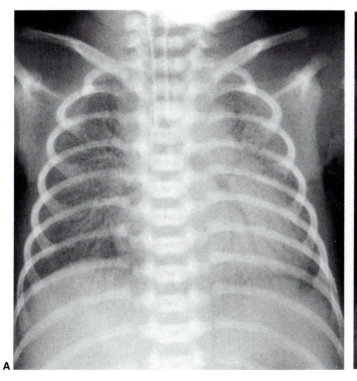
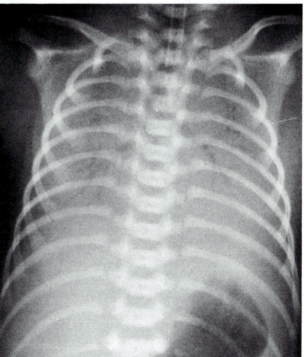

A   B

Fig. 19.3 Hyaline membrane disease. **A.** Mild changes aged 1 day — fine reticulonodular shadowing with accentuation of the air bronchogram. Endotracheal tube. **B.** More advanced changes aged 3 days — marked opacification with loss of diaphragmatic and cardiac contours.

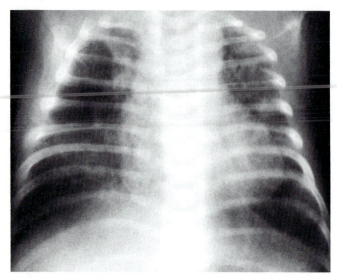

Fig. 19.4 Bronchopulmonary dysplasia. Patchy shadowing from areas of loss of volume and fibrosis, with areas of compensatory emphysema, especially in the right upper lobe.

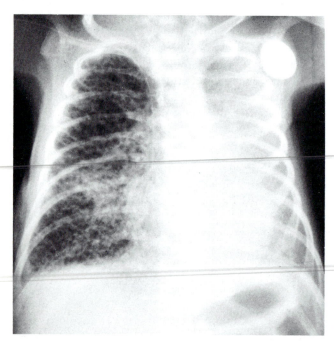

Fig. 19.5 Pulmonary interstitial emphysema. Fine reticular shadowing in the right lung with deviation of the mediastinum contra-laterally. Hyaline membrane disease in the left lung.

emphysema. Whereas hyaline membrane disease, if un-complicated, and transient tachypnoea of the newborn will quickly resolve, bronchopulmonary dysplasia can lead to severe respiratory distress lasting months and may end in respiratory failure and death.

Pulmonary interstitial emphysema (Fig. 19.5)

In this condition gas enters the interstitial tissues of the lungs and gives rise to multiple small lucencies

throughout the lung fields. Some of these lucencies are due to air passing from the interstitial tissue into the relatively large lymphatics of the newborn lungs. A lung affected by interstitial emphysema is frequently larger than the contralateral one and may lead to deviation of the mediastinum. If bilateral, venous return to the heart can be impeded. Interstitial emphysema is a frequent precursor of *pneumothorax* (Fig. 19.6) and pneumo-mediastinum. At times, the child being artificially ventilated for hyaline membrane disease will undergo marked deterioration, with the appearance of a bloodstained tracheal aspirate. This is frequently due to *pulmonary haemorrhage* and is accompanied by a marked increase in the opacification of the lungs as the alveoli become filled with haemorrhagic oedema. If the child's condition stabilizes, the oedema is usually quickly resorbed, but such a haemorrhage can frequently be a terminal event. It is important in the evaluation of neonatal respiratory distress to be adequately acquainted with the obstetric and maternal history. If there is a history of prolonged rupture of the membranes, patchy shadowing seen in the newborn lungs may well be due to *intrauterine pneumonia*. If there has been intrauterine respiratory distress, *aspiration of meconium* can lead to respiratory embarrassment. The lungs typically show bilateral, symmetrical, rather coarse shadowing, with frequent over-distention, complicated from time to time by pneumothorax and pneumo-mediastinum. Resolution of meconium aspiration can be prolonged. The *Mikity-Wilson syndrome* is essentially a radiological appearance consisting of diffuse interstitial infiltrations giving rise to a multicystic appearance. Onset is usually accompanied by apnoea and cyanosis in pre-

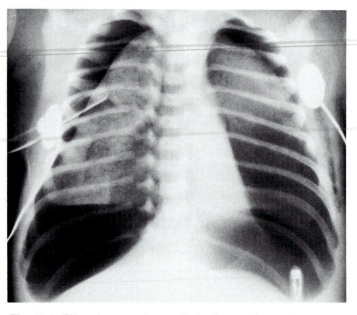

Fig. 19.6 Bilateral pneumothoraces in hyaline membrane disease. Right intercostal drain.

mature babies, later in the first week of life. Episodes of aspiration probably account for at least part of the syndrome, and if resolution does not occur, the condition can at times progress to bronchopulmonary dysplasia.

Pleural effusions

In the newborn these may be part of hydrops fetalis or of congestive cardiac failure. Chylothorax is the most common condition, causing a large pleural effusion; such effusions most frequently occur in the right pleural cavity when unilateral and can lead to respiratory distress with deviation of the mediastinum. With repeated pleural aspiration the effusion usually disappears over a period of a week or two.

Congenital lobar emphysema

Gross overinflation of an upper and middle lobe in this condition leads to infantile respiratory distress with contralateral deviation of the mediastinum, and compression of the other lobes of the same lung. Excision is often necessary. A similar but less florid appearance can be produced by a persistent ductus arteriosus obstructing the left upper lobe.

Cystic adenomatoid malformation

This rare congenital cystic anomaly can lead to deviation of the mediastinum and compression of adjacent normal lung, leading to neonatal distress, or may present as

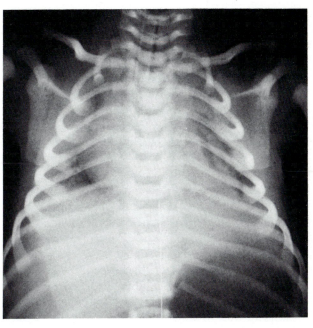

Fig. 19.8 Pulmonary hypoplasia. The rib cage shows the typical triangular configuration. An umbilical aortic catheter is present.

repeated localized pneumonia. The cysts, which may be filled with fluid in the neonatal period, are usually obvious.

Congenital diaphragmatic hernia (Fig. 19.7)

This is most frequently through the posterolateral part of the diaphragm, more frequently on the left. The hemithorax is filled with stomach or gut and as the newborn baby swallows gas, distension leads to respiratory embarrassment with contralateral deviation of the mediastinum. Surgical correction is urgently required; otherwise the condition is frequently fatal. The ipsilateral lung is usually hypoplastic. Congenital heart disease is an important association.

Pulmonary hypoplasia (Fig. 19.8)

This condition is frequently lethal, and is often associated with prenatal obstructive uropathy or renal aplasia. The lungs are small and the thoracic configuration triangular. Hypoplastic lungs are seen in several *skeletal dysplasias* such as asphyxiating thoracic dystrophy.

At times it is difficult to differentiate whether respiratory distress is due to lung disease or to congenital heart disease. However the clinical findings and the response to oxygenation and artificial ventilation will frequently allow such differentiation. Real-time cardiac ultrasound considerably facilitates diagnosis of structural anomalies of the neonatal heart, but at times resort must be made to formal cardiac catheterization.

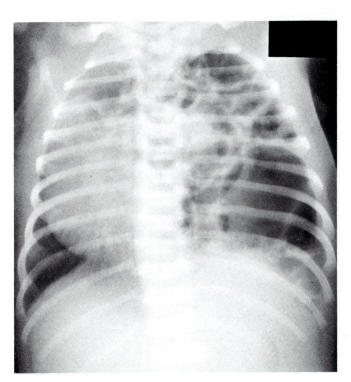

Fig. 19.7 Diaphragmatic hernia. Stomach and intestine occupy the left hemithorax with deviation of the mediastinum to the right.

CONGENITAL PULMONARY SEQUESTRATION
(Fig. 19.9)

This is an abnormality of development in which a portion of the lung shows separation from the normal bronchial tree and blood supply, though retaining some characteristics of lung tissue. Cases can be divided into intralobar, lying within the lung, and extralobar, in which the sequestrated segment develops enclosed in its own pleura (when it is termed by some 'an accessory lung'). In intralobar sequestration there is a nonfunctioning portion of the lung usually lying posteriorly in the left lower lobe. The right lower lobe is the next most common situation, and other lobes are rarely affected. Typically the segment is not connected with the normal bronchial tree, and when communication is established it is usually in association with infection. The radiological appearances are of a soft-tissue mass in the posterior part of the lower lobe, usually on the left contiguous with the diaphragm. If connection has been established with the bronchial tree, air-containing cystic masses with or without air-fluid levels will be seen. Bronchographic contrast medium rarely enters the lesion. The bronchial tree is spread round the mass and is typically complete in the number of its divisions. Extralobar sequestrations are much less common, and usually interposed between the interior surface of the left lower lobe and the diaphragm. They are frequently associated with other congenital anomalies and found incidentally during neonatal autopsies. Left-sided congenital diaphragmatic hernia may be associated.

Intralobar sequestrations typically derive their arterial blood supply from the aorta, usually the descending thoracic aorta, occasionally the abdominal aorta. Usually the venous drainage is via the pulmonary venous system, but occasionally via the inferior vena cava or azygos system. In contrast to the intralobar variety, venous drainage of extralobar sequestration is usually via the inferior vena cava, azygos or portal venous systems. The arterial supply is frequently from the abdominal aorta or one of its branches. The diagnosis of sequestrated segment should be borne in mind whenever an unusual abscess, cavity or cystic lesion is seen, particularly at the left base, and in all cases showing recurrent infection in one part of the lung.

CONGENITAL BRONCHIAL ATRESIA

This abnormality consists of an atresia of a lobar or smaller segment of bronchus, and particularly affects the apical posterior segment of the bronchus of the left upper lobe. Mucous secretions inspissated within the patent airways distal to the atresia can produce an elliptical mass. Peripheral to this, collateral air drift causes overinflation. Fluoroscopy will show expiratory air-trapping in the in-

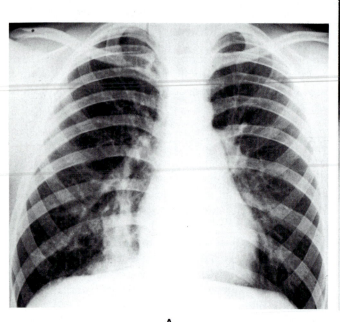

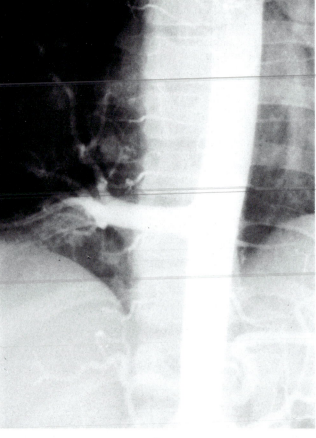

A   B

Fig. 19.9 Pulmonary sequestration. **A**. Consolidation in the right lower lobe was associated with absent bronchial filling on bronchography. **B**. Angiography demonstrated a large feeding artery arising from the right of the descending thoracic aorta.

volved segments and the vascular supply is diminished. Although the lesion may be associated with infection, it is usually discovered on routine chest radiography.

PULMONARY ARTERIOVENOUS FISTULAE

Arteriovenous fistulae are commonly asymptomatic, but some patients will show cyanosis, clubbing and polycythaemia and others will present with haemoptysis. About half of the patients with arteriovenous fistulae in the lungs (Fig. 19.10) will show such abnormal communications elsewhere in the skin and other organs (Rendu-Osler-Weber syndrome). Although the large fistulae typically present rounded homogeneous masses with enlarged serpiginous vessels radiating to the hilum, there is a high incidence of multiple lesions in the lungs and if resection is contemplated, careful angiographic evaluation of both lungs should be carried out preoperatively. Digital vascular imaging has facilitated this.

MUCOVISCIDOSIS (Cystic Fibrosis of the Pancreas)

Chronic suppuration in the lungs is an important feature of this condition, in which many organ systems are involved. The lungs appear normal at birth but poor clearance of bronchial secretions leads to obstruction, particularly of the smaller bronchi. In infancy this can lead to overdistension of the lungs, resulting in flattening of the diaphragms, sternal bowing and increased dorsal kyphosis. Infiltration of the bronchial walls by lymphocytes and plasma cells is seen radiologically as peribronchial thickening, particularly noticeable in bronchi seen end-on. Small discrete opacities are seen in later childhood in the periphery of the lung fields, due to small peripheral abscesses. When these burst into the bronchioles they remain as small thin-walled air spaces. Segmental bronchiectasis is seen consequent upon segmental collapse and consolidation. The upper lobes are more frequently involved in the bronchiectasis associated with cystic fibrosis than in other forms. Parabronchial abscesses can give rise to a more specific form of bronchiectasis, with characteristic rounded shadows arising close to the medium-sized bronchi with a widespread irregular distribution throughout the lung fields (Fig. 19.11). Pulmonary suppuration can lead to hilar lymph node enlargement. The hilar shadows may also be enlarged in the later stages of the disease, when pulmonary hypertension arises as a complication. In later childhood

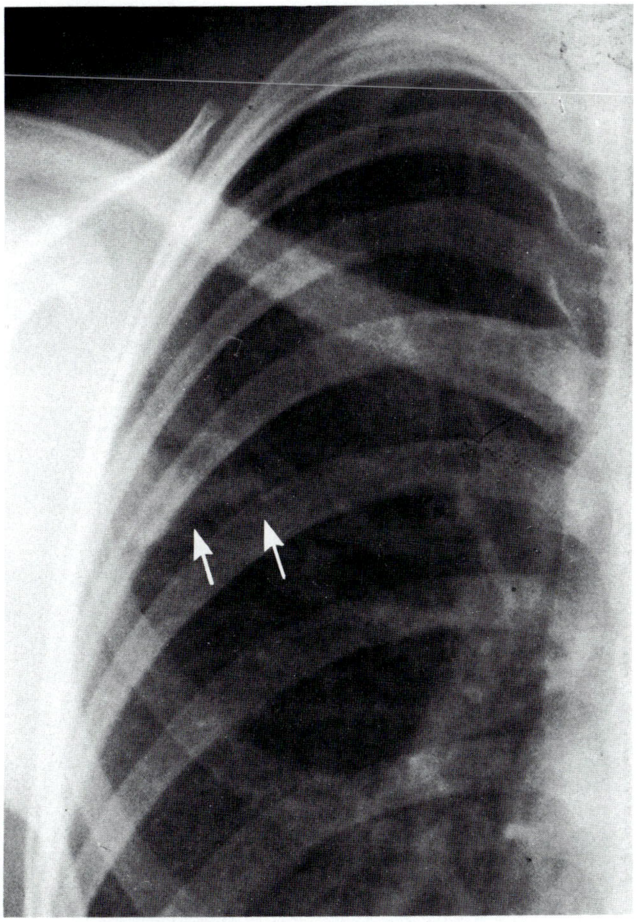

Fig. 19.10 Arteriovenous malformation. Peripheral serpiginous dilated blood vessels in the right upper lobe.

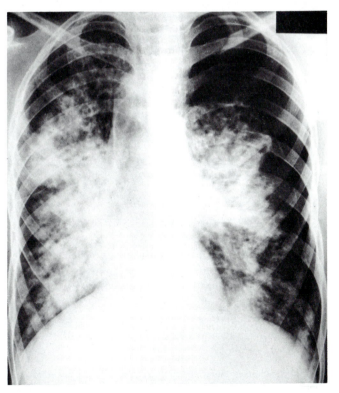

Fig. 19.11 Advanced cystic fibrosis (mucoviscidosis). Gross peribronchial shadowing with confluent pneumonic shadowing. There is a left pneumothorax with slight displacement of the mediastinum to the right.

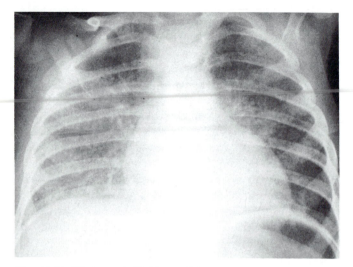

Fig. 19.12   Histiocytosis X. Fine nodularity in both lung fields.

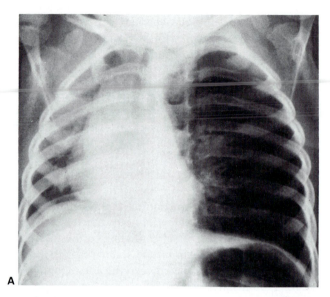

A

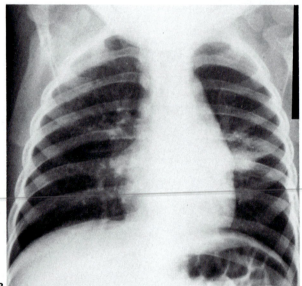

B

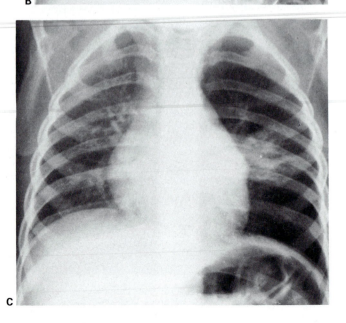

C

peripheral areas of emphysema arise as a result of the fibrotic changes occurring more centrally.

Pneumothorax is an important complication in the later stages of the disease and can lead to dramatic deterioration. The emphysematous changes are usually associated with a relatively narrow heart shadow, but cardiac enlargement in cor pulmonale is usually a sign of a poor prognosis. Although the infections associated are usually staphylococcal, *Pseudomonas* or other Gram-negative infections, superinfection with tuberculosis and *Aspergillus* can occur. In the latter this may be associated with total collapse of the lung or extensive variable areas of consolidation, sometimes with considerable parenchymal destruction. Repeated suppuration can lead to severe haemorrhage, and bronchial artery embolization has been used to control such life-threatening episodes.

Pleural disease is an uncommon feature, but is recognized as a late complication, when it can compromise selection for heart-lung transplantation, in which preoperative CT evaluation has proved useful.

LANGERHAN'S CELL HISTIOCYTOSIS
(*Histiocytosis X*)

In childhood, bone and central nervous system manifestations are frequently more prominent than lung involvement. Fine widespread nodularity can at times resemble miliary tuberculosis (Fig. 19.12), but often shows a reticular pattern which may progress to 'honeycomb' lung and complicating pneumothoraces.

Fig. 19.13   Foreign body inhalation. **A**. Obstructive emphysema from a foreign body in the left main bronchus. **B, C**. same child later; loss of volume in the left lung with patchy collapse in the apex of the left lower lobe; in inspiration (**B**) the mediastinum is slightly to the left; in expiration (**C**) the volume to the left lung changes little with the mediastinum swinging to the right.

BRONCHIOLITIS

This is often associated with the respiratory syncytial virus or pertussis. The lungs appear overinflated, with streaky peribronchiolar shadows. More confluent consolidation may complicate a frequently grave clinical condition.

INHALED FOREIGN BODIES (Fig. 19.13)

The variety of objects which children manage to aspirate is wide but peanuts are very common. There is a tendency to enter the more vertical right main bronchus. Complete obstruction will lead to peripheral collapse but partial obstruction can lead to obstructive emphysema. Films in expiration as well as inspiration, supplemented if necessary by fluoroscopy, will show mediastinal shift away from the obstructive emphysema on expiration. Bronchoscopy should be performed on strong clinical grounds even if the radiographs are normal.

TRAUMA

Contusion of the lung can occur without rib fracture. Patchy resulting haemorrhagic consolidation can cavitate or resolve uneventfully.

HYDROCARBON ASPIRATION

Petrol or paraffin, if accidentally swallowed, can enter the trachea and may cause patchy basal lung shadowing, sometimes with delayed onset and sometimes with pneumatocoele formation (Fig. 19.14).

IMMUNE COMPROMISE

A wide variety of common viruses, such as measles, or less common organisms such as *Pneumocystis* or cyto-megalovirus, cause extensive pulmonary shadowing in leukaemia or in children with immune deficiency or undergoing chemotherapy. At times biopsy may be necessary to establish the diagnosis, although *Pneumocystis* frequently has a typical appearance with gross opacification (Fig. 19.15) and an air bronchogram.

In *acquired immune deficiency syndrome* (AIDS) in childhood, in addition to those infections common to the immune-compromised, a widespread nodularity in the lung fields can represent lymphocytic infiltration.

IDIOPATHIC PULMONARY HAEMOSIDEROSIS
(Fig. 19.16)

This serious condition, frequently fatal in early adulthood, starts in childhood with repeated pulmonary haemorrhage, at first revealed as patchy shadowing with intervening clearing, but progressing to permanent linear and reticular shadowing.

ASTHMA

Prolonged episodic bronchospasm reveals itself radiologically as overdistension of the lungs with a low flat diaphragm, sternal bowing, peribronchial shadowing seen as 'rings' end-on or 'tramlines' longitudinally, with occasional patchy shadowing. *Aspergillus* colonization can lead to extensive parenchymal shadowing.

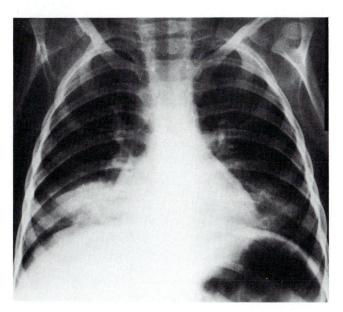

Fig. 19.14 Paraffin (kerosene) aspiration. Basal shadowing with early left basal pneumatocoele.

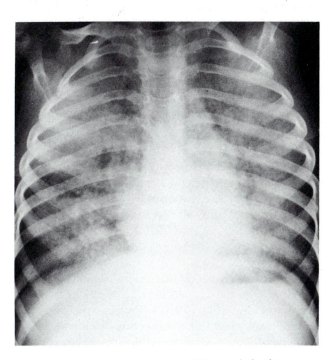

Fig. 19.15 Pneumocystis penumonia. Widespread alveolar shadowing.

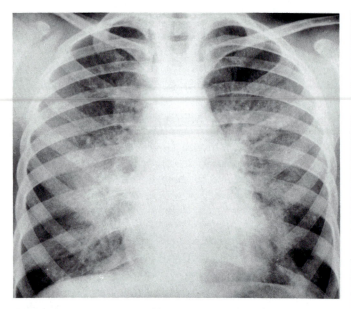

Fig. 19.16 Idiopathic pulmonary haemosiderosis. Perihilar shadowing with a reticulo-nodular pattern in the peripheral lung fields.

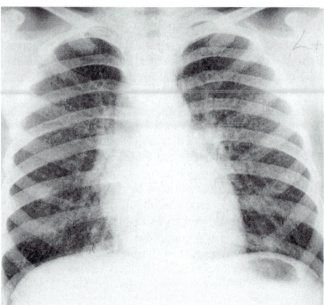

Fig. 19.17 Miliary tuberculosis. Fine nodularity throughout both lungs.

Pneumomediastinum is most usually associated with asthma in childhood; extension results in subcutaneous emphysema, particularly in the neck. Pneumothorax can at times also, but uncommonly, complicate.

TUBERCULOSIS

This is described in Chapter 15. In childhood, miliary tuberculosis is still too frequently seen, especially in immigrants. It can be congenital. A fine nodularity is evenly distributed throughout both lung fields (Fig. 19.17). At times, mediastinal lymph node enlargement is also apparent.

PNEUMONIA

Many childhood pneumonias are viral in origin, with non-specific features of patchy consolidation, overdistension and prominent hilar shadows (Fig. 19.18), because of the relatively narrow peripheral airways in the young.

An important complication is obliterative bronchiolitis. Decreased vascularity of the affected areas leads to radiolucency and relative failure of lung growth is associated with air-trapping (*MacLeod* or *Swyer-James syndrome*).

Staphylococcal pneumonia, in its earlier stages non-specific in appearance, can develop highly characteristic pneumotocoeles (Fig. 19.19) showing as thin-walled radiolucencies which can at times rapidly enlarge and lead to pneumothorax. Their resolution is frequently slow, with persistence long after pneumonic consolidation has resolved.

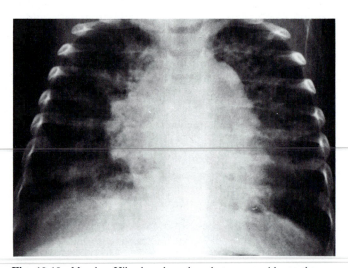

Fig. 19.18 Measles. Hilar lymph node enlargement with streaky shadowing radiating into the central lung fields.

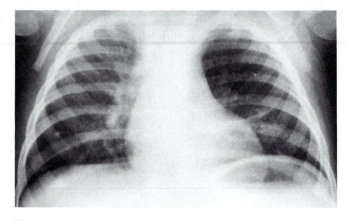

Fig. 19.19 Pneumatocele. Previous left staphylococcal pneumonia.

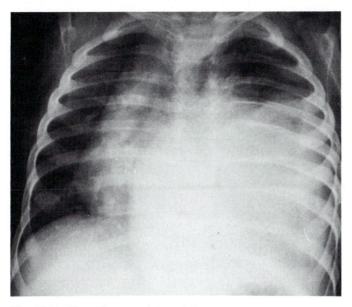

Fig. 19.20 Neuroblastoma. A large left posterior mass deviates the mediastinum to the right, with thinning and separation of the adjacent posterior ends of the ribs.

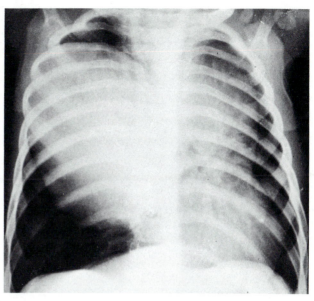

Fig. 19.21 Foregut duplication cyst with obstructive emphysema of the right lung.

INTRATHORACIC MASSES

Neurogenic tumours such as neuroblastoma (Fig. 19.20) and ganglioneuroma are typically posterior, frequently deforming ribs. Calcification within the tumour and pleural effusions may be present.

Foregut duplication and bronchogenic cysts are common middle mediastinal masses (Fig. 19.21) and can cause bronchial or oesophageal compression. Vertebral anomalies are frequent. Ectopic gastric mucosa may be demonstrated by technetium-99m in some of these cysts.

Cystic hygromas usually have a component in the neck as well as extension into the upper chest. Ultrasound is useful to demonstrate their characteristic massively cystic appearance.

Hilar lymph node enlargement occurs more obviously in pneumonia in childhood and is a feature of lymphoma and metastatic malignancies.

REFERENCES AND SUGGESTIONS FOR FURTHER READING

Avery, M. E., Fletcher, B. D., Williams, R. G. (1981) *The Lung and its Disorders in the Newborn Infant.* 4th edn. (*Major Problems in Clinical paediatrics*) W. B. Saunders, Philadelphia.

Felman, A. H. (1987) *Radiology of the Paediatric Chest. Clinical and Pathological Correlations.* McGraw-Hill, New York.

Griscom, N. T., Wohl, M. E. B., Kirkpatrick, J. A. (1978) Lower respiratory infections; how infants differ from adults. *Radiologic Clinics of North America,* **16**, 367–387.

Kaufmann, H. J. (ed) (1967) *Progress in Paediatric Radiology* Vol 1. *Respiratory tract.* Karger, Basel.

Kendig, E. L., Chernick, V. (1977) *Disorders of the Respiratory Tract in Children,* 3rd edn. W. B. Saunders, Philadelphia.

Phelan, P. D., Landau, L. I., Olinsky, A. (1982). *Respiratory Illness in Children.* 2nd edn. Blackwell, Oxford.

Silverman, F. (ed) (1985) *Caffey's Paediatric X-ray Diagnosis.* 8th edn. Year Book Press, Chicago.

Singleton, E. B., Wagner, M. L. (1971) *Radiologic Atlas of Pulmonary Abnormalities in Children.* W. B. Saunders, Philadelphia.

Swischuk, L. E. (1989) *Imaging of the Newborn Infant and Young Child.* 3rd edn. Williams and Wilkins, Baltimore.

Wesenberg, R. L. (1973) *The Newborn Chest.* Harper and Row, Hagerston, M. D.

PART 3

THE CARDIOVASCULAR SYSTEM

CHAPTER 20

THE NORMAL HEART: METHODS OF EXAMINATION

M. J. Raphael   R. M. Donaldson

PLAIN FILMS

The plain chest film, although it rarely provides a specific diagnosis of cardiac abnormality, is sufficiently important to be considered an integral part of the complete clinical assessment of the patient suspected of suffering from heart disease. It may indicate the nature of the functional derangement, and also its severity. To do this it should show the overall heart size, and evidence of selective chamber enlargement. It must also be of sufficient quality to enable the lung vessels to be studied. The standard cardiac series has consisted of a low-kV chest film to show lung parenchyma, a penetrated PA chest to see detail within the heart, and a left lateral film with barium in the oesophagus to show left atrial size. Today, a high-kV PA chest with an antiscatter system represents an excellent single frontal film compromise, enabling intracardiac details and lung vessel anatomy to be seen on one film. Combined with a high-quality lateral film, so that the left lower lobe bronchus may be identified, a two-film cardiac study is adequate for routine purposes, although calcification is difficult to perceive.

There is no place for routine oblique films in the examination of the heart. They are impossible to standardize and rarely give information which cannot be obtained more satisfactorily by other means.

FLUOROSCOPY

Image amplification fluoroscopy is easily performed but has only a limited place in the examination of the heart. Screening will show the relationship of any abnormal shadows to the heart. It is excellent for recognizing and locating intracardiac *calcification*, and may be of slight value in studying prosthetic valves.

Even in experienced hands it is of only limited value in the study of left ventricular aneurysm. The recognition of hilar dance in left-to-right shunts, and of systolic expansion of the left atrium in the diagnosis of mitral incompetence, are now of purely historical interest.

TOMOGRAPHY

Conventional tomography has virtually no place in present-day cardiac radiology but computed tomography has been used to demonstrate pericardial effusions and thickening and also has been able to recognize tumours of the heart and dissecting aneurysms of the thoracic aorta.

COMPUTED TOMOGRAPHY
Ian Isherwood and W. St. C. Forbes

Normal appearances. Computed tomography has provided an excellent means of studying the heart from an anatomical and even a functional basis. As well as details of cardiac anatomy and pathology, we can also obtain precise visual information concerning the surrounding anatomy related to the heart. The development of fast scan times in computed tomography, coupled with dynamic contrast enhancement, has increased enormously the opportunity and potential for cardiac imaging. The advantage that CT offers over the other imaging techniques, apart from high spatial resolution, is the ability to obtain clearer definition of cross-sectional anatomy without superimposition of structures. The cross-sectional anatomy of the heart and great vessels as seen on CT is quite straightforward (Figs 12.3, 20.1). Cardiac chamber size can also be determined on CT with dynamic contrast enhancement. Should there be any doubt about the precise size and limits of individual cardiac chambers, sequential scans obtained during a rapid bolus injection of contrast medium intravenously will demonstrate its transit through the right and left heart chambers (Fig. 20.1).

The structure and motion of valve leaflets are not well visualized on CT. Echocardiography is superior to CT in this respect and provides accurate assessment of valve motion with the option of variable imaging planes. However, due to the ability of CT to detect small calcium deposits, calcific disease of cardiac valves is well seen on CT.

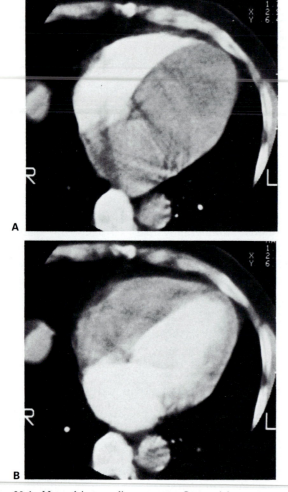

Fig. 20.1 Normal intracardiac anatomy. Sequential scans at same level demonstrate transit of contrast medium through (**A**) right ventricle and (**B**) left atrium and left ventricle.

Even without electrocardiographic gating it is possible to obtain detailed images of cardiac anatomy. Electrocardiographic gating allows visualization on CT of a particular phase of the cardiac cycle. This will allow some assessment of left ventricular function and myocardial wall motion.

Use of a high-speed cine CT scanner with an electron beam that is magnetically rather than mechanically deflected can provide sampling measurements of left ventricular dimensions, wall thickness and wall motion at 50 ms intervals. By obtaining 8 transverse sections on CT using the cine system, the entire heart can be scanned within 200 ms. Alternatively, dynamic spatial reconstruction can be performed by using multiple X-ray tubes and image intensifying chains to obtain multiple simultaneous cardiac sections, i.e. a real-time mode.

Myocardial infarction. Contrast-enhanced CT scanning allows visualization of inner endocardial walls as well as the epicardial surface; so that the thickness of myo-

cardial wall and of the interventricular septum can be determined accurately. Due to the relatively longer time interval of diastole as opposed to systole with ungated CT, myocardial wall dimensions are obtained in the diastolic phase of the cardiac cycle. Thinning of the left ventricular myocardium and also the interventricular septum can be directly visualized on CT after myocardial infarction (Fig. 20. 2B).

A frequent complication of myocardial infarction is mural thrombus in the left ventricle. By obtaining contrast enhancement of the left ventricle, intraventricular thrombi can be visualized. The precise position and extent of thrombi in cardiac chambers can thus be observed on CT (Fig. 20.2).

Left ventricular aneurysms. Left ventricular aneurysms are found at post-mortem in 3.5–20% of patients who have had a myocardial infarct. Aneurysms of the left ventricle are defined as a local area of total lack of wall motion or paradoxical wall motion. CT provides a very useful noninvasive means of detecting left ventricular aneurysms.

With contrast enhancement, the length of nonaneurysmal and aneurysmal myocardium can be assessed on each

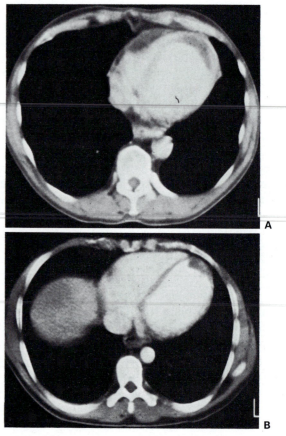

Fig. 20.2 Myocardial infarct and thrombus. Contrast enhancement. **A**. Low-density thrombus in left ventricle. **B**. Thinning of intraventricular septum anteriorly with mural thrombus near apex of left ventricle.

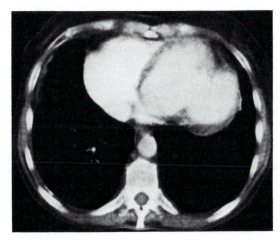

Fig. 20.3 Left ventricular aneurysm. Contrast enhancement demonstrates neck of apical and posterior aneurysm communicating with left ventricular cavity.

ography can be as accurate as selective coronary angiography in assessment of graft patency. Metallic clips on grafts will cause streak artefact on the image, making it difficult to assess graft patency. However if nonopaque materials are used bypass grafts will be successfully seen on CT.

By performing sections at the level of coronary artery bypass grafts during a rapid bolus injection of intravenous contrast medium, both enhancement and clearance of the graft will be observed on CT (Fig. 20.4). While the native coronary artery is not normally visualized, calcification within a diseased coronary artery will be detected on transverse section. It may frequently be necessary to obtain CT sections at more than one level to decide on patency or occlusion of a bypass graft.

section to the point of contour of the myocardium. The exact size of a left ventricular aneurysm can be determined, as well as its relationship to the remaining left ventricle. The neck of an aneurysm involving the left ventricle can usually be localized on CT (Fig. 20.3). Thrombus formation can be a complication of left ventricular aneurysms due to the akinetic myocardium, and CT will visualize thrombus within an aneurysmal sac.

Coronary artery bypass grafts. Information on the patency and function of bypass grafts to coronary arteries is important for the assessment of current and new surgical techniques and also in the management of patients with continuing and recurrent angina. Computed tom-

MRI OF THE NORMAL HEART
Ian Isherwood and Jeremy P. R. Jenkins

Cardiac MRI is now an established, although still advancing, technique providing information on morphology and function of the heart and cardiovascular system in both health and disease. Its attractions include a wide topographical field of view with visualization of the heart and its internal morphology and surrounding mediastinal structures, the capability of multiple imaging planes, and a high soft-tissue contrast discrimination between flowing blood and myocardium without the need for contrast medium or invasive technique. The multiplanar facility, including oblique sections, allows true long and short axis views of the heart (as used in echocardiography) and

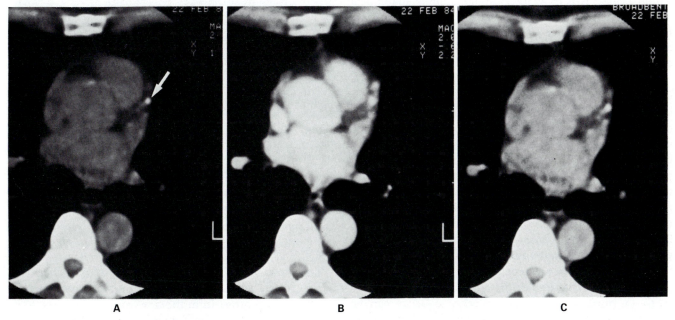

A   B   C

Fig. 20.4 Coronary artery graft. **A.** Unenhanced scan. Calcification in left anterior descending coronary artery (arrow). Left coronary artery graft anteriorly. **B, C.** Sequential scans demonstrate enhancement and clearance of the left coronary artery bypass graft.

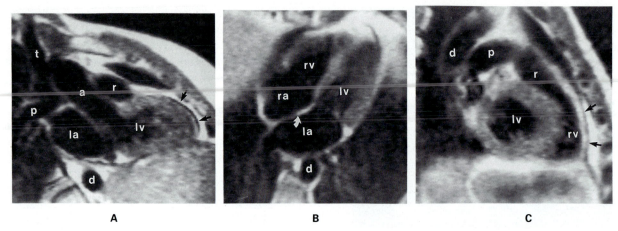

Fig. 20.5 **A**. Long-axis two-chamber view of the heart on a compound oblique ECG-gated spin-echo T_1-weighted image (TE = 26 ms). **B**. Four-chamber view on a compound oblique gated image using similar parameters. **C**. Short-axis view of the left ventricle using compound oblique planes with similar parameters. a = ascending aorta, d = descending aorta, la = left atrium, lv = left ventricle, r = outflow tract of right ventricle, ra = right atrium, rv = right ventricle, p = main pulmonary arteries, t = trachea, straight arrows = pericardium, curved arrow = interatrial septum.

long-axis images of the thoracic aorta to be obtained routinely (Fig. 20.5A–C).

The use of *ECG gating* of the RF pulse sequence, typically *spin-echo T_1-weighted*, allows for sequential images to be acquired at different times during the cardiac cycle, providing images of the internal morphology of the heart and great vessels with high spatial resolution. ECG gating initiates the RF pulse sequence to a constant point in the cardiac cycle, thus controlling the effects of heart motion and reducing flow-related artefacts. A *sequential* ECG-gated multislice T_1-weighted spin-echo sequence gives contiguous anatomical sections but with each image at a different phase of the cardiac cycle. This is a rapid way, within a single R-R ECG interval, of obtaining anatomical detail over a wide area (Fig. 20.6). Using *incremental* ECG-gated multislice imaging, each section can be obtained at a different spacing throughout the cardiac cycle at a designated anatomical level (see Fig. 20.7). The typical spacing between images is 50–100 ms (limited by a signal-to-noise ratio (SNR) constraint on some magnet systems). A repeat multi-set can be obtained with 25–50 ms gating delay from the R wave. These images can be interpolated, stacked in order and put into a cine display mode. This technique allows visualization of the beating heart, which helps to assess cardiac wall motion and also to evaluate blood flow. A fluctuation in myocardial signal, related to varying levels of phase-encoded noise in images obtained at different phases of the cardiac cycle, makes it difficult to evaluate changes in signal intensity from the walls. ECG gating, although relatively easy to instigate, reduces flexibility in the repetition time (TR) of the sequence which is controlled by the R-R interval of the ECG. A gated T_2-weighted spin-echo sequence can be performed by increasing the TR to twice the R-R interval and the TE to greater than 60 ms.

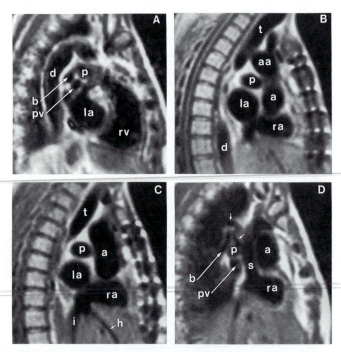

Fig. 20.6 Four sagittal multisection gated spin-echo images (TE 24 ms) (**A**) left to (**D**) right of the midline demonstrating normal anatomy, and the localized low- and high-signal artefacts from metallic sternal sutures following coronary artery bypass graft surgery. Same key as in Fig. 20.5 and including aa = aortic arch, b = bronchus, h = hepatic vein, i = inferior vena cava, pv = pulmonary vein, s = superior vena cava, small arrows in D = azygos vein. (Adapted with permission from Jenkins & Isherwood 1987.)

The *gated spin echo technique* clearly demonstrates internal cardiac anatomy and adjacent major vessels due to the intrinsic contrast from the flow void effect (Figs 20.5, 6, 7). Reasons why some images are not diagnostic are poor cooperation by the patient, an irregular heart rate

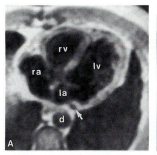
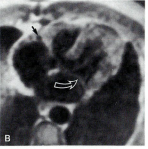

Fig. 20.7 Two transverse gated spin-echo images (TE 24 ms), (**A**) end-diastole and (**B**) end-systole. Same key as in Fig 20.5. Curved arrow = closed mitral valve leaflets, straight arrow in A = left circumflex artery, straight arrow in B = right coronary artery.

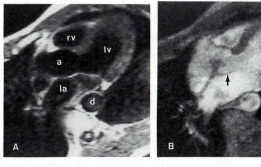

Fig. 20.8 Compound oblique gated images through the cardiac long-axis plane. **A**, spin-echo (TE 26 ms). **B**, gradient echo (TE 26 ms) scans. Same key as in Fig. 20.5. Arrow = mitral valve leaflet. (Adapted with permission from Mitchell et al 1989.)

or a low amplitude R-wave below the threshold sensitivity of the triggering device. In addition, difficulty in correct triggering can occur due to peaked T waves, simulating the R wave. Blood (which acts as a conductor) flowing in the aorta interacts with the magnetic field, producing a voltage which causes artefacts on the ECG. The myocardium and its endocardial surface can be delineated, although the latter may be obscured by signal from slow-flowing blood within the chamber during certain phases of the cardiac cycle. The interatrial and interventricular septa can be visualized, together with the papillary apparatus and the moderator band in the ventricles. The relatively thin and mobile cardiac valves are not consistently seen. The pericardium consists of fibrous tissue, and produces a linear low signal anterior to the right ventricle (see Ch. 21). Portions of the proximal coronary arteries can often be detected (see Figs 23.54, 23.56).

MRI can provide both anatomical and functional information about the heart. Using spin-echo techniques, global and regional right and left ventricular function as represented by stroke volumes and ejection fractions can be accurately obtained. Data from MRI are more accurate than those derived from left ventricular angiography, where the calculation is based on the assumption that the left ventricle is ellipsoid in shape. Volume measurement by MRI is independent of cavity shape, with the area from contiguous spin-echo sections integrated over the chamber of interest. *Gradient echo imaging* (also called *Cine* or *Cine-Flow MRI*), using gradient-refocused echoes (e.g. even-echo rephasing) and a low flip angle (typically 30–60°), can also provide a qualitative and quantitative assessment of valvular function and blood flow in vivo (see Ch. 23).

In spin echo imaging, the blood pool is usually demonstrated as a signal void. In contrast, the blood pool in gradient echo imaging has a high signal, with myocardium and stationary tissues retaining an intermediate mid-grey signal (Figs 20.8, 20.9). High contrast discrimination can thus be achieved between the blood pool

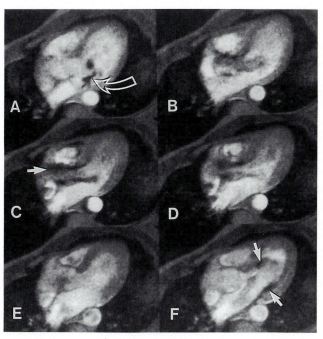

Fig. 20.9 Normal anatomy shown on six images in the same cardiac long-axis plane at 100 ms intervals through the cardiac cycle using the gradient echo sequence (TE 26 ms), with (**A**) 30 ms to (**F**) 530 ms after the R-wave of the ECG. Curved arrow in A = signal loss distal to the mitral valve at end-diastole, straight arrow in C = peripheral signal loss distal to aortic valve in mid-systole, straight arrows in F = signal loss adjacent to the mitral valve leaflets in diastole. (Adapted with permission from Mitchell et al 1989.)

and myocardial/vessel wall using either technique. The gradient echo sequence allows shorter timing intervals between scans (TR can be as low as 30 ms on some magnet systems) giving approximately 25 frames/acquisition with a typical R-R interval of 800 ms (the number of scans obtained is approximately the R-R interval divided by the TR). A further advantage of gradient echo imaging is its sensitivity to the disturbed flow and consequent signal loss associated with stenotic and regurgitant valves, shunts and vessel narrowings. The extent of signal loss associated with diseased valves or areas of stenosis is related to the severity of the lesion and correlates well with pressure gradient measurements at angiography (see Ch. 23). In addition, with gradient echo imaging both flow direction and a measurement of velocity can be derived by the use of 'phase mapping'. *Phase mapping* requires two sets of even-echo rephased scans to be obtained simultaneously. One set is phase-encoded, using a gradient profile to encode for flow in a selected direction. The two sets are subtracted producing a *velocity map* (see Fig. 25.82). The phase shift induced by flowing blood is proportional to its velocity and is detected as either a dark or light grey signal, depending on the direction of flow. Stationary tissue does not demonstrate any phase shift and thus remains mid-grey. Shortening of the TE of the gradient echo sequence (a reduction of the echo time of 3 ms has been achieved) allows reclamation of signal from areas of incoherent or turbulent flow (see Fig. 23.50). Flow velocity measurements can then be made.

Gradient echo imaging can also be used to provide quantitative evaluation of regional wall motion and systolic wall thickening to assess extent of regional myocardial ischaemia and infarction. A more sensitive method of quantifying myocardial motion and contraction is based on a novel technique termed '*cardiac tagging*'. Specified regions of the myocardium during diastole can be labelled by selective RF saturation of multiple thin grid lines which 'tag' points in the myocardium. This tagging is followed by incremental multislice SE imaging which allows sampling during the contractile phase of the cardiac cycle. The tagged regions appear as strips of low signal intensity and their pattern of displacement reflects the intervening myocardial motion. This technique allows easy evaluation of dyskinetic areas of the myocardium. In addition to the translational and rotational movement of the heart, more complex motions such as cardiac twist have been demonstrated. Further work with this method has provided a three-dimensional picture of myocardial motion and contraction.

In contrast to other techniques, including two-dimensional echocardiography (2DE, CSE) and angiography, anatomical information is easily defined on MRI. This is particularly valuable in the assessment of suspected congenital heart defects and abnormalities of the great vessels. The advantages of MRI over CSE are a wider topographical window and a superior contrast resolution. In obese patients, provided they fit into the magnet bore, good resolution images can be obtained. CSE can be limited by body habitus, and difficulties may arise in demonstrating the aortic arch, the descending thoracic aorta and the epicardial border of the left ventricular free wall.

Chemical shift imaging, which can separate and quantify the water and fat protons in vivo, is able to detect and study the composition of atheromatous plaques.

Echo planar imaging (EPI) is a different MR technique that offers virtual real-time, i.e. 'snapshot', imaging. It employs very short data acquisition times (milliseconds), and involves repeated sampling of the transverse magnetization in the presence of large, rapidly-switched field gradients, and requires specialized hardware and software. It offers great potential for the examination of the rapidly beating heart and the coronary arteries.

Magnetic resonance spectroscopy (MRS) can monitor the metabolism of intact organs noninvasively. Much of the work on MRS in the heart has been concerned with the assessment of myocardial ischaemia, and metabolic alterations have been demonstrated in these circumstances. Several major technical problems, including spatial resolution and localization, are currently being investigated and must be solved, before its clinical role can be established.

Safety aspects of cardiac MRI. Patients with pacemakers or pacing lines in situ should be excluded from the MRI unit and should not enter the 5-gauss (0.5 millitesla) line of the fringe field. Cardiac pacemakers can be damaged or change operation on exposure to switching magnetic field gradients. Although all pacemakers exhibit a torque when placed in the main field, this is unlikely to result in movement of the pacemaker within the chest or abdominal wall, due to the presence of surrounding fibrosis.

Patients with prosthetic heart valves (excluding the old Starr-Edwards valve replacement (pre-6000 model)), can be safely scanned without danger of valve displacement or significant image artefact (see Fig. 25.83). A localised loss of signal is to be expected close to prosthetic valves, so other imaging techniques are required to evaluate these implants. Surgical clips, including sternal wires, used in coronary artery bypass grafting and other cardiac surgery are not a significant problem, producing only local artefacts.

ECHOCARDIOGRAPHY

Ultrasonic imaging of the heart or 'echocardiography', based on pulsed echo techniques, allows the anatomy and movements of intracardiac structures to be studied non-invasively with ease and reproducibility. The echo signal indicates the presence and location of the structure in the ultrasound beam. Some details of intracardiac anatomy and pathology are much better documented by ultrasound than by X-ray or other imaging methods. There are three methods of cardiac ultrasound: one-dimensional scanning (M-mode echocardiography), two-dimensional scanning, known as cross-sectional echocardiography (CSE) (also described as the 2D-echogram, 2DE or real-time scan) and pulsed and

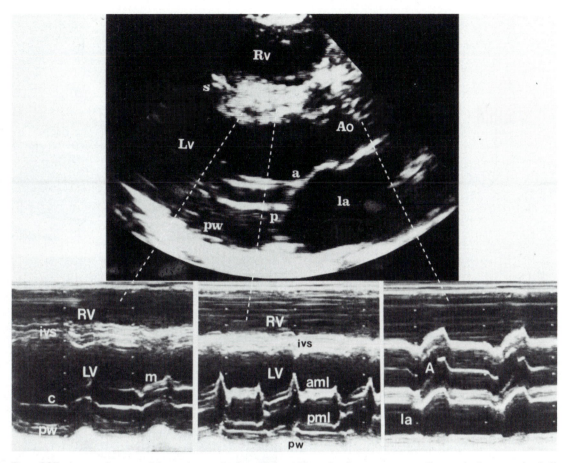

Fig. 20.10 Top. CSE picture of a normal heart, long-axis view. **Below**. M-mode pictures corresponding to the beam angles indicated on the CSE picture, made simultaneously on a modern machine. **Left-hand panel**: The beam goes through the left ventricular cavity below the level of the mitral valve. Both anterior and posterior walls of the left ventricle can be identified, together with their endocardial surfaces, and they move inwards together. Note that the cavity diameter can be measured in diastole and systole, as can the wall thickness. Without CSE control the exact level at which the beam intersects the left ventricular cavity would be uncertain. **Middle panel**: The characteristic M-shaped movement indicates that the beam is intersecting the anterior leaflet of the mitral valve. In addition, the posterior leaflet of the mitral valve can be identified as moving in the opposite direction in diastole. **Right-hand panel**: The box-shaped opening movement of the aortic valve leaflets can be seen, which confirms that the beam is going through the aortic root. The left atrium can be identified lying behind the aorta and its long diameter can be measured. Key to Figs 20.10–20.34: RV = right ventricle, LV = left ventricle, Ao [or A] = aorta, LA = left atrium, PW = posterior wall, a [or aml] = anterior leaflet mitral valve, p [or pml] = posterior leaflet mitral valve, c = chordae tendinae, ivs [or s] = interventricular septum, PA = pulmonary artery, RA = right atrium, L.ax = long-axis view, S.ax = short-axis view, e = endocardium, t = tricuspid valve, ias = inter-atrial septum, ED = end-diastole, ES = end-systole, AV = aortic valve, MV = mitral valve.

continuous-wave Doppler, which can be combined with both methods to provide information about blood flow velocity and direction. Doppler colour flow mapping (CFM) gathers Doppler shift information and visualizes abnormal flow patterns in relation to cardiac anatomy.

M-mode echocardiogram (Fig. 20.10). The echoes reflected from different interfaces are converted electronically into spots of light which fall on light-sensitive paper moving at constant speed, giving the position of the reflecting structures of the heart relative to the transducer plotted against time. Modern apparatus allows the plane of the M-mode echogram to be displayed on the CSE image (see below) so that the structures being studied can be clearly identified; the inability to do this was a

serious limitation of the isolated M-mode study. The present role of this combined M-mode study is simply to measure ventricular cavity dimensions and wall thickness. The many other applications of the technique are now of historic interest only.

Cross-sectional echocardiography (CSE) (Figs 20.10–20.13). By making the ultrasound beam oscillate automatically very rapidly backwards and forwards through an arc of 80°, the information from a large number of M-mode scans is combined. The series of images will produce an accurate moving picture of the structures within the heart. Thus lateral as well as range distances between structures can be appreciated, and the images obtained resemble heart structures. The CSE allows com-

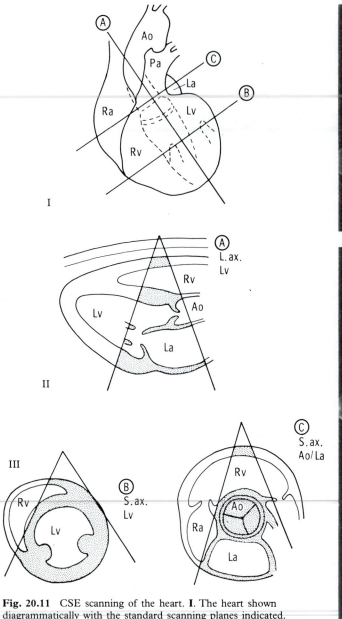

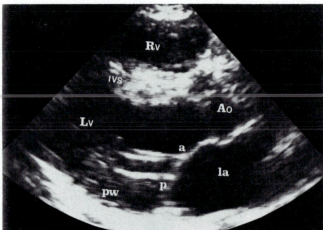

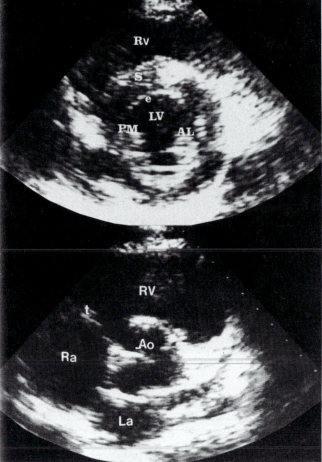

Fig. 20.11 CSE scanning of the heart. **I.** The heart shown diagrammatically with the standard scanning planes indicated. **A.** The long-axis view. **B.** Short-axis view through the cavity of the left ventricle below the level of the mitral valve. **C.** Short-axis view more cranially than in B. For key see Fig. 20.10. **II.** Long-axis view. **III.** Short-axis views.

plete visualization of all intracardiac structures. The structures shown on a CSE depend on the transducer position and the direction of oscillation. CSE images are effectively tomograms, showing structures in a slice of the heart. The most common planes used in adult echocardiography are shown in Figs 20.10–20.13.

Doppler echocardiography. The application of pulsed and continuous-wave Doppler principles to CSE permits blood flow direction and velocity to be derived. Using the CSE as a map, a sampling box can be positioned electronically by the operator adjacent to an abnormal valve, or tracked along the septum to observe

Fig. 20.12 CSE standard views corresponding to Fig. 20.11. **A.** Long-axis view. This is useful for orientation of the cardiac structures and good for acquired disease of the mitral and aortic valves. It is also useful in left ventricular disease. **B. Top** A short-axis cut through the left ventricle. The size and shape of the left ventricular cavity and wall thickness are demonstrated. **Below.** Short-axis cut at the level of the aortic valve. As the transducer is angled cranially from the left ventricle the beam leaves the papillary muscles and intersects the mitral valve which has a characteristic 'fish-mouth' appearance. More cranial angulation intersects the aortic valve and also reveals the right ventricular outflow and in children the pulmonary valve and pulmonary artery and its bifurcation.

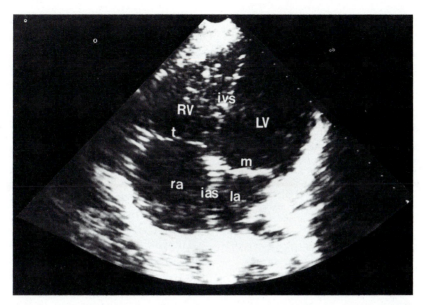

Fig. 20.13 CSE, the four-chamber view. To obtain this view the transducer is rotated as well as angled so that all four chambers can be identified simultaneously, together with both atrioventricular valves. This view gives one of the best demonstrations of the left ventricle and the ventricular septum and also of the atrioventricular valve. In acquired heart disease it enables structural abnormality to be seen. In congenital heart disease this view is excellent for identifying the opening of the valves into their respective ventricles. 'Drop-out' of echoes in the interatrial septum are common in this view, but by obtaining the view subcostally, more conclusions about the interatrial septum may be drawn.

turbulent flow. A flow profile of the direction, or the average flow velocity, may be derived, and provide insight into the physiological burden of valvular heart disease or intracardiac shunts.

Doppler colour-flow mapping (CFM). Pulsed and continuous-wave Doppler do not display flow images. They produce flow information from a very small area of interest indicated by the operator. Colour-flow mapping automatically gathers Doppler shift information from multiple sample volumes along each CSE scan line. Mean velocities are calculated from the Doppler shift and colour-coded electronically for display of direction and velocity.

Transoesophageal echocardiography (TEE). Conventional CSE is limited in certain situations because of poor depth penetration or because interference from anterior structures reduces the access window. TEE gives high-quality colour-flow images in all cases. The technique requires the passage of an oesophagoscope with an ultrasound transducer at its tip and this can be, to some degree, angled and advanced to different levels to visualize the aorta and the heart in multiple projections. Both CSE and CFM are available in current equipment. Current indications for TEE include the assessment of prosthetic valve dysfunction, endocarditis, thrombus in the left atrial appendage, aortic dissection, and monitoring of LV function during operations.

Summary. The M-mode echogram, now invariably combined with CSE, has only a small role in the quantitation of ventricular cavity size and wall thickness. The standard CSE provides decisive information on intracardiac anatomy in the vast majority of neonates and small children with congenital heart disease and in over 70% of adults with acquired heart disease. The limiting factor is usually the ultrasound window, and in these patients the TEE will usually give the required information, though it does require oesophagoscopy. Functional information is usually obtained initially using colour-flow mapping, which will reveal areas of abnormal flow such as intracardiac shunts and leaking valves, but it should be realized that the information is semiquantitative at best. Valvar stenoses may be quantified using continuous-wave Doppler sampling, which is required to demonstrate the very high flow rates caused by a valvar stenosis.

RADIONUCLIDES IN CARDIOLOGY

Ventricular function studies

Radionuclide techniques for monitoring global and regional ventricular functions fall into two major categories: 1. first-pass studies, in which the injected bolus dose is monitored during its first passage through the heart and great vessels; and 2. gated equilibrium studies, in which the tracer mixes with the blood pool before data collection. Both these nuclear studies can be performed at the patient's bedside using a mobile gamma camera; each technique has its own strength and weakness. (Table 20.1).

Following injection, the labelled radioactive tracer

Table 20.1 Comparison of the two methods of radionuclide angiography

	First-pass	Equilibrium
Radiopharmaceutical	^{99m}Tc pertechnetate (readily available). Bolus required	^{99m}Tc-labelled RBCs or HSA (preparation takes 15–20 min)
Camera	High count rate capability (multicrystal)	Conventional
Camera positioning	Before injection of agent any projection (RAO possible)	After administration of agent. LAO projection of choice
Imaging time	30 s	3–10 min
Measurements per injection	One	Multiple repeat measurements
Advantages	1. Minimal background activity 2. Temporal separation — optimal views of chambers 3. Visualization of inferior and anterior wall motion abnormalities slightly superior 4. Analysis of lung flow possible 5. Measurement of cardiac output 6. Quantification of shunts	1. Permits repeat studies after intervention over long periods 2. Estimation of severity of valvar regurgitation

settles in the heart, releasing energy in the form of gamma photons which traverse overlying tissues and interact with the imaging device (single-crystal or multicrystal gamma camera). A collimator permits only photons arising from specific areas of the heart to interact with the camera. The imaging device converts the energy of the gamma photons into an electrical signal that can be processed; an on-line computer records the information and permits the optimal visual or quantitive display of the data.

For cardiac nuclear imaging a number of heart cycles have to be averaged to provide data for accurate interpretation of structure and function. In first-pass studies, data are usually summed without regard to physiological signal; in the gated equilibrium technique, the start of each cardiac cycle is identified from a physiological marker (the R wave of the electrocardiogram) and data from each cycle are added in the correct temporal sequence ('gated'). Gated nuclear imaging is inaccurate if the cardiac rhythm is very irregular.

First-pass method. The first-pass method of radionuclide angiography consists of rapidly injecting a bolus of isotope (^{99m}Tc pertechnetate) into the antecubital vein and obtaining images as the bolus passes through

the right heart, lung fields and left heart chambers. A multi-detector gamma camera with high count rate (up to 250 000 per second) should be used, its disadvantage being its lack of mobility. The representative cycle can be played in cine format for quantitive evaluation of wall motion; superimposed end-diastolic and end-systolic perimeters are generated to evaluate regional wall motion further (Fig. 20.14).

Although single-crystal gamma cameras can also be used for this method, the count density obtained with them is limited and may hinder the accuracy of the values obtained. They have the advantage of mobility.

Gated equilibrium studies (Multiple Gated Acquisition, MUGA) (Fig. 20.15). An isotope which remains fixed within the vascular space (such as ^{99m}TC-labelled human serum albumin or red blood cells) is administered intravenously. This particular isotope permits the recording of data for up to four hours, thus allowing the acquisition of multiple images in various projections and also the study of the ventricular response to interventions. After equilibrium, the counts are synchronized in relation to a portion of the cardiac cycle, using the R wave of the electrocardiogram, and the cardiac cycle is divided by the computer into a fixed number of frames. This synchronization is called 'gated' imaging. Frame durations

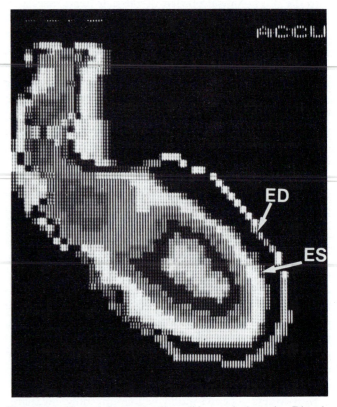

Fig. 20.14 Normal first-pass radionuclide ventriculography. Diastole and systole can both be identified, the shape of the ventricle determined and the pattern of contraction seen.

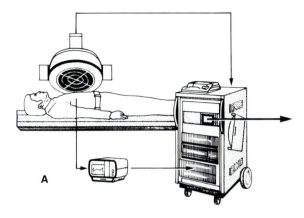

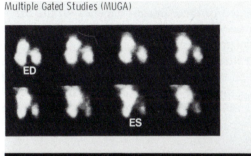

Multiple Gated Studies (MUGA)

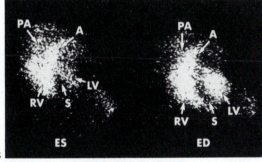

Fig. 20.15 A,B Gated equilibrium radionuclide ventriculography (MUGA = multiple gated acquisition). The gamma camera is positioned in the left anterior oblique position to obtain separation of right and left ventricles; data acquisition is synchronized ('gated') by the computer to the ECG signals.

the system. The difficulty with the probe method is how to position it correctly over the ventricular area of interest.

Quantitive data analysis

Ejection fraction. Semi-automatic methods for measuring cardiac ejection fraction have been in clinical use for many years. After data accumulation, the region of interest (e.g. the left ventricle) is identified and the computer generates a time/activity curve with a cyclic rise and fall in counts (Fig. 20.16). The counts are proportional to the volume of the chamber. The difference between peak counts at end-diastole (ED) and trough counts at end-systole (ES) reflects the stroke counts; stroke counts divided by ED counts (after appropriate background correction) determine the ejection fraction. This time/activity curve is independent of geometric assumptions inherent in the area–length technique utilized in contrast ventriculography and echocardiography.

Regional wall-motion analysis. The images are viewed in a cine film format on a continuous loop for evaluation of wall-motion abnormalities; by colour coding and by recycling the images over and over again a better perception of the ventricular function is obtained. The subjective interpretation of the images is complemented by the quantitive data; normal (Figs 20.14, 20.15) and

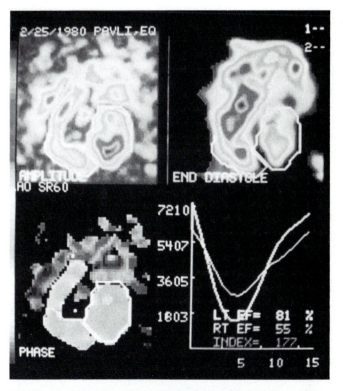

Fig. 20.16 Quantitative data analysis of the normal cardiac cycle (amplitude and phase analysis) made from a gated equilibrium scan. The phase image demonstrates uniform (normal) contraction. From the time activity curve, the ejection fraction of both ventricles (LT EF, RT EF) is calculated and expressed as a percentage.

of 40–50 ms are usually adequate. Most studies require 6–10 minutes to obtain enough counts for data analysis. Derived data are then processed by computer to determine the variables of left ventricular contraction, as with first-pass data.

Non-imaging methods. A single-crystal 'probe' coupled to a small processing unit is capable of producing beat-to-beat time/activity curves which permit the measure of ejection fraction and end-systolic and end-diastolic volumes from changes in left ventricular counts. This non-imaging device is small and readily portable. Ejection fraction may thus be measured over a long period of time if a non-diffusable indicator (such as labelled red cells) is used; the accuracy of the method is increased if electrocardiographic gating is incorporated in

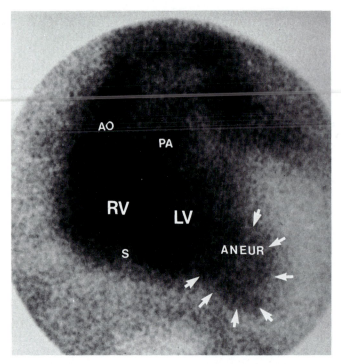

Fig. 20.17 Gated equilibrium scan in the left anterior oblique position. An apical left ventricular aneurysm has been demonstrated (arrows).

abnormal (Fig. 20.17) systolic wall motion in different areas of the ventricle can be assessed fairly accurately by this method. Wall motion can also be studied from the display of parametric data derived by computer analysis of the gated cardiac cycle. The cardiac cycle is divided into its various temporal frequency components, each frequency characterized by a specific amplitude and phase. The amplitude image represents the amount of contraction. The analysis of ventricular emptying and relaxation is derived from the phase image (Fig. 20.16); the degree of regional phase delay is generally related to the severity of contraction abnormalities and occurs in segments of the ventricle with no movement (akinetic) or in those moving paradoxically in systole (dyskinetic).

NUCLEAR TECHNIQUES FOR THE STUDY OF MYOCARDIAL PERFUSION AND INFARCT IMAGING

Assessment of myocardial perfusion. The use of thallium-201 myocardial scintigraphy for myocardial perfusion imaging has found wide acceptance in routine practice. Since thallium-201 uptake has been shown to depend mainly on myocardial blood flow and to a lesser degree on local cell metabolism, it can be used to assess the extent of hypoperfusion and hence ischaemic disease in the walls of the heart. Since the physical half-life of the isotope is 73 hours, transient myocardial ischaemia

can be detected by comparing the uptake data at the time of exercise with those obtained 3–4 hours later at rest. The thallium is injected at maximal exercise. Ten minutes after the exercise the patient is placed beneath the detector of the gamma camera and thallium scintigrams are made successively in the left anterior oblique 45° and anterior orientations (Fig. 20.18). Late imaging is performed in the same sequence after 3–4 hours. An area with reduced thallium uptake soon after exercise may be due to either transient uptake abnormalities (ischaemia) or a previous myocardial infarction (scar). While in an acute ischaemic area the uptake defect decreases or disappears with time (Fig. 20.18), the activity remains diminished or absent in an infarcted zone. The visual interpretation of these images depends on the experience of the observer, the quality of the image, the ratio of myocardial to background activity, and the medium by which the images are presented. To improve the reliability of the diagnosis, computer programs have been developed for the quantitative analysis of these images. The sensitivity and specificity of exercise ^{201}Tl myocardial imaging appear to be in the range of 85–95%, a moderate

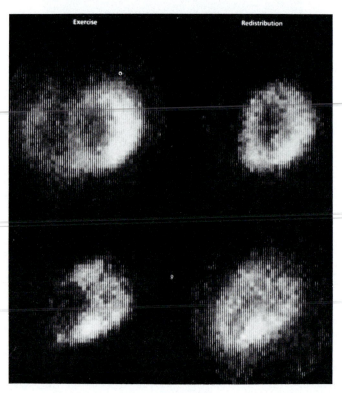

Fig. 20.18 Thallium-201 myocardial perfusion scanning. Above are the left anterior oblique views and below the lateral views of the same patient. Note the activity defect which is present in the septal aspect of the left ventricle on exercise but which fills in during the redistribution phase, seen on both views. The reversibility of the perfusion defect suggests that the myocardium is ischaemic but not necrotic. Note that the wall of the right ventricle is also demonstrated during exercise. The use of ^{201}Tl is one of the few ways of demonstrating abnormalities of right ventricular perfusion.

but definite improvement on the exercise electrocardiogram.

Infarct imaging agents. A variety of technetium-labelled phosphates are taken up by irreversibly damaged myocardium; a positive concentration gradient is therefore achieved between infarcted and normal tissue. The main application of these radiopharmaceuticals is in the serial evaluation of infarct size (usually overestimated by this method), in the differentiation between old and recent infarction (particularly in patients with bundle branch block on the ECG) and in the visualization of right ventricular infarction. The infarct may be detected as a positive focus 12 hours to one week after infarction.

ANGIOCARDIOGRAPHY

Angiocardiography is the X-ray imaging of the heart following the injection of radiopaque contrast medium. Selective angiocardiography — positioning the contrast medium injection, through a cardiac catheter, selectively in relation to the lesion to be demonstrated — is invariably employed. Selective angiocardiography is always combined with cardiac catheterization, so that intracardiac pressures (and if necessary oxygen saturations) can be measured. The aim is to delineate not only the types of abnormality which may be present but also their severity, so haemodynamic assessment is essential in other than coronary artery disease.

Filming is most commonly by cine from high-definition image amplifiers. 100 mm cut film may be employed in coronary arteriography, as the format is large enough for direct viewing by the surgeon. 14-inch square-cut film may be employed for pulmonary angiography or aortography where the large-field format is particularly useful. Direct digital imaging on a 512^2 matrix is now commercially available. Other advantages, besides its image quality, are instantaneous frame replay and stenosis quantitation.

Selective angiocardiography requires the site of the injection of contrast medium to be chosen for the best display of the lesion as suspected by clinical, echocardiographic or haemodynamic assessment. Contrast medium is injected downstream of leaking valves (cine angiography is still the best method of assessing the severity of regurgitation), upstream of obstructions, and in the chamber or vessel originating a shunt. The volume and rate of delivery of contrast medium are usually individually tailored to the problem to be investigated. For problems involving abnormal structure of the heart, where anatomical delineation is important, a volume of 1 ml/kg body weight should be delivered within 2 s, and the inevitable ectopic beats accepted for the sake of the high density of contrast which may be obtained. For functional cardiac studies such as left ventriculography in acquired heart disease, a slow injection should avoid

ectopic beats and a low density of opacification will be accepted. Here 8–16 ml/s over 3 s, (depending on the size and activity of the left ventricle and the quality of the X-ray equipment) will be adequate. An injector with rate and volume control is essential.

The choice of projection will also be influenced by the problem to be studied. Projections have become more complex. The standard biplane AP and lateral series gave way to the left anterior oblique and right anterior oblique views aimed at profiling the septal and atrio-ventricular valve planes; these have themselves partly given way to oblique views with the addition of cranial beam angulation, so that foreshortening of the profiled septum is reduced and septal and valve planes may be profiled in one view. These complex projections require ever more powerful X-ray equipment and ever more sophisticated tube suspensions.

Contrast medium. The standard ionic contrast media have pronounced effects on both the heart and the circulation. Passage of the contrast medium through the coronary circulation produces profound, though transient, changes in the ECG. These may be associated with demonstrable impairment of ventricular contraction and a rise in the left ventricular filling pressure, and associated left ventricular dilatation. The fall in blood pressure which is associated with angiocardiography is caused in part by the impairment of ventricular contraction associated with the perfusion of the coronary arteries by the contrast medium and in part by the peripheral vasodilatation which the contrast medium produces. Subsequently there is an increase in cardiac output due to haemodilution. Injection of contrast medium into the pulmonary artery may be associated with a rise in pressure in the pulmonary artery.

The low-osmolar contrast media are associated with much less subjective discomfort and significantly less haemodynamic abnormality than the standard media, though their viscosity and lack of anticoagulant properties are disadvantages. It seems likely that, in spite of their cost, these will be the agents of the future.

Angiocardiography is usually good at anatomical delineation of lesions but much less satisfactory in determining their severity and the degree of haemodynamic disturbance that they have produced. Angiocardiography can demonstrate an obstruction, be it valvar or subvalvar (or even supravalvar), but the severity of the obstruction must be assessed by the pressure gradient. This may be obtained by passing a catheter across the obstruction or by having catheters on either side. In the right heart the gradient across the pulmonary artery can usually be obtained by passing a catheter into the pulmonary arteries beyond the pulmonary valve and withdrawing it to the right ventricle. For tricuspid valve gradients it is customary to employ a double-lumen catheter because the overall pressures are low, pressure differences are very low and balancing the pressure recording system is critical. In the left heart an aortic gradient may be obtained by crossing the aortic valve retrogradely to the left ventricle from the aorta or by measuring aortic and left ventricular pressures separately, the latter from a transseptal catheter. Mitral gradients may be obtained by measuring an indirect left atrial pressure from a wedged pulmonary artery catheter, and by a catheter in the left ventricle.

When the significance of a gradient is not clear it may be necessary to measure the cardiac output (gradient depends not only on the severity of the obstruction but on the flow across it) and it may be necessary to increase the cardiac output by exercise to confirm the presence of a significant gradient.

The measurement of valvar regurgitation is difficult whatever measure is adopted. Aortic regurgitation is best assessed by cine aortography in the left anterior oblique projection, and mitral regurgitation by cine left ventriculography in the right anterior oblique projection. Quantification of the appearances is not really satisfactory but gives a general guide to the severity of the condition. An attempt may be made to assess pulmonary and tricuspid incompetence by cine angiography but the significance of the findings is never clear because of the presence of the catheter across the valve.

The number and size of shunts may be demonstrated by angiocardiography, but the degree of shunting requires either measurements of oxygen saturation changes or other more complex methods to measure shunt volumes.

Pulmonary vascular resistance, an important measurement in the management of congenital heart disease, requires knowledge not only of the pressure in the pulmonary artery and in the left atrium but also of the flow across the lungs.

The present method of studying left ventricular function, a key factor in the surgical management of patients with acquired heart disease, consists of studying the size of the left ventricle and the proportion of its content which it ejects with each beat (% ejection fraction, EF = stroke volume/end-diastolic volume $(SV/EDV) \times 100$). This can be measured by measuring the volume of the ventricle on cine angiograms, based on the assumption that the left ventricle is an ellipsoid of revolution, but most radiologists use visual assessment based on experience. Though the ejection fraction is the best method available for measuring ventricular function, it is widely influenced by factors outside the heart itself and may ultimately be replaced.

The era of catheterization and angiocardiography in every patient with heart disease considered for surgery is already drawing to a close. Any patient with acquired heart disease in whom the number and severity of the valvular lesions can be estimated on the basis of the clinical examination and echocardiography, and in whom

coronary artery disease is not suspected, can be operated on without this invasive investigation. An increasing number of patients with more complex congenital heart diseases are being subjected to surgery on the basis of the clinical and CSE examinations without angiocardiography. In some areas of anatomical delineation, particularly in the congenital abnormalities of the atrioventricular valves and their connections, CSE is demonstrably superior to angiography. In two areas however angiocardiography is still vital. In the investigation of coronary disease there are no simple noninvasive methods available. In disorders of the pulmonary circulation associated with congenital heart disease the standard CSE does not easily get beyond the main pulmonary artery, and to a lesser extent the same difficulty applies beyond the aortic valve; in these areas angiocardiography (or MRI) is still indicated in the absence of transoesophageal echocardiography.

NORMAL ANATOMY

Although the basic anatomy of the heart and its vessels is well known from the dissecting room, in situ in the closed thorax these structures may well appear unfamiliar when demonstrated by radiological methods. The normal *superior vena cava* (Fig. 20.19) forms the right border of the superior mediastinum. It is not normally visible as a discrete shadow. It may be visibly enlarged when distended, as in right heart cardiac failure.

A *persisting left superior vena cava* (which usually drains to the coronary sinus and thence to the right atrium) may be recognized as a low density shadow in the left superior mediastinum (Fig. 20.20).

The *inferior vena cava* is commonly recognized on good-quality lateral views of the chest by its straight posterior border rising from the diaphragm to join the back of the heart in the middle of the right atrium. It may also be seen in the frontal view in the right pericardiophrenic angle (Fig. 20.21) and may be visibly distended in heart failure.

The *azygos vein* rises in the posterior mediastinum on the right side and passes forward to join the superior vena cava before it enters the right atrium. Occasionally the normal azygos vein may be seen as a small 'end-on' shadow in the angle between the right main bronchus and the trachea. When an azygos lobe is present its fissure points to the azygos vein. The azygos vein may be quite large in the absence of pathology, when it may be confused with a paramediastinal mass. Contrast studies will serve to identify the shadow as vascular. It may be pathologically enlarged when the filling pressure in the right heart is increased from both cardiac and noncardiac causes, as in superior vena cava or portal obstruction. It reaches its largest size however when there is congenital interruption of the infrahepatic part of the inferior vena

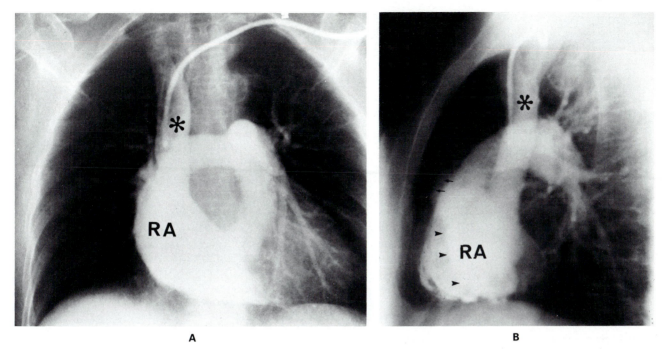

A **B**

Fig. 20.19 Normal right atrial angiogram. The injection has been made from a catheter in the superior vena cava. **A**. Frontal view.
B. Lateral view. The asterisk indicates the superior vena cava, and arrowheads mark the front border of the right atrium in the lateral view, overlapped by the right ventricle. Arrows indicate the front border of the right atrial appendage. The superior vena cava forms the right border of the superior mediastinum and the right atrium forms the border of the heart. Only the right atrial appendage forms part of the front border in the lateral view.

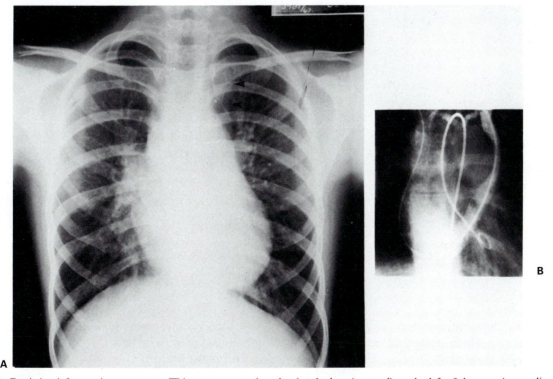

A **B**

Fig. 20.20 **A**. Persisting left superior vena cava. This appears as a low-density shadow (arrowed) to the left of the superior mediastinum in the plain film. **B**. The matching angiogram shows it to descend to the left of the aortic arch.

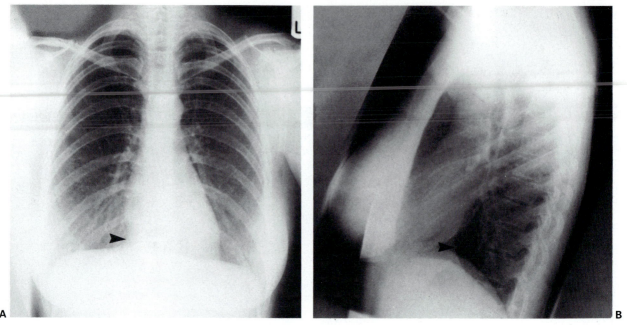

Fig. 20.21   Normal inferior vena cava (arrowed) seen in frontal (**A**) and lateral (**B**) views.

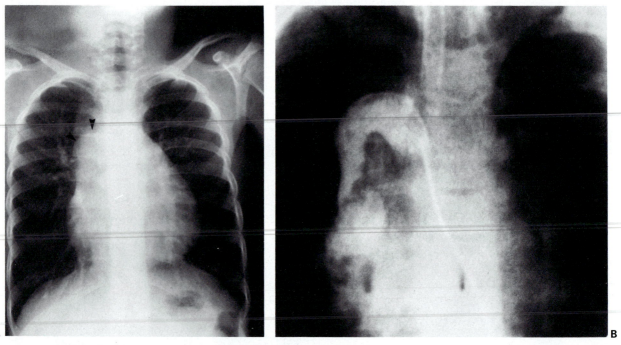

Fig. 20.22   Interruption of the inferior vena cava. **A**. The enlarged azygos vein (arrow) may resemble the aortic arch. **B**. Contrast studies in the same case show the azygos continuation of the inferior vena cava arching over the right main bronchus to enter the right atrium.

cava so that the distal inferior vena cava drains directly into the azygos vein which returns all the blood from the lower half of the body (Fig. 20.22). This arrangement always suggests the possibility of left isomerism or polysplenia.

A *left hemiazygos vein*, if present, may also be enlarged for similar reasons.

The right atrium (Fig. 20.19) is a globular chamber forming the right heart border in the frontal view. Its broad-based appendage passes forwards and to the left

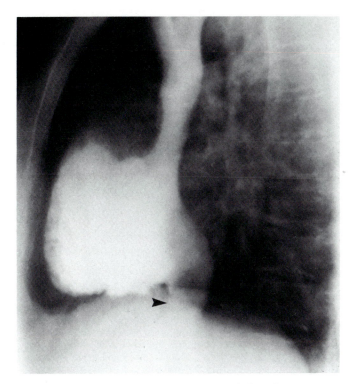

Fig. 20.23 Right atrial angiocardiogram, lateral view. Contrast medium has been injected into the superior vena cava and has refluxed down the inferior vena cava (arrow), showing it entering the back of the right atrium.

from its upper anterior aspect to sit on the front of the heart. The appendage is the only part of the right atrium seen anteriorly in the lateral view. The posterior wall of the right atrium is marked in the lateral chest film by the entrance of the inferior vena cava (Fig. 20.23).

When the right atrium is enlarged it makes the right heart border protrude to the right, and its radius of curvature, increases as the diameter of the spherical chamber increases (Fig. 20.24). A big right atrial appendage can fill in the space, seen in the lateral view, between the front of the heart and the back of the sternum.

Right atrial enlargement can occur in relation to both stenosis and incompetence in acquired tricuspid valve disease, and in both stenosis and incompetence in congenital anomalies of the tricuspid valve, more particularly in Ebstein's anomaly. The right atrium can also be enlarged when it carries a high flow, as in atrial septal defect.

The morphological characteristics by which the right atrium is distinguished as right, in complex congenital heart disease, are the presence of the limbus of the fossa ovalis on its septal aspect and its broad-based and squat atrial appendage.

The right ventricle (Fig. 20.25) is a chamber of complex shape. In the frontal view it appears triangular. The tricuspid valve enters from its right-hand posterior aspect and the ventricular apex lies at the left inferior part. At

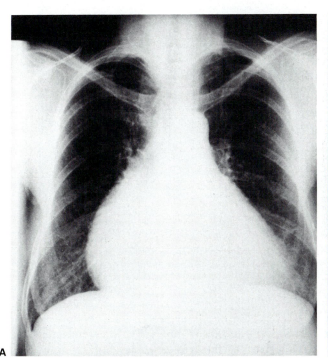
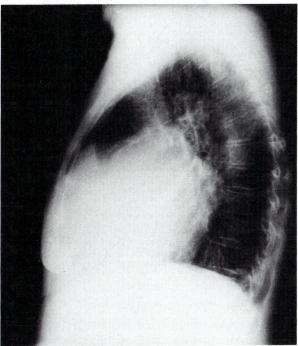

Fig. 20.24 Tricuspid stenosis. **A.** The right heart border has bulged to the right and its radius of curvature has increased. **B.** In the lateral view, the gap between the front of the heart and the sternum is filled in.

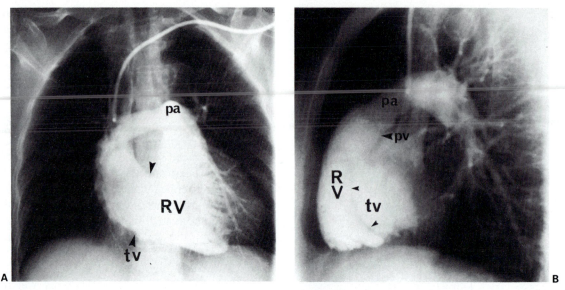

Fig. 20.25 Normal right ventricular angiocardiogram, superior vena cava injection. **A**. Frontal view. **B**. Lateral view. The right ventricle does not contribute to the cardiac silhouette in the frontal view except at the upper left border where its infundibulum reaches to the left border of the heart. It forms the front of the heart in the lateral view. These angiocardiograms indicate the position of the tricuspid valve, which because of its oblique lie is not seen in profile in either frontal or lateral views but its approximate position is indicated by the arrows. The pulmonary bay may be seen to be formed by the left border of the main pulmonary artery beyond the pulmonary valve and before it divides into right and left pulmonary arteries. The triangular shape of the right ventricle in the frontal view is obvious with the pulmonary artery sitting on its infundibulum. The flat shape in the lateral view is also obvious.

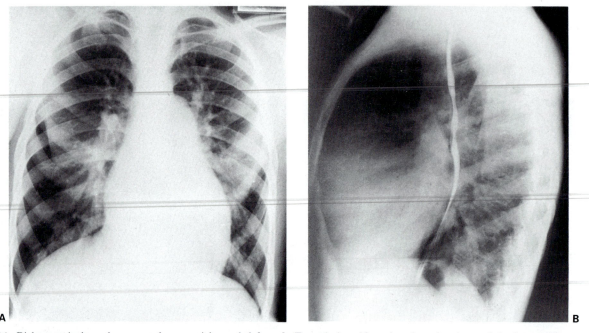

Fig. 20.26 Right ventricular enlargement due to atrial septal defect. **A**. Frontal view. Note the triangular shape of the heart with an indeterminate apex and a bulge of the left mid-heart border. There is also a convex pulmonary bay and pulmonary plethora (see below). **B**. Lateral view. This shows that there is slight bulging forward of the sternum but in addition there is increased area of contact between the front of the heart and the sternum.

the top of the right ventricle the pulmonary valve sits on the top of the muscular conus or infundibulum which separates it from the tricuspid valve. Seen from the side, the right ventricle is flattened with a meniscal cross-section produced by the large interventricular septum (really part of the left ventricle) bulging into the right ventricle. The right ventricle does not contribute to the cardiac outline in the frontal view but forms most of the

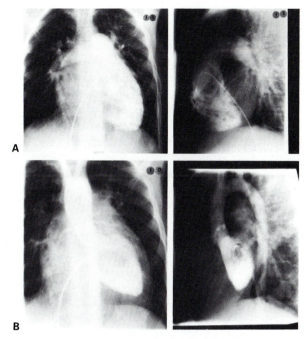

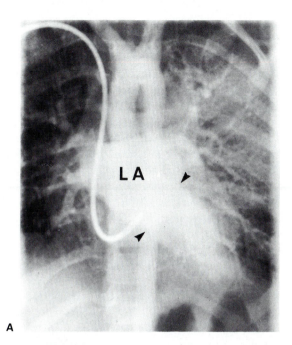

Fig. 20.27 Biventricular angiography in atrial septal defect. Same patient as Fig. 20.26. **A** (above). Frontal and lateral right ventricular angiogram. **B** (below). Frontal and lateral left ventricular angiogram. Note that the left border of the heart is now formed by the markedly enlarged right ventricle which also accounts for the increased contact of the heart with the sternum in the lateral view. The left ventricle, which has been pushed back by the large right ventricle, no longer contributes to the cardiac silhouette in the frontal view.

front of the heart in the lateral view. In the normally shaped chest only the lower half of the normal heart is in contact with the sternum.

Selective enlargement imposes the triangular shape of the right ventricle on the heart in the frontal view (Figs 20.26, 20.27). A bulge may be seen on the left heart border above the apex but below the expected position of the left atrial appendage where the large right ventricle, usually its infundibulum, forms part of the left heart border. Alternatively the bulge may be the large right ventricle lifting up a normal left ventricle. In the lateral view selective right ventricular enlargement may be recognized by the bulging forward of the front of the heart, increasing the area of contact with the sternum. A similar filling-in may also result if the right atrial appendage is very large.

Right ventricular enlargement may also occur as a result of pulmonary hypertension or pulmonary valve disease (usually pulmonary incompetence), tricuspid valve disease or left-to-right shunts.

The right ventricle is characterized morphologically by its muscular conus, (which separates its entry from its exit valves), by its coarsely trabeculated septal aspect, and by the direct attachment of part of its valve to the septum,

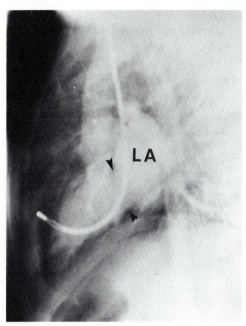

Fig. 20.28 Left atrial angiogram, follow-through angiogram. **A.** Frontal view. **B.** Lateral view. The left atrium forms a flattened structure, which is the upper posterior border of the heart in the lateral view, but does not contribute to the cardiac silhouette in the frontal view. The arrows indicate the position of the mitral valve which is not seen in profile.

either by chordae tendinae or by a papillary muscle of the conus.

The left atrium (Fig. 20.28) has an oval shape when seen from the front and is flattened when seen from the side. The four pulmonary veins enter its posterior aspect, two on each side. The left atrium forms the upper posterior border of the heart, although this border cannot clearly be seen as it is not in contact with air-containing lung. The position of the border can be identified in good-quality films as the air-containing left main bronchus lies in contact with the back of the heart; so does the oesophagus, and when this is opacified with barium it marks the back wall of the left atrium. The left atrial appendage is a narrow, finger-like protrusion from the left upper anterior border of the left atrium, passing forward round the upper left heart border to be buried in the epicardial fat. In the normal heart, neither the body of the left atrium nor its appendage make any significant contribution to the cardiac silhouette in the frontal view.

Left atrial enlargement (Fig. 20.29) may involve the appendage or the body or both. The enlarged appendage may be identified first by the straightening of the normally concave left heart border, then by the appearance of a discrete bulge below the pulmonary conus and above the left ventricle. Enlargement of the left atrial body may occur to the right, where it first appears as a double shadow through the heart progressing to form the right heart border. When gross it extends to the left. Enlargement may also occur posteriorly, displacing the left main bronchus and barium-filled oesophagus backwards. As most left atrial enlargement is associated with mitral valve disease the subject is considered again in Chapter 23, but enlargement may occur in any process causing either pressure or volume load to be transmitted to the left atrium, particularly left ventricular disease. The left atrium is the most sensitive chamber for the detection of chamber enlargement.

The morphological characteristics of a left atrium are the opposite of those of the right. It lacks a limbus to the fossa ovalis and its appendage is long, finger-like and narrow-based.

The left ventricle (Fig. 20.30) is a cone shaped structure whose base is formed by the fibrous skeleton of the aortic and mitral valves. The long axis of the ventricle points from the base, downwards, forwards and to the left to the apex of the left ventricle, which in turn almost invariably forms the apex of the heart. The left ventricle forms the left border of the heart in the frontal view and the lower posterior border, below the level of the mitral valve, in the lateral view.

Left ventricular enlargement is recognized in two ways. Left ventricular hypertrophy produces a rounding of the cardiac apex. Left ventricular dilatation (Fig. 20.31A) alters the shape of the heart in the frontal view by elongation of the cardiac apex either to the left or to the left and downwards, often combined with the rounding of the apex. Left ventricular enlargement may sometimes be identified in the lateral view when the soft-tissue shadow of the left ventricle protrudes behind the line of

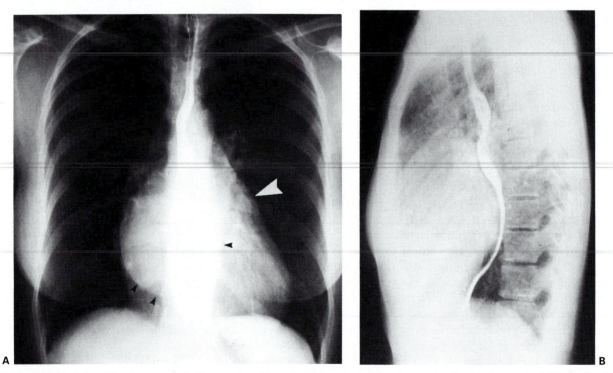

Fig. 20.29   Selective left atrial enlargement. **A**. Frontal view. The left atrial appendage produces a localized bulge on the left heart border (white arrow) below the pulmonary bay. The double shadow (paired arrows) of the left atrium is seen through the heart shadow. The displacement of the aorta to the left is indicated by the single arrow. Note that the right atrial shadow continues below the diaphragm as it is anchored by the inferior vena cava. **B**. Lateral view. Note the localized posterior displacement of the barium-filled oesophagus which returns to its normal position at the site of the mitral valve.

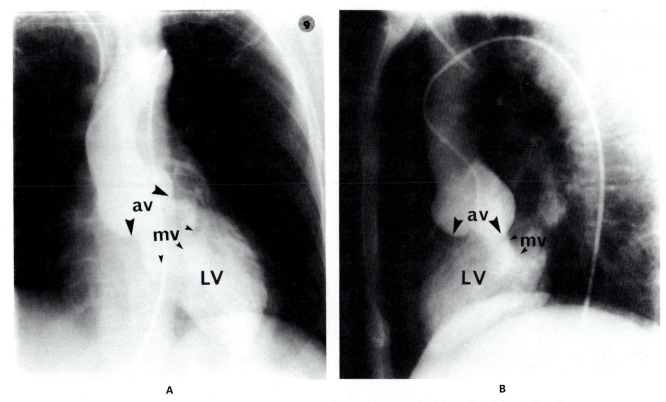

A B

Fig. 20.30 Left ventricular angiocardiogram. **A**. Frontal view. The left ventricle forms the left border of the cardiac silhouette and its apex forms the apex of the heart. The aortic valve lies approximately in the middle of the heart shadow. The mitral valve can be identified by the nonopaque blood entering and, with contrast medium, trapped under the posterior leaflet (small arrows). **B**. Lateral view. The left ventricle forms the lower part of the posterior border of the heart. The aortic valve lies approximately in the middle of the heart shadow. The anterior leaflet of the mitral valve (small arrows) is suspended from the noncoronary cusp of the aortic valve. The mitral valve lies obliquely and is not seen in profile in these views but its approximate position has been indicated. The aorta, beginning at the aortic valve, extends to the right of the superior mediastinum and then passes to the left of the oesophagus and trachea to reach the posterior mediastinum, and turns downwards as the descending aorta. On the right the aorta is concealed by the superior vena cava and its most posterior part forms the aortic knob of the frontal chest X-ray.

the barium filled oesophagus, or more than 2 cm behind the back of the right atrium as indicated by the entrance of the inferior vena cava (Fig. 20.31B).

Left ventricular enlargement may occur in any overload of pressure or volume in the left ventricle. Pressure overload results from hypertension, coarctation, aortic heart disease or any form of congenital aortic obstruction. Volume overload may be caused by mitral or aortic regurgitation or left-to-right shunt. Left ventricular enlargement may also result from diseases of heart muscle such as ischaemia or cardiomyopathy.

The morphological characteristics of the left ventricle are the lack of a muscular conus separating the entry and exit valves which are in fibrous continuity, a smooth septal aspect and a mitral valve which is not attached directly to the ventricular septum.

The aorta (Fig. 20.30) begins at the aortic valve, which lies just above the middle of the heart shadow in both frontal and lateral views. The aortic valve lies within the heart mass and does not usually cast a discrete shadow. Rarely, a faint small double shadow may be seen through the heart in the frontal view, rather resembling

that of the left atrium, though seen to be continuous with the ascending aorta. The normal ascending aorta does not form a discrete shadow in the right superior mediastinum, being covered by the superior vena cava. When dilated and elongated in old age or hypertension, the ascending aorta bulges to the right. Only the front wall of the ascending aorta is easily identified in the lateral view; the posterior wall, not being in contact with gas-containing lung, is imperfectly seen. The arch of the aorta passes in front of the trachea and then backwards on the left of the trachea and oesophagus. It can usually be seen indenting the left side of the trachea, in correctly penetrated films, and also the barium-filled oesophagus. In cases of doubt those signs indicate the side of the aortic arch. The shadow of the aortic knob is formed by the most posterior part of the aortic arch. The left border of a descending aorta can usually be identified in adult patients as a straight line passing downwards and towards the midline, lying to the left of the spine and in continuity with the arch of the aorta.

The main pulmonary artery (Fig. 20.25), that part of the pulmonary artery between the pulmonary valve and

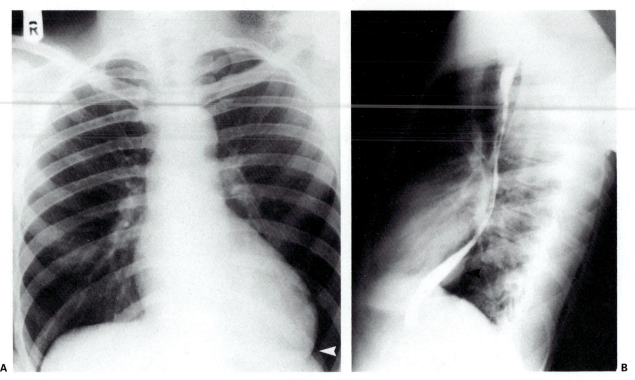

Fig. 20.31 Selective left ventricular enlargement in aortic incompetence. **A**. Frontal view shows that the left ventricle has enlarged along its long axis, taking the apex of the heart to the left and downwards (white arrow). **B**. Lateral view shows the left ventricle extending behind the line of the barium-filled oesophagus (arrow).

the bifurcation into the right and left pulmonary arteries, forms the floor of the pulmonary bay and lies on the left between the aortic arch and the heart proper. In the normal adult the floor of the pulmonary bay tends to be straight. In children and young women a convexity, indicating a prominent main pulmonary artery, may still be normal.

CARDIAC SIZE

The plain film is an important indicator of cardiac size, and the detection of cardiac enlargement is an important aspect of its use. The customary method of assessment is the measurement of the cardiothoracic ratio (Fig. 20.32). In adult white patients this should not exceed 50% (two standard deviations above the mean), but in black patients up to 55% may still be normal.

The cardiothoracic ratio is increased in the elderly; this may be due to an infolding of the ribs, reducing the thoracic component of the ratio, or due to heart disease. The cardiothoracic ratio may be increased in the neonate (see Ch. 19).

The transverse diameter of the heart may be measured directly on a radiograph taken at 1.83 m (6ft.). Upper

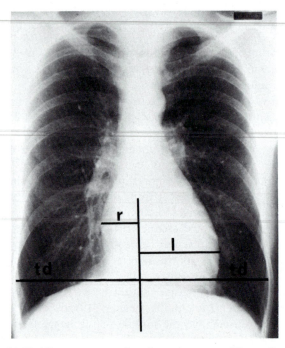

Fig. 20.32 The assessment of cardiac enlargement. The cardiac diameter should be the maximum cardiac diameter (r + l). The transverse thoracic diameter is measured in various ways; here it is measured as the maximum internal diameter of the thorax.

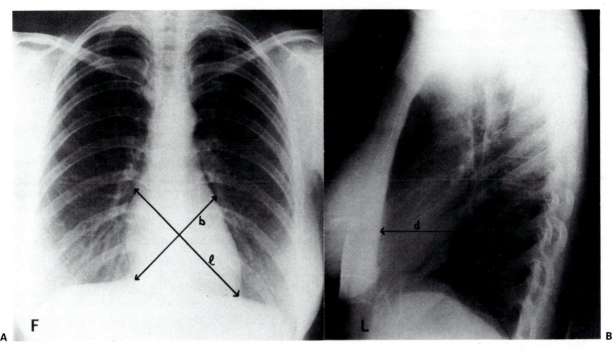

Fig. 20.33 A,B Measurement of cardiac volume. The volume of the heart may be measured on the assumption that the heart is an ellipsoid and if the lengths of its three axes can be determined, its volume $= 1 \times b \times d \times \pi/6 \times 1/m^3$ (where m is the magnification factor).

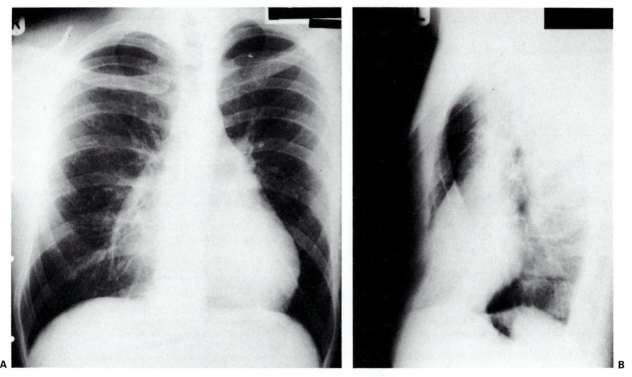

Fig. 20.34 Depressed sternum. **A.** Frontal view. The heart is displaced to the left. Its left border is straight and there is a prominence in the position of the main pulmonary artery. There is an ill-defined shadow to the right of the vertebral column. The clue to those appearances is given by the visualization of the intervertebral discs at the level of the lower thoracic spine where normally they would disappear.
B. Lateral view. This demonstrates the enormous sternal depression. This patient was thought to have a normal heart.

limits of 16 cm for men and 15 cm for women are usual. The advantage of a single measurement is that it may be compared in serial films. A difference of 2 cm is held to be a significant change. This applies only when the heart is originally normal, and physiological differences of almost that size may be encountered. In significantly enlarged hearts much less change in diameter will be significant.

The measurement of cardiac *volume* (Fig. 20.33), on the assumption that the heart may be represented as an ellipsoid, is not routinely performed, other than in Scandinavia.

In the neonate, the heart may be relatively larger compared to the thorax than in the adult, and a cardiothoracic ratio of up to 60% is not necessarily abnormal. Considerable care should be taken before diagnosing cardiomegaly radiologically, as much unnecessary investigation may follow. The neonatal chest is also difficult to study radiologically as the heart shape tends to be nonspecific because of the right ventricular preponderance which is present at birth. The mediastinal structures are frequently concealed by a large thymus so that identification of the side of the aortic arch and of the pulmonary bay may be difficult or impossible.

DEPRESSED STERNUM

Analysis of the size and shape of the heart may be made difficult or impossible in the presence of skeletal deformities, of which depressed sternum (Fig. 20.34) is the most common. The presence of odd murmurs, apparently related to the deformity, but resembling those of heart disease, may complicate the clinical examination. In the frontal view the heart shadow may appear overtly enlarged. Its left border is often straightened and the main pulmonary artery may appear prominent. The right border of the heart may bulge to the right if the heart is compressed against the spine, but most commonly it is not seen to the right of the sternum when the heart, as is usual, is displaced to the left. The central pulmonary vessels may appear prominent, and this together with the slightly odd murmurs may raise the possibility of an atrial septal defect. Ill-defined shadowing, often extensive, is frequently seen in the right pericardiophrenic angle, which the unwary might take for a pulmonary lesion. It does not show an air bronchogram. The easy visibility of the vertebral bodies and their intervertebral discs through the heart shadow of the standard frontal film always raises the possibility that the appearances of the heart are due to depressed sternum. If downward-sloping anterior ribs are present, this virtually confirms the diagnosis.

The appearances on the lateral view are often rather unimpressive, varying from a slight reduction in the anteroposterior diameter of the chest from flattening of the sternum to gross sternal depression with compression of the heart against the spine. The 'straight back syndrome', whose chief radiological feature is obvious from its name, also leads to a narrowing of the anteroposterior diameter of the chest, with squashing of the heart between sternum and spine, and similar, though less marked, cardiac appearances to those of depressed sternum in the frontal view. It may be associated with prolapse of the mitral valve.

REFERENCES AND SUGGESTIONS FOR FURTHER READING

Anderson, R. H., Becker, A. E. (1982) *Cardiac Anatomy: an Integrated Text and Colour Atlas.* Churchill Livingstone, Edinburgh.

Carr, D. H. (Ed.) (1988) *Contrast Media.* Churchill Livingstone, Edinburgh.

Elliott, L. P., Bargeron, L. M., Soto, B., Bream, P. R. (1980) Axial cine-angiography in congenital heart disease. *Radiologic Clinics of North America*, **18**, 515–546.

Feigenbaum, H. (1986) *Echocardiography.* 5th edn. Lea & Febiger, Philadelphia.

Fowler, N. O. (Ed.) (1983) *Non-invasive Diagnostic Methods in Cardiology.* F. A. Davis, Philadelphia.

Grossman, Z. D., Ellis, D. A., Brigham, S. C. et al (1984) *Cardiac Catheterisation and Angiography.* Lea & Febiger, Philadelphia.

Hatle, K., Angelson, B. (1985) *Doppler Ultrasound in Cardiology. Physical Principles and Clinical Applications.* Lea & Febiger, Philadelphia.

Higgins, C. B. (Ed.) (1983) *CT of the Heart and Great Vessels.* Futura, Mount Kisco, NY.

Netter, F. H. (1969) *The CIBA Collection of Medical Illustrations,* Vol. 5. *The Heart.* CIBA, London/Basel.

Raphael, M. J., Allwork, S. P. (1974) Angiographic anatomy of the left ventricle. *Clinical Radiology*, **25**, 95–105.

Raphael, M. J., Allwork, S. P. (1976) Angiographic anatomy of the right heart. *Clinical Radiology*, **27**, 265–272.

Underwood, R., Firmin, D. (1987) *An Introduction to Magnetic Resonance of the Cardiovascular System.* Current Medical Literature, London.

Walton, S., Ell, P. J. (1983) *Introduction to Nuclear Cardiology.* Current Medical Literature, London.

MRI

Brown, J. J, Scott, A. M., Sandstrom, J. C., Perman, W. H. (1990) MR spectroscopy of the heart. *American Journal of Roentgenology*, **155**, 1–11.

Henkelman, R. M. (1990) Technologic advances in magnetic resonance imaging and spectroscopy for cardiovascular applications. *Current Opinion in Radiology*, 2, 542–546.

Higgins, C. B. (1988) MR imaging of the heart: anatomy, physiology and metabolism. *American Journal of Roentgenology*, **151**, 239–248.

Jenkins, J. P. R., Isherwood, I. (1987) Magnetic resonance imaging of the heart: a review. In: D. J. Rowlands (Ed.) *Recent Advances in Cardiology 10*, Churchill Livingstone, Edinburgh, pp. 219–247.

Kanal, E., Shellock, F. G., Talagala, L. (1990) Safety considerations in MR imaging. *Radiology*, **176**, 593–606.

Mansfield, P., Morris, P. G. (1982) *NMR Imaging in Biomedicine.* Academic Press, New York.

Mirowitz, S. A., Lee, J. K. T., Gutierrez, F. R., Brown, J. J., Eilenberg, S. S. (1990) Normal signal-void patterns in cardiac cine MR images. *Radiology,* **176,** 49–55.

Mitchell, L., Jenkins, J. P. R., Watson, Y., Rowlands, D. J., Isherwood, I. (1989) Diagnosis and assessment of mitral and aortic valve disease by cine-flow magnetic resonance imaging. *Magnetic Resonance in Medicine,* **12,** 181–197.

Nayler, G. L., Firmin, D. N., Longmore, D. B. (1986) Blood flow imaging by cine magnetic resonance. *Journal of Computer Assisted Tomography,* **10,** 715–722.

Peshock, R. M. (1988) The heart and great vessels. In: Stark, D. D., Bradley, W. G. (Eds.) *Magnetic Resonance Imaging,* Mosby, St Louis, Ch. 36, pp. 887–920.

Pettigrew, R. I. (1989) Dynamic cardiac MR imaging: techniques and applications. In: Miller, S. W. (Ed.) Cardiopulmonary Imaging, *Radiologic Clinics of North America,* **27,** 1183–1203.

Rees, S. (1990) Magnetic resonance studies of the heart. (the George Simon Lecture) *Clinical Radiology,* **42,** 302–316.

de Roos, A., van Voorthuisen, A. E. (1989) Magnetic resonance imaging of the heart — morphology and function. *Current Opinion in Radiology,* **1,** 166–173.

Utz, J. A., Herfkens, R. J. (1988) Dynamic and physiologic cardiac MR. In: Stark, D. D., Bradley, W. G. (Eds.) *Magnetic Resonance Imaging,* Mosby, St Louis, Ch. 37, pp. 921–933.

Zerhouni, E. A., Parish, D. M., Rogers, W. J., Yang, A., Shapiro, E. P. (1988) Human heart: tagging with MR imaging — a method for non-invasive assessment of myocardial motion. *Radiology,* **169,** 59–63.

CHAPTER 21

THE PERICARDIUM

M. J. Raphael R. M. Donaldson

NORMAL ANATOMY

The pericardial sac consists of two layers separated by a potential space which is lubricated by a few millilitres of pericardial fluid. The parietal pericardium is a tough fibrous sac, enclosing the heart and attached to the central tendon of the diaphragm below. The visceral pericardium is closely applied to the surface of the heart. The two layers are fused next to the heart at the entry of the pulmonary veins to the left atrium posteriorly and at the entry of the inferior vena cava to the right atrium inferiorly. The two layers extend up the aorta, to fuse about half-way between the aortic valve and the origin of the innominate artery; they extend along the main pulmonary artery, fusing with it before its bifurcation, and along the superior vena cava.

Radiographic appearances

The pericardium has the same radiographic density as the heart. In spite of this it may be identified on the frontal film if there is a substantial amount of epicardial fat, which produces a low-density linear shadow, with a normal-density shadow of the pericardium appearing as a thin white line outside it.

The epicardial fat line is often best identified in the lateral view, and enables an estimate of the thickness of the pericardium to be made (see later).

The pericardial outline may be obscured by the pericardial fat pads, which may develop in the cardiophrenic angles as ill-defined low-density triangular shadows with their vertices in the cardiophrenic angles. The outline of the heart with its pericardium is often identifiable through them. The nature of these shadows is usually obvious from the lateral view, where they have a characteristically ill-defined triangular shape with the base of the triangle abutting on the anterior chest wall. Rather similar appearances may be produced by pleural thickening over the base of the middle lobe or lingula. Only rarely do these appearances lead to difficulties in differentiation from tumours or hernias occurring in the regions of the anterior cardiophrenic angles.

Ultrasound

The parietal pericardium produces strong echoes in both M-mode and cross-sectional echocardiography (CSE). In the absence of pericardial disease the strong echoes are continuous with the posterior wall of the left ventricle. The pericardium cannot be identified anteriorly unless it is abnormal.

CT scanning

Using modern high-speed machines the anterior and caudal part of the pericardium, where it is surrounded externally by the mediastinal fat and internally by epicardial fat, can be identified in almost all patients without the use of contrast medium. The normal pericardium appears as a fine line, 1–2 mm thick, in front of the lower part of the right and left ventricles and right atrium. Patchy areas of apparent pericardial thickening up to a few millimetres in thickness may be identified over the right ventricle in the apparently normal patient and are thought to be movement artefacts. The normal pericardium cannot usually be identified posteriorly.

MRI scanning

The pericardium is well-visualized on cardiac MR imaging (see below).

Angiocardiography

Opacification of the right atrium by contrast-medium injection into it or the vena cava, and frontal filming, will demonstrate the combined thickness of the pericardium and the wall of the right atrium, which is normally less than 3–4 mm. Later filming, as the contrast medium passes through the chambers of the heart, may also be helpful in detecting displacements and deformities of these chambers resulting from pericardial disease.

Pneumopericardium

The inner aspect of the pericardium may be outlined by gas introduced during pericardiocentesis, and the thickness of the pericardium determined.

DISEASES OF THE PERICARDIUM
CONGENITAL DEFECTS

These are rare and may be partial or complete, and usually involve the left side of the pericardium. Partial defects are usually asymptomatic, but may produce symptoms if the left atrial appendage herniates through the defect and then strangulates. They may be associated with nonspecific murmurs. Complete absence of the pericardium is not usually associated with specific clinical features. In both conditions, the plain films suggest the diagnosis.

In partial defects there is a bulge on the left heart border, usually in the position of the left atrial appendage and appearing to suggest that this structure is enlarged. However, there is no other radiological evidence of left atrial enlargement and no clinical features to suggest this, though the nonspecific murmurs may be confusing. Rarely the pulmonary artery may appear enlarged if it herniates through the defect and this (Fig. 21.1), combined with nonspecific murmurs, may suggest a diagnosis of pulmonary stenosis.

CT scanning reveals partial absence of the left pericardium and prominence and altered rotation of the main pulmonary artery.

Angiocardiography in the levophase of a pulmonary artery injection will confirm that the abnormal shadow is the left atrial appendage or an otherwise normal main pulmonary artery. In view of the danger of strangulation,

it has been suggested that the left atrial appendage should be amputated and the pericardial defect closed.

Complete defects of the left pericardium (Fig. 21.1) produce a characteristic appearance, with the whole heart displaced to the left with a prominent pulmonary artery shadow, perhaps a prominence of the left atrial appendage and with a slightly prominent left ventricular border. Gas-containing lung may be interposed between the heart and the left diaphragm if there is no connection between the pericardium and the diaphragm.

The diagnosis is usually made with confidence from the plain film and the absence of other features of heart disease. CT scanning may demonstrate the absence of the left pericardium and the altered axis of the main pulmonary artery to the left, and thus confirm the diagnosis. If there is still doubt, an artificial pneumothorax will allow gas to enter the pericardium and confirm its absence.

PERICARDIAL EFFUSION

This is the commonest abnormality of the pericardium to be encountered in routine radiological practice. The presenting features may be pain, when the cause is inflammatory, or malignant disease, or the clinical features of tamponade. Tamponade is characterized by shortness of breath, hypotension, pulsus paradoxus, and distended neck veins, and depends on the rapidity of fluid collec-

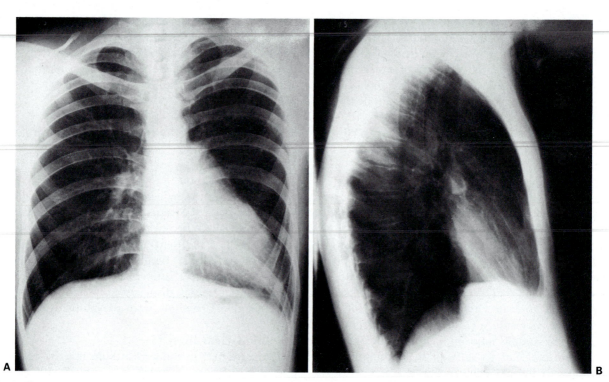

Fig. 21.1 Congenital absence of the left pericardium. **A**. Frontal view. Note that the heart is displaced to the left and there is a prominence in the position of the main pulmonary artery. Note also that the outline of the left diaphragm is clear as far as the spine.
B. Lateral view. This is unremarkable.

tion; over a litre may be present without symptoms if it collects slowly, whereas 200–300 ml collecting rapidly may cause symptoms. The fluid in the indistensible pericardial sac compresses the heart and obstructs the entry of blood through the vena cavae, leading to a fall in cardiac output.

The commonest disease of the pericardium, pericarditis, does not produce radiological abnormality unless an effusion is present.

Radiological appearances. The plain film appearances depend on the amount of fluid and its distribution. If there is sufficient fluid the heart shadow will be enlarged, and in larger effusions, grossly so. It may have a globular or nonspecific shape, but in large effusions there is very often a rather localized bulge in the left upper cardiac border which may lead to confusion (Fig. 21.2). Although the heart shadow appears enlarged, there are no features on the film to suggest selective chamber enlargement.

The accumulation and dispersal of fluid produces rapid changes in the heart size on serial films, and when these occur they always suggest pericardial fluid as the cause.

Displacement of the epicardial fat stripe inwards, when this can be identified, also points to a pericardial effusion. This is usually better seen on the lateral view, though in our experience it is rare. (Fig. 21.2).

Screening of the heart to show diminished pulsation and changes in shape from erect to supine posture, is of historical interest only.

The obstruction of venous return to the right heart rather than the left heart leads to a reduction in flow and pressure through the lungs, so that abnormalities of the pulmonary vasculature are striking by their absence.

These features lead to one of the characteristic appearances of a pericardial effusion: a large heart with clear lungs rather than congested lungs, which usually occur in heart disease. The other feature to suggest a pericardial effusion is a rapid change in heart size over serial films.

Other investigations. Once a pericardial effusion is suspected, *echocardiography* is the next step (Fig. 21.3). The CSE shows an echo-free space surrounding the heart, and if the effusion is large the whole heart can be seen swinging in it. CSE allows visualization of the aspiration needle during pericardiocentesis and thus avoids penetration of the myocardium. Several signs of cardiac tamponade have been described, such as right ventricular diastolic collapse, but the sensitivity of these is poor. Doppler examination shows an exaggerated inspiratory increase in tricuspid flow velocity, but again this feature is rather nonspecific.

CT scanning is also very helpful in medium and large pericardial effusions, showing a continuous layer of fluid surrounding the heart. The layer may be of either high or low density but this characteristic does not help in distinguishing the nature of the fluid.

Angiocardiography is now only rarely required, but right atrial angiography in the AP view will show an increase

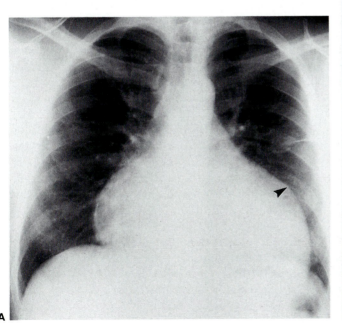
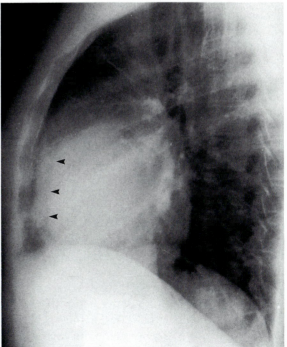

Fig. 21.2 Pericardial effusion. A chest film taken six months previously was normal. **A**. Frontal chest film. The heart silhouette has dramatically increased in size. There is an ill-defined bulge (arrow) above the cardiac apex. The lungs show no features of cardiac failure, which might be expected if this were a dilated heart. **B**. Lateral chest film. Epicardial fat is clearly identified (arrows), displaced away from the edge of the cardiac silhouette and indicating the presence of a pericardial effusion.

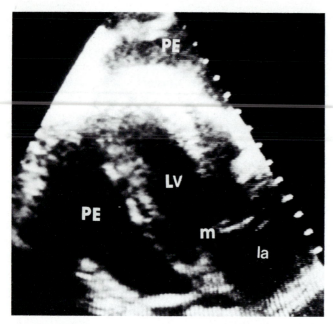

Fig. 21.3 Pericardial effusion, CSE study. In this long-axis view a large echo-free space of pericardial effusion (PE) is seen both behind and in front of the left ventricle (LV).

in the combined thickness of the right atrial wall and the pericardium to more than 4 mm. However it does not distinguish fluid from thickening. It would also show elevation of the floor of the right ventricle due to inferior fluid, and will show any localized fluid collecting over the left ventricle.

Aspiration. The nature of the pericardial effusion may be obvious on the basis of known clinical features, otherwise fluid may be aspirated and examined. *Gas* (or *contrast agent*) may be introduced into the pericardium at aspiration to outline the inside of the pericardium and indicate its thickness. A thin smooth pericardium suggests a transudate; a thick pericardium, an infection; and localized masses on the inside of the pericardium, a tumour. The heart structures are often clearly identified when there is gas in the pericardium.

A pneumopericardium may also result from chest or abdominal trauma or after cardiac surgery.

Aetiology. The following conditions may be associated with a pericardial effusion.

Malignant disease. Secondary malignant disease, usually from the breast, commonly produces a pericardial effusion and may lead to tamponade.

Inflammatory disease. Bacterial, tuberculous or viral infections may all lead to an exudative pericardial effusion.

Heart disease. A pericardial effusion may result from cardiac failure or may be associated with myocardial infarction when this is complicated by *Dressler's syndrome.*

Endocrine diseases. The best known of these is myxoedema, which frequently has a substantial though often asymptomatic pericardial effusion.

Collagen diseases. All the collagen diseases may be associated with a pericardial effusion, but in systemic lupus erythematosis it may be quite large.

Uraemia. A large pericardial effusion may be a feature of uraemia though it rarely leads to tamponade.

Haemopericardium. This may result from trauma, from rupture of the heart in the course of myocardial infarction, or a dissecting aneurysm leading into the pericardium.

CONSTRICTIVE PERICARDITIS

In this condition there is impairment of filling of the chambers of the heart, almost always involving mainly the right heart, and due to thickening and hence rigidity of the pericardium. Viral and tuberculous pericarditis are the commonest causes leading to constriction, but haemopericardium may lead to constriction, as may collagen disease involving the pericardium.

The patient presents with oedema and may have hepatomegaly and ascites. Shortness of breath is not a feature. The diagnosis of heart disease may not be obvious as there are no murmurs, and the neck veins may be so distended that pulsations are not visible, and the heart itself may not be enlarged. The diagnosis of constriction presents two problems: recognizing that the cause of symptoms is heart disease, and distinguishing constriction of the pericardium from a restrictive cardiomyopathy.

Radiological appearances. On plain film examination, the heart may be normal in size (Fig. 21.4A) or may be nonspecifically enlarged. Straightening of the right heart border with a smoothing-out of its contour from superior to inferior vena cava may be seen (Fig. 21.4A). There may be pleuropericardial adhesions roughening the outline of the heart. About half the cases have pericardial calcification, seen over the front and sides of the heart but not at the back where fluid cannot collect at the insertion of the pulmonary veins into the left atrium (Fig. 21.4B). Calcification may be seen on the plain film but is often better demonstrated by fluoroscopy, which is not only more sensitive but is also able to locate calcification to the pericardium. Calcification also develops in the atrioventricular groove and may encircle the heart. Calcification, however, does not invariably mean constriction.

Due to constriction over the right heart, the lungs are usually clear though there may be a pleural effusion. In those unusual cases where constriction in the atrioventricular groove obstructs left atrial emptying, pulmonary oedema may develop. Not all calcified pericardiums are constricted.

Investigations. These are usually devoted to confirming the presence of constriction, and distinguishing this condition from restrictive cardiomyopathy. The CSE

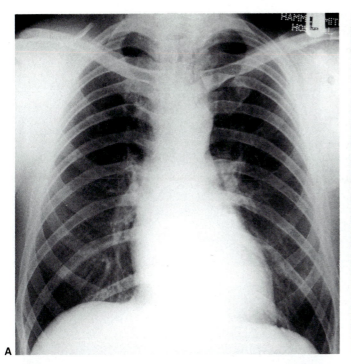
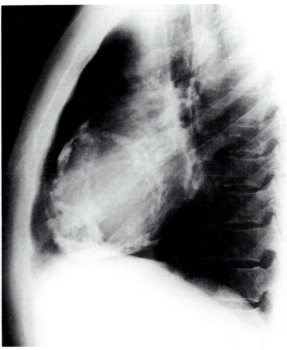

Fig. 21.4 Constrictive pericarditis. **A.** Frontal view. In this slightly light film the heart and lungs appear normal, apart from some possible straightening of the right heart border. **B.** Lateral view. This shows extensive pericardial calcification spreading over the front of the right ventricle and also encircling the heart in the atrioventricular grooves. There is no calcium at the back as fluid cannot collect there.

shows normally functioning chambers and may identify pericardial calcification by the dense echoes it produces. In the absence of calcification or pericardial fluid, the *CSE* may not demonstrate any abnormality of the pericardium. The *CT scan* will usually identify thickening of the pericardium and suggest a diagnosis of constrictive pericarditis (Fig. 21.5), but neither it nor the *MRI scan* can do other than show that the pericardium is abnormal, and this does not necessarily mean constriction is present. The demonstration of a normal pericardium (Fig. 21.6) virtually excludes the diagnosis of constrictive pericarditis.

Cardiac catheterization and angiocardiography. Right and left ventricular catheterization and simultaneous pressure records are required to establish a diagnosis of constriction. When constriction is present, the diastolic pressures in the right and left ventricle are identical. Thickening of the pericardium can be demonstrated by a right atrial injection, showing an increase in the thickness of the combined right atrial wall and pericardium above the normal 4 mm (Fig. 21.5C). The demonstration of thickening does not, however, inevitably point to constriction.

TUMOURS OF THE PERICARDIUM

These are relatively rare, the only common tumour encountered is the benign *spring-water cyst* (synonym *pleuropericardial cyst, pericardial coelomic cyst*). These cysts are unilocular and thin-walled and attached to the pericardium either intimately or by a pedicle, and are in some ways similar to pericardial diverticula, except that these communicate with the pericardial cavity. They are most commonly found in the pericardiophrenic angle, more often on the right than the left, though they can occur in any part of the lower half of the mediastinum. The smaller cysts may take up a rather 'tear-drop' shape and lie in an elongated fashion in the lower end of the oblique fissure, though the large ones are almost always spherical. On fluoroscopy they may be seen to change shape with respiration.

In the majority of cases the diagnosis is usually obvious on the plain radiograph, when they appear as rounded, sharply-defined cystic shadows anteriorly in the pericardiophrenic angle (Fig. 21.7). Rarely a Morgagni hernia, which may be filled only with omentum in the elderly, may cause confusion. Barium study will distinguish the two.

Secondary malignant involvement of the pericardium is common, producing a pericardial effusion and possibly tamponade. The breast is a common primary site.

MRI OF THE PERICARDIUM
Ian Isherwood and Jeremy P. R. Jenkins

The normal pericardium, demonstrated using ECG-gated T_1-weighted spin-echo sequences, is a thin (less than 2 mm) line of low signal intensity between the high signal

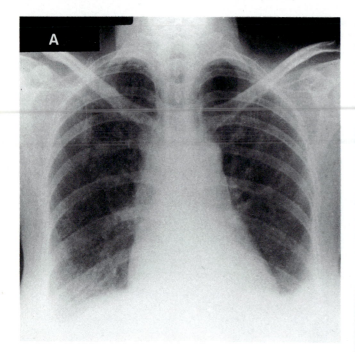

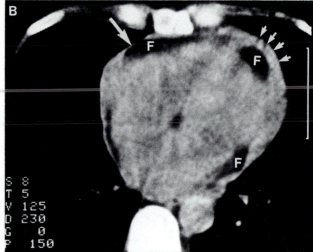

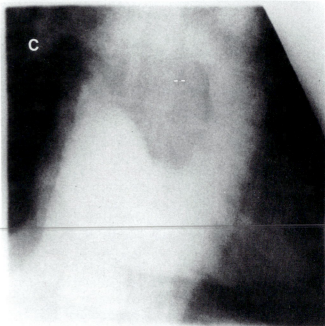

Fig. 21.5 Constrictive pericarditis. **A**. Frontal view. The heart is normal in size with some straightening of the right heart border. There are bilateral pleural effusions, larger on the left. There is also abnormal pulmonary shadowing due to active tuberculosis. This was the cause of the constriction. **B**. CT scan of the heart without contrast medium, same patient. Low-attenuation areas of pericardial fluid (F) surround the heart. The pericardium remains of normal thickness over the right ventricle (single arrow) but is grossly thickened over the left ventricle (multiple arrows). **C**. Right atrial angiogram, same patient. The increased thickness between the opacified right atrium and the outer aspect of the cardiac shadow is clearly visible. This indicates pericardial thickening but does not necessarily indicate constriction.

of pericardial fat and either the intermediate signal of myocardium or high signal of epicardial fat (Fig. 21.8). A variation in the clarity and thickness of the low-intensity line is observed during different phases of the cardiac cycle and in different anatomical regions. The low-intensity line is thicker in systole than in diastole and is best seen overlying the anterior part of the right ventricle. The variation in the thickness of this low-intensity line can be partly explained by a phase discontinuity artefact due to the shearing action between the visceral and parietal pericardium, produced in turn by the to-and-fro movement of the myocardium. This shearing action is most pronounced at the surface of the right ventricle, producing a loss of signal from the pixels spanning the

pericardium. The normal pericardial space also contains a small amount of fluid (up to 25–50 ml) and on T_1-weighted images this may make the pericardium appear slightly thicker. The variation in clarity of the low intensity line and its apparent absence over certain parts of the heart on MRI are due to chemical shift and motion artefacts.

MRI has been found to be a useful complementary procedure to CSE in the study of patients with suspected pericardial abnormalities. Pericardial effusions, thickening and tumours can be differentiated. MRI is the best modality for the characterization of pericardial fluid collections and the assessment of extrinsic invasion and compression of the pericardium.

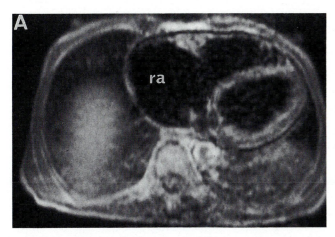
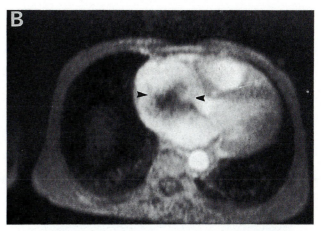

Fig. 21.6 Restrictive cardiomyopathy. **A**. MRI scan, spin-echo technique. The pericardium is clearly seen as a dark stripe outlined by the high signal from epicardial and pericardial fat and surrounding the front and left side of the heart. It is of normal thickness, virtually excluding the diagnosis of constrictive pericarditis, which, if present, would require surgery. Note the large right atrium (ra), compatible with tricuspid regurgitation. **B**. FEER (Field Even Echo Rephasing) sequence. Flowing blood is seen as a high signal. Note the signal drop-out from turbulent flow (arrows) produced by tricuspid regurgitation.

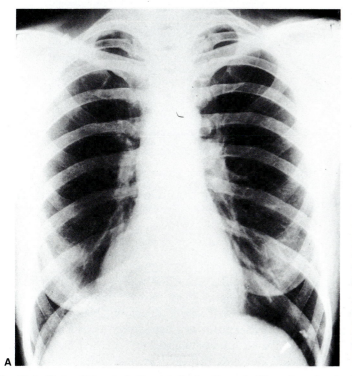
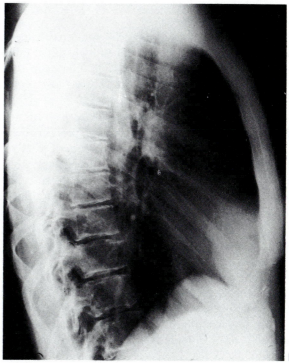

Fig. 21.7 Pericardial cyst. **A**. Frontal chest radiograph. There is a sharply defined abnormal shadow in the right pericardiophrenic angle. **B**. Lateral view. This is seen to lie anteriorly; this is one of the characteristic sites for a pericardial cyst.

Pericardial effusion. MRI correlates well with CSE in the assessment of size and distribution of pericardial effusions. It is more useful, however, in detecting small fluid collections and in differentiating between exudative and transudative effusions. Cross sectional echocardiography should nevertheless be used as the initial screening technique for the diagnosis and evaluation of pericardial effusions, reserving MRI for a problem-solving role when CSE results are inconclusive or there is a need for further tissue characterization.

The differentiation of an exudative from a transudative pericardial effusion is based on the signal intensity appearance relative to the myocardium. A transudative effusion has a lower signal, similar to that of normal pericardial fluid, whereas as exudative collection has a higher signal than that of myocardium (see Fig. 23.55).

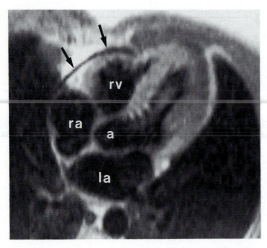

Fig. 21.8 Long-axis oblique gated T₁-weighted spin-echo image (TE 26 ms) of the left ventricle and aortic outflow tract demonstrating the pericardium (arrowed) as a low signal overlying the right ventricle. a = ascending aorta, la = left atrium, ra = right atrium, rv = right ventricle.

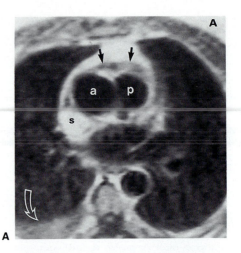

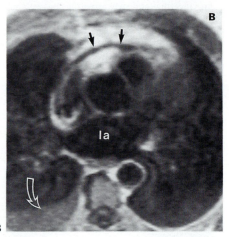

Fig. 21.9 A,B Constrictive pericarditis with a thickened pericardium (straight arrows) and a right pleural effusion (curved arrow) on two transverse T₁-weighted spin-echo images (TE 26 ms). Same key as in Fig. 21.8 and including p = pulmonary artery, s = superior vena cava.

Haemorrhagic effusions can be differentiated from other fluid collections by their medium-to-high signal intensity due to altered blood on T₁-weighted spin echo images. Non-haemorrhagic effusions usually give low signal on T₁-weighted spin echo images, whereas those associated with uraemia, trauma and tuberculosis give an heterogenous signal, related to a higher protein content. Effusions are usually differentiated from pericardial thickening by their morphological appearances rather than by changes in signal intensity (cf. Figs 21.9 and 23.55). Pericardial fluid, thickened fibrous pericardium and calcification all give a nonspecific low signal on MRI. CT, as might be expected, remains superior in the differentiation of fibrous and calcified tissue, and in the detection of pericardial calcification. In gradient echo images the pericardial space and any effusion are usually demonstrated as areas of high signal similar to moving blood.

Constrictive pericarditis. Thickening of the pericardium associated with constrictive pericarditis can be diagnosed and differentiated from restrictive cardiomyopathy by MRI. In restrictive cardiomyopathies the thickness of the pericardium is normal but there may be small pericardial effusions, whereas in constrictive pericarditis the pericardium is thickened (up to 5 mm or more) (Fig. 21.9). MRI assessment of myocardial wall thickness and cardiac function can also provide useful information. In constrictive pericarditis, in addition to pericardial abnormality, the end-diastolic volume is small, with a small compressed right ventricle and normal to increased systolic myocardial wall thickening. In restrictive cardiomyopathy there may be abnormal myocardial wall thickness and systolic thickening.

Pericardial tumours. Pericardial cysts can be readily differentiated from pericardial fat pads and Morgagni hernias on the basis of signal intensity and morphological appearances. A pericardial cyst has a low and high signal appearance on T₁- and T₂-weighted SE images respectively, whereas fat gives a high signal on both. A Morgagni hernia will show a defect in the diaphragm in connection with the peritoneal space and may contain liver or bowel. Infiltration of the pericardium by extrinsic tumour can be inferred from absence or loss of the pericardial low-intensity line.

REFERENCES AND SUGGESTIONS FOR FURTHER READING

Higgins, C. B. (Ed.) (1983) *CT of the Heart and Great Vessels.* Futura, Mount Kisco, NY.

Jefferson, K., Rees, S. (1980) *Clinical Cardiac Radiology.* 2nd edn. Butterworths, London.

Schiller, N. B. (1980) Echocardiography in pericardial disease. *Medical Clinics of North America*, **64**, 253.

Shabbetai, R., Mangierdi, L., Bhargava, V. et al (1979) The pericardium and cardiac function. *Progress in Cardiovascular Diseases*, **22**(2), 107–134.

Underwood, R., Firmin, D. (1987) *An Introduction to Magnetic Resonance of the Cardiovascular System.* Current Medical Literature, London.

MRI

Link, K. M. (1990) Noninvasive evaluation of the pericardium and myocardium. *Current Opinion in Radiology*, **2**, 586–594.

Miller, S. W. (1989) Imaging pericardial disease. *Radiologic Clinics of North America*, **27**, 1113–1125.

Mulvagh, S. L., Rokey, R., Vick, G. W., Johnston, D. L. (1989). Usefulness of nuclear magnetic resonance imaging for evaluation of pericardial effusions, and comparison with two-dimensional echocardiography. *American Journal of Cardiology*, **64**, 1002–1009.

Olson, M. C., Posniak, H. V., McDonald, V., Wisniewski, R., Moncada, R. (1989) Computed tomography and magnetic resonance imaging of the pericardium. *Radiographics*, **9**, 633–649.

CHAPTER 22

THE PULMONARY CIRCULATION

M. J. Raphael   R. M. Donaldson

The pulmonary circulation begins at the pulmonary valve, which sits on the infundibulum of the right ventricle. The valve cannot be identified specifically on the plain film but can be identified by cross-sectional echocardiography (CSE). Very rarely, it may calcify in middle-aged patients when the valve is congenitally abnormal or the seat of bacterial endocarditis, or in the presence of pulmonary hypertension.

The main pulmonary artery beyond the pulmonary valve may be identified on the frontal film, as its left border forms the floor of the pulmonary bay. This is the concavity on the left mediastinal shadow, below the knob-like shadow of the arch of the aorta, and above the shadow of the heart. In the normal adult the floor of the pulmonary bay is straight. In children and young women (Fig. 22.1A), a slight convexity is within normal limits.

Enlargement of the main pulmonary artery produces a convexity of the floor of the pulmonary bay. The main pulmonary artery is enlarged in left-to-right shunts, in pulmonary hypertension and in the post-stenotic dilatation of pulmonary valve stenosis; enlargement may be extreme in certain situations, such as when the Eisenmenger reaction occurs in rare association with an atrial septal defect, and in the pulmonary hypertension associated with bilharzia.

The main pulmonary artery divides, after a variable distance, into the right and left pulmonary arteries (Figs 22.1B, 22.2). The left pulmonary artery appears as the continuation of the main, passing backwards. It gives off the left upper lobe branches as it passes above the left main bronchus and then arches downwards as the branch to the left lower lobe, before dividing into the branches to the basal segments. The left pulmonary artery and its descending branch are silhouetted against the lung and can be identified on the plain film, as forming part of the left hilum and its continuation into the left lower lobe.

The right pulmonary artery appears as a sharply angled branch of the main pulmonary artery and passes to the right in the mediastinum. It divides within the mediastinum and its upper lobe branch leaves the mediastinum above the right hilum to supply the upper lobe. The

descending branch of the right pulmonary artery is the vessel first to be identified, as it forms the lower part of the right hilum where it is outlined against the lung (Figs 22.1A, B).

In the lateral view the right and left pulmonary arteries may be distinguished. The left pulmonary artery lies above and posterior to the radiolucency of the carina 'end-on'; the right pulmonary artery in front and slightly below (Fig. 22.2).

In the lungs the arteries lie within the parenchyma, roughly following the bronchial branching pattern. The short descending branches of both the right and left lower lobe arteries can usually be identified before they break up into the branches to the basal segments. The vessels to each lobe can be identified even though the branching pattern varies.

The arteries branch and taper smoothly out from the hilum and can be followed as discrete shadows to the outer third of the lung (Figs 22.1A, B).

The pulmonary arterioles, capillaries and pulmonary venules contribute to the lung radiopacity but cannot be identified as discrete structures.

The pulmonary veins form an inconstant arrangement (Fig. 22.1C). The pulmonary veins of the upper lobe collect into the superior pulmonary vein, those of the lower lobe into the basal veins which join to form the inferior pulmonary vein. The two veins on each side join the four corners of the left atrium.

The pulmonary veins may be distinguished from the arteries on the plain film (Fig. 22.3) by their course and position. The lower-lobe veins run horizontally to reach the left atrium and are usually visible and distinguishable from the more vertically running branches of the descending branch of the pulmonary artery. The upper-lobe veins, when visible, lie lateral to the upper lobe arteries, and run vertically to pass through the hilar shadow to reach the left atrium.

The hilar shadow has a concave outer aspect, formed by the superior pulmonary vein above and the descending branch of the pulmonary artery below.

The upper-lobe veins may not be visible on the erect

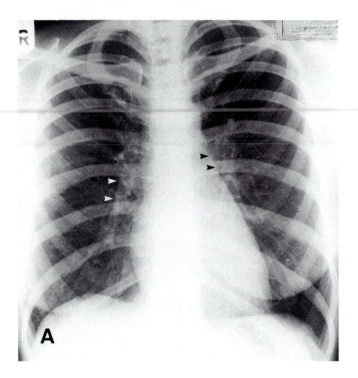

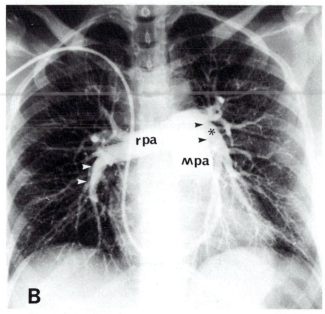

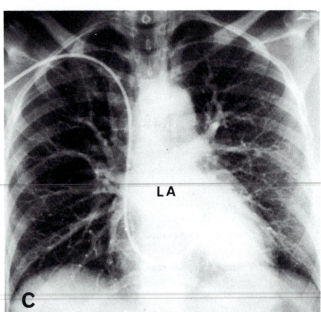

Fig. 22.1 A young woman with sudden onset of chest pain. **A.** Frontal film. The pulmonary artery beyond the pulmonary valve produces a slight convexity of the pulmonary bay (black arrows). The normal straight outer border of the descending right pulmonary artery may also be seen (white arrows). **B.** Pulmonary angiogram, arterial phase, same patient. The main pulmonary artery (MPA), beyond the pulmonary valve (black arrows), forms the floor of the pulmonary bay. The right pulmonary artery (RPA) appears as a branch of the main. It crosses the mediastinum and divides within it, so the arteries to the right upper lobe come out from the mediastinum above the hilum. The descending branch of the right pulmonary artery can be identified (white arrows) after it leaves the mediastinum and emerges to become silhouetted against the lung. The descending branch of the left pulmonary artery (asterisk) may also be seen silhouetted against the lung as it forms the left hilar shadow. **C.** Pulmonary angiogram, venous phase, same patient. The pulmonary veins are seen joining the left atrium. They converge to form four pulmonary veins, the superior and inferior pulmonary veins on each side, joining the four corners of the atrium.

film for two reasons. They are collapsed in the erect position, as the normal left atrial pressure is inadequate to distend them, and they carry little blood, as the normal pulmonary artery pressure is inadequate to perfuse the apices of the lungs. The normal upper-lobe vessels in the first interspace are rarely more than 3 mm in diameter.

The diameter of the descending branch of the right pulmonary artery does not normally exceed 15 mm in women and 16 mm in men. Normally it has a rather straight outer border. A convex outer border suggests that the vessel is abnormally large, a concave outer border that it is abnormally small. These features are probably more

helpful than measurements in evaluating pathology in the pulmonary circulation.

Rarely, the superior and inferior pulmonary veins may join each other, before entering the left atrium. This confluence can form a discrete rounded or oval shadow on the plain film (Fig. 22.4), on either side, and particularly so when there is an increase in pulmonary vein pressure. This shadow may resemble a tumour, but its nature is usually obvious because of its characteristic site right next to the left atrium, and once suspected can be confirmed by demonstrating its relationship to the pulmonary vein.

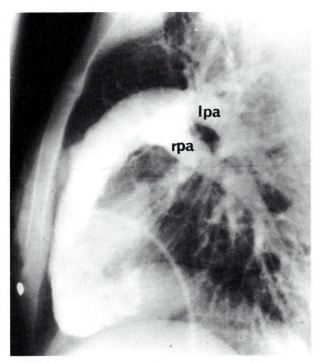

Fig. 22.2 Lateral angiogram to show the pulmonary arteries. The left pulmonary artery (LPA) lies above and behind the 'end-on' carina; the right pulmonary artery (RPA) lies below and in front.

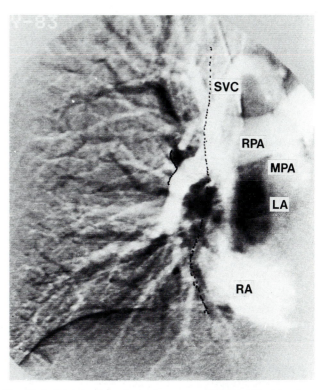

Fig. 22.3 Digital subtraction pulmonary angiogram. The use of computer techniques allows pulmonary arteries and veins to be displayed separately but simultaneously, in the same examination. The arterial phase appears in white, the venous phase in black; the right edge of the mediastinum has been dotted in. It is formed by the superior vena cava (SVC) above (the injection catheter, imperfectly subtracted due to movement misregistration, may be seen) and the right atrium (RA) below. The concavity of the outer aspect of the right hilum has been marked in ink. It is formed by the superior pulmonary vein above, descending vertically to reach the left atrium below the hilum, and the descending branch of the right pulmonary artery below. The upper-lobe artery is seen emerging from the mediastinum above the hilum and lying medial to the upper-lobe pulmonary vein. The lower-lobe vessels are less clearly seen, due to misregistration.

ABNORMALITIES OF THE PULMONARY CIRCULATION

The concept of pulmonary vascular resistance is derived by analogy from electricity. In the lung, PVR (pulmonary vascular resistance) is defined as P/F, where P is the pressure across the pulmonary vascular bed between the arteries and the veins, i.e. the pressure gradient (cf. voltage) in mmHg and F is the blood flow (cf. current) through the lungs in l/min. The normal pulmonary vascular resistance is one-sixth that in the systemic circulation, so that the normal pulmonary artery pressure (20/10 mmHg) is one-sixth that of the systemic circulation. The pulmonary artery pressure is easy to measure, and as pulmonary venous pressure is usually small, is taken to indicate the pressure gradient, unless there is evidence of pulmonary venous hypertension.

In normal lung, a marked increase in flow is accompanied by an increase in pulmonary artery pressure, even though pulmonary vascular resistance is normal; this is called 'hyperkinetic pulmonary hypertension'. When the increase in flow is reversed, pressure will fall to normal. An increase in pulmonary artery pressure may also occur if there is a rise in pressure in the pulmonary veins. This pressure will be transmitted directly back through the pulmonary vascular bed to the pulmonary artery, and this is called 'passive pulmonary hypertension'.

When a rise in pulmonary artery pressure is due to obstruction of the vessels within the lung, the condition is termed 'pulmonary hypertension'. It may be due to obstruction or destruction of the pulmonary capillary bed, to obstruction or vasoconstriction of the smaller arteries and arterioles, or to obstruction of the larger arteries.

CONGENITAL HEART DISEASE

Changes in the pulmonary circulation in congenital heart disease will be fully dealt with in Chapter 25, but the general patterns of abnormality are considered briefly here. Congenital heart disease may also show abnormalities and be associated with pulmonary changes similar to those in acquired heart disease.

Pulmonary plethora

This is the characteristic appearance of the lung vessels in the presence of increase in pulmonary flow, usually

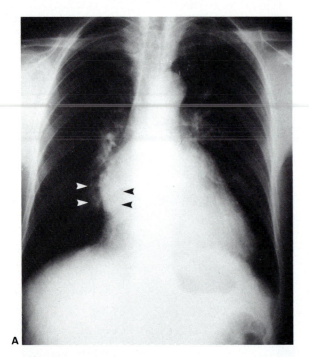

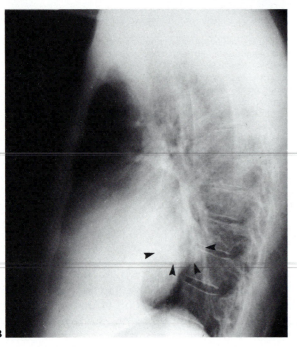

Fig. 22.4 Confluence of the pulmonary veins. In this patient with mitral valve disease, there is a large sharply-demarcated rounded shadow at the right corner to the left atrium (arrows). The nature of the shadow is suggested by its sharp definition and characteristic site, with pulmonary veins entering it. **A**. Frontal view. **B**. Lateral view.

from a left-to-right shunt, rarely from an increase in cardiac output. The main pulmonary artery is enlarged, producing a convex pulmonary bay. The pulmonary arteries and veins are increased in size and can be followed into the outer third of the lung. Upper- and lower-

lobe flow are equalized. Pulmonary oedema in association with large shunts may be superimposed on the appearances of pulmonary plethora.

If gross pulmonary plethora is present and an enlarged pulmonary artery cannot be identified, it may be: normally situated but concealed by the thymus; absent as in truncus arteriosus; or misplaced in the mediastinum as in transposition of the great arteries.

In the neonate the appearances of pulmonary plethora may be mimicked by an underexposed film. The following may produce the appearances of pulmonary plethora:

1. *Left-to-right shunts*
   a. Without cyanosis
      atrial shunts
      ventricular shunts
      aortopulmonary shunts
   b. With cyanosis
      All the following lesions are characterized by mixing of arterial and venous blood within the heart:
      transposition of the great arteries
      total anomalous pulmonary venous drainage
      truncus arteriosus
      common atrium
      single ventricle
      double outlet right ventricle
2. *Increased cardiac output*
   Pregnancy
   Anaemia
   Thyrotoxicosis
   Beriberi
   Systemic arteriovenous fistulae
   Chronic liver disease
   Polycythaemia
   Paget's disease

PULMONARY ARTERY PRUNING

High-pressure left-to-right shunts are associated with obstructive changes in the smaller pulmonary arteries and arterioles, which lead to an increase in pulmonary vascular resistance and a rise in pulmonary artery pressure, which ultimately reaches systemic levels, and hence to a reduction and then reversal of a shunt: the 'Eisenmenger reaction'. The characteristic but not invariable appearance in this situation is of a large main, and large central pulmonary arteries which taper down rapidly to very small vessels over a few orders of branches, giving a 'pruned tree' appearance. Unless the appearances are gross, the level of the increase of pulmonary vascular resistance cannot be judged by the plain film appearances.

In long-standing Eisenmenger reaction patients, calcification may develop in the main and central pulmonary arteries. The Eisenmenger reaction is a common complication of large ventricular septal defects and large patent ductus arteriosus defects, but is rare in atrial septal defects. Rise in pulmonary vascular resistance may also occur in association with similar communications in transposition of the great arteries or in syndromes allied to ventricular septal defect such as double-outlet right ventricle and single ventricle.

Pulmonary oligaemia

Reduced blood flow from obstruction proximal to the main pulmonary artery may produce characteristic radiological appearances. The main pulmonary artery is small and often displaced medially (as in the tetralogy of Fallot), producing an empty or concave pulmonary bay. The pulmonary vessels are small and the lungs are hypertranslucent. These appearances can be mimicked in the neonate by overexposure of the film, and are then difficult to assess, and the pulmonary bay itself may be obscured in the neonate by a large thymus.

Asymmetrical perfusion

The plain film may demonstrate abnormal asymmetrical perfusion. There is a normal perfusion gradient from above downwards, and the reverse perfusion gradient of pulmonary venous hypertension is considered below. Differences in perfusion on the two sides, as evidenced by differences in the size and extent of the blood vessels on the two sides, are a common feature of congenital heart disease, either as a result of revascularization surgery such as Blalock or Waterston shunt operations, or with congenital abnormalities of pulmonary flow. Localized abnormalities of perfusion, scattered throughout the lungs, are always strongly suggestive of complex pulmonary atresia (see below).

Bronchial circulation

An increase in the bronchial circulation, which usually develops as a response to severe obstruction of the pulmonary circulation, leads to an enlargement of the bronchial arteries. The enlargement may be suspected from a curious spotty appearance of the lungs, spreading out from the hilum. Pulmonary oligaemia can often be seen in association with this appearance of the bronchial circulation.

PULMONARY VENOUS HYPERTENSION

Impairment of function of the valves or chambers of the left heart commonly leads to a rise in pressure in the left atrium, which is transmitted back into the (valveless) pulmonary veins, producing pulmonary venous hypertension. This increase in pressure leads to the distention of the normally collapsed upper lobe veins. These veins may be recognized on the erect plain film (Fig. 22.5), as enlarged and rising up towards the apex of the lung. They may

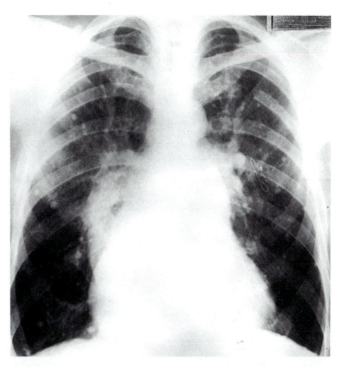

Fig. 22.5 The end result of long-standing severe pulmonary venous hypertension. There has been a closed mitral valvotomy through the left 6th rib. There is very marked upper-lobe blood diversion, with very large upper-lobe pulmonary veins and almost no veins visible in the lower lobes. There is also severe pulmonary arterial hypertension, with gross enlargement of the main and central pulmonary arteries with peripheral tapering. In addition, note the characteristic densities of pulmonary ossific nodules.

enlarge alone or there may be some enlargement of the arteries which accompany them, so that the vessels above the hilum appear larger than those below. The positive identification of *upper lobe blood diversion* almost invariably indicates disorder of the left side of the heart, though basal emphysema may rarely produce similar appearances without the explanation being obvious. Rarely, local lung disease involving the upper lobes may prevent its radiological recognition. However, it is common to see the changes of pulmonary oedema (see later) indicating severe functional impairment of the left heart, without recognizing upper-lobe blood diversion.

The explanation for the development of upper-lobe blood diversion is not clear. It has been suggested that perivascular oedema surrounding the lower lobe veins in the erect position leads to their compression and produces the redistribution of flow to the upper lobe.

As the pulmonary venous pressure rises above 25 mm Hg it exceeds the plasma osmotic pressure and reaches the threshold level for pulmonary oedema. This appears initially as **interstitial lines** (Fig. 22.6). *B lines* are horizontal basal peripheral non-branching fine lines visible on the frontal and lateral film. They are thought to be due to oedema of the interlobular septa through which the lymphatics pass. *A lines* are irregular lines

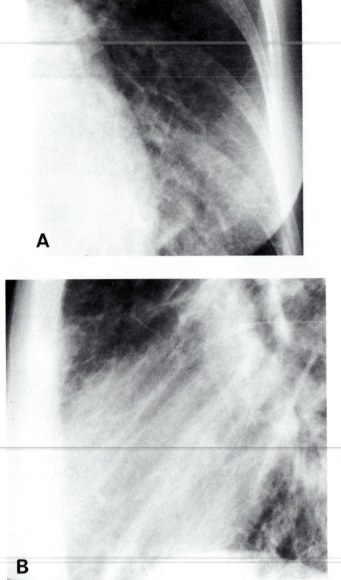

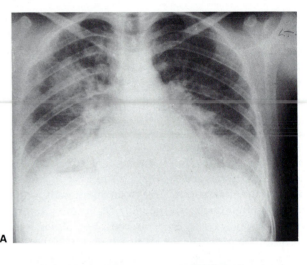

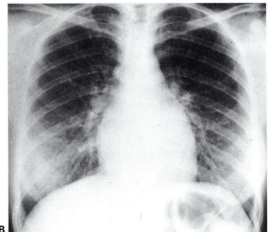

Fig. 22.7 Acute pulmonary oedema in mitral stenosis. The heart shadow is not large but shows the features of selective left atrial enlargement, compatible with mitral valve disease. **A**. On admission there was extensive bilateral pulmonary shadowing, primarily perihilar, and associated with loss of definition of the outline of the hila and vessels. **B**. Within one day this shadowing had cleared. The extensive nature of the shadowing, its perihilar rather than segmental distribution, and the rapidity with which its appearance changed, are the features which point to the diagnosis of pulmonary oedema.

Fig. 22.6 Pulmonary interstitial oedema. **A**. Localized frontal view of the left base. **B**. Localized lateral view of the front of the chest. The horizontal basal peripheral line shadows are the B lines, probably due to oedema of the interlobular septa. The lines running in apparently random directions are the A lines. In the lateral view, the B lines can be seen running horizontally at the back of the sternum, together with A lines. In addition, the fissures are thickened, indicating fluid within them.

spreading out from the hilum and thought to be due to oedema of the intercommunicating lymphatics. They are less frequently seen but have the same import as the B lines. They may also be seen behind the sternum, rising up the chest on the lateral view.

Interstitial oedema is mainly seen in association with a rise in left atrial pressure from any cause; mitral valve disease — either stenosis or incompetence, or obstruction at the mitral valve from a left atrial myxoma, will lead to a rise in left atrial pressure which is transmitted back to the pulmonary veins. *Left ventricular failure*, either from aortic disease, hypertension or disease of heart muscle, may be associated with the rise in left ventricular and hence left atrial pressure and pulmonary oedema. The non-failing left ventricle of *hypertrophic cardiomyopathy* may become so stiff that the high pressure required to distend it in diastole is transmitted back to the left atrium and leads to pulmonary venous hypertension. Rarely, the obstruction may lie in the pulmonary veins in unusual forms of *constrictive pericarditis* or in *pulmonary veno-occlusive disease*. In this last condition the plain film illustrates the characteristic appearances of interstitial and alveolar oedema, but there is no overt upper-lobe blood diversion or evidence of left heart disease. Unless a lung biopsy is taken, the diagnosis becomes one of exclusion. Interstitial lines are also a feature of a number of primarily lung diseases (see Part 2 of this book).

Once the left atrial pressure rises beyond the level at which the distended lymphatics can clear oedema fluid from the lungs, overt **alveolar pulmonary oedema** develops (Fig. 22.7). The classical appearance of this is of a confluent alveolar shadowing, developing in both lungs and having a perihilar or 'bat's wing' appearance. The densest shadow appears around the hilar regions, spreading off to an ill-defined periphery and sparing the bases of the lungs. Less commonly it may be localized to one lung, or part of the lung when its typical situation is in the right upper lobe. It may develop in the lung bases, or it may appear as a rather granular shadowing throughout the lungs without any overt perihilar concentration, or even as a peripherally distributed abnormal shadowing. Its association with a large heart, its rapid onset, rapid change with diuretic therapy, and often its extent, together with lack of fever, usually serve to differentiate it from infection.

Other features which may be seen in pulmonary oedema are blurring of the outline of the slightly distended hilum and blurring of the outlines of the central pulmonary vessels, due to perivascular oedema. Similar blurring may be seen around bronchi taken end-on in the frontal chest X-ray, the so-called 'endobronchial cuffing'. These features go to support the diagnosis of pulmonary oedema.

The development of **pleural effusion** is common in the evolution of pulmonary oedema and may go to support the diagnosis. Pleural effusions may be of considerable size, and have their characteristic appearances in the costophrenic angles; however, when very small they may appear as the lamellar shadow of a small parietal effusion lying against the outer wall of the thorax deep in the costophrenic angles. Fluid in the fissures of the lung may be recognized as thickenings of the fissures in both the frontal and lateral view and may go to support the diagnosis. Although pleural fluid may be distributed anywhere, it is relatively common for quite large effusions to collect in the fissures in the pulmonary oedema of cardiac failure, where they may appear to resemble tumour masses on the frontal film. The nature of these 'disappearing tumours' is quite clear when a lateral view is taken.

Once diuretic therapy has begun, the relationship between rise in pulmonary venous pressure and radiological demonstration of pulmonary oedema is lost.

A sustained rise in left atrial pressure leads not only to distension of the upper lobe veins but also to constriction of the lower lobe veins and then the arteries, so that flow through the lungs is virtually confined to the upper lobes. These appearances are most commonly seen in long-standing mitral valve disease, the 'stag's antlers' appearance (Fig. 22.5).

Initially, pulmonary venous hypertension is associated with a rise in pulmonary artery pressure equivalent to the rise in the pressure in the pulmonary veins, so that the pressure gradient across the lungs is normal: *passive pulmonary hypertension*.

Ultimately, obliterative changes in the pulmonary arterioles develop, leading to superimposed active pulmonary arterial hypertension, which is thought to be some form of protective reaction to the lungs. This can be seen on the plain film (Fig. 22.5) when the main pulmonary artery and the central pulmonary arteries begin to enlarge, the changes being particularly marked in the upper lobe. When such changes are present, they indicate pulmonary arterial hypertension but their absence does not exclude it.

Long-standing pulmonary venous hypertension may be associated with the development of **haemosiderosis** (Fig. 22.8) which appears on the plain film as a series of fine punctate calcifications scattered throughout the lungs.

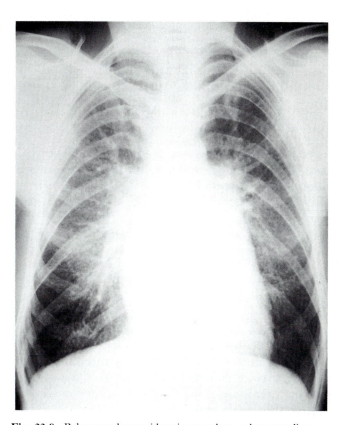

Fig. 22.8 Pulmonary haemosiderosis secondary to long-standing mitral valve disease. The fine granular background pattern to the lung is typical of haemosiderosis. In addition, note changes suggestive of mitral valve disease: straightening of the left heart border and some upper-lobe blood diversion.

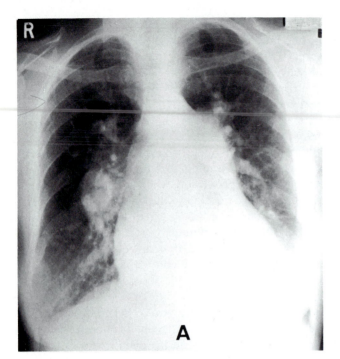

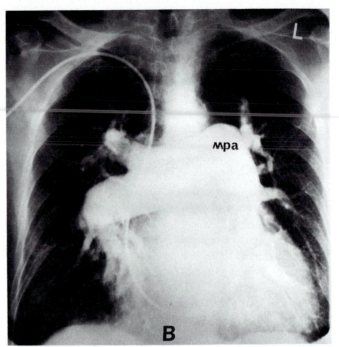

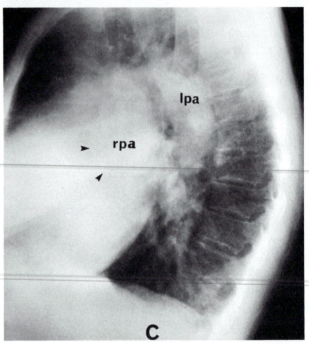

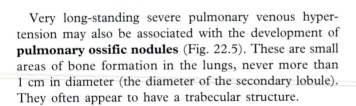

Fig. 22.9 Primary pulmonary hypertension. **A.** Frontal chest film. The heart is enlarged, with the triangular outline suggestive of right heart enlargement. The main pulmonary artery and central vessels are large but taper rapidly to the periphery. The enlarged right hilum is made up of an enlarged descending branch of the right pulmonary artery. **B.** Frontal pulmonary arteriogram, same patient. This enables the main pulmonary artery to be identified, confirms the make-up of the right hilum, and illustrates the dramatic peripheral pruning of the pulmonary arteries. **C.** Lateral chest film, same patient. This shows the enlarged right pulmonary artery (rpa) (arrows) and left pulmonary artery (lpa) and the right heart enlargement against the sternum.

Very long-standing severe pulmonary venous hypertension may also be associated with the development of **pulmonary ossific nodules** (Fig. 22.5). These are small areas of bone formation in the lungs, never more than 1 cm in diameter (the diameter of the secondary lobule). They often appear to have a trabecular structure.

PULMONARY ARTERIAL HYPERTENSION
This is defined as pulmonary artery pressure over 30 mm Hg in systole (and the pulmonary venous pressure is normal). In the absence of a shunt, the pulmonary artery pressure can rise above the systemic levels.

When the pressure in the pulmonary artery approaches systemic levels, a number of consequences develop. The right ventricle is unable to increase its output against this high pressure, so that any fall in peripheral vascular resistance, such as that produced by exercise, leads to a fall in systemic blood pressure and may lead to syncope. This is the mechanism of hypotension and death associated with angiocardiography, which produces a profound peripheral systemic vasodilatation. Low fixed cardiac output may lead to an anginal type of chest pain. Shortness of breath may be a feature. The high pulmonary artery pressure leads ultimately to right ventricular failure, with dilatation and peripheral oedema. This clinical picture will of course be modified according to the nature of the underlying causative lung disorder.

Radiographic appearances. The plain film (Fig. 22.9) characteristically shows a large and often triangular heart.

THE PULMONARY CIRCULATION

The main pulmonary artery and central pulmonary arteries are usually large, and may be very large, but taper rapidly to the periphery. Rarely, the pulmonary vessels or heart may appear normal, but it is very rare for the main pulmonary artery to be inconspicuous.

Lung scanning usually shows normal perfusion and ventilation, though rarely, small peripheral perfusion defects may be seen.

PULMONARY EMBOLISM

This may lead to a variety of clinical pictures, according to the size and number of the emboli and the underlying state of the circulation.

Acute massive pulmonary embolism

This occurs when one or more large pulmonary emboli, usually consisting of detached thrombus from the larger veins of the lower limb, impact in the central pulmonary arteries. It leads to the rapid onset of severe pulmonary obstruction, but this is usually associated with only a modest rise in pulmonary artery pressure, as right ventricular dilatation and failure quickly ensues. The clinical onset is usually with some shortness of breath, hypotension and tachycardia and perhaps chest pain. A history suggestive of deep-vein thrombosis of the legs may be present. The physical signs of a loud P2 on auscultation and the ECG evidence of right ventricular strain may suggest the diagnosis, but the clinical picture could fit with myocardial infarction, concealed haemorrhage or other cause of shock.

Radiographic appearances. The plain film may be helpful in this situation if it is of good quality and if the patient is otherwise fit (Fig. 22.10A). There may be a moderate increase in the heart size. The characteristic feature is the demonstration of *localized areas of under-perfusion* of the lung. These may be brought into relief by an apparent increase in perfusion of other segments. Large areas of one or both lung may be affected. Increased density of the main pulmonary artery associated with peripheral cut-off vessels, though well recognized, is exceptionally rare. Comparison with previous radiographs may be helpful in recognizing changes in the pulmonary vascular supply to the lungs. The characteristic changes are usually not recognized in poor-quality films such as produced by most portable X-rays; or when there is underlying heart disease, which is extremely frequent in association with pulmonary embolism; or if the embolization is extensive, when it produces an overall diminution in pulmonary perfusion rather than localized hypoperfusion with compensatory hyperperfusion elsewhere. When the characteristic features *are* present they are helpful in diagnosis, but this is rather an infrequent finding.

The investigation of acute massive pulmonary embolism depends on the facilities available, the time of day

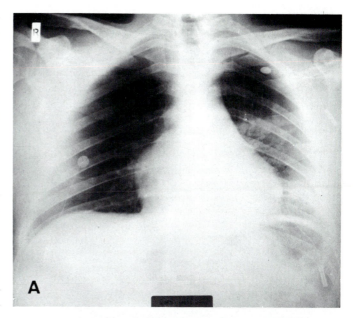

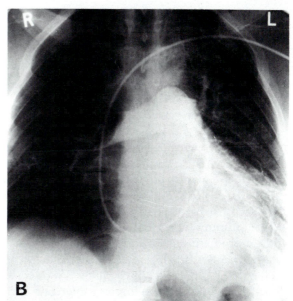

Fig. 22.10 Acute massive pulmonary embolism. **A**. Frontal chest film (portable). The right lung and the left upper zone are hypertransradiant due to oligaemia, and there is overperfusion of the left mid and lower zones. **B**. Pulmonary arteriogram, same patient. The leading edge of an embolus is seen impacted in the right pulmonary artery, producing virtually complete obstruction. Another embolus is seen in the supply to the left upper lobe which is also impaired. Only the left lower lobe fills adequately with contrast medium.

at which the clinical picture develops and the clinical certainty of the clinician. The situation clinically may be so precarious and the diagnosis so certain that little more than an ECG and a plain X-ray may be taken before beginning treatment with anticoagulants. The fatal pulmonary embolus is often not the one which brought the patient to medical attention, but one which follows soon

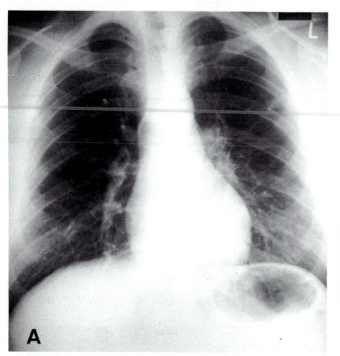
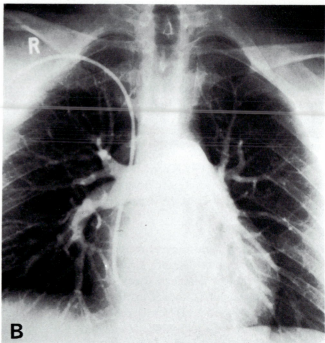

Fig. 22.11 The pulmonary embolism of Fig. 22.10, four months later, after effective treatment. **A**. Frontal film. This is now entirely normal. **B**. Pulmonary arteriogram. The pulmonary emboli have completely resolved.

after; if this can be prevented the patient should recover completely (Fig. 22.11). If the diagnosis is in doubt, it is usually quicker in most departments to organize emergency pulmonary angiography than pulmonary scanning, and this should be the investigation of choice (Fig. 22.10B).

Sub-acute pulmonary embolism

When the emboli are smaller and fewer so that acute cor pulmonale does not develop immediately, changes have time to develop in the lungs. As the lungs have a second, bronchial, circulation, overt pulmonary infarction is rare. It usually occurs when a large vessel is occluded and there is impairment of the bronchial circulation, a feature which commonly occurs in association with heart failure. The usual sequence of events following occlusion of a pulmonary artery (Fig. 22.12) is that the unperfused lung ceases to aerate properly, and this is associated with some reduction in volume, which is commonly seen on the plain film as an elevation of the diaphragm on the affected side. Over the next few days this hypoventilation may lead to areas of collapse, which usually re-expand if the patient survives. Infarction itself may develop to some degree in the affected vascular segment, of which the obstructed artery forms the apex and the pleural aspect the base. The infarction may be barely visible, but may lead to a haemorrhagic pleural effusion, and this may be seen as a small fluid collection in the costophrenic angle. The infarction very rarely appears as the characteristic

triangular shadow described in older textbooks. More commonly it appears as an area of rather nondescript consolidation whose chief characteristic is that it is associated with a pleural surface. This may only be apparent on the lateral view, and includes the surfaces of the fissures as well as the periphery of the lungs. These infarctions are usually partial and reversible in the course of time. They may disappear entirely or may heal to a linear scar. However if the infarction is large and there is impairment of bronchial perfusion, it may be irreversible and heal ultimately by scarring and fibrosis in the lungs.

The plain film appearances of pulmonary embolism with infarction are largely confined to the lung bases, the right side being more commonly involved than the left.

Pulmonary embolism with infarction is associated with a sudden onset of chest pain, with haemoptysis and with progressive increase in shortness of breath, as emboli arrive progressively and occlude the lung bed. A normal chest X-ray, even if of good quality, does not exclude the diagnosis, which may be clinically difficult. It should be suspected in any case of what appears to be a chest infection which does not respond to antibiotics, or in which the shortness of breath seems excessive. It should be considered with any patient with chest pain and clinical indications of possible deep-vein thrombosis. It may also be suspected in any patient — particularly in patients with heart failure — in whom the possibility of complicating pulmonary embolism arises, and whose shortness of breath appears to be out of proportion to the underlying

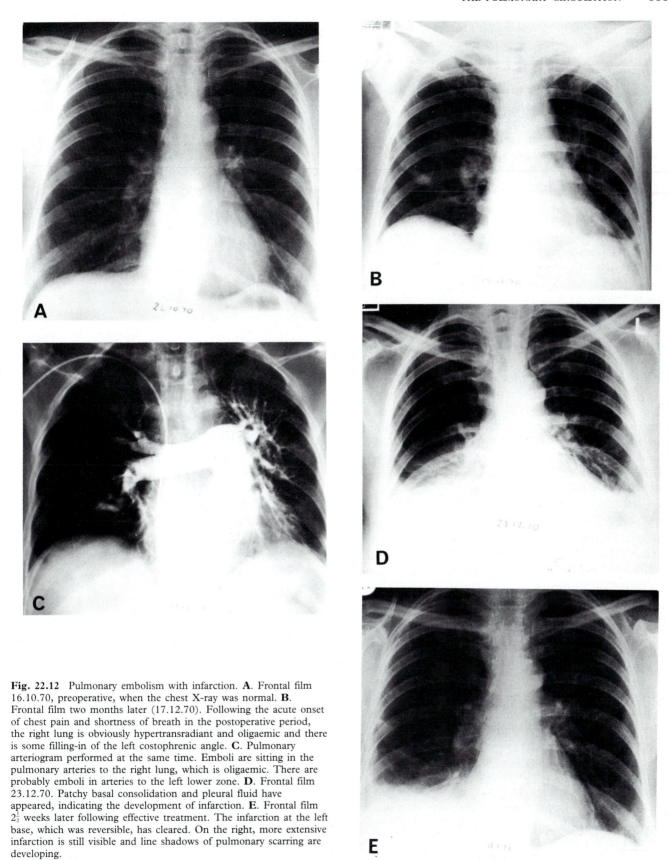

Fig. 22.12 Pulmonary embolism with infarction. **A**. Frontal film
16.10.70, preoperative, when the chest X-ray was normal. **B**.
Frontal film two months later (17.12.70). Following the acute onset
of chest pain and shortness of breath in the postoperative period,
the right lung is obviously hypertransradiant and oligaemic and there
is some filling-in of the left costophrenic angle. **C**. Pulmonary
arteriogram performed at the same time. Emboli are sitting in the
pulmonary arteries to the right lung, which is oligaemic. There are
probably emboli in arteries to the left lower zone. **D**. Frontal film
23.12.70. Patchy basal consolidation and pleural fluid have
appeared, indicating the development of infarction. **E**. Frontal film
$2\frac{1}{2}$ weeks later following effective treatment. The infarction at the left
base, which was reversible, has cleared. On the right, more extensive
infarction is still visible and line shadows of pulmonary scarring are
developing.

condition. It is in the subacute pulmonary embolism that radionuclide lung scanning plays its major part.

Radionuclide lung scanning

Modern methods of radionuclide imaging of the lung using a large crystal gamma camera have enormously improved diagnostic accuracy in pulmonary embolism. Technetium-labelled albumin macroaggregates or microspheres injected intravenously will impact in the lung in the absence of any right-to-left shunt, either cardiac or extracardiac. The distribution of these microspheres may be recorded by the gamma camera. A normal perfusion radionuclide lung scan excludes the diagnosis of pulmonary embolism from venous thrombus. If the perfusion lung scan shows the characteristic wedge-shaped localized perfusion deficits, then pulmonary embolism becomes a possibility. Perfusion deficits can be caused by localized lung pathology such as infections or areas of emphysema, or they can be part of a pattern of diffuse obstructive airways disease of the chronic bronchitis type. Multiple perfusion deficits, involving part of the lung which appear normal on the chest X-ray, increase the suspicion of pulmonary embolism. At this stage it is desirable to perform a ventilation scan; much the most effective is the inhalation of krypton-81m until equilibrium is reached and then recording the ventilation pattern with a gamma camera (Fig. 22.13). When the localized deficiencies of perfusion can be matched with deficiencies of ventilation, the likely underlying cause is some form of lung disease; and if a chest film appears normal, then obstructive airways disease is most likely (Fig. 22.14). When the ventilation remains normal yet a localized perfusion deficit is present, pulmonary embolism is highly likely; if the mismatch is definite and the perfusion deficits typical (Fig. 22.15), then the diagnosis may be taken as proven and treatment instituted.

Pulmonary angiography

If the ventilation/perfusion findings are not typical, or a full study cannot be performed, then it is desirable to proceed to angiography. Pulmonary angiography is usually performed by passing a catheter from a vein in the elbow through the heart to the main pulmonary artery. The pulmonary artery pressure can be recorded and then a pulmonary angiogram performed. A bolus of 50 ml at 25 ml/s is usually satisfactory and a large-film format

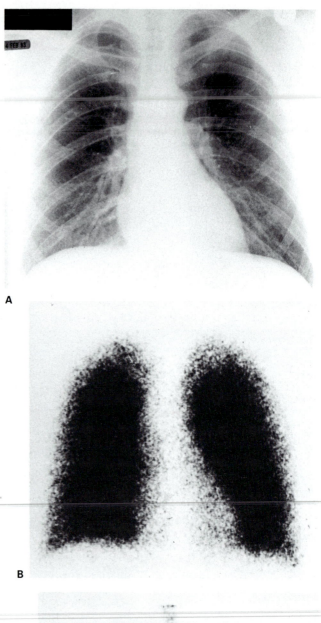

A

B

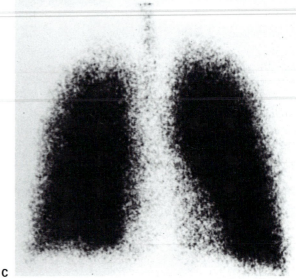

C

Fig. 22.13 Normal lung scan in a patient with acute chest pain. **A**. Frontal film. Normal. **B**. Frontal perfusion scan. This shows even perfusion over the whole of both lungs. **C**. Krypton-81 m ventilation scan. This shows even ventilation over both lungs. Note the activity in the trachea which can be recognized in this type of ventilation scan. The even and matched distribution of radionuclide with perfusion and ventilation excludes the diagnosis of pulmonary embolism.

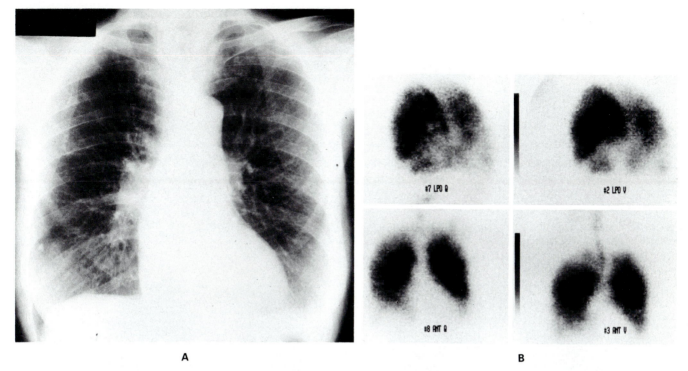

Fig. 22.14 Chronic obstructive airways disease. **A**. Frontal film. Apart from a slight 'streakiness' of the lung markings, which always raises the possibility of obstructive airways disease, the appearances are normal. **B**. Computer reconstructions of perfusion and ventilation scans. Perfusion is on the left and ventilation on the right. Note that in the left posterior/oblique (LPO) view there is a very large but matched defect of perfusion at the left base. The matching suggests that this is due to obstructive airways disease and not to pulmonary embolism.

rapid-film changer with rapid early and slow delayed films gives whole lung cover and adequate definition.

Venous angiography using a catheter in a peripheral vein and a larger bolus may give adequate visualization of the pulmonary arteries, and this technique has now been upgraded by the use of digital subtraction angiography, so that a fine catheter placed in the superior vena cava, using a mechanical injector to give a large bolus of contrast medium, gives adequate opacification of each lung in turn. This technique is best suited to the recognition of large central emboli.

The right lung is usually well seen in the frontal view; the direct posterior inclination of the left pulmonary artery means that it, and its proximal branches, may be too foreshortened, and a right posterior oblique, which is usually obtained by raising the left shoulder towards the overhead tube, will unfold them. With sophisticated apparatus the AP film may be taken with cranial angulation of the X-ray tube to reduce the foreshortening of the central pulmonary vessels within the mediastinum.

Pulmonary emboli can usually be directly demonstrated as sharply demarcated intraluminal filling defects in the pulmonary arteries filled with contrast medium (Figs 22.10B, 22.12C). When these are seen the diagnosis is certain. The presence of emboli reduces blood flow in the affected vessel, so that parts of the lung may appear

underperfused, but similar appearances may be produced by abnormal lung and are only suggestive rather than specific. Reabsorbed pulmonary emboli from previous episodes may appear as irregular narrowings of vessels without the demonstration of the intraluminal filling defects. Normal pulmonary arteries (down to the usual limits of the pulmonary arteriogram vessels of about 2–3 mm) excludes recent pulmonary embolus.

Pulmonary emboli may be lysed rapidly by the local infusion of streptokinase, which may be necessary if the patient is in extremis as in massive pulmonary embolism. More usually, the simple prevention of further pulmonary emboli by anticoagulation therapy is enough to save the patient's life and to promote the complete reabsorption of emboli. This takes place over a period of several weeks, and the subsequent pulmonary arteriogram may appear entirely normal (Fig. 22.11B). Further venous emboli may be prevented by the percutaneous insertion of a vena cava filter device if anticoagulant therapy proves ineffective.

CHRONIC PULMONARY THROMBOEMBOLISM
Established and irreversible pulmonary hypertension may develop as the result of continuing release of small emboli into the circulation. The patient presents with the clinical

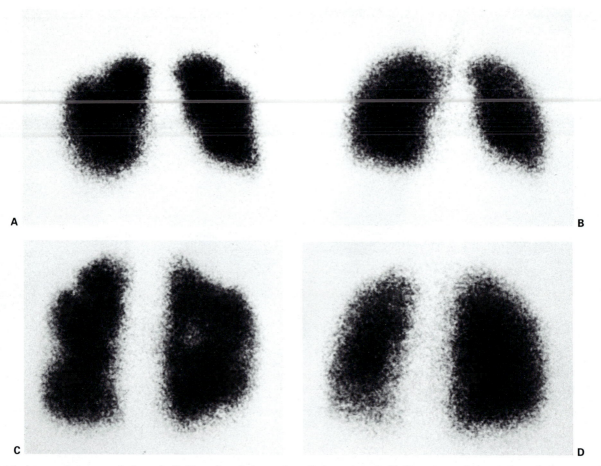

Fig. 22.15 Acute pulmonary embolism. **A, B**. Frontal perfusion and ventilation scans. **C, D**. Posterior perfusion and ventilation scans. Note the multiple wedge-shaped deficits on both the frontal and posterior perfusion scans but the entirely normal distribution of the radionuclide in the frontal and posterior ventilation scans. These appearances are typical of acute pulmonary embolism. The plain film was normal.

features of pulmonary hypertension and right heart failure, though in the history there may be episodes of recurrent chest pain and haemoptysis and of deep vein thrombosis in the legs. This form of pulmonary embolism is characterized commonly by the presence of widespread small-vessel disease in the lung and by associated localized obstructions of larger vessels.

The *plain film* will show the large main pulmonary artery which is usually seen in pulmonary hypertension, and also enlargement of central vessels and peripheral pruning. This is of a patchy nature, with some vessels remaining obviously enlarged and others small or absent and associated with hypertranslucent areas of the lungs (Fig. 22.16A).

The *radionuclide lung scan* will show widespread perfusion deficits with normal ventilation. *Cardiac catheterization* will reveal a pulmonary artery pressure which is markedly raised and may reach systemic levels, and *pulmonary angiography* shows several large vessels blocked proximally and with no distal perfusion of that

segment of the lung, whereas other vessels are obviously enlarged and perfusing the remaining part of the lung. The disease may be so advanced that only one lobe of a lung appears to be adequately perfused (Fig. 22.16B).

Chronic pulmonary thromboembolism may also occur as a complication of bilharzia. The plain film changes are often exceptionally gross, with very extreme dilatation of the main and central pulmonary arteries and with marked pruning peripherally (Fig. 22.17).

Pulmonary hypertension may also result from tumour emboli, and the usual source is choriocarcinoma.

Fat embolism
Fat embolism following major bone trauma may be associated with respiratory symptoms and a miliary or perihilar shadowing in the lungs. Fat globules may be seen in the sputum. However, the respiratory symptoms are more usually due to cerebral embolization occurring at the same time.

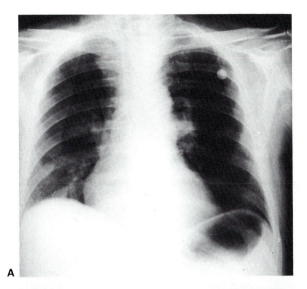

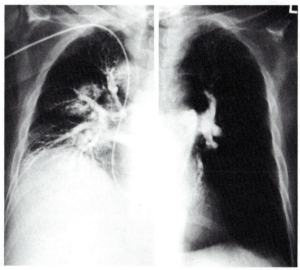

Fig. 22.16 Chronic pulmonary thromboembolism of the large-vessel variety. **A.** The frontal film shows a hypertransradiant left lung with areas of hypertransradiancy mixed with areas of increased perfusion in the right lung. **B.** The pulmonary arteriogram of this patient shows obstructions of many of the large branches of the left pulmonary artery with irregularity and rapid tapering of the arteries of the right lung, leading to patchy perfusion.

OTHER CAUSES OF PULMONARY ARTERIAL HYPERTENSION

Chronic bronchitis

Chronic bronchitis is defined as excessive sputum production associated with hypertrophy of the mucus glands of the bronchi. Acute infective exacerbations are extremely common. Superadded bronchospasm is also extremely frequent. In addition, infection of the abnormal bronchial mucosa leads to airways obstruction, and in long-standing severe cases to hypercapnia and hyoxia with cyanosis, which in turn lead to a rise in pulmonary artery pressure, and also to right heart failure with peripheral oedema, the so called 'blue bloater' type of patient.

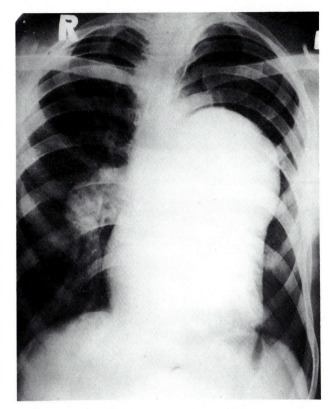

Fig. 22.17 Bilharzial pulmonary hypertension. Note the enormous enlargement of the main pulmonary artery. Some of the largest main pulmonary arteries are seen in this condition.

Between acute attacks the plain film may look relatively normal, though the lungs are often overinflated. The heart appears small but the main and central pulmonary arteries often appear rather large. There may be evidence of emphysema, with bullae and diaphragmatic adhesions, and there may be scars of previous infections within the lung. In the acute phase the diaphragms rise and the lungs are no longer overdistended. The heart shadow increases in size and the main and central pulmonary arteries also enlarge. The increase in vessel size may occur out to the periphery of the lungs so that the appearances almost resemble those seen in a shunt. There may be fresh pulmonary consolidation. If the patient recovers these changes reverse and the appearances revert to those before the infection (Fig. 22.18).

Special investigations to make the diagnosis of chronic bronchitis are rarely indicated, though its presence may complicate the interpretation of lung scans, if these have been performed to exclude pulmonary embolism. Perfusion deficits are common but they are usually associated with ventilation defects, and in experienced hands the exclusion of pulmonary embolism is not difficult.

Emphysema

Emphysema, the destruction of the terminal air spaces of the lung, often complicates chronic bronchitis but may

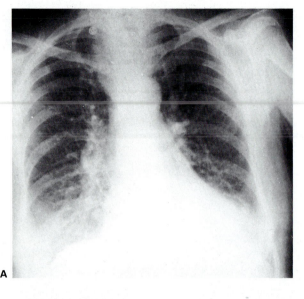

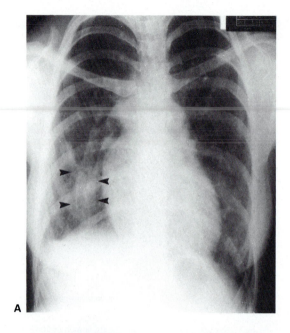

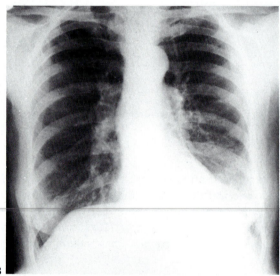

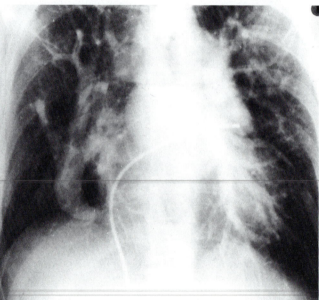

Fig. 22.18 Chronic obstructive airways disease with an acute exacerbation. **A.** The heart is large and the pulmonary vessels increased in size and apparently in number, almost resembling a shunt. **B.** Six weeks later, after resolution of the acute episode, both the heart and the pulmonary vessels have reduced in size. Note however that the central vessels still remain quite large.

Fig. 22.19 Scimitar syndrome, the heart normally situated. **A.** In the frontal film the scimitar is indicated by arrows. **B.** It can be clearly identified in the levophase of the pulmonary angiogram. Almost the entire right lung drains anomalously to this vessel, which is passing below the diaphragm.

occur alone. The usual pattern is of a dyspnoeic but not cyanosed patient, the so called 'pink puffer'. Rarely, emphysema, especially when gross, may lead to hypercapnia and pulmonary hypertension and cor pulmonale.

Cystic fibrosis

With modern treatment many patients are surviving the inevitable severe respiratory infections to reach adolescence or beyond. In some of these patients, characteristic cor pulmonale and pulmonary hypertension may develop, with a large main and central pulmonary vessels against

a background of overinflated lungs with the characteristic features of cystic fibrosis.

Other conditions

Pulmonary hypertension and right heart failure may be associated with severe *kyphoscoliosis* of the thoracic spine, particularly when it occurs in the high thoracic region. Hypercapnia and hypoxia may occur. The problem is primarily one of hypoventilation, due to a combination of respiratory muscle difficulty and underdevelopment of lung. In severe kyphoscoliosis the chest deformity is often so gross that no effective conclusions about the state of the lungs can be drawn from the usual plain films.

The *Pickwickian syndrome* consists of somnolence in an extremely obese patient. Polycythaemia is present and there may be right ventricular hypertrophy with right ventricular failure and associated pulmonary hypertension.

Ondine's curse is *idiopathic hypoventilation*. It occurs in young men and presents with lack of energy, somnolence, headache, shortness of breath on exertion and polycythaemia. The sufferers often stop breathing intermittently when they are asleep and this produces cyanosis. There may be pulmonary hypertension. The lungs are normal. A rather similar syndrome may occur in children with hypertrophy of the adenoids.

Pulmonary hypertension may also develop in patients who live at *high altitudes*.

CALCIFICATION OF PULMONARY ARTERIES

Calcification in pulmonary arteries can occur as a result of *atheroma* of the arterial wall, or in *thrombus* within arteries. Atheroma is almost always due to long-sustained severe pulmonary hypertension, and thus calcification may occur in the pulmonary arteries in those conditions in which this situation occurs. In addition, the majority of cases of pulmonary artery thrombosis occur in conditions where pulmonary hypertension is a major manifestation, and hence on occasions pulmonary artery atheroma and thrombosis occur together. The characteristic appearance of pulmonary artery calcification is that of curvilinear calcifications, demonstrable by films of appropriate penetration, in the position of what are obviously enlarged central pulmonary arteries, with peripheral pruning in addition. Differentiation of pulmonary artery calcification from the so-called 'eggshell calcification' of hilar glands is usually not in doubt.

PULMONARY ARTERY THROMBOSIS

Thrombosis of the main pulmonary artery or its branches is an uncommon complication of a variety of lung, heart and blood diseases. It may occur in association with parenchymal lung disease, rheumatic or congenital heart disease, sickle cell anaemia, polycythaemia, or even trauma to the lung. It may be found at post-mortem or demonstrated unsuspectedly by pulmonary angiography. There are no specific symptoms or signs, the occurrence being just part of the natural history of the underlying disease process.

The *radiological appearances* depend on the extent of the thrombosis. Where a lobar or segmental artery alone is involved the plain chest radiograph will probably not reflect any change. Where a main pulmonary artery is entirely thrombosed the hilar shadow is thought to be dense and rather sharply defined, and slightly large. There will be marked reduction of the peripheral lung markings. It may be difficult to recognize these changes if the appearances of the lung are disorganized by the underlying precipitating disease.

The appearances at *pulmonary angiography* will vary according to the extent of the obstruction. Occlusion of a lobar or segmental vessel will be manifested by the non-filling of this vessel, but without the classical leading edge of an embolus sign. Thrombosis of the main pulmonary artery will be revealed by a failure of any peripheral filling, and often by the demonstration of a filling defect within the main pulmonary artery, the thrombus itself. Again, contrast medium will probably not trickle pass the intraluminal mass, pointing to this as an intrinsic thrombosis rather than an ill-fitting embolus.

ANEURYSM OF THE PULMONARY ARTERIES

Dilatations of the pulmonary arteries are common in situations of altered pulmonary haemodynamics. They may occur in association with increased flow, as in atrial septal defect; with increased pulmonary artery pressure, as in long-standing mitral valve disease; or when these factors are combined, particularly in patent ductus arteriosus. These dilatations may be visualized radiographically, but rarely exert a specific influence over the course of the underlying disease. Aneurysms of the pulmonary arteries — dilatations associated with abnormalities of the wall of the pulmonary artery — are rare. They may be due to syphilis, atheroma, mycotic embolization or other local disease of the arterial wall, or to trauma. These aneurysms may be asymptomatic, or may lead to recurrent chest pain and haemoptysis, presumably by peripheral embolization of the aneurysmal contents. It is this latter group of aneurysms which presents problems in differential diagnosis, because they are unilateral and also have therapeutic implications.

Radiological appearances. In virtually all cases in which radiological examination of the chest has been performed, the aneurysm has been recognized as a rounded shadow in the hilum. It may grow to a large size, and be visible in the lateral view extending anterosuperiorly from the hilum. Curvilinear calcification may be demonstrated in its wall. Secondary lung abnormalities may be seen. In the cases where aneurysmal dilatation is associated with alterations of pulmonary haemodynamics due to heart disease, the pulmonary artery dilatations are commonly bilateral, and evidence of underlying cardiopulmonary abnormalities will usually be obvious. The chief differential diagnosis on plain-film radiography is from a localized aortic aneurysm, which usually affects an older age group and has a male sex preponderance. Bronchogenic carcinoma, or more rarely other lung or mediastinal masses, may also be considered in the differential diagnosis.

The diagnosis is confirmed by contrast examination. Any apparent increase in wall thickness is likely to be due to clot lining the aneurysm. Obstructions of peripheral arteries in relation to the aneurysms may be evidence of embolization. In the investigation of hilar mass by angiography it is important that filming should be carried on into the levophase, so that if a mass fails to fill from the pulmonary artery it may be possible to determine its relationship to the opacified aorta.

SCIMITAR SYNDROME

The degree of haemodynamic abnormality associated with anomalous insertion of the pulmonary veins depends on the number of pulmonary veins which are abnormally draining, and the site into which they insert. Total anomalous pulmonary venous drainage usually presents as a cardiac emergency. The majority of forms of partial anomalous venous drainage are associated with atrial septal defect, and are considered in Chapter 24. An abnormal pulmonary vein draining the right lower lobe and inserting below the diaphragm, usually into the inferior vena cava, may be found in the absence of significant heart disease and will be considered separately. The condition may present with recurrent respiratory infection involving the right lower lobe of the lung, and physical findings may reveal some crowding of the ribs of the right hemithorax and the presence of adventitial

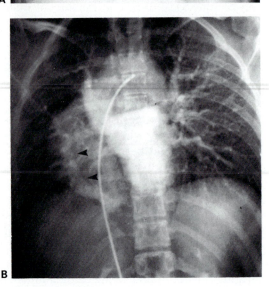

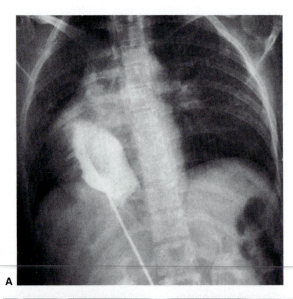

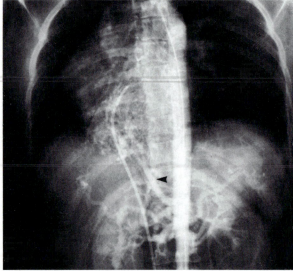

Fig. 22.20 Scimitar syndrome associated with dextroposition of the heart. **A.** In the plain film the scimitar shadow (single arrow) is overlapped and largely concealed by the misplaced heart. **B.** In the venous phase of the pulmonary angiogram, it can be clearly identified (paired arrows) passing below the diaphragm.

Fig. 22.21 Scimitar syndrome. **A.** A venous catheter has been passed from the inferior vena cava into the abnormal vein. **B.** Aortogram shows a systemic blood supply (arrow) ascending from the lumbar aorta through the diaphragm to supply part of the right lower lobe.

sounds in the right lung. The murmur of any associated *atrial septal defect* may also be heard, as the condition commonly occurs in association with atrial septal defect.

Radiological appearances. The characteristic findings are those which give the syndrome the name; the abnormal pulmonary vein is visible as an inverted scimitar-shaped shadow of soft-tissue density in the right lower zone, terminating at or below the diaphragm. The shape is so characteristic that when seen, the diagnosis of the nature of the abnormal shadow is rarely in doubt (Fig 22.19). Where the right lower lobe is hypoplastic, as it may be when drained by an anomalous vein, and particularly when supplied by a systemic artery, the diagnosis may be complicated by displacement of the heart and mediastinal structures to the right — *dextroposition* of the heart. This may be so marked as to obscure the characteristic scimitar shadow unless good-quality over-penetrated films are taken (Figs 22.20, 22.21). The condition is not of course a true dextrocardia, as the apex of the heart still remains pointing to the left. Scimitar syndrome is one of several causes of dextroposition of the heart.

The appearances of the scimitar are pathognomonic. Investigation is only indicated to elucidate the presence of any associated intracardiac malformation, or prior to surgery to determine which parts of the lung are drained by the abnormal vein, and how the arterial supply of the abnormal part of the lung is derived. For this reason the preoperative assessment, in addition to selective pul-

monary angiography filmed into the levophase to demonstrate the scimitar and its drainage, must also include descending aortography to determine any element of systemic supply to the abnormal lung (Fig. 22.21B).

When the condition presents in the neonatal period it may lead to very severe symptoms and be difficult to treat.

RIGHT PULMONARY ARTERY–LEFT ATRIAL COMMUNICATION

This congenital malformation usually occurs as an isolated abnormality unassociated with other cardiac abnormalities. The communication is usually a saccular aneurysm of the descending branch of the right pulmonary artery which opens into the left atrium, though pulmonary venous abnormalities may also occur. Patients

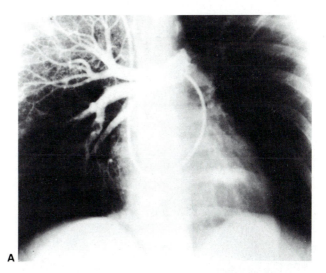

A

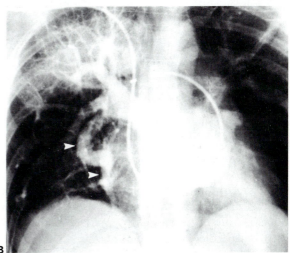

B

Fig. 22.23 A,B Right pulmonary artery to left arterial communication, pulmonary angiogram. In the venous phase the dilated right pulmonary artery (white arrows) has been opacified and is seen to be draining into the left atrium.

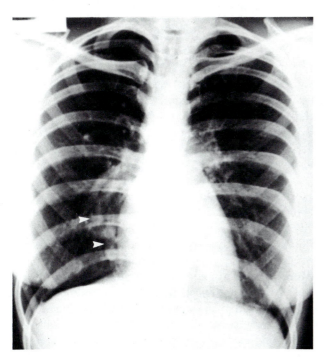

Fig. 22.22 Right pulmonary artery to left atrial communication. The white arrows indicate the abnormal density at the right heart border.

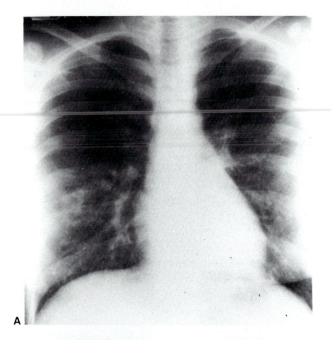

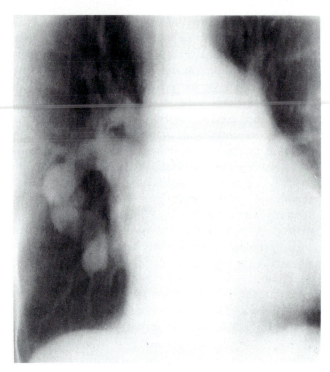

Fig. 22.25 Pulmonary varix. The AP tomogram shows the multiple rounded densities associated with the pulmonary veins which are typical of pulmonary varices. The venous nature of these was confirmed by angiography.

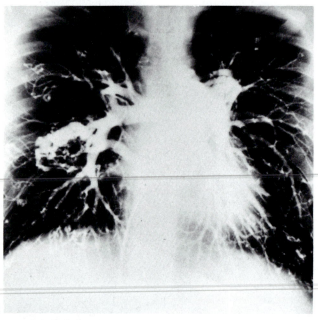

Fig. 22.24 Pulmonary arteriovenous malformations. **A.** Frontal chest film. Abnormal pulmonary shadows, typically elongated, can be identified in the right mid zone. **B.** Pulmonary arteriogram. The pulmonary arteriovenous malformations in the right mid zone, associated with premature venous filling, can be identified. Additional abnormal pulmonary vessels are clearly visible in the right upper zone and throughout the left lung.

may present at any time from infancy to middle age. Symptoms are usually those of cyanosis and exertional dyspnoea. Emboli occur only rarely. About half of patients have rather nonspecific murmurs.

Over 75% of patients (Figs 22.22, 22.23) have an abnormal density, visible at chest radiography and fluoroscopy, at the right heart border, below and behind the right hilum, and this is the aneurysmal dilatation of the pulmonary artery. A cardiac catheter may be passed through the fistula to the left atrium. Pulmonary angiography will opacify the aneurysm and demonstrate its communication with the left atrium.

PULMONARY ARTERIOVENOUS MALFORMATIONS

These are direct communications between the smaller pulmonary arteries and veins. The right-to-left shunt produced leads to dilatation of the terminations of these vessels. The lesions may be multiple in one-third of cases and may show progressive enlargement. Also in one-third of cases they are associated with telangiectasis elsewhere — Osler-Weber-Rendu disease.

The pulmonary lesions may be asymptomatic, or lead to dyspnoea or haemoptysis. The right-to-left shunt may be complicated by polycythaemia, cyanosis and cerebral abscess. These may worsen as the lesions increase in size.

Radiological appearances. If the lesions are large and have led to dilatation of the peripheral pulmonary artery and vein, a soft-tissue density will be seen (Fig. 22.24A) which may be seen to change size if studied fluoroscopically during extremes of respiration. *Tomography* should be carried out to confirm the vascular nature of the lesion by demonstrating the supplying vessels, and reveal other small lesions not suspected on the standard chest X-ray.

Their vascular nature may be apparent at enhanced CT.

The definitive investigation is *pulmonary angiography*, which is claimed to be both easy and helpful in this condition, as the high flow through the lesions aids in the opacification. It demonstrates enlargement of feeding arteries and draining veins and the direct connection between the two (Fig. 22.24B). There is no enlargement of the main pulmonary artery in uncomplicated arteriovenous malformations. Investigation should be performed if the condition is suspected prior to surgery, as if its nature is known, only a limited resection is required; also unsuspected lesions may be demonstrated. Embolization may alleviate symptoms.

PULMONARY VARIX

Localized dilatations of the pulmonary veins may occur with acquired or congenital heart disease, or may occur in asymptomatic patients, unassociated with cardiac abnormality. They are usually recognized as rounded or lobulated shadows, often near the hila, on the chest X-ray, which may be mistaken for other lesions. Some may be seen to change size with respiration on fluoroscopy. Tomography may demonstrate the draining vein (Fig. 22.25), thus suggesting the diagnosis. Confirmation of the nature of the abnormal shadow is obtained by selective pulmonary angiography. The shadows show delayed filling with contrast medium after pulmonary artery injection, and impaired drainage of the isolated vein. The appearances differ angiographically from those of arteriovenous malformation, which shows early shunting and enlarged drainage veins. The difference is due to the by-passing of the capillary bed in arteriovenous malformations.

REFERENCES AND SUGGESTIONS FOR FURTHER READING

Alderson, P. O., Martin, E. C. (1987) Pulmonary embolism; Diagnosis with multiple imaging modalities. *Radiology* **164**: 297–312.

Fazio, F., Lavender, J. P., Steiner, R. E. (1978) Krypton 81 m ventilation and $^{99}Tc^m$ perfusion scans in chest disease. *American Journal of Roentgenology* **130**: 421–428.

Ferris E. J., Holder, J. C., Lim, W. N. et al. (1984) Angiography of pulmonary emboli: Digital studies and balloon occlusion cine angiography. *American Journal of Roentgenology*, **142**: 369–373.

Grossman Z D, Ellis D A, Brigham S L et al (1984) Digital subtraction angiography of the pulmonary arteries for the diagnosis of pulmonary embolism. *Radiology*, **150**: 843–844.

Harris P, Heath D. (1986) *The Human Pulmonary Circulation*. 5th edn. Churchill Livingstone, Edinburgh.

Jefferson K, Rees S. (1980) *Clinical Cardiac Radiology*. 2nd edn. Butterworths, London.

Raphael M J. (1970) Pulmonary angiography: *British Journal of Hospital Medicine*, pp. 377–390.

Rees S. (1981) Arterial connection of the lung. *Clinical Radiology* **32**: 1–15.

CHAPTER 23

ACQUIRED HEART DISEASE

M. J. Raphael   R. M. Donaldson

VALVULAR HEART DISEASE

RHEUMATIC FEVER

This condition, now decreasing in incidence in the West, but still a major problem in developing countries, results from an abnormal response to group A streptococcal infection. The major clinical feature, flitting pains in the large joints, comes on about two to three weeks after a sore throat. There is no radiological evidence of joint destruction. Clinical evidence of carditis may be present and there may be radiological cardiomegaly, due either to carditis or to pericardial effusion. The acute phase usually regresses to an asymptomatic or quiescent phase lasting for many years, as chronic valve damage develops. The mitral is the commonest valve to be affected, followed by the aortic and then tricuspid valves. A history of rheumatic fever can be elicited in about half the patients with rheumatic valve disease. A similar valve disease may be seen after chorea.

MITRAL VALVE DISEASE

Mitral stenosis

Much the commonest cause of obstruction at the mitral valve is rheumatic fever. Stenosis develops by fusion of the leaflet commissures, thickening of the valve leaflets and shortening and thickening and adherence of the chordae tendineae, all of which restrict valve opening. Until the orifice is critically narrowed symptoms are few; then shortness of breath on exertion develops. Overt cardiac failure may not appear until the onset of atrial fibrillation. The clinical diagnosis is usually obvious, once the characteristic apical diastolic murmur is heard; however, a similar murmur may be heard in torrential aortic incompetence (the Austin-Flint murmur), in atrial septal defect (the patient, if elderly, may also be in atrial fibrillation), and in other forms of mitral obstruction (left atrial myxoma, and congenital obstructions). The murmur may be inaudible in low-output states or with tachycardia.

Radiographic appearances. The plain film signs are those of selective *left atrial enlargement*, which may vary

from trivial to gross (Figs 23.1, 23.2). Enlargement of the left atrial appendage is almost universally present as part of the left atrial enlargement and always suggests rheumatic mitral disease (as opposed to non-rheumatic). This enlargement may vary from a simple straightening of the left heart border to a very gross local protrusion (Fig. 23.3).

Mitral valve calcification indicates long-standing and usually severe mitral valve disease (Fig. 23.4). It is not commonly seen on the plain film. It is best seen in the lateral view, between the left atrium and the left ventricle, and is more rarely seen in the frontal view on an adequately penetrated film, in the position of the mitral

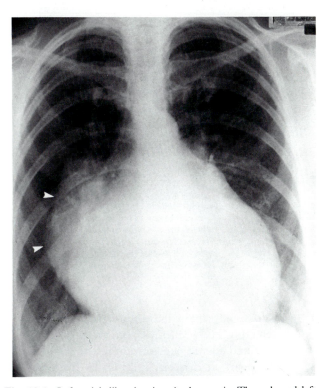

Fig. 23.1 Left atrial dilatation in mitral stenosis. The enlarged left atrium (arrows) extends beyond the right heart border. Note that the border of the right atrium can be identified where it is joined by the inferior vena cava coming up through the diaphragm.

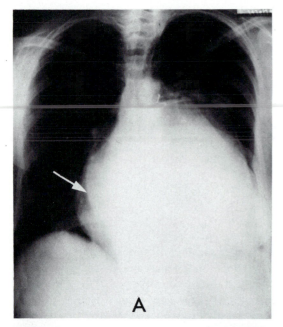

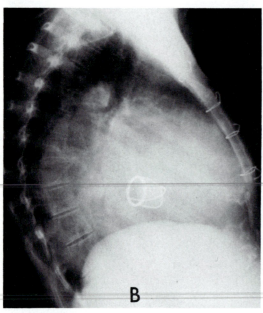

Fig. 23.2 Gross left atrial enlargement in association with a prosthetic mitral valve. **A**. Frontal view. The double shadow of the left atrium, seen to the right of the spine, is indicated by an arrow. Note that the left atrium has so lifted up the left bronchus that it now goes upwards. **B**. Lateral view. The prosthetic valve is more clearly seen. Again, the left bronchus goes upwards. The right bronchus can also be seen in its normal position.

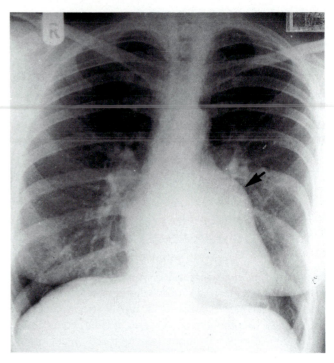

Fig. 23.3 Rheumatic mitral stenosis. This frontal film shows marked enlargement of the left atrial appendage (arrow).

valve. Image amplification fluoroscopy is much the best way of detecting such calcification, locating it to the mitral valve, and identifying its movement towards the apex of the heart in diastole. It must be distinguished from the characteristically 'C' or 'J'-shaped calcification which may occur in the mitral valve ring in the elderly. This may also be associated with a murmur but is of little haemodynamic importance (Fig. 23.5).

Calcification may occur in the left atrium in long-standing mitral valve disease with atrial fibrillation (Fig. 23.6).

Marked *changes in the pulmonary circulation* resulting from the chronically raised left atrial pressure may be present (Ch. 22). Upper-lobe blood diversion is seen in its most florid form, and is brought into prominence by lower-lobe vascular constriction. Enlarged main and central pulmonary arteries and peripheral pruning indicate pulmonary arterial hypertension. Long-standing interstitial oedema with acute alveolar pulmonary oedema may be seen. *Haemosiderosis* and *ossific nodules* are mainly seen in rheumatic valve disease.

A very large or aneurysmal left atrium (one which reaches to within an inch of the chest wall) may be associated with segmental or lobar collapse from bronchial compression, usually on the right (Fig. 23.7). The consolidation of pulmonary infarction may also occur. Tracheobronchial calcification is also common in rheumatic mitral valve disease.

Echocardiography. The distinctive motion in the cross-sectional echocardiographic (CSE) image of the mitral valve leaflets is due to their tethering by chordal and commissural fusion (Fig. 23.8). A pretty reliable estimate of mitral valve area can be obtained from Doppler recordings of mitral valve flow. The presence of left atrial thrombus can also be documented (Fig. 23.9); the left atrial appendage, however, can only be visualized by transoesophageal echocardiography.

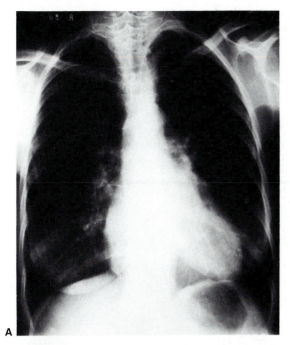

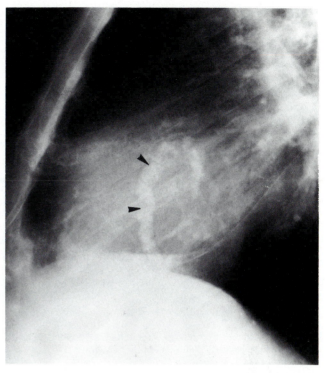

Fig. 23.5 Calcification in the mitral ring. In this lateral view the calcified mitral valve ring (arrows) appears as a characteristic C-shape; it may take a J-shape.

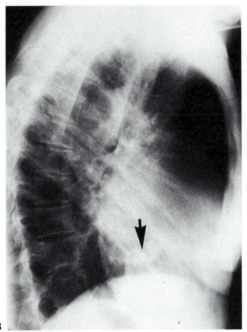

Fig. 23.4 A,B Calcified mitral valve in rheumatic mitral stenosis. The calcification is best seen in the lateral view (arrow).

Rheumatic mitral incompetence

Rheumatic mitral incompetence results from: 1. destruction of cusp tissue, mainly at the free edges, so that these do not meet and seal off the orifice; and also 2. shortening of the chordae, so that they hold the valve in the open position. The clinical presentation is with shortness of breath and the hallmark of the condition is the apical pansystolic murmur radiating to the axilla. Symptoms may be precipitated by the development of atrial fibril-

lation. The murmur may be confused with that of non-rheumatic mitral incompetence or ventricular septal defect. When there is a murmur of associated mitral stenosis, or additional aortic valve disease, and a history of rheumatic fever, the diagnosis is obvious. Many patients have been diagnosed as having rheumatic fever when a murmur is first heard in childhood following an atypical febrile illness, and may turn out to have congenital heart disease.

The commonest result of rheumatic mitral valve disease is a valve which is both stenosed and incompetent, failing to open properly in diastole, and failing to adequately seal the mitral orifice in systole. The valve cannot be both severely stenosed and severely incompetent as stenosis limits the degree of incompetence that can develop.

Radiographic appearances. The plain film findings resemble those of mitral stenosis, though the heart, and particularly the left atrium, is in general larger; the left atrium may be very large or aneurysmal in mitral incompetence. It is not usually possible to identify specifically associated left ventricular enlargement due to mitral incompetence. If present, left ventricular enlargement is usually due to aortic valve disease. It is not possible to diagnose mitral incompetence by fluoroscopic demonstration of systolic expansion of the left atrium.

Echocardiography. The echocardiographic assessment of mitral incompetence consists mainly in

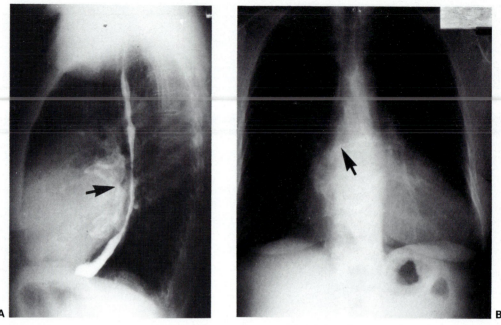

Fig. 23.6   Calcified left atrium in chronic rheumatic mitral valve disease. In both lateral and frontal views curvilinear calcification (arrow) is identified in the position of the wall of the left atrium.

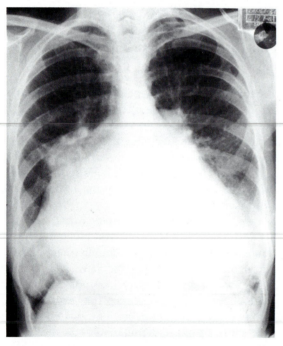

Fig. 23.7   Lobar collapse in association with left atrial enlargement. In this patient, with a very large left atrium, there is segmental collapse of the middle and part of the lower lobe on the right, due to bronchial compression.

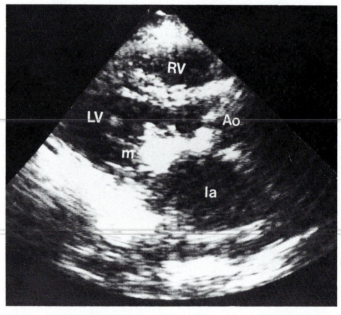

Fig. 23.8   Rheumatic mitral stenosis. The CSE shows marked fibrosis and tethering of the mitral (m) leaflets due to chordal and commissural fusion. Ao = aorta, la = left atrium. RV = Right ventricle, LV = Left ventricle.

determining its aetiology. The severity of the regurgitation cannot be assessed by the appearances of the valve itself. Mitral regurgitation caused by chronic rheumatic carditis is usually associated with thickened, deformed and often calcified cusps. Regurgitation through the mitral valve can be determined and quantified into mild, moderate, and severe by Doppler colour-flow mapping (Fig. 23.10). Quantitation depends on measuring the size of the regurgitant jet and relating it to the size of the atrium.

Non-rheumatic mitral incompetence

Two patterns of abnormality are commonly seen. In the commoner variety, *myxomatous degeneration of the valve*

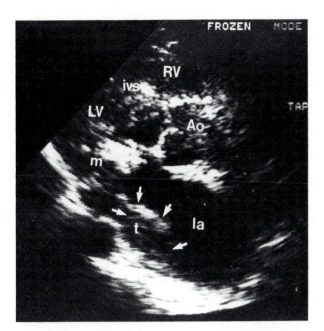

Fig. 23.9 Mitral stenosis. The CSE demonstrates a large left atrial (la) cavity and the presence of atrial thrombosis (arrows). There is fibrosis and calcification of the mitral leaflets. ivs = interventricular septum. Other lettering as in Fig. 20.8.

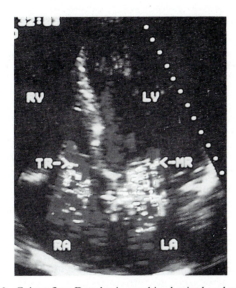

Fig. 23.10 Colour-flow Doppler in combined mitral and tricuspid regurgitation. This figure is reproduced in colour in the colour plate section at the front of this volume. The extensive red colouring in the left atrium indicates marked mitral regurgitation (MR), the lesser colouring in the right atrium indicates a lesser but still significant degree of tricuspid regurgitation (TR).

leaflets allows redundant valve tissue to balloon into the left atrium in systole, and the same process may lead to elongation of the chordae. The ballooning of the valve produces an audible systolic click, and if chordal elongation is severe enough to impair apposition of the leaflets, mitral incompetence results.

Chordal rupture may also precipitate mitral incompetence by producing a flail leaflet (or part of a leaflet)

so that apposition fails. This condition often progresses jerkily, with groups of chordae rupturing and producing mitral incompetence, followed by compensatory left ventricular dilatation and then another episode of rupture.

Both types of mitral involvement may lead to cardiac failure, which may be steadily or intermittently progressive and may lead to death. There is a characteristic mid- or late-onset systolic murmur which may be initiated by a click. Atrial fibrillation is rarer than in rheumatic carditis. The differential diagnosis includes other causes of a late systole murmur combined with left ventricular hypertrophy on the ECG, i.e. aortic stenosis and hypertrophic cardiomyopathy. Mitral incompetence in the course of ischaemic heart disease is considered below.

Radiographic appearances. The plain film appearances are very different from those in rheumatic mitral incompetence. In the acute phase the heart may be virtually normal in size and shape, even in the presence of pulmonary oedema or other evidence of a high left atrial pressure (Fig. 23.11). If the patient survives to enter the chronic phase, the heart enlarges, with a left ventricular configuration. Left atrial enlargement is slight and the left atrial appendage is very rarely enlarged. Calcification does not occur. In the prolapsed mitral valve associated with the Marfan syndrome, aortic root dilatation may be present.

Rarer causes of non-rheumatic mitral incompetence are those associated with a *left atrial myxoma* damaging the mitral valve, with *bacterial endocarditis* involving the mitral valve, with *cardiac trauma* damaging the mitral valve, with *ischaemic heart disease* involving the papillary muscles and with *cardiomyopathy* leading to mitral incompetence. *Congenital causes* are dealt with in Chapter 26.

Echocardiography. CSE is very useful in the diagnosis of non-rheumatic mitral incompetence. It shows virtually all cases of prolapse of the mitral valve leaflet (Fig. 23.12) and also the flail mitral leaflet associated with chordal rupture. The essential feature is that the anterior and posterior leaflets do not oppose properly in systole, usually because one or the other has prolapsed back into the left atrium. Doppler sampling and Doppler colour-flow mapping again serve to localize and to quantify the valvar regurgitation (Fig. 23.10).

Cardiac catheterization and angiocardiography. Investigation is indicated for the diagnosis in those rare cases where it is in doubt, even after echocardiography.

Severity. Catheterization and angiocardiography are better able to assess the severity of the valve lesion than echocardiography. When the severity is in doubt, or with associated lung disease as a possible cause of dyspnoea, and especially when more than one valve is abnormal, haemodynamic and angiographic investigation may be indicated. Additionally, they may help when it is not clear whether valve disease or impaired left ventricular function is the cause of the patient's symptoms, particularly after valve replacement.

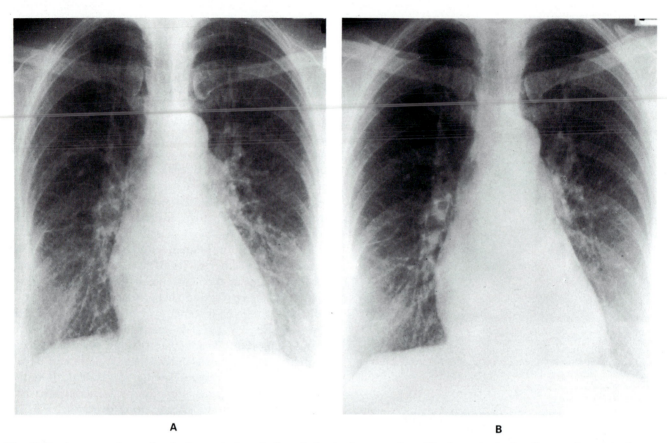

A   B

Fig. 23.11 Acute non-rheumatic mitral regurgitation. **A.** Frontal view in the acute phase. The heart size is virtually normal, even in the presence of high left atrial pressure as evidenced by the preferential dilation of the upper-lobe vessels and interstitial oedema. **B.** Frontal film two weeks later. This shows clearing of the oedema though upper-lobe blood diversion can still be seen.

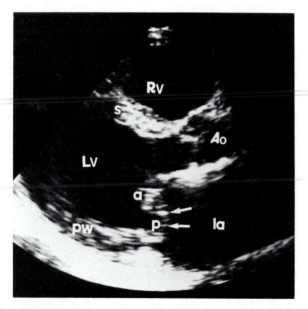

Fig. 23.12 Mitral valve prolapse. The CSE shows striking bowing of the posterior (p) mitral leaflet into the left atrium (la) (arrows). Other lettering as in Fig. 20.8.

Associated coronary artery disease. Coronary arteriography is routinely performed before surgery in patients with chest pain or ischaemic changes on the ECG, or aged over 55. The severity of mitral valve obstruction is assessed by measuring the gradient across the mitral valve between simultaneously-recorded indirect left atrial (wedged) pressure (or direct left atrial pressure recorded by transeptal catheter) and the left ventricular pressure obtained by retrograde catheterization of the left ventricle across the aortic valve. The flow across the valve must also be measured by determining the cardiac output. If the gradient is low at rest, in patients clinically suspected of having significant mitral obstruction, it is usual to increase the cardiac output by exercise and check the gradient again.

Mitral incompetence is assessed by **cine left ventriculography** in the right anterior oblique projection. This projection brings the mitral valve into profile, and separates the left ventricle from left atrium. The severity of mitral regurgitation is estimated by the rapidity with which contrast medium passes across the mitral valve from left ventricle to left atrium to opacify the left atrium. Rapid passage of large quantities of contrast medium indicates that regurgitation is severe. In non-rheumatic mitral incompetence this feature can be misleading, as

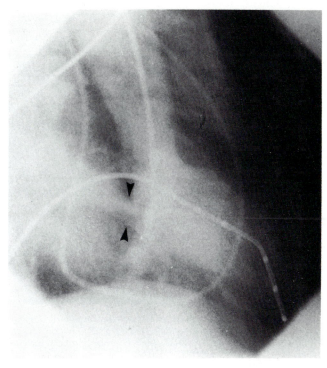

Fig. 23.14 Rheumatic mitral regurgitation. Left ventriculography in the RAO projection, systole. A discrete jet of mitral regurgitation (arrowed) passes through the closed mitral valve into the left atrium.

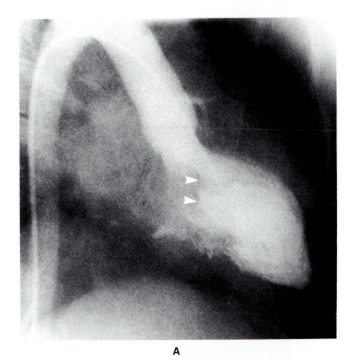

A

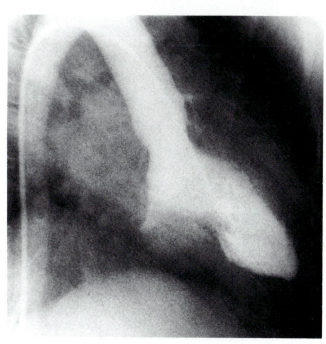

B

Fig. 23.13 Left ventriculography in mitral stenosis. **A**. Right anterior oblique diastole. **B**. Right anterior oblique systole. The mitral valve has closed normally in **B**. In **A** the stenosed valve is outlined by nonopaque blood on its atrial side so that it domes (arrows) into the ventricle in diastole.

the atrium is commonly small and opacifies rapidly, with only slight regurgitation. In this situation pulmonary artery and left atrial pressures, if normal, suggest that regurgitation is not severe. The angiographic appearances of the mitral valve are of interest but rarely of significance. The normal mitral valve is flung widely open in diastole, allowing an ill-defined broad front of nonopaque blood to enter the opacified left ventricle. If the valve is stenosed it is outlined by opaque blood on its ventricular aspect and nonopaque blood on its atrial aspect, producing a domed valve if examined in profile (Fig. 23.13), or appearing as a filling defect under the aortic valve if seen en-face.

The regurgitation of rheumatic mitral disease usually appears as one or more discrete jets of contrast medium passing through the mitral valve directly back into the left atrium (Fig. 23.14). Non-rheumatic mitral regurgitation appears as a jet of contrast medium escaping under the flail mitral valve and passing in a circular fashion around the wall of the left atrium.

A prolapsing mitral valve can be seen to balloon backwards into the left atrium during ventricular systole, but it must be distinguished from the various crevices which appear in the left ventricle in the mitral valve area, by the fact that it must disappear entirely in ventricular diastole (Fig. 23.15).

Left ventricular function may be assessed from the cine left ventriculogram by the size of the ventricle and the

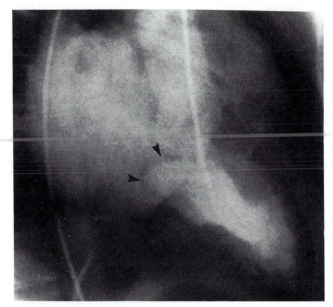

Fig. 23.15 Prolapse of the mitral valve. Systolic left ventriculogram in RAO projection. Part of the mitral valve, probably middle scallop of posterior leaflet, is clearly visible (arrows) prolapsing back into the left atrium.

degree of emptying that occurs with each beat, although in the presence of atrial fibrillation assessment may be difficult.

Coronary arteriography will exclude or demonstrate associated atheromatous coronary artery disease. It may also demonstrate blood vessel formation in left atrial thrombus, which is not uncommonly found when arteriography is performed for the investigation of long-standing rheumatic heart disease.

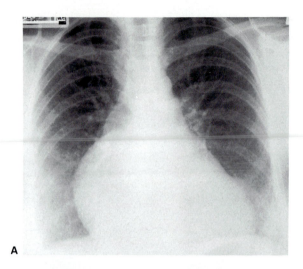

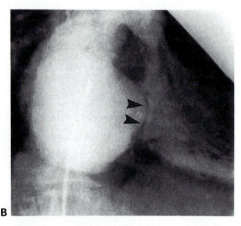

Fig. 23.16 Tricuspid stenosis developing in the course of rheumatic valvular heart disease. **A.** The frontal chest film shows a bulge of the large right atrium to the right. **B.** The right atrial angiogram in RAO projection confirms the enlargement of the right atrium and demonstrates its cause, a stenosed tricuspid valve (arrows).

TRICUSPID VALVE DISEASE

This most commonly occurs late in the course of *rheumatic heart disease*. Tricuspid stenosis or tricuspid incompetence may be due to involvement of the valve by the rheumatic process, or tricuspid incompetence may be *functional*. Tricuspid disease may be suspected clinically when the jugular venous pressure is raised and its form abnormal, and the liver is enlarged and pulsatile, though the murmurs closely resemble those of mitral valve disease.

The **plain film** shows enlargement of the right atrium bulging the heart shadow to the right (Fig. 23.16). Right atrial enlargement can usually be distinguished from left atrial enlargement due to mitral disease by the entry of the inferior vena cava, which limits its extent below.

The development of the characteristic murmur in a patient with a known *carcinoid syndrome* indicates the well-recognized development of tricuspid stenosis in this condition. It may be associated with a large right atrium on the plain film.

Bacterial endocarditis on the tricuspid valve is a common complication of *intravenous drug abuse*. The majority of the infections are staphylococcal, and the main clinical and radiological manifestations appear in the lungs, with extensive areas of consolidation often progressing rapidly to cavitation. In those patients who survive and develop significant tricuspid incompetence, right atrial enlargement may be detected on serial chest films.

Echocardiography. CSE visualizes the tricuspid valve, and in the majority of cases it is able to show thickening of the valve when it is stenosed. Vegetations on the leaflets are visualized by CSE in cases of bacterial endocarditis. The Doppler is useful in assessing tricuspid stenosis; colour-flow mapping is particularly effective in visualizing the retrograde systolic flow into the right atrial cavity in tricuspid regurgitation (Fig. 23.10). An indirect estimate of pulmonary artery systolic pressure can be obtained from the Doppler-derived transtricuspid valve gradient.

Cardiac catheterization and angiocardiography may be difficult to perform and interpret in tricuspid valve disease. Tricuspid stenosis is measured by simultaneous recording of right ventricular and right atrial pressures. As the pressures in diastole are low and the pressure gradients, even when significant, are small, pressures must be measured very carefully.

Right atrial angiography may reveal the large right atrium and thickened domed tricuspid valve leaflets, confirming that the tricuspid valve is abnormal. Right ventriculography will show tricuspid incompetence, but the significance of the findings must be assessed carefully, as some regurgitation may occur through the tricuspid valve during right ventriculography simply because the catheter, passed through the tricuspid valve, holds it open.

AORTIC VALVE DISEASE

The aortic valve may be stenotic or incompetent or both.

Aortic stenosis

This may occur as a congenitally stenotic valve or may develop in adult life, either on the basis of a congenital bicuspid valve or from inflammatory commissural fusion, which develops in the course of rheumatic heart disease.

Calcific aortic stenosis. This usually develops on the basis of a congenitally bicuspid valve, which may be detected in its mobile, pre-stenotic phase by its ejection click, there being no murmur. With deposition of calcium on the abnormal valve, beginning in the fourth decade, mobility (and the click) are lost, and stenosis develops. Valve calcification is invariable, as it is the cause of the stenosing process (not, as in mitral stenosis, a result of the stenosis). Calcification makes the cusps rigid and impedes the flow of blood.

Presentation is with shortness of breath, angina or syncope. The diagnosis is made on the basis of the slow rising plateau pulse, the ejection systolic murmur and thrill and the presence of left ventricular hypertrophy in the ECG.

Plain films may show rounding of the left ventricular apex indicative of left ventricular hypertrophy, post-stenotic dilatation of the ascending aorta, and, on the lateral film, calcification in the position of the aortic valve (Fig. 23.17).

In older patients, when the aorta has become unfolded and slightly dilated, localized post-stenotic dilatation may be difficult to detect. Significant aortic stenosis may be present with a virtually normal heart shadow, though it is rare not to detect some evidence of ventricular enlargement in either frontal or lateral views.

Echocardiography. CSE shows a thickened immobile aortic valve with dense echoes indicative of calcium deposition. It may also show thickened ventricular walls

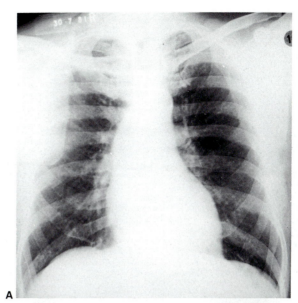

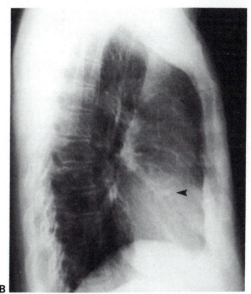

Fig. 23.17 Aortic stenosis. **A.** Frontal film, showing rounding of the left ventricular apex indicative of left ventricular hypertrophy, and also poststenotic dilatation of the ascending aorta. **B.** Lateral film, showing calcification (arrowhead) in the position of the aortic valve.

and permit the detection of various forms of subvalvular or supravalvular stenosis. Doppler studies require continuous-wave measurements because of the high blood-flow velocities reached in the aortic root in aortic stenosis. By recording the maximal velocity of blood flow in the ascending aorta, it is possible to recognize left ventricular outflow tract obstruction and also to estimate the severity with great reliability (Fig. 23.18).

The clinical diagnosis is usually obvious when the characteristic murmur is heard, though, rarely, hypertrophic cardiomyopathy and non-rheumatic mitral

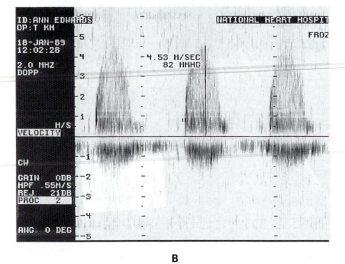

Fig. 23.18 Aortic stenosis. **A**. CSE study visualizing a thickened immobile valve with dense echoes indicative of calcium deposition (arrow). **B**. Continuous-wave Doppler sampling from the aortic jet of a patient with aortic stenosis. The peak velocity of over 4 m/s indicates a predicted pressure gradient of 82 mmHg.

regurgitation may have similar murmurs and also show left ventricular hypertrophy on the ECG.

In serious doubt, *fluoroscopy* will show valve calcification or exclude it. Note that the amount of calcium correlates only very roughly with the severity of the aortic stenosis.

Difficulty may be encountered when congestive cardiac failure has developed and cardiac output is so low that the characteristic murmur is not audible; the clinical picture may then resemble congestive cardiomyopathy; the presence of valve calcification on the lateral plain film may be the first indication of the diagnosis.

Rheumatic aortic stenosis. This is due to commissural fusion immobilizing the cusps. Calcification is frequently visible at image amplification fluoroscopy but is rarely more than a few flecks and is almost never seen on the plain film. Left ventricular hypertrophy may be seen on the plain film but post-stenotic dilatation is rare. A history of rheumatic fever and evidence of mitral valve involvement either clinically or on echocardiography point to the diagnosis.

Aortic incompetence

This is most commonly due to damage to the aortic cusps by *rheumatic fever* or *endocarditis* and it may occur in association with aortic stenosis. More rarely, it may be due to primary disease of the aortic wall when this is involved by *aortitis* of any aetiology (syphilis being the best known), or due to an *aortic root aneurysm* occurring either alone or as part of Marfan's syndrome. *Dissecting aneurysm* reaching to the ascending aorta and valve ring may also precipitate aortic incompetence. The diagnosis is made clinically on the basis of the collapsing pulse and the detection of an early diastolic murmur.

Radiographic appearances. The appearances will vary depending on whether the aortic incompetence is chronic or of acute onset. In the chronic form the plain film shows a large heart with left ventricular configuration, and the heart size is commensurate with the severity of the aortic incompetence (Fig. 23.19). The aorta is often large in both the ascending part and the arch. Calcification of the aortic valve is not a feature of pure aortic incompetence but may be seen if aortic incompetence is combined with stenosis on a calcified congenitally abnormal valve. Aortic root abnormalities may show a localized aortic deformity, or what may appear to be simply a large ascending aorta bulging to the right of the mediastinum, or less often to the left. Sometimes the frontal film appears normal but an abnormal forward bulge of the root of the aorta may be seen on the lateral view (Fig. 23.20). Rarely, no aortic abnormality may be detectable.

In *acute aortic incompetence*, usually due to bacterial endocarditis or aortic dissection, there may be congestive

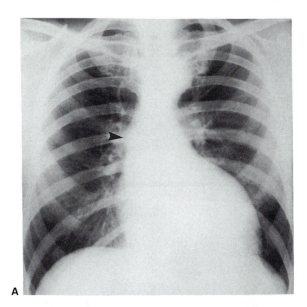

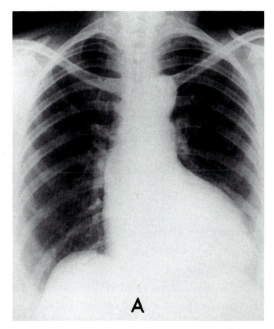

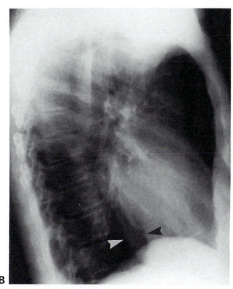

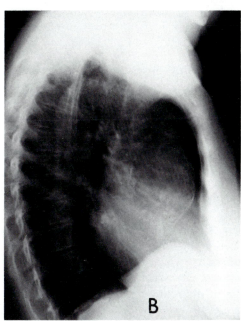

Fig. 23.19 Gross left ventricular dilatation from chronic aortic incompetence. **A**. The axis of the heart is elongated to the left with rounding of the apex. There is slight prominence of the ascending aorta (black arrow). **B**. The body of the left ventricle (white arrow) can be seen bulging behind the line of the right atrium (black arrow)

Fig. 23.20 Aortic incompetence due to syphilitic aortic root aneurysm. **A**. Frontal view, showing left ventricular dilatation extending to the left and only a slight prominence in the position of the ascending aorta, with a barely visible rim of calcium. **B**. Lateral view, showing a large saccular aortic root aneurysm clearly outlined by calcification.

cardiac failure with a virtually normal-sized heart, when this has not had time to dilate.

The diagnosis of aortic incompetence is usually obvious once the early diastolic murmur has been heard. Only in acute aortic incompetence may this be inaudible.

Echocardiography. *CSE* may show an abnormal aortic valve and a large hyperdynamic left ventricle. Abnormalities of the aortic root may also be picked up by the CSE, which may recognize aortic root abscess and vegetations in endocarditis. *Pulsed Doppler* and *Doppler colour-flow mapping* are sensitive in distinguishing the severity of the aortic regurgitation, although precise

volumetric measurements are not possible at present. *Transoesophageal echocardiography* is of particular value when aortic dissection is suspected. Aortic incompetence, often of acute onset, may be due to disease of the wall of the aorta, such as the aortic root aneurysm which occurs often in association with Marfan's syndrome, or dissections which have spread to involve the root of the

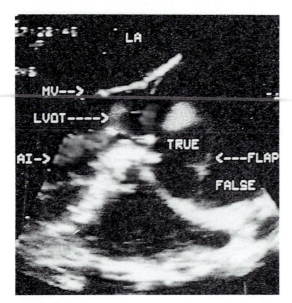

Fig. 23.21 Transoesophageal echocardiography in aortic dissection. This figure is reproduced in colour in the colour plate section at the front of this volume. True and false lumens, and the intimal flap, are all visualized. Colour-flow Doppler indicates significant aortic incompetence.

aorta. More recently, *transoesophageal echocardiography* has become a definitive technique for studying dissections of the aorta non-invasively (Fig. 23.21).

CT scanning has been extensively utilized in the recognition of both dissections and aortic aneurysms, and more recently **Magnetic Resonance Imaging** has been used for the same purpose. Both techniques are able to make a diagnosis of aneurysmal dissection but neither is able to demonstrate reliably the haemodynamic consequences of involving the aortic valve or the anatomical consequences of involving the coronary arteries, for which catheterization and angiography are required.

Angiography, which is invasive and not infallible, will reveal contrast medium tracking between the intima and the media in dissecting aneurysms (see Ch. 25). Aortic root aneurysms will be seen as rather symmetrical fusiform dilatations of the aortic root involving the valve ring and often the cusps of the aortic valve (the so-called triple sinus aneurysm) but the dilatation usually stops short of the origin of the innominate artery. In Marfan's syndrome small intimal dissections may not be seen at aortography, and attacks of acute chest pain probably represent small dissections even in the presence of a non-diagnostic arteriogram.

Cardiac catheterization and angiocardiography
(Fig 23.22)
The severity of aortic stenosis is assessed by measuring the gradient across the aortic valve, and knowing the cardiac output. The left ventricular pressure may be obtained if the valve can be crossed retrogradely, or measured by

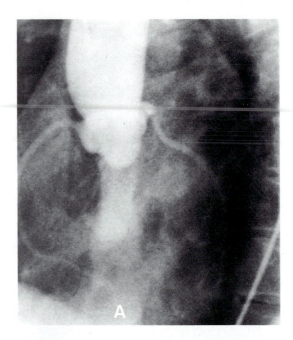

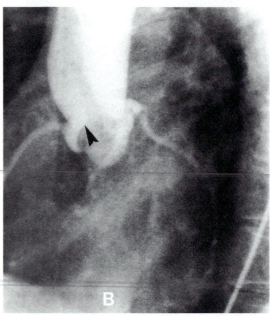

Fig. 23.22 Aortography in aortic stenosis. LAO projection. **A**. Diastole. **B**. Systole. In **A** the aortic valve appears largely normal and there is slight aortic regurgitation. In **B** the domed aortic valve (arrow) is clearly seen, and passing through its centre is a negative jet of nonopaque blood, indicating the size of the orifice.

a trans-septal approach. The aortic pressure is obtained by retrograde catheterization.

The angiographic visualization of the aortic valve is by retrograde root aortography, using cine-radiography in the left anterior oblique projection.

The normal aortic valve has three sinuses of Valsalva with three valve cusps which close in diastole, so that no contrast medium leaks past them into the left ventricle;

in systole they fly open against the side of the aorta where they usually cannot be seen. The lowermost sinus of Valsalva seen on the aortogram is always the non-coronary one.

Aortic stenosis. In lone calcific aortic stenosis, calcification can almost invariably be seen and may be extremely gross. Even in rheumatic aortic stenosis, small flecks of calcification are commonly seen in good-quality cine-angiograms. The stenosed valve (Fig. 23.22) may be domed or simply show restricted opening. It is usually thickened so that the cusps can be seen well. The densely calcified valves are almost immobile during the cardiac cycle. The aortic root is often pinched in rheumatic aortic valve disease.

The severity of aortic stenosis can only be estimated angiographically when a discrete negative jet of non-opacified blood is seen. In the absence of a recognizable negative jet at root aortography (or positive jet at left ventriculography), no conclusions can be drawn, as the density of calcification correlates only very roughly with the severity of stenosis. A small negative jet indicates severe stenosis and a large negative jet insignificant stenosis.

Aortic incompetence. Aortic incompetence is categorized from the left anterior oblique cine aortic root angiogram in four grades:

1. A small puff of contrast medium enters the left ventricle in diastole and is cleared immediately in systole.
2. The left ventricle is outlined with contrast in diastole but it is still cleared away in systole.
3. Progressively increasing opacification of the left ventricle occurs with each beat.
4. Massive immediate opacification of the left ventricle occurs.

Unfortunately there is no close correlation between this radiological assessment and the degree of aortic incompetence quantitated by measurement of the regurgitant flow by ventricular volume studies.

In disease of the aortic cusps the appearances of the aortic regurgitation are largely nonspecific, except when there is a pinhole jet of regurgitation through a valve cusp. This always raises the possibility of cusp perforation. Patients with rheumatic aortic incompetence may show evidence of 'doming' of the valve with commissural fusion. In acute bacterial endocarditis, the nature of the pathological process may be suspected by recognizing paravalvar abscesses tracking into the septum (it is these that produce heart block, an indication for immediate surgery) or between the left ventricle and the left atrium.

When aortic wall disease is suspected, investigation is always indicated. Dissections may be diagnosed by the tracking of contrast medium between the aortic wall and the elevated flap of intima (see Ch. 25). An aortic root aneurysm will be seen as a rather symmetrical fusiform dilatation of the aortic root involving the valve ring and often the cusps of the aortic valve (the so-called triple sinus aneurysm) but the dilatation usually stops short of the origin of the innominate artery.

ISCHAEMIC HEART DISEASE

CORONARY ARTERIOGRAPHY

This is the radiological visualization of the coronary arteries by direct selective injection of contrast medium. It is the most sensitive and accurate method of studying disease in the coronary arteries and the effects of this disease on the heart.

Technique. Two approaches are available to cannulate the coronary arteries. The more popular is the percutaneous femoral Seldinger technique using pre-shaped catheters, different for each coronary artery and for the left ventricle. Different configurations have been described by Judkins, Amplatz and Bourassa.

The earlier technique, that of Sones, required an arteriotomy of the right brachial artery, and used a single soft-tipped catheter which was buckled against the aortic valve and introduced into each coronary artery in turn, and into the left ventricle.

Filming. High-quality high-resolution cine filming at 25 to 50 frames per second is the current method of recording the image. *Digital subtraction angiography* can however visualize a left ventricle either by central intravenous injection or by direct injection of low doses of contrast medium into the ventricle in the course of coronary arteriography. Direct digital recording of selective coronary arteriograms will be the future imaging method, allowing image processing, instantaneous replay and computer analysis.

Normal coronary anatomy. The left coronary artery (Fig. 23.23) comes off its sinus of Valsalva, which is on the left and slightly posterior. The main stem, whose length varies, passes to the left and divides into two.

The *anterior descending* coronary artery passes forward over the surface of the heart in the anterior interventricular groove (which marks the interventricular septum) and reaches to, and beyond, the apex of the heart to reach the inferior interventricular groove on the undersurface. Parallel *septal branches* descend from the anterior descending artery into the septum and diagonal branches to the free wall (as opposed to the septum) of the left ventricle pass to the left. The *circumflex artery* passes to the left in the left atrioventricular groove (which marks the atrio-ventricular valvar plane, separating atrial from ventricular part of the heart). It gives off forward-running obtuse *marginal branches* to the left ventricular free wall, and normally terminates above the crux.

The *right coronary artery* (Fig. 23.24) comes off its sinus of Valsalva, in front and only slightly on the right, and

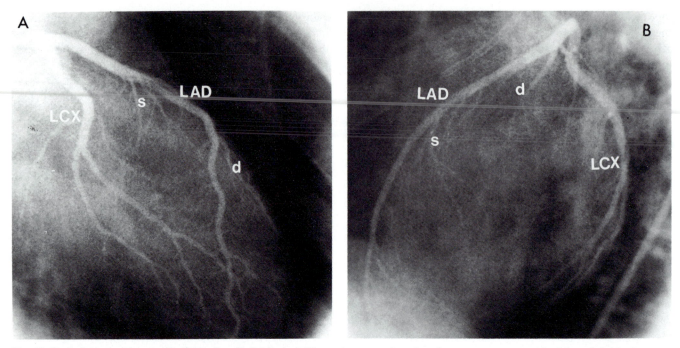

Fig. 23.23 Left coronary artery. **A**. RAO view. **B**. LAO view. The main stem, whose length can vary, passes to the left and divides into the anterior descending (LAD) and circumflex (LCX) branches. s = septal branch, d = diagonal branch.

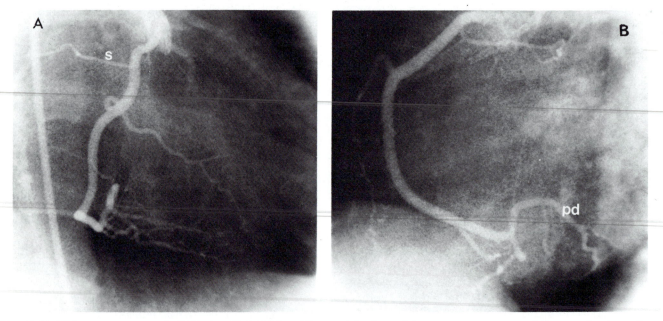

Fig. 23.24 Right coronary artery. **A**. RAO view. **B**. LAO view. The usual dominant right coronary artery gives off the posterior descending (pd) branch immediately before the crux of the heart. s = sinus node artery.

passes forward and to the right to reach the right atrioventricular groove in which it encircles the right side of the heart. Its first branch, the *conus branch*, is to the conus of the right ventricle; its second, which runs posteriorly, is the *sinus node artery* to the sinus node in the interatrial septum. Then come right ventricular branches. The usual, dominant, right coronary artery reaches the crux (the junction of the atrioventricular plane and the interventricular plane on the undersurface of the heart). Immediately before the crux it gives off the *posterior descending coronary artery* which runs forward in the inferior interventricular groove to supply the posterior septum. At the crux the right coronary artery loops into the myocardium, giving off the *atrioventricular node artery* at the apex of the loop before emerging back onto the surface of the heart. The right coronary artery then continues in the left atrioventricular groove, supplying posterolateral *left ventricular branches* to the left ventricular free wall.

Normal variants. Variation of balance of the coronary arteries can make interpretation of the angiogram difficult. The common variation is *left dominance*. The circumflex branch of the left coronary artery is very large and extends around the back of the heart in the left atrioventricular groove until it reaches the crux, where it supplies the posterior descending and atrioventricular nodal branches. The right coronary artery is consequentially small and supplies only the right ventricle, and may appear abnormal.

The circumflex branch may, rarely, be so large as to entirely replace the right coronary artery, or the right coronary artery may be so large that there is virtually no circumflex. Both may be large and the anterior descending artery very small.

Congenital anomalies. These abound in the coronary circulation. The circumflex may arise from the right coronary artery or from the right sinus of Valsalva; rarely, the anterior descending may do this. Circumflex and anterior descending may have separate origins from the left coronary sinus of Valsalva. These anomalies lead to difficulties in catheterization but do not in themselves produce symptoms. Origin of the left coronary artery from the right sinus of Valsalva or of the right coronary artery from the left sinus of Valsalva may lead to symptoms if the artery is compressed.

Coronary disease

On angiography the normal coronary artery is seen as a smoothly outlined, gently tapering structure. *Atheroma* appears as an irregularity of outline (Fig. 23.25A). When atheromatous plaques spread around the artery to form a stricture, this can be identified and its severity evaluated (Fig. 23.25B). Angiography understates the extent of atheroma and the severity of strictures. Complete occlusions may be detected and the patency of the vessel beyond the complete occlusion identified as it opacifies by collateral flow (Fig. 23.26).

Spasm may also be seen during coronary arteriography. Catheter-induced spasm generally occurs as a smoothly tapered narrowing, usually in the right coronary artery, at the catheter tip. It is not usually associated with symptoms and may be relieved by nitroglycerine. Spontaneous or drug-induced (ergot preparations) spasm often begins at a rather minor atheromatous plaque and may progress to occlusion of the whole artery, often with the development of the patient's symptoms and ECG changes. It is usually relieved by nitroglycerine.

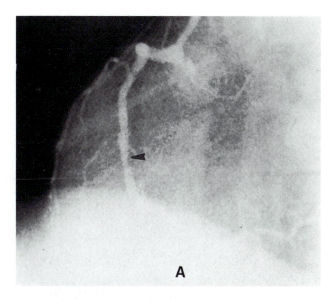

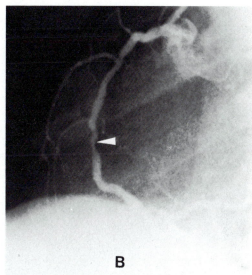

Fig. 23.25 Coronary artery disease, right coronary artery, LAO view. **A**. Atheromatous lesion in mid third of right coronary artery appearing as irregularity of outline (arrow). **B**. Same patient 14 months later, visualizing a severe stricture (arrow).

Left ventriculography

The normal left ventricle is a cone-shaped structure with the aortic and mitral valves at its base (Fig. 23.27). It contracts concentrically, with its anterior wall, apex and inferior wall all moving equally inwards. Ischaemic heart disease (Fig. 23.28) produces localized abnormalities of wall movement (Fig. 23.27): hypokinesia (reduced movement), akinesia (no movement) and dyskinesia (paradoxical movement). Wall-movement abnormalities are associated with overall impairment of function, which can be seen on the angiogram as ventricular dilatation and poor emptying. Emptying is measured as the *ejection fraction* (stroke volume/diastolic volume × 100), the

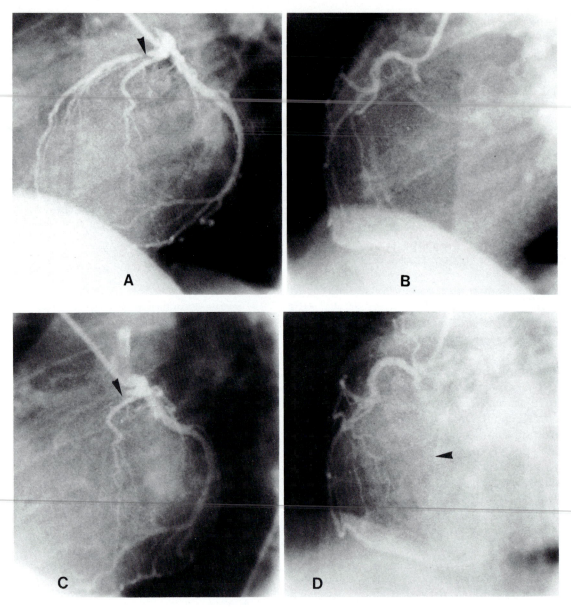

Fig. 23.26 Progression of coronary disease. LAO views. **A.** Left coronary artery. There is a critical narrowing at the origin of the anterior descending branch (arrow). **B.** Right coronary artery. **C** and **D** were taken 7 months later following an anterior infarction (see Fig. 23.28). The left coronary artery has become completely occluded (C, arrow) and fills via collaterals from the right coronary artery (D, arrow).

proportion of the ventricle which empties with each beat; in normal people this fraction is two-thirds (66%). Significantly impaired function would be represented by an ejection fraction of under 50%, proceeding to the very severest impairment, 10–20%.

ANGINA PECTORIS

This is an episodic pain occurring almost anywhere above the diaphragm and thought to be due to transient myocardial ischaemia. Classical angina is a crushing chest pain, often radiating to the left arm, brought on by exercise,

and relieved by rest or trinitrin. The ECG becomes abnormal during pain with ST segment depression. This condition is almost invariably associated with obstructed coronary arteries.

Prinzmetal's variant angina is an anginal pain, often coming on spontaneously, and associated with ST segment elevation on the ECG. The coronary arteries develop spasm during the pain but show no atheromatous narrowing when the patient is symptom-free.

Diagnosis of angina pectoris may be difficult when the pain develops in a bizarre site, such as the jaw, or when its relationship to exercise and relief by rest is unclear,

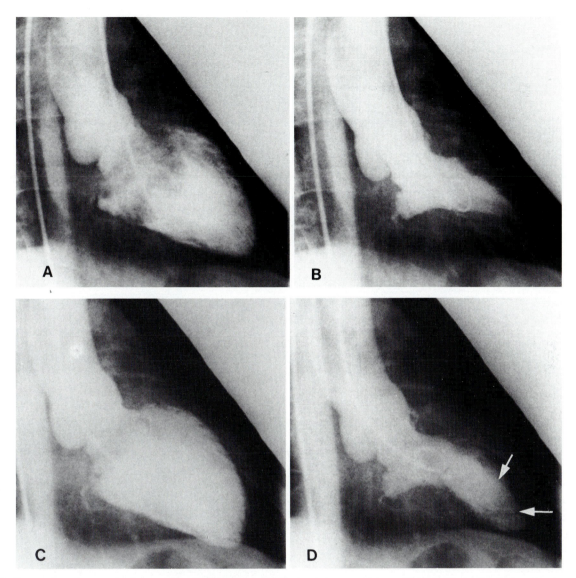

Fig. 23.27 Progression of coronary disease. Left ventriculogram (RAO views) (same patient as Fig. 23.26). **A, B** Initial study visualizes normal left ventricle which is shaped like an upside-down carrot (with the aortic and mitral valves in its base) and contracts concentrically. **C, D**. 7 months later, following anterior infarction and occlusion of the left anterior descending coronary branch (see Figs. 23.26C and 23.28). The left ventriculogram shows localized abnormality of wall movement in the anteroapical wall of the heart (arrows).

as may occur in the many mixed patterns of angina which may be encountered.

^{201}*Thallium scanning*, performed during the ischaemic episode, may show a perfusion deficit which fills in at rest, supporting the idea that a localized area of myocardium becomes ischaemic, and that this is the cause of symptoms. Unfortunately thallium scanning is neither sensitive nor specific enough to be a particularly useful test in excluding the diagnosis of coronary artery disease, though if its results are very positive it does support the diagnosis.

The *plain film* is normal in patients with uncomplicated angina pectoris unless there has been a previous myocardial infarction.

MYOCARDIAL INFARCTION

When ischaemia is severe enough to lead to death of muscle the syndrome of myocardial infarction results. The clinical features depend on the size of the infarction, the presence of arrhythmias and the development of the mechanical complications of myocardial infarction.

Radiographic appearances. The *plain films* are initially taken on a portable X-ray unit, in the ward, anteroposteriorly, at short distance and often with low-power apparatus. They are thus usually of poor quality, and with distorted geometry and heart size difficult to assess. The size of the heart will depend on the size of the current infarct and the effects of any previous infarctions. It may be small if the present infarct is the only

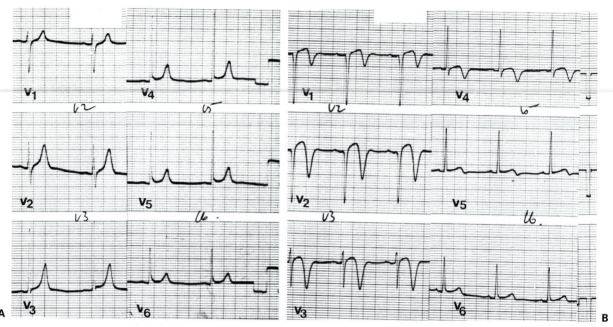

Fig. 23.28 Electrocardiographic tracings corresponding to Figs. 23.26 and 23.27. **A**. Normal ECG obtained at the time of the initial angiographic assessment (precordial leads V1–V6). **B**. The ECG shows an evolving anterior infarction following occlusion of the left anterior descending vessel (see Fig. 23.26C).

one and is small, and large if the present infarct is large or there have been previous infarcts. The pulmonary vessels will reflect the haemodynamic disturbance with upper-lobe blood diversion, interstitial and alveolar oedema, reflecting progressively more severe disturbance with higher left atrial pressure. Persisting pulmonary oedema or a large heart are both bad prognostic features.

In the convalescent phase a number of features may be seen. Ill-defined basal shadows beginning within a day or two of infarction and developing into broad basal-line shadows are probably areas of collapse due to diaphragmatic splinting from pain (Fig. 23.29). *Dressler's syndrome* of pleuritis, pneumonitis and pericarditis comes on after 10 days with chest pain and fever (Fig. 23.30). Small effusions may be seen in the costophrenic angle, with ill-defined basal shadows resembling pulmonary infarcts, but the prompt response to aspirin or steroids usually makes the diagnosis obvious. Rarely a pericardial effusion may be so large as to cause tamponade. Dressler's syndrome may remit and relapse.

As the patient recovers, films may be taken in the Radiology Department. *Coronary calcification* may be identified by its parallel-line appearance, usually best seen in the lateral view, in the position of the anterior descending or right coronary artery. It is much better seen on image-amplification television fluoroscopy. Calcification may also be seen in old infarcts, as a curvilinear density in the position of the wall of the left ventricle. Multiple infarctions produce congestive failure, 'ischaemic cardiomyopathy'. The heart is large with a left

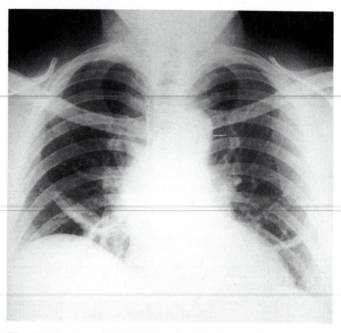

Fig. 23.29 Myocardial infarction. The chest X-ray demonstrates broad basal line shadows, probably areas of collapse due to diaphragmatic splinting from pain.

ventricular configuration, though all chambers are involved to some extent. Pulmonary oedema may be seen in untreated cases.

Ventricular aneurysm may develop about two months after a large infarction. Patients may present with

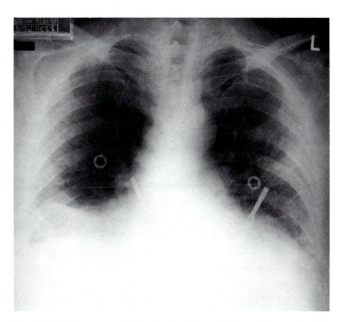

Fig. 23.30 Postmyocardial infarction (Dressler's) syndrome. Small effusions are seen in both costophrenic angles, together with ill-defined basal shadows resembling pulmonary infarcts.

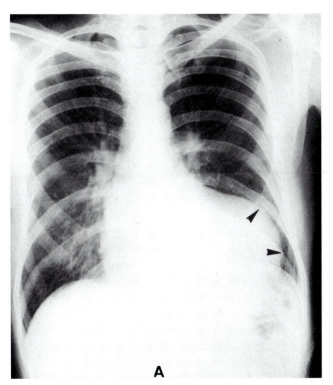

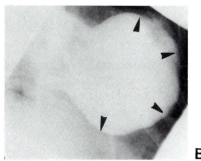

Fig. 23.31 Ventricular aneurysm. **A.** The chest radiograph shows an enlarged heart with a localized bulge. **B.** The aneurysm is clearly defined in the left ventriculogram which visualizes a large anteroapical dyskinetic area (arrows).

congestive cardiac failure, angina or arrhythmias, or may be asymptomatic. A variety of appearances may be seen, varying from an apparently normal heart shadow (rarely) to left ventricular enlargement, and to a localized bulge of the apex of the heart (Fig. 23.31). The lungs will reflect the effects of treatment on the haemodynamic disturbance. In some cases curvilinear mural calcification may be seen, which always suggests an aneurysm and one of long standing (Fig. 23.32). The diagnosis may be confirmed by *radionuclide ventriculography*, (either first-pass or multiple gated studies), *cross-sectional echocardiography* (which also shows thrombus — Fig. 23.33), or *CT scanning* which demonstrates the aneurysm and may also show intraventricular clot as can MRI. *Left ventriculography* and *coronary arteriography* are usually performed preoperatively.

Perforation of the ventricular septum following anterior myocardial infarction is marked by clinical deterioration and the development of a systolic murmur. The heart is usually large and the lungs show gross pulmonary oedema. Echocardiography shows not only the large and dyskinetic left ventricle but usually reveals the site of the perforation (see Fig. 23.34). The abnormal jet can be visualized by Doppler CFM and this technique will also differentiate septal perforation from the clinically similar post-infarction mitral regurgitation.

Left ventriculography and coronary arteriography are usually attempted preoperatively if the patient's clinical condition permits. Pulmonary plethora may be seen in those few patients who survive long enough to develop it.

Post-infarction mitral incompetence may be trivial if there is slight ischaemia of the papillary muscle, or

catastrophic if the papillary muscle necroses and ruptures. This event is marked by sudden clinical deterioration and the development of a systolic murmur. The heart may be moderately enlarged but left atrial enlargement is not seen. There is usually gross pulmonary oedema. CSE may demonstrate the size and function of the left ventricle in the presence of a flail mitral leaflet. The mitral regurgitation is visualized by Doppler CFM. Coronary angiography is usually performed preoperatively.

CORONARY ARTERY SURGERY

The standard surgical procedure for the treatment of ischaemic heart disease is saphenous-vein aortocoronary bypass graft. The vein is attached end-to-side to the ascending aorta above and end-to-side to the coronary

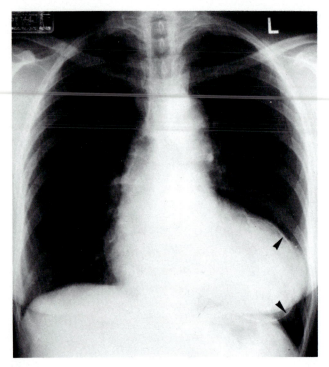

Fig. 23.32 Ventricular aneurysm. Cardiac enlargement and apical calcification (arrows) in a patient with a long-standing left ventricular aneurysm.

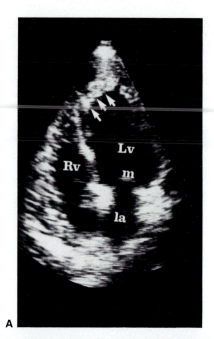

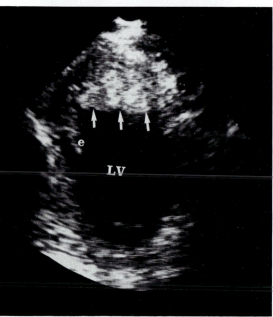

Fig. 23.33 A,B Ventricular aneurysm. The CSE study (apical and short-axis views) visualizes an anteroapical thinned-out aneurysmal area with mural thrombus (arrows). e = endocardium. Other lettering as in Fig. 20.8.

artery below, beyond the obstruction. Distal variations are used with Y grafts or jump grafts.

The indication for surgery, and hence the indications for preoperative coronary arteriography, are:

1. Angina unresponsive to medical treatment.
2. Post-infarction ischaemia, either anginal or on exercise testing.
3. Mechanical complications.
4. Before valve surgery in patients with chest pain or aged over 50.

Coronary arteriography is also used postoperatively to study the state of the grafts and the state of the native coronary circulation, in cases where angina recurs. Blocked grafts, strictured grafts and progress in the disease of the native circulation are all causes of unsuccessful relief of ischaemia.

NON-SURGICAL INTERVENTIONS

Percutaneous transluminal coronary angioplasty is a significant advance in the management of coronary artery disease. The technique consists of using a large-diameter guide catheter to introduce a small balloon dilatation catheter into the coronary artery and through the stricture to dilate it (Fig. 23.35). The main indications for the procedure should be similar to those for coronary bypass surgery, as this may be needed to manage the complications. Severe single-vessel non-occlusive strictures remain the classic indication for the procedure and respond well, with a high success rate (90%) initially and a low complication rate (3% emergency surgery). About one-third of strictures will recur and can be re-dilated. The indications are currently more relaxed, with multivessel disease being attempted, and in certain situations one vessel — that causing the symptoms, the so-called culprit lesion — will be dilated in the presence of other blocked vessels, though this is obviously more hazardous.

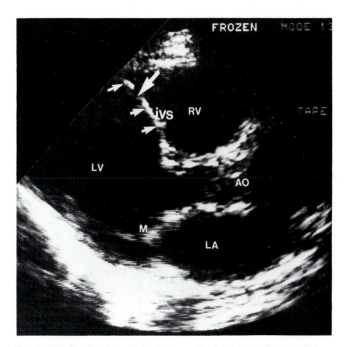

Fig. 23.34 Perforation of the interventricular septum in association with anterior myocardial infarction. The CSE study reveals an anteroseptal (ivs) thinned-out segment corresponding to the infarction (small arrows) and reveals the site of the perforation (long arrow). Other lettering as in Fig. 20.8.

Thrombolytic therapy. A great deal of research has demonstrated that the immediate exhibition of thrombolytic therapy in acute myocardial infarction (preferably in under 4 hours) will result in lysis of the causative thrombus in about 60% or more of blocked arteries. The effects of this are to limit the extent of infarction, to improve ventricular function in the long term, and a lower mortality compared to control. Thus, in the absence of contra-indications, and if the infarction is taken early enough, *intravenous* thrombolytic therapy is the treatment of choice.

HEART MUSCLE DISEASE

When heart failure occurs without recognizable mechanical cause the fault is presumed to be in the heart muscle itself. Heart muscle disease occurring in recognized association is so described, e.g. alcoholic heart disease (see below). When there is no recognizable cause the condition is termed cardiomyopathy. Three varieties are recognized: *congestive (dilated)*, *hypertrophic* and *restrictive*.

CONGESTIVE (DILATED) CARDIOMYOPATHY

The hallmark of this condition is dilatation of the left ventricle with impairment of emptying, i.e. a reduction

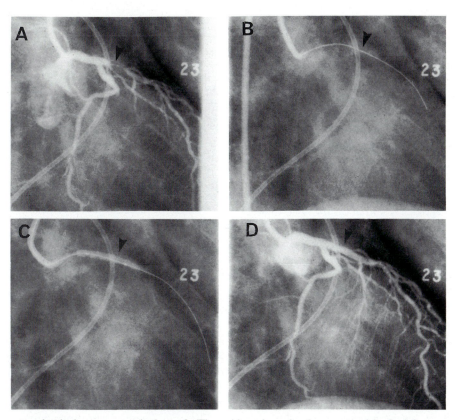

Fig. 23.35 Percutaneous transluminal coronary angioplasty. **A.** The guide catheter has been engaged in the left coronary ostium and a pre-procedure angiogram serves to demonstrate a severe proximal stenosis of the anterior descending coronary artery (arrow). **B.** The steerable guide-wire has been passed through the guide catheter into the left coronary artery. It has entered the anterior descending coronary artery and crossed the stenosis (arrow). **C.** The balloon catheter has been passed over the guide-wire and into the stenosis and inflated (arrow). The two studs indicate the position of the balloon before inflation. **D.** After balloon catheter and wire have been removed, a post-procedure angiogram shows that the stenosis has been almost entirely relieved (arrow).

in the ejection fraction. Asymptomatic dilatation may be present for years, symptoms only developing when congestive cardiac failure supervenes.

Presentation may be with congestive cardiac failure, often manifesting as an attack of bronchitis, as an arrhythmia or, rarely, with chest pain or even embolism from clot in the left ventricle. The clinical findings of a third sound gallop and an abnormal ECG indicate left ventricular disease.

The usual differential diagnosis is from other forms of congestive cardiac failure, particularly ischaemic heart disease, left ventricular aneurysm, silent aortic stenosis or even silent mitral stenosis. Ventricular dilatation may be associated with slight mitral regurgitation and a systolic murmur, and occasionally it may be difficult to distinguish between congestive cardiomyopathy with some mitral regurgitation and mitral regurgitation leading to severe cardiac failure.

Radiographic appearances. The plain film almost always shows cardiac enlargement, which may be restricted to the left ventricle (Fig. 23.36), or all chambers may be involved, resulting in a globular heart. Very rarely, left ventricular enlargement may only be seen in the lateral view. The lungs will show evidence of raised left atrial pressure in the untreated patient. Patients usually respond to treatment with considerable clinical improvement, a reduction in heart size (rarely to normal) and the clearing of the lungs. Relapse however, is usual and response to treatment less satisfactory with each relapse.

Radionuclide ventriculography usually demonstrates the dilated and poorly but concentrically contracting left ventricle. It will also exclude the surgically treatable possibility of left ventricular aneurysm.

Echocardiography using CSE (Fig. 23.37) will demonstrate the large and overall poorly contracting left ventricle and exclude silent aortic and mitral stenosis, and ischaemic heart disease.

Cardiac catheterization and *angiocardiography* are only indicated when the diagnosis is still in doubt. The dilated, poorly but concentrically contracting cavity of the left ventricle is usually obvious (Fig. 23.38); mitral and aortic stenosis and left ventricular aneurysm can all be excluded. In those cases complicated by mitral regurgitation, the severity of this may be assessed, and, taken together with the degree of impairment of left ventricular contraction, it is usually possible to distinguish between congestive cardiomyopathy and mitral regurgitation. The coronary arteries may also be studied at the same time.

HYPERTROPHIC CARDIOMYOPATHY

In this condition there is inappropriate hypertrophy of the myocardium occurring in the absence of any recognized stimulus. The hypertrophy is usually asymmetrical, and often concentrated in the upper septum, though all types

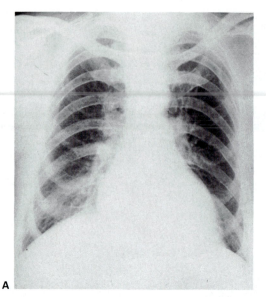

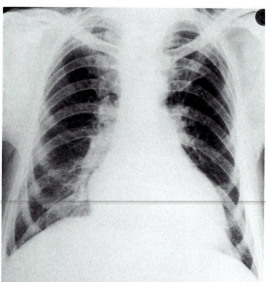

Fig. 23.36 Congestive cardiomyopathy. **A**. The heart is only slightly large. **B**. Significant dilatation involving mainly the left ventricle has developed 16 months later.

of distribution of hypertrophy may be seen. The excessive muscle apparently contracts well.

The condition may present as sudden death; with shortness of breath due to difficulty in filling the hypertrophied stiff left ventricle; with angina; or with arrhythmias. The pulse is characteristically jerky and the apex beat left-ventricular with an atrial beat. Auscultation reveals a late systolic murmur and a fourth heart sound. The ECG usually shows gross left ventricular hypertrophy.

The *plain film* findings range from an apparently normal heart through a heart showing obvious left ventricular hypertrophy, often with a rather chunky outline to it (Fig. 23.39), to a globular heart with all chambers involved.

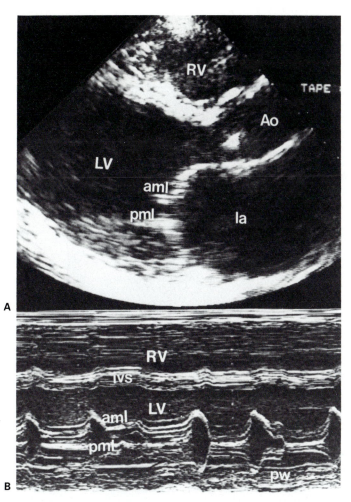

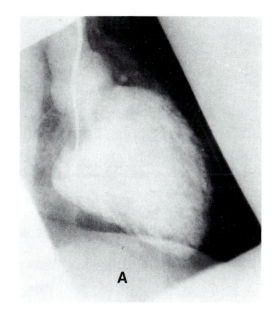

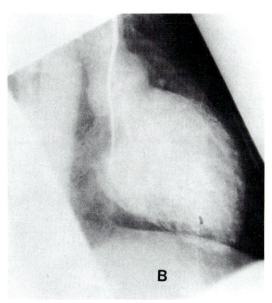

Fig. 23.37 A,B Congestive cardiomyopathy. The CSE demonstrates a large left ventricular cavity with poor wall movement, together with limited opening of the mitral valve leaflets (aml, pml) due to the low cardiac output.

Fig. 23.38 Congestive cardiomyopathy. Left ventricular cine-angiogram (RAO view) corresponding to Fig. 23.36B. **A**. Diastolic and **B**. systolic frames demonstrate a large ventricular cavity with generalized reduction in wall motion.

Evidence of raised left atrial pressure may be seen in the lungs.

The differential diagnosis usually lies between ischaemic heart disease, fixed aortic stenosis, non-rheumatic mitral regurgitation and hypertrophic cardiomyopathy.

Echocardiography. CSE will provide diagnostic information by visualizing the localized 'asymmetric' or generalized septal hypertrophy, the obstruction to the left ventricular outflow, the small left ventricular cavity and abnormal mitral valve movements (Fig. 23.40). A Doppler study will estimate the outflow tract gradient.

Cardiac catheterization may reveal a high filling pressure and a variable intracavity gradient, which may be provoked by post-ectopic beats. *Angiocardiography* reveals a range of abnormalities from a left ventricle indistinguishable from normal, to one which is of normal size but empties excessively and with prominent papillary muscles and septum (Fig. 23.41), through to the grossly distorted ventricle almost resembling a myocardial tumour.

RESTRICTIVE CARDIOMYOPATHY

Mild forms of this may be encountered in patients being investigated for nonspecific chest pain and found to have a high end-diastolic filling pressure in the left ventricle with no other abnormality.

The most florid example is seen in the condition of *endocardial fibrosis*, which is usually identified in Africans, but is seen sporadically in Europeans under the name of *Loeffler's endocarditis*. The pathological process is the laying-down of fibrous tissue on the inner aspects of the ventricles, beginning at the apices and spreading to involve the inlet valves.

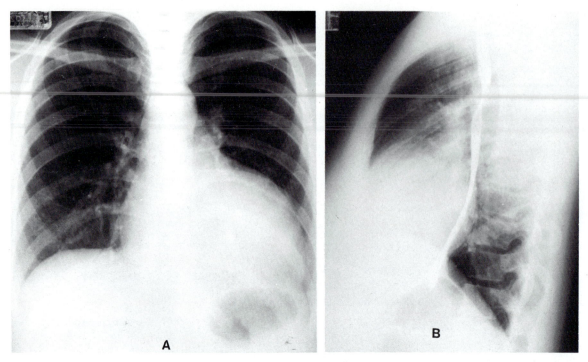

Fig. 23.39 Hypertrophic cardiomyopathy. **A**. Frontal film. The heart shadow is markedly enlarged with an elongation of its axis to the left and rounding of the apex but with a rather bulky and irregular outline. **B**. Lateral film. The enlarged left ventricle bulges back beyond the line of the barium-filled oesophagus. In this patient the cavity of the ventricle (see Fig. 23.41) is normal in size and the bulk of the heart shadow is due to an enormous increase in thickness of the wall of the heart.

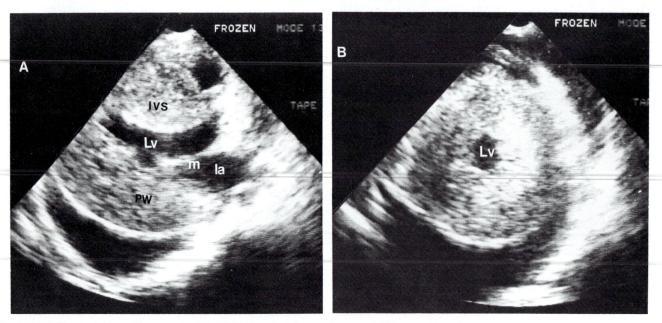

Fig. 23.40 Hypertrophic cardiomyopathy. The CSE visualizes the massive septal and posterior wall hypertrophy, almost obliterating the ventricular cavity. **A**. Long-axis view. **B**. Short-axis view.

On the left side this leads to difficulty in filling the ventricle (but not in contraction or emptying) and mitral incompetence. On the right side there is a high filling pressure in the right ventricle and tricuspid incompetence and there may be a pericardial effusion. In left-sided involvement the heart tends to be normal in size unless mitral regurgitation is severe. With right-sided involvement the heart shadow is large and globular.

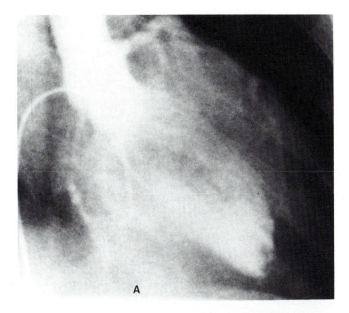

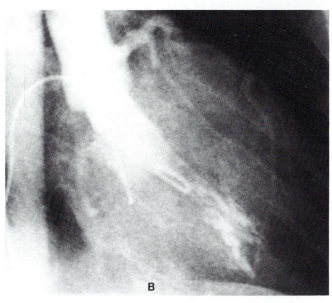

Fig. 23.41 Hypertrophic cardiomyopathy. Left ventricular cine-angiogram (RAO views). **A**. Diastolic frame. **B**. Systolic frame. Note the systolic obliteration of the ventricular cavity which results from the massive muscle hypertrophy.

Findings of *angiocardiography* are characteristic, with amputation and smoothing off of the apices of the ventricles and atrioventricular valvar regurgitation.

SPECIFIC HEART MUSCLE DISEASE

Abnormalities of heart muscle leading to a clinical syndrome similar to that of congestive cardiomyopathy may occur in a large variety of conditions.

Infections and collagen disorders

Viral myocarditis. This may be suggested when con-gestive cardiac failure occurs in relation to an obvious viral pyrexia (usually Coxsackie), particularly when there is a high, rising, antibody titre. However, cardiomyopathy may apparently begin with an influenza-like illness, or myocarditis may have no antecedent pyrexia. Endocardial biopsy, showing inflammatory cells eroding myocardial fibres, is the most satisfactory diagnostic tool, and may indicate appropriate treatment.

Bacterial myocarditis. A toxic myocarditis may occur with severe bacterial infections and is a well-known complication of the exotoxin of diphtheria. Myocarditis may also occur in the course of bacterial endocarditis.

Parasites. Chagas' disease, due to infection by *T. cruzi*, leads to a patchy fibrotic destruction of the myocardium, causing left ventricular failure after a long latent period. The oesophagus may be involved, producing appearances similar to those of achalasia. The disease is confined to Latin America.

Collagen diseases. Collagen diseases, including rheumatic fever, may involve the heart in their acute phase, leading to arrhythmias or congestive cardiac failure. Systemic lupus erythematosus usually produces a pericardial (and pleural) effusion. It may also produce sterile vegetations (Libman-Sacks) on the mitral and aortic valves.

Myocardial infiltrations

Haemochromatosis. The deposition of iron in the heart in this condition leads to congestive cardiac failure and is the cause of death of about one-third of patients.

Sarcoidosis. Involvement of the heart by sarcoidosis is rare, but may precede the appearance of sarcoidosis elsewhere in the body by several years. The usual manifestation is an *arrhythmia* but *congestive cardiac failure* may occur and rarely there may be *mitral incompetence* from papillary muscle involvement.

Amyloid heart disease. Amyloid may involve the heart alone or as part of a generalized disorder. There is severe cardiac failure, with low cardiac output and a low volume pulse. The patient is often murmur-free. The diagnosis may be suspected when echocardiography demonstrates a left ventricle only slightly enlarged. It may be confirmed by endomyocardial biopsy.

Glycogen storage disease. This condition usually presents in the neonatal period with characteristic muscle weakness, but rarely the heart failure may appear first. The condition may be suspected by echocardiography or left ventriculography, which shows a moderate cavity dilatation associated with gross wall thickening.

Metabolic disorders

Thyroid disease. Both forms of thyroid disease may lead to cardiac abnormalities. *Myxoedema* usually produces a pericardial effusion, but there may be involvement of the heart muscle with cardiac dilatation.

Thyrotoxicosis usually produces atrial fibrillation and should be suspected when this condition develops in the absence of mitral valve disease. Cardiac dilatation may also occur if thyrotoxicosis leads to high-output cardiac failure.

Acromegaly. There is generally held to be a specific dilated cardiomyopathy in association with acromegaly, but there is also a very high instance of hypertension and coronary artery disease.

Beri-beri. This condition, due to a deficiency of thiamine, leads to a high-output, or much more rarely a low-output, cardiac failure. It usually responds to thiamine.

Drugs and poisons

Alcoholic heart disease. Alcoholic heart disease may be manifest by arrhythmias or overt congestive cardiac failure. A history of excessive intake of alcohol, and improvement when alcohol is forsaken, suggest the specific diagnosis.

Drugs. *Beta-blocking drugs* in large doses may lead to cardiac dilatation or overt cardiac failure. It is not clear whether this only occurs in the presence of heart disease or could occur in a normal heart. The *anthracycline antimitotic agents* may lead to irreversible congestive cardiac failure. The effect is critically dose-related.

Other conditions

Congestive cardiomyopathy may develop in a variety of *heredo-familial neuromuscular disorders* and may be the cause of death. Congestive cardiomyopathy may also develop after pregnancy (*post-partum cardiomyopathy*). It usually responds to treatment but may relapse with subsequent pregnancies.

MISCELLANEOUS CONDITIONS

TUMOURS OF THE HEART

Secondary tumours, which commonly originate from *breast* or *bronchus*, are much commoner than primary tumours. They are often silent and only recognized at necropsy. Involvement of the pericardium leading to pericardial effusion and tamponade is much commoner.

Primary tumours of the heart are rare and the majority are benign, consisting mainly of *myxomas* (50%), *rhabdomyomas* and *fibromas*. The clinical manifestations often depend on the site of origin. Intracavity tumours are often pedunculated and cause obstruction, whereas intramural tumours may infiltrate, leading to arrhythmias or cardiac failure.

Myxomas

The vast majority of these occur in the left atrium, originating from a pedicle attached to the left side of the interatrial septum. Three groups of symptoms may occur:

1. *Obstructive*. Presentation is with shortness of breath. Examination reveals the physical signs of mitral valve disease, though with normal rhythm. The physical signs may vary from day to day or with the position of the patient.
2. *Embolic*. Parts of the tumour may embolize, causing stroke or limb ischaemia. On occasion, the first diagnosis of myxoma has been histological examination of an embolectomy specimen.
3. *Systemic*. Fever, anaemia, a raised ESR, and sometimes finger clubbing, may suggest the possibility of infective endocarditis, though blood cultures are sterile and splenomegaly does not occur.

Radiographic appearances. The plain film appearances may vary from a normal chest X-ray to an enlarged heart with selective left atrial enlargement, and the left atrial appendage may also be enlarged (Fig. 23.42). If obstruction is severe, upper-lobe blood diversion or pulmonary oedema may be seen. Very rarely, myxomas may be calcified and such calcification may be visible moving up and down in the atrium at fluoroscopy.

Echocardiography. Correctly performed CSE should invariably identify the tumour in the left atrium (the commonest site) (Fig. 23.43) or anywhere else in the heart. The mobility of the pedunculated tumour descending into the mitral valve in ventricular diastole is very typical. In cases where the echo window is poor, the *transoesophageal*

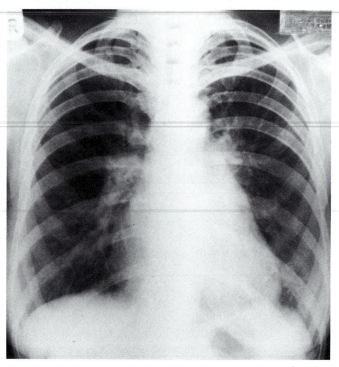

Fig. 23.42 Left atrial myxoma. The chest X-ray shows selective enlargement of the left atrium; the left atrial appendage is also enlarged.

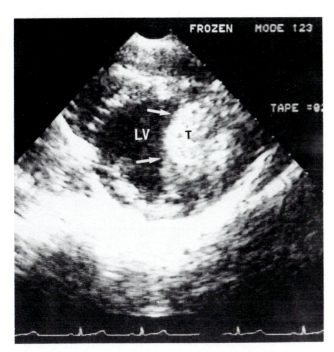

Fig. 23.43 Myocardial tumour. The CSE (short-axis view) demonstrates the presence of an intracavitary echo-dense mass (T) (arrows). LV = left ventricle.

echocardiogram will almost invariably be diagnostically decisive.

Both *CT scanning* and *Magnetic Resonance Imaging* have been used to visualize myxomas and other cardiac tumours. With the introduction of the transoesophageal echogram they have little role in diagnosis, but may be able to elucidate the extent of tumours (Figs 23.44, 23.45).

Cardiac catheterization and *angiocardiography* are no longer indicated if echocardiography is adequately performed. Occasionally cavity opacification may be required

to determine the extent of a tumour and coronary angiography may be valuable, not only in demonstrating the coronary anatomy prior to surgery, but also in showing a pathological circulation, which is not an infrequent feature of myxomas but is also seen in left atrial thrombus, in long-standing rheumatic mitral disease, and also in malignant cardiac tumours.

TRAUMA TO THE HEART

Trauma to the heart may be either penetrating or blunt.

Penetrating injuries usually lead to haemopericardium and tamponade, and require emergency drainage and possibly open surgery. Penetrating wounds may also damage the coronary arteries, producing myocardial infarction, or disrupt the valves of the heart.

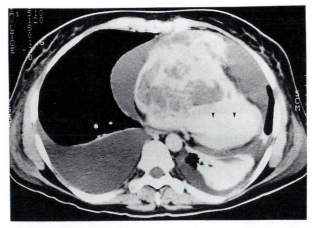

Fig. 23.45 Malignant angiosarcome — CT scan with contrast. The tumour mass appears as an irregular filling defect in the right atrium and ventricle. The left ventricle is displaced posteriorly (arrows). A large pericardial effusion surrounds the heart.

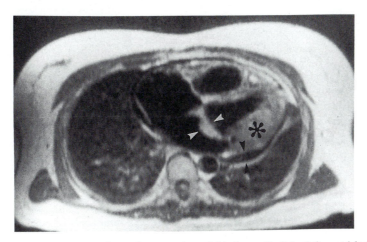

Fig. 23.44 Myocardial tumour. Spin echo MR scan shows the expansion of the free wall of the left ventricle by a tumour, (asterisk) and its spread onto the mitral valve which is seen to be grossly thickened (white arrows). The tricuspid valve is seen at this level to be of normal thickness. There is a small pericardial effusion (black arrows).

Blunt trauma may lead to myocardial contusion, producing a similar clinical finding to myocardial infarction. The coronary arteries may be injured, leading to the syndrome of myocardial infarction. The valves may be disrupted, producing incompetence.

False aneurysms may result from trauma to the heart. They are characterized by an unusual origin from the left ventricle and a narrow neck. They require surgery as they may rupture.

ENDOCARDITIS

Bacterial (or *rickettsial*) infections may settle on abnormal valves on either side of the heart, or in congenital heart lesions such as the right ventricle opposite a ventricular septal defect; or on a patent ductus arteriosus. Resultant infection produces a protracted and, unless treated, fatal febrile illness.

Vegetations are best assessed by CSE, where they appear as rapidly oscillating masses that are either attached to or replace normal valve tissue. These masses can be localized to the individual leaflet, and the size and mobility of the lesion readily assessed.

An extremely small vegetation may be missed by CSE

and improper gain settings may result in a false positive diagnosis. Furthermore, severely fibrotic, calcified or redundant valves may be incorrectly diagnosed as bacterial vegetation, and many patients have normal echocardiograms in the presence of confirmed infective endocarditis. The presence of a visible mass in the clinical setting of infective endocarditis does not always require surgical intervention; approximately 50% of the patients with this situation have been successfully treated medically.

Excavating abscesses may be identified by angiography or by CSE on transoesophageal echocardiography.

MRI OF ACQUIRED HEART DISEASE
Ian Isherwood and Jeremy P. R. Jenkins

Valvular heart disease
Accurate measurement of left and right ventricular stroke volumes using spin-echo images allows small discrepancies to be highlighted. In the absence of a shunt this indicates a regurgitant fraction. In the presence of dysfunction of two or more valves, gradient echo imaging can be used (see Ch. 20). The area of signal loss in the high signal blood pool proximal to an abnormal valve relates to the degree of regurgitation (Fig. 23.46). The severity of valvular stenosis can also be assessed by the length of signal loss distal to the valve (Fig. 23.47). Good concordance has been observed between this signal loss and pressure gradients measured at angiography or by Doppler ultrasound. Aortic sclerosis, with thickened and abnormal aortic valve leaflets on CSE but no pressure gradient at angiography, produces loss of signal distal to the valve (using TE values 22–28 ms) but to a lesser

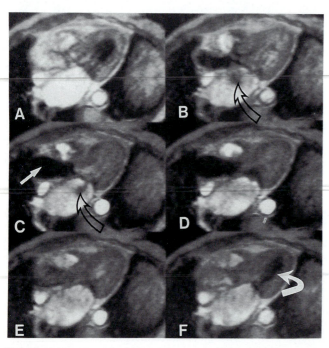

Fig. 23.46 Aortic and mitral stenosis and mitral regurgitation demonstrated on six oblique gated images in the cardiac long-axis plane using the gradient echo sequence (TE 26 ms) with timings at 100 ms intervals from (**A**) 30 ms to (**F**) 530 ms after the R wave of the ECG. Straight arrow = signal loss distal to the aortic valve in systole from aortic stenosis; curved open arrows = signal loss proximal to the mitral valve in systole from mitral regurgitation; curved solid arrow in **F** = signal loss distal to the mitral valve in diastole due to mitral stenosis (reproduced with permission from: Mitchell et al, 1989).

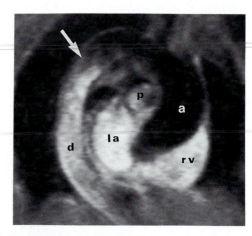

Fig. 23.47 Aortic stenosis on an oblique gated gradient echo image (TE 22 ms) through the aortic arch during peak systole. Note signal loss, with a maximum measured length of 16 cm, extending to the descending aorta (arrowed), due to turbulent flow distal to the stenosed aortic valve (on cardiac catheterization the pressure gradient across the valve was 80 mmHg). a = ascending aorta, d = descending aorta, la = left atrium, p = pulmonary artery, rv = right ventricle.

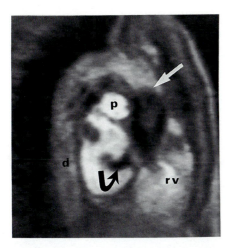

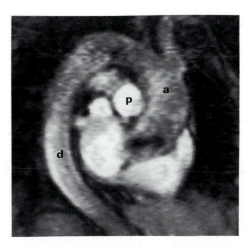

Fig. 23.48 Aortic sclerosis (no pressure gradient across the valve) on an oblique gated gradient echo image (TE 22 ms) through the aortic arch at peak systole, where the signal loss (maximum length 5 cm) distal to the aortic valve is confined to the ascending aorta (straight arrow). Note the coincidental mitral regurgitation (curved arrow). Key as in Fig. 23.47.

Fig. 23.50 Aortic stenosis on an oblique gated gradient echo (TE 12 ms) image through the aorta at peak systole. Note reclamation of signal in the aorta using the shorter echo time which can allow direct measurement of flow velocity. (Same patient as in Fig. 24.47.)

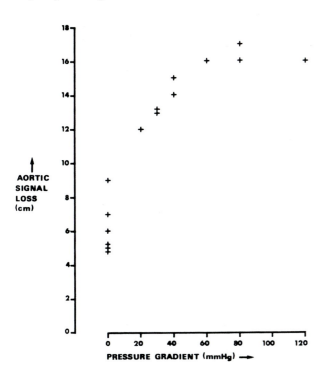

Fig. 23.49 Graph of peak aortic valve pressure gradient against maximum length of signal loss distal to the valve on gradient echo imaging (reproduced with permission from Mitchell et al, 1989).

where G = pressure gradient in mmHg and v = peak velocity through stenosis in m/s as used in Doppler US.

It is important that the normal appearances on gradient echo imaging where partial signal losses can be observed adjacent to valves in different phases of the cardiac cycle be appreciated and not mistaken for valvular dysfunction (see Fig. 20.52).

Ischaemic heart disease

Several reports, using both animal and human data, have shown that MRI is accurate in the estimation of acute myocardial infarct size. On T_2-weighted spin-echo images a high signal is produced from the infarcted myocardium. This area is less well visualized as a low signal on T_1-weighted scans but shows marked enhancement following intravenous gadolinium-DTPA with improved conspicuity as compared with T_2-weighted spin-echo imaging (Fig. 23.51). Unenhanced T_1-weighted spin-echo scans are, however, useful in demonstrating wall thinning and other complications of infarction including left ventricular aneurysm, pericardial effusion, cardiac chamber enlargement and septal rupture producing a VSD. The accuracy in the detection of myocardial infarction on MRI was 87%, using the criteria of abnormal high signal and reduced wall thickening. In acute infarction, some reduction in systolic wall thickening can usually be demonstrated on MRI within 24 hours of the onset of chest pain. No differences in signal intensity have been found between reperfused and non-perfused infarcted myocardium. There is conflicting evidence as to whether the contrast agent gadolinium-DTPA can aid in this separation.

Gradient echo imaging allows dynamic scanning with qualitative and quantitative assessment of ventricular function, including an accurate measure of myocardial

degree than with stenosis of the valve (Fig. 23.48). The length of signal loss, which does not reach the aortic arch in sclerosis, allows differentiation between the two conditions (Fig. 23.49). By using shorter TE values the signal can be reclaimed in the area of disturbed flow, allowing peak blood-flow velocity measurements to be made (Fig. 23.50). A pressure gradient can then be calculated by the modified Bernoulli equation (viz. G = 4v^2,

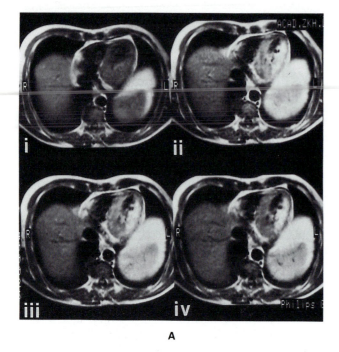

A

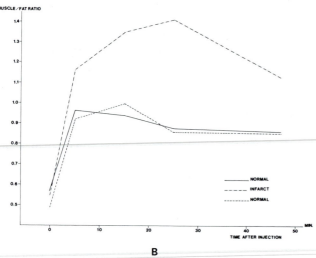

B

Fig. 23.51 **A**. Acute myocardial infarction of 7 days duration on transverse gated T$_1$-weighted images (i) before and (ii–iv) after gadolinium-DTPA. (ii) was performed immediately post-injection, (iii) 10 min and (iv) 20 min later. The posterolateral wall infarct shows marked enhancement and is clearly delineated. Note the lesser degree of enhancement of the normal myocardium in the early post-contrast phase. **B**. Graph of signal intensity vs. time in the same patient, demonstrating maximal contrast between the infarcted region and two areas of normal myocardium approximately 20–30 min after gadolinium-DTPA administration. (Reproduced with permission from: De Roos et al, 1988 (prints kindly supplied by Dr. A de Roos))

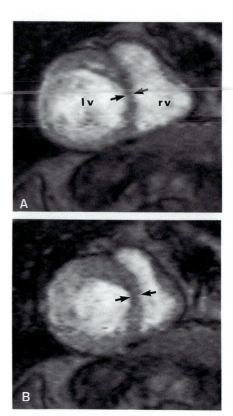

Fig. 23.52 Chronic myocardial infarction producing marked septal wall thinning (arrowed) on two gated short-axis gradient echo images (TE 26 ms) **A**. end-diastole. **B**. end-systole. lv = left ventricle; rv = right ventricle.

mass, together with evaluation of the end-diastolic and end-systolic wall thickness (Fig. 23.52). The distinction between flowing blood and thrombus is more consistently demonstrated using gradient echo images than on conventional spin-echo scans. On gradient echo imaging there is a high contrast between the high signal from flow-ing blood and the low signal from thrombus (Fig. 23.53). In addition, the cine-loop display improves identification of the dyskinetic segment of the infarcted segment. Viable myocardium can be distinguished from scar or chronic infarction by assessment of systolic wall thickening. The former shows some thickening of the myocardium in sys-tole, whereas the latter can be identified as an area of absent systolic thickening and diastolic wall thinning.

In the evaluation of coronary artery bypass grafts, the accuracy in the detection of graft patency is 90% using the spin-echo technique. The grafts appear as small areas of signal voids due to flowing blood, with errors in diag-nosis due to surgical clips in situ and small size of grafts (Fig. 23.54). A disadvantage of the spin-echo technique is that the presence of a signal void infers patency, in-dicating some, but not necessarily effective, blood flow down the graft. Gradient echo imaging not only enables graft patency to be more accurately detected but is also able to measure the flow velocity through the graft.

Heart muscle disease

Cardiomyopathies. Whilst MRI can clearly demon-strate ventricular hypertrophy and wall thickness, it is unlikely to replace CSE in the routine evaluation of these changes. A clear distinction between the hypertrophic and

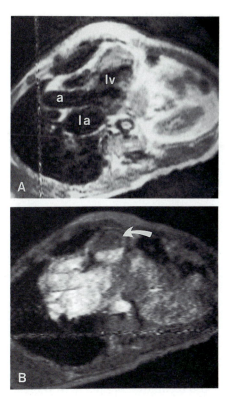

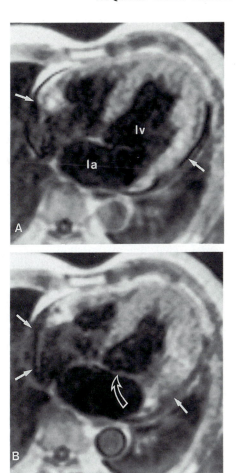

Fig. 23.53 Thrombus (arrowed) in a left ventricular aneurysm on two gated long-axis scans. **A.** Spin echo (TE 26 ms). **B.** Gradient echo (TE 28 ms). Key as in Fig 23.47.

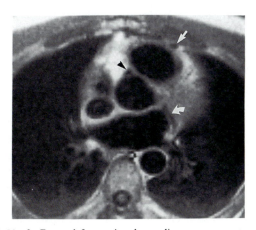

Fig. 23.54 A. Patent left anterior descending coronary artery bypass graft (straight arrow) is demonstrated on a transverse gated spin-echo image (TE 26 ms). The native right coronary (arrowhead) and left circumflex (curved arrow) arteries are also visualized. (Reproduced with permission from Jenkins et al 1988).

Fig. 23.55 Hypertrophic cardiomyopathy on transverse gated spin-echo images (TE 40 ms). **A.** End-diastole. **B.** End-systole. The myocardium is markedly thickened, with an associated pericardial effusion (straight arrows). Key as in Fig. 23.47. (Adapted with permission from Jenkins and Isherwood 1987.)

congestive groups of cardiac muscle disease can be observed with MRI, with delineation of the extent and distribution of muscle involvement (Fig. 23.55). In the unusual form of apical hypertrophic cardiomyopathy, MRI is useful in showing the extent of involvement. Gradient echo imaging can be used to evaluate the functional consequences of hypertrophic cardiomyopathy

as well as defining any associated myocardial ischaemia.

Cardiac sarcoidosis. MR appears to be the most sensitive imaging technique in the detection of cardiac involvement by sarcoidosis. Infiltration of the left ventricular myocardium and interventricular septum can be demonstrated as patchy high signals on T_2-weighted spin-echo images, allowing correct localization for myocardial biopsy and histological confirmation.

Amyloid infiltration. In amyloid heart disease, MRI has demonstrated a thickened atrial septum and myocardium with reduced wall thickening during systole.

Cardiac transplant. MRI is of limited value in the detection of acute and chronic cardiac transplant rejection, based on currently-used tissue characterization parameters including intravenous gadolinium-DTPA. Acute rejection induces an increase in the myocardial wall thickness, predominately of the left ventricle. Myocardial wall thickening, best evaluated by gradient echo imaging, could in principle be used to detect rejection. This parameter, however, is more readily and repeatably assessed on CSE.

Cardiac masses

Whilst CSE is the mainstay technique used in the diagnosis of left ventricular thrombi and other mass lesions (including right atrial myxoma), a significant number of patients cannot be adequately assessed by this method due to body habitus or proximity of the lesion to the cardiac apex. In a recent study, only 15 of 25 (60%) patients with *left ventricular thrombus* secondary to chronic anterior myocardial infarction were diagnosed correctly by CSE — six (24%) were inadequate CSE studies compared with none on MRI or CT. On spin-echo imaging some abnormal signal, due to slow flow, can be noted in the blood pool of the ventricular chambers, mimicking thrombus formation. The introduction of gradient echo imaging has overcome this disadvantage; the blood pool is shown consistently as a high signal fluctuating with time against the constant intermediate mid-grey signal of thrombus (Fig. 23.53). In addition, functional information can be gained in the demonstration of the dyskinetic segment adjacent to the thrombus.

MRI can distinguish some mass lesions such as lipomas and fibromas which give high (similar to surrounding fat) and low (due to a paucity of mobile protons) signals respectively. Cystic lesions usually give a high signal on T_2-weighted spin-echo scans, greater than those of adjacent fat. Some difficulty, however, may occasionally be encountered on MRI in differentiating between cystic and solid lesions, a distinction that can easily be made on CSE. Lymphomas give a higher signal and myxomas a signal similar to myocardium on spin-echo imaging. Myxomas can be diagnosed by their characteristic appearance and position. The use of gadolinium-DTPA enables enhancing tumour to be separated from non-enhancing thrombus (Fig. 23.56). Calcified intracardiac lesions cannot be clearly visualized and a heavily calcified mass may be missed due to the low signal obtained from such tissue. The use of gradient echo imaging can improve the sensitivity in the detection of such lesions. CT,

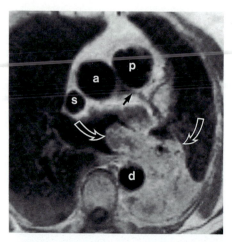

Fig. 23.56 Enhancing bronchial carcinoma (curved arrows) invading the left lower lobe bronchus, left atrium and descending aorta on a transverse gated T_1-weighted post-gadolinium-DTPA spin-echo image (TE 26 ms). Note the associated lower lobe collapse, which is difficult to differentiate from the tumour. The left coronary artery (straight arrow), with its anterior descending and circumflex branches, is shown. Key as in Fig. 23.47; s = superior vena cava.

however, is the technique of choice in the assessment of cardiac calcification. In patients suspected of having an atrial myxoma, sufficient information is usually gained on CSE making MRI unnecessary. MRI does have a role in the further assessment of suspected intracardiac filling defects suspected on CSE, and in clearly defining normal structures such as a prominent moderator band in the right ventricle or fat pad in the atrioventricular groove. Comparative studies of transoesophageal ultrasound and MRI in the evaluation of cardiac masses are needed.

On MRI, intra- and extracardiac masses can be directly visualized, together with their relationship to surrounding structures. Paracardiac masses are best evaluated by spin-echo imaging because of its high soft-tissue contrast resolution and discrimination. MRI can complement CSE in defining the extent of metastatic disease, with its wider topographical view more easily delineating thoracic and abdominal involvement.

REFERENCES AND SUGGESTIONS FOR FURTHER READING

Donaldson, R. M., Raphael, M. J. (1982) Missing coronary artery. *British Heart Journal*, **42**, 62–70.
Hurst, J. J. (1990) *The Heart*. 7th edn. McGraw-Hill, New York.
Jefferson, K., Rees, S. (1980) *Clinical Cardiac Radiology*. 2nd edn. Butterworths, London.
Julian, D., Camm, A. J., Fox, K. M., Hall, R. J. C., Poole-Wilson, P. A. (Eds) (1989) *Diseases of the heart*. Baillière Tindall, London.
King, S. B. IIIrd., Douglas, J. S., Jr. (1985) *Coronary Arteriography and Angioplasty*. McGraw-Hill, New York.
Miller, G. (1989) *Invasive Investigation of the Heart*. Blackwell Scientific Publications, Oxford.

Raphael, M. J., Hawkin, D. R., Allwork, S. P. (1980) The angiographic anatomy of the coronary arteries. *British Journal of Surgery*, **67**, 181–187.
Reiber, J. H. C., Serruys, P. W. (1988) *New Developments in Quantitative Coronary Arteriography*. Kluwer, Dordrecht.

MRI
Freedberg, R. S., Kronzon, I., Rumanick, W. M., Liebeskind, D. (1988) The contribution of magnetic resonance imaging to the evaluation of intracardiac tumour diagnosed by echocardiography. *Circulation*, **77**, 96–103.

Higgins, C. B. (1987) The heart: acquired disease. In: Higgins, C. B., Hricak, H. *Magnetic Resonance Imaging of the Body*. Raven Press, New York, Ch. 13, pp. 239–265.

Higgins, C. B. (1990) Nuclear magnetic resonance (NMR) imaging in ischemic heart disease. *Journal of the American College of Cardiology*, **15**, 150–151.

Jenkins, J. P. R., Isherwood, I. (1987) Magnetic resonance imaging of the heart: a review. In: Rowlands, D. J. (Ed.) *Recent Advances in Cardiology 10*. Churchill Livingstone, Edinburgh, pp. 219–247.

Jenkins, J. P. R., Love, H. G., Foster, C. J., Isherwood I., Rowlands, D. (1988) Detection of coronary artery bypass graft patency as assessed by magnetic resonance imaging. *British Journal of Radiology*, **61**, 2–4.

Johnston, D. L., Mulvagh, S. L., Cashion, R. W., O'Neill, P. G., Roberts, R., Rokey, R. (1989) Nuclear magnetic resonance imaging of acute myocardial infarction within 24 hours of chest pain onset. *American Journal of Cardiology*, **64**, 172–179.

Lund, J. T., Ehman, R. L., Julsrud, P. R., Sinak, L. J. (1989) Cardiac masses: assessment by MR imaging. *American Journal of Roentgenology*, **152**, 469–473.

Mitchell, L., Jenkins, J. P. R., Watson, Y., Rowlands, D. J., Isherwood, I. (1989) Diagnosis and assessment of mitral and aortic valve disease by cine-flow magnetic resonance imaging. *Magnetic Resonance in Medicine*, **12**, 181–197.

Peshock, R. M. (1988) Heart and great vessels. In: Stark, D. D., Bradley, W. G. (Eds.) *Magnetic Resonance Imaging*, C. V. Mosby, St Louis, Ch. 36, pp. 887–920.

Pettigrew, R. I. (1989) Dynamic cardiac MR imaging techniques and applications. In: Miller, S. W. (Ed.) Cardiopulmonary Imaging. *Radiologic Clinics of North America*, **27**, 1183–1203.

Rees, S. (1990) Magnetic resonance studies of the heart. (The George Simon Lecture) *Clinical Radiology*, **42**, 302–316.

de Roos, A., Matheijssen, N. A., Doornbos, J., van Dijkman, P. R. M., van Voorthuisen, A. E., van der Wall, E. E. (1990) Myocardial infarct size after reperfusion therapy: assessment with Gd-DTPA-enhanced MR imaging. *Radiology*, **176**, 517–521.

Sechtem, U., Jungehulsing, M. (1990) Nonivasive imaging of cardiac masses. *Current Opinion in Radiology*, **2**, 575–580.

Stanford, W., Galvin., J. R., Skorton, D. J., Marcus, M. L. (1990) The evaluation of coronary bypass graft patency: Direct and indirect techniques other than coronary arteriography. *American Journal of Roentgenology*, **156**, 15–22.

Underwood, R., Firmin, D. (Eds.) (1990) *Magnetic Resonance of the Cardiovascular System*. Blackwell Scientific Publications, Oxford.

CHAPTER 24

CONGENITAL HEART DISEASE

Peter Wilde

The incidence of congenital heart disease in live births is estimated at between 0.5% and 1.0% in various large series. Many of these recorded abnormalities are relatively simple, with only a small proportion of cases having very complex abnormalities. The common congenitally *bicuspid aortic valve* (2% incidence in the population) is not included in these figures, nor is the increasingly recognized *patent ductus arteriosus* in premature infants.

This relatively low incidence means that many radiologists will see only a small number of congenital heart disease cases each year, particularly if they are not working in a centre with special paediatric or cardiac interests. It is not possible for a general radiologist or even a general paediatric radiologist to be familiar with the detailed radiology of all forms of congenital heart disease. It is essential however that all radiologists are sufficiently well informed in this field to be able to recognize possible cardiac problems and guide further investigation. They should also be able to assist in basic medical management and be aware of the changing patterns of disease seen in the natural history or surgical management of many of these conditions.

Over the last two decades the progress in treatment of congenital heart disease has been spectacular and, in particular, operative management has led to the survival of many patients who would previously have died from their congenital malformations. In many cases surgery is able to achieve complete or nearly complete anatomical correction of the abnormality and in many other cases a high level of palliation can be achieved. An increasing number of patients will return for routine radiological assessment following surgery.

The treatment of congenital heart disease is generally undertaken in large specialist centres and in these there will usually be a team approach to diagnosis and management. The best centres will have close co-operation between cardiac physicians, surgeons and radiologists. The specialist radiologist will be able to offer a range of investigations, particularly echocardiography and angiocardiography and increasingly in the future, magnetic resonance imaging. More recently the radiologist has also had a role to play in the management of cases requiring interventional treatment, particularly balloon dilatation of stenotic valves and vessels and less commonly the embolization and occlusion of abnormal communications and channels.

Radiologists may deal with congenital heart disease at various stages and in various ways. These include:

1. Recognition that congenital heart disease is present. A preliminary diagnosis or general diagnosis is frequently possible from the *chest radiograph* but it is rare that the plain film will give a precise, accurate and reliable diagnosis of the intracardiac abnormality.
2. Detailed diagnosis by *echocardiography* with the possible addition of *cardiac catheterization*, *angiography* and other techniques.
3. Detailed evaluation of investigation results, usually at a joint case conference in which the full clinical picture is assessed and management is discussed.
4. Management, which can be continued medical management, palliative surgery, corrective surgery, or *interventional catheter techniques*. The radiologist may well have an important role in the interventional techniques, as well as in monitoring management by the use of plain chest radiography and other non-invasive imaging techniques.
5. Follow-up. This will usually be done jointly between the specialist centre and the referring centre.

The two most obvious ways in which **cardiac surgery** has changed in recent years are the increasing number of total anatomical corrections that are possible and the decreasing age at which these operations are performed. In many large units a high proportion of congenital heart abnormalities are now completely corrected before the age of one year. In other cases early palliative surgery precedes later definitive surgery. This has a particular effect on the practice of cardiac radiology, because the classical appearances of long-standing congenital heart abnormalities on the chest radiograph are becoming increasingly uncommon and their practical importance less.

Cardiac surgery is considered to include the heart and great vessels and can be divided into two major types; closed heart surgery and open heart surgery. In *closed heart surgery* the operation is performed whilst the heart continues to function, and for this reason most closed heart operations are limited in terms of intracardiac repair. This type of procedure is most commonly carried out for abnormalities of the aorta and pulmonary arteries and palliation of other conditions. The procedures include *repair of coarctation*, insertion of a *systemic-to-pulmonary shunt* or *banding of the main pulmonary artery*.

Open heart surgery requires that the cardiac function must cease. During this time the patient is maintained on cardiopulmonary bypass or is cooled to low temperatures to facilitate a safe period of cardiac standstill. In this situation it is vital that the cardiac surgeon has full knowledge of the nature of the abnormality or abnormalities before undertaking the operation, so that the time taken for the repair is kept to an absolute minimum. This reduces the risks of operative mortality or morbidity, which increase progressively with the length of time the heart is taken out of circulation.

The practice of **preoperative assessment** has changed considerably in recent years. Nowadays the *clinical*, *radiographic* and particularly *echocardiographic* data is frequently adequate to make a complete diagnosis of the intracardiac abnormality. *Cardiac catheterization* and *angiography* are still required in a significant number of patients with a full echo diagnosis, because additional details may be required for precise management decisions to be made. In some cases this detail is of a haemodynamic nature. It is often necessary to measure the pulmonary vascular resistance in patients with large left-to-right shunts to exclude the possibility of irreversible pulmonary damage. Certain pressure gradients and absolute intracardiac pressures are also needed if they are not obtained by Doppler echocardiography.

It is sometimes necessary to clarify anatomical detail by *angiocardiography*, often with a view to excluding known pitfalls that may be encountered by the surgeon. For example, coronary anatomy cannot adequately be assessed by echocardiography whilst it can be clearly assessed using cineangiography. The pulmonary artery anatomy is often crucial to the management of many patients and it is often not possible to visualize the left and right pulmonary arteries beyond their origins by echocardiography due to surrounding intrapulmonary air. Other fine details of anatomy are often obtained by cardiac catheterization and angiography, such as the assessment of small or multiple ventricular septal defects (unless high-quality Doppler colour-flow mapping is available) and the visualization of systemic to pulmonary collaterals or shunts. There will also be cases where the echo study has been technically difficult for one reason or another and the angiogram is essential.

Finally the cardiac catheterization procedure is sometimes accompanied by an interventional procedure. These include *Rashkind balloon septostomy* for transposition of the great arteries, *dilatation of pulmonary valve* or *coarctation*, and more recently *ductal closure, occlusion of abnormal fistulae* and *blade septostomy*. These techniques are developing rapidly but require expert knowledge of intracardiac anatomy to ensure their success.

CLASSIFICATION AND DESCRIPTION OF CONGENITAL HEART DISEASE

A number of different attempts have been made to classify congenital heart disease, but whichever approach is adopted there is a large array of differing conditions which must be recognized.

The first and most important requirement is for accurate description of what is being seen. It is therefore vital to recognize the morphological appearance of each cardiac chamber and each great vessel wherever possible so that abnormal connections are unambiguously described. It is frequently helpful to use the phrase *morphologically left ventricle* to describe a ventricular chamber which has all the characteristics of the left ventricle irrespective of where it is in the patient and irrespective of which connections it makes. It is for example possible to have a morphologically left ventricle that lies on the right side of the body or to the right of the other ventricle.

The **morphological features** of important structures are described in detail in Ch. 20, and are here briefly reviewed.

1. **Right atrium**. The appearance of the atrial appendages has long been fundamental in the accurate determination of atrial morphology and is particularly suited to angiocardiography or, on occasion, to pathological or surgical examination. It is not possible to determine this information from plain films and it is very difficult to achieve using echocardiography. The right atrial appendage is broad-based and triangular in shape. The inferior vena cava almost always enters the right atrium, and though this rule is not invariable, it is a clinically important guide. The site of drainage of the inferior vena cava can be demonstrated by angiocardiography or echocardiography. The latter technique can also be very helpful in assessing the anatomy of the atrial septum to determine morphology; the septum secundum lies to the right of the septum primum and its lower margin forms the upper edge of the foramen ovale. This is frequently patent in early life, but even in later life the closed fossa ovale remains as a marker of the right side of the atrial septum.

2. Left atrium. This chamber can be defined most precisely by its atrial appendage which is long and narrow, usually curling around the left side of the heart. The left atrium cannot reliably be defined by the presence of pulmonary veins as these can often be anomalous.

3. Right ventricle. This is rhomboid in shape and shows heavy bands of trabeculation throughout the chamber. There is often a prominent band crossing the main cavity of the ventricle, the 'moderator band'. The trabecular pattern is particularly suited to demonstration by angiocardiography, but can sometimes be deduced using echocardiography. In the assessment of trabecular pattern by any technique it is important to look comparatively at both ventricles because the typical patterns may be a little distorted in some complex cases.

The papillary muscles arise from multiple groups in the right ventricle and there is usually some attachment of chordae to papillary muscle or muscles on the septum which itself is heavily trabeculated. The atrioventricular valve of the right ventricle is by definition the tricuspid valve, and is inserted slightly more towards the apex of the heart than the atrioventricular valve of the left ventricle (mitral valve). This particular feature is very well demonstrated by echocardiography. There is normally an outflow muscular tube known as the conus or infundibulum which leads up to the exit semilunar valve. The semilunar valves (pulmonary and aortic) are named in accordance with the appropriate great artery, so the exit valve of the right ventricle is not necessarily the pulmonary valve.

4. Left ventricle. This is the ventricular chamber with a more symmetrical oval shape and fine lattice-like trabeculation. The basal half of the interventricular septum is smooth, without any trabeculation. There are normally two large papillary muscles in this ventricle, both of which arise from the free wall and not from the interventricular septum. Both papillary muscles give attachment to chordae from both mitral valve leaflets.

The atrioventricular valve entering the left ventricle is by definition the mitral valve, and the insertion of the mitral valve is further towards the base of the heart than the atrioventricular valve of the right ventricle, the tricuspid valve. In the left ventricle there is usually fibrous continuity between the inflow and outflow valves, although this is not always the case. The fibrous continuity is well demonstrated on the two-dimensional long-axis view, where the anterior leaflet of the mitral valve is seen arising from the posterior wall of the aortic root.

5. The pulmonary artery is the great artery which bifurcates into two branches after a short distance, each branch supplying one lung. If two great arteries are present then it is often easier to define the aorta first. It is also important to distinguish true pulmonary arteries arising from the pulmonary trunk from abnormal aorto-pulmonary vessels.

6. The aorta is the great artery which supplies branches to the head and neck. The aorta cannot be defined in terms of its connection to the heart (in transposition of the great arteries the aorta arises from the right ventricle) or the presence of coronary branches (anomalous coronary vessels can arise from the pulmonary artery).

CLASSIFICATION OF CARDIAC ABNORMALITIES

In recent years a reasonably standardized approach has been achieved in the description of congenital cardiac abnormalities. Although this is not necessarily used in the description of very simple abnormalities, it is invaluable in the description of complex abnormalities as it avoids confusion or ambiguity. The approach is one with five major descriptive steps:

1. Situs.
2. Cardiac connections.
3. Looping.
4. Positions.
5. Malformations.

These will be described in turn.

1. Situs. The abdominal and thoracic viscera are asymmetrical, and for this reason normal situs can be recognized by obvious features such as the liver and inferior vena cava lying on the right side and the spleen and heart lying on the left side. The very high association with the inferior vena cava draining into the right atrium has led to the development of the term '*viscero-atrial situs*'. This essentially means that the atrial situs in almost all cases conforms to the situs of the upper abdominal viscera, irrespective of the situs or position of the remainder of the heart. A transverse upper abdominal ultrasound scan will allow definition of the viscero-atrial situs by showing variations in position of the inferior vena cava, aorta and sometimes the azygos vein.

It is also important to recognize the presence of asymmetry in the lungs, which is usually apparent in the form of *bronchial situs*. The right main bronchus is shorter, wider and more vertically orientated than the left main bronchus, which is usually at least $1\frac{1}{2}$ times as long as the right from bifurcation to first major branch (Fig. 24.1). The bronchial situs nearly always corresponds to the visceroatrial situs. Special filtration techniques of chest radiography may be needed for the assessment of bronchial situs.

From time to time situs abnormalities will occur and it is important to describe variations accurately.

a. Situs solitus. This describes the normal situation with normal visceroatrial situs (liver, inferior vena cava and right atrium on the right side) and normal bronchial situs. The 'position' of the cardiac mass and/or cardiac

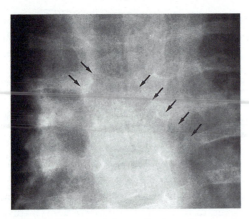

Fig. 24.1 Plain radiograph of the mediastinum showing normal bronchial anatomy. Arrows indicate the length of left and right bronchi.

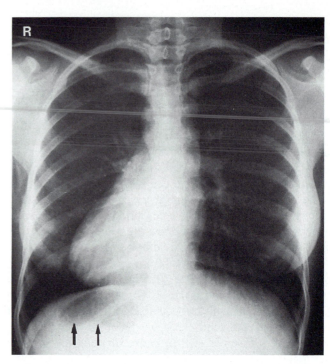

Fig. 24.3 Chest radiograph of a patient with total situs inversus (gastric bubble arrowed).

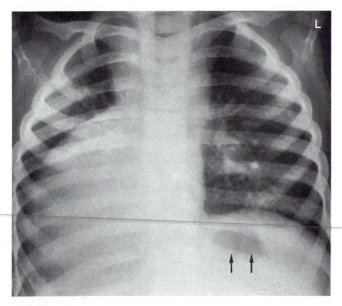

Fig. 24.2 Chest radiograph of a patient with visceroatrial situs solitus (gastric bubble arrowed) and isolated dextrocardia.

apex is not directly related to visceroatrial situs and may not correspond with it. The apex can occasionally be directed towards the right side even with normal visceroatrial situs, this sometimes being described as *isolated dextrocardia* or dextrorotation of the heart (Fig. 24.2).

b. *Situs inversus*. In this condition there is complete reversal of the visceroatrial situs and the bronchial situs. The condition is not necessarily associated with any other cardiac abnormality. An example of this is shown in Figure 24.3. Meticulous technique in the use of radiographic side markers is of paramount importance. If films are marked up after processing, then cases of total situs inversus are almost certainly going to be marked wrongly. Once again the cardiac apex may not lie in the expected position. Thus in most cases of situs inversus the cardiac

apex lies on the right side but occasionally it will lie on the left (*isolated levocardia*).

c. *Situs ambiguus*. This describes a situation in which the left- and right-sided nature of abdominal or thoracic organs and the atria are not clearly distinct. A number of variations of this can be recognized. The first of these is most easily understood as '*bilateral right-sidedness*'. In this condition there is a mid-line liver running across the upper abdomen (Fig. 24.4), the spleen is absent, the stomach is usually centrally positioned and the bronchial anatomy shows right-sided morphology of both major bronchi. Both atrial chambers have right-sided characteristics and, not surprisingly, there is a frequent association with abnormalities of pulmonary venous drainage. Often many other cardiac abnormalities are also associated with this condition. '*Bilateral left-sidedness*' is also associated with a mid-line liver, often smaller, but there is frequently polysplenia and bilateral left atrial morphology, and the two main bronchi both show left morphology. Again, there is an association with major cardiac abnormality. The final form of situs ambiguus is one in which the morphological characteristics of the various structures are very hard to determine and a left- or right sided nature cannot easily be determine. In this case again many cardiac anomalies can be associated.

2. Cardiac connections. Once the cardiac chambers have been identified in morphological terms it should be possible to state which vessel or chamber is connected to which. For example, in transposition of the great arteries

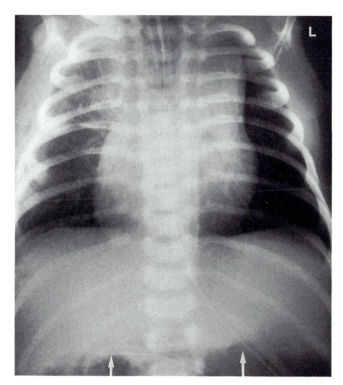

Fig. 24.4 Chest radiograph of an infant with situs ambiguous. A centrally positioned cardiac apex and transverse liver (arrowed). There were complex intracardiac anomalies.

it can be stated that the aorta arises from the morphologically right ventricle and the pulmonary artery arises from the morphologically left ventricle. In this situation there is said to be *ventriculoarterial discordance*. From time to time there will be *atrioventricular discordance* which will occur when the morphologically right atrium drains into the morphologically left ventricle and vice versa.

In some cases the connections will not be completely distinct as, for example, in the *tetralogy of Fallot* where the aorta partially overrides onto the right ventricle from its position above a large ventricular septal defect. Complete overriding of great arteries can occur in the presence of a ventricular septal defect, most typically in *double-outlet right ventricle*.

If there is a large ventricular septal defect lying between the atrioventricular valves there can also be partial or total override of the mitral or tricuspid valve. Double-inlet ventricle is thus a recognized occurrence. Although it is a simple matter to state that an atrioventricular valve is related to one or other or both ventricles, the diagnosis of the exact relationship may not be easy. The complex curving nature of the interventricular septal anatomy and the limitations of all the imaging techniques make precise diagnosis very difficult in some cases. Surgical or pathological inspection does not provide an unequivocal diagnosis in every case either. In spite of these difficulties, it should be the aim of any intracardiac examination in

complex congenital heart disease to obtain a clear idea of the basic relationships of the chambers, with any difficulties in description or nomenclature being stated clearly.

3. Looping (or topology). This term relates to the ventricular loop which has been formed during cardiac development. If the heart is well enough developed to have two ventricles, each with an inlet and an outlet, and an interventricular septum lying between them, then it will be possible to define the loop. D-loop and L-loop configurations are stereo-isomers of each other, the difference between the two types of loop being analogous to the difference between the left hand and right hand. Each hand is uniquely different, being defined by the relationship of the fingers and thumb with the palm and back of the hand. Whichever position a hand is in, it can always be distinguished as a right or left hand. Looping is also independent of cardiac situs or position.

The normal *ventricular D-loop* can be understood most simply using the analogy of the *right hand rule* devised by Van Praagh. In this description the morphological right ventricle is likened to a right hand. The inflow is represented by the thumb, the outflow is represented by the fingers and the interventricular septum will lie on the palmar side of the hand. This can be appreciated by placing one's right hand near another person's heart. If, however, the morphologically right ventricle is configured in such a way that the relationship of inflow, outflow and interventricular septum can only be represented by a left hand, this infers that the ventricle is actually a stereo-isomer (mirror image) of a normal D-loop ventricle.

L-looping is most frequently seen in association with transposition of the great arteries in the condition known as anatomically corrected transposition or commonly just 'corrected transposition'.

4. Position. Although the position of the heart in the chest is the first thing to be seen on a chest radiograph, the absolute position is of secondary importance in describing the fundamental nature of the congenital heart abnormality. The position is of course of practical importance in planning surgical procedures. If one imagines that the heart is a model made out of extremely flexible elastic material then it is easy to see that the position of even a completely normal heart can be considerably distorted by twisting, stretching or turning various chambers into different positions, whilst the heart still maintains absolutely normal situs, cardiac connections and ventricular looping. Similarly, the presence of particular situs, connection or looping arrangements does not necessarily indicate what the final cardiac position will be.

A complex positional variation is the 'criss-cross' heart. In this abnormality there is, in addition to any other abnormalities of situs or connection, an additional twist of the ventricular mass. This results in the ventricles lying in unexpected positions given the particular situs and connection. Sometimes the ventricles adopt a supero-inferior relationship but occasionally their positions can be completely reversed. The simplest example to understand would occur in a heart with normal situs and connections; in this case twisting of the ventricular mass could lead to the morphologically left ventricle lying anterior to the posteriorly displaced morphological right ventricle.

It is important to note the position of the *aortic arch* relative to the trachea. The normal aortic arch is left-sided but some congenital abnormalities are associated with a higher than normal incidence of right-sided arch. There are a number of variations in aortic branching patterns which will be considered later. The recognition of a right-sided aortic arch is of course important for surgical planning. A right-sided arch may also occur in isolation (Fig. 24.5).

5. Malformations. This refers to the specific deformities or abnormalities within the heart, such as *stenotic* or *atretic valves*, *abnormal communications* and *narrowed vessels*. These malformations are often the most obvious abnormality and they are commonly used as the overall descriptive term for a particular abnormality (e.g. *ventricular septal defect*, *pulmonary atresia* or *coarctation of the aorta*). Some malformations are a little more complex, for example atrioventricular septal defects, and in some cases there are multiple associated malformations as in tetralogy of Fallot (ventricular septal defect and pulmonary stenosis).

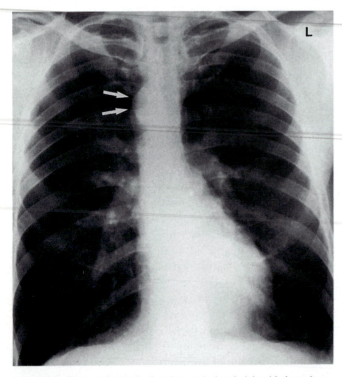

Fig. 24.5 Chest radiograph showing an isolated right-sided aortic arch (arrows indicate aortic knuckle).

In many cases the malformations are the only abnormality and in this situation the full description of situs, connection, looping and position is omitted for simplicity in general discussion, the implicit assumption being made that all these other aspects are normal. This is acceptable in normal practice, provided that the full descriptive nomenclature is used as soon as the congenital heart abnormality is anything other than straightforward.

Malformations also occur commonly in association with the more complex abnormalities and in fact they are frequently associated with major abnormalities of situs, looping or connection.

HAEMODYNAMIC AND FUNCTIONAL PRINCIPLES

A thorough understanding of the radiology of congenital heart disease must include not only structural abnormalities but also functional abnormalities. Normal cardiac anatomy and physiology must be understood before the developmental, functional and pathological consequences of the abnormalities can fully be appreciated.

Developmental aspects

1. Development of chambers and vessels. The blood flowing through a chamber or vessel is a powerful stimulus for the growth of the cavity. Conversely, if there is no flow then the structure will be hypoplastic or absent. It is the chamber size that is affected by flow, not usually the wall thickness (hypertrophy). This is seen most dramatically in the condition of *hypoplastic left heart* in which the left ventricle fails to develop beyond a tiny size because there is aortic and/or mitral atresia which prevents normal flow through the left ventricle and aorta. It is also seen in some cases of *pulmonary atresia* when the low pulmonary blood flow predisposes to very small pulmonary arteries. The converse is also true, high flow leading to a large cavity size, as is seen in right heart dilatation with an atrial septal defect.

The pressure generated by a chamber stimulates the development of the muscular wall rather than the size of the cavity. Thus in pulmonary atresia with an intact ventricular septum, there is a high-pressure obstructed ventricle with very low flow through it. In this situation the chamber is usually very small but very hypertrophied. In tetralogy of Fallot, the right ventricle is subjected to high pressure and high flow (most of which passes down the aorta) and thus the chamber shows both dilatation and hypertrophy. Some surgical procedures are directed at increasing flow through structures in order to encourage their growth.

2. Physiological changes at birth. In fetal life the right-sided cardiac pressures and the pressure in the pulmonary artery remain high because the postnatal low-resistance pulmonary capillary bed has not yet developed.

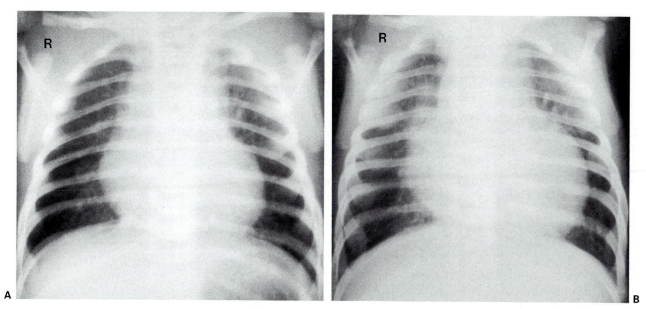

Fig. 24.6 A. Chest radiograph of an infant aged one day. The heart is only slightly enlarged and the child was asymptomatic. **B**. Chest radiograph of the same infant after one month. The heart size has increased and the pulmonary vasculature is now plethoric. The child had developed feeding difficulties and a VSD was diagnosed.

At birth, the first breath of the infant initiates the rapid decrease in pulmonary vascular resistance which in turn leads to a rapid decrease in right-sided cardiac pressures. This causes the interatrial foramen to close by acting like a valve, and will also stimulate closure of the patent ductus arteriosus. Ductal closure is a complex phenomenon and may take some hours or days or even weeks in premature infants. It is important to realize, however, that the consequential drop in pulmonary artery pressure can take several hours or days to be complete and this will have important consequences on the clinical and radiological presentation of certain conditions in early life.

Signs and symptoms of left-to-right shunts will tend to increase in the early days and weeks of life as the pulmonary resistance falls (Fig. 24.6). On the other hand some conditions (e.g. pulmonary atresia) are 'ductus dependent', and the closure of the ductus in early life will lead to progressive pulmonary oligaemia and consequent cyanosis.

Pathological circulations

1. Left-to-right shunt. In the normal postnatal situation the pressure in the right ventricle and pulmonary artery will be much lower than that on the left side because of the lower vascular resistance in the lungs. If any communication between the left and right side of the heart exists, there will be a left-to-right shunt. This can be measured by catheter oximetry, or noninvasively by radionuclide studies and Doppler techniques. The ratio of pulmonary to systemic flow (often called the QP/QS ratio) can vary from less than 2:1 (a small shunt) to 4:1 (a moderate shunt) or as much as 10:1 or over (a very large shunt). It is generally held that a shunt of 2:1 or less is difficult to detect on the chest radiograph by either pulmonary plethora or increased heart size.

If the left-to-right shunt is at *atrial level* then the pressure in the left and right ventricles will not necessarily be affected. The right ventricle can tolerate a significantly increased flow of blood by increasing its cavity size and contractility whilst maintaining normal or slightly raised pressures. On the chest X-ray the lung fields will be *plethoric* (generalized enlargement of all the vessels) and the dilated right-sided chambers will manifest themselves as an increased heart size (Fig. 24.7). If this situation exists for many years the continuing large flow in the lungs can gradually damage the pulmonary circulation, and will eventually lead to right-sided pressure increase and ultimately equalization of left- and right-sided pressures. Thus simple atrial septal defects do not often cause trouble in childhood or early adult life but may cause pulmonary hypertension or heart failure in middle age or later.

If the *ventricular septal defect* is small this will increase the flow through the lungs but will not necessarily raise the pressure on the right side. It is highly probable that small ventricular septal defects will close in the early years of life.

If there is a large ventricular septal defect, then the left and right ventricles will immediately be at the same pressure, and the lower resistance of the lungs will induce a large left-to-right shunt. In this situation the combination of increased flow and increased pressure in the lungs will produce progressive pulmonary vascular damage at a much earlier age than would occur with atrial mixing.

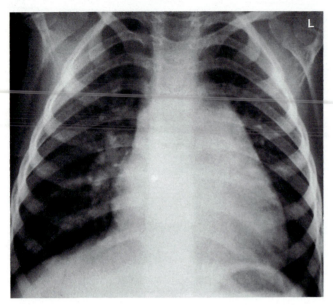

Fig. 24.7 Chest radiograph of a child with a moderately large ASD. The main pulmonary artery segment is large and the lung vessels are large.

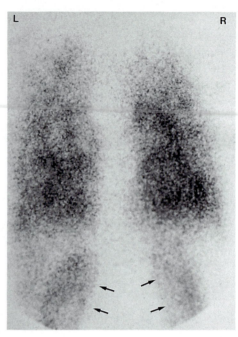

Fig. 24.8 Posterior view of a ^{99m}Tc microsphere lung scan in a patient with Eisenmenger's syndrome. Renal uptake (arrowed) is due to right-to-left shunting in the heart.

Irreversible pulmonary damage will occur in this situation, and ultimately the right-sided pressure elevation will cause reversal of the shunt with the development of cyanosis (the *Eisenmenger syndrome*). The development of this condition is associated with a reduction in the left-to-right shunt with consequent reduction in heart size and pulmonary plethora. Thus the chest radiograph that is 'improving' or has returned to 'normal' may actually be showing the development of progressive irreversible damage. A similar situation can occur with any other high-pressure mixing situation such as might occur with a large *patent ductus arteriosus* or other *aortopulmonary connection*. The right-to-left shunting is occasionally demonstrated by radionuclide techniques (Fig. 24.8).

2. Circulation in transposition. Complete transposition of the great arteries with no other intracardiac abnormality is incompatible with life unless there is mixing of the two circulations at some point. It is useless to have a large amount of well-oxygenated blood returned to the left atrium if it is subsequently redirected to the left ventricle and then to the pulmonary artery and lungs again. There is usually a small amount of shunting across the foramen ovale which sustains life in the early post-natal period but it is essential to improve mixing at an early stage. In line with the principles outlined above, the obligatory shunting is best at an atrial level where the pressure is low, and it is thus common practice to perform a *Rashkind balloon septostomy* as soon as possible in cyanosed infants with transposition of the great arteries. This procedure ruptures the thin septum primum covering the foramen ovale which facilitates increased atrial shunting (which must of course be in both directions).

Although the total amount of shunting from left to right and right to left must be equal, there is overall much more blood flowing in the pulmonary circuit than the systemic circuit, so that the small proportion of this oxygenated pulmonary flow which passes across the atrial septum will be adequate to sustain the systemic requirements.

Patients with complete transposition frequently have other communications between pulmonary and systemic circuits, ventricular septal defects and patent ductus arteriosus being common examples. These communications will be advantageous in increasing the mixing but disadvantageous in that they will predispose to high pulmonary pressures which might permanently damage the lungs.

3. Common mixing circulation. This can occur with a number of different conditions. A *common atrium* or *total anomalous pulmonary venous drainage* to the right atrium will produce this at atrial level. An *atretic tricuspid valve* will lead to obligatory right-to-left shunting into the left atrium and consequent common mixing. At ventricular level a very *large ventricular septal defect* or any of the *'single ventricle'* variants will produce common mixing. At great arterial level there will be common mixing in *pulmonary atresia* and *common truncus arteriosus*.

In all these situations the aorta and pulmonary artery will both be supplied with partially desaturated blood. The lungs will be at little disadvantage if they receive adequate flow (unless they are subjected to an excessively high pressure/flow combination) but the systemic supply will be significantly affected and the patient will be cyanosed, the degree depending on the particular haemodynamic details. If there is very rapid circulation through the lungs, then there will be a high proportion of saturated blood returned to the common mixing pool, and the cyanosis will be slight (as in truncus arteriosus). If pulmonary blood flow is low, then the common mixing pool will be very desaturated (for example in pulmonary atresia).

4. Pulmonary atresia. In many congenital cardiac abnormalities there is complete obstruction of the pulmonary artery or valve which may be associated with atresia or narrowing in the right ventricular outflow tract. In this situation no blood will enter the pulmonary circulation in the normal way and the only flow in the pulmonary circuit will be that produced by *ductal flow* or by *systemic to pulmonary collaterals*, the latter being small or absent at birth.

In patients in this category, closure of the patent ductus arteriosus at birth can lead to rapid progressive cyanosis and it is therefore necessary to increase the blood supply to the lungs. In the short term this is done by *medical therapy* to keep the patent ductus open, but as soon as practicable a *systemic-to-pulmonary shunt* is performed to improve the blood flow into the lungs. Patients surviving this early stage without surgical palliation will go on to develop *aortopulmonary collateral communications*. These vary considerably and can enter the lungs in many sites. Some of these vessels may be of bronchial artery origin but it is not always clear what their morphological origins are. Supply is most frequently from the descending aorta but subclavian, internal mammary and intercostal arteries may give rise to collaterals.

5. Left-sided obstruction. *Coarctation of the aorta* and *aortic valve stenosis* are two common obstructive lesions which, if severe, can lead to left-sided heart failure in early life. This will be radiographically manifest as enlargement of pulmonary vessels (due to pulmonary venous hypertension, not plethora), possible interstitial or alveolar pulmonary oedema and cardiomegaly. Obstruction at *mitral* or *left atrial* level is less common but will give the pulmonary changes with less cardiomegaly because the left ventricle is not working against the obstruction.

6. Right-sided obstructions. Severe obstruction to the outflow into the lungs is usually a less serious problem than severe systemic outflow obstruction but it can still have important effects. Right ventricular failure can be caused by *very severe pulmonary stenosis*, but commonly this does not occur because a ventricular septal defect will also be present (e.g. tetralogy of Fallot) which will allow decompression of the elevated right-sided pressures by right to left shunting.

7. Birth asphyxia. Obstetric problems which lead to severe birth anoxia can have serious cardiac effects. These are most commonly manifest as heart failure with cardiomegaly and pulmonary changes. If resuscitation is achieved successfully, the chest radiograph may revert to normal over a few days.

IMPORTANT CONGENITAL CARDIAC ABNORMALITIES

A number of conditions will be discussed in detail and are presented in order of frequency of occurrence as shown below. The data is taken from the Bristol Registry of Congenital Heart Disease and represents all live births presenting with congenital heart disease to the centre from 1977 to 1987.

Condition	%
Ventricular septal defect	36.1
Atrial septal defect	8.2
Patent ductus arteriosus	7.9
Pulmonary stenosis	6.9
Coarctation of the aorta	5.9
Aortic stenosis	5.7
Tetralogy of Fallot	4.6
Transposition of the great arteries	3.8
Atrioventricular septal defect	3.6
Pulmonary atresia	2.6
Single ventricle	2.2
Tricuspid atresia	1.5
Mitral valve abnormalities	1.4
Hypoplastic left heart syndrome	1.4
Cardiomyopathy	1.3
Anomalous pulmonary venous connection	1.2
Total	94.3

The following conditions with a reported incidence of less than 1% are also discussed.

Truncus arteriosus
Ebstein's anomaly
Sinus of Valsalva fistula
Double-outlet ventricle
Great arterial anomalies
Coronary anomalies
Arteriovenous malformations
Cardiac tumours

Systemic venous anomalies are also discussed. These are quite commonly associated with other forms of congenital heart disease, occurring in 10% of cases with diagnosed congenital heart disease.

VENTRICULAR SEPTAL DEFECT (VSD)

This abnormality is the commonest of all and can occur alone or be associated with other simple or complex congenital heart conditions. The interventricular septum has a complex curved shape and defects can occur in any part of it. Various descriptive classifications have been proposed but the following classification (or a modification of it) is generally accepted.

Perimembranous defect. This is the commonest type of VSD, involving the membranous septum and adjacent muscular tissue below the aortic root and close to the upper margin of the tricuspid valve annulus. Sometimes this can be large and extend round towards the outlet part of the septum.

Muscular defects. a. *Inlet* or basal muscular defect lying in the muscular septum between the mitral and tricuspid valves. b. Mid muscular or *apical* defect between the main right and left ventricular chambers. Sometimes called apical trabecular defect. c. *Outlet* defect. This involves either the high anterior trabeculated part of the septum or the band of muscle immediately below the pulmonary valve forming the conus of the right ventricle (the term 'conal' defect is sometimes used in the latter situation).

It is possible for single or multiple VSDs to be present at any site throughout the large and complex shape of the interventricular septum. In diagnosis and investigation of this condition it is not only important to confirm the presence of interventricular communication but to localize the exact site and size of the communication and to determine if there are any additional communications. The latter point is essential if corrective surgery is to be successful.

If defects are of the large inlet or outlet type, it may be possible to over-ride the inlet or outlet valves. The over-riding aorta in the tetralogy of Fallot is a good example of this. The term *malalignment VSD* is sometimes used in this situation. Extreme forms of malalignment will result in such conditions as double-inlet or double-outlet ventricle. These will be considered elsewhere.

The *Gerbode defect* is a communication through the small portion of the basal septum that separates the left ventricular outflow tract from the right atrium (the atrioventricular septum). This defect is very rare and must be diagnosed with care, because it can easily be confused with a perimembranous defect and coexistent tricuspid regurgitation.

Many other congenital heart defects are associated with a VSD and these will be considered in the appropriate sections. Of particular importance is the association of VSD with *coarctation of the aorta* which can produce a particularly severe form of infantile cardiac failure. The remainder of this description will deal with the various forms of 'simple VSD', i.e. unassociated with other anomalies.

Clinical presentation. The presentation of this condition depends on the overall size of the interventricular communication. The condition does not normally present in the first few days of life unless the interventricular septal defect is very large. This is because the pulmonary vascular resistance drops markedly in the first days and weeks of life and thus prevents the early development of pulmonary plethora. The characteristic systolic murmur may take even longer to develop. Thus even with large VSDs the patient may be asymptomatic, with a normal chest radiograph at birth. A large VSD will present after a few days or weeks, with breathlessness and feeding difficulties, and the chest X-ray will usually show moderate enlargement of the heart with prominence of the main pulmonary artery, the hilar pulmonary arteries and the peripheral pulmonary arteries (Fig. 24.6). In severe cases there will be cardiac failure also.

With smaller VSDs, the presentation can be much later in life and may occur with the detection of an asymptomatic murmur. In these cases the chest X-ray can range from normal (if the communication is very small) to mild or moderate cardiac enlargement with mild or moderate pulmonary plethora.

It is not an easy matter in paediatric practice to distinguish ventricular septal defect from other left-to-right cardiac shunts (e.g. patent ductus arteriosus, aortopulmonary communication or even large atrial septal defect) on the basis of the chest X-ray alone, particularly in the young infant. Distinction becomes easier with increasing age, due to the differing natural histories of the conditions, but this is obviously of little immediate value in individual infants or children. It is important to point out, however, that a large VSD with a big shunt presenting early in life will inevitably lead to severe pulmonary damage and pulmonary hypertension in the first few years of life. It is thus essential to recognize the abnormality and treat the condition as soon as possible. *Echocardiography* is vital in the differential diagnosis of these conditions and must be performed as soon as the condition is clinically or radiographically suspected.

Non-invasive imaging. The diagnosis of VSD can frequently be confirmed on *two-dimensional echocardiography* (Fig. 24.9). It is most important that the full extent of the interventricular septum is examined in any case of suspected VSD. The examination will include, as an absolute minimum, the *parasternal long- and short-axis views*

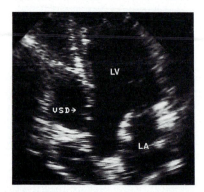

Fig. 24.9 Two-dimensional echocardiogram taken from the apex in a child with a small perimembranous ventricular septal defect — VSD. The margins of the defect act as distinct echogenic structures. LV = left ventricle, LA = left atrium.

and the *apical four-chamber views* (Fig. 24.10). Each view will include a sweep along the heart in the particular plane being examined. Sometimes the defect is easier to identify because the edges of the septal hole act as strong ultrasonic reflectors and highlight the defect. In some parts of the septum the trabecular pattern will produce multiple reflections which can obscure small defects. In some cases of perimembranous VSD there is associated tissue in or near the defect which can partially obstruct it, the growth of this probably being one of the mechanisms of spontaneous closure of moderate or small defects. Sometimes there is prominent bulging of this tissue into the right ventricle, the so-called '*aneurysmal perimembranous VSD*'.

It may be necessary to use *Doppler flow assessment* to detect the presence of small defects, using the turbulent jet passing through the defect as a marker. Careful searching along the right ventricular surface of the septum with the pulsed Doppler sample volume will usually reveal any abnormal jet. In this situation the addition of *colour-flow mapping* has been very valuable in speeding and simplifying the detection of small or multiple ventricular septal defects (Fig. 24.11). Colour-flow imaging will also show the direction of the jet, which is particularly important if a continuous-wave Doppler beam is to be aligned with the jet to measure the peak jet velocity and calculate the pressure drop across the VSD. This is an important non-invasive method for deducing the right ventricular pressure.

Mild tricuspid regurgitation is frequently associated with perimembranous VSDs, and Doppler techniques are particularly useful in detecting this, though care must be taken to avoid confusion with the VSD jet itself.

Magnetic resonance imaging has been used with success to demonstrate VSDs but at present the technique is only sufficiently accurate to detect large defects and cannot be

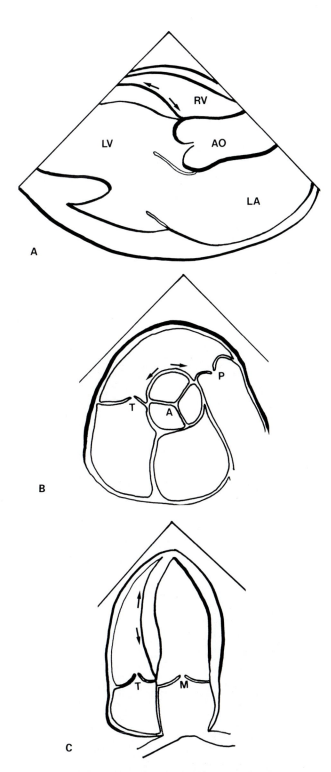

Fig. 24.10 A. Diagram showing a parasternal long-axis echocardiogram. The arrows indicate the region for seeking a ventricular septal defect on Doppler examination. LV = left ventricle, RV = right ventricular outflow tract, AO = aortic root, LA = left atrium. **B**. Parasternal short-axis echocardiogram at the level of the aortic root. The arrows indicate the area which should be examined just below the aortic valve to detect a perimembranous ventricular septal defect. T = tricuspid valve, A = aortic valve, P = pulmonary valve. **C**. Apical four-chamber echocardiogram. The arrows indicate where a muscular ventricular septal defect might be sought using Doppler techniques. T = tricuspid valve, M = mitral valve.

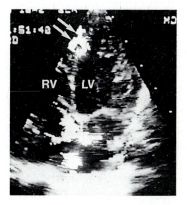

Fig. 24.11 Colour-flow Doppler study taken in an apical four-chamber view. This figure is reproduced in colour in the colour plate section at the front of this volume. The arrows indicate the orange flow pattern (towards the transducer) of an apical muscular defect. LV = left ventricle, RV = right ventricle.

used reliably to detect small defects in uncommon positions. Conventional *CT scanning* is not of practical use in the detection of VSDs.

Defects cannot be visualized with any clarity using *nuclear medicine* techniques, but first-pass studies are useful in calculating pulmonary-to-systemic flow ratios and in conjunction with echocardiography they can produce a very full noninvasive assessment of a VSD.

Cardiac catheterization and angiography. Cardiac catheterization is still frequently undertaken if there is any doubt about the intracardiac anatomy or about the nature of the pulmonary vascular resistance. Cardiac angiography must be performed in such a way that the interventricular septum is completely examined in its entirety. There is no such thing as 'the view that profiles the septum'; rather, there are many views which profile different parts of the septum, and they must be used in a logical fashion not only to locate the site of the known VSD but to confirm or exclude the possibility of additional VSDs.

If biplane cinéangiocardiography is available, the best two views to select for initial examination of the septum are:

1. 65° left anterior oblique with 20°–25° cranial tilt
2. 30° right anterior oblique

These two views will demonstrate the majority of the perimembranous, inlet, and mid muscular septum (LAO) and the high anterior and conal septum (RAO). The outflow region will not be demonstrated adequately by the LAO view because the region will be obscured by contrast medium in the ventricle and aorta.

If the VSD or VSDs demonstrated by these views is small and clearly localized then no additional view is necessary. If the VSD is large, however, it may be obscuring additional defects and its dimension in the foreshortened plane may not be apparent. If multiple defects are shown, at least one additional view may be necessary to localize the defects precisely. With biplane studies the following additional two views may be helpful:

1. 55° left anterior oblique with 10°–15° caudal tilt
2. 40° right anterior oblique with 15° caudal tilt

The LAO view will distinguish high from low defects in this view, whereas the previous cranial tilt will distinguish basal from apical defects. The RAO view will profile the portion of the septum between the inflow and outflow portions.

A full series of four views is not of course mandatory, and the potential hazards of radiation and contrast medium must always be considered. Nevertheless it is not in the patient's best interests if the study is completed with inadequate localization for proper surgical management. If single plane studies are being performed, the

first two views are essential and two ventricular injections are necessary.

The study of a VSD should not be concluded before consideration of the possible coexistence of a *patent ductus arteriosus*. A moderate or large VSD will give rise to simultaneous aortic and pulmonary opacification and with some overlapping of structures it is not always possible to exclude a patent ductus with certainty. A separate aortogram (RAO 30°, LAO 60°) is thus required.

The most common VSD is in the membranous or perimembranous region and is often associated with some form of associated fibrous tissue which is often closely related to the tricuspid valve (Fig. 24.12). In some cases the VSD is aneurysmal, with a bulging structure being pushed towards the right ventricle with each systolic contraction of the left ventricle, and this can occasionally cause obstruction in the outflow tract of the right

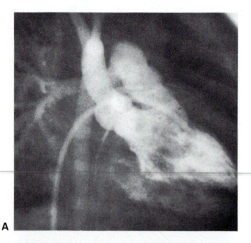

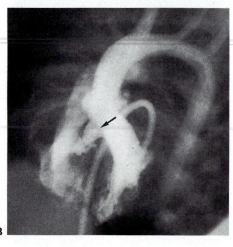

Fig. 24.12 A. Left ventricular cineangiogram taken in a right anterior oblique view. There is simultaneous filling of the aorta and pulmonary artery, indicating the presence of a ventricular septal defect which is not profiled in this projection. **B**. Simultaneous view of the angiogram in (A). shown in the cranially angled left anterior oblique view. An aneurysmal perimembranous ventricular septal defect is profiled (arrowed).

ventricle. Often a large VSD can be virtually occluded with such a large membranous aneurysm. Large VSDs in this region can also be associated with *aortic regurgitation* due to prolapse of the aortic root into the defect and this is another reason for performing an aortogram in the complete assessment of a VSD.

Surgical treatment. Treatment of a VSD is most commonly surgical but small defects may be left for some years (as long as there is no significant pulmonary hypertension) to see if spontaneous closure occurs. During this period precautions must be taken against the development of infective endocarditis.

It has been common practice to place a *band around the pulmonary artery* as a palliative operation in small infants with large VSDs, so that a definitive closure of the VSD can take place at a later age (often 3 or 4 years). This approach is giving way to earlier and earlier primary closure of the VSD, which is now done under the age of one year in many cases. *Primary closure* is a more complex operation in the very small infant but has the advantage that the pulmonary artery anatomy is not distorted and a second operation is not required. If banding is undertaken, a cardiac angiogram is usually necessary to assess the pulmonary artery anatomy prior to definitive closure, because reconstruction of the pulmonary artery will need to be planned carefully. Angiography of the main pulmonary artery is best performed in the following two views:

1. Lateral view (usually left lateral).
2. Steep cranially tilted (30° if possible) anterior view.

The latter view avoids the foreshortening of the main pulmonary artery seen in the normal anterior view.

Closure of VSD is usually performed using a prosthetic patch, although sometimes the defect is closed by direct suture. Wherever possible the surgeon will close the defect from an approach via the right atrium and tricuspid valve. This avoids the need for any incision into the ventricle, but underlines the need for accurate diagnosis, because the entire septum cannot be inspected from this approach.

Recent studies using colour-flow Doppler show that in the early postoperative period there is often leakage through or around the patch, which soon ceases as the patch endothelializes. The patch itself is usually easy to see in two-dimensional imaging as it is very echogenic.

ATRIAL SEPTAL DEFECT (ASD)

This abnormality can be divided into two major categories, the *ostium primum* atrial septal defect (which will be considered separately under the heading of atrioventricular septal defects) and the *ostium secundum* atrial septal defect which is the more common type. The ostium secundum defect is usually at the level of the

foramen ovale and does not involve the tissues of the septum primum or the atrioventricular valves. A third form of atrial septal defect is less common and is known as the *sinus venosus* defect. This is very high in the atrial septum near the insertion of the superior vena cava. This type of defect is often associated with some form of partially anomalous pulmonary venous drainage.

Atrial septal defect must be distinguished from *patent foramen ovale*. The latter condition is a normal finding in small infants because in the first few weeks or months of life the flap valve mechanism across the foramen ovale has not finally fused shut. In abnormalities where the atrial chambers are enlarged, this can cause stretching of the foramen ovale which can sometimes regress after appropriate treatment. In practical terms, the patent foramen ovale is distinguished from a true atrial septal defect by the persisting interatrial pressure difference in the former condition. This can be detected in some adults as an incidental finding, particularly when using colour-flow Doppler mapping (Fig. 24.13).

The low-pressure shunting that occurs with atrial septal defect is usually accommodated very well by the right ventricle and patients with an isolated ASD very rarely present with significant problems in the early years of life. Presentation later in childhood or adolescence is quite common, when mild abnormalities are detected on routine medical examination or chest X-ray. The *chest X-ray* is usually normal if the pulmonary-to-systemic flow ratio is less than 2:1 but if it exceeds this level there will be pulmonary plethora and cardiac enlargement (Fig. 24.7). The cardiac enlargement is mainly due to right atrial and right ventricular dilatation, both these chambers taking increased flow.

From time to time atrial septal defect will present in the middle-aged or elderly, when heart failure or pulmonary hypertension can finally develop and cause symptoms for the first time. In patients with significant

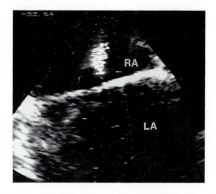

Fig. 24.13 Colour-flow Doppler study taken from the subcostal position in an adult with mitral valve disease. This figure is reproduced in colour in the colour plate section at the front of this volume. The patent foramen ovale is seen as an orange jet (towards the transducer). This was an incidental finding. LA = left atrium, RA = right atrium.

pulmonary arterial hypertension (usually the elderly un-treated patients), the chest X-ray will show dramatic appearances of centrally dilated pulmonary arteries and peripheral pulmonary vascular 'pruning' (Fig. 24.14). There is a risk of these patients with pulmonary hypertension having a paradoxical embolus from a systemic venous thrombosis. These patients may be inoperable.

Atrial septal defect occurs quite commonly in association with many other cardiac abnormalities and in some conditions it is an obligatory communication that sustains life, as in the case of tricuspid atresia or total anomalous pulmonary venous drainage.

Non-invasive diagnosis. *Echocardiography* is the cornerstone of diagnosis in this condition. Two-dimensional imaging will show the defect in almost all cases (Fig. 24.15). The typical *secundum defect* is best seen from the subcostal view, which places the interatrial septum at a significant angle to the examining beam and reduces the chance of an artefactual false-positive diagnosis. The latter can occur in the apical view when the interatrial septum lies parallel to the beam and reflects poorly, causing 'drop-out' and an apparent defect. The characteristic dilatation of the right-sided chambers is well seen and the dominance of the right ventricular volume overload will often be seen as 'paradoxical' septal motion (Fig. 24.16). This is an abnormal anterior movement of the interventricular septum during ventricular systole.

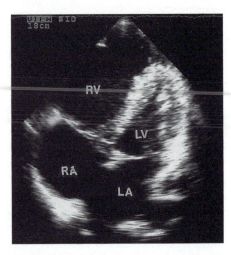

Fig. 24.15 Modified apical four-chamber echocardiogram of a patient with a secundum atrial septal defect. The right-sided chambers are considerably enlarged. LA = left atrium, RA = right atrium, LV = left ventricle, RV = right ventricle.

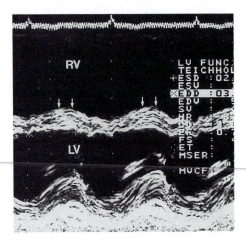

Fig. 24.16 M-mode echocardiogram in a patient with an atrial septal defect and right ventricular volume overload. There is 'paradoxical' motion of the interventricular septum (arrowed). LV = left ventricle, RV = right ventricle.

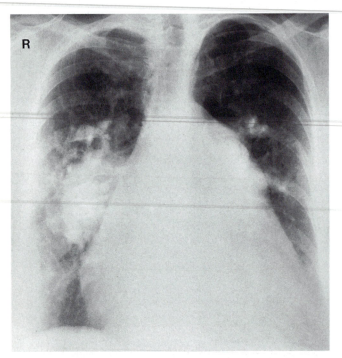

Fig. 24.14 Chest radiograph of an elderly women with an atrial septal defect and severe pulmonary hypertension. The main pulmonary artery and hilar pulmonary arteries are very large, with peripheral vascular attenuation.

The *ostium primum defect* (also known as partial atrioventricular septal defect) is also well seen, as is atrioventricular valve anatomy. The less common *sinus venosus defect* is harder to visualize as it lies high in the atrium near the termination of the superior vena cava. Transoesophageal studies have recently been used to demonstrate this difficult lesion. All studies of atrial septal defect must be accompanied by a thorough examination of the pulmonary and systemic venous connections as these are quite often abnormal.

Doppler studies will often complete the diagnostic information. *Colour-flow mapping* is particularly helpful in the diagnosis of the defect and any venous anomalies (Fig. 24.17). A short acceleration time in pulmonary artery flow can sometimes point to the presence of pulmonary

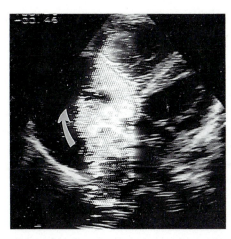

Fig. 24.17 Colour-flow Doppler study in a patient with a secundum atrial septal defect in the same orientation as Fig. 24.15. This figure is reproduced in colour in the colour plate section at the front of this volume. Flow through the defect towards the tricuspid valve is in red (towards the transducer).

hypertension, as will a high-velocity jet of tricuspid regurgitation. Pulmonary-to-systemic flow ratios can be calculated using Doppler techniques, but these are very time-consuming and are prone to error. Simpler and more accurate noninvasive assessment of the degree of left-to-right shunting can be achieved by first-pass *radionuclide studies*.

Cardiac catheterization and angiography. A comprehensive echocardiographic diagnosis will often eliminate the need for invasive investigation but there will be occasions when there is a need for catheterization, either to calculate the shunt ratio accurately or to confirm or exclude some anatomical detail. A left atrial injection of contrast medium is occasionally helpful, but usually angiography is used to assess abnormal venous anatomy or to assess left ventricular function. Atrial septal defect is of course commonly associated with other forms of congenital heart disease which might require cardiac catheterization for diagnosis.

Treatment. The condition requires surgical closure in patients with a significant shunt. *Surgical treatment* is relatively straightforward, and so surgery for atrial septal defect is often also carried out in patients with relatively mild symptoms, because the operation has a very low mortality and complications in later life can be avoided. *Transcatheter occlusion* of ASD is being developed and may become practical in the future.

PATENT DUCTUS ARTERIOSUS (PDA)

The patent duct is a vital part of the fetal circulation and this communication usually closes within the first few days of life. The ductus arteriosus often remains open rather longer in premature infants, but in the majority of cases it still closes spontaneously. If there is a persistent

failure of closure of the duct, then the consequences will depend on the size of the communication. A tiny residual patent ductus arteriosus can remain undiagnosed throughout life as it will produce minimal effects. A large patent ductus arteriosus will have similar effects to a large ventricular septal defect, with pressure and volume overloading of the pulmonary circulation. In most diagnosed cases the patent ductus arteriosus is closed surgically to avoid the risk of endocarditis, whether or not there is a large shunt. Patent ductus arteriosus is commonly associated with many other congenital cardiac abnormalities, and no investigation of congenital heart disease is complete without diagnosis or exclusion of a coexisting patent ductus arteriosus.

The clinical sign of a continuous murmur is classically associated with a PDA but *coronary artery fistulae* and *ruptured sinus of Valsalva* can also give a continuous murmur and must be distinguished from patent ductus arteriosus by echocardiography or angiography.

The *chest X-ray* will show pulmonary plethora if the shunt is large and there will be mild to moderate cardiac enlargement. The normally smooth outline of the aortic knuckle and upper descending aorta will often be interrupted by the 'bump' of the ductus, but this is often difficult to detect in young infants in whom the normal aorta is hard to visualize. In an older child or adult it is probably true to say that the presence of a well-defined aortic knuckle leading into a straight and uninterrupted descending aorta will almost certainly exclude the presence of a patent ductus arteriosus. Later in life there may be some *calcification* present in a PDA. The ascending aorta and aortic arch carry greater flow than normal in this condition and consequently the aortic knuckle is sometimes enlarged, but this cannot be regarded as a reliable sign.

The presence of a ductal communication can often be life-saving in neonates with pulmonary atresia. The physiological closure of the ductus will lead to increased cyanosis and the use of *prostaglandin therapy* is directed towards maintaining ductal patency until a definitive palliative or corrective operation can be performed. In this situation the anatomy of the ductus arteriosus is different to normal, with the angulation of the communication being opposite to normal. This is due to the abnormal ductal flow, being from aorta to pulmonary artery in fetal life.

Non-invasive imaging. *Echocardiography* will show clearly the persistent communication on two-dimensional scanning in many cases. The best view for demonstration of the patent ductus arteriosus is a modification of the parasternal short-axis view, sometimes called the '*ductus cut*'. The imaging plane in this view is orientated anatomically through the main pulmonary artery, the left pulmonary artery, the ductus itself and the descending aorta. A patent ductus arteriosus can also be imaged from

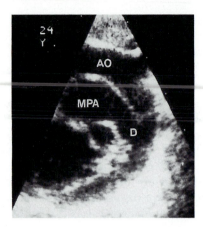

Fig. 24.18 Suprasternal echocardiogram in a patient with transposition of the great arteries and a patent ductus arteriosus (D). The great arteries lie parallel in this condition. AO = aorta, MPA = main pulmonary artery. (Courtesy Dr. R. Martin.)

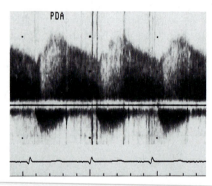

Fig. 24.19 Continuous-wave Doppler study taken from the parasternal position. Continuous flow through the patent ductus arteriosus is shown above the baseline — towards the transducer. (Courtesy Dr. R. Martin.)

other views, particularly the suprasternal view, which will show the same structures (Fig. 24.18). The images can sometimes be misleading if there is particular prominence of the diverticulum at one or both ends of the ductus arteriosus. The aortic and pulmonary diverticula can both be large even when there is no actual continuity and thus visualization of complete continuity of the duct on the images is essential for a reliable diagnosis.

Doppler echocardiography is of great value in the diagnosis of this condition. Careful positioning of the pulsed Doppler sample volume in or near the duct will reveal the characteristic continuous turbulent signal of ductal flow. This can also be shown on continuous-wave Doppler (Fig. 24.19) and of course the flow can be mapped clearly using *colour-flow imaging*. In older patients imaging of the duct itself often proves difficult, and in this situation Doppler evaluation is of particular importance and is sometimes the only definite sign of the abnormality. Haemodynamic circumstances will affect the nature of

ductal flow. In particular, if there is pulmonary hypertension with equal pulmonary and systemic pressures, then ductal flow will be much reduced and Doppler techniques will be of limited use. In this situation angiography can also be difficult. There are a number of conditions that will cause unusual flows in the pulmonary arteries, for example, pulmonary hypertension or pulmonary valve stenosis, and so the accurate diagnosis of patent ductus arteriosus depends on detection of flow in the communication itself, not just an abnormal flow pattern in the pulmonary arteries.

Aortopulmonary window is a rare condition that can present similarly to a large patent ductus arteriosus. There is usually a large direct communication from the ascending aorta to the pulmonary artery. Echocardiographers must be certain that the condition is not overlooked and colour-flow Doppler techniques will doubtless make this easier.

CT scanning and *nuclear medicine* studies have relatively little part to play in the assessment of the condition. *Magnetic resonance imaging* may play an increasing role in the future but it is not currently an important investigational technique in this condition.

Cardiac catheterization and angiography. Angiography is a reliable method of diagnosing the condition, and a well-placed aortic injection will show the abnormality. This is often achieved with an arterial catheter, but frequently the venous catheter can be passed via the right heart chambers to the pulmonary artery and then to the aorta via the actual patent ductus. Passage of the catheter through the communication can of course be diagnostic in itself but it is important to advance the catheter well down the descending aorta below the diaphragm to avoid confusion with a position in a lower lobe pulmonary artery. This method does not show the size of the duct itself, and on occasion a catheter can be passed across the obstructed lumen of a recently closed ductus.

Standard cardiac oblique views, RAO 30° and LAO 60°, are usually best for the demonstration of the abnormality. Ideally both views are recorded because each has its own advantages. The RAO view clearly separates the main pulmonary artery from the ascending aorta and is excellent for the detection of very small shunts, but the view may foreshorten the duct itself. The LAO view will usually profile the duct well but sometimes the superimposition of a large main pulmonary artery and the aorta can obscure detail. Angiographers must be careful not to miss an *aortopulmonary window* as it can often be out of profile if inappropriate projections are selected and may not be shown at all if the ascending aorta is not opacified.

It is important not to overlook a patent ductus arteriosus in the presence of other important left-to-right shunts. In the case of a *large ventricular septal defect*, a left ventricular injection will produce almost simultaneous opacification of the aorta and pulmonary artery. In these circumstances, the ductal communication can often be hard to diagnose with certainty and a separate aortic injection is necessary to exclude the condition. *Coarctation of the aorta* is commonly associated with a patent ductus arteriosus.

There are variations in the site of the ductus arteriosus which depend on variations in the development of the sixth arch. The ductus can be right-sided and may occasionally form part of a vascular ring. There may be a bilateral ductus arteriosus in rare cases. Very rarely the ductus itself may become aneurysmal.

Treatment. In the majority of cases there is *spontaneous closure* but in a few children there is a clinical need to close the communication. This is usually performed through a left thoracotomy incision which allows the communication to be ligated and sometimes also divided. *Simple ligation* can sometimes be inadequate, with persistent communication being detectable in later life in a proportion of cases.

More recently the prospect of transcatheter occlusion has become a reality with the *Rashkind duct occluder*. The device takes the form of two small stainless steel 'umbrellas' mounted 'back to back', with foam material fixed to the spokes of each umbrella. In appropriately selected cases the folded device can be loaded into a catheter delivery system whence it can be introduced into the ductus arteriosus via the right heart chambers. The umbrellas stabilize the device between aorta and main pulmonary artery (Fig. 24.20). The technique is still new and can be complicated by accidental displacement of the device, but as experience grows this is likely to be the treatment of choice for most cases of persistent patent ductus arteriosus that require closure.

PULMONARY STENOSIS

The most common form of pulmonary stenosis is *isolated pulmonary valve stenosis* in which there is fusion and thickening of the pulmonary valve leaflets. There may also be *infundibular stenosis* with right ventricular hypertrophy causing increased contractility and systolic narrowing of the outflow tract. *Distal pulmonary stenosis* involving the main pulmonary artery or its branches is also recognized.

The severity of this condition varies greatly, and in mild cases the abnormality is of little clinical importance and may not present until late in life or not at all. Many cases of mild pulmonary stenosis present at routine medical examination with a heart murmur or with an abnormal chest radiograph or electrocardiogram.

More severe cases may present with tiredness and breathlessness, and the most severe cases may be associated with cyanosis and heart failure. In cases of moderate to severe stenosis, it is not reduction of cardiac output but the strain on the right side of the heart which

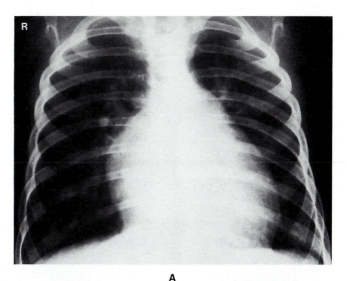

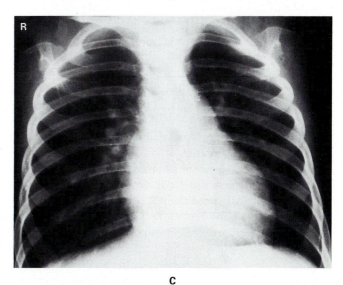

Fig. 24.20 A. Chest radiograph of a child with a patent ductus arteriosus immediately before closure. The heart is large and there is pulmonary plethora. **B.** Localized view of the Rashkind duct occluder in position in the same patient. **C.** Chest radiograph in the same patient 24 h after ductal occlusion. The heart has decreased considerably in size.

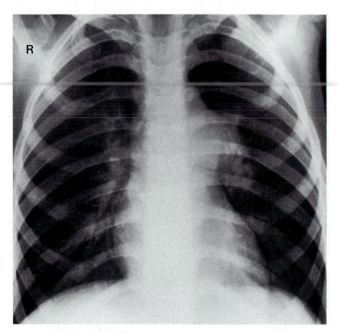

Fig. 24.21 Chest radiograph in a child with pulmonary valve stenosis. The main pulmonary artery and left pulmonary artery are considerably enlarged but pulmonary vascularity is otherwise normal.

causes problems. The *chest X-ray* often shows a prominent main pulmonary artery which is caused by post-stenotic turbulence and consequent dilatation, and the proximal left pulmonary artery is also dilated in many cases because it lies in a direct line with the main pulmonary artery (Fig. 24.21). The right pulmonary artery is not usually so dilated because it branches quite sharply from the main pulmonary artery and turbulence from the stenotic valve is not carried down into it. Peripheral pulmonary vascularity is normal or slightly oligaemic. In cases where infundibular stenosis predominates, the main pulmonary artery may not be recognized as abnormally dilated on the chest X-ray because the turbulence caused by the obstruction is not carried into the main pulmonary artery.

Non-invasive imaging. Diagnosis is usually possible by *echocardiography*, particularly if a Doppler examination with continuous-wave techniques is available. Two-dimensional imaging can be difficult, as the pulmonary valve lies partially behind the left sternal border, but turning the patient well to the left and keeping the transducer close to the sternum will frequently give a satisfactory short-axis view. Good-quality images are needed to distinguish simple leaflet fusion from a thickened and dysplastic valve. *Doppler studies* are the key to diagnosis, not only detecting the high-velocity flow through the stenotic valve but also to quantify the severity of the lesion. Infundibular stenosis (often dynamic with marked systolic narrowing) and pulmonary artery stenosis can both be diagnosed using echocardiography. The pressure

drop or 'gradient' across the stenotic valve can be estimated using continuous-wave Doppler measurements.

Cardiac catheterization and angiography. Contrast medium injection into the right ventricle will normally give an excellent demonstration of pulmonary valve anatomy, the best two views being the lateral projection and a steeply cranially tilted (20–25°) anterior view. The cranial tilt is necessary to minimize the foreshortening of the infundibulum and main pulmonary artery segment. Passage of the catheter across the valve will of course allow measurement of the pressure drop caused by the stenosis.

Treatment. Treatment has changed considerably in recent years. Mild forms of pulmonary stenosis (up to a pressure drop of approximately 40 mm Hg) do not normally require surgery. More severe cases have traditionally had *pulmonary valvotomy* performed surgically but recent interventional techniques have been very successful and in most cases of pulmonary valve stenosis a *balloon dilatation* technique is now the treatment of choice (Fig. 24.22). Excellent results are obtained using this approach (Fig. 24.23). Occasionally the valve is too dysplastic (thickened, deformed and irregular) for balloon valvuloplasty to be indicated. Successful balloon valvuloplasty requires careful measurement of the pulmonary

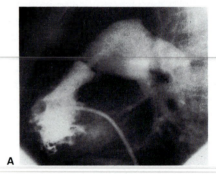

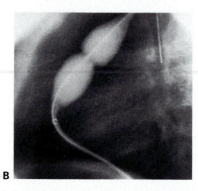

Fig. 24.22 A. Lateral view of a right ventricular angiogram in a child with pulmonary valve stenosis. The doming of the stenotic valve and the central jet of contrast medium are seen. There is post-stenotic dilatation of the main pulmonary artery. **B**. Lateral view of pulmonary valve dilatation in the same patient. The indentation in the balloon indicates that the valve is not yet fully dilated.

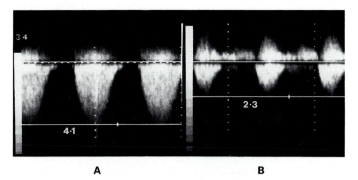

Fig. 24.23 A,B Continuous-wave Doppler traces taken from a patient immediately before and after pulmonary valve dilatation. Peak velocity in m/s is indicated and can be used in the modified Bernoulli equation (pressure in mmHg = 4 × velocity in m/s²) to show a predilatation pressure drop of 67 mmHg reduced to 21 mm Hg.

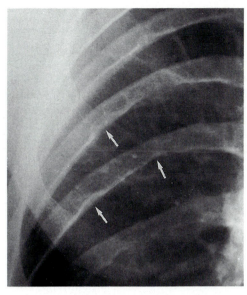

Fig. 24.25 Localized view of the ribs showing notching (arrowed) in an adult patient presenting with coarctation of the aorta.

valve annulus from the preliminary angiogram and selection of an appropriate-sized balloon, usually slightly larger than the annulus itself. Pulmonary regurgitation may develop or increase after the procedure but it is rarely a problem.

COARCTATION OF THE AORTA

In this condition there is a characteristic shelf-like narrowing of the aorta which usually occurs just beyond the origin of the left subclavian artery. The severity of this narrowing can vary considerably and it is this severity which determines the age of presentation.

Severe coarctation of the aorta can present in the first few days or weeks of life with cardiac enlargement and cardiac failure (Fig. 24.24). Physiological closure of the

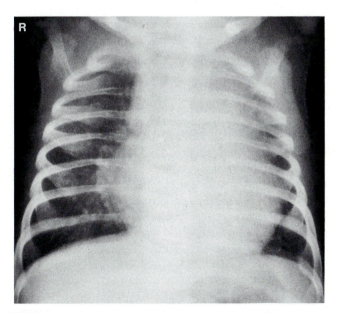

Fig. 24.24 Chest radiograph of an infant with coarctation of the aorta. There is cardiomegaly and evidence of left heart failure.

patent ductus arteriosus presents a potential hazard in severe coarctation in infancy as it may impair renal and other vital perfusion.

Lesser degrees of coarctation may present later in life with abnormal physical signs or abnormality on the chest X-ray. The classic late appearances on the chest X-ray are a small or irregular contour of the upper descending aorta and rib notching, which is caused by the prominent intercostal collateral vessels which are bypassing the narrowing (Fig. 24.25). Rib notching is rare in the first five years of life and it is increasingly common for the condition to be detected and treated before this age. There is an association with abnormalities of the aortic valve, in particular a *bicuspid aortic valve* which can develop in later life to a stenotic aortic valve.

Coarctation of the aorta has numerous variations in severity but the *site* of the coarctation itself can also vary. Occasionally the narrowing can occur between the left common carotid and the left subclavian artery and in this situation the rib notching is likely to be unilateral, being generated only on the right side from the right subclavian distribution into the right intercostal vessels. Sometimes there is quite severe hypoplasia of the aortic arch, particularly between the left common carotid artery and the left subclavian artery.

Interruption of the aortic arch is the most severe variant of the condition. In this condition both carotid arteries and sometimes one or both subclavian arteries arise from the ascending aorta before the interruption. The patent ductus supplies the lower half of the body, which becomes severely compromised as the ductus arteriosus closes. There may be a substantial gap between the two parts of the aorta.

Non-invasive diagnosis. In experienced hands *echocardiography* is reliable in the diagnosis of the condition, but it becomes increasingly difficult in older patients because of difficult ultrasonic access from the suprasternal notch, the best site for imaging. Care must be taken to avoid misdiagnosis due to the aorta passing out of the plane of the scan. An associated patent ductus arteriosus must always be sought. Doppler studies can help by demonstrating the abnormal persistent diastolic flow through the narrowing, but this also depends on good ultrasonic access. The 'gradient' across the coarctation can, in theory, be measured using Doppler techniques but practical experience has shown this to be somewhat unreliable. *Magnetic resonance imaging* can be used very successfully to demonstrate coarctation (Fig. 24.26).

In some cases the anatomy of the bypassing collaterals needs to be assessed for surgical planning. This is hard to achieve by echocardiography, and *angiography* is often necessary, although MRI is proving increasingly successful in the demonstration of these collaterals.

Cardiac catheter and angiography. Catheter access for an ascending aortic injection of contrast medium to demonstrate the aortic arch and coarctation can sometimes be a problem. A severe coarctation can prevent an arterial catheter from crossing from below, and in older patients without an atrial or ventricular septal defect, access to the left side of the heart from the right heart chambers may not be possible. Left-sided access may be achieved by trans-septal puncture or by brachial arterial approach but these offer a higher risk of complications than usual.

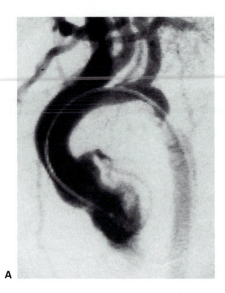

A

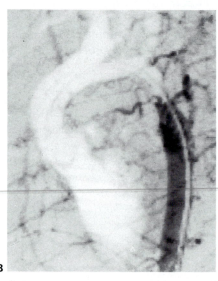

B

Fig. 24.27 **A**. Digital subtraction study of a left ventriculogram in the left anterior oblique (LAO) projection. A severe coarctation of the aorta is seen in the typical position. **B**. Late image from the study shown in (A) shows delayed filling of the descending aorta by collaterals.

Alternative angiographic approaches may be used. A pulmonary artery injection may be followed through to the left side, and with good equipment excellent detail of the coarctation and collateral vessels may be achieved. Digital subtraction angiography offers the opportunity for even better contrast enhancement in this situation (Fig. 24.27). Peripheral or central venous contrast injection causes considerable dilution of contrast medium and images are not usually of satisfactory quality.

Treatment. There is a long-term risk of severe systemic hypertension in the upper body and this is the indication for repair even in asymptomatic patients. In severely ill infants the operation is often carried out as an emergency, frequently following ultrasound diagnosis alone.

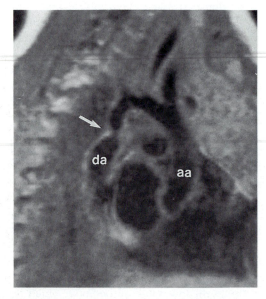

Fig. 24.26 Oblique sagittal gated spin-echo MR image in a child with coarctation of the aorta (arrowed). aa = ascending aorta, da = descending aorta. (Courtesy of the Trustees of the Bristol MRI Centre.)

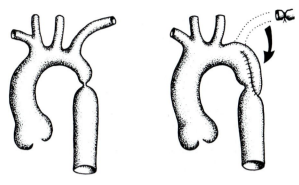

Fig. 24.28 Diagram showing the subclavian flap repair for coarctation of the aorta. (Reproduced with permission from Jordan & Scott, 1989.)

Surgical repair is carried out by various techniques which include the incorporation of the left subclavian artery as a flap (Fig. 24.28) or direct anastomosis of the aorta after resection of the narrow segment. Occasionally prosthetic patch material is incorporated into the repair. It should be noted, however, that surgical correction of coarctation carries a small but definite risk of paraplegia developing as an operative complication in older patients. Recent attempts at correction using *balloon dilatation* have been attempted but it has not yet been established as a definitive technique. Balloon dilatation has been more successful in the treatment of a proportion of patients who develop restenosis after initial surgical repair. Repair of aortic interruption is of course more complex and it carries a higher mortality.

AORTIC STENOSIS

Congenital aortic stenosis has a variety of forms, varying from a simple malformation in which the leaflets of the aortic valve remain partially fused, to a complex dysplastic valve which may be bicuspid or even unicuspid. There are also various forms of *subaortic stenosis*, ranging from a simple diaphragm to more complex tubular narrowing or obstructive fibrous tissue in the left ventricular outflow tract. Distinctly different is the dynamic narrowing of the left ventricular outflow tract caused by *hypertrophic cardiomyopathy*.

Supravalvular aortic stenosis occurs above the sinuses of Valsalva and is less common but can nevertheless be considered under the heading of congenital aortic stenosis. This most commonly occurs in *Williams' syndrome* in which there is severe hypoplasia of the ascending aorta above the sinuses of Valsalva. The condition may be associated with vascular abnormalities elsewhere, including peripheral pulmonary artery stenosis and renal artery stenosis. Associated features are a typical *'elfin facies'* and vitamin-D hypersensitivity. In suitable cases surgery can enlarge the aorta at the point of stenosis.

The degree of obstruction is extremely variable and the severity will determine the mode of presentation. *Severe cases* present in infancy with heart failure and left ventricular dilatation with impaired function. Severe aortic stenosis presenting in early infancy carries a high mortality and early operation is required to divide the fused commissures. *Milder degrees* of aortic stenosis carry a better prognosis and can be operated on electively in childhood. Recently a number of critical cases have been detected by fetal echocardiography.

The condition can be recognized on *chest X-ray* if there is a dilated ascending aorta due to poststenotic dilatation but this is usually seen in older children only. Heart failure and cardiomegaly may be recognized in infancy, and in this situation there is little to distinguish the X-ray from that of severe coarctation or other forms of left ventricular failure.

Congenital bicuspid valves are not normally stenotic but they can lead to 'acquired' calcific aortic stenosis in adult life. They are present in up to 2% of the 'normal' population. The abnormality can be recognized clearly on *two-dimensional echocardiography* (Fig. 24.29). There is an association between coarctation of the aorta and congenital bicuspid aortic valve. There is also an increased incidence of 'left dominant' coronary circulation with bicuspid aortic valve.

Non-invasive diagnosis. The diagnosis of aortic stenosis can be made easily with *echocardiography*. Good-quality images of the left ventricle and aortic valve are usually possible from standard views. It is important to examine the subaortic and supra-aortic regions as carefully as the valve itself (Fig. 24.30). The most typical type of aortic stenosis shows thin (or only slightly thickened) leaflets that 'dome' in systole due to the narrow opening between the fused commissures. The presence of left ventricular hypertrophy should be noted as well as the overall contractility of the left ventricle. The aortic valve gradient can be measured using *continuous-wave Doppler*, the peak velocity of flow across the valve being used to calculate the peak pressure drop using the modified Ber-

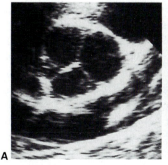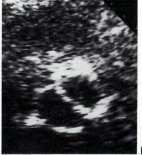

Fig. 24.29 A. Short-axis echocardiogram of a normal aortic valve showing three leaflets. **B.** Short axis echocardiogram of a bicuspid aortic valve.

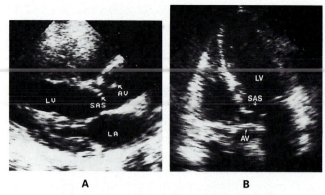

Fig. 24.30 A. Parasternal long-axis echocardiogram showing an obstructive subaortic membrane. LV = left ventricle, LA = left atrium, AV = aortic valve, SAS = subaortic stenosis. **B**. Apical four-chamber echocardiogram of the same case showing the obstructive subaortic membrane. LV = left ventricle, AV = aortic valve, SAS = subaortic stenosis.

noulli formula. *Colour-flow Doppler* will show the stenotic jet, any subaortic obstruction and any coexisting aortic regurgitation.

The detail of qualitative and quantitative information available from echocardiography means that surgery can often be performed on the basis of a good ultrasound study.

Cardiac catheterization and angiography. This is still an important technique and is used to measure valve 'gradient' and left ventricular pressures. Left ventricular angiography will allow assessment of ventricular function as well as assessing the function of the mitral valve. A supraaortic injection is usually performed to detect or exclude coexistent aortic regurgitation.

Left ventriculography is best performed in RAO 30° projection and LAO 60° with 20° cranial tilt.

The cranial tilt allows better profiling of the left ventricular outflow tract to exclude subaortic stenosis. Aortography is best performed in the same projections but without the cranial tilt.

Treatment. Minor degrees of stenosis can be observed for many years till there are signs of deleterious left ventricular effects. Echocardiography is useful as a routine check for early signs of left ventricular dilatation or impairment. Valve replacement is not practical in small infants and children as there are no suitable prostheses. Thus severe cases in early life are usually treated by *surgical valvotomy*. This can be very successful but will almost always be followed by *valve replacement* in later life. The introduction of *balloon valvuloplasty* has altered the management of some cases of congenital aortic stenosis and the procedure has been life-saving in some critically ill infants. There are potential complications with the technique, however, one of which is the development of severe aortic regurgitation.

The surgical treatment of a localized diaphragm and a tubular hypoplasia of the outflow tract are substantially

different and vary from case to case. Interventional techniques have played little part as yet in the treatment of subaortic stenosis.

TETRALOGY OF FALLOT

This abnormality is a complex of four related abnormalities which are part of a fundamental malformation of the heart. A large ventricular septal defect (1) is associated with malalignment of the great arteries, such that the aortic root overrides the ventricular septal defect (2) and is thus partly related to the right ventricle. There is associated stenosis of the right ventricular outflow tract (infundibulum) and pulmonary valve (3), together with a variable degree of hypoplasia of the pulmonary valve annulus and pulmonary arteries. The infundibular stenosis may have a dynamic component to the obstruction, being maximal in late systole. Finally there is right ventricular hypertrophy (4), which develops as a response to the systemic pressure in the right ventricle. In some cases the hypertrophied muscle bundles in the right ventricle can produce an additional intraventricular obstruction.

This abnormality is expressed in different ways, which depend mainly on the severity of the pulmonary stenosis. In mild cases of pulmonary stenosis the abnormality behaves much like a simple ventricular septal defect, with possible benefit caused by the restriction of blood flow into the lungs (as in pulmonary artery banding). These patients form the *acyanotic* end of the spectrum. More typically presenting cases are *cyanosed* because the pulmonary stenosis is sufficiently severe to restrict pulmonary blood flow. These children will present in childhood with varying degrees of cyanosis and fainting spells on exertion, which are usually caused by increasing infundibular obstruction to pulmonary flow with increasing cardiac work.

The most severe end of the spectrum is represented by critical pulmonary stenosis and severe pulmonary artery hypoplasia with very little flow into the lungs through the pulmonary valve. In this situation life must be sustained by alternative flow into the pulmonary vascularity and this occurs by *ductal flow* or by *aortopulmonary collaterals* that develop in early life. The severe cases in this spectrum will present shortly after birth with progressive cyanosis as the ductus arteriosus closes. These babies will need urgent palliation by systemic shunting to maintain pulmonary blood flow.

Approximately 25% of patients with tetralogy of Fallot (or pulmonary atresia and ventricular septal defect — a closely related condition) have a *right-sided aortic arch*. This type of right arch is usually associated with mirror imaging branching (i.e. left brachiocephalic, right common carotid, and right subclavian in order of branching).

The *chest X-ray* is not always typical (Fig. 24.37A) but in the classic developed appearance there will be con-

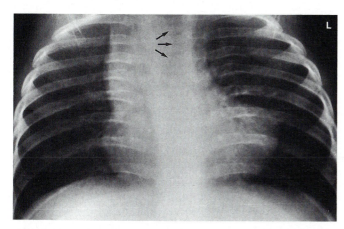

Fig. 24.31 Chest radiograph of an infant with tetralogy of Fallot. The trachea is indented by the right-sided aortic arch (arrowed), the cardiac apex is angled upwards and the lung fields are oligaemic.

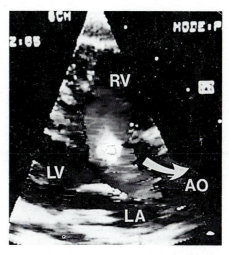

Fig. 24.32 Colour-flow Doppler study in a child with tetralogy of Fallot. This figure is reproduced in colour in the colour plate section at the front of this volume. In this parasternal long-axis view there is right-to-left flow from the right ventricle (RV) to the aorta (AO). The majority of the flow is encoded blue (away from the transducer) but the fastest moving central flow shows aliasing (orange). LV = left ventricle, LA = left atrium.

cavity in the left heart border in the region of the hypoplastic main pulmonary artery, upward prominence of the cardiac apex due to the distortion by the large right ventricle, pulmonary oligaemia and in some cases a right-sided aortic arch (Fig. 24.31). Whilst these signs are almost diagnostic, many cases of tetralogy of Fallot have a nearly normal chest film.

Non-invasive imaging. *Echocardiography* is very useful in diagnosing the condition and will show the ventricular septal defect, the overriding aorta and the right ventricular hypertrophy very clearly. The pulmonary valve and pulmonary artery anatomy is often more difficult to assess by ultrasound as these areas lie deeply and are partially surrounded by air, but it is still possible to measure the proximal parts of the vessels in many cases. The right ventricular outflow gradient and the pulmonary valve gradient can both be estimated using *Doppler techniques* but there are many possible inaccuracies due to the many levels at which obstruction can occur. Right-to-left shunting across the VSD can be seen on colour-flow Doppler examination (Fig. 24.32).

Other noninvasive imaging techniques have little to add in most cases but there are occasional applications, for example the occasional use of *thallium-201 scanning* to demonstrate the degree of right ventricular hypertrophy (Fig. 24.33).

Cardiac catheterization and angiography. This is often required in addition to echocardiography because precise assessment of anatomy is essential in surgical planning. The size of the pulmonary valve annulus as well as the size and anatomy of the more distal pulmonary arteries must be determined.

Left ventricular angiography should be performed in views similar to those selected for a simple ventricular septal defect (Fig. 24.34) but a steeper LAO view (e.g. 70°) is sometimes helpful, due to the rotation of the heart produced by the large right ventricle. Right ventriculo-

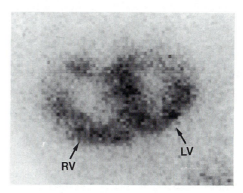

Fig. 24.33 ²⁰¹Thallium scan in the left anterior view. In this adult patient with long-standing tetralogy of Fallot without complete correction there is marked right ventricular hypertrophy, with activity equalling that in the left ventricular wall.

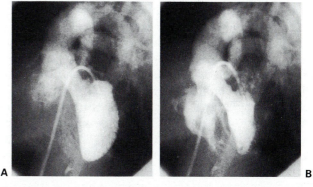

Fig. 24.34 **A.** Cranially angled AO ← AO left ventriculogram in a child with tetralogy of Fallot. There is early passage of contrast to the right ventricle across the ventricular septal defect. Aortic over-ride is seen. **B.** Later image from the same study. The right ventricle is now well filled. The hypoplastic pulmonary arteries can be seen.

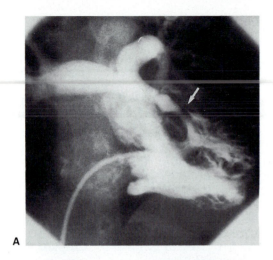

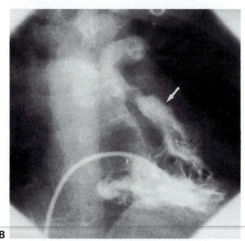

Fig. 24.35 **A**. Cranially angled anterior view of a right ventriculogram in a patient with tetralogy of Fallot. Severe infundibular stenosis is seen in systole (arrowed). The hypoplastic pulmonary annulus and main pulmonary artery can be seen. **B**. Diastolic image from the same study. The right ventricular infundibulum is now much wider (arrowed).

(using an oblique patch) and reconstruction of the right ventricular outflow tract and pulmonary arteries. In the latter situation a transannular patch may be incorporated into the repair to widen the outflow. In most cases the pulmonary valve function is destroyed by the reconstruction of the right ventricular outflow tract but the pulmonary regurgitation that follows appears to be of little clinical significance.

In severe cases presenting in early life a palliative shunt may be performed if the child is too small or too ill for definitive repair. This is usually achieved with a *Blalock shunt* from the subclavian artery to the pulmonary artery. The classic procedure involves division of the subclavian artery and forming an end-to-side anastomosis with the ipsilateral pulmonary artery. The more recent 'modified Blalock' shunt uses an interposed prosthetic graft which allows continued patency of the subclavian artery (Fig. 24.36).

Postoperative appearances on the chest X-ray may be characteristic. Not only should the pulmonary oligaemia revert to normal, but the right ventricular outflow tract and main pulmonary artery may look unusually large, due

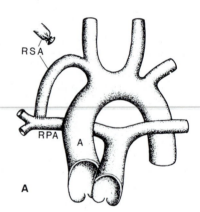

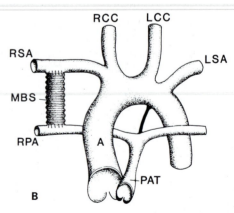

Fig. 24.36 **A**. Diagram showing the classic Blalock shunt. **A**. Aorta RPA. Right pulmonary artery RSA. Right Subclavian artery **B**. Diagram showing a modified Blalock shunt. MBS. Modified Blalock shunt, RCC. Rt. common carotid artery, LCC L. common carotid artery, LSA L. subclavian artery, PAT. Pulmonary artery trunk. (Both diagrams reproduced with permission from Jordan & Scott 1989.)

graphy is best performed in a very steep LAO (e.g. 80–90°) and a cranially tilted (20°) anterior view to show the right ventricular outflow and pulmonary valve (Fig. 24.35). An aortogram performed in 30° RAO and 60° LAO oblique views will show a patent ductus arteriosus, aortopulmonary collaterals, aortic arch anatomy, brachiocephalic and coronary anatomy.

The most common *coronary artery variant* occurring with tetralogy of Fallot is the anomalous origin of the left anterior descending coronary artery from the right coronary artery. This vital artery runs over the surface of the right ventricle just where the surgeon might make the incision to enlarge the right ventricular outflow tract and so it is extremely important to detect this in advance.

Treatment. Surgical treatment will depend on the severity of the condition, but the long-term aim will be total correction by closure of the ventricular septal defect

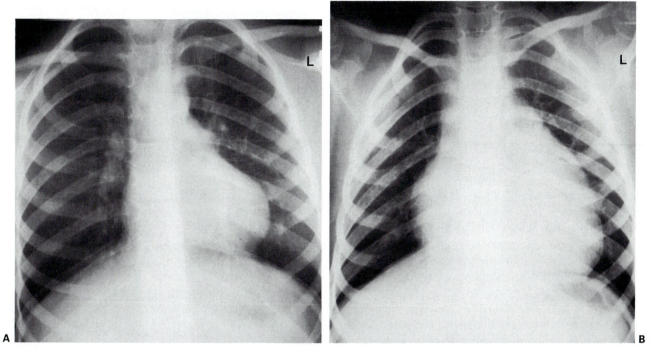

Fig. 24.37 A. Preoperative chest radiograph in a child with classic tetralogy of Fallot. The appearances of mild oligaemia and mild pulmonary artery hypoplasia do not allow definitive diagnosis from this film. **B.** Postoperative chest radiograph of the same patient. The left heart border is much more prominent, mainly due to the right ventricular outflow patch.

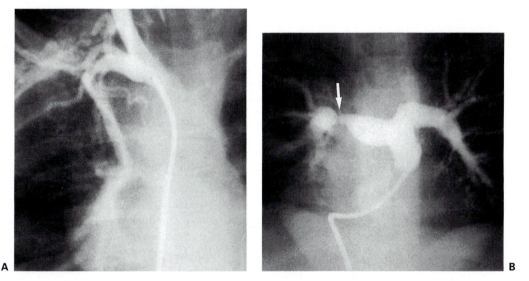

Fig. 24.38 A. Anterior view of a selective angiogram of a right Blalock shunt. The right pulmonary artery is opacified. **B.** Anterior view of a pulmonary arteriogram in the same patient. There is a severe stenosis at the site of insertion of the Blalock shunt.

to the presence of an outflow patch (Fig. 24.37). In cases palliated with a Blalock shunt there may be a difference in pulmonary blood flow in the two lungs, particularly if anatomical abnormalities prevent satisfactory central connection between the two pulmonary arteries. The Blalock shunt itself may cause troublesome narrowing of the pul-

monary artery into which it is inserted and this can be recognised on angiography (Fig. 24.38).

Interventional techniques do not as yet have a major part to play in the treatment of this condition although a few centres have tried palliative *balloon dilatation* of the pulmonary stenosis.

TRANSPOSITION OF THE GREAT ARTERIES
(TGA)

The common form of this abnormality is **D-loop transposition** in which the atrial and ventricular anatomy is normal. There is a simple reversal of connection of the great arteries, with the aorta arising from the morphologically right ventricle and the pulmonary artery arising from the morphologically left ventricle. The exact orientation of the great arteries varies, but the most common arrangement is with the aortic valve arising from a high anterior position from the right ventricle, and the pulmonary valve arising from the lower posterior position above the left ventricular outflow tract. There is loss of the normal arrangement where the right ventricular outflow twists around the left ventricular outflow. The two great arteries run parallel upwards from their respective chambers (Fig. 24.39). This leads to the formation of a relatively narrow pedicle which can frequently be recognized on the chest X-ray.

These infants usually present in the first few weeks of life with cyanosis and breathlessness. Cyanosis depends on the exact degree of mixing at atrial or ventricular level. Although the condition can be diagnosed simply by echocardiography, cardiac catheterization is commonly performed so that the Rashkind balloon septostomy can be performed at the same time. In this technique an inflated balloon is used to rupture the thin part of the septum primum covering the foramen ovale in order to improve the atrial mixing and thus allow a higher proportion of oxygenated blood to pass from the left atrium to the right atrium and right ventricle and then to the systemic circulation. Recently this procedure has been performed under echocardiographic control (Fig. 24.40).

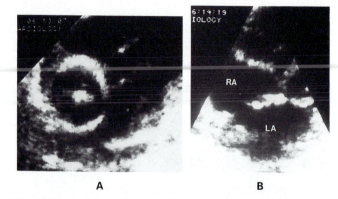

A   **B**

Fig. 24.40 **A**. Subcostal echocardiogram showing a Rashkind balloon being drawn from the right atrium (RA) to the left atrium (LA) to rupture the atrial septum. (Courtesy Dr. R. Martin.) **B**. Taken immediately after (A), showing an atrial septal defect created by the balloon septostomy. (Courtesy Dr. R. Martin.)

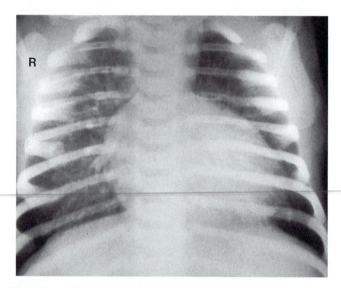

Fig. 24.41 Chest radiograph of an infant with D-transposition of the great arteries. The pedicle (mediastinum) is narrow and there is cardiomegaly and pulmonary plethora.

The *chest X-ray* is often, but not always, characteristic. The heart is sightly enlarged and rounded and there is pulmonary plethora. The pedicle remains narrow because the main pulmonary artery is behind the aorta (Fig. 24.41). The condition may give a similar appearance on chest X-ray to truncus arteriosus, where there is again loss of the normal twisting arrangement of the main pulmonary artery around the aorta. There are many associated conditions, the most common of which are *ventricular septal defect, patent ductus arteriosus* (Fig. 24.18), *coarctation of the aorta* and *pulmonary* (or *subpulmonary*) *stenosis*, the latter being particularly important as it can be difficult to treat surgically.

L-loop transposition of the great arteries is distinctly different to the more usual D-loop TGA but it still conforms to the morphological definition of transposition (or

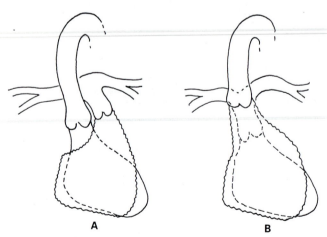

A   **B**

Fig. 24.39 **A**. Diagram showing normal great arterial connections in the anterior view. The morphological left ventricle (smooth outline) lies posteriorly to the morphological right ventricle (wavy outline) as shown by the interrupted line. **B**. Diagram showing connections in D-transposition of the great arteries in the anterior view. Compare with (A). The great arteries have an antero-posterior relationship which gives the narrow pedicle.

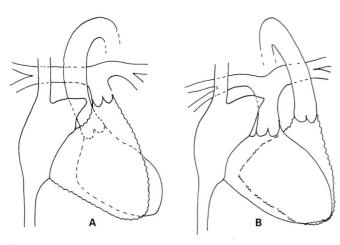

Fig. 24.42 **A**. Normal cardiac connections in the anterior view. The morphological left ventricle (smooth outline) lies posterior to the morphological right ventricle (wavy outline) as shown by the interrupted line. **B**. Connections in L-transposition of the great arteries ('corrected transposition'). The morphological right ventricle (wavy line) lies behind the morphological left ventricle (smooth line) as shown by the interrupted line. The aorta has a leftward origin which accounts for the long curved left heart border seen in some cases.

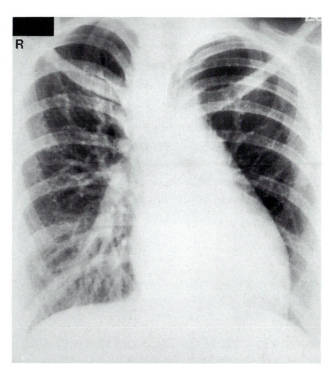

Fig. 24.43 Chest radiograph of a patient with L-transposition of the great arteries. There is a long smooth curve to the left heart border due to the abnormal leftward origin of the aorta.

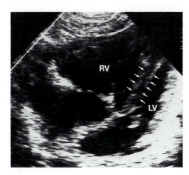

Fig. 24.44 Subcostal echocardiogram of a patient with D-transposition of the great arteries. The morphological right ventricle (RV) is much larger than the morphological left ventricle (LV) and the interventricular septum (arrowed) is curved towards the left ventricle.

ventriculoarterial discordance). This condition is also known as 'anatomically corrected transposition' or just 'corrected transposition'. The cardiac apex is normally directed to the left, but the morphologically left ventricle lies anterior and to the right of the posterior ventricle which is of right morphology. Visceroatrial situs is normal, which means that there is atrioventricular discordance as well as ventriculo-arterial discordance (Fig. 24.42). Thus the abnormal connections result in a *physiologically corrected circulation*. Patients with this abnormality will usually have symptoms only if there is an associated abnormality, and the symptoms, treatment and prognosis will all depend on the nature of the additional malformations. Common associations are *ventricular septal defect* and *conduction abnormalities*.

The *chest X-ray* may show a characteristic long curve to the left heart border due to the abnormal leftward origin of the aorta (Fig. 24.43) but this is not reliable in all cases as the positions of the great arteries are somewhat variable. A significant proportion of these patients have chest X-rays indistinguishable from normal.

Non-invasive imaging. *Echocardiographic* diagnosis is relatively straightforward in both types of TGA but care must be taken to identify correctly the two parallel great arteries as they may not lie in typical positions. The aorta can be identified specifically if the vessel is traced up to the brachiocephalic artery origins. It is essential to avoid the pitfall of assuming which great artery is which simply by position. Two-dimensional imaging will show the smaller left ventricle in D-TGA, which pumps to the pulmonary circuit, and the reversed curve of the

interventricular septum will usually be apparent (Fig. 24.44). Associated conditions must be sought. In the case of L-loop TGA, the reversal of the morphologically left and right ventricles can be demonstrated by the reversed insertions of the antrioventricular valves (Fig. 24.45).

Cardiac catheterization and angiography. Angiography will show clearly the abnormal connections (Fig. 24.46) and will also be useful for clarifying details of anatomy concerning associated anomalies. It is again important to assess *coronary anatomy* for surgical planning, particularly when the great arterial switch procedure is being contemplated. Left ventriculography is probably

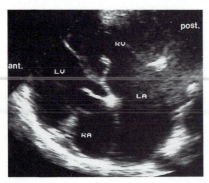

Fig. 24.45 Modified apical four-chamber view in a patient with L-transposition of the great arteries. The morphological left ventricle (LV) lies anteriorly and the morphological right ventricle (RV) lies posteriorly, as shown by the insertions of their respective atrioventricular valves. The tricuspid valve in the right ventricle is inserted more apically than the mitral valve. ant. = anterior, post. = posteiror, RA = right atrium, LA = left atrium. (Compare the valve insertions with the diagrams in Fig. 24.10C and 24.50A.)

best for assessment of possible ventricular septal defects, even though the cavity is usually at a lower pressure than the right ventricle. This is because of the relatively simpler contours of the morphological left ventricle. It is also essential to examine the left ventricular outflow to exclude obstruction and this is best achieved using a 20° cranially tilted LAO 60° projection which profiles the outflow well. Right ventriculography in standard oblique views (LAO 60° and RAO 30°) will confirm the diagnosis, show right ventricular function and demonstrate the coronary arteries. An aortic injection may be helpful to exclude a patent ductus arteriosus and to show coronary anatomy in more detail.

Treatment. Initial palliation by *Rashkind septostomy* is frequently performed in the neonatal period as described above. Definitive surgical treatment is of two types. The more traditional approach is to use an *atrial baffle operation* (Mustard or Senning) in which the venous returns are redirected at atrial level so that systemic venous return is directed to the left ventricle and pulmonary artery with pulmonary venous return being directed to the right ventricle and aorta via an intra-atrial conduit (Fig. 24.47). This operation provides a satisfactory physiological circulation but it leaves the right ventricle performing the systemic pumping function, and this can from time to time cause problems in later life. There are also problems with stenosis developing in the surgically formed systemic venous pathways, particularly in the earlier Mustard procedure in which a large prosthetic patch is incorporated into the atrial repair (Fig. 24.48). The Senning procedure makes better use of the native tissues.

A more recent approach has been to use the *great arterial switch operation*. This is complicated by the need to transpose the coronary arteries as well as the great arteries themselves (Fig. 24.49). Early results of this operation have shown a higher mortality than the atrial baffle approach but it is thought that the longer-term outlook may be better. This has not as yet been definitely proved. The great arterial switch operation cannot be performed in patients where the morphologically left ventricle has become accustomed to functioning at low pressure function over a long period. The procedure should thus be performed in the first few days or weeks of life or later in life in those patients with a large ventricular septal defect and equalization of the ventricular pressures.

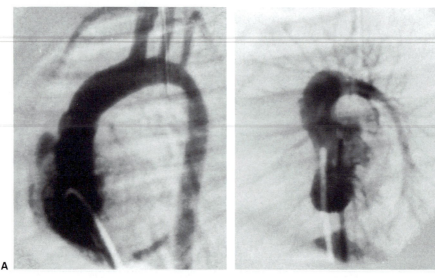

Fig. 24.46 **A**. Digital subtraction angiogram of a right ventricular injection recorded in the AO projection. The anteriorly placed morphological right ventricle gives rise to the aorta, indicating D-transposition of the great arteries. **B**. Digital subtraction left ventriculogram in the same patient and projection. The pulmonary artery arises from the morphological left ventricle.

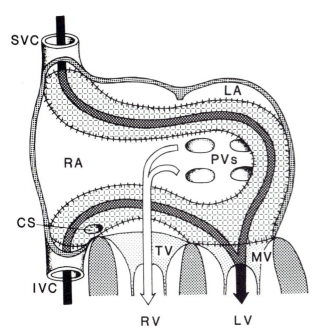

Fig. 24.47 Mustard procedure for D-transposition of the great arteries. A prosthetic intra-atrial conduit leads the systemic venous return from the superior vena cava (SVC) and inferior vena cava (IVC) to the left ventricle (LV) through the mitral valve (MV). Flow from the pulmonary veins (PVs) passes over the conduit to reach the right ventricle (RV) through the tricuspid valve (TV). RA = right atrium, LA = left atrium and CS = coronary sinus.

If there is D-TGA with a large VSD, the *Rastelli procedure* may be indicated. In this operation the VSD is closed with an oblique patch, directing left ventricular flow to the aorta through the VSD. An external conduit, sometimes with a prosthetic or homograft valve, is used

to connect the right ventricle to the main pulmonary artery. In this way normal circulation is effectively reconstituted.

ATRIOVENTRICULAR SEPTAL DEFECT (AVSD)

This group of conditions has also been known as *atrioventricular canal defect*. All the variations of the condition have the same fundamental cardiac abnormality. The base of the interventricular septum in the region of the membranous septum is normally in continuity with the atrial septum primum. This central portion of the cardiac structure is missing in all types of atrioventricular septal defect. The *partial* type of atrioventricular septal defect results in only an interatrial communication and leads to the so-called 'ostium primum' atrial septal defect. The *total* atrioventricular septal defect leads to interventricular and interatrial communications with a large common atrioventricular valve. There is also an '*intermediate*' type in which the interventricular communication is relatively small, due to partial tethering of the common atrioventricular valve to the septal crest.

Figures 24.50A–D show the difference between normals, partial AVSD and complete AVSD, comparing them with a secundum ASD.

The atrioventricular valves are commonly malformed and produce regurgitation of varying degrees. This is not invariably present but when it is, it will lead to exacerbation of any symptoms produced by left-to-right shunting. In the case of the partial defect (ostium primum ASD) the anterior leaflet of the mitral valve has a cleft, which can be an important cause of regurgitation.

There is an increased association of this condition with

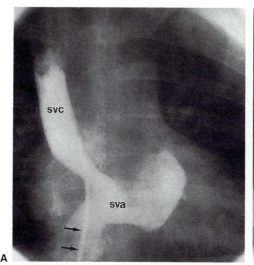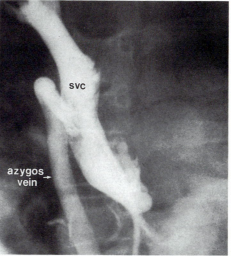

Fig. 24.48 **A**. Anterior view of an angiogram performed with the venous catheter (arrowed) passed to the superior vena cava (svc) in a patient with a previous Mustard operation. Contrast medium flows to the systemic venous atrium (sva) before its passage to the left ventricle. **B**. Similar angiogram to that in (A), but there is severe postoperative narrowing at the point of entry of the superior vena cava to the systemic venous atrium. Flow bypasses the obstruction through a dilated azygos vein.

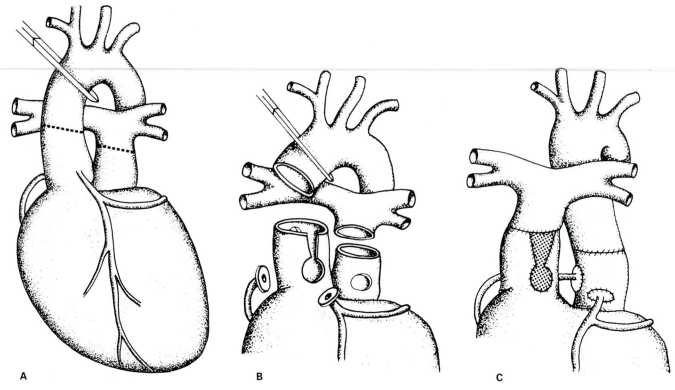

Fig. 24.49 A. Cross clamping of the aorta prior to the great arterial switch procedure for D-transposition of the great arteries. **B**. Division of the great arteries and excision of the origins of the coronary arteries with a small 'button' of aortic wall. **C**. Re-anastomosis of the great arteries and coronary arteries. Systemic arterial blood flows into the coronaries from the newly created 'aortic root', previously the main pulmonary artery. (Reproduced with permission from Jordan & Scott 1989.)

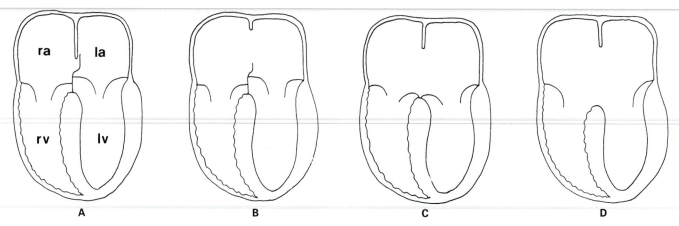

Fig. 24.50 A. Normal relationships of the interventricular and interatrial septa with the atrioventricular valves. The atrioventricular valves are inserted into the septum primum (thin line). Right atrium (ra), left atrium (la), right ventricle (rv) and left ventricle (lv). **B**. Ostium secundum atrial septal defect. The atrioventricular valves and left ventricular outflow tract are normal. **C**. Ostium primum atrial septal defect. The septum primum is absent and the atrioventricular valves are inserted in a low position into the crest of the muscular interventricular septum. **D**. Total atrioventricular septal defect. A large common valve separates the atrial cavities from the ventricular cavities. There is an ostium primum atrial septal defect and a large ventricular septal defect in continuity.

Down's syndrome. The presentation varies, depending on the precise nature of the abnormality, but tends to be earlier and more severe than with conventional atrial and ventricular septal defects of similar size. There is no specific abnormality that can be detected on chest X-ray to differentiate these conditions from the more usual type of atrial or ventricular septal defects although the cardiac enlargement, pulmonary plethora and cardiac failure are often all more prominent. The presence of only eleven pairs of ribs may be a clue to an underlying Down's syndrome aetiology.

Non-invasive diagnosis. *Echocardiography* is the key

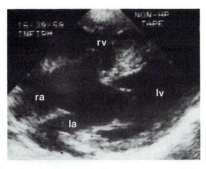

Fig. 24.51 Subcostal echocardiogram showing an ostium primum atrial septal defect lying between the left atrium (la) and the right atrium (ra). There is no ventricular septal defect between the left ventricle (lv) and the right ventricle (rv).

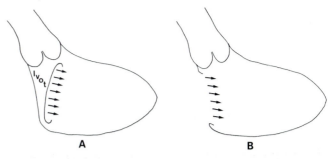

Fig. 24.52 A. Normal left ventricular angiogram in the right anterior oblique projection. Diastolic inflow does not wash out contrast medium lying below the aortic root in the left ventricular outflow tract (lvot). **B**. Left ventricular angiogram performed in a patient with an atrio-ventricular septal defect. The normal left ventricular outflow region is missing due to the absent septum primum, and so the contrast medium in the sub-aortic region is washed out by the incoming mitral flow. This produces the frequently misinterpreted 'goose-neck' appearance.

to diagnosis in this range of conditions. The atrioventricular valve anatomy can clearly be seen (Fig. 24.51) and the presence of a ventricular component to the defect is usually obvious. There is often considerable enlargement of the right-sided cardiac chambers and the right atrium may be particularly large if there is accompanying atrioventricular valve regurgitation. *Doppler studies* will clearly demonstrate the presence of atrioventricular valve regurgitation and this is particularly well seen on *colour-flow studies*. This regurgitation is more commonly seen through the mitral valve in ostium primum ASD and the regurgitant jet is often directed across the interatrial defect to the right atrium.

Cardiac catheter and angiography. Angiography is also capable of demonstrating the anatomy clearly. The most obvious abnormality seen on angiography is the absence of the usual left ventricular outflow tract. The mitral valve hinges directly from beneath the aortic root (Fig. 24.52) and when open creates a distinct appearance that has been likened to a 'goose-neck', a misleading term that is open to misinterpretation; it does not indicate narrowing of the left ventricular outflow tract in systole but merely reflects the washout of contrast medium during ventricular diastole as the abnormally positioned mitral valve is open.

Views can be the same as for assessing a straightforward ventricular septal defect but the large right-sided chambers may necessitate a more steeply angled left anterior oblique view to profile the basal septum. A conventional LAO view will show the common valve well as the non-opaque atrial blood passing through it, but a cranial tilt will aid in exclusion of additional defects and can help in detecting small interventricular communications in the 'intermediate' type. Both the cleft mitral valve and variable degrees of mitral prolapse are well shown on angiography. Atrioventricular valve regurgitation is well assessed by angiography but it should be remembered that the catheter may have been passed into the left ventricle through the valve and so might itself produce regurgitation.

Treatment. Surgery in this condition is somewhat more complex than with conventional atrial or ventricular septal defects as the repair usually involves some form of reconstruction of the atrioventricular valves as well as patch closure of one or both septal defects. It is for this reason that corrective surgery is sometimes performed at a slightly later age, with palliative banding of the main pulmonary artery being performed initially to protect the lungs. There is no place for interventional therapy in this condition at present.

PULMONARY ATRESIA

The presence or absence of a VSD with pulmonary atresia will markedly affect the expression of the condition.

1. Pulmonary atresia with ventricular septal defect. In these circumstances the anomaly is essentially the same as a very severe form of tetralogy of Fallot. The obstructed outflow of the right ventricle, together with the usual over-ride of the aorta, means that the right ventricle can empty into the aorta although it must do this at the same systemic pressure as the left ventricle. Flow thus continues through the right ventricle, and the chamber remains large and its walls become hypertrophied due to the systemic pressure in it. The pulmonary arteries are often very small and they receive their blood supply from the patent ductus arteriosus initially and then subsequently through aorto-pulmonary collateral vessels of various sorts.

The *chest X-ray* shows a slightly enlarged heart, often with a slightly upturned apex due to the right ventricular enlargement, the pulmonary bay is small and the lung fields are oligaemic. There is a right aortic arch in about 25% of cases (Fig. 24.53). In older patients the multiplicity of aorto-pulmonary collaterals can give a complex vascular pattern, particularly near the hilar regions, and this can sometimes be mistaken for pulmonary plethora.

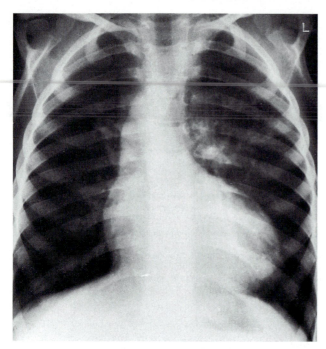

Fig. 24.53 Chest radiograph of a child with pulmonary atresia and a ventricular septal defect. There is a right-sided aortic arch indenting the trachea which accentuates the concave pulmonary bay. The left heart border does not show an upturned apex as seen in Fig. 24.54.

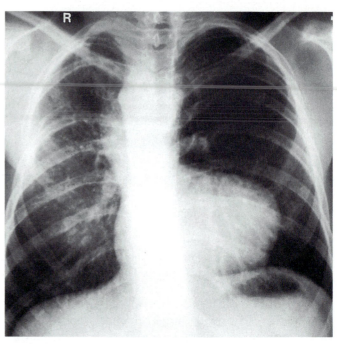

Fig. 24.54 Chest radiograph of an adult with long-term palliation of pulmonary atresia. There is a right-sided aortic arch and an upturned cardiac apex. The vascularity in the right lung is more prominent due to the presence of a right sided shunt.

Palliation with various types of shunt is often required in early life and this may give rise to uneven vascularity in the lungs (Fig. 24.54).

Angiography is commonly required in the diagnosis of this condition because successful definitive surgery depends on careful planning of a reconstructed outflow from the right ventricle to the pulmonary arteries, which themselves often need reconstruction. It is usually not possible to determine all the details of the anatomy of the hypoplastic pulmonary arteries and the collaterals using echocardiography. A good-quality aortogram, together with a series of selective angiograms to different collaterals, is usually required. In difficult cases where there is very poor collateral flow to the pulmonary arteries it may be helpful to perform a wedged pulmonary venous injection to opacify the hypoplastic pulmonary arteries.

Surgery may be similar to that required for a severe form of the tetralogy of Fallot but this is only possible if there is a reasonably-sized pulmonary artery. In some cases complex reconstructions of hypoplastic pulmonary arteries are attempted, but often long-term palliation with multiple shunting procedures is the only option. If the main pulmonary artery is of good size, the VSD may be closed and an external conduit, usually with a valve, is placed from the right ventricle to the pulmonary artery, the *Rastelli procedure* (Fig. 24.55).

2. Pulmonary atresia with intact ventricular septum. In this situation there is no outlet for the right

ventricle and thus no way that it can decompress. The cavity is usually very small but often generates very high pressures (supra-systemic), especially if there is a small but functionally competent tricuspid valve. Under these circumstances the unusual problem of abnormal coronary communications can occur. Blood may shunt from right to left through the abnormal vessels and this can cause myocardial ischaemia and sometimes infarction. The *chest X-ray* will show a small pulmonary segment and pulmonary oligaemia but the cardiac contour will show a more rounded left ventricular contour, often similar to that seen in tricuspid atresia. Imaging techniques are particularly important in this condition as the size and function of the right ventricle must be estimated.

Palliative shunting may be needed in early life, but a successful surgical correction is dependent on the degree of underdevelopment of the right ventricular cavity. If the right ventricle is extremely hypoplastic, then the condition must be considered as a form of 'single-ventricle', but if there is reasonable development of the right ventricular cavity, a full correction might be possible, although this is often a high risk procedure. Patients with very severe pulmonary valve stenosis are considered in a similar way.

SINGLE VENTRICLE (primitive ventricle)

There are many complex variants in this category and they must all be assessed carefully on their individual

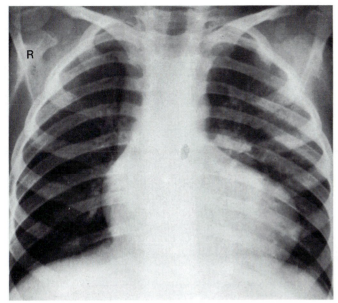

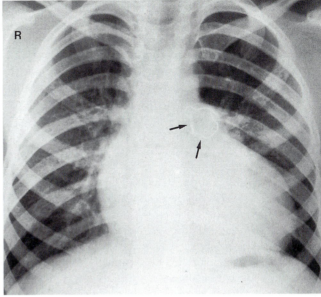

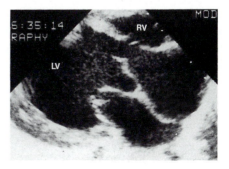

Fig. 24.55 A. Chest radiograph of a child with pulmonary atresia and a left-sided aortic arch. **B.** Chest radiograph of the same patient following closure of the ventricular septal defect and insertion of an external valved conduit (arrowed) from the right ventricle to the main pulmonary artery. **C.** Lateral view of (B), showing the metallic frame of the prosthetic valve in the conduit.

The following situations may lead to a 'single ventricle':-

1. *Double-inlet ventricle* — both atrioventricular valves enter the same ventricle (Fig. 24.56), or there is considerable override of one valve across a VSD.
2. *Common inlet valve* — a single large atrioventricular valve enters a large ventricular chamber.
3. *Atresia of one atrioventricular valve*, mitral or tricuspid — may be indistinguishable from 2.
4. *Very large ventricular septal defect* with little residual septal tissue, effectively a single chamber.

Multiple abnormalities are common and nothing must be taken for granted in the assessment of the cases. Great arterial connections may be abnormal and must be assessed carefully. Atrial anatomy may be abnormal and there may be a single common atrium. The positions of the chambers may be distorted or twisted and this must also be taken into careful consideration. Other malforma-

Fig. 24.56 Left parasternal echocardiogram in a patient with 'single ventricle'. Both atrioventricular valves enter the large left ventricle (LV) from two distinct atria. Outflow to the aorta is via a restrictive ventricular septal defect and a small outflow chamber of right ventricular type (RV).

merits. The conditions are commonly referred to as 'single ventricle', but this is not always an easy description to understand, because often a second small or rudimentary ventricular chamber is present; but according to accepted morphological classifications, the small chamber may not be entitled to the name 'ventricle'. The second small chamber often acts, via a ventricular septal defect, as an outlet chamber.

tions such as pulmonary stenosis, coarctation or patent ductus arteriosus may well be present.

In all these cases there is common mixing of the pulmonary and systemic venous return in the heart, and the clinical presentation depends particularly on the presence or absence of *pulmonary stenosis*. If pulmonary stenosis is present the patient may be cyanotic with pulmonary oligaemia, and if absent, the patient may have heart failure and pulmonary plethora.

There is no 'typical' *chest X-ray* but the heart is often enlarged, with the pulmonary vascularity depending on the presence of other abnormalities. The size and position of the great arteries will help to determine the overall cardiac configuration. *Angiography* and *ultrasound* must be used, as appropriate for the circumstances, but in these complex cases it is often useful to assess the anatomy by both techniques to ensure maximum diagnostic accuracy. Work with *magnetic resonance imaging* suggests that this modality may become the technique of choice for 'unscrambling' these complex cases.

In the presence of only one useful ventricle surgical options are often palliative, using shunts or pulmonary artery banding, but reconstructive surgery using the single ventricular chamber is increasingly carried out. This is normally achieved by the use of the *Fontan procedure* or one of its variants. This operation uses the single ventricle to pump systemic blood to the aorta whilst redirecting systemic venous return to the lungs without the use of a second ventricle. This is often achieved by the direct anastomosis of the right atrial appendage to the main pulmonary artery. The details of the technique will vary with individual cases but the success of the procedure depends on a well-functioning systemic ventricle and low pulmonary vascular resistance. Occasionally *cardiac transplantation* can be offered to these patients.

TRICUSPID ATRESIA

In this condition there is no tricuspid orifice, the valve having either fused leaflets or a mass of obstructive tissue in the expected valve plane (Fig. 24.57). There is obligatory flow of the systemic venous return across an atrial septal defect to the left atrium and the left ventricle. The left ventricle is large as it carries both pulmonary and systemic venous return. Some of the blood in the left ventricle then crosses a ventricular septal defect to reach the right ventricle and the pulmonary artery whilst the remainder passes out in the normal way through the aortic valve.

The VSD is often restrictive (small size with a pressure drop across it and a low-pressure right ventricle) and there may be associated pulmonary stenosis. The right ventricle is often so underdeveloped that the condition is considered as one of the 'single ventricle' group. There is often relatively low pulmonary blood flow, although

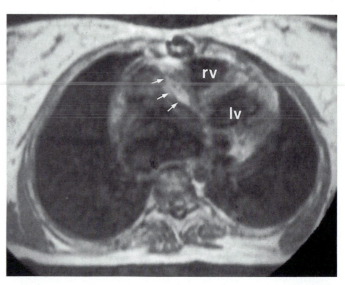

Fig. 24.57 Transverse gated spin-echo MR image of a patient with tricuspid atresia. A wedge-shaped segment of tissue (arrowed) lies in the expected position of the tricuspid valve. Right ventricle (rv) and left ventricle (lv). (Courtesy of the Trustees of the Bristol MRI Centre.)

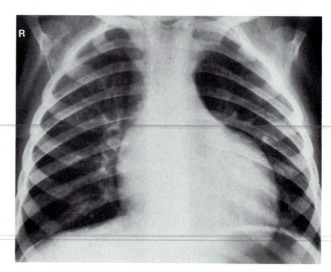

Fig. 24.58 Chest radiograph of a patient with tricuspid atresia. There is pulmonary oligaemia, a small pulmonary artery and a prominent rounded left ventricular curve to the left heart border.

this is not invariable, and the condition may be expressed in various ways, depending on the state of the VSD and right ventricular outflow.

The *chest X-ray* commonly shows pulmonary oligaemia, a small pulmonary bay and a moderately large heart with a rounded contour due to the downward and leftward enlargement of the left ventricle (Fig. 24.58). *Echocardiography* will show the anatomy clearly with Doppler studies adding information about flow across the interatrial septum and the pressure drops across the VSD and the pulmonary valve.

Cardiac angiography will show the anatomy well. Left ventriculography should be modified by the use of a shallower than usual LAO projection (e.g. 40–50° LAO) to take account of the alteration of the position of the interventricular septum by the large left ventricle and small right ventricle.

Surgical treatment will depend on the details of the individual case. If the VSD is relatively small and the right ventricle is poorly developed then correction can only be achieved by the use of a Fontan procedure.

MITRAL VALVE ABNORMALITIES (including supramitral ring and cor triatriatum)

Obstructive lesions in or near the mitral valve include *congenital mitral stenosis*, *supramitral ring* and *cor triatriatum*. The first resembles rheumatic stenosis with fusion of the valve leaflets and doming of the valve. A supramitral ring is an obstructive diaphragm lying very close to the mitral valve on the left atrial side. Cor triatriatum is a condition in which there is an obstructive membrane in the left atrium which divides it into a high- and a low-pressure portion with a small and restrictive communication between the two (Fig. 24.59).

The *chest X-ray* is similar in all cases, showing a normal-sized heart with increased pulmonary vessel size, due to pulmonary venous hypertension similar to that seen in the obstructed form of totally anomalous pulmonary venous drainage. There will often be pulmonary oedema. *Echocardiography* will show the obstructive detail well, often better than angiography. Doppler studies may indicate the degree of obstruction.

Mitral regurgitation can form part of a complex abnormality such as atrioventricular septal defect but it can also occur alone. In the latter case there may be abnormal papillary muscle formation such as a single papillary muscle giving a 'parachute' mitral valve. The chest X-ray

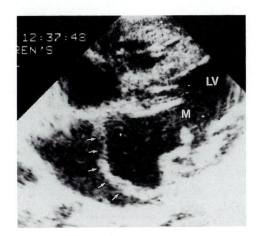

Fig. 24.59 Subcostal echocardiogram of a patient with cor triatriatum. A prominent membrane runs across the left atrium (arrowed). M = mitral valve, LV = left ventricle.

will show signs of pulmonary venous hypertension and possibly pulmonary oedema. The heart will be larger than with obstructive mitral lesions because of the ventricular volume overload.

HYPOPLASTIC LEFT HEART SYNDROME (aortic atresia)

At the most severe end of the spectrum of aortic stenosis lies aortic atresia. If there is no flow through the aortic valve the left ventricle itself will not develop, being only a rudimentary slit-like cavity. The aortic atresia may also be associated with mitral atresia. This abnormality is known as hypoplastic left heart syndrome.

In this condition the right ventricle performs the entire systemic pumping function, with the systemic blood supply being directed through the ductus arteriosus. The brachiocephalic branches are supplied retrogradely and the ascending aorta is diminutive in size, carrying only reverse flow from the patent ductus arteriosus and aortic arch sufficient to fill the coronary arteries. The condition is uniformly fatal and this probably explains why the condition appears relatively low on the list of incidence of congenital heart disease. Many cases probably die before being recognized at a paediatric cardiology referral centre. Patients with hypoplastic left heart are often born in good condition but deteriorate very rapidly in the first few days of life as the life-sustaining ductus closes.

In the case of hypoplastic left heart, the diagnosis can almost always be made by *echocardiography*. The key feature to identify is the diminutive ascending aorta and the single functional ventricle because these are the features associated with the uniformly poor prognosis. *Cardiac catheterization* may be required if high-quality echocardiography is unavailable. In this situation the best approach is to perform a normal catheter study from the venous approach and pass the angiographic catheter to the pulmonary artery or, if possible, through the patent ductus arteriosus to the descending aorta. An *angiogram* performed from either of these positions will immediately show the retrograde flow down the diminutive ascending aorta and the diagnosis will be confirmed. The condition can now be recognized by *antenatal echocardiography*.

Some experimental approaches to surgery are being investigated at present, with radical multistage reconstructions being attempted in a few cases. The only surgical successes achieved so far have been with *neonatal heart transplantation* in a few specialized centres.

CARDIOMYOPATHY

Hypertrophic cardiomyopathy with left ventricular outflow obstruction can occur in infants and children and is thought to be dominantly inherited in a proportion of cases. There are also associations with *Noonan's syndrome*

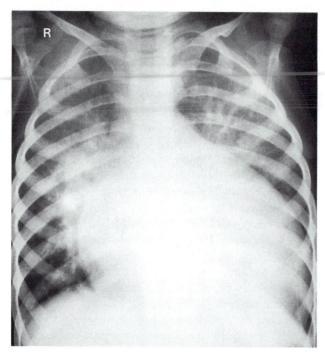

Fig. 24.60 Chest radiograph of a child with a severe dilated cardiomyopathy. There is marked cardiomegaly and left heart failure.

and *maternal diabetes*, but in the latter circumstance the condition tends to resolve, whereas it tends to be progressive in the remainder. There is an association with arrhythmias and sudden death in a minority of cases. Diagnosis is classically made on the *echocardiogram* which may show asymmetrical hypertrophy of the interventricular septum and obstruction of the left ventricular outflow tract by anterior motion of the mitral valve.

Dilated cardiomyopathies (alternatively called *endocardial fibroelastosis*) occur occasionally in infancy and are most commonly related to intrauterine infections. Occasionally they are due to inherited factors or are secondary to valvular or coronary anomalies. The aetiology of the conditions is often hard to determine. The chest X-ray will show a large heart with pulmonary signs of cardiac failure (Fig. 24.60) and other imaging modalities will be capable of demonstrating the poor ventricular function. This is particularly clearly seen on two-dimensional echocardiography which will also demonstrate the characteristic endocardial thickening. Occasionally the condition can be detected by fetal echocardiography.

Endomyocardial fibrosis is a tropical condition in which there is endocardial thickening which leads to cavity obliteration.

ANOMALOUS PULMONARY VENOUS CONNECTION

This abnormality of cardiac connection can take various forms. **Partial anomalous pulmonary venous connection** (PAPVC) can occur when one or more individual pulmonary veins drain to the right side of the atrial septum, either into the right atrium itself or into the superior or inferior vena cava. This abnormality is commonly associated with atrial septal defect, in particular the sinus venosus type of defect, and it is important to check pulmonary venous connections when performing echocardiographic or angiographic examination. The anomalous veins can often be redirected correctly at surgery, providing the surgeon is aware of the problem.

Sometimes an anomalous pulmonary vein can drain down to the inferior vena cava below the diaphragm, more commonly on the right side (Fig. 24.61). This vein can sometimes be identified on the chest X-ray as a curved vessel in the right lower zone, widening as it approaches the right cardiophrenic angle (Fig. 24.62). This is sometimes referred to as the *scimitar syndrome*. The condition is frequently associated with hypoplasia of the right lung and sometimes there is a shift of the heart to the right.

Total anomalous pulmonary venous connection (TAPVC) is a more serious condition which can take three forms, *supracardiac*, *cardiac* or *infracardiac*. In all three types the major pulmonary veins come to a confluence behind the left atrium but do not communicate directly with it (Fig. 24.63). In the case of *supracardiac TAPVC* there is a large ascending vein on the left side which is a remnant of the embryological left superior vena cava. This connects into the left brachiocephalic vein which then passes down the right-sided superior vena cava into the right atrium (Fig. 24.64). The *cardiac type* of abnormality drains into the right side of the heart,

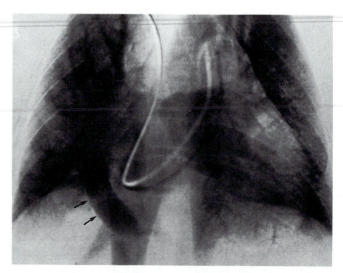

Fig. 24.61 Digital angiogram of a follow-through pulmonary artery injection in a patient with partial anomalous pulmonary venous drainage. A large vein (arrowed) is seen draining from the right lung to the inferior vena cava below the diaphragm.

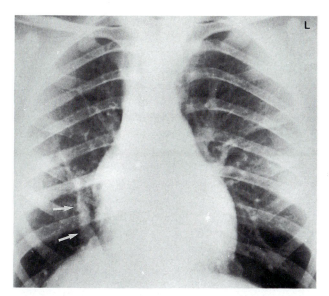

Fig. 24.62 Chest radiograph of the patient as in Fig. 24.61. The anomalous vein (scimitar sign) is seen in the right lower zone (arrowed).

usually via the enlarged coronary sinus. In the case of *infracardiac TAPVC* the confluence of pulmonary veins drains downwards in a descending vein which passes through the diaphragm, often obstructed at this point, into either the portal venous system or the inferior vena cava. The portal venous system is usually at a higher pressure than other venous systems and this fact may also contribute to the 'obstruction' in this condition (Fig. 24.65). The pulmonary venous blood then returns to the right atrium through the inferior vena cava.

In all of these conditions there is total cardiac mixing at right atrial level and the patient remains partially cyanosed. In the case of supracardiac or cardiac TAPVC the *chest X-ray* shows that the heart is enlarged and there is pulmonary plethora, which is obligatory due to the need for a higher pulmonary flow in the mixed circulation (Fig. 24.66). The supracardiac TAPVC will often show wide mediastinum due to the left-sided ascending vein, and in long-established cases the classic *cottage loaf* heart will be evident. This will become less common because these cases are now usually diagnosed and treated in infancy. The infracardiac type of abnormal drainage will often be associated with little or no cardiac enlargement and the obstruction of the pulmonary circulation will lead to interstitial oedema and heart failure. The findings of a normal heart size with severe heart failure usually indicate infracardiac TAPVC (Fig. 24.67).

Non-invasive diagnosis. The three types of TAPVC may be diagnosed by *echocardiography*, the abnormal venous confluence being visible behind the left atrium. The abnormal course of drainage can usually be traced. The left atrium is usually small and there is right-to-left flow across the atrial septal communication. The flow in

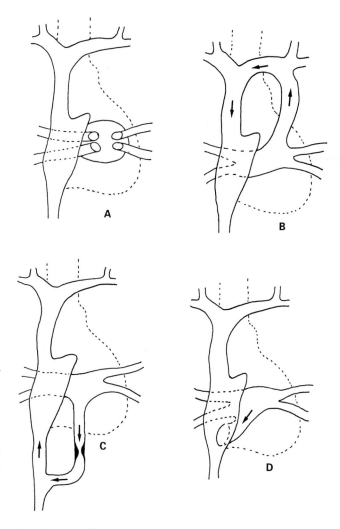

Fig. 24.63 A. Normal pulmonary venous drainage to the left atrium. **B**. Totally anomalous pulmonary venous connection of the supracardiac type draining to a left-sided ascending vein and then to the left brachiocephalic vein. **C**. Totally anomalous pulmonary venous connection of the infracardiac type showing obstructed drainage to the inferior vena cava. **D**. Totally anomalous pulmonary venous connection of the cardiac type draining to the coronary sinus.

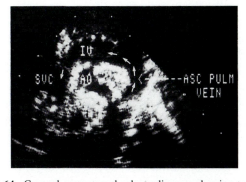

Fig. 24.64 Coronal suprasternal echocardiogram showing totally anomalous pulmonary venous connection of the supracardiac type draining as shown in Fig. 24.63b. IV = brachiocephalic vein or innominate vein, SVC = superior vena cava, AO = aorta. (Courtesy Dr. R. Martin.)

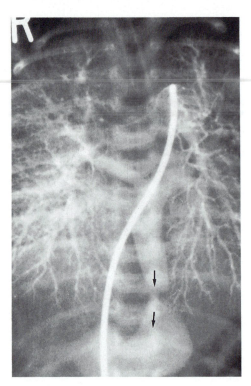

Fig. 24.65 Follow-through pulmonary arteriogram in a child with obstructed totally anomalous pulmonary venous connection of the infracardiac type draining past an obstruction at diaphragmatic level (arrows) to a dilated vein connecting to the inferior vena cava.

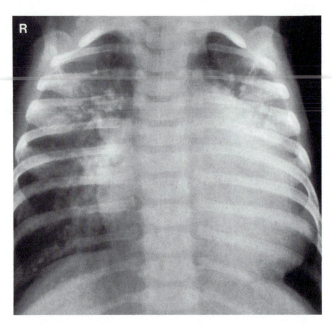

Fig. 24.66 Chest radiograph in a child with totally anomalous pulmonary venous connection of the cardiac type draining to the coronary sinus. There is marked cardiomegaly and pulmonary plethora but the upper mediastinum is not wide because the drainage is directly to the heart.

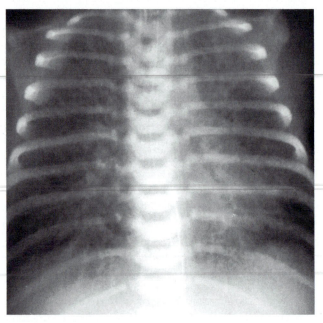

Fig. 24.67 Chest radiograph of a child with obstructed totally anomalous pulmonary venous connection of the infracardiac type. The heart borders are obscured by diffuse interstitial oedema but there is no significant cardiomegaly.

the venous confluence and drainage channels can often be shown using *Doppler colour-flow mapping*.

Partial anomalous pulmonary venous connection can be diagnosed by the visualization of the individual veins draining to the right atrium, but the diagnosis can be more difficult if the site of drainage is to the inferior or superior vena cava rather than to the right atrium.

Cardiac catheterization and angiography. Angiography will also show these features but it may not be necessary if high-quality ultrasound results are available. A large and rapid injection of contrast medium to the main pulmonary artery will opacify the pulmonary venous system well. The anterior view is the clearest for demonstrating the venous pathways. Infants presenting with this condition are often seriously ill and the morbidity of catheterization and angiography is significant.

The delineation of the individual pulmonary veins in partial anomalous pulmonary venous connection can be more difficult and may require separate injections to the left and right pulmonary arteries in oblique views. Sometimes the direct injection of contrast medium to the suspected abnormal veins can be diagnostic, but this approach can be surprisingly difficult to interpret as the contrast medium is rapidly diluted and the atrial anatomy is often unclear. In either case oblique views are preferable to PA and lateral views as they will separate the two atria more effectively.

Treatment. Surgery is directed towards reanastomosing the pulmonary venous confluence with the left atrium, dividing the abnormal connection and closing the atrial septal defect that is present. In spite of its apparently straightforward nature the operation carries a high mortality. Surgical treatment of partial anomalous venous connection usually consists of closing the associated atrial septal defect with a patch that incorporates all the pulmonary veins into the left atrium but surgery may not be necessary at all for this condition.

TRUNCUS ARTERIOSUS

In this condition a single great artery arises from the heart, due to a failure of division of the embryonic common truncus arteriosus. The common truncus arises from above a large ventricular septal defect (Fig. 24.68) and the pattern of division of the common truncus varies. A single common pulmonary artery with a well-developed main pulmonary artery segment may arise from the common truncus before it divides into left and right pulmonary arteries — *Type 1 truncus arteriosus*. In *Type 2 truncus arteriosus* the length of the main pulmonary artery segment is negligible, but the two pulmonary arteries arise close together just above the truncal valve. In *Type 3 truncus arteriosus* the left and right pulmonary arteries arise independently from the main truncus at a higher level, usually one from each side of the main artery. Type 3 truncus is the least common form. Various intermediate forms have also been classified. Pulmonary atresia with large aortopulmonary collateral vessels has sometimes been called pseudotruncus, but this is misleading as the condition is developmentally quite different.

In all cases there is common mixing across the ventricular septal defect and the flow in the pulmonary arteries is very large, because it originates directly from the common truncus which is at systemic pressure. In many cases a fully developed main pulmonary artery segment does not develop in its usual position and so the *chest X-ray* shows marked pulmonary plethora with a relatively narrow mediastinal shadow (as in transposition of the great vessels). With truncus arteriosus there is also an increased incidence of *right-sided aortic arch*. In many patients the heart is moderately enlarged and there may be cardiac failure. *Echocardiographic* diagnosis is relatively straightforward (Fig. 24.69), which is helpful, as it is difficult to perform good angiography on these patients due to the very fast blood flow through the heart which dilutes the contrast medium. The patients are often very ill, and catheterization with angiography produces significant morbidity. There may still be difficulties in obtaining good detail of the truncal branching pattern and MRI shows great promise in such cases.

Palliation by banding of the pulmonary artery is sometimes carried out, but the preferred operation is a complete correction with closure of the VSD. This will allow the left ventricle to empty through the truncal valve and a separate prosthetic or homograft valved conduit must be placed from the right ventricle to the pulmonary arteries (Fig. 24.70).

EBSTEIN'S ANOMALY

This condition is an anomaly of the tricuspid valve. It has often been described as a displacement of the tricuspid valve towards the apex of the right ventricle which produces a larger right atrium and a smaller right ventricle. This is in effect what is present, although the more precise descriptions of cardiac morphologists detail a condition in which the tricuspid annulus is normally positioned and the valve leaflets are larger and more redundant than normal, being adherent to the right ventricular walls, particularly the septum, for some distance into the ventricular cavity.

The result of this anomaly is a larger right atrium than normal (the so-called 'atrialized' portion of the right

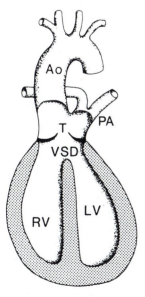

Fig. 24.68 Anatomy of truncus arteriosus. VSD = ventricular septal defect, RV = right ventricle, LV = left ventricle, T = common truncus arteriosus, PA = pulmonary artery, AO = aorta. (Reproduced with permission from Jordan & Scott 1989.)

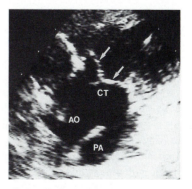

Fig. 24.69 Modified subcostal echocardiogram in truncus arteriosus. CT = common truncus, AO = aorta, PA = pulmonary artery. The truncal valve is arrowed.

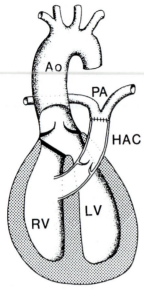

Fig. 24.70 Correction of common truncus arteriosus using the Rastelli procedure. RV = right ventricle, LV = left ventricle AO = aorta, HAC = homograft aortic conduit, PA = pulmonary artery. (Reproduced with permission from Jordan & Scott 1989.)

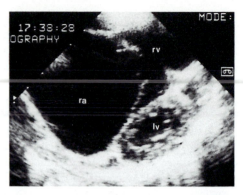

Fig. 24.72 Subcostal echocardiogram in a child with Ebstein's anomaly. This view shows the marked right atrial enlargement (ra) and the prominent tricuspid valve. In spite of the displacement of the valve, the right ventricle (rv) is still larger than the left ventricle (lv).

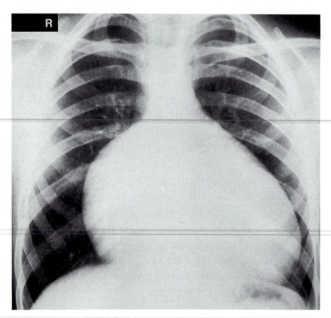

Fig. 24.71 Chest radiograph of a child with severe Ebstein's anomaly. There is marked globular cardiomegaly and pulmonary oligaemia.

ventricle) and a relatively small right ventricle which is relatively ineffective in pumping blood to the lungs. There is often associated infundibular narrowing. The function of the tricuspid valve itself is variable, sometimes being normal, but often showing significant regurgitation. The clinical presentation varies considerably, severe cases presenting in infancy with right heart failure and poor forward flow to the pulmonary artery. The chest X-ray in these cases may show massive globular cardiomegaly with pulmonary oligaemia (Fig. 24.71). The mildest expression occurs in some adults who present with mild signs or symptoms and a virtually normal chest X-ray.

Ultrasound studies show the abnormal tricuspid valve as a very prominent feature (Fig. 24.72) and many of the functional aspects can be derived from Doppler studies. The need for catheterization depends on the clinical severity and the quality of the echocardiogram.

SINUS OF VALSALVA FISTULA

In this condition there is usually enlargement of one of the sinuses of Valsalva in the aortic root, commonly the right sinus. This may rupture into the right ventricle and produce a left-to-right shunt. There will be continuous flow from the higher-pressure aorta to the right ventricle and the murmur may be mistaken for a patent ductus arteriosus, a coronary fistula or the recognized association of ventricular septal defect with aortic regurgitation.

The *chest X-ray* may show typical features of a left-to-right shunt but the aneurysmal sinus itself is rarely visible on the cardiac contour. *Echocardiography*, particularly with colour-flow Doppler mapping, will show the abnormality (Fig. 24.73). An aortic root *angiogram* will also show the lesion.

It is important to distinguish this condition from the *perimembranous ventricular defect*. The communications are in very similar positions, one above and one below the aortic valve. Besides visualization of the defect, differentiation can be achieved using continuous-wave Doppler studies, which will show that there is prominent continuous flow through the aortoventricular defect, which is due to the persistent differential pressure between the two chambers.

The principles of surgical repair are relatively straightforward but it may be complicated by aortic regurgitation due to the distortion of the aortic valve by the abnormality and the repair.

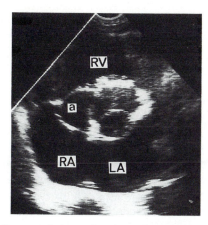

Fig. 24.73 Parasternal short-axis echocardiogram showing a sinus of Valsalva aneurysm (a). RV = right ventricle, RA = right atrium, LA = left atrium.

DOUBLE-OUTLET VENTRICLE

Double-outlet right ventricle is the most usual type of double-outlet ventricle. Once again each case must be assessed individually, but accurate anatomical assessment is vital. Corrective surgery is often possible but this depends on detailed knowledge of the intracardiac anatomy. There are usually two well-developed ventricles with a ventricular septal defect and so the positions of the great arteries and the septal defect must all be determined accurately. A double-outlet right ventricle with a large subaortic ventricular septal defect can be corrected by closing the ventricular septal defect with an oblique patch, allowing the left ventricle to empty to the aorta through the VSD. If the ventricular septal defect is subpulmonary, a similar operation will produce 'transposed great arteries' and this condition then has to be corrected using an atrial baffle procedure. The latter situation with a subpulmonary defect is often termed a *Taussig-Bing anomaly*.

The chest radiograph will give clues about the nature of the anomaly but echocardiography and cardiac angiography are both very important diagnostic techniques for the determination of the precise intracardiac anatomy.

GREAT ARTERIAL ANOMALIES (including vascular rings)

The commonest major variation in the aortic arch and its branching is the **anomalous right subclavian artery** occurring with a normal left-sided arch. The subclavian artery is the last brachiocephalic branch of the aorta, arising from the descending portion of the arch. The anomaly causes inconvenience for surgeons and those performing right brachial artery catheterization, but it does not normally produce symptoms. The vessel runs obliquely behind the oesophagus and its indentation can be recognised on the barium swallow.

There are two common forms of **right-sided aortic arch**. The first is the so-called *mirror image type* with the brachiocephalic branches being the mirror image of normal. This type is the most usual form of right arch to be found in association with the various types of cyanotic heart disease (25% incidence in tetralogy of Fallot and pulmonary atresia). The second form of right arch is that with an *anomalous origin of the left subclavian artery*. This is almost the mirror image of the anomalous right subclavian type but the anomalous vessel often arises from a prominent *diverticulum* which can make a prominent indentation in the posterior part of the oesophagus. This type is the most likely to be found as an isolated anomaly (approximately 0.1% of the population). Common aortic arch variations are shown in Figures 24.74A–D.

Double aortic arch is more serious as it can form a vascular ring that compresses the trachea or major bronchi and causes stridor in infancy. It can be diagnosed occasionally on the chest X-ray or barium swallow by evidence of bilateral compression on the trachea or oesophagus. Echocardiography may also be useful in making the diagnosis but it can be difficult to identify with confidence the two separate arches. Magnetic resonance imaging can show the condition clearly and

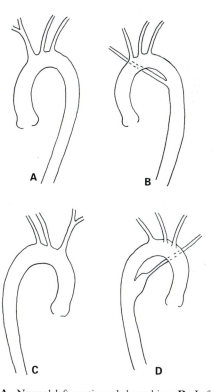

Fig. 24.74 A. Normal left aortic arch branching. **B.** Left aortic arch with an anomalous origin of the right subclavian artery. **C.** Right aortic arch with 'mirror image' branching. This is the commonest type associated with cyanotic congenital heart disease. **D.** Right aortic arch with an anomalous origin of the left subclavian artery arising from a posterior diverticulum. This is the commonest type of right aortic arch to occur as an isolated abnormality.

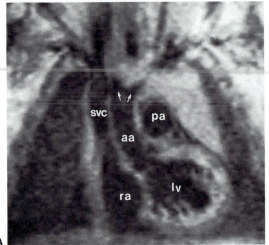

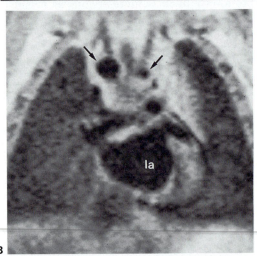

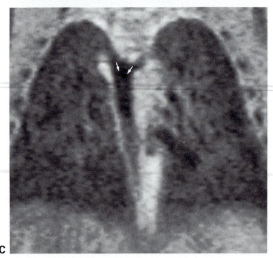

Fig. 24.75 A. Coronal gated spin-echo MR image from a child with a double aortic arch. The ascending aorta (aa) bifurcates at its upper end (arrows). lv = left ventricle, pa = pulmonary artery, svc = superior vena cava (svc), ra = right atrium. **B**. A more posterior coronal section from the same study. The large right and small left arches are shown in cross section (arrows) with brachiocephalic arteries arising from them. **C**. A yet more posterior coronal section of the same study, showing confluence of the two arches to form the descending aorta. The findings were confirmed at surgery with no angiography being necessary. (Courtesy of the Trustees of the Bristol MRI Centre.)

may become the investigation of choice in the future (Fig. 24.75). At present angiography is essential for definitive confirmation.

Anomalous origin of the left pulmonary artery (pulmonary artery sling) is another important cause of stridor in infancy. The left pulmonary artery arises as a branch of the right pulmonary artery and runs posteriorly to the right of the trachea, reaching its destination in the left hilum as it passes leftwards behind the trachea. This is one of the few conditions where the abnormal vascular structure runs anterior to the oesophagus (between oesophagus and trachea). This can occasionally be recognized as an abnormal soft-tissue structure on the lateral chest X-ray between the oesophagus and trachea. This condition is difficult to treat surgically as there may be distortion and narrowing of the trachea or bronchii.

Diagnosis may involve barium swallow and bronchography, but once again echocardiography and MRI may add more information, and arteriography will produce the definitive diagnosis.

There are very many other vascular anomalies, some of which can cause tracheal compression. Sometimes a vascular ring is formed by *rudimentary vascular bands* which are not demonstrated angiographically and this possibility must always be considered. Any vascular ring can potentially cause major airway obstruction, and thus stridor in infancy is a serious problem which must always be investigated thoroughly, usually with angiography (see Appendix B).

CORONARY ANOMALIES

There are many variants of coronary anatomy and most cause no problems. The most common is the '*left dominant*' system in which the posterior descending artery arises from the circumflex artery rather than the right coronary artery, this occurring in 5–10% of the normal population. Numerous other variants in the course of the vessels have been documented. There is one anomalous course with theoretical clinical consequences, namely the left coronary artery which runs between the aorta and main pulmonary artery where it may be compressed, but it has been hard to document this problem precisely.

Clinically important abnormalities include *anomalous origin* of one or both coronary arteries *from the pulmonary artery*. This leads to desaturated coronary perfusion and/or reversed coronary flow and can cause myocardial ischaemia, myocardial infarction or sudden death in infancy. Surviving infants can have marked cardiomegaly due to severe ischaemic cardiomyopathy.

Coronary fistulae to cardiac chambers or the pulmonary artery occur occasionally and often present asymptomatically with a continuous murmur. 90% drain to the right side of the heart, most often from the right coronary artery, and function as a right-to-left shunt. The shunt itself is often less of a worry in younger patients than the

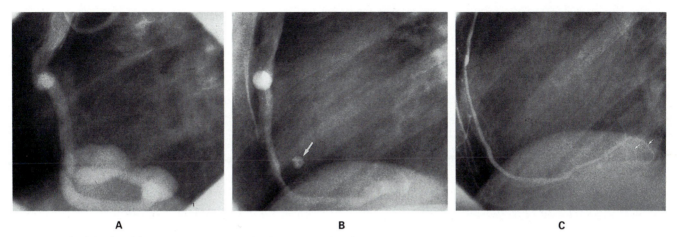

Fig. 24.76 A. Selective right coronary arteriogram in the L → L AO AO projection in a child with an aneurysmal fistula to the right ventricle. **B**. Angiogram in the same projection as (A) immediately after embolization with a detachable balloon (arrowed). **C**. Angiogram in the same projection taken one year later. The fistula remains closed, the right coronary artery has decreased in size and the distal myocardial branches are now seen (arrowed). (Courtesy Dr. G. Hartnell.)

other potential complications such as coronary ischaemia ('steal' phenomenon) or endocarditis. In later life the shunt may become symptomatic. The fistulous communications can dilate to aneurysmal proportions with the development of unusually positioned bumps on the heart border seen on *chest X-ray*. The aneurysmal fistulae may calcify and in theory they can rupture, but this latter has rarely been reported. These lesions may be diagnosed or suspected on *ultrasound* examination but *angiography* is essential for precise evaluation. The communications are commonly closed surgically to prevent complications but more recently, interventional occlusion techniques have been employed to close them (Fig. 24.76).

Kawasaki's disease is not a congenital abnormality but is acquired in childhood. It is probably infective in origin and has systemic features which give it the alternative name of '*mucocutaneous lymph node syndrome*'. A relatively mild illness in young children may be followed by the development of aneurysmal dilatation of the proximal coronary arteries. These can often be seen on *echocardiography* and there is generally no indication for angiography, because there is no specific therapy for the coronary abnormalities apart from general medical measures and observation. The coronary dilatations can resolve in many cases but in a minority, they can dilate and rupture or become stenotic.

ARTERIOVENOUS MALFORMATIONS (Systemic and pulmonary)

Both types of arteriovenous malformation are uncommon. **Systemic** arteriovenous malformations may cause local problems but can also produce high-output cardiac failure. A shunt through an *aneurysmal vein of Galen* in the skull is a possibility that must always be remembered when considering heart failure of unknown cause in in-

fancy. An intracranial bruit is often a key sign and a left ventricular or aortic injection must be followed to the skull to exclude this condition if it is seriously considered.

Pulmonary arteriovenous malformations can sometimes be obvious on the chest X-ray, but this is not always the case as they may be obscured by other structures or they may be of the complex (plexiform) type with no large vessel or aneurysm present. These abnormalities can produce profound central cyanosis and they require angiography for definitive diagnosis.

In some situations, systemic or pulmonary arteriovenous malformations are amenable to closure by transcatheter embolization, but frequently surgical treatment is necessary.

CARDIAC TUMOURS

It is debatable whether cardiac tumours can be described as congenital abnormalities but they occur occasionally in the newborn and have even been detected antenatally. The commonest tumour in children is the *rhabdomyoma*. This is usually histologically benign, a hamartoma, but can sometimes cause fatal obstruction within the heart. They are commonly multiple and are frequently associated with *tuberous sclerosis*. Surgery is best avoided as they do not grow with the heart and so become less of a problem as the child becomes older.

Teratomas and *fibromas* are occasionally diagnosed. The *myxoma* is a commoner tumour in the older child and has well-known features, particularly when it occurs in its commonest site, the left atrium. The presentation may be with a murmur, malaise and pyrexia, obstructive symptoms and signs or with a systemic embolus. All tumours, but particularly the left atrial myxoma, are well suited to diagnosis by *echocardiography* and the latter condition should always be treated by urgent surgical removal.

SYSTEMIC VENOUS ANOMALIES

Bilateral superior vena cava is the commonest systemic venous anomaly, being present in about 10% of patients with congenital heart disease. Many of these are small left-sided connections, only about half being large enough to be of haemodynamic significance. In a proportion of cases there is an intercommunicating vein between the two venae cavae at the root of the neck (Fig. 24.77). The left superior vena cava usually drains into the coronary sinus. It is not normally of clinical importance, but is surgically important, as the venous connections need to be correctly placed in instituting cardiopulmonary bypass, and in some complex procedures the presence of a left-sided superior vena cava is a positive benefit for construction of the final repair.

The condition cannot be diagnosed easily on the plain chest radiograph but is generally recognizable on a good-quality *echocardiogram*. The condition is often signalled by an unusually large coronary sinus entering the right atrium. *Angiography* will provide a definitive diagnosis and this can be performed via the inferior vena cava (during cardiac catheterization) or by a left subclavian vein injection.

Interruption of the inferior vena cava just before it reaches the heart is an uncommon anomaly. The venous drainage from the lower body continues into the azygos system, draining into the superior vena cava through the azygos vein on the right side. The hepatic veins usually drain directly to the right atrium. The abnormality rarely produces symptoms but can be very inconvenient if catheterization is being performed via the inferior vena cava.

FETAL ECHOCARDIOGRAPHY

The routine 16–18 week antenatal ultrasound scan has now expanded considerably to include assessment of a wide range of organs. The heart can be clearly visualized at this stage with good equipment, and the 'routine' examination should include assessment of the 'four-chamber view'. More detailed cardiac scanning starts with this view and includes other assessments as described below. This detailed cardiac assessment is only available in certain specialist centres at present but the technique is becoming more widely available as experience develops.

Protocol for fetal cardiac scanning

The transverse section of the fetal chest shows a four-chamber view with normal orientation of the cardiac apex to the left (Fig. 24.78). (The left side should be determined using the overall orientation of the fetus, not by comparison with adjacent organs which might also be malpositioned.)

The fetal heart should occupy about a third of the area of the thorax.

Both ventricles should be of similar size (Fig. 24.79). Both atria should be of similar size.

Mitral and tricuspid valves should be seen, in their normal offset relationship, the tricuspid valve being positioned slightly closer to the cardiac apex than the mitral valve.

The valve of the foramen ovale should be visible as a thin mobile structure on the left side of the atrial septum.

Adjustment of the transverse section should show normal connections of the pulmonary artery and aorta.

M-mode tracings of cardiac valve movements can often be recorded (Fig. 24.80).

The schedule described above is possible in most cases and can be used to exclude most major structural abnormalities, depending on the experience of the operator. If abnormalities are detected, decisions regarding future

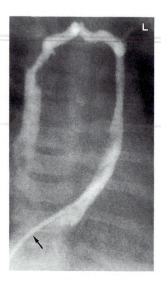

Fig. 24.77 Bilateral superior vena cava. A venous catheter (arrowed) has been used for an angiogram in the left superior vena cava which drains to the coronary sinus. There is a large intercommunicating vein between the left and right vena cavae.

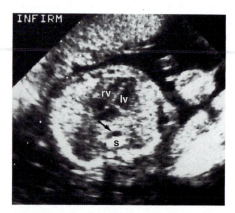

Fig. 24.78 Transverse echocardiogram of a 20-week fetus showing the 'four-chamber view'. rv = right ventricle, lv = left ventricle, s = spine. The descending aorta is arrowed.

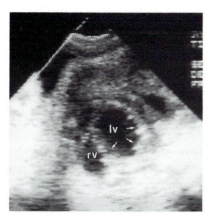

Fig. 24.79 Fetal echocardiogram in a fetus with a left ventricular cardiomyopathy due to critical aortic stenosis. The left ventricle (lv) is much larger than the right ventricle (rv), was visibly less contractile and showed endocardial fibroelastosis (arrowed) as an echogenic endocardium.

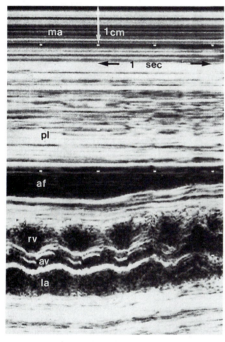

Fig. 24.80 M-mode echocardiogram across the normal aortic valve of a 20 week fetus. ma = maternal abdomen, pl = placenta, af = amniotic fluid, rv = right ventricle, av = aortic valve, la = left atrium. Depth and time markers are shown indicating that the heart rate is 150/min and the aortic root diameter is 4 mm.

management can be made and these include termination of pregnancy, treatment of the mother with drugs (fetal cardiac failure) and referral to a specialist centre for delivery. Defects with minor anatomical derangements such as small ventricular septal defect or isolated stenosis of the pulmonary valve cannot be detected reliably.

The technique can be extended further. The long and short axis planes of the heart can be shown to confirm the anatomy and connections of the great arteries. The aortic arch can usually be visualized. Systemic and pulmonary venous connections can often be seen. Doppler studies can be used to confirm normal flow through valves and vessels and this can sometimes demonstrate pathology such as a regurgitant valve.

Heart rate and rhythm, as well as more detailed assessment of ventricular function, can be derived from the fetal M-mode examination. The normal fetal heart rate is well in excess of 100 beats per minute (usually 150–180/min at 18 weeks' gestation). Persistent bradycardia below 100/min is associated with a high chance of structural cardiac abnormality. Transient periods of bradycardia (30–60 seconds only) are of no prognostic significance.

Most patients scanned are mothers who have had a previous child with congenital heart disease. In this group there is a two to three fold increase in the chance of congenital heart disease in the fetus. This should be seen in the context of overall incidence, and even in these mothers the chance of congenital cardiac abnormality being present is still only 2–3%. Thus the great majority of scans are normal and are reassuring for the parents. There is a small but increasing group of parents with congenital heart defects, in whom the risk of congenital heart disease in the fetus is slightly greater — 3–4%.

Referrals are also made in cases when a less experienced operator suspects an abnormality in a routine scan or a scan performed for another reason. It is not surprising to find that detailed cardiac scanning will reveal a much higher incidence of abnormality in this group, hence the importance of checking the four-chamber view as part of the protocol in the 'routine' antenatal scan. Detailed cardiac scans may also be helpful when other congenital abnormalities have been detected.

If a cardiac abnormality is detected it is essential to discuss the findings with the obstetrician and paediatric cardiologist so that proper advice can be given to the mother. In some cases of major abnormality, such as hypoplastic left heart syndrome, termination might be considered, but in other cases careful management of the pregnancy and early cardiological attention for the infant might be considered more appropriate. In many cases however, the outcome is poor even with careful management.

SUMMARY OF CHEST X-RAY APPEARANCES IN CONGENITAL HEART DISEASE

Particular points should be considered in the assessment of the chest film in the case of known or suspected congenital heart disease.

1. Note abdominal and cardiac *situs* at the start. If possible, assess the bronchial situs. Beware the handwritten side-marker: the radiographer may have been fooled too!

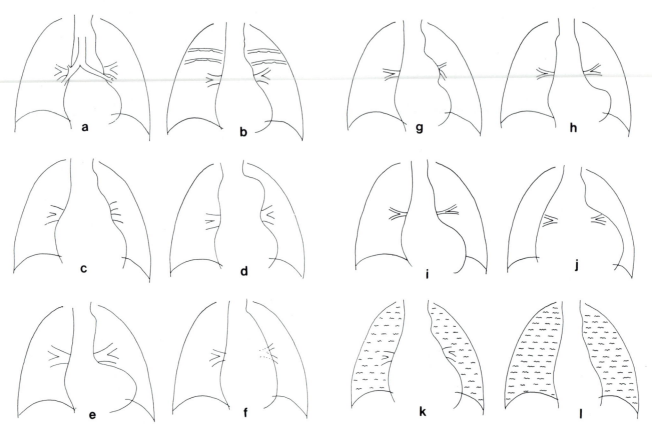

Fig. 24.81 a. Normal cardiac contour and normal pulmonary artery size. Normal bronchial anatomy is superimposed. **b**. Normal heart size and pulmonary vessels with a small and irregular aortic knuckle and rib notching. Established coarctation in an older child or adult. **c**. Cardiomegaly and large pulmonary vessels. Left-to-right shunt, particularly ASD or VSD. Also consider patent ductus arteriosus and partially or totally anomalous pulmonary venous connection of the cardiac type (draining directly to the heart). A left-to-right shunt alone rarely gives massive cardiomegaly. **d**. Cardiomegaly and large pulmonary vessels with a very wide upper mediastinum. Totally anomalous pulmonary venous connection of the supracardiac type. A large thymus will widen the mediastinum also. **e**. Moderate cardiomegaly and large pulmonary vessels with a small pulmonary artery segment. Pulmonary arteries must be anatomically abnormal so consider D-transposition of the great arteries and truncus arteriosus. The latter is more likely if the aortic arch is right-sided. **f**. Large smooth curve to the left heart border. L-transposition of the great arteries with an abnormal leftward position of the aorta. The appearance may also be due to other complex malpositions. L-TGA may occasionally have a virtually normal chest X-ray. **g**. Prominent main pulmonary artery with normal or small pulmonary vessels. Pulmonary valve venosis. The left pulmonary artery also may be dilated. The dilatation is not prominent in subpulmonary stenosis and is not invariably present in valvar stenosis. **h**. Upturned cardiac apex, right-sided aortic arch and small pulmonary vessels. Almost diagnostic of tetralogy of Fallot but can be seen in pulmonary atresia with a VSD and in a few cases of double outlet right ventricle (similar haemodynamics). **i**. Small pulmonary artery and pulmonary vessels with a large rounded left heart border. Tricuspid atresia. The condition is variable and there can be normal or occasionally increased vascularity depending on the haemodynamics of the VSD and pulmonary valve. Sometimes pulmonary atresia can give this appearance. **j**. Very large heart with normal or small pulmonary vessels. Ebstein's anomaly, dilated cardiomyopathy (including anomalous coronary origin from the pulmonary artery) and pericardial effusion. There may be associated left heart failure with cardiomyopathy. **k**. Cardiomegaly with large pulmonary vessels and pulmonary oedema. Left to right shunt with failure, left heart obstruction (aortic stenosis or coarctation) severe mitral regurgitation (alone or with other conditions) and cardiomyopathy. **l**. Small heart with pulmonary oedema. Obstruction before the heart. Totally anomalous pulmonary venous connection of the obstructed infracardiac type, cor triatriatum, congenital mitral stenosis. Pulmonary conditions must be distinguished.

2. Note the overall *cardiac size*. It is generally unhelpful to read too much into this unless comparing serial films. Consider only normal, moderately enlarged or very enlarged.

3. Look at the *mediastinum*. Is the pulmonary artery segment absent, small, normal or enlarged? Is the aortic arch visible, is it normal in appearance, on which side is it? (Note tracheal indentation and descending aorta as part of this). If a thymic shadow is present then assessment can be difficult.

4. Look at the *pulmonary vascularity*. First decide if the vessels are clearly visible or not. If not, consider heart failure (interstitial of alveolar pulmonary oedema), complex collateral vasculature, or pulmonary disease. These are not always easy to distinguish.

If vessels are distinct, are they:-
Definitely oligaemic
Normal to oligaemic

Normal
Normal to plethoric
Definitely plethoric
(Abnormal vascular distribution in the lung is generally unhelpful in infants and small children unless very marked — e.g. unilateral plethora with a shunt)

5. Is there any characteristic *unusual shape* to the heart contour that suggests a particular diagnosis?
6. Is there any *evidence of previous surgery*? (e.g. thoracotomy, sternal wires or implanted prosthesis)
7. Note *skeletal or other abnormalities*. (e.g. 11 pairs of ribs suggests Down's syndrome, which in turn suggests atrioventricular septal defect)

Figures 24.81a–l summarize major patterns to be seen in a number of well-recognized congenital cardiac abnormalities. The recognition of these patterns will not lead to a definitive diagnosis in many cases but it will usually help to classify the type of abnormality present, often allowing the radiologist to highlight key functional and anatomical features which will be of vital importance in further diagnosis and management of the patient.

SUMMARY OF IMAGING TECHNIQUES IN CONGENITAL HEART DISEASE

Plain chest radiograph
Essential in initial assessment but not necessarily fully diagnostic.
Essential in continuing management of patients.
Standard supine AP film in small children and infants.
Standard erect PA and lateral films in older children and adults.
Localized view for bronchial anatomy.

Fluoroscopy
Rarely needed for diagnostic purposes.
An essential part of diagnostic and therapeutic catheter techniques.

Barium swallow
Occasionally helpful in the assessment of vascular anomalies.
Otherwise superseded by other techniques.

Echocardiography
The most important noninvasive diagnostic technique.
Two-dimensional imaging uses three main echocardiographic windows (left parasternal, apical and subcostal) to examine the heart in three main planes (long-axis, short-axis and four-chamber). Modified views are also used as well as the suprasternal approach for assessing the great vessels.

M-mode imaging (one-dimensional imaging) is useful for accurate measurement of distances and timing within the heart.
Doppler echocardiography. Pulsed Doppler allows measurement of flow at a specific point selected within an image but is limited in its ability to record high-velocity flow accurately, with aliasing being a common problem. Continuous-wave Doppler can be used to measure the highest velocities but has no depth resolution along the beam. The high velocities in pathological flows can be used to deduce pressure drops by means of the modified Bernoulli equation. *Colour-flow mapping* is similar to pulsed Doppler examination but the image as a whole is analysed, flow towards and away from the transducer being coded in different colours. Colour-flow mapping is also limited in its ability to record high-velocity flow accurately.
Transoesophageal echocardiography. This technique can produce very high resolution images and is particularly suited to larger patients in whom good-quality imaging is hard to achieve. Paediatric-sized transducers are now available. The technique has increasingly important applications in the operating theatre and intensive care unit.

Nuclear medicine
Myocardial perfusion imaging is rarely indicated.
Ventriculography, particularly using first pass studies is useful for measuring pulmonary to systemic flow ratios. The normal decay of activity in the right ventricle as the activity moves on to the lungs is interrupted by additional peaks of activity as left-to-right shunting occurs. In complex cyanotic cases it can occasionally be useful to compare pulmonary and systemic blood flow by using *radionuclide-labelled microparticles*.

Computerized tomography (CT)
Normal scan times are too slow to allow accurate recording of intracardiac detail (typically no less than 2 s). In addition to this, contrast medium is needed to outline cardiac chambers. The technique is sometimes useful for the assessment of mediastinal masses which may be close to the heart. A few very sophisticated 'fast scanners' are in use in some specialist centres. These use an accelerator to produce an electron beam which can be moved very fast around the patient to give scan times of 50 milliseconds or less.

Magnetic Resonance Imaging (MRI)
This technique is in its infancy as far as the study of congenital heart disease is concerned but it holds enormous promise. Temporal and spatial resolution are limited at present but as equipment and techniques improve and become more widely available, MRI will

probably equal or even exceed echocardiography as the most important noninvasive cardiac imaging technique.

The advantages of cardiac MRI can be summarized as follows:-

1. Short scan times or gating can 'freeze' cardiac motion;
2. Scans can be taken in transverse, coronal or sagittal planes and complex combinations of these planes can also be achieved.
3. Cardiac chambers and walls can be distinguished clearly without the use of contrast media.
4. Blood flow patterns can be recognized. It will soon be possible to quantify stenotic and regurgitant lesions as well as volume flow (cardiac output, shunts etc.)
5. Three-dimensional reconstructions of complex anatomy will soon be possible.

Cardiac angiography

It will be some time yet before cardiac angiography is superseded as one of the mainstays of cardiac imaging. As noninvasive techniques replace catheter techniques in more and more cases, there is a parallel increase in interventional therapies, which need the full resources of a catheterization and angiography laboratory.

Most angiography is performed using 35-mm cine film recording techniques from the image intensifier. Equipment suspensions must allow a full range of oblique views, as well as cranial and caudal angulation, so that appropriate structures can be profiled. Biplane cine techniques are commonly in use in paediatric cardiology as they allow more views to be taken for smaller doses of contrast medium to the patient. *Digital recording* of images has now reached a stage where it is potentially better than cine film recording. Manipulation of contrast and other image detail is possible and radiation doses can be reduced significantly. Only the best (and most expensive) digital equipment is adequate, however, because image acquisition at 50 frames per second on a 512×512 matrix is an ideal requirement. This type of system requires a very large storage capacity and this has been one of the main factors limiting the development of cardiac digital studies. Digital recording of the radiographic image is the key requirement, subtraction of the digital image being only of secondary importance. Intravenous injections of contrast medium have not proved adequate, so digital techniques do not dispense with intracardiac catheters.

Contrast medium can put a major load on the circulation of a sick child and thus great care must be taken with its use. Nevertheless, it must be used properly, and inadequate volumes or rates of injection which produce poor angiograms are of no benefit to the patient. Wherever finances permit, nonionic media should be used and iodine concentrations of 350–400 mg/ml are necessary. Lower concentrations may be possible with good-quality digital equipment. Contrast medium should be administered fast enough to prevent unnecessary dilution, and catheter size must be selected appropriately for the anticipated injection.

The following is a guide to contrast medium doses for use with nonionic media of 370 mg iodine/ml, when using conventional cine film technique.

Start with 1 ml/kg, suitable for a normal ventricle in a neonate

Reduce by 25–50%, for hypoplastic chambers or a small aorta

Increase by 50–100%, for large chambers with large flow or shunts

Also reduce progressively with increasing weight, as follows:

2–10 kg, no change
10–20 kg, reduce by 20%
20–30 kg, reduce by 30%
30–50 kg, reduce by 40%

The contrast medium must be delivered in $1\frac{1}{2}$–2 cardiac cycles to avoid excessive dilution. Thus neonates with heart rates of 150–180/min will need it delivered in 0.5–0.7 second. This may not be possible if a relatively large dose is to be delivered through too small a catheter. If a child weighing 4 kg with a very large VSD and a heart rate of 180/min is to be studied by left ventriculography, a dose of 8 ml contrast medium should be delivered at 16 ml/s. This cannot be achieved through a 5 French catheter, and a 6 French size must be used.

Total dose limits are hard to state with accuracy, as they depend on the condition of the child and the sequence of the injections. 4 ml/kg is a safe limit for divided doses of 370 mg iodine/ml nonionic medium, provided the child is reasonably well and not dehydrated. With care and proper hydration this arbitrary limit can be exceeded. As with all diagnostic radiology, the potential benefits must be weighed against the potential hazards in any individual cases.

REFERENCES AND SUGGESTIONS FOR FURTHER READING

Anderson R. H., MacCartney F. J., Shinebourne E. A., Tynan M. J. (1987) *Paediatric Cardiology*. Churchill Livingstone, Edinburgh.

Freedom, R. M., Culham, J. A. G., Moes, C. A. F. (1984) *Angiocardiography of Congenital Heart Disease*. Macmillan, London.

Jordan, S. C., Scott, O. (1989) *Heart Disease in Paediatrics*. 3rd edn. Butterworths, London.

Sutton, M. St J., Oldershaw, P. (1989) *Textbook of Adult and Pediatric Echocardiography and Doppler*. Blackwell Scientific, Oxford.

Wilde, P. (1989) *Doppler Echocardiography*. Churchill Livingstone, Edinburgh.

CHAPTER 25

ARTERIOGRAPHY AND THERAPEUTIC ANGIOGRAPHY

David Sutton

Historical

It is a remarkable fact that the history of arteriography began only a few weeks after the discovery of X-rays. Roentgen announced his discovery of X-rays in December 1895 and the first arteriogram was produced within a month, when Haschek and Lindenthal in Vienna published the picture of the arteries of an amputated hand in January 1896.

Realizing the enormous potential of Roentgen's work they had immediately begun experimenting with the injection of radiopaque substances into the arteries of amputated limbs. Even by today's standards of rapid communication this was an outstanding achievement.

Unfortunately the absence of a safe intravascular contrast medium for in-vivo work and the prolonged exposures then necessary (about 60 minutes) meant that this work could not be put into clinical practice.

It was to be another 27 years before the first successful in-vivo arteriograms were achieved (Sicard & Forestier, 1923; Berberich & Hirsch 1923; Brooks, 1924). Soon afterwards, Moniz carried out his classical work on cerebral angiography which was published in 1928, and in 1929 Dos Santos described lumbar aortography.

Cardiac catheterization was first carried out by Forssman in Germany in 1929 and in 1936 Amiaille first opacified the heart chambers by catheterization. In 1937 Castellanos, Pereiras and Garcia described the use of right-heart angiocardiography in the diagnosis of congenital heart disease and in 1941 Farinas first described retrograde catheter angiography.

Although all the basic work had now been done, it was not till the 1950s that arteriography became widely used in medicine. This was because arteriography was still an investigation which required surgical intervention, and Scandinavian workers did not develop percutaneous techniques of arteriography till the 1940s. The percutaneous technique of catheterization was not developed till 1953 (Seldinger). It was these innovations which, together with the development of organic iodinated contrast media, set the stage for the more widespread use of angiography.

TECHNIQUES OF IMAGING ARTERIES

The vast majority of arterial investigations continue to be carried out by direct percutaneous needle puncture, or by percutaneous catheterization of arteries followed by conventional cut film radiography or by DSA. These will be discussed below.

Other imaging techniques, however, have made important and increasing contributions to the study of arterial pathology.

Ultrasound. This has long been used to demonstrate aneurysms of the abdominal aorta and is the simplest and cheapest method of diagnosing such lesions and measuring their size (Fig. 25.1). It is also an ideal method for monitoring the clinical progress of such aneurysms, and it can be used to diagnose and assess peripheral aneurysms as well.

The method can also be used to assess arterial stenosis and thrombosis of accessible vessels such as the internal carotid origins. The use of Doppler ultrasound for this and other purposes is discussed below.

Radionuclide angiography. Though resolution is too poor to compare with conventional angiography, the

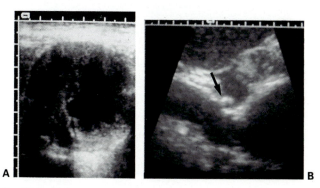

Fig. 25.1 Abdominal aortic aneurysm shown by ultrasound. **A**. Transverse section showing irregular intramural thrombus. The aneurysm diameter measures 5 cm. **B**. Coronal section. The right renal artery is clearly shown proximal to the upper end of the aneurysm (arrow). The coronal plane is essential for clear visualization of this area.

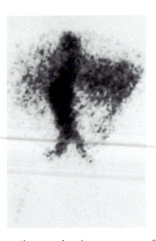

Fig. 25.2 Nuclear angiogram showing aneurysm of the abdominal aorta. This method gives a good idea of the lumen but not of the wall of clot.

method will readily show aortic aneurysms (Fig. 25.2) or major arterial occlusions. It has also been used to show the patency of arterial grafts; and is particularly useful in dealing with patients with known iodine sensitivity which precludes the use of conventional contrast media.

CT. This is a noninvasive method of demonstrating major vascular lesions such as thoracic or abdominal aneurysms. It is usual however to inject an i.v. bolus of contrast medium prior to the examination to show intraluminal clot and other abnormalities. With this technique large aneurysms are well shown and their dimensions accurately measured (Fig. 25.3). Dissecting

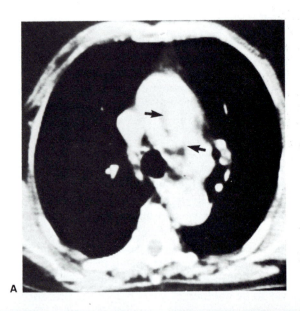

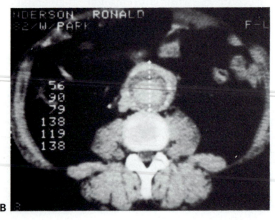

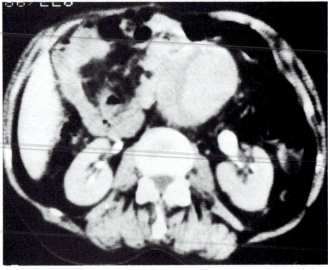

Fig. 25.3 A. CT scan of lower abdomen shows a huge abdominal aneurysm with a diameter of 8.5 cm and a calcified wall. **B**. CT scan of lower abdomen in another patient after i.v. contrast medium shows the lumen of a medium-sized aneurysm with a wall of clot. The diameter as measured by the electronic cursor is 5.6 cm. The wall is thickened and irregular and enhances with contrast medium, features of so-called 'inflammatory' aneurysms or perianeurysmal fibrosis.

Fig. 25.4 A. Dissecting aneurysm shown by CT after contrast medium; both true and false lumen are opacified but are separated by displaced intimal flaps (arrows) in the dilated ascending aorta (W512 L60). **B**. Dissection involving abdominal aorta, which shows fusiform aneurysmal dilatation. Contrast in both true and false lumens separated by intimal flap (W512 L38).

aneurysms can be diagnosed (Fig. 25.4) and the anatomy of a coarctation demonstrated. The patency of coronary or other arterial grafts can also be shown by CT.

MRI. This is an ideal noninvasive method for demonstrating lesions of the major vessels. The absence of intraluminal signal from rapidly-flowing blood provides a high degree of contrast between lumen and vessel wall and its surrounding tissues (Fig. 25.5). Thrombus and haematoma can be easily differentiated by their relatively high signal (Fig. 25.33), and major branches can be identified. Nevertheless ultrasound, as an equally noninvasive and radiation-free method of routine screening for such lesions as abdominal aortic aneurysms, remains the method of choice in the abdomen and limbs because it is so much cheaper and more readily available than MRI. The latter however is now of considerable importance in the brain and thorax and in the difficult and problem cases which are not readily resolved by ultrasound, e.g. some cases of suspected dissecting aneurysm. Recent advances in technique have also greatly improved the resolution and potential of MR angiography (see below).

Venous arteriography was used in the past as a method of showing major vessels such as the aorta without the hazards of direct arteriography. A large i.v. bolus of contrast medium was used and subtraction films of the appropriate area obtained to acquire images of the aorta and great vessels. These were often adequate for the demonstration of major lesions though the resolution was not comparable with that obtained by direct arteriography. This method was the forerunner of the more sophisticated digital subtraction angiography.

Digital subtraction angiography (DSA) is similar to the technique just described but uses the image intensifier and computers to obtain rapid digital information as the bolus of contrast medium passes through the arteries. The computer is able to subtract the bones and other tissues, leaving on the analogue images obtained only the vessels filled with contrast medium.

Using intravenous injections this method can be performed on an outpatient basis and has been widely used as a screening procedure for such lesions as carotid stenosis and thrombosis and renal artery stenosis. DSA has also proved useful as a less invasive technique for left ventriculography and for postoperative angiography. Thus it has been used to check the patency of grafts, in the follow-up of angioplasty, and in the postoperative assessment of aneurysms.

The technique is also now widely applied to direct arteriography. Here its main function is to reduce the dose and volume of contrast medium used for intraarterial injections and to permit the use of smaller and safer catheters. Catheters as small as 3F have been used, sometimes on an outpatient basis.

DIRECT ARTERIOGRAPHY

Two basic techniques are widely used for direct arteriography:

1. Percutaneous needle puncture.
2. Percutaneous arterial catheterization.

The sites for arterial puncture and arterial catheterization are illustrated in Figure 25.6.

PERCUTANEOUS NEEDLE PUNCTURE

In the past the method was applied to most vessels in the body, though percutaneous catheterization has now taken over many of the areas where it was once so widely used (e.g. carotid angiography). Investigations practised for different areas include or have included —

1. Head and neck
   a. Common carotid arteriography
   b. Vertebral arteriography
2. The upper limb
   a. Subclavian arteriography
   b. Axillary arteriography
   c. Brachial arteriography
3. The abdomen
   Lumbar aortography
4. The lower limb
   Femoral arteriography

For most practical purposes, direct needle puncture has now been superseded by percutaneous catheterization in the head and neck, upper limb and abdomen, though it is still widely used for femoral arteriography and to a lesser extent for lumbar aortography. It may still be used as a back-up method in the other areas when catheterization fails or is impractical for technical reasons.

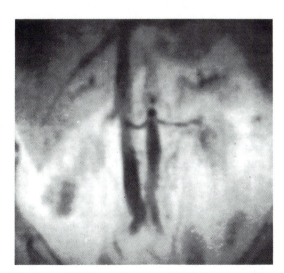

Fig. 25.5 Coronal MR scan showing abdominal aorta and renal arteries, IVC, hepatic and right renal veins.

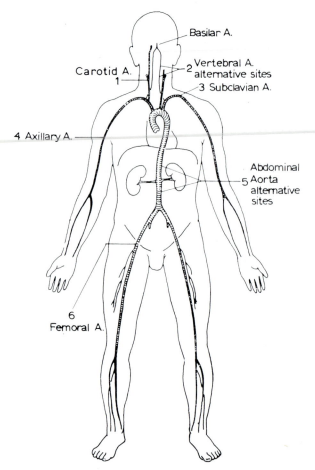

Fig. 25.6 Sites of arterial puncture: 1. Carotid artery; 2. Vertebral artery, showing alternative sites; 3. Subclavian artery; 4. Axillary artery; 5. Abdominal aorta showing alternative sites; 6. Common femoral artery. Sites of percutaneous catheterization: 6. Common femoral artery; 4. Axillary artery; 1. Carotid artery (rarely used).

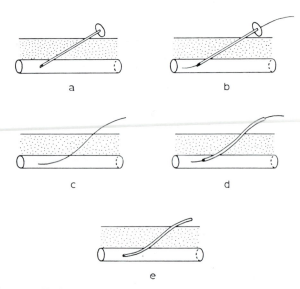

Fig. 25.7 Technique of percutaneous catheter insertion using the Seldinger-Sutton needle. a. Needle inserted into artery. b. Guide passed through needle into artery. c. Needle withdrawn leaving guide in artery. d. Catheter passed over guide into artery. e. Guide withdrawn leaving catheter in artery.

PERCUTANEOUS ARTERIAL CATHETERIZATION

Percutaneous arterial catheterization is based on the original work of Seldinger (1953) in Stockholm. The use of a special needle and guide-wire permits the percutaneous introduction of a catheter into a superficial and palpable vessel such as the femoral artery. The basic technique is illustrated in Figure 25.7. The most useful sites for the insertion of catheters into the arterial tree are:-

1. The femoral artery in the groin.
2. The axillary artery in the axilla.

Catheters have also been inserted from the brachial artery just above the elbow, from the common carotid artery in the neck, and from the abdominal aorta using a translumbar approach. In practice, the femoral and axillary arteries permit investigation of most areas and the other sites of insertion are little used.

Selective and superselective arterial catheterization

This is a refinement of the standard technique in which specially shaped catheters are introduced into branches or sub-branches of the aorta. Arteries which are frequently catheterized include most major branches of the abdominal aorta (renal, coeliac axis, superior and inferior mesenteric arteries), major branches of the aortic arch (subclavian, innominate and left common carotid arteries and their major branches, including the vertebrals, internal and external carotid arteries). Superselective catheterization is frequently performed on branches of the coeliac axis, including the splenic, hepatic and gastroduodenal arteries, and on branches of the external carotid such as the internal maxillary.

Most catheterizations are now performed with relatively small catheters, usually of 5 French gauge.

TECHNIQUE OF ARTERIAL PUNCTURE

The technique used for arterial needle puncture is similar for most of the arteries used.

The common femoral artery is readily palpable in the groin and is usually punctured just below Poupart's ligament. The axillary artery is palpable with the arm held in abduction and is punctured in its lower part. The common carotid artery was punctured with the neck slightly extended, though as noted above this is now rarely done.

In all the above cases the artery is palpated and fixed by the index and middle fingers of the operator's left hand whilst the needle is inserted with the right hand.

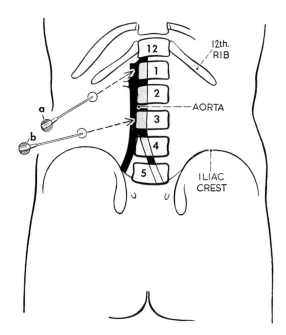

Fig. 25.8 Lumbar aortography — site of puncture. a. High puncture. b. Low puncture.

For lumbar aortography the abdominal aorta is approached from the left lumbar region with the patient lying prone. A preliminary X-ray film with markers is usually taken to localize the vertebral levels. Depending on the purpose of the investigation, the aorta is punctured either at L1 (for renal angiography, aortic thrombosis, or abdominal aneurysms) or below the renals at L3 (for low aortic or iliac or peripheral vascular disease) (Fig. 25.8).

Successful puncture of an artery is marked by rapid pulsation of arterial blood through the needle into the transparent plastic connecting tubing. This is the signal for immediate flushing of the system with saline, which is then sealed off by the tap between tubing and syringe. Saline flushing is continued intermittently throughout the procedure except during the contrast medium injections. The aim is to keep the needle and tubing free of blood (except momentarily) so that no stasis or clotting can occur in the system.

TECHNIQUE OF PERCUTANEOUS CATHETERIZATION

A simplified Seldinger technique routinely used by the author is illustrated in Figure 25.7, and consists of the following consecutive steps:

1. The artery (usually the femoral and less commonly the axillary) is punctured by a thin-walled needle exactly as described above;
2. Once the needle tip is firmly in the vessel lumen the connecting tubing is detached, allowing blood to spurt back (Fig 25.7A). The guide-wire is then immediately passed through the needle into the vessel and its tip advanced 5–8 cm (two or three inches) along the lumen (Fig. 25.7B). Holding the guidewire firmly in position, the needle is then withdrawn along it and off the guide wire (Fig. 25.7C).

   Meanwhile firm manual pressure is maintained with gauze swabs at the puncture site to prevent oozing of blood and haematoma formation.
3. The catheter, with a two-way tap attached to its hind end, is now passed along the guide-wire and into the artery. The guide-wire is longer than the catheter and protrudes from its back end once the catheter tip reaches beyond its front end (Fig. 25.7D). It can then be removed, leaving the catheter safely in the artery (Fig 25.7E). Saline can now be perfused through the catheter exactly as with needle puncture.

The catheter can now be passed along the artery to any desired level. In tortuous or atheromatous arteries it may be necessary to use special guides with 'J' or more flexible tips in order to advance catheters through difficult areas.

Saline infusion of the catheter is maintained either by slow hand injection or by an automatic drip system. Unless contraindicated for clinical reasons, heparinized saline is routinely used to counteract any tendency to clot formation in or around the catheter tip.

RADIOGRAPHIC APPARATUS

Arteriography requires rapid serial films of the area under investigation to capture the flow of contrast medium through the arteries and in some cases through the capillary bed and drainage veins as well. In some areas (e.g. the lower limb) four serial films taken within 5 to 8 seconds may be adequate; in others (e.g. the aortic arch) films taken at 3 or 4 per second for 4 seconds may be necessary. In certain situations such as large AV fistulas or angiomas, multiple rapid serial films will also be required to define the full anatomy of the lesion.

Many types of commercial serial film changers are on the market and choice will depend on local availability and preferences. The Schonander cut-film changers allow speeds up to 6 films per second and the Elema roll film faster speeds up to 12 frames per second. For most purposes the versatile Puck changers, allowing speeds of 3 films per second, are adequate.

Fine-focus high-power X-ray tubes are essential for rapid serial films and to facilitate *magnification* techniques. *Subtraction* techniques are also widely used in angiography.

Arteriography is now widely practised using DSA. This has many advantages, including lower doses and volumes of contrast medium and automatic electronic subtraction. Resolution is less than can be obtained with the best film techniques but is adequate for most practical purposes.

Injections of contrast medium can be performed by hand for many forms of angiography, but pressure injection using specialized apparatus is essential for thoracic aortography, abdominal flush aortography and angiocardiography. It is also essential for DSA using intravenous injection.

ANAESTHESIA

Most angiographic procedures can be carried out under local anaesthesia, but basal sedation may be necessary with the more complex investigations. Some drugs such as *pethidine* are more likely than others to produce a hypotensive reaction and must therefore be used with caution, particularly if arterial stenosis is suspected.

General anaesthesia is usually necessary with children and may be required with difficult or very nervous patients or those unable to cooperate. Besides prolonging the investigation and increasing its cost, it undoubtedly adds to the hazards, since the patient is unable to react to misplaced injections or other mishaps. With a conscious patient, symptoms and untoward reactions are at once apparent and the procedure can be stopped immediately.

CONTRAST MEDIA

The earliest vascular contrast media mentioned above were far from ideal. They included lipiodol injected into veins in small quantity (Sicard & Forestier); strontium bromide (Berberich & Hirsch), and sodium iodide (Brooks), which were the first contrast agents injected into arteries. Thorium dioxide (Thorotrast) was used by Moniz and became the standard medium in the 1930s. Unfortunately it was retained indefinitely by the reticuloendothelial system, and being radioactive gave rise to delayed malignancy. Abdominal films taken years after injection showed a characteristic stippling in the spleen resembling miliary calcification.

Organic iodide preparations stemmed from the work of Swick (1929) who developed uroselectan (Iopax) (containing one atom of iodine per molecule) as a reliable agent for intravenous urography. Later, organic iodides were developed, first with two and then with three atoms of iodine per molecule. The standard media widely used in the 70s and 80s are listed in Table 25.1.

The ideal contrast medium should be completely non-toxic and completely painless to the patient in the high concentrations used for angiography. A further advance towards this ideal was the introduction in the eighties of *low-osmolality contrast media*. These agents are relatively painless, compared with their high-osmolar predecessors,

Table 25.1 Intravascular contrast media

Product	Formula	Iodine content, g/ml	viscosity, mPa.s, at 37°C
Hypaque 45	a. Sodium diatrizoate 45% w/v	0.27	2.1
Hypaque 65	b. Sodium diatrizoate 25% w/v and N-methylglucamine salt of diatrizoic acid 50% w/v		8.4
Hypaque 85	As Hypaque 65 but mixture is: (1) 28.33% w/v; and (2) 56.67% w/v	0.44	12.2
Urografin 290	Mixture of the sodium and the methylglucamine salts if diatrizoic acid in the proportion 10 : 66	0.44	8.4
Urografin 370		0.37	8.5
Urografin 310 (Angiografin)	Meglumine amidotrizoate 65%	0.306	5.1
Conray 280	Meglumine iothalamate 60% w/v	0.28	4.0
Conray 325	Sodium iothalamate 54% w/v	0.375	2.7
Conray 420	Sodium iothalamate 70% w/v	0.42	5.4
Cardio-Conray	Meglumine iothalamate 52%, sodium iothalamate 26% w/v	0.40	8.6
Triosil 280	Meglumine metrizoate 59% w/v (with Ca)	0.28	4.0
Triosil 370	Meglumine metrizoate (with Na and Ca)	0.37	8.5
Triosil 350	Sodium metrizoate 52% w/v (with meglumine, Ca or Mg)	0.35	3.4
Triosil 440	Sodium metrizoate 66% w/v (with meglumine, Ca or Mg)	0.44	6.6

and are claimed to produce fewer toxic side-effects. Both these benefits are related to the low osmolality, which is closer to that of normal plasma than was that of their predecessors. At an iodine concentration of 280 mg/ml the osmolality measures about 480 mmol/kg H_2O. This compares with 1500 for the equivalent Conray (high-osmolar) preparation and 300 for plasma (Table 25.2).

Further low-osmolality contrast media introduced in recent years include Ultravist (Schering) (= iopromide) and Iopentol (Nycomed, Oslo). Also recently introduced is Isovist (iotrolan) (Schering), a dimeric nonionic low-osmolar contrast medium.

Osmolality is proportional to the ratio of iodine atoms to the number of particles in solution. In the older hyperosmolar contrast media, this ratio was 3 : 2, whereas the new low-osmolar agents have a ratio of 3 : 1 and do not ionize in solution. Ioxaglate, which is a monoacid dimer, does ionize in solution but has a similar iodine : particle ratio (6 : 2 or effectively 3 : 1) and therefore enjoys the same benefits of low osmolality. To date the only drawback to the new media is that they cost a good deal more than their predecessors, and this remains an important factor inhibiting their more widespread use.

Table 25.2 Low-osmolality contrast media

Product	General formula	Iodine atoms: particles in solution	Iodine content mg/ml	Viscosity at 37°C
Iopamidol (Niopam), non-ionic		3 : 1	200	2.0
			300	4.7
			370	8.6
Iohexol (Omnipaque), non-ionic	Similar to above but with different radicles R_1, R_2 or R_3	3 : 1	240	3.3
			280	4.8
			300	6.1
			350	10.6
Ioxaglate (Hexabrix), ionic		6 : 2 [= 3 : 1]	320	7.5

Dosage

Peripheral and smaller arteries. As a general principle, the dose of contrast medium injected is related to the flow rate in the vessel being injected. Small vessels with low flow rates require small amounts at low pressures, whilst large vessels with high flow rates require larger volumes at high pressures. The recommended doses for different smaller arteries are listed in Table 25.3, and in most arteries the recommended dose can safely be repeated after a short interval. In each case the injection is made in about 1 to 2 seconds.

Of the high-osmolar contrast media, we regarded Urografin 310 as the best for cerebral angiography and Triosil 370 as preferable for coronary angiography, since there is experimental evidence that these agents are less toxic than other high-osmolar products at these sites. The quantity used for coronary artery injections varies from 4 to 8 ml, depending on the state of the patient and the flow rate in the individual vessel.

As already explained, the new low-osmolar contrast media are preferable to the older high-osmolar products and should be used routinely whenever cost is not a major inhibiting factor.

Larger arteries. *1. Arch aortography.* For injections into the aortic arch, which has the highest flow rate in the body, 40 ml of high-concentration contrast medium

Table 25.3 Recommended doses (ml) of Conray 280 or equivalent (smaller arteries)

Femoral artery	20
Subclavian (or axillary) artery	20
Carotid artery	10
Vertebral artery	8
Renal artery	10
Inferior mesenteric artery	15
Intercostal artery	3
Bronchial artery	5

is injected by pressure machine at 20 ml/s. Triosil 370 or 440 or Conray 420 were high-osmolar products widely used for this purpose, though they are now largely replaced by the new low-osmolar agents such as iopamidol 370, iohexol 350 or Hexabrix 320.

2. Abdominal aortography. Whether performed by catheter or by lumbar injection, 30 ml of a high-concentration contrast medium (Conray 420, Hypaque 350, Hexabrix 320 or iohexol 350), delivered in 1.5–2 seconds, is regarded as a safe dose for high aortic injection — i.e. above the renal arteries — and provided both kidneys are functioning normally. However if there is severe renal impairment or only one kidney functioning, caution should be observed and the dose reduced to a maximum of 20 ml. Similar precaution is necessary if there is an aortic thrombosis present which would result in a higher dose to the kidneys.

For a low aortic injection — i.e. below the renal arteries — 25 ml injected in 1.5 seconds is usually adequate.

The normal coeliac axis and superior mesenteric arteries both have high flow rates and can tolerate injections of 30 ml of Hypaque 350 or equivalents at one injection. Some workers recommend doses as high as 50 ml where it is desirable to show the portal circulation. Speed of injection, however, is relatively low at 8 ml/s.

Contrast medium reactions

Reactions to the intravascular injection of contrast media, whether intravenous or intra-arterial, are not uncommon (about 12% in one major i.v. series using high-osmolar contrast media). Fortunately the vast majority are trivial or of minor importance. Reactions can be classified as mild, intermediate or severe. The latter are potentially fatal but formed less than 0.25% of the series just quoted.

The mechanism of these reactions is debated, though many factors have been postulated, including anxiety, histamine and serotonin release, antigen antibody formation, activation of the complement and coagulation systems, and interruption of the blood–brain barrier.

Mild reactions include sneezing, mild urticaria, nausea and vomiting, feelings of heat or cold, tachycardia or bradycardia, and arm pain following intravenous injections. Recovery is rapid and requires no treatment except reassurance.

Intermediate reactions include widespread urticaria, bronchospasm and laryngospasm, angioneurotic oedema, and moderate hypotension. Immediate treatment is required but response is rapid.

Severe reactions are rare but can be fatal. They include cardiopulmonary collapse with severe hypotension, pulmonary oedema, refractory bronchospasm and laryngospasm. The *mortality* from hyperosmolar intravenous contrast medium injections is estimated at 1 case per 40,000 injections. Arterial injections probably carry a similar risk.

The risk from the newer low-osmolar media appears to be significantly lower for minor and intermediate reactions (about 3% as against 12%); it also appears to be significantly lower for severe reactions, but is not yet accurately quantified for fatal reactions, where the evidence remains inconclusive.

Major risk factors associated with the use of contrast media include: 1. allergy, especially asthma; 2. extremes of age (under 1 year and over 60 years); 3. cardiovascular disease; and 4. history of previous reaction to contrast medium. Minor risk factors include diabetes mellitus, dehydration, impaired renal function, haemoglobinopathy and dysproteinaemia.

Previous minor reactions to contrast medium are not a contraindication to a repeat examination, but patients with previous severe reactions should be examined by other means. Patients with previous intermediate reactions should be carefully assessed and the examination abandoned or, if essential, only repeated under careful control. This implies pretreatment for three days with oral prednisone (50 mg) 8-hourly. Ephedrine (25 mg) and diphenhydramine (50 mg) are also given one hour before the examination and only a low-osmolar contrast medium should be used.

Pretesting for allergy with small doses of contrast medium was once widely performed but has now been abandoned as completely unreliable. Fatalities have occurred after previous negative test doses and test doses have resulted in fatalities.

Treatment. Emergency drugs and equipment should be immediately available wherever contrast media are used. Intermediate and severe reactions usually involve hypotension, which is treated by elevation of the legs and may require rapid intravascular fluid. Oxygen may also need to be administered, and it is essential to distinguish a vasovagal reaction (characterized by hypotension with *bradycardia*) from an allergic or anaphylactoid reaction (characterized by hypotension with *tachycardia*). The former requires *atropine*, whilst the latter requires *epinephrine* (adrenalin).

Iodism. The radiologist should be aware that free iodine present in contrast media will interfere with the performance of radioactive iodine tests of thyroid function. Salivary gland enlargement ('iodine mumps') may follow several days after the injection and hyperthyroidism may be induced.

Nephrotoxicity. Intravascular contrast media may have a nephrotoxic effect. The pathogenesis is debated but may be multifactorial due to vasoconstriction, a direct toxic effect on tubular cells and cast formation in tubules with intrarenal obstruction. Acute renal failure due to nephrotoxicity is claimed to occur in 5% of patients with chronic renal failure but in less than 1% of patients with normal function. Clinically the patient may be asymptomatic with rapid recovery, show non-oliguric renal dysfunction, or, rarely, show severe oliguric renal failure.

Risk factors include large doses of contrast medium, dehydration, diabetes mellitus, pre-existing renal insufficiency and multiple myeloma. Caution in administering contrast media is desirable in diabetic patients with impaired renal function, in multiple myeloma patients with Bence-Jones proteinuria and in hyperuricaemic patients. Dehydration is definitely contraindicated in patients at risk.

PHARMACOANGIOGRAPHY

This refers to the use of vasoactive drugs to modify blood flow to target organs. The procedure was once very popular but is now less frequently used.

Vasodilators were used to reverse vasospasm, to increase the size of arterioles and collaterals, and to improve the visualization of the venous return. They will also enhance the outline of nonvascular lesions such as cysts, by contrast with the enhanced parenchyma. They were once widely used in arterioportography for better visualization of the portal circulation. They were also used in peripheral arteriography to improve visualization of poorly filling distal vessels.

The vasodilators used were *Priscoline* (tolazoline) for the splanchnic, femoral and brachial arteries, *prostaglandin E1* in the femoral artery and *bradykinin* in the renal and superior mesenteric arteries.

In healthy patients Priscoline was given as a 25-mg bolus in the splanchnic vessels and as a 12-mg bolus into limb vessels. It must be used with caution in cardiac patients as it can produce hypotension and cardiac arrhythmias.

Vasoconstrictors can help to distinguish tumour from normal circulation since the latter reacts to them but the former does not and thus stands out more clearly. Epinephrine (adrenaline) was once widely used for this purpose in both renal and splanchnic arteriography. It is administered as a 3–6 µg bolus into the renal artery and as a 5–8 µg bolus into splanchnic vessels. Vasopressin and angiotensin have also been used as vasoconstrictors.

Epinephrine increases blood pressure and peripheral resistance and must therefore be used with great caution in patients with cardiac disease, where it may be contraindicated.

Hyperventilation can be used in cerebral angiography to produce similar effects, since normal cerebral vessels react to hyperoxaemia and hypocapnia by vasoconstriction whilst tumour vessels are unaffected. Hyperventilation was performed by the anaesthetist in cerebral angiograms conducted under general anaesthesia.

COMPLICATIONS

Many complications have resulted from arteriography and these are summarised in Table 25.4. This formidable list of complications emphasizes that arteriography should not be undertaken lightly and that it is best performed by radiologists with considerable training and experience in this field. The complication rate is also significantly lower at centres where large numbers of arteriograms are routinely performed than at centres where they are only occasionally seen.

A full discussion of the complications of arteriography will be found in specialist monographs, but attention is drawn below to some of the more important complications.

Damage to arterial walls. This may result from a traumatic needle or catheter puncture. Local subintimal stripping may result, particularly if contrast medium or saline is accidentally injected subintimally (Figs 25.9, 25.10). In small vessels this can result in actual occlusion and thrombosis (see below). The use of short bevelled needles, together with skill and experience, is the main means of preventing these accidents.

Perivascular injection of contrast medium can also occur (Fig. 25.11), but is relatively harmless apart from local pain and discomfort to the patient being examined under local anaesthesia.

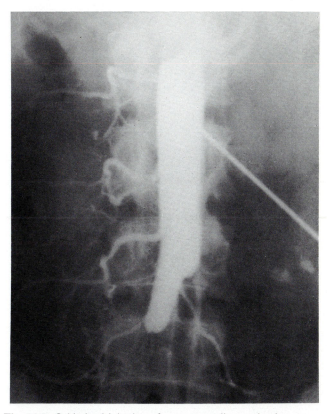

Fig. 25.9 Subintimal injection of contrast medium at lumbar aortography. Most of the contrast medium lies in the wall of the aorta and right common iliac artery. A small amount is intraluminal and outlines lumbar arteries. Contrast medium in the aortic wall persists on serial films.

Table 25.4 Complications of contrast arteriography

A. General
  1. Contrast reactions
    a. Severe life-threatening
    b. Intermediate
    c. Minor (coughing, sneezing, mild, urticaria)

  2. Embolus
    a. Catheter clot
    b. Cholesterol
    c. Cotton fibre
    d. Air

  3. Septicaemia

  4. Vagal inhibition

B. Local
  1. Puncture site
    a. Haemorrhage and haematoma
    b. False aneurysm
    c. AV fistula
    d. Perivascular or subintimal contrast injection
    e. Local thrombosis
    f. Local infection
    g. Damage to adjacent nerves

  2. Damage to target or other organs due to
    a. Excess of contrast
    b. Catheter clot embolus

  3. Fracture and loss of guide-wire tip

  4. Knot formation in catheters

  5. Embolization accidents (see below)

  6. Angioplasty accidents (see below)

Thrombosis of arteries. As just noted, this can result from trauma to the arterial wall at arterial puncture, or from subintimal stripping from injections of contrast medium or saline with formation of a local dissecting aneurysm. Another well-documented mechanism is formation of clot at the end of a catheter. This is then stripped off as the catheter is withdrawn through the puncture hole and forms a focus for local thrombosis. Another causative or contributory factor is a severe hypotensive reaction (see below). Whatever mechanism or combination of mechanisms is responsible, there is also a direct relationship with the experience of the operator and with the adequacy of the patient's cardiovascular system. Patients with cardiovascular insufficiency and severely atheromatous vessels are at greater risk, and should only be examined by experienced operators.

Systemic **heparinization** is generally recommended to counter catheter clot formation and thrombosis. As soon as the catheter has been passed into the aorta, 3000 units of heparin are injected. The procedure is useful in prolonged catheterization procedures and rarely causes any problem. If there is excessive oozing from the puncture site at completion, heparinization can be reversed by

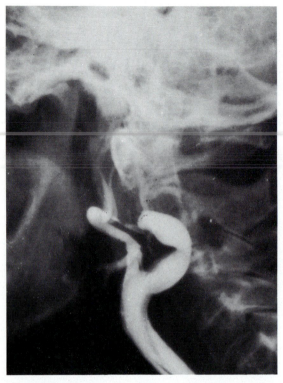

Fig. 25.10 Subintimal injection of contrast medium at needle common carotid arteriogram. Contrast medium persists in the arterial wall on serial films. Note linear translucencies caused by displaced intima.

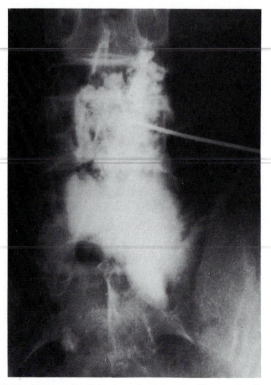

Fig. 25.11 Perivascular injection of contrast medium at lumbar aortography.

injecting 10 mg protamine sulphate per 1000 units of heparin used.

Allergy. The minor allergic contrast reactions (see above) rarely give rise to concern and patients can be reassured that sneezing, coughing or urticaria will rapidly subside. However, radiologists must be aware of the danger of the very rare major hypersensitivity reaction, and be prepared for its prompt treatment. This requires dexamethasone 10–20 mg i.v., and if necessary artificial respiration with positive pressure and oxygen. For oedema of the glottis, 0.5 mg adrenaline subcutaneously or intramuscularly is recommended, together with slow intravenous injection of an antihistamine. Arrangements should also be ready beforehand for the emergency treatment of such catastrophies as cardiac arrest, ventricular fibrillation and collapse with circulatory insufficiency.

Hypotension. Severe hypotensive reactions may occur with any arteriographic procedure, but particularly with complex or prolonged investigations. Blood pressure should be monitored and it should be remembered that patients with vascular disease, particularly atheromatous stenosis, may have lesions in many vessels and that hypotension can precipitate a thrombosis. Coronary infarction or hemiplegia from a carotid thrombosis are potential complications.

Hypotension has also been recorded several hours after a major procedure and the patient must be monitored on the ward for several hours after arteriography.

Catheter clot embolus. Clot may form in and around the tip of a catheter, particularly during a prolonged procedure, and such clot may be detached by a contrast medium injection. The main danger is with catheters lying in or proximal to the cerebral vessels, when detached clot may be directed to the brain. Left ventriculography, coronary arteriography, arch aortography and 'headhunter' catheterization of the cerebral and subclavian vessels are all procedures which carry this risk. The use of small catheters and speedy and skilled angiography help to minimize the risk, as does systemic heparinization.

Cholesterol embolization may occur spontaneously in patients with severe atheromatous disease. It may also occur after surgery, and is occasionally precipitated by arterial catheterization. A large shower of cholesterol crystals can produce disastrous results, particularly if vital organs are involved. Postmortem studies suggest that minor degrees of cholesterol crystal embolism are commoner than is generally appreciated.

Air embolus has undoubtedly been a cause of fatalities in the past, particularly when large steel syringes were used for major injections. Air could easily enter a large opaque syringe and could be injected without the operator being aware of the mishap, especially if the nozzle was horizontal or pointing upwards. Even with the translucent plastic syringes now in general use, great care must be taken not to include air when loading with contrast medium or saline solution and all injections should be made with the nozzle pointing down.

Haematomas and **false aneurysms** at the puncture site should be relatively uncommon, provided small needles are used and the tips of larger catheters are well tapered. They are seen most frequently with hypertensive patients. After an arterial puncture, firm manual pressure transmitted through gauze swabs should be maintained on the puncture site till all oozing has stopped. The puncture site should also be inspected before the patient leaves the department (an hour or two later) and the following morning, and the patient warned to report immediately if there is any further swelling or oozing.

False aneurysms (pulsating haematomas) will require surgical treatment.

It is important to ensure that any patient is taken off anticoagulant drugs before arteriography and that the prothrombin time has fallen to normal before the investigation.

Damage to nerves. Transaxillary catheterization carries the particular risk of damage to branches of the brachial plexus since the artery is closely related to its distal part. This can result in severe disability. Most of the reported cases were due to nerve compression by haematomas or false aneurysms, though direct damage by needle puncture may be responsible in some cases. Transaxillary catheterization should only be undertaken by senior and experienced angiographers, and observation for signs of haematoma or nerve damage should be maintained for 24 hours after the investigation. If symptoms of paresis appear and progress, they are usually due to compression by a haematoma, and urgent surgical decompression of the neurovascular sheath is essential if permanent paralysis is to be prevented.

Vagal inhibition may occur after a major contrast-medium injection and has been encountered after intravenous urography and intravenous cholangiography. It is characterized by collapse of the patient with bradycardia. This helps to distinguish it from circulatory collapse in acute allergy, which is usually associated with tachycardia. The distinction is of vital importance, since the latter is often treated with adrenalin, a drug which is contraindicated in vagal inhibition, where atropine is the drug of choice and may be life-saving.

Damage to organs. Since angiography often targets vital organs, including heart, brain, kidneys and bowel, it is not surprising that damage to such organs can result, followed by death or serious morbidity. In most cases the cause has been arterial thrombosis from the causes mentioned above or organ damage from an excessive dose of contrast medium.

Non-fatal *brain damage* has resulted in hemiplegia, both transient and permanent. Cortical blindness — occasionally permanent, but fortunately in most case transient — has resulted from vertebral angiography.

Spinal cord damage is a rare and tragic complication of arteriography, usually due to an excessive dose of contrast medium entering a main artery of supply to the spinal cord. Thus paraplegia has been recorded after both lumbar and abdominal aortography, presumably from injection of the artery of Adamkewicz which supplies the cord from D8 downwards and arises from one of the upper lumbar or lower intercostal arteries.

Tetraplegia has resulted from vertebral angiography and from thyroid axis angiography. In the latter case, an excess of contrast medium has entered the deep cervical artery which supplies the cervical cord. It has been suggested that such cases should be treated by replacement of CSF with isotonic saline and by systemic steroids, though others doubt the value of this.

Coronary angiography carries the special dangers of vagal inhibition, ventricular fibrillation, cardiac systole and myocardial infarction. All of these are potentially fatal unless immediate treatment is at hand.

Embolization and **angioplasty** carry special hazards which are discussed below.

THERAPEUTIC ANGIOGRAPHY

The following procedures involving angiographic techniques are used for therapeutic rather than diagnostic purposes:

1. Transluminal angioplasty
2. Embolization
3. Intra-arterial drug therapy
4. Balloon valvoplasty (see Ch. 24)
5. Septostomy (see Ch. 24).

TRANSLUMINAL ANGIOPLASTY

A percutaneous technique for dilating arterial stenoses and recanalizing arterial occlusions was first suggested by Dotter and Judkins in 1964, using a guide-wire and coaxial catheters of increasing size. The major advance in this field was the introduction of the dilatable double-lumen balloon catheter (Gruntzig 1975).

Dilatable balloon catheters (Fig. 25.12) were first used in the femoral and iliac arteries, but their use was soon extended to renal and coronary arteries and to splanchnic and other vessels. The type of vascular stenosis most suitable for dilatation by a balloon catheter is a localized one, but multiple stenoses and even localized occlusions can also be treated by the method.

More recently, promising results have been obtained both with laser angioplasty and with so-called dynamic

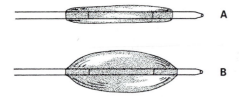

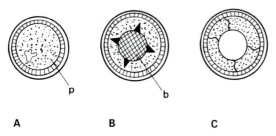

Fig. 25.12 Double-lumen balloon catheter. **A**. Deflated. **B**. Inflated.

Fig. 25.13 Mechanism of angioplasty. **A**. Before angioplasty. p = atheromatous plaque. **B**. Dilated balloon (b) dilates lumen and artery, allowing fissuring of plaque and redistribution around dilated lumen. Volume of plaque is unchanged. **C**. Late result.

angioplasty, using a flexible catheter with a motor-driven rotating cam at the distal tip. In both case the instruments can be inserted percutaneously using the normal guide-wire and catheter technique.

Laser angioplasty is performed using either a water-cooled 1–100 W Nd-YAG laser (Living Technology) or an air-cooled 1–60 W Nd-YAG laser (Surgical Laser Technology) with a quartz fibre tipped with a rounded-ended sapphire. For *dynamic angioplasty* the Cordis 'Kensey' system uses a flexible 8F catheter incorporating the rotating cam with speeds of 20 000–80 000 rpm.

Percutaneous *video angioscopy* using a high-resolution thin angioscope has also been used to examine the arterial lumen directly but is still in the research phase. *Intra-vascular stents* have now been designed which can be introduced by percutaneous catheter. These are undergoing trials at several centres and in a variely of clinical settings where they act as a mechanical brace helping to preserve pakeney.

At the time of writing, balloon angioplasty remains the most widely accepted and the most widely used technique.

Originally it was thought that balloon angioplasty acted by compressing and redistributing atheromatous material against the arterial wall. However, experimental work on animals and on human cadavers showed that the increase in size of the arterial lumen was due to splitting of the intima followed by retraction of the plaque on either side over the next few weeks. This was associated with slight stretching of the media and dilatation of the arterial wall, resulting in a permanent slight local increase in arterial diameter (Fig. 25.13).

Intra-arterial pressure recording is an essential part of the procedure, both to confirm that the stenosis is producing a significant pressure gradient and to monitor its successful abolition or improvement following the procedure. Pressures are recorded both proximal and distal to the lesion before and after its dilatation. It is important that the lesion is only traversed once by the guide-wire. If a catheter has to be withdrawn for exchange or other purposes it should always be done with the guide-wire left traversing the lesion as this greatly reduces the risk of damaging the intima by repeated manipulations.

Femoral and popliteal angioplasty. A high ante-grade femoral puncture is used. There is a tendency for the guide-wire to enter the profunda rather than the main

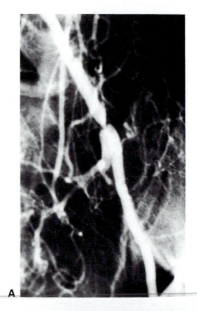

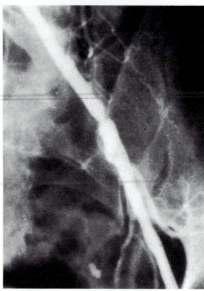

Fig. 25.14 Gruntzig catheter dilatation of iliac arterial stenosis. **A**. Before. **B**. After. Slight narrowing persists but the pressure gradient was abolished.

femoral artery; this is countered by abduction and external rotation of the limb or by the selection of the superficial femoral with a 6-mm J guide wire or both.

Iliac angioplasty (Fig. 25.14). A standard retrograde femoral puncture is used and this is usually possible even with a markedly damped or absent pulse.

Renal artery angioplasty and *splanchnic angioplasty*. These are best performed with Simmons-type 'sidewinder' balloon catheters (Fig. 25.15). The catheters are turned in the aortic arch and then brought down to the abdominal aorta where they are engaged in the appropriate artery. Stenosis at the anastomosis of a renal artery transplant or of a renal segmental artery can be treated in a similar way.

Aortic angioplasty can be performed by using two 8-mm balloons positioned side by side.

Coronary angioplasty is now a routine procedure and is discussed in Chapter 23.

Carotid and vertebral angioplasty are relatively easy to perform but are little used because of the more serious consequences of embolization or other accidents, and the possible limited and unpredictable tolerance of the brain to even temporary balloon occlusions.

Anticoagulants. In order to reduce the possibility of thrombosis or embolus, 5000 units of heparin are injected through the catheter once the lesion has been traversed. For coronary angioplasty the dose is increased to 10 000 units. Aspirin therapy is usually recommended for 24 hours before and for 6 months after an angioplasty, and some workers also recommend long-term Warfarin therapy from the second postoperative day.

Contrast medium. It is desirable that nonionic contrast media should be used for the control angiograms taken before and after angioplasty, since they are less likely to irritate the intima, besides being more tolerable to the patient.

Results of angioplasty

There has now been widespread experience of balloon angioplasty at vascular centres throughout the world and many published reports confirm a primary success rate in the femoral and iliac arteries of over 90% with a 3-year patency rate of over 70% in the femoral and over 80% in the iliac. These are as good as can be achieved by surgery but without the significant surgical mortality of 1–4%. Complications requiring further surgery are the same for angioplasty and surgery, at 3%.

The results for renal angioplasty are again similar to those for direct surgery. Both are performed mainly for significant hypertension which cannot be adequately controlled by drugs. As measured by restoration of normal blood pressure, success is obtained in 75% of patients with fibromuscular stenosis but in less than 50% of those with atheromatous stenosis. However, once again there is

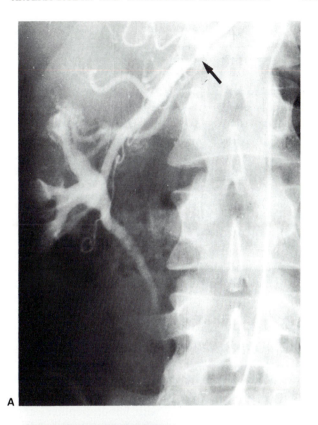
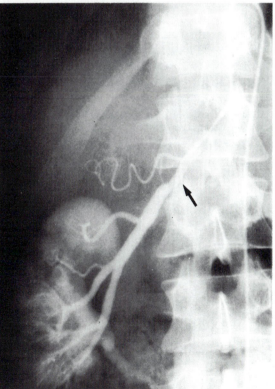

Fig. 25.15 **A**. Renal angioplasty. Before dilatation there is a severe localized stenosis about 4 cm from the origin of the right renal artery. **B**. After dilatation only slight narrowing remains. Note the 'sidewinder' balloon catheter withdrawn proximal to the stenosis. The deflated balloon lies between the two metal markers. The pressure gradient was abolished and blood pressure fell to normal.

a significant morbidity with surgery but not with angioplasty. Surgery has the further disadvantages of requiring general anaesthesia and much longer hospitalization.

Complications

Local dissection. The guide-wire or catheter may be passed subintimally, producing a local dissection; this may be further complicated by local thrombosis.

Embolization may occur, particularly during the recanalization of occluded vessels, and atheromatous fragments or clot transmitted distally.

Arterial perforation has been recorded, especially when trying to pass the guide-wire through a difficult and irregular stenosis or an occluded segment.

Balloon rupture may occur, though modern balloons can usually withstand very high pressures. Balloons with longitudinal tears can usually be withdrawn without much difficulty but a transverse tear may lead to the balloon peeling back along the catheter, and require surgical intervention for its removal.

Local *arterial trauma* at the site of puncture with *haematoma, false aneurysm* or *thrombosis* as described above may all occur, particularly with large catheters or coaxial sheaths.

Spasm is not uncommon with femoropopliteal angioplasty if the guide-wire is passed below the knee. It can be guarded against by giving 50 mg of lignocaine intra-arterially before the catheter passes through the stenosis. Tolazoline, 10–20 mg, can also be administered if spasm is encountered.

These complications emphasize that the procedure should not be undertaken lightly and that surgical help must always be available if required. In the case of renal or coronary angioplasty, immediate emergency surgery may be required.

EMBOLIZATION

Deliberate transcatheter arterial occlusion has now become an important branch of interventional radiology.

Clinical indications. These include:

1. Haemorrhage difficult to control by conventional means;
2. Occlusion of arteriovenous malformations;
3. Occlusion of arteriovenous fistula;
4. Occlusion of aneurysms;
5. Infarction of neoplasms or reduction of their blood supply;
6. Organ ablation (e.g. kidney or spleen) as an alternative to major surgery;
7. Treatment of varicocoele.

Embolic agents. A wide variety of particulate materials has been used for this purpose, and some are listed in Table 25.5.

Table 25.5 Embolic agents

Biological	Muscle slips
	Fibrous tissue
	Fat
	Autologous clot
Gelatin	Gelfoam
	Oxycel
	Avilene
Fibre	Ivalon
Metallic	Stainless steel balls
	Silastic-coated metal balls
	Carbon microspheres
	Metal filings
	Barium particles
Plastic	Polyvinyl alcohol
	Silastic spheres
	Acrylic spheres
	Polystyrene spheres
	Sephadex particles
Steel coils with attached fibre strands	
Bucrylate (an organic adhesive, or 'superglue')	
Sclerosing agents	Hyperosmolic contrast media
	Alcohol
Detachable balloons	

Of all the substances in Table 25.5, those which have been most widely used include autologous clot, Gelfoam, Avilene and polyvinyl alcohol. Others which have been fairly widely used include steel coils, bucrylate and absolute alcohol. The agent used in a particular case depends to some extent on local experience and preferences, and whether a permanent or temporary occlusion is desired.

The permanence of the vascular occlusion varies with the substances used. Autologous clot is rapidly re-absorbed and its effect lasts only hours or days. It was also of little use in patients with poor blood clotting. Though it was once widely used for patients with gastrointestinal haemorrhage it was later replaced by longer-lasting agents. Gelfoam and Avilene produce effects lasting many days or weeks, but in most cases are resorbed in three months or so. Polyvinyl alcohol, steel coils, bucrylate and absolute alcohol produce more permanent results.

Haemorrhage

Upper gastrointestinal haemorrhage can be treated by endoscopy or by vasopressin infusion as described below. However, when vasopressin fails to control the bleeding, embolic therapy should be considered. A rich collateral blood supply normally protects from the danger of local infarction, but great caution is necessary in the postoperative situation where major vessels have already been ligated or where surgery with vascular ligation is likely to follow.

The site of bleeding must first be demonstrated by superselective angiography, and, depending on this, embolization of the left gastric, gastroduodenal or pancreaticoduodenal artery will be performed.

Embolization has also been undertaken in bleeding from the territories of the superior and inferior mesenteric arteries, but is more difficult and dangerous because of the difficulties of superselective catheterization. Normally lesions in these areas are best treated by vasopressin infusions.

Pelvic haemorrhage can be difficult to control in carcinoma of the bladder or of the cervix, or in a postradiation or post-trauma situation. Such haemorrhage can be controlled by embolization of one or both internal iliacs or their branches.

Renal haemorrhage, either from neoplasm or trauma, can also be treated by superselective embolization (Fig. 25.16), as can hepatic haemorrhage (Fig. 34.23).

There are many other sites where haemorrhage can be treated by embolization as a simpler and safer alternative to major surgery, e.g., in the external carotid territory for bleeding from *head and neck tumours* or even for *severe epistaxis*, and in the bronchial arteries for uncontrollable *haemoptysis*. In all cases great care must be taken that the procedure is as superselective as possible and that the dangers of backflow and infarction are guarded against. In some situations temporary balloon catheter occlusion of the major feeding vessel may offer a simpler alternative.

Angiomatous malformations

Large angiomatous malformations were difficult or impossible to treat in the past and the treatable cases usually required major radical surgery. Such cases are being increasingly treated by embolization but still remain a major challenge owing to the multiplicity of feeding vessels and the rapid arteriovenous shunting. More than one embolization session is often required and even then success may be only partial. Smaller lesions respond well however, provided a good superselective approach to the major feeding vessels can be obtained.

Arteriovenous fistula

Small arteriovenous fistulas can be closed with emboli provided that the main feeding vessel can be superselectively catheterized (Figs 25.16, 25.17). With larger fistulas there is a danger of pulmonary emboli, and these are usually treated with detachable balloons.

Aneurysms

Aneurysms and false aneurysms of nonvital arteries can be occluded by embolization of the aneurysm or its artery of supply, and the technique has been successfully used in patients with aneurysms of a renal or hepatic artery branch (Fig. 34.23). In such cases there is little danger even if the arterial branch is occluded, but there is considerable danger with more vital arteries. Nevertheless the

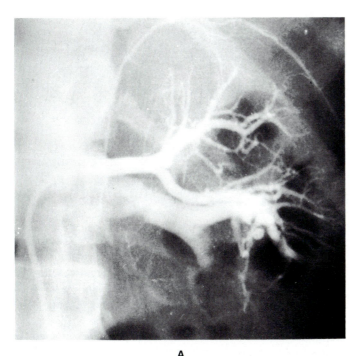

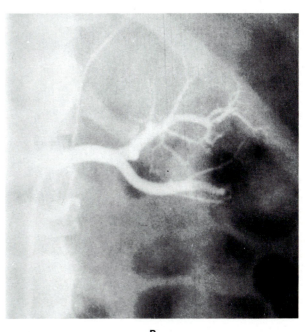

A   B

Fig. 25.16 Patient with severe haematuria following renal biopsy. **A.** Angiogram shows traumatic AV fistula. **B.** Fistula closed following embolization.

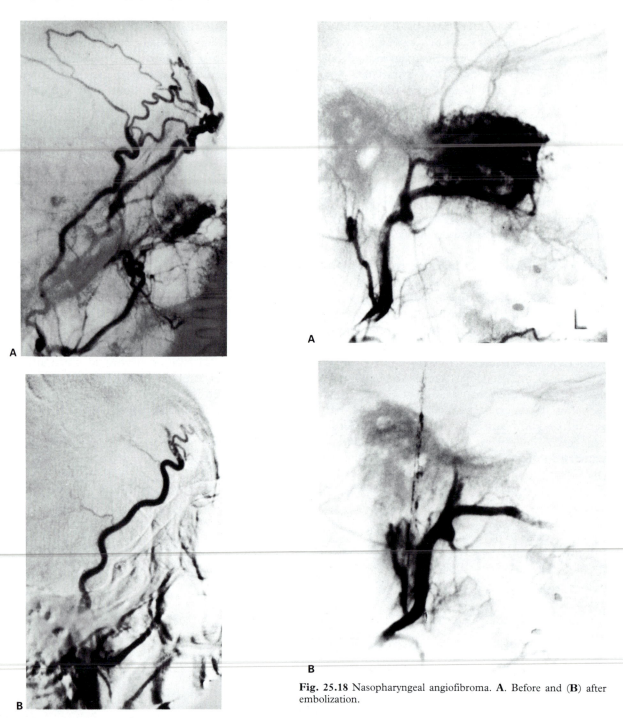

Fig. 25.17 AV fistula of scalp with drainage to superior ophthalmic vein. **A**. Before and (**B**) after embolization.

Fig. 25.18 Nasopharyngeal angiofibroma. **A**. Before and (**B**) after embolization.

technique has been used in neuroradiology (see Ch. 56), and even with aneurysms of the abdominal aorta.

Neoplasms

Embolization has also been used in the treatment of tumours, either to cause infarction of the tumour or to reduce the blood supply of a vascular tumour prior to operation (Fig. 25.18). The most widespread use has been in *renal carcinoma*. It has been suggested that even in inoperable cases the embolization of renal tumours may stimulate an immune response. It also reduces tumour bulk and may stop haematuria. Embolization of renal tumours is usually followed by flank pain lasting some 48 hours and requiring relief by narcotics. There may also be mild fever for several days, accompanied by nausea or vomiting, and transient hypertension may be seen. Other complications are discussed below.

Liver tumours, both primary and secondary, have been

treated by embolization (see Fig. 34.24). This liver is extremely vascular and in addition to the double blood supply (hepatic and portal) has multiple collateral pathways. Normal liver receives some 75% of its blood supply from the portal system and only 25% from the hepatic. In liver neoplasms the situation is reversed and 95% of the tumour blood supply comes from the hepatic artery. Selective hepatic artery embolization is thus a relatively safe procedure in inoperable primary carcinoma or other tumours, or as a preoperative measure in operable cases (Figs 34.24, 34.25). It is also useful in patients with multiple liver deposits not responding to chemotherapy.

Embolization has also been used with a variety of other neoplasms, including bone tumours. Small adrenal tumours have been infarcted by retrograde venous injection of an excess of hyperosmolar contrast medium, and parathyroid adenomas have also been destroyed by superselective arterial contrast injections.

Organ ablation
Embolization of both the kidney and the spleen have been used as alternatives to surgical nephrectomy and splenectomy. The latter procedure however has been complicated by a high incidence of postinfarction splenic abscess.

Varicocoele
This condition may be associated with infertility, and successful treatment is claimed by some workers after embolization of the left testicular vein. A percutaneous catheter is passed from the femoral vein in the groin to the left renal vein and thence to the left testicular vein. The latter is then occluded, either with a sclerosant or with a detachable balloon.

Complications
Apart from the usual complications of percutaneous angiography there are special hazards associated with embolization. The main dangers are undesired *ischaemia* and even *tissue necrosis* in the target area, or even in a different area. The latter can occur from back-flow of particles or even from misplacement of the catheter tip. It should be guarded against by careful monitoring of the particulate injections on the intensifier screen, using contrast medium with the injections and using multiple small injections rather than one or two large doses. The danger of particle reflux is greatest near the end of the procedure as the capillary bed becomes progressively occluded. A further safeguard is the use of a balloon catheter to block the afferent vessel whilst delivering particles.

Among the complications recorded are lower-limb ischaemia and gangrene; gut necrosis; splenic and hepatic infarction and abscess; renal infarction, abscess and anuria; spinal cord infarction; and pulmonary infarction.

There are special dangers associated with the use of steel coils and bucrylate. These include loss of coils to the aorta or other vessels and arterial perforation, whilst bucrylate has resulted in internal catheter gluing. Neuroradiological embolization carries further special hazards because of the particular vulnerability of cerebral tissue (see Ch. 56).

BALLOON CATHETER ARTERIAL OCCLUSION
Double-lumen balloon catheters with inflatable balloons near their tips are available for percutaneous introduction by the routine Seldinger technique. These can be used for temporary occlusion of blood vessels and then deflated and withdrawn. The method has been used for the control of internal haemorrhage as described above. We have also used it as an alternative to embolization of highly vascular hypernephromas before surgery. The catheter is introduced and the balloon inflated immediately prior to surgery, enabling the surgeon to operate in an almost bloodless field (Fig. 25.19). The balloon is deflated and the catheter removed immediately following surgery.

Detachable balloons were introduced by Debrun (1974) and are illustrated in Figure 25.20. They are widely used in the treatment of arteriovenous fistulas, particularly caroticocavernous fistula (see Ch. 56). They are also used in the embolization of aneurysms, particularly intracranial aneurysms (see Ch. 56).

INTRA-ARTERIAL DRUG THERAPY
Chemotherapy. Maximal doses of cytotoxic drugs can be delivered directly to tumours by selective arterial catheterization. The technique has been widely used for the treatment of inoperable tumours, particularly liver metastases (Fig. 25.21) and for presurgical treatment of large tumours. The catheter is usually left in situ for some time and it is vital to check by contrast-medium injection before each drug injection that the tip remains correctly sited.

Vasoconstrictors. Slow intra-arterial infusion of vasoconstrictors has been mentioned above as an effective treatment for gastro-intestinal haemorrhage. Vasopressin is mainly used after angiographic demonstration of contrast-medium extravasation at the bleeding point. Selective infusion into the left gastric artery is used to control bleeding from Mallory-Weiss tears or from gastritis and stress ulcers in the upper part of the stomach. Infusion into the common hepatic artery is used to control antral lesions and into the gastroduodenal artery in duodenal bleeding. The superior mesenteric and inferior mesenteric arteries can be used for bleeding in their respective territories.

Dosage for vasopressin is 0.2 units/min and for epinephrine 8–30 µg/min. Initial duration is 20–40 min

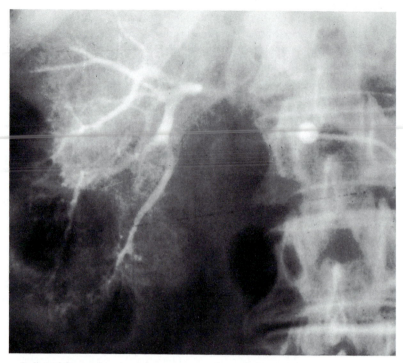

Fig. 25.19 Balloon catheter occluding right renal artery prior to surgery. A small dose of contrast medium is lingering in the arteries 10 s after injection, confirming occlusion of lumen.

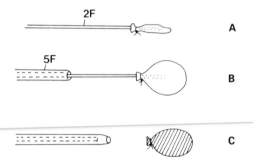

Fig. 25.20 Principle of Debrun detachable balloon. **A**. A latex balloon is attached to the end of a 2F Teflon catheter by a latex ligation. **B**. The balloon can be inflated with contrast medium after introduction through a 5F catheter. **C**. Before detachment, balloon is filled with liquid silicone. Once the silicone has hardened the balloon is detached by advancing the 5F catheter to push it off the smaller 2F catheter.

but may have to be prolonged, particularly in older arteriosclerotic patients.

The method is very successful in controlling small-vessel and capillary haemorrhage as in mucosal tears, stress ulcers and colonic diverticula, but less so when large arteries are involved, as in chronic peptic ulcers or where haemocoagulation defects exist.

Venous bleeding from oesophageal or gastric varices in portal hypertension can also be treated by superior mesenteric infusion. The aim in these cases is to try to stop the bleeding by reducing portal flow and hence portal pressure, and thus avoid emergency surgery. The

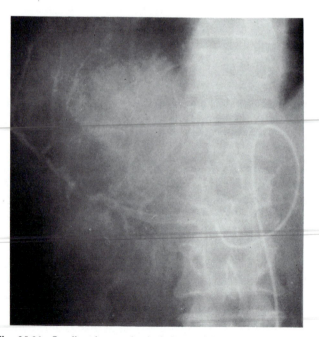

Fig. 25.21 Small catheter selectively inserted into right hepatic artery arising from superior mesenteric artery. The catheter was left in site for several days for infusion of cytotoxic drugs. Multiple liver secondaries. The site was confirmed by a small injection of contrast medium.

technique may succeed in the presence of normal haemocoagulation, but not in patients with severe cirrhosis and clotting defects.

Complications of vasopressin therapy include water

retention (ADH effect) which may require treatment by diuretics and electrolyte replacement. Abdominal cramp and diarrhoea may also occur, as may cardiotoxic effects (hypertension, bradycardia or arrhythmia). The drug must therefore be used with caution in patients with cardiac disease.

Thrombolysis. Intra-arterial infusions of thrombolytic drugs have been used to treat acute embolic and acute thrombotic occlusions of peripheral vessels. The lower limbs are usually involved and the procedure is usually undertaken as an alternative to surgical intervention or amputation, which are known to have a high morbidity and significant mortality. Streptokinase or the more expensive TPA (Tissue Plasmogen Activator) may be used as a low-dose infusion with the site of the catheter tip just proximal to the hind end of the clot. The procedure is monitored by serial angiography undertaken every few hours. Successful results are usually apparent within 24 hours and if there is no improvement after 48 hours success is unlikely.

INDICATIONS

VASCULAR LESIONS
The vascular lesions investigated by angiography will be discussed under the following headings:

1. Congenital
2. Aneurysms
3. Thrombosis and stenosis
4. Embolus
5. Angiomatous malformation
6. Arteriovenous fistula
7. Haemorrhage.

CONGENITAL
Congenital anomalies of the arterial system are not uncommon. Those involving the aortic origin and the *ascending aorta* have been described in Chapter 24. The major *coronary* abnormalities are also discussed in the cardiac section. *Anomalies of the great vessels* are noted in the neuroradiology section (Ch. 55), as are the commoner anomalies of the *cerebral arteries*. Anatomical variations of the peripheral arterial system are well described in anatomical texts but some of those with clinical implications will be noted here.

The *brachial artery* occasionally divides into its radial and ulnar branches at a high level, and this had some practical importance when brachial arteriography was more widely practised. In the lower limb the *popliteal artery* sometimes divides into its anterior and posterior tibial branches above the knee joint. The *femoral artery*, which normally arises from the external iliac, may occasionally be replaced by a large branch of the dilated hypogastric artery passing through the greater sciatic notch and behind the femoral neck, the so-called *persistent primitive sciatic artery*. In these cases the true femoral artery is hypoplastic and may terminate in the profunda femoris.

Congenital anomalies of the *renal* supply are very common and some 25% of kidneys have an accessory artery supplying them. For this reason arteriography is performed on live renal donors to check that the proposed kidney is suitable for grafting. Occasionally three renal arteries are found, but four arteries are very rarely seen. Horseshoe and ectopic kidneys frequently have accessory arteries, often arising from the aortic bifurcation or iliac artery.

Anomalies of the arterial supply to the liver are also frequently seen. The classical anatomical description of the *common hepatic artery* arising from the coeliac axis and dividing into right and left hepatic arteries is only seen in some 50% of cases. Some 20% have a right hepatic artery or an accessory right hepatic arising from the superior mesenteric artery. A further 20% have a left hepatic or accessory left hepatic artery arising from the left gastric artery. In about 2% of patients the common hepatic artery arises from the superior mesenteric.

Other major branches of the coeliac axis, i.e. the *splenic* and *left gastric arteries*, may sometimes arise directly from the aorta.

The *bronchial arteries* which arise on the anterior surface of the aorta just below the level of the carina are double on the left in 60% of cases and on the right in 30%.

Coarctation of the aorta. The condition has been described above, in Chapter 24. Post-stenotic aneurysm occurs as a complication in some 4% of cases (see Fig 25.37). It should also be realized that the condition may also occur at more distal sites than the classic level in the distal arch and can involve the lower thoracic or abdominal aorta. So-called *abdominal coarctation* usually affects the upper abdominal aorta and may involve a short or long segment. Splanchnic vessels and the renal artery origins may also be involved in the lesion (Fig. 25.22).

Pseudocoarctation or lateral buckling of the aortic arch is an unusual condition which can simulate a rounded mass in the region of the aortic knuckle. There is a sharp kink in the aorta at the junction of the arch and descending aorta in the region of the ligamentum arteriosum. Buckling of the aorta may also occur in the

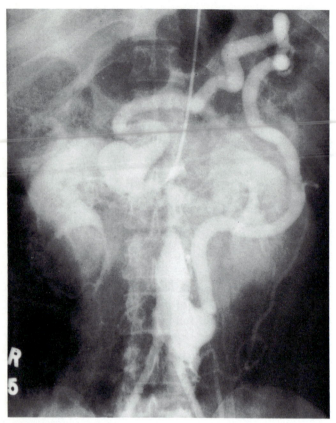

Fig. 25.22 Abdominal coarctation with involvement of the superior mesenteric origin. There is a collateral circulation through the artery of Drummond from the left colic branch of the inferior mesenteric to the middle colic branch of the superior mesenteric. Owing to the increased flow, aneurysms have developed at both ends of the collateral. (Courtesy of Dr R. Eban.)

mid-arch and this is best identified in the lateral view.

Vascular rings around the oesophagus can be of many types and the commonest lesions are illustrated in Appendix B. Study of the barium-filled oesophagus is helpful in elucidating these lesions.

Hypoplasia of the aorta is sometimes encountered as a chance finding. It may be associated with Marfan's syndrome, where there is a mesodermal defect and medial degeneration of the aorta. However in Marfan's syndrome the aorta will eventually dilate because of the medial defect and dissecting aneurysms may develop, particularly in the ascending aorta.

ANEURYSMS

Aneurysms can be classified on an aetiological basis as follows:

1. Congenital
2. Infective
3. Degenerative
4. Traumatic
5. Dissecting
6. Necrotizing vasculitis
7. Poststenotic.

Congenital aneurysms. These are commonest in the intracranial vessels, where they have in the past been termed 'congenital berry aneurysms'. Whilst these aneurysms are basically due to a defect in the muscular coat at points of arterial bifurcation, it is clear from clinical experience that other factors such as age, atheroma and hypertension are also important in their pathogenesis, as is the fact that they usually arise where the arteries lie in the subarachnoid space unsupported by surrounding soft tissues. They are discussed in more detail in Chapter 55. Congenital aneurysms have been described elsewhere in the body but are relatively rare, a fact which supports the importance of the local cerebral anatomy in their aetiology.

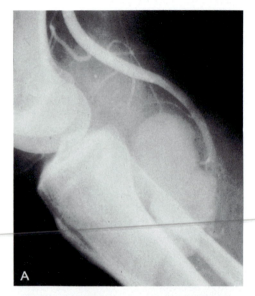

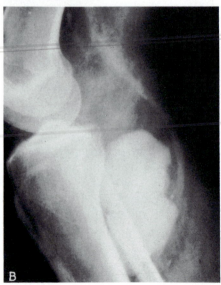

Fig. 25.23 A,B Mycotic aneurysm in the lower popliteal artery.

Infective aneurysms. Infective aneurysms may be classified as mycotic or syphilitic.

Mycotic aneurysms are nearly always secondary to bacterial endocarditis. They may involve any artery in the body and we have encountered examples in the abdomen and pelvis, in the brain and in the limbs (Figs 25.23, 25.24, 25.25). They can grow in size very rapidly and usually require urgent surgery to prevent rupture. Mycotic aneurysms are occasionally secondary to involvement of the arterial wall by an adjacent infection such as a pyogenic or tuberculous abscess.

Syphilitic aneurysms were once extremely common but with the advent of antibiotics they are now rarely seen in developed countries. They can involve arteries in any part of the body but are commonest in the ascending aorta and arch where they can reach a large size (Fig. 25.26).

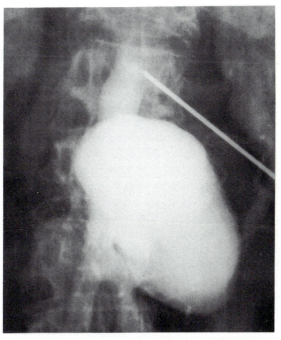

Fig. 25.25 Mycotic aneurysm at the origin of the inferior mesenteric artery.

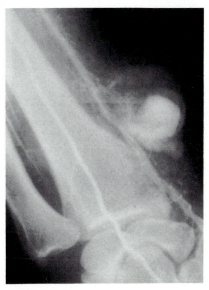

Fig. 25.24 Mycotic aneurysm of the lower end of the ulnar artery.

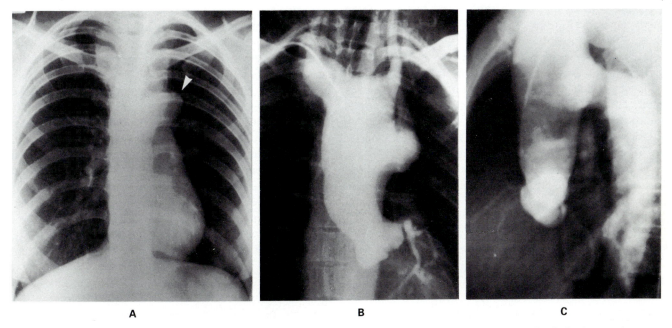

A   B   C

Fig. 25.26 **A**. Chest film showing aortic knuckle (arrow) apparently displaced downwards by supra-aortic mass. **B, C**. Angiogram shows that this is due to an aneurysm of the arch and innominate artery.

Angiography is usually required as a prelude to surgery with most mycotic aneurysms, though the diagnosis can be made with noninvasive imaging in most areas. CT or MRI will characterize large thoracic aneurysms which can stimulate mediastinal masses at simple radiography.

Degenerative aneurysms. Degenerative aneurysms result from atheroma. They are commoner in males and are seen most frequently in the abdominal aorta. Other common sites are the iliacs and the popliteal arteries. They are also becoming more frequent in the thoracic aorta, where they have replaced syphilis as the main type of aneurysm in developed countries. Degenerative thoracic aneurysms affect mainly the descending aorta and distal arch and rarely involve the ascending aorta. Atheromatous aneurysms may also occur in the splenic artery, in the renal artery, and in cerebral arteries, including the internal carotid and basilar arteries where they can be fusiform or saccular. Atheroma is also thought to be a major contributory factor to the development of the smaller so-called 'congenital' berry aneurysms.

Degenerative aneurysms are often fusiform, resulting in generalized dilatation of the artery, but they may become saccular, particularly in the sites of election mentioned above. Such saccular aneurysms may rupture with disastrous or even fatal consequences. They may also form a nidus for intraluminal clot which can embolize to more distal vessels.

Imaging. *Simple radiography* often shows characteristic curved linear calcification in the wall of large aortic aneurysms or of atheromatous aneurysms at other sites.

Ultrasound is the simplest method of confirming a suspected diagnosis of abdominal aortic aneurysm (Fig. 25.1) and monitoring any growth. It can also be used to diagnose popliteal and other peripheral aneurysms.

Nuclear angiography will show the lumen of an aneurysm well (Fig. 25.2), but not the clot which may be between it and the outer wall.

CT has the advantage of showing both the lumen and the extent of any intraluminal clot. It can also show evidence of leakage and the important relationship of the renal arteries to the upper limit of an abdominal aneurysm. Direct measurement of the aneurysm in all planes is possible (Fig. 25.3A). CT can also characterize the so-called 'inflammatory aneurysm' (Fig. 25.3B) or perianeurysmal fibrosis. This has a thickened irregular and enhancing wall, probably due to slow periarterial haemorrhage, and should be differentiated from retroperitoneal fibrosis.

MRI can also easily define large aneurysms and their relationships as well as imaging them in all planes.

Traumatic aneurysms can occur wherever an arterial wall is subject to injury (Fig. 25.27). Such aneurysms are commonest in the limbs but can occur in the thorax, abdomen, and head and neck. They may follow direct penetrating injury from a knife, missile or foreign body,

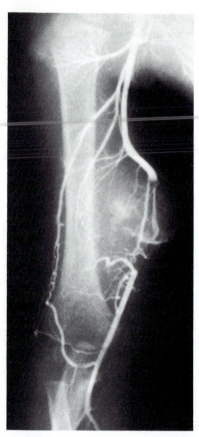

Fig. 25.27 Traumatic false aneurysm with rupture of the brachial artery in a child, following a fall while carrying a glass milk bottle.

or they may result from closed injury. Trauma to the femoral artery in the groin is a well-recognized occupational hazard in the butchering trade.

Traumatic aneurysm of the aortic arch is a frequent and potentially fatal result of chest injury in automobile accidents. It can easily be missed, with disastrous results, if not specifically suspected and looked for, since many of these patients have other injuries. The shearing effect of an acute deceleration injury usually involves the distal arch in the region of the ligamentum arteriosum. In most cases the injury is rapidly fatal but some 20% of cases survive the acute episode by the formation of a periaortic haematoma and false aneurysm or because the adventitia has not yet ruptured.

It is vital to recognize these cases since secondary rupture will follow within 24 hours in 30%, and within a week in most of the remainder. Only 2% will survive to chronic aneurysm formation, according to a study of 262 cases at the American Armed Forces Institute of Pathology.

Imaging. *Simple chest X-ray* may show broadening of the mediastinum but this will be difficult to assess on portable or emergency films. *CT* may show periaortic haemorrhage.

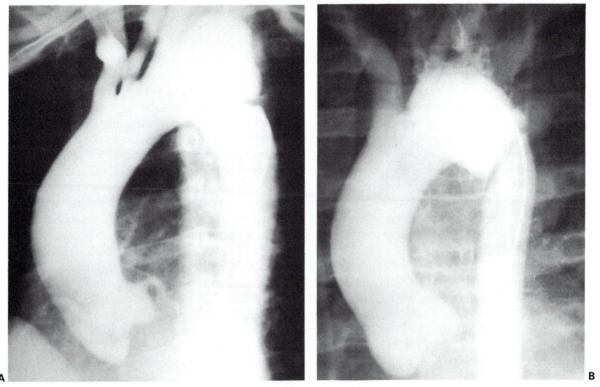

Fig. 25.28 A,B Traumatic false aneurysms of the aortic arch; two different cases. Note intimal flaps.

Aortography will show the false aneurysm, usually near the isthmus (Fig. 25.28), but the signs may be more subtle, consisting merely of an intimal flap or mural irregularity at the site of the tear. A small ductus diverticulum may occur near this site but should be differentiated by its smooth wall and inferomedial position.

Dissecting aneurysms. Dissecting aneurysms are mainly encountered in the aorta and hypertension is the main predisposing cause. The incidence in the USA has been estimated at 5–10 cases annually per million population. Men are mostly affected, usually aged between 50 and 70 years. Only 5% of case are under 40 and these are usually associated with rare causes such as Marfan's syndrome or, in women, with pregnancy. Other rare associations are with coarctation, aortic stenosis and bicuspid aortic valves.

Dissections usually commence in the aortic arch or ascending aorta and extend distally. De Bakey has classified them into three groups (Fig. 25.29). Type I commences in the ascending aorta and extends through the arch and descending aorta to the iliacs. Type II commences in the ascending aorta but does not extend beyond the arch. Type III commences in the distal arch and extends down to the iliacs.

Type II is the least common and is often associated with Marfan's syndrome. It forms 10% of the cases with Types I and III representing 45% each.

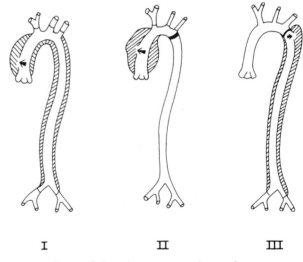

Fig. 25.29 Types of dissecting aneurysms (see text).

From the surgical viewpoint a more practical classification is into two groups: Type A, including all cases involving the ascending aorta (i.e. Types I and II above), and Type B, including those not involving the ascending aorta (i.e. Type III above); since the former are best treated surgically and the latter medically (see below).

The clinical features in classic cases are well known and include sudden agonizing pain in the chest. It is important to realize however that many cases are atypical and easily missed or misdiagnosed, since symptoms may vary considerably depending on the aortic branches involved. Hemiplegia and vertebral symptoms may result from involvement of great vessels and their cerebral branches; paraplegia can follow occlusion of intercostal or lumbar arteries supplying the cord; in the abdomen the coeliac axis and mesenteric arteries can be affected, giving rise to abdominal pain, mesenteric ischaemia or pancreatitis; renal artery occlusion may precipitate acute hypertension or anuria; the iliac vessels may be obstructed with lower-limb ischaemia; retrograde spread of the dissection in the ascending aorta can lead to coronary involvement, causing cardiac ischaemia or rupture into the pericardium with cardiac tamponade.

Dissecting aneurysms carry a grave prognosis: 30% are fatal within 24 hours and a further 50% of sufferers die in the next few days or weeks. Only 20% are likely to survive beyond 6 weeks and half of these will die later from rupture of the aneurysm. Some of the late survivals are associated with a large re-entry of the dissection into the true lumen in the lower abdominal aorta, giving rise to the so-called 'double bore' aorta. We have diagnosed cases of this type by aortography, where the true diagnosis was completely unsuspected by the referring physician.

The best prognosis rests with Type III cases not involving the ascending aorta, and present opinion favours medical treatment in these, since the survival rate is not significantly affected by surgery. However, surgery is recommended for Types I and II or Group A which involve the ascending aorta. In one series of Group A cases treated surgically, survival was 64% as against a medically-treated survival rate of 22%. There is thus some urgency in establishing the diagnosis and case type as rapidly as possible.

Imaging. *Simple radiographs* of the chest may show widening of the mediastinum, though this may be difficult to assess on portable films. More characteristic is localized dilatation of the aortic knuckle and upper descending aorta, which may give rise to a prominent 'hump' sign due to lateral projection of the knuckle (Figs 25.30A, 25.31A). Lateral and anterior displacement of the trachea has also been described, and the descending aorta often bulges to the left and is sometimes lobulated. A recent chest film, if available, is most helpful, as a change in contour then becomes obvious. Medial displacement of the calcified intima at the aortic knuckle has been described but is rarely clear-cut, and a pleural effusion (haemothorax) is present in about 20% of cases. In patients with Marfan's syndrome, localized bulging of the ascending aorta to the right may be recognized.

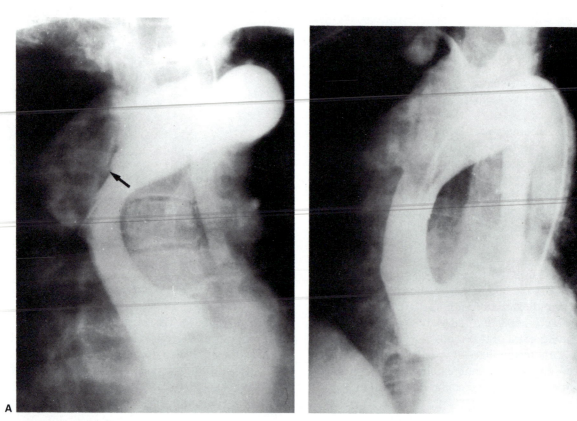

Fig. 25.30 Type I dissections; two cases. **A.** The dissection is compressing the true lumen of both the ascending and descending aorta. A small amount of contrast medium is seen entering the dissection through the tear in the intima of the ascending aorta (arrow). **B.** Contrast medium is entering the false lumen, separated by intimal flap in descending aorta.

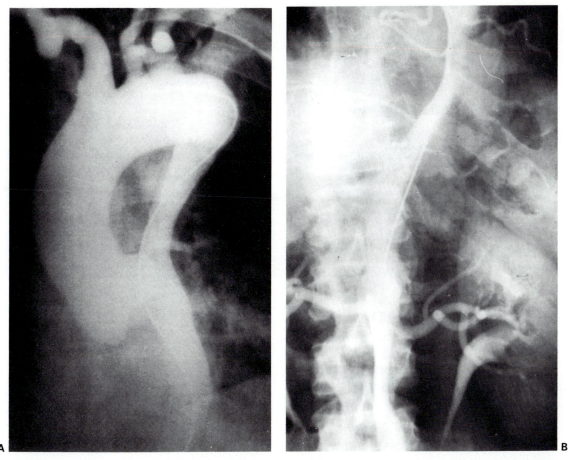

Fig. 25.31 Type III dissection. **A**. The dissection commences in the distal arch and compresses the descending aorta. **B**. Irregular compression of the lower thoracic and abdominal aorta. Both renal arteries fill well but the coeliac and superior mesenteric arteries are not identified and appear compressed. They are probably perfused by the dissection, which shows faint opacification.

CT or *MRI* can both be used to confirm or refute a diagnosis of dissecting aneurysm. CT requires intravenous contrast enhancement, provided the patient's renal and cardiovascular state permits. In typical cases the dilated aorta is well shown, with the true and false lumens separated by a linear intimal flap (Fig. 25.32). MRI fulfills the same function without contrast (Figs 25.33, 25.81 and 25.82) and has the further advantage of easy sagittal and coronal imaging.

Aortography has been widely used in the past to confirm the diagnosis, and can provide much vital anatomical information, provided the patient is well enough for a thorough examination which may involve multiple areas. The transfemoral route is usually used, though the right transaxillary route can be used in cases where this is difficult. The catheter tip is passed into the aortic root so that the whole of the ascending aorta can be visualized and contrast medium can enter the false lumen if the tear is a proximal one (Fig. 25.30). It also allows aortic insufficiency and regurgitation to be recognized.

Usually both the true and false lumens will fill with contrast medium and the displaced intima appears as a linear band separating the two (Fig. 25.30B). The intimal tear lies at the point where contrast medium enters the false from the true lumen (Fig. 25.30). In some cases only the true lumen fills, even with the catheter tip proximal to the tear (Fig. 25.31), implying that the false lumen contains blood clot or stagnant blood with no re-entry into the true lumen at a lower level. Such patients have a much better prognosis and in one series had a 90% survival rate. In these cases only the true lumen is outlined by contrast, but it is compressed and distorted by the false lumen ('twisted tape' sign). This appearance is similar to that seen when injections are made with the catheter tip distal to the tear. Such injections are made deliberately with an abdominal series in order to show the lower limits of the dissection and involvement of the splanchnic and renal arteries (Figs 25.31B, 25.34).

The thoracic aorta is the commonest site for dissection but the lesion is occasionally encountered in more peripheral vessels. In our material we have encountered examples in the abdominal aorta, the iliacs and the renal arteries. Localized dissection in the internal carotid artery is also well documented.

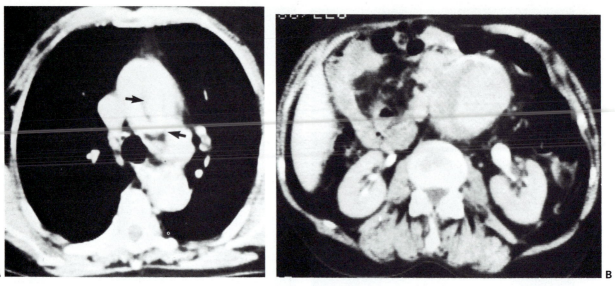

Fig. 25.32 A. Dissecting aneurysm shown by CT after contrast. Both true and false lumens are opacified but are separated by displaced intimal flaps (arrows) in the dilated ascending aorta (W512 L60). **B**. Dissection involving abdominal aorta, which shows fusiform aneurysmal dilatation. Contrast medium in both true and false lumens separated by intimal flap (W512 L38).

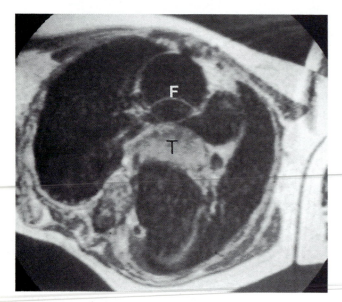

Fig. 25.33 Axial MRI section of thorax shows a dissecting aneurysm. In the ascending aorta both lumens are patent and separated by an intimal flap (F). In the descending aorta the false lumen contains thrombus (T). (Courtesy of Dr Peter Wilde and Bristol MRI Centre.)

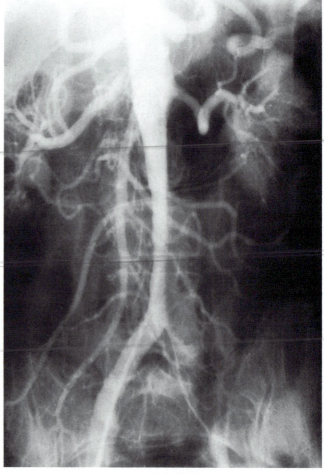

Iatrogenic arterial dissection as a complication of angiography has been mentioned above. Such events are usually minor in degree and resolve spontaneously, particularly where they are produced by retrograde catheterization so that blood flow flattens rather than fills the intimal flap.

Necrotizing vasculitis. The mysterious disease *poly-arteritis nodosa* is associated with necrotizing vasculitis. The process involves the walls of small vessels, and as

Fig. 25.34 Dissecting aneurysm. Abdominal series shows good filling of splanchnic and renal vessels but the lower abdominal aorta and left common iliac artery are obstructed. The latter forms the lower limit of the dissection.

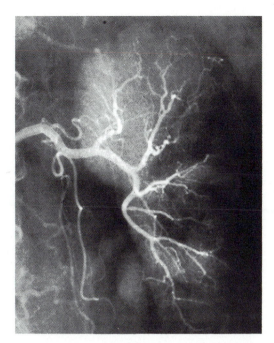

Fig. 25.35 Polyarteritis nodosa showing multiple microaneurysms.

the disease progresses these weaken and aneurysms develop. The nodose lesions have a predilection for arterial bifurcations but can occur anywhere along the artery. Any artery in the body may be involved, including the vasa vasorum, which accounts for the protean clinical manifestations.

The kidneys are very frequently involved and hypertension is seen in 70% of cases. Multiple small aneurysms may be identified at angiography and are characteristic, though not always seen (Fig. 25.35). The small aneurysms can rupture, giving rise to perirenal haematomas. Aneurysms of other splanchnic vessels can also rupture, leading to retroperitoneal or other abdominal haemorrhages. The demonstration of multiple small aneurysms is almost diagnostic, so that renal and visceral angiography is a valuable tool.

Other rarer causes of similar small aneurysms are *Wegener's granulomatosis* and *systemic lupus erythematosus*. *Atrial myxoma* embolization can also give rise to small peripheral aneurysms, as can necrotizing arteritis resulting from abuse of drugs, particularly *metamphetamine*. *Acute pancreatitis* may involve small vessels adjacent to the pancreas and lead to aneurysms which can rupture with serious consequences (Fig. 25.36).

Post-stenotic aneurysms. These are probably due to turbulence and eddy flows affecting the vessel wall distal to the arterial stenosis. They are a well-recognized complication of *coarctation*, occurring in some 4% of cases (Fig. 25.37). They may also be seen in the subclavian artery in the *thoracic inlet syndrome* (see below), and in the renal artery with *fibromuscular hyperplasia*. They can also complicate *atheromatous stenosis* in any artery.

STENOSES AND THROMBOSES

Congenital stenoses of major arteries as in thoracic and abdominal coarctation of the aorta have been described above. Abdominal coarctation may also involve the origins of splanchnic or renal arteries. Congenital stenoses have also been described in other vessels, including the pulmonary arteries.

Extrinsic pressure from tumours, cysts or other masses can also involve arteries and obstruct flow; in these cases the cause is usually obvious. Less commonly, localized arterial obstruction is due to a fibrous band, as may sometimes occur in the thoracic inlet syndrome, in renal artery stenosis or in the coeliac compression syndrome. An anomalous tendon can obstruct the popliteal artery in popliteal entrapment, as can a developmental cyst in the popliteal wall (see below).

Arteritis of inflammatory or unknown aetiology may also lead to arterial stenosis as in Takayasu disease.

Atheroma is far and away the commonest cause of arterial stenosis and thrombosis in clinical practice, and, depending on the site, can give rise to a variety of clinical syndromes. It is found most often in males, though females are also frequently affected, particularly in the older age groups. Lesions of the greatest clinical importance involve:

1. Internal carotid and vertebral origins, giving rise to transient ischaemic attacks and cerebrovascular insufficiency (see Ch. 55)

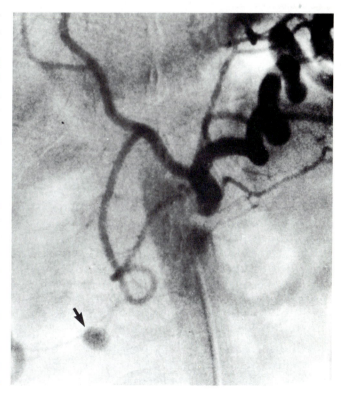

Fig. 25.36 Aneurysm of the pancreatico-duodenal arcade (arrow) secondary to acute pancreatitis (subtraction film).

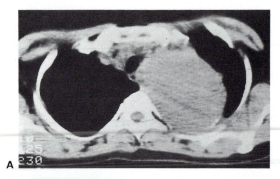

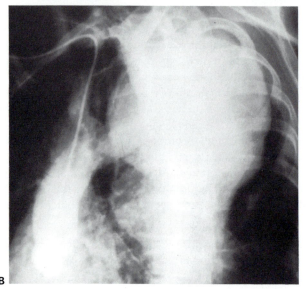

Fig. 25.37 **A**. CT of a large mediastinal mass presenting in a young woman. **B**. Transaxillary aortogram confirms giant post-stenotic aneurysm and previously unrecognized mild coarctation.

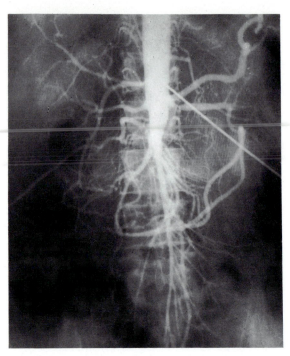

Fig. 25.38 Aortic thrombosis. There is also atheromatous stenosis of the left renal artery and filling of the inferior mesenteric from the artery of Drummond.

2. Coronary artery lesions causing cardiac ischaemia (see Ch. 23)
3. Renal arteries, with resulting hypertension
4. The abdominal aorta
5. Iliac and femoral arteries.

Intermittent claudication is the cardinal symptom of stenosis and thrombosis of the aorta, iliacs and femorals. Atheromatous stenosis also involves the major vessels to the upper limb but is of less clinical significance because of the excellent collateral circulation.

Atheromatous stenosis of the abdominal aorta is frequently seen, as is its successor aortic thrombosis (*Leriche syndrome*). Lesions usually commence near the aortic bifurcation, and thrombosis extends upwards but usually stops short of the renal arteries (Fig. 25.38). Occasionally the origin of a renal artery is involved, with secondary hypertension ensuing.

The iliacs are among the commonest sites for atheromatous stenosis and thrombosis (Fig. 25.39), as are the femoral and popliteal arteries.

So-called '*primary popliteal thrombosis*' occurs in young males, and though atheroma at a young age is occasionally responsible, most cases are due to rare congenital anomalies, namely popliteal cysts and popliteal entrapment.

Popliteal cysts usually present with calf claudication in men with an average age of 36. Angiography shows a healthy smooth-walled femoral artery and either a smooth narrowing suggesting external compression or a localized thrombosis in the popliteal artery. The cyst secretes mucin and lies in the wall of the artery. It is claimed to be due to developmental inclusion of mucin-secreting synovial capsular cells from the knee joint. Similar lesions have been described in other vessels including the iliac, radial and ulnar arteries. The diagnosis has been made by CT of the popliteal artery and could also be suggested by ultrasound or MRI.

Popliteal entrapment also occurs mainly in young males and may present in boys or adolescents either with calf claudication or, more commonly, acute popliteal thrombosis. The condition is due to an anomalous tendon of the medial head of gastrocnemius passing over and trapping the artery. Angiography shows either a characteristic linear external compression or thrombosis of the popliteal.

Coeliac or *superior mesenteric stenosis* from atheroma is quite common, particularly at the origins of these arteries (Fig. 25.40). Other causes include fibromuscular hyperplasia and involvement by arteritis as in Takayasu

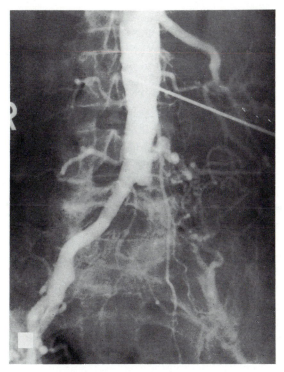

Fig. 25.39 Iliac thrombosis due to atheroma.

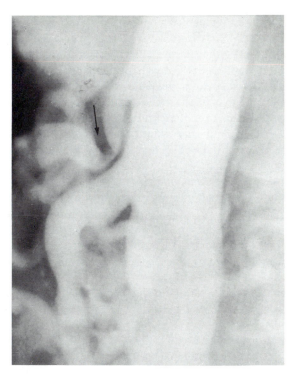

Fig. 25.40 Coeliac stenosis shown by lateral aortogram (arrow).

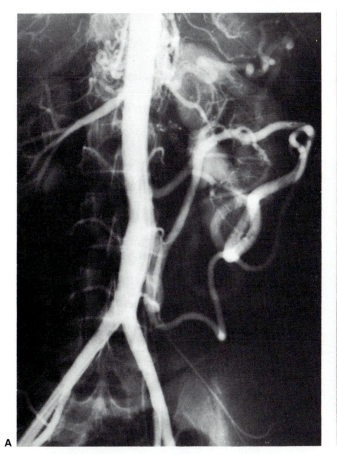

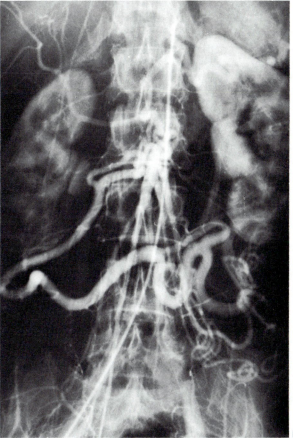

Fig. 25.41 **A**. Occlusion of coeliac and superior mesenteric arteries. Separate origin of splenic artery. Artery of Drummond arising from inferior mesenteric. **B**. Artery of Drummond supplies superior mesenteric origin and then hepatic artery through pancreatic arcades.

disease, or by congenital coarctation or external coeliac compression. Such lesions have been cited as causing dyspepsia and other gastrointestinal symptoms. However it should be realized that the collateral circulation between the splanchnic vessels is so good that even total occlusion of two of the three main vessels (coeliac axis superior and inferior mesenteric) can be easily tolerated (Fig. 25.41) and the inferior mesenteric is usually occluded in the Leriche syndrome without referrable symptoms.

Coeliac compression syndrome is the term used for gastrointestinal symptoms associated with narrowing of the coeliac at its origin by external compression. This is due either to the median arcuate ligament of the diaphragm or to coeliac plexus fibrosis. As implied above, this is more likely to be a chance association than a true syndrome.

Coronary stenosis and *thrombosis* due to atheroma and their investigation and treatment have been discussed in Chapter 23.

Renal artery stenosis is an important and sometimes remediable cause of renal ischaemia and hypertension. Atheroma is the main aetiological cause (Fig. 25.42) but in younger, mainly female, patients fibromuscular hyperplasia is also important (Fig. 25.43). This is a rare disease of unknown aetiology leading to irregular beading of the vessel; it is further discussed below. Other rare causes of renal artery stenosis include *extrinsic pressure* by fibrous bands or sympathetic chain fibres, neurofibromatosis, and *arterial stretching* or compression by tumours. Aortic involvement by abdominal coarctation or by arteritis can also affect the renal artery, as can aortic thrombosis.

Whatever the cause of the renal ischaemia, secondary hypertension may result and the kidney can develop changes recognizable at both plain X-ray and urography. The affected kidney becomes smaller than normal but remains smooth in contour, unlike the irregular contour of the small kidney of chronic pyelonephritis. At urography, the excretion of contrast medium is slightly later than from the normal side, but as the investigation proceeds contrast becomes denser on the affected side and shows small spindly calices.

The radiological treatment of renal artery stenosis by percutaneous angioplasty has been discussed above (see Fig. 25.15). The anatomy of renal artery stenosis is best shown by catheter arteriography but screening for the condition can be accomplished on an outpatient basis by intravenous DSA.

Subclavian stenosis. Compression of the subclavian artery at the root of the neck is seen in the *thoracic inlet syndrome* and may be associated with various congenital anomalies. Some, like cervical rib or an anomalous first rib, will be readily diagnosed on a plain film, but others, like fibrous bands or compression by the scalenus anticus muscle, will only be manifest at angiography.

Clinically these patients may present with ischaemic hands, with Raynaud's phenomenon or with digital emboli. The latter derive from clot arising at the level of the lesion or in a poststenotic aneurysm. These are a frequent complication and are usually fusiform, though they can also be saccular (Fig. 25.44). Thrombosis of the subclavian artery can also result (Fig. 25.45).

Arteriography in these patients may appear normal or equivocal with the arm in neutral position, and Adson's

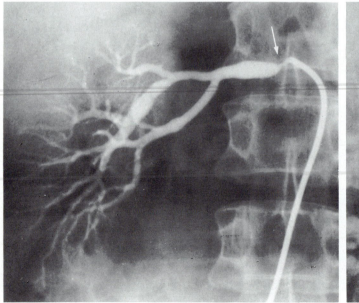
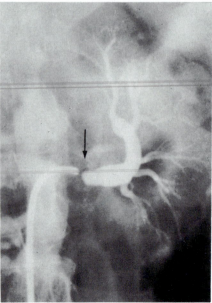

Fig. 25.42   **A**. Renal artery stenosis due to atheroma. **B**. Renal artery stenosis. Note post-stenotic dilation of the renal artery.

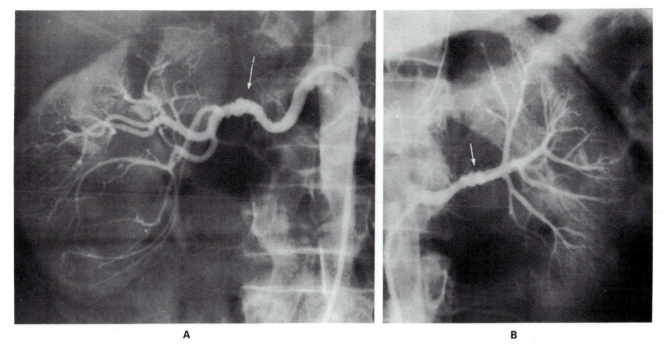

Fig. 25.43 A,B   Renal artery fibromuscular hyperplasia (arrows).

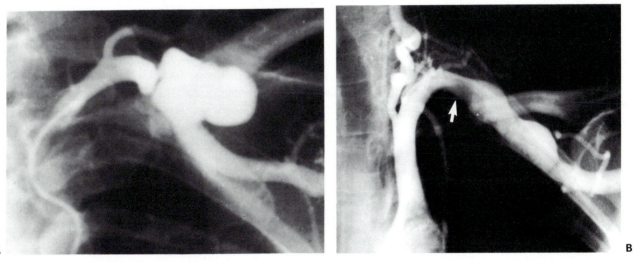

Fig. 25.44   Subclavian stenosis with post-stenotic aneurysm formation. **A.** Saccular. **B.** Fusiform aneurysm.

manoeuvre may be necessary to confirm the lesion. This consists of fully abducting the arm with the head fully turned to the opposite side. These patients can also be investigated less invasively by intravenous DSA (Fig. 25.46).

Raynaud's phenomenon. This frequently occurs in normal healthy individuals as an abnormal response to cold. In these cases it appears to be purely due to a spastic response of the small vessels. Apart from this *primary* type, the condition may also be *secondary* to a variety of conditions which impair blood flow and includes major and minor vascular lesions. Table 25.6 lists the numerous

diseases which have been associated with digital ischaemia and Raynaud's phenomenon.

Atheromatous lesions in the subclavian, axillary and brachial arteries are quite common but are often asymptomatic because of the excellent collateral circulation at the root of the neck, shoulder and elbow. Thus thrombosis of the first part of the subclavian artery is often encountered by chance during arch or headhunter angiography, when the vertebral artery on the affected side is demonstrated to supply the distal subclavian by reversed flow (*subclavian steal* — see Ch. 55).

Atheromatous occlusions are also encountered in the

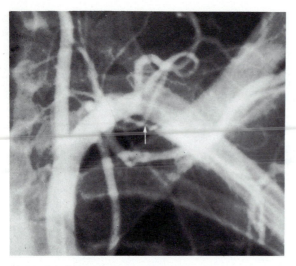

Fig. 25.45 Subclavian thrombosis (arrow).

Table 25.6 Digital ischaemia and Raynaud's phenomenon

1. Lesions of major vessels (often with small-vessel emboli)
   Atheroma
   Takayasu's disease
   Non-specific arteritis
   African idiopathic aortitis
   Thoracic inlet syndrome
   Buerger's disease
   Fibromuscular hyperplasia

2. Collagen disorder
   Scleroderma
   DLE
   Rheumatoid arthritis
   Polyarteritis nodosa

3. Blood disorders
   Polycythaemia
   Sickle-cell disease
   Cryoagglutination
   The contraceptive pill
   PVC poisoning

4. Specific conditions
   Raynaud's phenomenon (spastic type)
   Vibrating tools
   Ergotism

distal vessels of the upper limb. In the digital vessels they can give rise to severe localized ischaemia which may require amputation. In elderly men most cases of localized digital ischaemia are due to atheroma.

Generalized digital ischaemia is usually due to a generalized disease such as scleroderma.

Buerger's disease

This has remained a controversial subject since the condition was first described in 1908. The diagnosis of Buerger's disease or 'thromboangiitis obliterans' was once widely applied to a variety of vascular thromboses including the first cases of internal carotid thrombosis described by Moniz, as well as to the lower limb lesions originally

described. As a healthy reaction to the overdiagnosis of Buerger's disease, Wessler et al (1960) pointed out that most of the cases examined by them were indistinguishable pathologically from atheromatous disease with thrombosis. This led some to the view that Buerger's disease was a myth and that most cases were in fact due to atheromatous disease.

Angiographic studies show that whatever the pathological nature of the lesions, Buerger's disease does appear to be a separate clinical entity. It occurs in a much younger age group than typical atheromatous vascular dis-

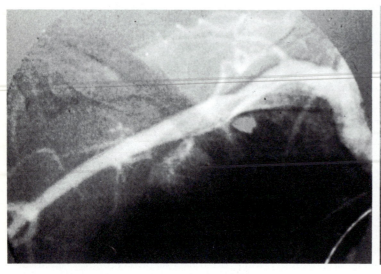

A

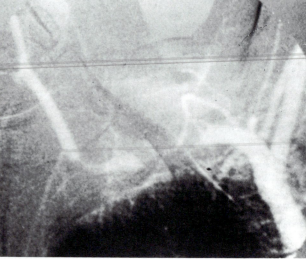

B

Fig. 25.46 Right subclavian artery shown by DSA. **A**. In neutral position there is slight fusiform aneurysmal dilatation, but no obvious stenosis. **B**. With Adson's manoeuvre there is marked obstruction.

ease, the patients being mainly in their twenties or early thirties. It also has a much higher male sex incidence than has atheroma, female patients being extremely rare; and there is a much stronger association with heavy cigarette smoking, the patients usually showing strong addiction, sometimes maintained despite the threat of amputation.

Unlike atheroma, the major vessels (aorta, iliacs and femorals) usually appear smooth-walled and healthy and the disease starts in the foot vessels and spreads retrogradely up the calf vessels. The typical angiographic appearance is of healthy femoral and popliteal arteries, with the calf vessels largely occluded and replaced by fine collaterals (Fig. 25.47). Long tortuous collaterals following the course of the occluded anterior and posterior tibials or peroneal are sometimes seen and may represent hypertrophied vasa vasorum.

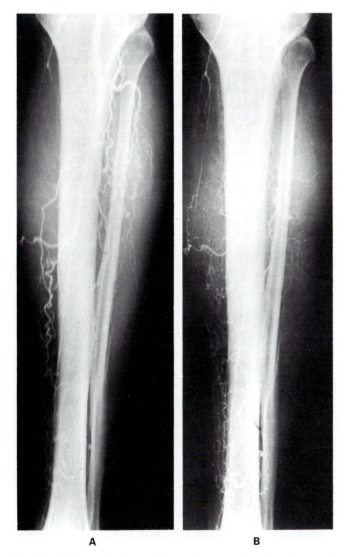

Fig. 25.47 Buerger's disease. Femoral arteriography showed normal smooth-walled femoral and popliteal arteries, but occlusion of the calf vessels with collaterals.

Spasm. *Ergot poisoning* may occur in migraine patients who have overdosed themselves with ergotamine tartrate, of which there are several proprietary preparations. This results in peripheral vascular spasm, presenting as ischaemic lower limbs. Such patients are easily misdiagnosed unless an adequate history is obtained, and we have been asked to perform angiography on several such patients without the referring physician suspecting the true diagnosis. The angiographic appearances are unusual but are diagnostic, consisting of spastic contraction of the vessels below the common femoral (the superficial femoral, popliteal and peripheral vessels), which are uniformly narrowed, so that they appear more like narrow threads than normal vessels. Upper-limb vessel involvement has also been described, as has spasm of splanchnic and renal vessels. If the condition is correctly diagnosed, withdrawal of the offending drug brings a rapid reversal of the spasm.

Localized spasm of peripheral arteries may be induced at *angiography*, usually in small vessels with a prominent muscular coat, either by the guide-wire or catheter tip or by a local high concentration of contrast medium. It may be observed on the angiogram just distal to the tip of the catheter and should not be mistaken for a local stenosis. Any doubt can be resolved by repeating the contrast injection with the catheter tip withdrawn to a more proximal position.

Beaded spasm is a term used for an unusual appearance usually seen in the femoral and popliteal arteries and less commonly in other arteries such as the iliacs and splanchnics. The condition has also been referred to as 'standing' or 'stationary arterial waves' or 'arterial beading'. Its nature remains controversial but it is generally thought to represent a physical phenomenon due to arterial pressure waves. In our experience it has been seen most frequently in the femoral arteries of patients with Buerger's disease and high peripheral resistance from obliterated calf vessels. The regular and perfectly symmetrical nature of the beading has been likened to a chain of pearls and helps to distinguish it from the asymmetrical and less regular beading of fibromuscular hyperplasia.

Fibromuscular hyperplasia is an unusual arterial disease first described in the renal arteries as a rare cause of renal artery stenosis and occurring mainly in young women. The diagnosis is made by angiography, which shows an irregular beaded appearance of the affected artery (Fig. 25.43). The lumen of the artery, when examined pathologically, exhibits both stenoses and sacculations and the latter may become aneurysmal.

The lesions are presumably congenital, though usually presenting in early adult life, and they have been described in many other arteries, though commonest in the renals. We have encountered examples in the iliac and splanchnic arteries as well as in the internal carotid artery, which is now a well-recognized site for the lesion.

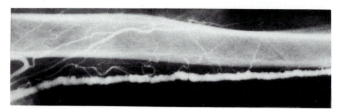

Fig. 25.48 Fibromuscular hyperplasia of the brachial artery in a woman of 50 presenting with digital ischaemia.

It appears to be extremely rare in limb vessels though we have previously reported a case in the brachial arteries of a middle-aged woman (Fig. 25.48).

ARTERITIS

Takayasu's arteritis. This is a rare condition first described in Japan in 1908 but now recognized to have a worldwide distribution. It manifests mainly in young women aged 20 to 30 and the incidence in the United States is 0.11%. The aorta is attacked by a granulomatous inflammation of the media proceeding to fibrosis and atheroma-like changes with involvement of the main branches which can become thrombosed. The main pulmonary artery and its major branches may also be involved. The aetiology is unknown but an autoimmune mechanism has been postulated by some workers.

Clinical manifestations depend on the major aortic branches most affected and include upper-limb ischaemia, ocular and cerebral symptoms, renovascular hypertension, coronary disease and lower-limb ischaemia. The *aortic arch syndrome* of progressive occlusion of the great vessels of the arch is a common complication.

Angiography shows a surprising irregularity of the aorta, which resembles that of an elderly atheromatous person, together with stenoses or occlusions of the origins of the major branches.

Giant-cell arteritis. This is a vasculitis affecting people above the age of 50 or 60 and usually involving smaller or middle-sized arteries. It is not clear whether the cause is inflammatory or whether an autoimmune mechanism is involved. Temporal arteritis is common, as is involvement of intracerebral vessels, and blindness is a complication in some 10% of cases. Large-vessel vasculitis is very uncommon but is occasionally seen and can give rise to lower-limb ischaemia or an aortic arch syndrome. Angiography of the temporal artery may show irregular stenotic areas with intervening normal areas (skip lesions).

EMBOLUS

Major embolus to the systemic arterial system is most commonly *cardiac* in origin, being seen in patients with atrial fibrillation and intra-atrial clot, or following clot formation in the left ventricle after cardiac infarction. Another cardiac cause is clot forming on prosthetic valves after cardiac surgery.

Embolus may also follow clot formation in a large aneurysm which is then detached and carried distally.

The rare paradoxical embolus is carried from the venous system through a patent foramen ovale. This is present in one-third of the population but remains closed unless right atrial pressure exceeds left atrial pressure, as in chronic lung disease or pulmonary embolus, when clots may pass through to the left heart and systemic circulation.

Ulcerated atheromatous plaques in major vessels can also give rise to emboli from *cholesterol* showers or debris, which being smaller lodge in small peripheral vessels in the limbs and are usually less serious. However when they affect the brain they can give rise to transient ischaemic attacks or more serious strokes (see Ch. 55).

Finally, clot embolus is a well-recognized complication of catheter angiography, as previously described.

75% of large emboli lodge at the aortic bifurcation, iliac bifurcation, or major vessels of the lower limb. The clinical diagnosis is usually obvious from the acute onset of pain, numbness, pallor and coldness, with loss of peripheral pulses in the context of cardiac disease, aneurysm or previous cardiac surgery. If however the onset is more insidious it may be difficult to differentiate from arterial thrombosis.

Angiography shows a sharp cut-off at the point of occlusion (Fig. 25.49) with sometimes a characteristic convex upper margin (meniscus sign). Larger emboli af-

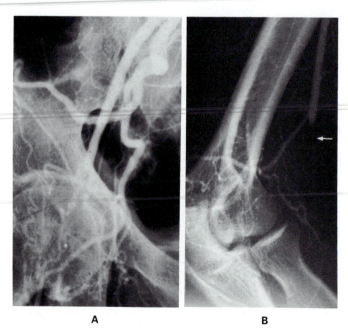

A   **B**

Fig. 25.49 A. Embolic occlusion of the common femoral artery. **B.** Embolic occlusion of the brachial artery (←).

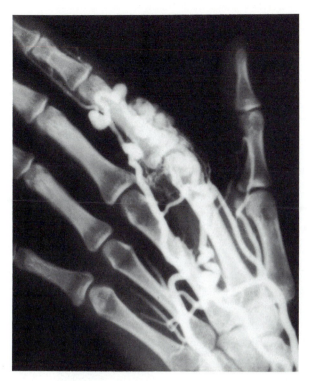

Fig. 25.50 Angioma of the hand.

fecting the aortic, iliac or femoral bifurcation are usually removed surgically with a Fogarty balloon catheter. They should be treated as surgical emergencies since delay of more than 24 hours leads to a significantly higher amputation rate. Smaller and more distal emboli and those in the arm have a better prognosis but if the limb is at risk treatment by intra-arterial thrombolysis may be attempted as described above.

Mesenteric embolism should be suspected in patients with acute abdominal pain and coexisting atrial fibrillation, mitral stenosis or a recent cardiac infarction.

ANGIOMATOUS MALFORMATIONS

These lesions, also referred to as *angiomas* and *congenital arteriovenous fistulas*, represent direct communications between arterioles and venules without the interposition of a capillary bed. They are presumably congenital but often present in adults, probably due to increasing size after adult blood pressure is established. They are common in the cerebral circulation (see Ch. 55) but can present anywhere in the body. They should be distinguished from acquired communications between arteries and veins — arteriovenous fistulas — which are described below.

Figures 25.50, 25.51 and 25.52 show the angiographic appearances in lesions presenting in the hand, vulva and

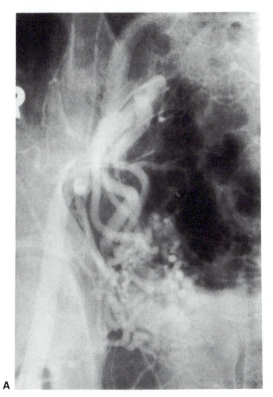

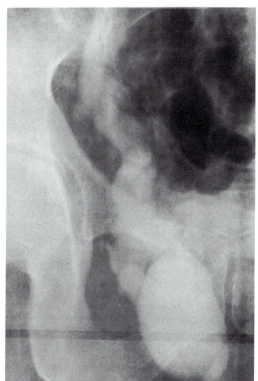

Fig. 25.51 A,B Angioma of the pelvis, presenting as vulval swelling. Aneurysmal dilatation of draining vein.

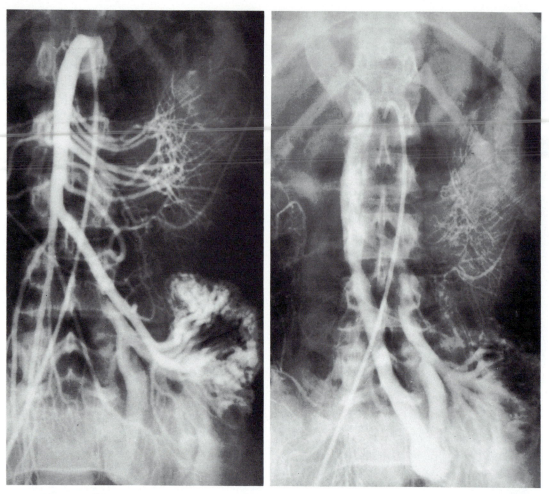

Fig. 25.52   Angioma of the small bowel with high-volume shunting into the portal system in a woman of 24 with repeated attacks of melaena. In the previous ten years she had had four barium enemas and five barium follow-throughs with negative findings. Large angiomas like this are unusual, small areas of dysplasia being more common.

bowel respectively. In all cases there are hypertrophied arteries leading to the lesion and hypertrophied veins draining it, their size depending on the degree of shunt present. Both arteries and veins fill rapidly and before contrast medium has passed through normal capillaries in the adjacent regions. Some smaller angiomas and those at very fine vessel level are more difficult to demonstrate and may require superselective angiography of the feeding vessels to show their full extent. Treatment by angiographic embolization has been discussed above.

ARTERIOVENOUS FISTULA

This term is best limited to the condition where there is a single communication between an artery and a vein, and is mainly of traumatic origin, particularly following gunshot or other penetrating wounds. Occasionally it may result from a closed injury (Fig. 25.53). Traumatic fistula may occur anywhere in the body and we have encountered cases in all anatomical sites from the scalp to the foot.

Spontaneous arteriovenous fistula is also occasionally encountered, resulting from rupture of an aneurysm into an adjacent vein (Fig. 25.54). A site of election for this is the cavernous sinus, where rupture of an aneurysm can give rise to pulsating exophthalmos (see Ch. 55). Another well-documented site is the abdominal aorta, where rupture of an aneurysm into the inferior vena cava leads to aortocaval fistula (Fig. 25.55). These intra-abdominal cases can give rise to difficult diagnostic problems, and the larger shunts can give rise to high-output cardiac failure without the true cause being suspected.

So-called congenital arteriovenous fistulas are sometimes seen in infants and children but it is usually difficult or impossible to exclude trauma in these cases.

Iatrogenic AV fistulas, apart from those deliberately induced for dialysis, can arise from many procedures, particularly orthopaedic operations on the hip, ankle and spine. Aortocaval and ilioiliac fistula have followed lumbar disc operations when the rougeur has been passed through the anterior spinal ligament, and renal arteriovenous fistula is a common complication of renal

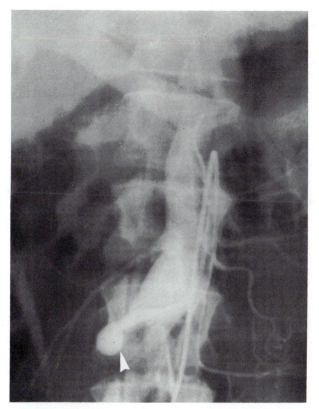

Fig. 25.53 Mesenteric-portal fistula (arrowed) shown by selective superior mesenteric injection. There is rapid filling of dilated superior mesenteric and portal veins. The lesion followed a crush injury to the abdomen.

biopsy (Fig. 25.16). Arteriography has given rise to arteriovenous fistula at the site of puncture, usually of small arteries (brachial and vertebral) but it has also been recorded in the femoral artery.

Because of the grossly hypertrophied drainage veins carrying arterial blood, a fistula may be very difficult to locate at surgery, and prior angiography with localization of the fistula is essential. As with angiomas, the dilated feeding artery fills early, as do the dilated drainage veins, and large amounts of contrast medium with rapid serial films are necessary to clearly define the anatomy and the site of the fistula.

A large arteriovenous fistula throws an extra burden on the heart because of the large amount of shunt and can result in cardiac failure from high cardiac output unless successfully treated. As noted above many fistulas, particularly smaller ones, are now treated successfully by embolization.

HAEMORRHAGE

Arteriography can be extremely useful in the diagnosis and treatment of internal haemorrhage. Serious or life-threatening haemorrhage can be due to many causes including trauma, peptic ulceration, ruptured aneurysms, neoplasms or inflammatory lesions involving blood ves-

sels, radiation and blood disorders. In many situations previously requiring surgical intervention, percutaneous catheterization and embolization as described above offers a simpler and safer alternative to surgery.

Upper gastrointestinal tract haemorrhage. The common causes are oesophageal varices, Mallory-Weiss tears, gastritis, gastric ulcer, and duodenal ulcer. Endoscopy is now widely used for both diagnosis and treatment, and angiography and embolization have played a diminishing role in recent years.

Haemorrhage from the small bowel is much less common and more difficult to diagnose. *Scintigraphy*, as described below, may be useful in demonstrating the site, and *arteriography* will occasionally demonstrate rare causes such as angioma (Fig. 25.52). Other rare causes are jejunal diverticulum, Meckel's diverticulum, neoplasms and typhoid enteritis.

Lower gastrointestinal tract haemorrhage. Radionuclide scintigraphy is the technique of choice for the investigation of acute lower GI tract bleeding. ^{99m}Tc sulphur colloid or ^{99m}Tc-labelled red cells may be used to localize the approximate source of the haemorrhage, provided the patient is still bleeding (Ch. 30).

Diverticulosis is the commonest cause and, rather surprisingly, most bleeding diverticula lie in the ascending colon, though diverticula are much less common here than in the sigmoid and descending colon. *Angiodysplasia*, the second commonest cause, also involves mainly the caecum or ascending colon, and these lesions can be multiple.

Colonoscopy is less successful in identifying these lesions than arteriography, which is often necessary. Bleeding from colonic diverticula can be controlled by vasopressin though success may only prove temporary. Some cases have been controlled by embolization, though this requires difficult superselective catheterization. The alternative of emergency colectomy carries a high mortality, and even temporary control may permit a later elective colectomy. Angiodysplasias are often small and require high-quality angiograms for their demonstration, as bleeding is less severe than with diverticula. Arteriovenous shunting with early venous filling should raise suspicion. These lesions are usually treated surgically.

NEOPLASMS AND MASS LESIONS

Arteriography was once widely used for the characterization of tumours, cysts and other mass lesions but with the advent and constant improvement of the noninvasive techniques of ultrasound, CT and MRI the method has become largely obsolete as a purely diagnostic tool. Where angiography is still used, its purpose is either to complement the noninvasive investigations by providing anatomical information to the surgeon about the vascularity and blood supply of a tumour, or in some cases to permit embolization of inoperable tumours or of highly

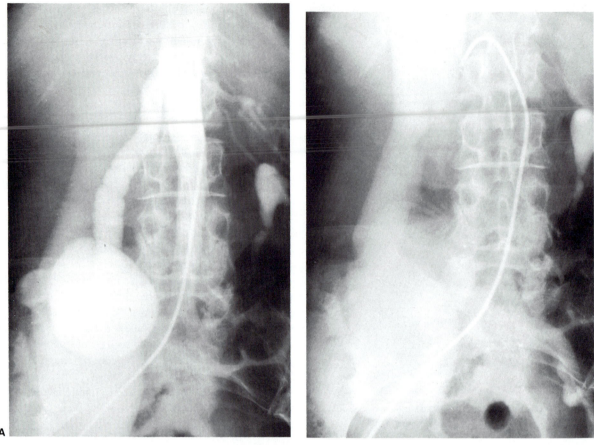

Fig. 25.54 Giant renal AV fistula, possibly due to rupture of an aneurysm associated with fibromuscular hyperplasia. The patient presented with heart failure and a pulsating mass clinically thought to be pelvic because of ptosed kidney. **A**. Arterial phase. **B**. Venous phase showing dilated IVC.

vascular tumours prior to surgery. In rare cases it may be used to help establish the correct diagnosis where ultrasound and CT have proved equivocal or inconclusive.

The value of angiography in tumour diagnosis arose from three facts. *First*, tumours often have circulations different from those in the tissues in which they arise. This results in abnormal or 'pathological' vessels being outlined by contrast and thus localizing and characterizing the neoplasm. Arteriovenous shunting with early opacification of drainage veins is a frequent feature of the more malignant neoplasms which tend to be more vascular than benign tumours. *Second*, the growth of the tumour may displace and stretch the normal vessels at its margins, thus enabling less vascular tumours to be located. *Third*, tumours may actually involve adjacent arteries, leading to 'cuffing' or irregular narrowing of the affected arteries.

RENAL MASSES

Hypernephromas are usually highly vascular tumours and the demonstration of typical pathological vessels in a renal mass is diagnostic (Fig. 25.56). Occasionally these tumours are so vascular as to simulate angiomatous malformations (Fig. 25.57). Conversely, they are also occasionally nonvascular, simulating cysts. However such cases will sometimes show tortuous or irregular vessels entering the periphery of the mass, a feature not seen with cysts.

Renal cysts are typically rounded avascular masses best shown in the nephrogram phase. The cortex at the margin of the cyst is compressed and displaced, producing a pointed projection of opacified cortex, the so-called 'beak sign' (Fig. 25.58). Further, the normal arteries at the margins of the cyst are stretched and displaced.

Carcinoma of the renal pelvis is much less vascular than hypernephroma, but high-quality angiograms will show one or more abnormal fine tortuous vessels leading to the tumour, and similar appearances may be seen in carcinoma of the ureter.

Wilms' tumour (nephroblastoma) occurs in children below the age of 5, though occasionally presenting at an older age and even in an adult. These tumours can reach a very large size and 10% are bilateral. At angiography they may show only limited neovascularity.

Angiomyolipoma (hamartoma) is a benign tumour but

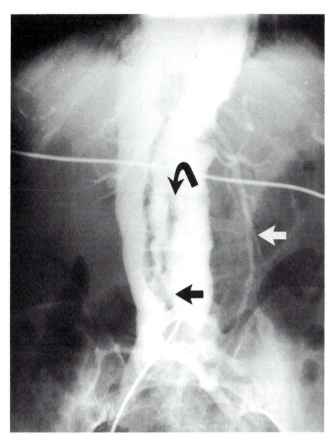

Fig. 25.55 Aortocaval fistula following spontaneous rupture of an abdominal aortic aneurysm. The superior mesenteric is displaced by the aneurysm containing mural thrombus (white arrow). The fistula into the IVC is marked by the black arrow. The curved arrow suggests an intimal flap in the aneurysm. (From Gregson et al. (1983) by permission of the Editor of *Clinical Radiology*.)

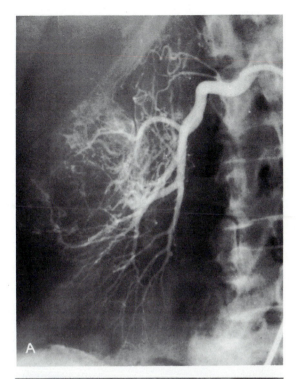

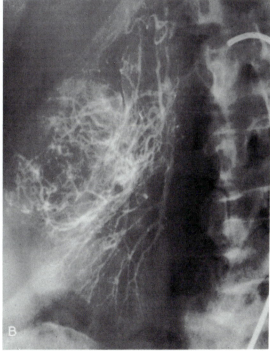

Fig. 25.56 A,B Renal carcinoma showing pathological vessels.

the angiogram shows a vascular lesion which can be mistaken for a carcinoma. Such tumours are common in *tuberous sclerosis* when they may be multiple. *Xanthogranulomatous pyelonephritis* is a chronic inflammatory condition which can also produce a vascular angiogram resembling that of a malignant tumour.

Renal oncocytomas have been described as rare benign tumours resembling hypernephromas but well encapsulated and sometimes showing a 'spoke-wheel' pattern at angiography. The existence of this entity remains controversial and they are considered by some to be low-grade hypernephromas.

Benign tumours of the kidney are rare but important in differential diagnosis. *Adenomas* are usually small and subcapsular in situation. A rare form of *giant benign renal adenoma* has been described which at angiography is well circumscribed and separate from adjacent normal renal tissue. There is no arteriovenous shunting or other feature to suggest malignancy.

The rare renin-secreting *juxtaglomerular cell tumour* is found in hypertensive patients. At angiography it shows as a small cortical defect in the nephrogram phase, resembling a small cyst. A few fine vessels to the tumour may be identified, as may the slight bulge in the surface of the kidney. *Renin assay* from the renal veins helps to confirm the diagnosis by demonstrating higher concentrations on the affected side.

Renal angiography has also been used in the past to confirm such benign conditions as *pseudotumours* (e.g.

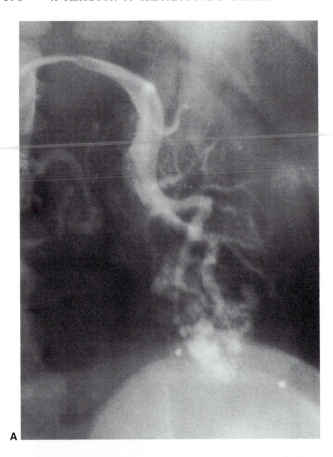

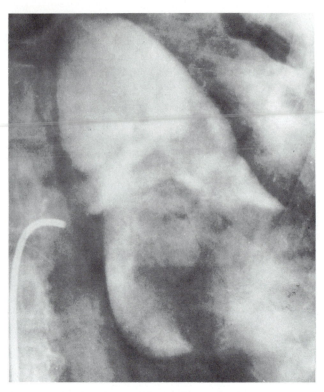

Fig. 25.58 Renal angiogram. Nephrogram shows large cyst displacing cortex ('beak sign').

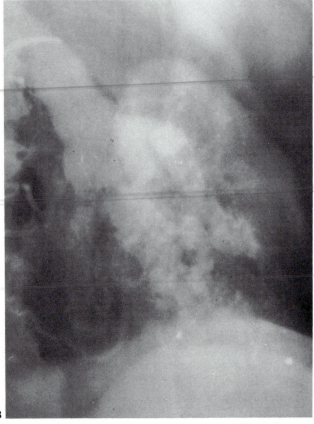

Fig. 25.57 A,B Highly vascular renal carcinoma resembling angioma. Note huge drainage vein in nephrogram phase.

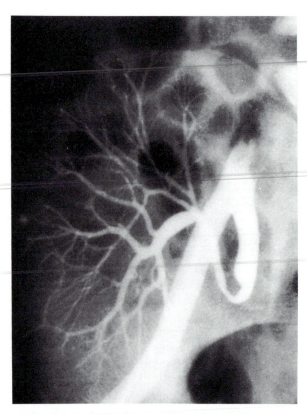

Fig. 25.59 Renal graft arteriogram. The patient developed secondary hypertension and a bruit. The arteriogram shows an unusual stenosis of the proximal segment of the graft artery.

enlarged column of Bertin, dromedary hump, congenital polar enlargement, suprahilar and infrahilar lips, and areas of compensatory hypertrophy).

Renal graft angiography. Multiple arteries occur in 25% of kidneys and it is therefore necessary to perform angiography on live kidney donors to ensure that the proposed kidney has only one artery of supply. The grafted kidney is usually placed in the right iliac fossa with its artery anastomosed to the patient's internal iliac artery.

The commonest cause of failure of a transplant kidney is renal rejection, which can be early or delayed. Sometimes it is difficult to differentiate clinically between rejection of the graft and other complications affecting renal function.

A graft arteriogram will show whether the kidney is perfusing normally and will demonstrate such complications as stenosis at the anastomosis (Fig. 25.59). Generalized small-vessel occlusions, which are usually due to rejection, will be shown, as will thrombosis of the main artery or impaired perfusion. Kidney transplant arteriography can be performed by injection of a large bolus of contrast medium into the common iliac artery (20 ml of iopamidol 300 or equivalent of other contrast media). Selective angiography of the internal iliac artery will give better resolution and intra-arterial DSA will permit low doses of contrast medium.

HEPATIC TUMOURS

The primary investigation of liver masses is by ultrasound, with scintiscanning, CT and MRI all able to provide fur-ther help in characterizing lesions. Angiography now has little place in such diagnostic studies, but it can still be used for therapeutic purposes such as intra-arterial chemotherapy or embolization or for the elucidation of the occasional problem case (see Ch. 34).

Selective hepatic angiography can demonstrate both *primary* and *secondary carcinoma* of the liver. Such malignant tumours usually show a well-marked pathological circulation (Fig. 25.60), but are occasionally poorly vascularized and difficult to differentiate from benign masses. The latter tend merely to displace and stretch branches of the hepatic artery, though some are more vascular.

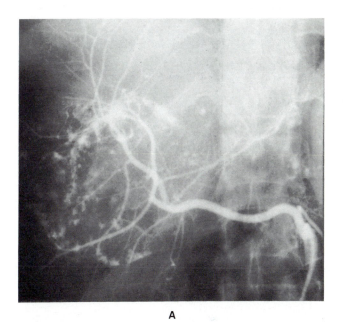

A

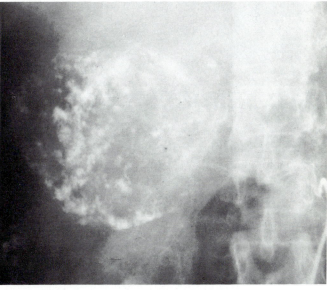

B

Fig. 25.60 Selective hepatic arteriogram. A large vascular tumour is shown in the lower part of the right lobe of the liver. Histology : primary hepatoma.

Fig. 25.61 A,B Vascular lesion simulating tumour in the liver. Haemangioma. Note absence of drainage veins or AV shunting and persistence of contrast medium in late phase. (**B.**)

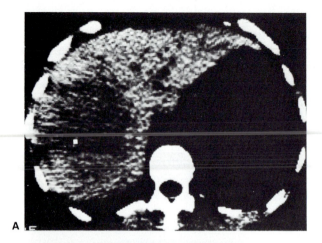

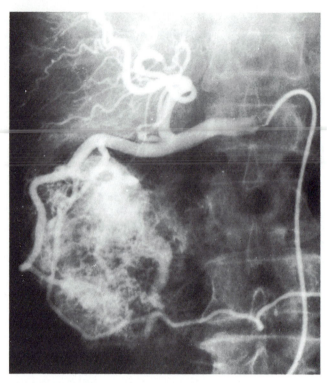

Fig. 25.63 Pancreatic cystadenoma showing florid pathological circulation in the head of the pancreas.

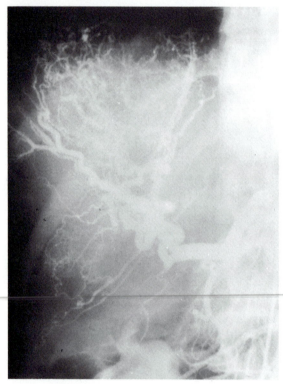

Fig. 25.62 Hepatic adenomas. **A**. CT shows large low-density mass in right lobe of liver (Wl34 L67). **B**. Angiogram shows large vascular mass with smaller mass in lower part of right lobe.

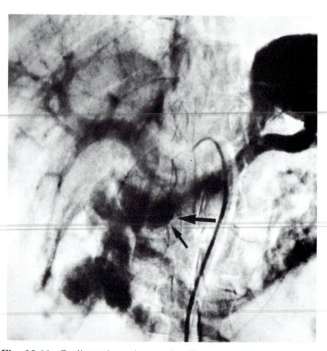

Fig. 25.64 Coeliac axis angiogram (capillary and venous phase). Subtraction film. The well-defined blush in the pancreatic head (arrowed) was an insulinoma. (Courtesy of Dr R. Dick.)

Haemangioma is the commonest benign tumour of the liver to show an abnormal circulation. These lesions are sometimes multiple and can then be suspected as deposits at ultrasound or other noninvasive investigations. Differentiation is possible on the angiogram since the lesions, though vascular, show a typical sluggish circulation, with persistence of contrast medium in the venous phase (Fig. 25.61). This is quite unlike the rapid arteriovenous shunting seen in malignant tumours.

Hepatic *adenomas* may also occur and have been described as a complication of hormonal treatment with contraceptive pills or with androgens. At angiography they are vascular tumours but their vascular pattern is more regular than that of a malignant tumour and they stand out as encapsulated tumours in the hepatogram phase (Fig. 25.62).

PANCREATIC TUMOURS

Ultrasound, CT and ERCP are now the methods of choice for the diagnosis of pancreatic tumours. Angiography, once widely used for this purpose, is now obsolete except for the elucidation of suspected small endocrine tumours.

Pancreatic *carcinoma* is relatively avascular and tumours were recognized by displacement of vessels supplying the pancreas or by invasion of their walls with cuffing or occlusion.

Cystadenoma of the pancreas however can be highly vascular and shows a florid pathological circulation (Fig. 25.63).

Islet-cell adenomas of the pancreas may be quite small and difficult to diagnose by noninvasive imaging techniques. At superselective angiography, however, they can be identified as a rounded blush of contrast in the venous or capillary phase (Fig. 25.64). Large islet-cell adenomas are occasionally seen and can be highly vascular.

Pancreatic hormone-producing tumours can also be identified by *venous blood sampling* and *assay* from the pancreatic drainage veins. The samples are obtained by transhepatic portal vein catheterization as described below (Ch. 35).

ADRENAL TUMOURS

Angiography is no longer used for the diagnosis of adrenal tumours and CT is now the primary imaging method (see Ch. 36).

TUMOURS OF BONE AND SOFT TISSUE

The newer imaging techniques, particularly CT and MRI, are now the investigations of choice for tumours involving bone and for soft-tissue tumours in all parts of the body. Angiography is now rarely undertaken in these cases except for embolization or other therapeutic purposes.

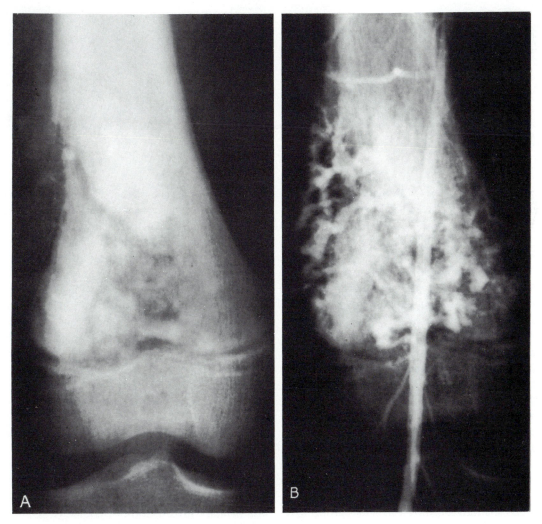

Fig. 25.65 A,B Osteogenic sarcoma showing pathological vessels with arteriovenous shunting.

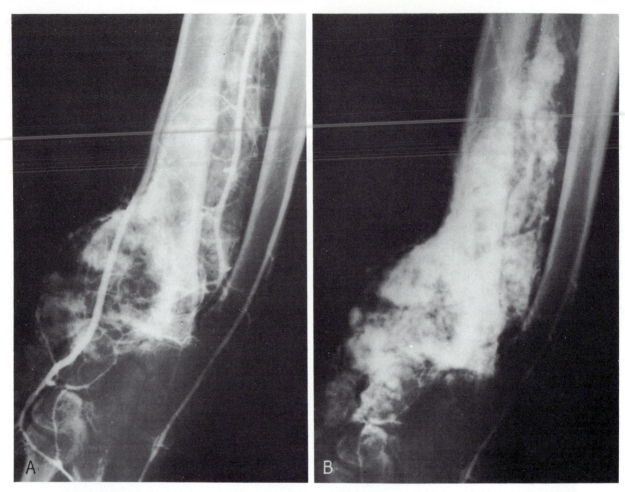

Fig. 25.66 A,B Malignant osteoclastoma. Note spread outside bone.

Malignant bone tumours are usually highly vascular and the angiographic appearances are pathognomonic (Fig. 25.65). Prior to the advent of CT, angiography was widely used to demonstrate the extraosseous spread of such tumours (Fig. 25.66). Secondary deposits in bone vary in their vascularity, ranging from the highly vascular to the relatively nonvascular. Hypernephroma and thyroid metastases have been amongst the most vascular encountered and such deposits in the soft tissues can simulate pulsating aneurysms.

Sarcoma of the soft tissues, when highly malignant, usually shows abundant pathological vessels (Fig. 25.67) but low-grade fibrosarcomas may be relatively nonvascular.

Chromaffinoma (chemodectoma). These tumours are most frequently found at the carotid bifurcation where they are known as *carotid-body tumours*. They are extremely vascular and show a characteristic appearance at angiography (Fig. 25.68). Occasionally they are familial, when they can also be bilateral. Clinically they have been mistaken for local aneurysms, and conversely, rare aneurysms at this site have been mistaken for carotid body tumours.

Another common site for chromaffinoma is the glomus jugulare at the base of the skull (*glomus jugulare tumour*). Here they are also very vascular and the angiographic appearance is similar to that of the carotid body tumour. Careful superselective angiography of the external carotid feeding branches may be required to show their full extent or for embolization, which may be required prior to surgery or in inoperable cases (see Ch. 56). The *glomus tympanicum tumour* lies in the middle ear, and will require high-quality subtraction films for its demonstration.

These tumours occur less commonly in other sites, but the angiographic appearances are similar. The *glomus vagale tumour* lies between the carotid body and glomus jugulare sites, whilst the *aortic body tumour* lies in the mediastinum above the aortic arch. Pelvic tumours are also described.

Nasopharyngeal angiofibroma (juvenile angiofibroma). These highly vascular tumours present as swellings arising from the nasopharynx of adolescent boys. They may invade the antrum and produce swelling of the cheek. They are best shown by CT which is now the primary investigation of choice (Fig. 25.69), but they are also well shown by superselective angiography of the external carotid artery. Surgery, which may otherwise be

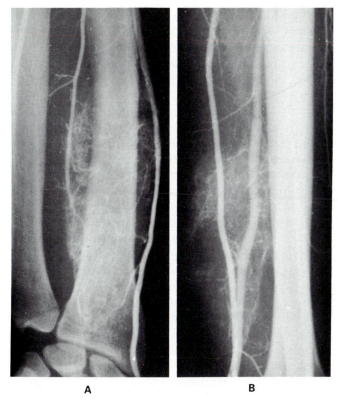

Fig. 25.67 Malignant tumour of the forearm (rhabdomyosarcoma). **A**. AP view. **B**. Lateral view.

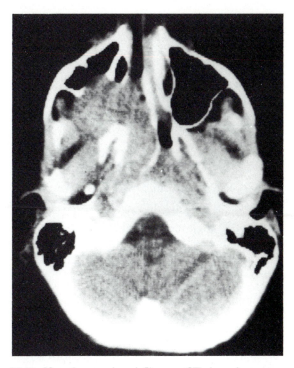

Fig. 25.69 Nasopharyngeal angiofibroma. CT shows large mass deforming right antrum and nares (W256 L36). Same case as Fig. 25.18.

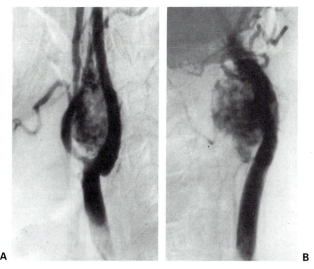

Fig. 25.68 A,B Carotid-body tumour.

hazardous, can be aided by prior embolization of the main feeding vessels (Fig. 25.18).

Haemangiopericytoma. These rare tumours of small blood vessels may occur anywhere in the body where there are capillaries but are mainly seen in the soft tissues. They may be benign but they can also be highly malignant. In our experience the latter type are very vascular (Fig. 25.70), and malignancy may be related to the degree of vascularity. Specific diagnosis however depends on biopsy and is made by the histopathologist.

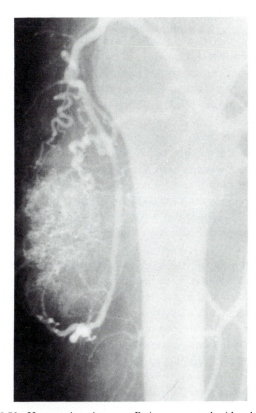

Fig. 25.70 Haemangiopericytoma. Patient presented with a lump in the thigh. The vascular tumour was highly malignant and metastasized rapidly.

DOPPLER ULTRASOUND OF THE VASCULAR SYSTEM
W. R. Lees and W. K. Chong

Doppler ultrasound of the vascular system utilizes the basic physical principle that the frequency of reflected sound waves increases if the reflector (flowing blood) is moving towards the source and decreases if the reflector is moving away.

The Doppler equation represents this as:-

$$\text{Frequency shift} = 2FV \cos \theta / c$$

where F = transducer frequency, V = velocity of moving blood, θ = the angle between the ultrasound beam and flow direction, and c = the speed of sound in the tissues.

Clinically it is employed and presented in three different ways:

1. Continuous-wave Doppler
2. Pulsed Doppler
3. Colour flow mapping.

Duplex Doppler combines pulsed Doppler with a real time B-scan image.

Continuous-wave Doppler uses two transducer crystals mounted side by side, one continuously emitting and the other continuously receiving sound waves. Very high velocities can be recorded and peak velocities obtained but significant depth resolution, which is easy with pulsed Doppler, is not possible.

Pulsed Doppler utilizes a single transducer to emit short bursts of energy which are received and recorded in the intervals between emission. This method permits precise focusing of the ultrasound beam on sample volumes as small as 2 or 3 mm diameter. However the necessity for repeated pulses renders the method less accurate than continuous-wave Doppler for measuring high velocity flows and recording high peak velocities.

Colour flow mapping is based on the principle of pulsed Doppler and the system allows assessment across the full field of a two-dimensional image. The results are coded in colour, with flow towards and away from the transducer recorded in a contrasting range of colours and permitting immediate visual recognition.

Doppler examination of the carotid arteries

Duplex ultrasound is an accurate and reliable technique for evaluating carotid stenosis. It is useful for initial screening of patients with symptoms of carotid disease, enabling better selection of patients for angiography, when the intracranial carotid or the roots of the great vessels will be shown in full (Bluth 1988 and Hartnell 1989).

Frequencies of 5–10 MHz are used for the B-mode image. The patient is placed in the supine position with the head turned away from the side to be examined. The common carotid artery is examined low in the neck and by directing the transducer downwards it is possible to get close to the origins of the great vessels. The common carotid is then scanned longitudinally and transversely. Where plaques are seen the luminal diameter is assessed by studying the vessel transversely and Doppler recordings are made. Samples should be taken from the centre of the lumen. A variable degree of widening takes place at the carotid bifurcation (the carotid bulb) and in the proximal 1–2 cm of the internal carotid artery. A longitudinal image of the bifurcation should be obtained. The external carotid lies anterior and medial to the internal carotid. Its branches may sometimes be seen and the two vessels have characteristic Doppler waveforms. Representative spectra are recorded from disease-free portions of the external, internal and common carotid arteries. (Fig. 25.71). The examination can be performed much more quickly if colour Doppler is available.

The arterial lumen should be free of echoes. Thrombus or plaques with a predominantly fatty content are poorly echogenic while fibrous (collagen) plaque is moderate to strongly echogenic without acoustic shadowing. Heterogeneous plaques are suggestive of intraplaque haemorrhage or a mixture of lipid and collagen. Strongly echogenic plaque with acoustic shadowing indicates calcification. Plaque can be anechoic and will only be seen with colour Doppler by appearing as a filling defect in the colour image. Ultrasound is not sensitive enough to detect plaque ulceration.

To assess the extent and severity of a plaque accurately the vessel must be imaged transversely as longitudinal imaging alone may give rise to error. (see above). Heavily calcified plaque may completely obscure the lumen and the sonographer must then rely on Doppler recordings taken proximal and distal to the lesion to assess its significance (Fig. 25.72).

Spectral broadening is the earliest sign of stenosis and can be seen with minor lesions (up to 15% diameter reduction). As a stenosis becomes more severe the peak systolic velocity (PSV) will increase and the spectrum will broaden until the whole systolic 'window' is filled in. There is dispute about the exact PSV value corresponding to a 50% stenosis, but most authorities accept 120 cm/s. Careful positioning of the cursor in the middle of the stenotic jet is required to detect the highest velocities. In severe stenoses (90% or greater) there is simultaneous forward and reversed flow and the PSV can exceed 300 cm/s (Fig. 25.73).

PSV can be altered by other factors; it is reduced by low cardiac output or another more proximal stenosis. If one carotid artery is occluded the flow (and peak velocity) on the other side will increase. Reliance on PSV alone to estimate the severity of a stenosis will therefore lead to

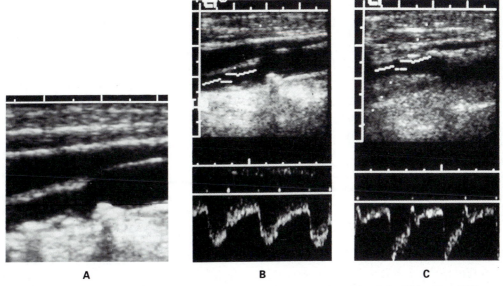

A   B   C

Fig. 25.71 **A**. A longitudinal section of the carotid artery showing a dense plaque at the origin of the ICA with a 30% stenosis. **B**. Pulsed Doppler spectrum of the ICA just beyond the bifurcation showing slight spectral broadening compared with the normal ECA. **C**. Normal flow pattern in the ECA.

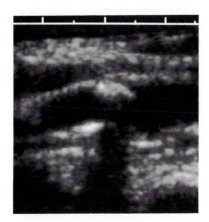

Fig. 25.72 Calcified plaque in the carotid bulb. Note that the acoustic shadow obscures the lumen behind.

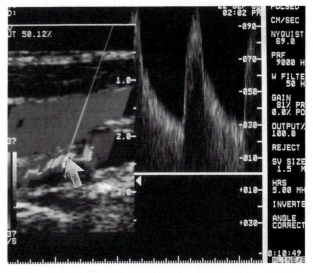

Fig. 25.73 Triplex study. B-scan, colour flow map and pulsed Doppler waveform all operating simultaneously. Real-time frame rates for all three are not yet available. The image shows the spectral broadening from a sample gate (arrow) within a haemodynamically significant stenosis of the internal carotid artery.

errors. These can be avoided by using relative velocities, and one of the most widely used is the ratio of PSV to the peak velocity in the common carotid (VCCA). A ratio of 1.5 corresponds to a 50% stenosis. A completely obstructed ICA will show no flow.

The common carotid pulse profile provides much valuable information. It is most easily assessed by comparison with the profile of the contralateral artery (provided that is disease-free!). Reduction of diastolic flow is highly suggestive of distal obstruction. If no significant abnormality is shown in the neck this suggests disease in the intracranial carotid artery. A severe stenosis will reduce the VCCA while a major proximal stenosis will result in overall damping of the waveform. Low cardiac output,

tachycardia and hypertension lead to abnormal but symmetrical CCA spectra; asymmetrical abnormality suggests obstruction.

Potential pitfalls. The Doppler sample should be taken in midstream. Spectral broadening occurs if the pulse profile is taken too close to the vessel wall, thus leading to overestimation of a stenosis. The change in calibre of the CCA at the carotid bulb gives rise to flow

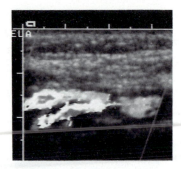

Fig. 25.74 Colour-flow study of a more than 50% stenosis of the common carotid bifurcation and internal carotid origin. This figure is reproduced in colour in the colour plate section at the front of this volume.

reversal, which may be misread as an abnormality. A severe stenosis can be mistaken for a complete occlusion if the cursor is not placed in the narrow high-velocity jet emerging from it. Heavily calcified plaques may make sampling from the correct site impossible. Consistent results will only be obtained if the angle of insonation is constant, which may be difficult in tortuous vessels. As has already been mentioned, abnormalities of cardio-vascular physiology will alter arterial pulse profiles (Fig. 25.74).

Colour flow imaging enables many of these pitfalls to be avoided. It overcomes the principal limitation of duplex imaging, namely that flow information is only obtained from the small area where the Doppler cursor is positioned. Turbulence and jets of increased velocity are easily identified and this is particularly useful for distinguishing a completely occluded from a severely stenosed artery. The examination time is shorter. As the entire image is being 'sampled', the problem of obtaining Doppler information with the same angle of insonation at each site does not arise.

Doppler examination of the renal arteries

Doppler can be used to assess renal artery stenosis and to evaluate the viability of renal transplants.

The renal arteries can be difficult to visualize by B scan and even experienced operators report failure rates of up to 18% due to obesity, abdominal aortic aneurysms, bowel gas and arterial calcification. The origins of the renal arteries may be found by scanning inferior to the coeliac axis. A 2–3.5 MHz transducer is used. The left and right arteries are rarely in the same transverse plane. Colour Doppler is very helpful for locating the arteries and a pulse profile can be obtained even if the vessel is not visualized. If adequate samples cannot be obtained from the proximal renal arteries then signals can be obtained from the renal hilum by scanning in the prone and decubitus positions.

Interpretation. The normal renal artery has a pulse profile similar to that of the internal carotid, with forward flow during diastole, reflecting its low peripheral resistance. Renal artery stenosis produces an increase in the peak velocity at the stenosis and a value greater than 100 cm/s or a ratio of renal to aortic peak velocities greater than 3.5 are taken as abnormal. Spectral broadening and bidirectional flow due to turbulence will be seen distal to the stenosis. A reduction in diastolic flow velocity at the hilum is suggestive of a more proximal stenosis. The absence of a Doppler signal within the renal artery indicates complete occlusion.

Pitfalls. The optimum criteria for diagnosing RAS have not yet been established. Renal parenchymal disease increases vascular resistance, thus reducing diastolic flow. Complete occlusion can only be diagnosed if no flow is seen in a clearly imaged renal artery, otherwise an erroneous positive diagnosis will be made. Collaterals can be mistaken for patent renal arteries. Two renal arteries will complicate Doppler interpretation.

Doppler evaluation of renal transplants

Doppler has been found to be reliable in diagnosing the vascular complications of renal transplantation. Recordings are taken from the main, segmental and arcuate arteries as well as from the renal vein. The arcuate arteries are rarely seen on the real-time image but can be located by placing the cursor at the corticomedullary junction. The main renal artery is frequently not visualized.

Complete or segmental occlusion from thrombosis can be shown by absence of Doppler signal from all or part of the kidney. Renal vein thrombosis will result in absence of normal venous signal. Renal artery stenosis can be diagnosed in the same way as in native arteries.

In 60% of graft rejections there is increased peripheral resistance due to vascular obstruction with inflammatory debris. This results in decreased, absent or even reversed flow in diastole. This can be quantified as the pulsatility index (PI):

$$\frac{\textit{Peak systolic frequency shift} - \textit{lowest diastolic frequency shift}}{\textit{mean frequency shift}}$$

A PI of greater than 1.5 was found diagnostic of rejection with a sensitivity of 75%, and no normals had an index above 1.8. Acute tubular necrosis also leads to increased vascular resistance, although not as much as vascular rejection. Serial measurements of PI are very useful for monitoring progression or recovery of rejection or ATN.

Other applications of Doppler ultrasound

Peripheral arteries. Pseudoaneurysms (Fig. 25.75) and AV fistulas are easily shown on colour Doppler. Stenoses in the femoral and popliteal vessels are also well

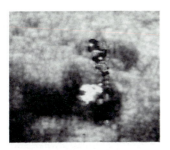

Fig. 25.75 False aneurysm of the femoral artery caused by arterial catheterization. High flow in the artery is shown in yellow and the jet into the aneurysm is largely red. This figure is reproduced in colour in the colour plate section at the front of this volume.

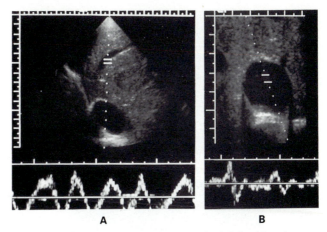

A   B

Fig. 25.76 A. Reciprocal flow pattern in the left hepatic vein. The normal flow pattern is exaggerated by tricuspid incompetence. **B**. Complex flow in the IVC.

demonstrated although the time required for a complete Doppler study of the peripheral arteries makes it unlikely that it will replace angiography.

Gastrointestinal. Colour Doppler is extremely useful for differentiating bile ducts from vessels, and flow can be assessed in the hepatic and portal veins. Diagnosis of portal vein thrombosis or the Budd-Chiari syndrome is as effective as by angiography. The direction of flow can be determined in the portal vein but spectral analysis is usually unhelpful in patients with portal hypertension.

By studying the transmission of the right atrial pressure waves into the hepatic veins we can gain information about the compliance of the liver parenchyma. In the normal patient there is reverse flow during systole (Fig. 25.76). Continuous forward flow throughout the cardiac cycle is indicative of liver disease if there are no other complicating factors such as ascites (Fig. 25.77).

Both colour flow mapping and duplex Doppler are used in liver transplant assessment as for the kidney (Fig. 25.78).

Doppler is potentially useful for evaluating mesenteric ischaemia but its clinical value has still to be established.

Testes. Reduced or no flow in the testicular arteries is a reliable sign of testicular torsion.

Vascular impotence. *Impotence* affects at least 10% of males and is of organic origin in over 70% of cases. The blood flow within the cavernosal artery can be monitored by duplex Doppler after injection of 40–80 mg of papaverine directly into the corpora cavernosa. There is immediate dilatation of the arteries within the corpora, leading to a massive inflow of blood. As the pressure gradually rises the flow in diastole diminishes to zero as a full erection is obtained. The peak systolic flow then should be in excess of 35 cm/s. In patients with psychogenic or neurological impotence a normal response is obtained. Patients with arteriogenic impotence show a diminished peak systolic velocity with a damped waveform. Venous leakage as a primary cause can be determined by continuous high flow in diastole despite a

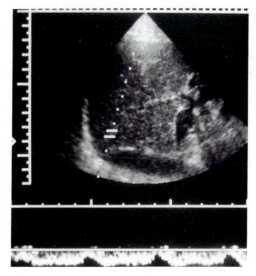

Fig. 25.77 Chronic liver disease with no flow reversal in systole.

good arterial response. This is a simple test which can successfully elucidate many of the causes of impotence.

Tumour blood flow. Colour flow mapping is very effective at identifying abnormal flow patterns within malignant tumours. This may be helpful in differential diagnosis. For example: *liver haemangiomas* show no significant flow even with the most sensitive instruments, but *hepatocellular carcinomas* consistently show high flow and thus the two can be distinguished. Neoplastic involvement of the portal venous system can be reliably detected with colour flow mapping, as can invasion of the renal veins and IVC by renal tumours.

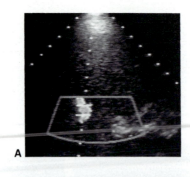

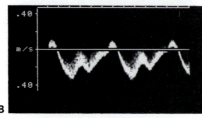

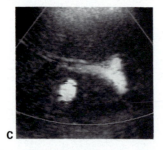

Fig. 25.78 A. Colour flow map of portal vein flow. **B**. Pulsed Doppler study after optimal positioning of the cursor on the colour map **C**. Flow in portal branches colour coded for direction. Yellow is high velocity flow. Parts **A**. and **C**. of this figure are reproduced in colour in the colour plate section at the front of this volume.

MR ANGIOGRAPHY

Ian Isherwood and Jeremy P. R. Jenkins

MRI is inherently sensitive to the detection of flow, and applications in the noninvasive assessment of vascular structures are increasing. This has been brought about by the development and implementation of multiplanar data acquisitions, sophisticated radiofrequency (RF) pulse sequences and postprocessing of data into 2- and 3-dimensional display formats. The ability to acquire not only morphological but functional information noninvasively is an important advantage. Further developments are to be expected in improving spatial resolution and the postprocessing capabilities for 3-dimensional display of the data. MR angiography is unlikely, however, to compete with conventional X-ray angiography in spatial resolution, vessel selectivity and therapeutic (interventional) options.

An understanding of the basic processes involved in flow phenomena is required in order to interpret the MR images obtained. Only a brief review will be given. The appearance of flowing blood is essentially a balance between those effects that produce a decrease or an increase in signal intensity. A decrease in the intensity of flowing blood can be achieved by *saturation, dephasing,* and *washout* effects, whereas an increase occurs with *flow-related enhancement* and *rephasing* of spins.

Protons exposed to repeated RF pulses become saturated (have a low magnetization) and produce a low signal. Unsaturated (i.e. fully magnetized) protons give a high signal when excited by an RF pulse. The *saturation* effect relates to the longer T_1 (and thus lower signal intensity) of blood compared with adjacent tissue. With appropriate T_1 weighting the intraluminal signal would be expected to be lower than that from the surrounding tissues. In conventional spin echo imaging this saturation effect is often opposed by the *flow-related enhancement* or *entry* phenomenon. This results from fresh blood (unsaturated protons) entering the imaging volume and producing a high intraluminal signal. In a multislice sequence this enhancement is more pronounced in sections nearest the entry point of the vessel into the imaging volume.

The most important process leading to a reduction in intraluminal signal is the *washout* effect. In order to generate a spin echo signal protons must receive both the 90° and 180° RF pulses. Since these pulses are usually 'slice selective' their effect is limited to the image sections. Blood flowing at above a certain velocity will have passed through the plane of section in the interval between the 90° and 180° RF pulses and thus produce a signal void. For this to occur the average velocity within the vessel has to be equal to or greater than the slice thickness of the section divided by the time interval between the two RF pulses (TE). In conventional spin echo imaging, rapidly flowing (arterial) blood is usually demonstrated as a *signal void* with slow-flowing (venous) blood as a *high signal*.

Another cause of intraluminal signal loss, particularly for inplane flow, is the spin *dephasing* effect. The moving spins in flowing blood are subjected to magnetic field gradients which lead to phase differences that are constantly changing relative to adjacent stationary spins. The greater the flow the larger the phase differences, which are also dependent on the strength and duration of the magnetic field gradients. There is thus a direct relationship between flow velocity and phase shifts which can be exploited to allow precise measurements of the former. Dephasing effects can reduce the intraluminal signal sufficiently to mask any flow-related enhancement that might be present.

Under certain circumstances, the phase differences induced by blood flowing through magnetic field gradients can be partially corrected, leading to an increase in signal from flowing blood. This *rephasing* effect is termed even-echo rephasing (gradient refocused echo imaging) and allows both the display and quantification of flow (Ch. 20).

From the preceding discussion, it is clear that the signal intensity appearance of flowing blood is complex and dependent on several factors. These include flow velocity, repetition time (TR), echo time (TE), type of echo produced, slice thickness and position of the section in the multislice set.

A number of MR angiographic methods which have exploited the above-mentioned phenomena are currently being investigated for the display and quantification of blood flow. The two techniques most widely studied are *time-of-flight* and *phase shift*. Each has advantages and disadvantages and can be implemented in either a 2- or 3-dimensional mode. Different techniques will be required for specific applications. In the *time-of-flight* (*saturation*) method the blood is modified by a selective RF pulse which then enters the region of interest. The effect is dependent on the T_1 relaxation rate of blood, which is short. This technique is thus best suited for studies of defined regions containing tortuous vessels with fast-flowing blood, such as the carotid arteries and the circle of Willis (Fig. 25.79). *Phase shift* (*gradient refocussed*) methods rely on velocity-induced phase differences to discriminate flowing blood from surrounding stationary tissue. These techniques are sensitive to the detection of

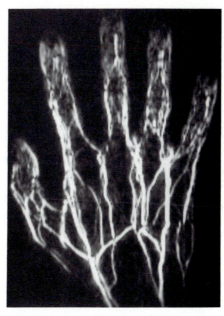

Fig. 25.80 Two-dimensional projection gradient refocused (phase shift) MR angiogram of the hand showing vessels as small as 0.2 mm in diameter. (Courtesy of IGE.)

slow flow in small vessels and produce a more efficient suppression of the stationary background tissue (Fig. 25.80). A further advantage of the phase-sensitive methods is that a precise measure of blood flow velocity can be made (see Ch. 20). *Subtraction* techniques (analogous to digital subtraction angiography) can be used to provide high signal from blood with the elimination of the background signal from stationary tissue. The use of *saturation RF pulses* allows tagging of particular vascular areas in order to visualize venous and arterial anatomy separately. Further studies are currently under way to compare the various MR angiographic techniques with conventional X-ray angiography and ultrasound.

Aorta

MRI, including MR angiographic techniques, has significant advantages over X-ray angiography and CT in the evaluation of *aortic aneurysms* and *dissections* (Fig. 25.81). The use of phase-sensitive methods (gradient refocused echo imaging) allows clear separation between the true and false lumens and assessment of the re-entry site to be made in aortic dissection (Fig. 25.82). Knowledge of normal anatomy (e.g. location of the left brachiocephalic vein and superior pericardial recess) and awareness of artefacts that can mimic aortic dissection are important in order to avoid any possible misinterpretation. MRI is superior to CT in the assessment of the postoperative patient (Fig. 25.83). Perigraft collections and aneurysms at the graft site can be

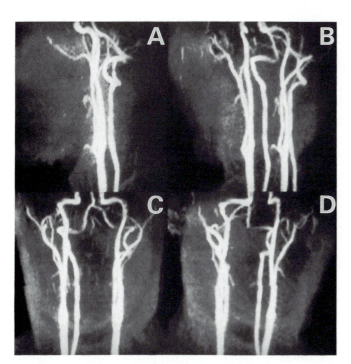

Fig. 25.79 Projection images. (**A**) Sagittal, (**B**) LAO, (**C**) Coronal and (**D**) RAO planes, from a time-of-flight MR angiogram showing normal neck and basal arteries. (Courtesy of IGE.)

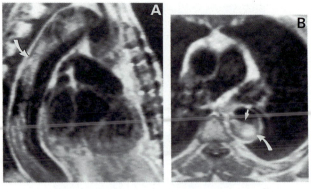

Fig. 25.81 Chronic descending aortic dissection on (**A**) sagittal and (**B**) transverse gated T_1-weighted spin echo (TE 26 ms). Note the signal from the slow-flowing blood in the false lumen (curved arrow), and the intimal flap (straight arrows).

demonstrated in the majority of cases without significant postoperative signal artefact.

The precise location, extent and severity of *aortic coarctation* can be assessed with MRI, providing information equivalent to that from X-ray angiography. The whole of the thoracic aorta can usually be demonstrated by oblique sagittal scanning along the line of the aortic arch (Fig. 25.84A). In some instances the aorta is more tortuous and multislice imaging is required for complete assessment. On MRI, the degree of stenosis of the coarctation segment, compared with the normal, correlates well with measurements made on X-ray angiography. A precise measurement of the pressure gradient and velocity across the coarctation segment can be obtained using MR angiographic techniques, (Fig. 25.84B). A pressure gradient can be calculated from the measured peak flow velocity at the stenosis using the modified Bernoulli equation. Collateral vessels, including the internal mammary, intercostal and posterior mediastinal arteries, can be visualized (Fig. 25.85). The evaluation of the descending aorta below the isthmus, which can be difficult on 2DE, is also important in the preoperative assessment and can be well demonstrated on MRI.

Pulmonary arteries

The normal dimensions of the pulmonary arteries can be well shown on transverse and coronal ECG-gated spin echo and gradient refocused images. High signals can be seen in peripheral small branching pulmonary arteries on gated spin echo images due to slow blood flow towards end-diastole. Similar high signals can be seen in the main pulmonary arteries and aorta. These signals clear with the onset of systole. Abnormal persistence of signal in the

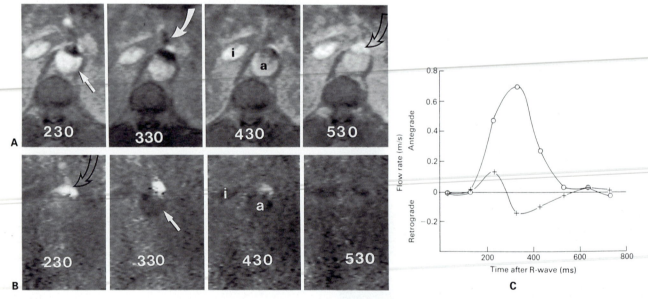

Fig. 25.82 Chronic aortic dissection on: (**A**) a set of four transverse cine gradient refocused (TE 28 ms) MR angiograms through the upper abdomen at the same anatomical level; (**B**) flow velocity maps derived from (**A**); and (**C**) a plot of the maximum flow rates in the true and false lumens at different times in the cardiac cycle, showing reversal of blood flow in the false lumen (0 — 0 = true lumen; + — + = false lumen). (Same patient as in Fig. 12.10.) In (**A**) images have been taken at 100 ms intervals from the R-wave of the patient's ECG (indicated by the number on each image). There is a high signal within the false lumen (straight arrow) of the aorta (a) and inferior vena cava (i). Note signal loss in the true lumen (curved open arrow) and superior mesenteric artery (curved closed arrow) during systole due to high flow rates, with return of signal at 530 ms as the flow rate reduces. In (**B**) flow direction and velocity can be derived. Antegrade flow appears as light grey, absence of flow as mid-grey (similar to background) and retrograde flow as dark grey. The true lumen (curved arrow) shows antegrade flow during systole, whereas the false lumen (straight arrow) shows initial antegrade flow with flow reversal at 330 ms (see **C**). Flow in the inferior vena cava (i) is consistently caudocranial. (Reproduced with permission from Mitchell et al. 1988.)

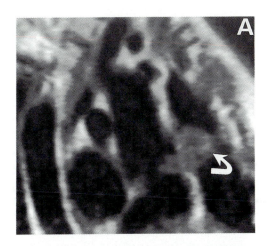

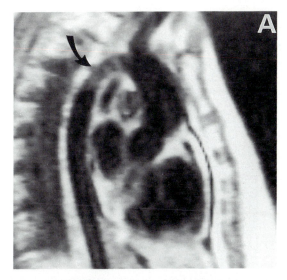

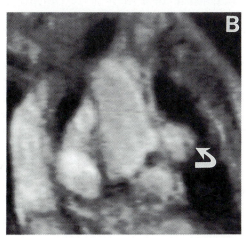

Fig. 25.83 Pseudoaneurysm of the aortic root associated with an aortic valve prosthesis on oblique-sagittal gated (**A**) T$_1$-weighted spin echo (TE 26 ms) and (**B**) gradient refocused (TE 22 ms) MR angiogram at the same anatomical level. The pseudoaneurysm (curved arrow) is clearly shown to contain flowing blood in (**B**).

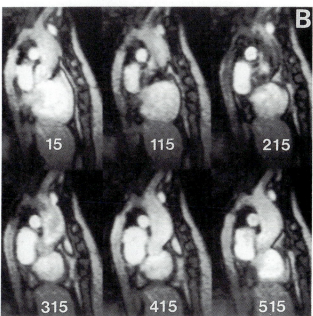

Fig. 25.84 Coarctation of the aorta, arrowed, previously repaired. **A**. Oblique gated T$_1$-weighted spin echo (TE 26 ms). **B**. A set of six cine gradient refocused echo (TE 12 ms) MR angiograms at the same anatomical level, spaced at 100 ms intervals from 15 ms from the R-wave of the ECG. At peak flow rates during systole, there is some signal reduction at the repaired coarctation site (arrowed) indicating turbulence. Velocity maps (not shown) were performed at this site giving a peak velocity (v) of 2 m/s (pressure gradient = $4v^2$ making a calculated gradient of 16 mmHg). This compared favourably with the value of 20 mmHg obtained from Doppler ultrasound.

pulmonary arteries during systole, on gated spin-echo images, has been used to identify patients with pulmonary arterial hypertension.

On gradient refocused images the normal pulmonary arteries are characterized by a rapid increase in intraluminal signal intensity and diameter in systole, with a consequent decrease in diastole. In addition, branch vessels down to the subsegmental level and beyond can be delineated, extending the range of pulmonary vessels accessible to examination. In contrast to the appearance of normal pulmonary arteries, the normal *pulmonary veins* have a distinctive signal intensity peak in both systole and diastole. These different appearances allow distinction to be made between pulmonary arteries and veins. In *pulmonary arterial hypertension* there is reduction in the normal compliance, with loss of the pulsatile systolic increase and diastolic decrease in diameter and signal intensity of the proximal pulmonary arteries.

MRI is gaining acceptance as the preferred technique for assessing pulmonary arteries in patients with pulmonary artery *atresia* or *obstruction* (Fig. 25.86). In neonates and infants, thin sections (< 5 mm) are required. Gated spin echo imaging can clearly demonstrate hypoplastic pulmonary arteries to the level of the first

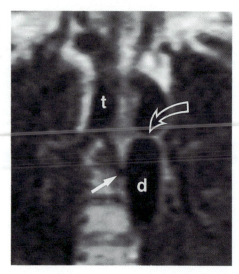

Fig. 25.85 Coarctation of the aorta on an oblique-coronal gated spin echo T₁-weighted image (TE 26 ms) demonstrated as a narrowed diaphragm (curved arrow). Note a dilated bronchial (straight arrow) supplying the descending aorta (d) beyond the coarctation. t = trachea.

size, because of magnetic susceptibility effects between the vessel wall and adjacent lung, which may lead to signal loss at the edge of the vessel. The combined use of gated spin echo imaging should overcome this problem. Difficulties in evaluating pulmonary arteries in patients with obstructive lesions have been encountered with both cine angiocardiography and 2DE, and MRI should have a useful role here.

Pulmonary emboli as small as 3 mm diam. can be detected experimentally on spin echo imaging, but may be difficult to interpret due to flow-related artefacts and poor differentiation between thrombus and areas of atelectasis or endobronchial mucous plugs. In addition, this technique does not allow acute and chronic pulmonary emboli to be distinguished. In a study of 11 patients with pulmonary embolic disease, acute and chronic emboli were distinguished using MR angiographic techniques. On gradient refocused echo imaging, acute pulmonary embolus was recognized as a persistent low signal intraluminal filling defect (due to the magnetic susceptibility effect of haemosiderin) with a curvilinear capping by the high signal intensity vascular column. Abrupt vessel cutoff without capping or the presence of webs or a narrowed and irregular vessel were interpreted as due to a chronic pulmonary embolus. No emboli distal to lobar branches, however, were demonstrated. MR angiographic techniques may have a useful role in the assessment of pulmonary embolic disease, with advantages over current imaging modalities. In addition, it is possible using MRI to examine for the presence of deep vein thrombosis.

hilar branch. The use of MR angiographic techniques extends the range for assessment of more peripheral branches, overcoming the limitation of 2DE in depicting distal pulmonary artery branch stenoses (Fig. 25.86). Important clinical determinants in the management of patients with right ventricular outflow obstruction are the size of the pulmonary artery and the presence or absence of a pulmonary confluence. Assessment of pulmonary artery growth following correction surgery is required to monitor and detect any developing stenoses. It should be noted that calculating vessel diameters from the intraluminal high signal obtained by MR angiographic techniques could lead to an underestimate of true vessel

Carotid arteries

The normal carotid bifurcation can be reliably imaged on MR angiography (see Fig. 25.79). Both carotid bifurcations can be imaged simultaneously in less than

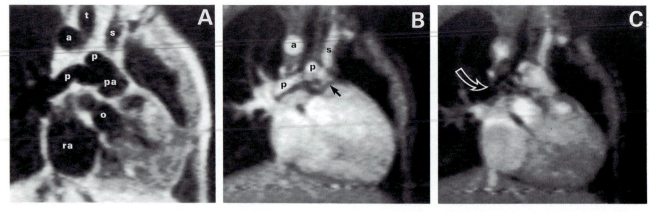

Fig. 25.86 Congenital branch pulmonary artery stenosis in an 11-year old child with corrected Fallot's tetralogy and persistent pulmonary artery hypertension. **A**. Oblique-coronal gated T₁-weighted spin echo (TE 26 ms) image. **B,C**. Gradient-refocused echo (TE 12 ms) MR angiograms at the same anatomical level. **B**. End-diastole. **C**. In systole, showing signal loss, due to turbulence, in the right pulmonary artery (curved arrow). a = right-sided aortic arch, o = outflow tract of the left ventricle, p = right and left pulmonary arteries, pa = main pulmonary artery, ra = right atrium, s = left-sided superior vena cava, t = trachea, straight arrow in (B) = position of pulmonary valve.

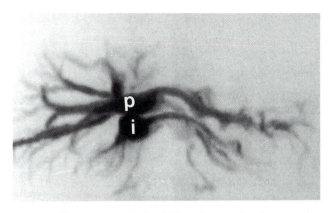

Fig. 25.87 Transverse projection MR angiogram showing venous anatomy of the portal system (p) and inferior vena cava (i) at the level of the left renal vein.

10 minutes by using a multi-slab 3-dimensional sequence. Subsequent images can be reformatted in multiple orientations to optimize the demonstration or show both bifurcations. Patients who have undergone recent carotid endarterectomy can also be evaluated noninvasively. As indicated in the assessment of aortic coarctation, short TE values are essential to demonstrate carotid artery stenoses. In severe stenosis there may, however, be profound signal loss mimicking occlusion. Recent developments, including the use of an intravascular space contrast agent, should help to resolve this problem. In order to demonstrate the circle of Willis, images are usually acquired in the transverse plane, where detail of the basal arterial tree and small branches can be obtained.

On MR angiography aneurysms and arteriovenous malformations (including intraspinal angiomas) can be visualized together with the relative flow contribution of the individual feeding vessels, allowing improved treatment planning.

The relationship and effect of tumours on adjacent vascular structures can be more easily appreciated than with conventional spin echo imaging.

Abdominal vessels. Respiratory motion artefacts have limited the early application of MR angiography to the chest and abdomen. Recent developments have overcome these problems, making it possible to detect renal artery stenosis and suspected portal vein thrombosis (Fig. 25.87).

Peripheral vessels. The absence of physiological motion in the extremities makes them ideal areas for vascular study (see Fig. 25.80). Normal and occluded popliteal trifurcation vessels can be reliably imaged using MR angiographic techniques. Stenotic lesions of this area, however, cannot be consistently portrayed. MR angiography can be used to investigate patients with claudication and in the noninvasive follow-up of patients who have undergone angioplasty, but further refinements are required if it is to compete with the more accessible and less expensive technique of ultrasound.

REFERENCES AND SUGGESTIONS FOR FURTHER READING

See end of Chapter 26.

CHAPTER 26

PHLEBOGRAPHY

David Sutton

The types of contrast phlebography used in clinical practice include:

1. Phlebography of the lower limb
2. Pelvic phlebography and inferior vena cavography
3. Hepatic, renal and adrenal phlebography
4. Phlebography of the upper limb and superior vena cava
5. Portal phlebography.

Intraosseous phlebography and spinal phlebography were once fairly widely practised but are now obsolete.

The investigations listed use direct contrast phlebography. Indirect phlebography can be achieved by serial filming following arteriography. The latter method is the one routinely used for the demonstration of the cerebral veins following cerebral angiography and commonly for the demonstration of the renal veins following selective renal arteriography. It is also used for portal phlebography following selective coeliac or splenic arteriography — so-called *arterioportography.* Other imaging techniques have been used in the investigation of the venous system but most have only limited application.

Radioisotope phlebography can be performed as a prelude to a perfusion lung scan in suspected pulmonary embolus. Half the dose of ^{99m}Tc is injected into each foot simultaneously and the passage of the isotope up the legs and through the abdomen recorded. The resulting images may show evidence of venous obstruction or a normal deep venous system. Delayed scans are also obtained of the calf and thigh to demonstrate local hold-up suggesting venous obstruction. Radioisotope phlebography offers an alternative technique in patients with iodine sensitivity or other contraindications to formal phlebography.

^{125}I-fibrinogen has also been widely used to diagnose deep vein thrombosis. In this case, however, the isotope is injected into an arm vein and is later taken up by the developing thrombosis. Recordings are made over the calf, popliteal and femoral veins and will demonstrate local increase of uptake. False positives may be obtained over wounds, haematomas and cellulitis, but the test has a high degree of accuracy with large recent thrombi and is relatively easy to perform.

Doppler ultrasound has major attractions as a non-invasive technique for diagnosing venous thrombosis. Doppler flow signals can be recognized over the femoral, popliteal and posterior tibial veins. Deep vein thrombosis is suggested when signals are absent or when muscle compression of the thigh does not produce the expected increase in femoral vein blood flow. In expert hands and with the addition of colour Doppler, a high degree of accuracy is claimed, though smaller lesions in the calf are more difficult to identify by this method (see below).

Real-time or B scan ultrasound will demonstrate well such deep-seated structures as the inferior vena cava or portal vein but, generally speaking, has little place in the investigation of most of the lesions discussed in this chapter.

CT will demonstrate the major veins well, but usually requires contrast injections for the confirmation of such lesions as caval thrombosis, and in view of its cost can hardly be justified for routine use.

MRI (discussed in Ch. 25) also shows major veins well and does not require contrast media injections. It is further discussed below.

DSA is limited in the area that can be examined at one time but will reduce contrast-medium dosage in areas where it can be used.

Liquid crystal thermography, which uses simple portable equipment, has a sensitivity of some 80% in deep venous thrombosis and a specificity of 57%.

C-reactive protein assay is a simple blood test which has been shown to have a sensitivity of 100% and a specificity of 52% in deep vein thrombosis. A normal result can therefore exclude DVT and prevent further unnecessary investigation.

THE LOWER LIMB

Indications. Phlebography of the lower limb is practised at most medical centres for the following purposes:

1. To demonstrate deep vein thrombosis in the calf, thigh, pelvis or inferior vena cava;

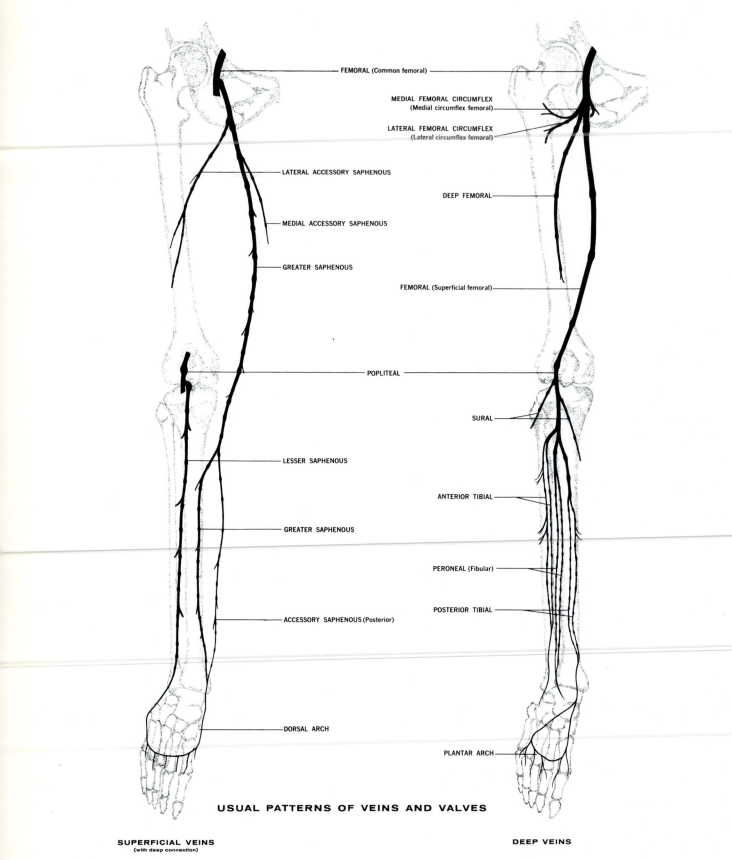

USUAL PATTERNS OF VEINS AND VALVES

SUPERFICIAL VEINS
(with deep connection)

DEEP VEINS

Fig. 26.1 Diagram of the deep and superficial veins of the lower limb. (Copyright Eastman Kodak Co. Reprinted courtesy of Health Sciences Division, Eastman Kodak Co.)

2. To show suspected venous obstruction by tumour or extrinsic pressure;

3. To investigate secondary or recurrent varicose veins thought to be associated with an abnormality of the deep venous system such as post-thrombotic destruction of valves and associated incompetent perforators, or with inadequate surgery;

4. To investigate swollen legs where the differential diagnosis between lymphoedema, cellulitis, and venous incompetence (or obstruction) is not clear;

5. To investigate varicose ulcers in the post-thrombotic syndrome.

6. To outline venous malformations.

Suspected deep vein thrombosis is the commonest cause for patient referral and in most cases there is strong clinical evidence for the lesion. In some cases, however, e.g. in patients with repeated pulmonary emboli but no obvious source, the investigation may be undertaken to exclude the lower limb as a source of emboli.

Normal anatomy. The venous drainage of the lower limb can be divided into two separate systems, the deep veins and the superficial veins. These are connected by the communicating veins (Figs 26.1, 26.2).

The *deep* veins in the calf follow the same distribution as the main arteries but are usually double, forming the anterior tibial, posterior tibial, and peroneal veins. The calf veins, or sural veins, arise in calf muscles and emerge from them to join the peroneal, posterior tibial or popliteal veins.

The communicating veins are usually small and paired and connect the superficial and deep veins. Normally they are extremely narrow, but they can become quite large when hypertrophied. They are valved so that blood only flows from the superficial to the deep veins. Under pathological conditions they can become incompetent, permitting reverse flow from the deep to the superficial veins (Fig. 26.3). They are most numerous and important in the calf, though there is usually one in the mid-thigh and sometimes two or three at different levels (Fig. 26.4).

The popliteal vein is a smooth large vessel lying behind the knee and passing up into the femoral vein which follows the course of the femoral artery. The femoral vein is sometimes double, or the profunda vein, which usually lies in the upper two-thirds of the thigh, may connect in its lower part with the femoral or popliteal vein. Perforating or communicating veins in the thigh are normally small, but if incompetent may be demonstrated connecting the superficial and deep veins (Fig. 26.4).

The *superficial* leg veins drain into the saphenous veins. The short saphenous vein passes up the lateral side of the leg to the knee, where it passes deeply to join the popliteal vein. The long saphenous passes up the medial

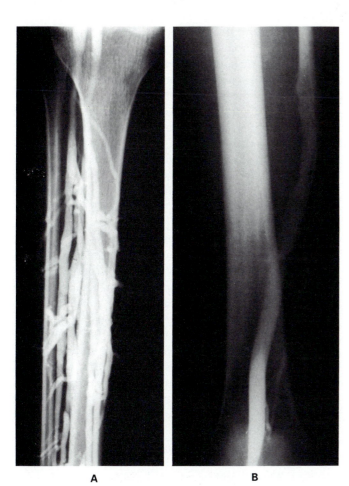

A   **B**

Fig. 26.2 Normal ascending phlebogram of the deep veins.

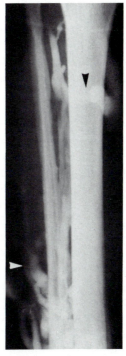

Fig. 26.3 Incompetent perforating veins in the calf (arrows).

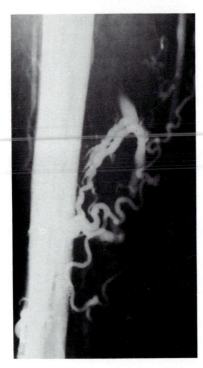

Fig. 26.4 Incompetent perforating veins in the thigh.

side of the calf and thigh and then joins the femoral vein below the groin.

The venous system can be regarded as a blood reservoir and normally contains some two-thirds of the body blood, largely in the lower limbs. Flow to the heart depends on the pressure gradient between the veins and right atrium, and is assisted by the muscle contractions, particularly in the calf, acting as a pump. The veins themselves can also actively contract and help onward flow of blood. The valves are also of great importance in preventing retrograde flow, and their destruction or damage by thrombosis has serious haemodynamic consequences leading to venous incompetence.

Technique

1. Ascending phlebography. A large number of different techniques have been described in the literature. No standard technique has been generally accepted. The technique used by us has been modified over the years and is as follows. A small needle is inserted percutaneously into a vein on the dorsum of the foot. Occasionally this may prove impossible and the needle may have to be inserted by cut-down. If the foot is swollen or oedematous, prior bed rest with the foot elevated is desirable to reduce the swelling. Once the needle is in position, compression is applied just above the ankle and also just above the knee by tourniquets or by inflatable cuffs. The pressure used is just sufficient to occlude the superficial veins completely without affecting the patency of the deep veins.

Contrast medium (40–50 ml) is then injected by hand pressure. In some cases more may be required to obtain adequate filling of the femoral and iliac veins, but it should rarely be necessary to use more than 80–100 ml. In the past, 65% Hypaque or equivalent other media has been used. However, the newer contrast media with low osmolality are now increasingly used (see Ch. 25) and these are better tolerated by the patient and less likely to produce complications.

Since the foot veins are usually punctured with small butterfly needles (21 British standard wire gauge) the injection can take 20–30 seconds. Flow is monitored by observation with an image intensifier and films obtained at appropriate moments as the veins are sequentially filled. Whilst some workers conduct the examination with the patient supine, others insist that the patient should be tilted on the table into a 30°–60° feet-down position. This is mainly to prevent layering of contrast medium posteriorly, which gives rise to artefactual filling defects, and to ensure mixing of blood and contrast medium. The foot and leg should be medially rotated to separate the tibia and fibula and the deep veins of the calf. The weight should not be borne by the foot being injected, so that the calf muscles remain relaxed and their veins can be filled with contrast.

2. Descending phlebography. This is less frequently practised but is occasionally used, with the patient supine on a tilting table and his feet against the footrest. The femoral vein is punctured at the groin and, with the needle in situ, the patient is then tilted to the erect or near erect position and contrast medium injected. If the patient performs the Valsalva manoeuvre, contrast medium will reflux down an incompetent femoral vein into the popliteal vein. It has been claimed, however, that contrast will sometimes flow past competent valves, though it is usually possible to assess the degree of true incompetence and show the valves clearly, particularly when they are competent (Fig. 26.5).

Complications. With the older contrast media, a few patients tolerated the procedure badly and complained of pain and discomfort in the calf with ascending phlebography. Nausea, vomiting and minor allergic reactions were also occasionally seen, as with all contrast media. The new low-osmolality contrast media are better tolerated and give rise to little discomfort.

Care should be taken to ensure there is no contrast medium extravasation at the site of puncture as this can be quite painful, and with a large volume of extravasation the consequences, particularly in an ischaemic or oedematous foot, can be serious. Skin necrosis has been recorded from this accident.

Phlebitis and postphlebography venous thrombosis can occur where large volumes of high-concentration contrast are used. This should be guarded against by flushing out residual contrast agent with saline at the end of the pro-

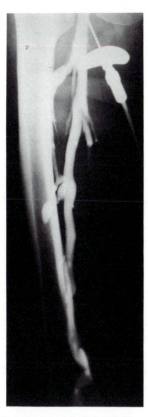

Fig. 26.5 Descending phlebogram showing incompetent valves and reflux down to the popliteal vein.

cedure, and by using the new low-osmolality contrast media.

Radiological findings. In the normal patient the deep veins of the calf are outlined by contrast at ascending phlebography with cuffs inflated; three paired veins accompanying the peroneal, posterior and anterior tibial arteries can be recognized, the last being smaller than the others. There is no filling of the superficial or communicating veins (Fig. 26.2), but with progressive injections of contrast medium there will be varying degrees of filling of the soleal muscle veins, which are typically large and valveless and drain into the peroneal and posterior tibial veins. There may also be filling of the gastrocnemius veins, which are valved and usually multiple, running a downward course from their points of entry into the upper popliteal vein.

The popliteal vein is single and commences near the knee joint, passing upwards to become the femoral vein. Views of the calf are usually obtained in both AP and lateral projections. Valves are usually obvious in the distended veins but can be accentuated by the patient performing the Valsalva manoeuvre.

A good-quality ascending phlebogram will also demonstrate the iliac veins and inferior vena cava, but these are best shown by releasing the tourniquet and manually compressing the calf to improve the upward flow of contrast medium at the same time as the pelvic exposure is made. This ensures a good bolus of contrast medium entering the iliac veins. If the suspected lesion affects only the pelvic veins or inferior vena cava direct pelvic phlebography is to be preferred (see below).

Deep vein thrombosis (DVT)
Venous thrombosis appears to be multifactorial in origin and is associated with slowing of the blood flow and an increased liability to blood coagulation. Conditions known to predispose include malignant disease, age, obesity, trauma and surgery, as well as prolonged immobilization, myocardial infarction and congestive heart failure. A rare but frequently fatal condition is Hughes Stovin syndrome, usually seen in young boys, where recurrent DVT is associated with haemoptysis from a ruptured segmental pulmonary aneurysm.

The risk of deep vein thrombosis is particularly high after abdominal and pelvic surgery, and even higher after operations on the hip, knee or femur. It becomes even greater if there is associated myocardial infarction or congestive heart failure. The thrombosis may be bilateral in some 30% of patients.

Clinically, symptoms are present only if there is significant obstruction or inflammation produced by the thrombosis, and it is claimed that 50% or more of cases are silent and symptomless.

The main danger is pulmonary embolus, and the incidence in the USA of this complication is over 500 000 cases per annum. The mortality in different series ranges from 10 to 30%.

The vast majority of these emboli arise from the leg veins. As already noted, half the cases show no prodromal leg symptoms before the embolus occurs.

Acute thrombosis of the deep veins appears as filling defects within the veins, the defect often being outlined by a marginal layer of contrast. Views in more than one plane may show that the clot is adherent to the vein at some point in one or other plane. Upward extension of the clot may be seen lying more freely in the lumen, and such a floating tail is likely to embolize. Adherent clot is regarded as relatively less dangerous. Clot may be identified in calf veins only, or involving the popliteal and femoral veins, or in the iliac veins and inferior vena cava (Figs 26.6–26.9).

True clot defects should be distinguished from

1. artefacts due to layering,
2. streaming from the entry of large non-opacified tributary veins, and
3. turbulence around valves.

Films in more than one plane, the Valsalva manoeuvre and multiple films all help in this respect, as do large doses of contrast medium and the semi-erect position.

Acute thrombosis is later followed by clot retraction,

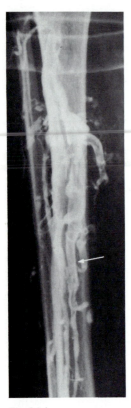
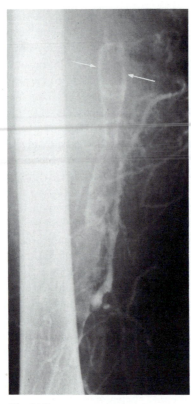

Fig. 26.6   *Fig. 26.7*

Figs 26.6 and 26.7 Phlebogram showing venous thrombosis (Fig. 26.6) in deep veins of the calf, and (Fig. 26.7) in the femoral vein. The clot shows as central filling defects with marginal contrast (arrows).

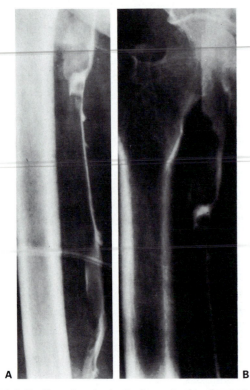

Fig. 26.8 A,B Extensive clot in the femoral vein adherent in part.

thrombolysis and recanalization, but the venous valves are damaged and destroyed so that the vein becomes irregular and incompetent. Some veins are severely stenosed or occluded and in these cases venous return is largely by dilated collaterals. In either case a *post-thrombotic syndrome* may develop, characterized by swelling and pain in the affected leg. Eventually this may lead to induration and ulceration. This is usually on the medial aspect of the ankle, but is occasionally lateral in position. This is related to the fact that the medial aspect of the lower third of the leg just above the ankle is the site for a group of communicating veins, usually three in number. As these are at the most dependent part of the limb the increased pressure from incompetence and partial obstruction is greatest here and is accentuated by the pressure from calf muscle contractions.

Phlebography in patients with post-thrombotic states will show involved veins to be irregular and incompetent. In severe cases the major veins may be occluded in whole or in part and replaced by numerous collateral veins.

Recurrent varicose veins. The recurrence of varicose veins after surgery is a frequent clinical problem and may occur several years later. In these patients a useful procedure is direct injection of one or more of the superficial thigh varicose veins to demonstrate their distribution and the pattern of recurrences at the groin following the previous high ligation of the long saphenous vein. There are several mechanisms but the most usual is a tortuous leash of recanalized vein and not a missed tributary of the long saphenous or a missed perforating vein (Fig. 26.10). The procedure may have the additional bonus of sclerosing the recanalized trunk and producing a clinical cure.

CONGENITAL ANOMALIES

Duplication of the popliteal or femoral vein or of both is not infrequent, as is duplication of the long saphenous vein. Congenital *absence* of the posterior tibial veins is another anomaly that is not infrequent. In this case veins are usually seen passing laterally above the ankle to drain into the peroneal veins.

Congenital absence of the venous valves is described in the major veins giving rise to venous stasis (*primary deep venous insufficiency*) and should be considered when children or teenagers present with varicosities or chronic leg swelling. However, such a diagnosis should be made with caution as previously unrecognized deep vein thrombosis with recanalization cannot always be excluded. It is claimed that such recanalization can sometimes result in apparently normal-looking veins without the usual irregularities seen in the post-thrombotic syndrome.

Klippel-Trenaunay syndrome. This is characterized by a naevus with hypertrophy of bones and soft tissues of affected limbs, usually legs, though arms may also be

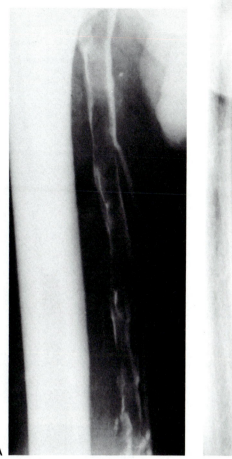
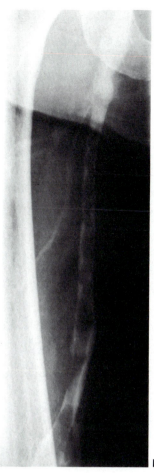

Fig. 26.9 A,B Extensive clot in the femoral vein.

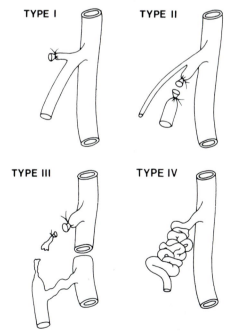

Fig. 26.10 The four types of recurrence in the thigh are shown diagrammatically. More than one type may apply in a given patient. (Reproduced with permission from Starnes et al., 1984.)

affected. There is venous dysplasia and the normal venous return is replaced by persistence of a more primitive system, usually a large lateral venous channel in the leg, or a single large medial venous channel in the arm (Fig. 26.27). These can be associated with superficial varicosities. The large drainage vein is often valveless and shows very sluggish flow.

Other anomalies. A large *varix* or venous aneurysm can occur anywhere in the venous system. Such lesions are not uncommon at the termination of the long or short saphenous veins. Superficial or deep venous varices or *venous angioma* are sometimes seen, such lesions having no obvious connection with an arterial lesion. Their anatomy is well shown by simple phlebography.

THE PELVIS AND ABDOMEN

As noted above, the iliac veins and inferior vena cava are quite well shown by good-quality ascending phlebograms from the foot, and their demonstration should be part of all such investigations. However, they can be more constantly and clearly demonstrated by direct femoral phlebography, which is the technique of choice where the

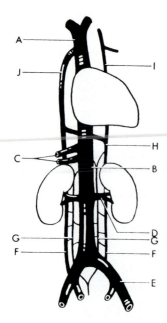

Fig. 26.11 Diagram showing venous drainage and connections of the inferior vena cava. A = superior vena cava. B = inferior vena cava. C = hepatic veins. D = renal veins. E = iliac veins. F = ascending lumbar veins. G = vertebral venous plexus. H = hemiazygos vein. I = ascending hemiazygos vein. J = azygos vein.

lesion is known to be intra-abdominal. The method is also used in the occasional cases where ascending phlebography from the foot has failed to clearly exclude or confirm clot in the iliacs or inferior vena cava because of poor contrast for technical or other reasons.

The lesions shown by pelvic and inferior caval phlebography include:

1. Acute thrombosis with recent clot, or post-thrombotic sequelae with partial obstruction and collateral circulation.
2. Obstruction by neoplastic or glandular masses, usually by extrinsic pressure, but also by tumour invasion as in hypernephromas
3. Extrinsic pressure from large benign tumours or other lesions, e.g. lymphocoele, aneurysms, retroperitoneal fibrosis, haematoma
4. Obstruction of the left common iliac vein by pressure from the right common iliac artery (so-called 'lymphoedema praecox')
5. Post-traumatic or radiotherapy venous damage
6. Pelvic varicosities
7. Congenital anomalies.

Technique. The iliac veins and inferior vena cava are well shown by direct injection into the femoral veins of 30–40 ml of contrast medium on each side. Both veins are injected at the same time unless only one iliac vein is obstructed and it is desired to show collateral and bypass drainage pathways clearly (Fig. 26.16). A unilateral injection will also suffice if only the inferior

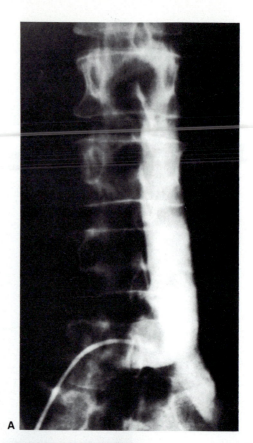

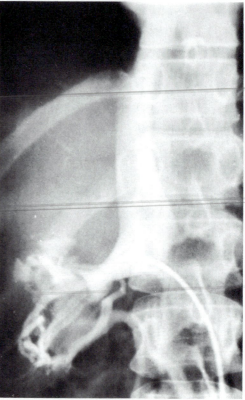

Fig. 26.12 A. Left-sided inferior vena cava as a chance finding in a patient undergoing renal vein catheterization. **B**. The catheter has passed over to the right renal vein through the left IVC where it joins the left renal vein; the upper part of the IVC is normally sited.

vena cava is under examination. The injection is made through a large needle inserted into the femoral vein at the groin, or after percutaneous insertion of a catheter which is passed 5–8 cm up the vein.

To obtain good filling, contrast medium is injected rapidly as a bolus, taking 2–4 seconds for the 40 ml on each side. Serial films of the abdomen are obtained at the rate of 1 per s for 5 s as normal flow is rapid. Better and more prolonged filling can be obtained if the patient performs the Valsalva manoeuvre.

Radiographic appearances. The normal external and common iliac veins and inferior vena cava are valveless and appear as large contrast-filled tubes. There may be a slight extrinsic pressure defect at the termination of the left common iliac where it is crossed by the overlying right common iliac artery. Occasionally the artery can partially obstruct venous flow (see below). The internal iliac veins do contain valves and are not normally demonstrated. The Valsalva manoeuvre will fill their terminations and sometimes provides better filling, but this is unusual. Stream-lining by nonopacified blood may be seen where large veins such as the renal veins enter the inferior vena cava. Figure 26.11 illustrates the normal inferior vena cava and its connections.

Congenital anomalies of the inferior vena cava occur in less than 1% of patients, but the incidence is higher in patients with congenital heart disease.

Left sided inferior vena cava is the commonest of these anomalies. In these cases the left-sided vena cava terminates in the left renal vein, which then usually drains into a normally sited terminal segment of the inferior vena cava (Fig. 26.12). Less frequent is a *double inferior vena cava* with the right larger than the left, or both equal in size. The left vena cava again terminates in the left renal vein (Fig. 26.13). Occasionally a left inferior vena cava may drain into the lumbar and hemiazygos systems, the coronary sinus or the left atrium. The suprarenal segment of a normal or abnormal infrarenal IVC occasionally drains into the azygos vein and hemiazygos vein instead of passing through the liver. This anomaly has been recognized at CT, when the dilated veins are shown behind the diaphragmatic crura adjacent to the aorta as it enters the thorax.

Both *agenesis* and *hypoplasia* of the inferior vena cava have been described. In these cases blood from the pelvis and lower limbs drains mainly into the lumbar, hemiazygos and azygos veins, which act as collaterals.

Thrombosis of the iliacs or inferior vena cava in the acute phase shows similar appearances to those described above in lower limb thrombosis, i.e. clot defect occupying most of the lumen with attachment to the vein wall (Fig. 26.14A), or, more dangerously, with a tail of clot extending into the lumen. In the latter case surgery may be indicated to prevent emboli passing to the lung. In the past this consisted of plication of the inferior vena

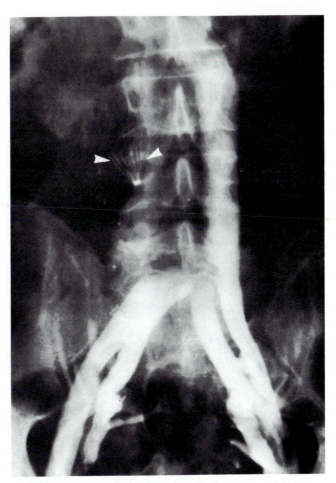

Fig. 26.13 Double inferior vena cava. A Mobin-Uddin umbrella (arrowed) has been inserted in the normal right-sided IVC. Postoperative phlebogram shows an unsuspected double inferior vena cava with the right side now occluded.

cava, an operation superseded by the transvenous insertion of filters (see below). Collateral bridging vessels will be seen, dependent on the site and extent of obstruction.

Complete thrombosis of the inferior vena cava is occasionally seen and there is then a collateral circulation utilizing a wide variety of collaterals including the lumbar and azygos veins, the vertebral plexus, the anterior abdominal wall veins, the retroperitoneal or even mesenteric veins (Figs 26.14B and 26.15). Such complete thrombosis usually extends to the level of the renal veins which remain patent. The upper limit can be demonstrated by retrograde phlebography from above a catheter being passed from the arm through the right auricle to the upper inferior vena cava.

Recanalization of the iliacs veins and inferior vena cava may occur after complete thrombosis when the vessels will appear smaller and more irregular with evidence of collateral vessels (Fig. 26.16).

Glandular and neoplastic masses can produce considerable distortion of the iliac veins and inferior vena

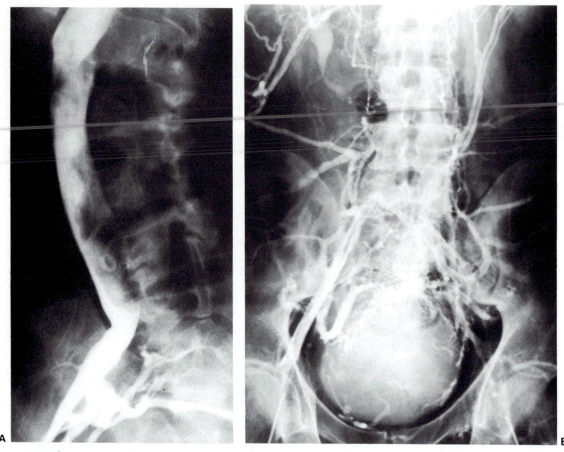

Fig. 26.14 A. Recent clot obstructing left common iliac and partially obstructing lower inferior vena cava. **B**. Thrombosis of IVC and common iliacs with collateral circulation. Some irregular recanalization of common iliacs.

cava. Large benign masses can produce marked displacement with little obstruction when only the inferior vena cava is affected (Fig. 36.26), but the iliacs are more easily obstructed by extrinsic pressure (Fig. 26.17). In the past, inferior vena cavography was widely used to assess para-aortic glandular involvement in reticulosis with conjunction in lymphangiography, but with the development of CT and ultrasound this is no longer indicated.

Renal vein invasion by hypernephroma is quite common and tumour may then spread into the inferior vena cava. Such tumour spread is well shown by inferior vena cavography (Fig. 26.18) or by CT.

Spontaneous iliac vein rupture is a very rare condition which has been reported in patients with proximal iliac obstruction (several by the common iliac artery). In one fatal case the rupture was precipitated by straining at stool. The patient presented with severe groin pain and circulatory collapse from the internal haemorrhage. Ruptured calf veins with haematoma formation are also well documented.

THERAPEUTIC INTERRUPTION OF THE INFERIOR VENA CAVA

Pulmonary embolus is a major cause of death. It is estimated that there are 630 000 cases per annum in the USA with some 200 000 deaths. In untreated cases the recurrence rate is said to be 60% with a significant further mortality rate (22%). Most cases are treated by anticoagulation, with thrombolysis by streptokinase or pulmonary embolectomy indicated in cases of massive pulmonary embolus. If anticoagulation is contraindicated, or fails to prevent recurrence, then caval interruption should be considered, since over 90% of emboli arise from the leg veins.

Therapeutic interruption of the inferior vena cava to prevent further pulmonary emboli was first practised in 1945 by operative occlusion. Later operative partial interruption was practised by suture partition, bead compression and external fenestrated clipping. Because of the risks involved to seriously ill patients from general anaesthesia and laparotomy, these operations were gradually

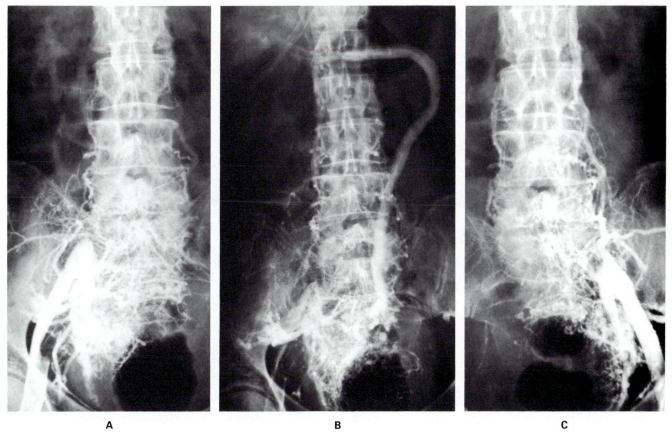

A   B   C

Fig. 26.15 A,B Thrombosis of IVC and common iliacs. Collateral drainage from the right leg via internal iliacs and haemorrhoidal plexus → inferior mesenteric vein → portal vein. **C.** Same patient. Collateral drainage from the left leg mainly via ascending lumbar veins and vertebral venous plexus.

replaced by a simpler technique. This involved transvenous insertion of devices from the right internal jugular vein after operative cut-down under local anaesthesia. The devices used included:

1. The Mobin-Uddin umbrella filter (1967) (see Fig. 26.13)
2. The Kimray-Greenfield filter (1973)
3. The Hunter detachable balloon (1975).

A preliminary inferior vena cavogram is necessary to confirm patency, to demonstrate possible anomalies and to show the level of the lowest renal vein. The device is passed down below the renal veins before being detached and stabilized. In some cases filters can be introduced percutaneously from a femoral vein approach, e.g. the 'bird-nest filter' (Cook Inc.) devised by Roehm et al. This can be introduced through a sheath and an 8F catheter. It consists of four stainless steel wires 0.18 mm wide and 25 cm long. The filter has two fine wire hooks at each end which can be fixed to the caval wall. The whole procedure can be rapidly performed by a radiologist but requires preliminary phlebography to ensure that the iliacs and IVC are free of clot.

MISCELLANEOUS ABDOMINAL CONDITIONS

Vulval varices are seen in pregnancy in 1 or 2% of patients and persist in a small proportion, some of whom complain of discomfort requiring surgery. In some cases phlebography by direct injection of the varix will be required to show the anatomy and drainage. This is mainly into the internal pudendal and obturator veins and thence to the internal iliac, but there may be partial drainage to the external pudendal and femoral veins.

Lymphoedema praecox was the term used for swelling of the left leg, usually occurring in young females and sometimes associated with partial obstruction of the left common iliac vein by the right common iliac artery passing over it (Fig. 26.17A).

Pelvic varicosities in the uterovaginal plexus and in the broad ligament are said to be fairly common and have been cited as a cause of the 'pelvic congestion syndrome'. They can also be associated with vulval varices. High-dose bilateral femoral phlebography with simultaneous compression of the inferior vena cava has been recommended to demonstrate these pelvic varicosities, but is not always successful.

Gonadal veins (ovarian and testicular veins). The

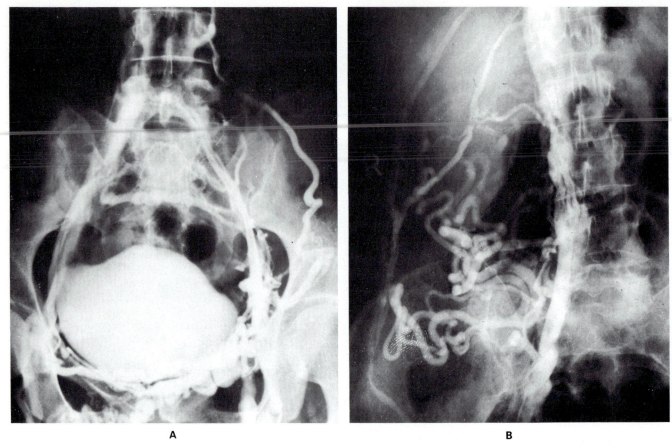

A   **B**

Fig. 26.16 A. Thrombosis of left iliac veins with partial recanalization and drainage of the left leg mainly by collaterals to the right iliacs via pubic veins. **B**. Thrombosis of IVC with recanalization and collateral circulation.

right gonadal vein crosses in front of the ureter at the level of L4 as it passes up and medially to enter the inferior vena cava below the right renal vein. When hypertrophied the ovarian vein can cause obstruction to the ureter giving rise to the so-called *ovarian vein syndrome*. This remains a controversial subject and the existence of this entity is not generally accepted.

The left gonadal vein usually drains into the left renal vein. Both gonadal veins can be demonstrated by passing a catheter into their upper ends from a transfemoral vein approach and injecting contrast medium. *Varicocoeles*, which occur mainly on the left side, have been treated by percutaneous embolization of their drainage veins. Considerable success has been claimed for this procedure in the treatment of varicocoele associated with male infertility. Another rare indication for the procedure is the localization of an *ectopic testis* which the noninvasive techniques of US, CT or MRI have failed to locate.

Hepatic vein obstruction (Budd-Chiari syndrome). Following the passage of a catheter into the upper part of the inferior vena cava, the hepatic veins can often be demonstrated by a forced injection of contrast medium, particularly if the patient performs the Valsalva manoeuvre during injection. Failure to fill the hepatic

veins provides some evidence of thrombosis as occurs in the Budd-Chiari syndrome. In this condition the hepatic venous drainage is obstructed by tumour or thrombosis and a collateral circulation develops through the peri-umbilical veins. At inferior vena cavography, the upper inferior vena cava may be seen to be compressed or obstructed (Fig. 26.19) when a tumour is responsible.

Direct *hepatic phlebography* is performed by passing a catheter from the arm through the right auricle and into a hepatic vein. In the Budd-Chiari syndrome the normal wedged hepatic vein pattern is replaced by fine collateral vessels ('spider's web network'), or actual occlusions may be shown (see Ch. 34 — Figs 34.40 and 34.41).

Renal phlebography. The renal veins can be selectively catheterized using the Seldinger percutaneous technique. A forced injection of 10 ml of contrast medium will show the venous drainage of most of the kidney and will thus confirm or exclude a renal vein thrombosis (Fig. 27.12B). The method has also been used to demonstrate mass lesions in the kidney, but these are better shown by other techniques.

The renal veins can also be shown by serial films taken after selective renal arteriography. The normal renal veins usually show well by this method. If they do not and a

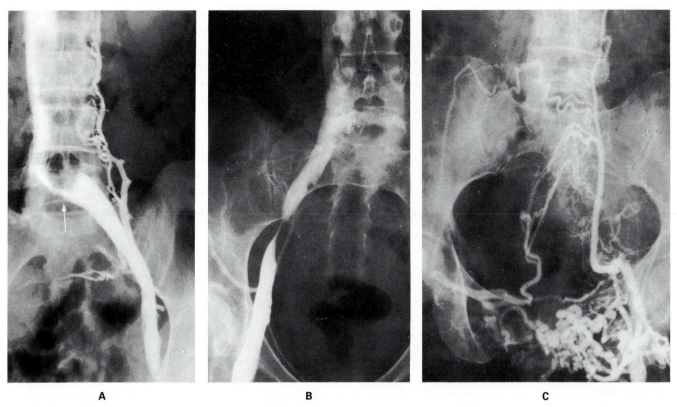

A   B   C

Fig. 26.17 **A**. Obstruction of the left common iliac vein by pressure from the right common iliac artery (arrow). Note collateral circulation via ascending lumbar vein. **B**. Iliac vein obstruction by glandular mass. **C**. Obstruction of left iliac veins in a patient with carcinoma of the cervix treated by radiotherapy.

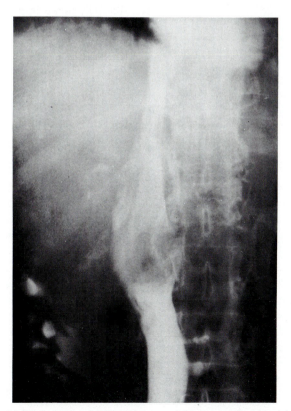

Fig. 26.18 Invasion of IVC by hypernephroma spreading up right renal vein.

collateral venous drainage is also shown, this is good presumptive evidence of main renal vein occlusion.

It is important to realize that there may be more than one renal vein on either side, and attempts should always be made to identify and catheterize accessory veins. On the left side 7% of individuals have a lower accessory vein which is smaller than the normal upper vein and is retroaortic in position. The two veins form a circumaortic ring with the lower one usually entering the inferior vena cava at L3–4 (Fig. 26.20).

Renal vein thrombosis has also been investigated by inferior vena cavography. In the normal inferior vena cavagram 'streamlining' effects are usually visible when the large renal veins enter the inferior vena cava. Absence of this normal streamlining effect is thought to be very suggestive of renal vein thrombosis, particularly when unilateral. Direct renal phlebography will prove the diagnosis conclusively.

Renal vein thrombosis is common in dehydrated infants with diarrhoea. It also occurs in adults in association with inferior vena caval thrombosis, or thrombotic disease elsewhere. Occasionally it is seen with pyelonephritis or other renal disease. The affected kidney is usually enlarged from venous engorgement and the nephrotic syndrome may result. The vein itself is narrowed and irregular and the small peripheral veins may be occluded.

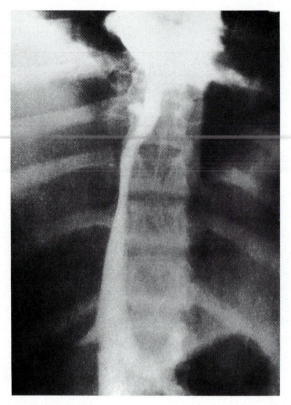

Fig. 26.19 Obstruction of hepatic veins with compression and distortion of upper IVC by liver neoplasm resulting in Budd-Chiari syndrome. The patient was performing the Valsalva manoeuvre. Note reflux filling of renal veins.

Adrenal vein phlebography. The adrenal veins can be selectively catheterized using special catheters. Small tumours have been demonstrated by this means when other methods have failed. In our experience the method has proved of most value in the diagnosis of small Conn's tumours in primary hyperaldosteronism. The method is discussed in greater detail in Chapter 36, but has now been superseded by CT. The technique is sometimes used for deliberate infarction of adrenal tumours.

UPPER LIMB AND SUPERIOR VENA CAVA

The usual indications for investigation of the venous drainage of the arm and superior vena cava are:

1. Oedema of the upper limb thought to be associated with venous thrombosis or obstruction, in order to demonstrate the site of obstruction, in either the axillary, subclavian or innominate veins.
2. Superior vena caval obstruction.
3. Demonstration of the full anatomy of venous angiomas or varices.
4. Demonstration of congenital venous anomalies as in the Klippel-Trenaunay syndrome.

Technique. A vein at the elbow is catheterized and a catheter advanced several inches up the arm. This can be done percutaneously in most cases though occasionally a cut-down exposure may be necessary. It is best to use the median basilic vein, since this will make it possible

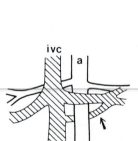

Fig. 26.20 Circumaortic ring formed by renal veins. a = aorta, IVC = inferior vena cava.

As noted above, hypernephroma frequently involves the renal vein and tumour may extend into the inferior vena cava (Fig. 26.18). The renal vein may also be occluded or compressed by extrinsic tumour masses by aneurysm, or by retroperitoneal fibrosis.

Renal vein renin. In cases of renal artery stenosis or suspected renal ischaemia it is helpful to assay the renin in the renal venous blood from the suspected kidney. This is obtained by percutaneous catheterization of the renal veins using the Seldinger technique. Samples are obtained from an arm vein at the same time so that comparisons can be made with peripheral venous blood. A renal vein renin ratio greater than 1.5:1 is usually significant.

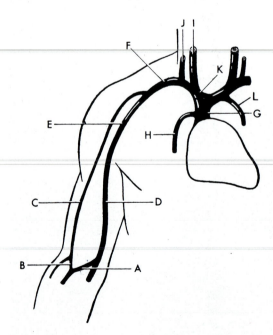

Fig. 26.21 Diagram showing venous drainage of the arm. A = median basilar vein. B = median cephalic vein. C = cephalic vein. D = basilic vein. E = axillary vein. F = subclavian vein. G = superior vena cava. H = azygos vein. I = internal jugular vein. J = external jugular vein. K = innominate vein. L = hemiazygos vein.

to opacify the axillary vein. Use of the median cephalic vein will of course bypass the basilic and axillary veins, since the cephalic vein does not join the subclavian vein until it has pierced the clavipectoral fascia (Fig. 26.21).

Some 30 ml of contrast medium are injected within 2 seconds, using a pressure injector if necessary. A rapid rate of injection is essential, since otherwise the contrast will fail to show the superior vena cava well. It is rapidly diluted in the thorax by the large blood flow from the head and neck and contralateral upper limb.

Serial films are taken at speeds of 1 or 2 films per second.

Another technique which can be used where percutaneous puncture of an elbow vein proves difficult is similar to that used for ascending phlebography of the lower limb. A vein on the dorsum of the hand is percutaneously punctured with a fine needle of the type routinely used by anaesthetists (SWG 21 or 23).

A tourniquet is applied just above the elbow and some 30 ml of contrast medium injected. The tourniquet is then released and the forearm massaged to ensure that a good bolus of contrast medium is delivered to the large veins in 2 s.

Radiographic appearances. The normal findings are illustrated in Figure 26.22.

Left-sided superior vena cava is an important congenital anomaly in which the superior vena cava lies on the left and drains into the coronary sinus. It may occur alone or in association with congenital heart disease. Occasionally there is a *double superior vena cava*, the right draining normally to the right auricle, and the left into the coronary sinus (Fig. 26.23).

Where a localized thrombosis is present in a major drainage vein, such as the axillary or subclavian vein, the blockage is usually well shown, together with the collateral circulation which develops to bypass the lesion (Fig. 26.24).

Superior vena caval obstruction. This is characterized by venous engorgement of the head, neck and arms. The involvement of the superior vena cava by malignant glands can be recognized well before clinical evidence of superior vena caval obstruction is seen. In these cases extrinsic pressure defects on the vein will be seen. In the past, superior vena cavography has been used to assess the suitability of cases of bronchial carcinoma for surgery, and to exclude clinically silent mediastinal glandular involvement. However, CT now provides a less invasive method of assessing mediastinal glandular involvement. DSA will also enable the superior vena cava to be checked using only a small amount of low-concentration contrast medium. Radioisotope scanning can also confirm caval obstruction.

The majority of patients (over 95%) with superior vena caval obstruction are suffering from *malignant neoplasm* (Fig. 26.25). Of these, about 80% have carcinoma of the lung and about 20% are suffering from lymphomas.

The small group of patients with *benign* superior vena caval obstruction are usually suffering from *fibrosing mediastinitis* (Fig. 26.26). These patients present with a relatively slow onset permitting the development of multiple collaterals. The aetiology is either unknown (idiopathic) or it is granulomatous. In this country the latter cases are usually *tuberculous*, but in North America *histoplasmosis* is also a cause of the syndrome. Very rarely thrombosis of the superior vena cava is seen as a complication of ventriculo-atrial shunts. Compression of the

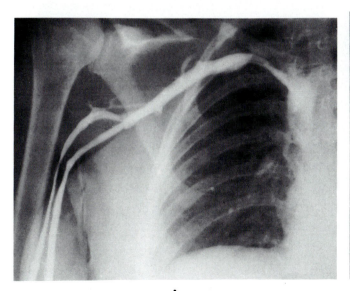
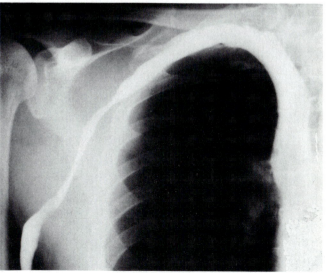

A **B**

Fig. 26.22 **A**. Arm phlebogram showing normal appearances. **B**. Normal arm phlebogram (different case).

superior vena cava may also be occasionally seen with aneurysm and other non-malignant mediastinal masses.

The *Klippel-Trenaunay syndrome* has been noted above. The appearances in the affected upper limb of a patient with this condition are illustrated in Figure 26.27. Multiple phleboliths were present in addition to the venous dysplasia.

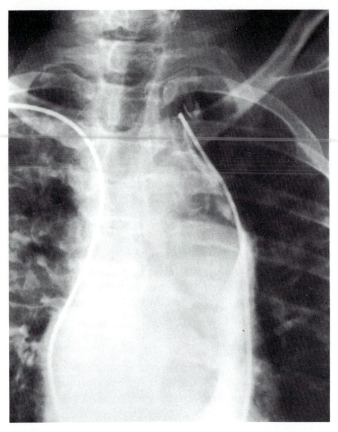

Fig. 26.23 Double superior vena cava. A catheter has been passed from the right arm for pulmonary angiography. Instead of entering the ventricle it has passed through the dilated coronary sinus and into the left superior vena cava draining into it, as evident on contrast injection. Note the widened mediastinum.

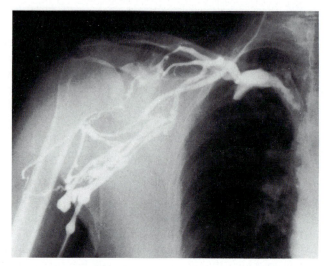

Fig. 26.24 Arm phlebogram showing obstruction in the axillary and subclavian veins.

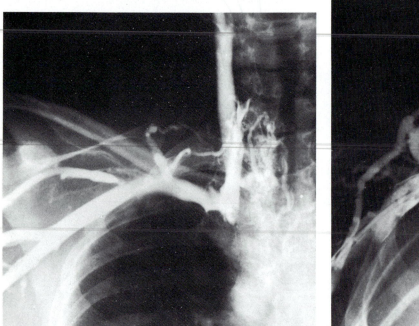

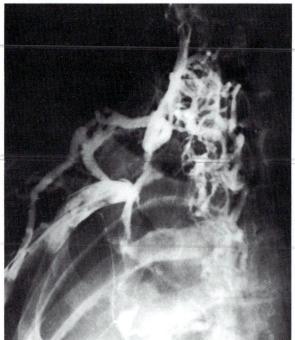

Fig. 26.25 **A**. Right arm phlebogram confirms malignant occlusion of innominate and SVC with reflux up right internal jugular, and vertebral collaterals. **B**. Occlusion of SVC innominate and termination of right subclavian vein. Collaterals to the vertebral vein and vertebral plexus.

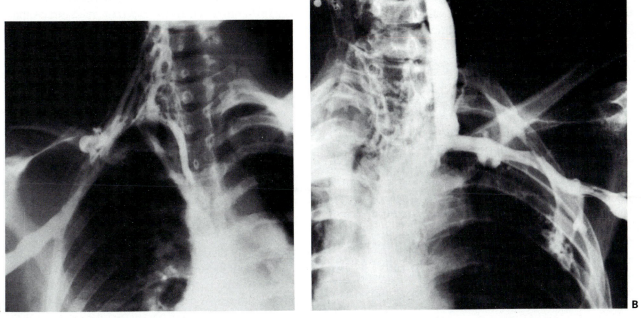

Fig. 26.26 **A**. Right arm phlebogram in fibrosing mediastinitis with involvement of SVC and right innominate vein. **B**. Left arm phlebogram in patient with fibrosing mediastinitis (tuberculous). Note kinked trachea. SVC and left innominate occluded. Collateral circulation via left internal jugular and vertebral plexus.

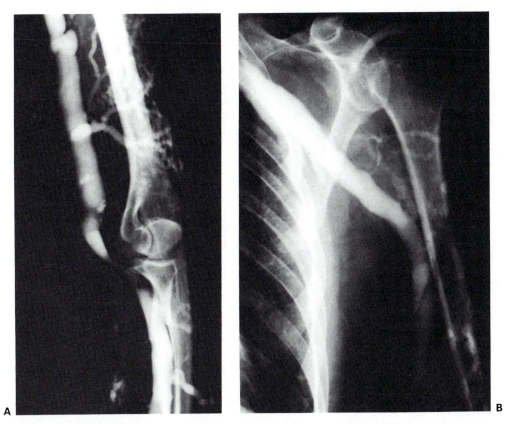

Fig. 26.27 A,B   Klippel-Trenaunay syndrome involving left arm. Drainage is via a single medial vein which appears valveless with very sluggish flow.

PORTAL PHLEBOGRAPHY

The portal circulation, which is illustrated diagrammatically in Figure 26.28, can be outlined by four different methods:

1. Percutaneous splenic puncture
2. Operative mesenteric phlebography
3. Arterioportography
4. Transhepatic portal phlebography.

1. Percutaneous splenic puncture

This technique has been widely used in the past in the investigation of portal hypertension or suspected portal hypertension. It was also used in some cases of splenic enlargement where thrombosis in the splenic vein or portal system was thought to be a factor.

Technique. The usual landmark for percutaneous puncture of the spleen is in the 10th or 11th interspace in the mid-axillary line. The needle is passed inwards and upwards, and where the spleen is enlarged puncture is fairly easy. Usually the needle point can be felt puncturing the splenic capsule, and once it is in the splenic pulp a backflow of blood into the connecting tubing takes place. If portal pressure is very high the reflux of blood may be at considerable pressure. It is possible to measure the intrasplenic pressure by attaching the connecting tubing to a manometer and many workers practice this routinely.

For the contrast injection 20–50 ml of water-soluble iodide contrast medium is used. Better contrast is obtained by using high concentrations such as 85% Hypaque, or 440 Triosil, though lower concentrations can also be used.

Serial films are taken commencing about half-way through the injection of the contrast medium. Rates of 1 to 2 films per second for up to 10 seconds are generally adequate.

Where needle puncture is practised the needle is kept in the spleen for the minimum period necessary to complete the investigation. This is normally not more than 2 or 3 minutes. The procedure can be aided by the use of an image intensifier. This enables a small test dose to be given before the main injection and so permits more accurate siting of the needle tip. It also prevents the occasional accident of subcapsular extravasation of the contrast medium. Whilst the needle is in situ the patient is warned not to breathe too deeply and use only shallow respiration.

Some workers prefer to introduce a catheter into the spleen, either of polythene or of Teflon. This is done in the same way as for percutaneous needle puncture. The catheter is fitted tightly over the puncture needle, and the latter is withdrawn once its tip is in the correct position. If a catheter is inserted percutaneously it can of course remain in the spleen for a longer period than a needle.

Complications. Rupture of the spleen requiring splenectomy has been reported following the procedure. Therefore, unless laparotomy is to be proceeded with immediately after the splenic phlebogram, the patient should be carefully observed for a few days after the investigation for any sign of splenic rupture.

Occasionally the needle tip has been badly positioned and a major injection of contrast medium has been made into the subcapsular region of the spleen. Less commonly, injections have been made into the peritoneum, and even into the colon. Apart from localized pain, these accidents appear to have had no serious consequences.

Indications. The main value of splenic phlebography is in the investigation of portal hypertension. Most cases are due to cirrhosis of the liver, but it is sometimes impossible to differentiate clinically between intrahepatic and extrahepatic portal obstruction. Where this problem arises, portal phlebography will often provide a clear-cut and unequivocal answer by showing a patent portal vein (Fig. 26.29).

If surgery is contemplated it will also provide the surgeon with valuable information by demonstrating the size of the portal vein and whether or not it is possible to anastomose it to the inferior vena cava. It will also show the size and shape of the splenic vein if the alternative operation of a splenorenal anastomosis is being considered.

Postoperative splenic phlebograms were occasionally performed to demonstrate the patency of a surgical anastomosis (Fig. 26.30).

Extrahepatic portal obstruction can result from tumours primary or secondary at the liver hilum. It can also result from portal vein thrombosis and this can occur

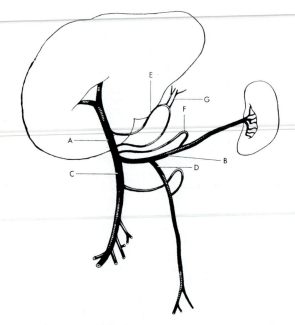

Fig. 26.28 Portal circulation. A = portal vein, B = splenic vein, C = superior mesenteric vein, D = inferior mesenteric vein, E = left gastric vein, F = gastroepiploic vein, G = oesophageal vein.

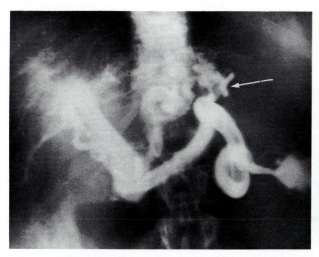

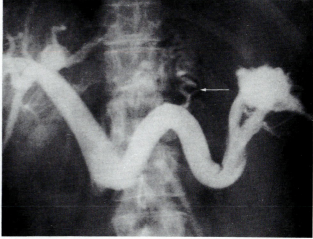

Fig. 26.29 Splenic phlebogram showing gastric and oesophageal varices. The portal vein is patent.

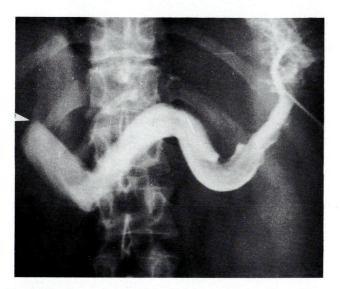

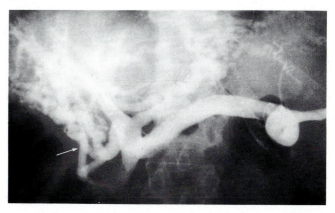

Fig. 26.31 Splenic phlebogram showing gastric varices. The portal vein is thrombosed and replaced by collaterals (arrow).

Fig. 26.30 Postoperative splenic phlebogram showing shunt of contrast from portal vein into inferior vena cava (arrow).

in cases of cirrhosis, as can splenic vein thrombosis. A thrombosed or partially thrombosed portal vein can result in the development of collateral veins (Fig. 26.31), a condition once thought to be congenital and termed 'cavernoma' of the portal vein. It is thus clear that non-visualization of the portal vein at splenic phlebography can be due to several causes and does not exclude a diagnosis of cirrhosis.

It is also important to realize that the portal vein may occasionally fail to outline, even when patent, if there is a major collateral circulation into which the splenic blood is being diverted. In these cases most of the portal blood is derived from the mesenteric circulation. Thus, where the portal vein failed to show at a splenic phlebogram, or where the splenic vein itself appeared obstructed, it was necessary to perform arterial portography or even an

operative mesenteric phlebogram to decide whether or not the portal vein was patent (Fig. 26.32). This can now be done non invasively by US.

Umbilical sepsis in infants is another cause of portal vein thrombosis. Recanalization may follow, with a collateral circulation resulting in so-called cavernoma of the portal vein as described above.

Splenic phlebography has also been used in the past for demonstrating the morphology of the liver, in particular its vascular pattern in suspected neoplasms (both primary and secondary) and in cases of cirrhosis.

Radiological appearances. In cases of portal hypertension due to cirrhosis of the liver or to posthepatic portal obstruction the splenic and portal veins are normally well demonstrated, the latter being large in calibre. The collateral circulation is usually well shown also, and where gastric or oesophageal varices are present these can be clearly outlined (Fig. 26.29). In most cases, portal venography gives a better and more accurate demonstration of oesophageal varices than does the simpler

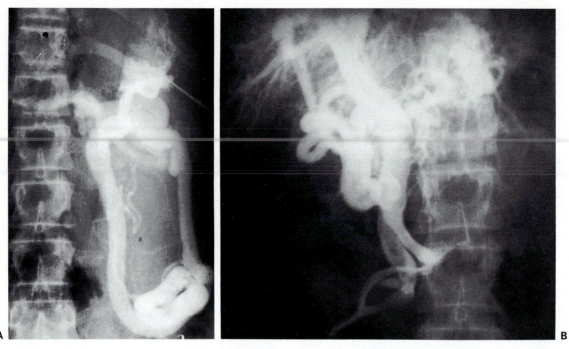

Fig. 26.32 A. Splenic phlebogram showing collateral circulation through huge inferior mesenteric vein. The splenic vein was occluded distally. **B.** Operative superior mesenteric phlebogram showing patent portal vein in the same case.

examination of barium swallow. Sometimes, however, cases occur with excellent demonstration of oesophageal varices by barium swallow where these failed to show well at portal venography.

Distortion of the intrahepatic vascular pattern may be seen in cases of cirrhosis, but this can be difficult to interpret.

The widespread use of splenic venography has demonstrated the existence of numerous other collateral venous channels beside the well-recognized ones.

2. Operative mesenteric phlebography

In this method the portal system is demonstrated by injecting a mesenteric vein at laparotomy. As noted above the technique was required to prove patency of the portal vein where the findings by other techniques were inconclusive (Fig. 26.32).

Some early workers used the operative technique as a routine, but most preferred the percutaneous technique as the primary procedure.

3. Arterioportography

Advocates of this method prefer it because it obviates the dangers of direct splenic puncture and because the information obtained comprises both arterial and venous phases and can show the whole portal system. It can also contribute to the planning of shunt surgery. The normal technique is to catheterize the coeliac axis and then inject from a superselective position of the catheter tip in the splenic artery. 30–60 ml of contrast medium are injected

at a rate of 10 ml/s and serial films obtained in the arterial and venous phase. If the patient's condition permits, the common hepatic artery can also be injected to show the state of the liver and pancreas, with late films to demonstrate any possible hepaticofugal flow in the portal veins. If required, the left gastric artery can be injected to show varices and the superior mesenteric artery can also be injected to demonstrate the superior mesenteric vein. It may be essential to show this if mesocaval shunting is being considered.

There is no doubt that thorough arterioportography provides more information than simple splenic phlebography but it can be a more prolonged and technically difficult procedure than simple direct splenic phlebography. It also requires good-quality subtraction films to show the portal circulation well (Fig. 26.33). Even with these, definition is never as clear as with the direct splenic method.

DSA considerably improves the definition of arterioportography. It also permits adequate visualization with much smaller doses of contrast medium.

4. Transhepatic portal phlebography

The main collateral venous supply of gastro-oesophageal varices may be visualized by percutaneous transhepatic catheterization of the portal vein (Fig. 26.34). Apart from being demonstrated by injection through the percutaneous catheter, the varices can be selectively catheterized and obliterated by embolization (Lunderquist & Vang 1974, Viamonte et al 1977). The major indication

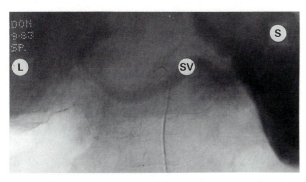

Fig. 26.33 Arterioportography — subtraction film. Venous phase of selective splenic angiogram. The portal vein is compressed by a mass of malignant glands. The spleen is grossly enlarged. SV = splenic vein, L = liver, S = spleen. (Courtesy of Dr Janet Murfitt.)

is severe cirrhosis in patients in whom surgery is contraindicated. After successful obliteration of varices, surgery may be performed electively or deferred.

The method of transhepatic portal phlebography has also been used for the purpose of obtaining venous samples for assay from the pancreatic drainage veins into the splenic and superior mesenteric veins. These assays are helpful in the localization of pancreatic hormone-producing tumours. The method is discussed in greater detail in Chapter 35.

ULTRASOUND PHLEBOGRAPHY
W. R. Lees and W. K. Chong

Although contrast phlebography remains the 'gold standard' for the diagnosis of deep vein thrombosis it is uncomfortable for the patient and can itself induce thrombosis. Ultrasonography with Doppler studies is proving a reliable alternative.

Ultrasound signs of venous patency

1. *Compressibility.* The iliac, femoral and popliteal veins and most of the deep veins of the calf are readily visualized by ultrasonography, particularly using a linear array transducer. Clot can be seen within the lumen of the vein but the echogenicity of the thrombus depends on its age: very fresh thrombus may be isoechoic with blood and may not be visualized. However, clot renders the vein incompressible to gentle pressure from the transducer.
2. *Detection of flow.* Normal blood flow in the veins of the leg is slow and may cease during diastole. To be useful, duplex or colour Doppler devices must be sensitive to such slow flows. Augmentation is often required to show flow in the calf veins. Flow can be augmented by squeezing the calf distal to the measuring point or by release of a proximal cuff.

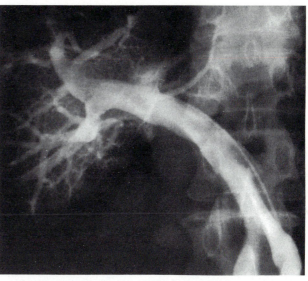

A

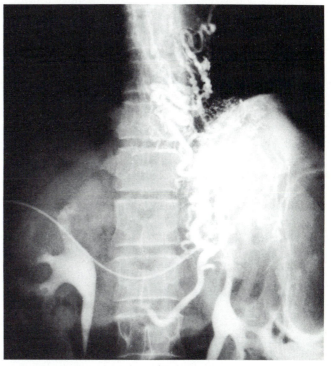

B

Fig. 26.34 A. Transhepatic portal phlebogram showing main portal vein and mesenteric tributaries. (Courtesy of Dr Janet Murfitt.) **B.** Varices demonstrated by transhepatic portal vein catheterization.

Colour Doppler imaging (CDI) is capable of showing blood flow around a clot. (Figs 26.35, 26.36)

3. *Phasicity of flow.* Flow in the main veins of the lower limbs is modulated by pressure changes in the thorax and will therefore vary with the phase of respiration or during a Valsava manoeuvre.

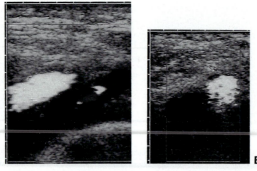

Fig. 26.35 A. Longitudinal CDI scan of the common femoral vein showing partially occluded flow (blue). **B.** Transverse scan. This figure is reproduced in colour in the colour plate section at the front of this volume.

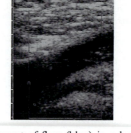

Fig. 26.36 Small amount of flow (blue) in a largely occluded popliteal vein. The vessel is incompressible and flow is only demonstrated after augmentation. This figure is reproduced in colour in the colour plate section at the front of this volume.

Using these three signs in conjunction, ultrasound phlebography is over 98% reliable down to and including the popliteal vessels. Accuracy in the deep veins of the calf is less good and although patent veins may be demonstrated it is impossible to exclude small thrombi in the smaller veins.

MRI OF VEINS

Ian Isherwood and Jeremy P. R. Jenkins

An understanding of the flow phenomena, and MRI techniques for assessment (given in detail in the preceding chapter) are applicable to the MRI study of venous structures. *Thrombi* in abdominal and pelvic veins can be identified on T_1- and T_2-weighted spin-echo sequences. MR angiographic (MRA) techniques have been found to be more sensitive than conventional spin echo imaging in detecting thrombosis in the femoral and iliac veins. A good correlation with conventional X-ray venography has been observed. The distinction between an acute and chronic thrombus can be made by evaluating the signal intensity appearance of the clot. A homogeneous signal, probably indicative of an acute clot, has been noted in more proximal thrombi. Heterogeneity in appearance, with a peripheral lower and a central higher signal, of distal portions of thrombi are in keeping with their greater age. MRI is limited, however, in the demonstration of small calf vessels. Advantages of MRI over X-ray phlebography are that it is painless, non-invasive, relatively quick to perform, able to demonstrate central veins and other diseases when a deep vein thrombosis is not present, and uses non-ionizing radiation. It is unlikely, however, that MRI will replace Doppler US in the assessment of thrombosis of leg veins, but it may be useful in depicting pelvic and upper limb venous thromboses.

REFERENCES AND SUGGESTIONS FOR FURTHER READING (Chapters 25 and 26)

Major textbooks

Abrams, H. L. (Ed.) (1983) *Angiography*. 3rd edn. Little Brown, Boston.

Athanasoulis, C. A., Pfister, R. C., Greene, R. E., Roberson, G. H. (Eds.) (1982) *Interventional Radiology*. Saunders, Philadelphia.

Reuter, R. S., Redman, R. H. (1977) *Gastro-intestinal Angiography*. 2nd edn. Saunders, Philadelphia.

References of historical interest

Berberich, J., Hirsch, S. (1923) Die roentgenographische Darstellung der Arterien und Venen am lebenden Menschen. *Klinische Wochenschrift*, pp. 2226–2228.

Brooks, B. (1924) Intra-arterial injection of sodium iodide. *Journal of the American Medical Association*, **82**, 1016–1019.

Doby, T. (1976) *Development of Angiography*. Publishing Sciences Group, Littleton, MA.

Dos Santos, R., Lamas, A. C., Caldas, J. P. (1931) *Arteriographie des membres et de la aorte abdominale*. Masson, Paris.

Farinas, P. L. (1941) A new technique for the arteriographic examination of the abdominal aorta and its branches. *American Journal of Roentgenology*, **46**, 641–645.

Forssman, W. (1929) Die Sondierung der rechten Herzens. *Klinische Wochenschrift*, **8**, 2087–2089.

Gruntzig, A. (1978) Transluminal dilatation of coronary artery stenosis. *Lancet*, **i**, 263.

Gruntzig, A. et al. (1978) Treatment of renovascular hypertension with percutaneous transluminal dilatation of a renal artery stenosis. *Lancet*, **i**, 801.

Haschek, E., Lindenthal, T. O. (1896) Ein Beitrag zur praktischen Verwerthung der Photographie nach Röntgen. *Wiener Klinische Wochenschrift*, **9**, 63–64.

Moniz, E. (1931) *Diagnostic des Tumeurs Cérébrals et Epreuve de l'Encephalographie Artérielle*. Masson, Paris.

Orrin, H. C. (1920) *X-ray-Atlas of the Systemic Arteries of the Human Body*. Baillière Tindall & Cox, London.

Seldinger, S. (1953) Catheter replacement of the needle in percutaneous arteriography. *Acta Radiologica*, **39**, 368–376.

Serbinenko, F. A. (1974) Balloon catheterization and occlusion of major cerebral vessels. *Journal of Neurosurgery*, **41**, 125–145.

Sicard, J. A., Forestier, J. (1923) Injections intravasculaires d'huile iodée Sous contrôle radiologique. *Comptes Rendus de la Société de Biologie*, **88**, 1200.

Sicard, J. A., Forestier, J. (1932) *The Use of Lipiodol in Diagnosis and Treatment.* Oxford University Press, London.

Sutton, D. (1962) *Arteriography.* Livingstone, Edinburgh.

References

Ansell, G., Wilkins, R. A. (Eds.) (1987) *Complications in Diagnostic Radiology.* 2nd edn. Blackwell, Oxford.

Bell, A. M., Cumberland, D. C. (1989) Percutaneous atherectomy. *Clinical Radiology,* **40**, 122–126.

Bluth, E. I., Stavros, A. T., Marich, K. W. et al (1988) Carotid Duplex Sonography: a multicenter recommendation for standardized imaging and Doppler criteria. *Radiographics,* **8**, 487.

Carr, D. H. (Ed.) (1988) *Contrast Media.* Churchill Livingstone, Edinburgh.

Chuang, V. P., Wallace, S. (1981) Hepatic artery embolization in the treatment of hepatic neoplasms. *Radiology,* **140**, 51–58.

Debrun, G., Legre, J., Kasbarian, M. et al. (1979) Endovascular occlusion of vertebral fistulae by detachable balloons with conservation of vertebral blood flow. *Radiology,* **130**, 141–147.

Ekelund, L., Gerlock, J., Ogoncharenko, V. (1978) The epinephrine effect in renal angiography revisited. *Clinical Radiology,* **29**, 387–392.

Godwin, J. D., Herfkens, R. L., Skiöldebrand, C. G., Federle, M. P., Lipton, M. J. (1980) Evaluation of dissections and aneurysms of the thoracic aorta by conventional and dynamic CT scanning. *Radiology,* **136**, 125–133.

Gregson, R. H. S., Sutton, D., Brennan, J. et al. (1983) Spontaneous aortocaval fistula. *Clinical Radiology,* **34**, 683–687.

Hallam, M. J., Reid, J. M., Cooperberg, P. L. (1988) Colour flow Doppler and conventional duplex scanning of the carotic bifurcation: prospective, double blinded, correlative study. *American Journal of Roetgenology,* **152**, 1101.

Hartnell, G. C. (1989) Controversies in radiology: Doppler of the carotid arteries. *Clinical radiology,* **40**, 117.

Henderson, M. J., Manhire, A. R. (1990) Cholesterol embolisation following angiography. *Clinical Radiology,* **42**, 281–282.

Herlinger, H. (1978) Arterioportography. *Clinical Radiology,* **29**, 255–275.

Hill, S., Billings, P. J., Walker, R. T. et al. (1990) True spontaneous rupture of the common iliac vein. *Journal of the Royal Society of Medicine,* **83**, 117.

Hobbs, J. T. (Ed.) (1977) *The Treatment of Venous Disorders.* Lippincott, Philadelphia.

Hughes, J. P., Stovin P. G. I. (1959) Segmental pulmonary aneurysms with peripheral deep vein thrombosis Brit J. Dis. Chest 53: 19–27

Lang, E. K. (1981) Transcatheter enbolization of pelvic vessels for control of intractable haemorrhage. *Clinical Radiology,* **35**, 85–93.

Lea Thomas, M. (1982) *Phlebography of the Lower Limb.* Churchill Livingstone, Edinburgh.

Lunderquist, A., Vang, J. (1974) Transhepatic catheterization and obliteration of the coronary vein in patients with portal hypertension and oesophageal varices. *New England Journal of Medicine,* **291**, 646–649.

Merritt, C. R. B. (1987) Doppler colour flow imaging. Journal of Clinical Ultrasound, **15**, 591.

Mandell, V. S. et al. (1985) Persistent sciatic artery. *American Journal of Roentgenology,* **144**, 245–249.

Miller, D. C., Stinson, E. G., Oyer, P. E. et al. (1979) Operative treatment of aortic dissections: experience with 125 patients. *Journal of Thoracic and Cardiovascular Surgery,* **78**, 365.

O'Halpin, D., Legge, D., MacErlain, D. P. (1984) Therapeutic arterial embolisation: report of five years experience. *Clinical Radiology,* **35**, 85–93.

Royal, S. A., Callen, P. W. (1979) CT evaluation of anomalies of the IVC and left renal vein. *American Journal of Roentgenology,* **132**, 759–763.

Starnes, H. F., Vallance, R., Hamilton, D. N. H. (1984) Recurrent varicose veins: a radiological approach to investigation. *Clinical Radiology,* **35**, 95–99.

Thomas, E. A., Cobby, M. J. D., Rhys Davies, E. et al. (1989) Liquid crystal thermography and C-reactive protein in detection of deep venous thrombosis. *British Medical Journal,* **299**, 951–952.

Viamonte, M., Jr., Pereiras, R., Russell, E., Le Page, J., Hudson, D. (1977) Transhepatic obliteration of gastro-oesophageal varices. *American Journal of Roentgenology,* **129**, 237–241.

Wallace, S., Chuang, V. P., Swanson, D. et al. (1981) Embolization of renal carcinomas: experience with 100 patients. *Radiology,* **138**, 563–570.

Wells, I. P., Hammonds, J. C., Franklin, K. (1983) Embolization of hypernephromas: a simple technique using ethanol. *Clinical Radiology,* **34**, 689–692.

Whitehouse, G. H. (1990) Venous thrombosis and thrombo-embolisms. *Clinical Radiology,* **41**, 77–80.

Wilbur, A. C., Woelfel, G. F., Meyer, J. P., Flanigan, D. P., Spigos, D. G. (1985) Adventitial cystic disease of the popliteal artery. *Radiology,* **155**, 63–64.

Ultrasound

Baxter, G. M., McKechnie, S., Duffy, P. (1990) Colour Doppler ultrasound in deep vein thrombosis. *Clinical Radiology,* **42**, 32–36.

Chong, W. K., Raphael, M. J. (1991) The significance of haemodynamic significance: general considerations. *British Journal of Radiology* (in press).

Jaffe, C. (Ed.) (1984) *Vascular and Doppler Ultrasound.* Churchill Livingstone, Edinburgh, pp. 1–50.

Polak, J. F., Dobkin, G. R., O'Leary, D. H., Wang, A. Y., Cutler, S. S. (1989) Internal carotid artery stenosis: accuracy and reproducibility of color Doppler-assisted duplex imaging. *Radiology,* **173**, 793–798.

Rigsby, C. M., Burns, P. N., Weltin, G. G. et al. (1987) Doppler signal quantification in renal allografts: comparison in normal and rejection transplants, with pathologic correlation. *Radiology,* **162**, 39–42.

Scoutt, L. M., Zawin, M. L. Taylor, K. J. W. (1990) Doppler US. II. Clinical applications. *Radiology,* **174**, 309–319.

Symposium on Image-directed Doppler Ultrasound (1987) *Journal of Clinical Ultrasound,* **15**.

Taylor, J. W., Holland, S. (1990) Doppler US. I. Basic principles, instrumentation and pitfalls. *Radiology,* **174**, 297–307.

Zweibel, W. J. (1987) A primer of cerebrovascular ultrasound. *Seminars in Ultrasound, CT and MR,* **8**, 2–57.

MRI: arteries

Alfidi, R. J., Masaryk, T. J., Haacke, E. M. et al. (1987) MR angiography of peripheral, carotid, and coronary arteries. *American Journal of Roentgenology,* **149**, 1097–1109

Bradley, W. G. (1988) Flow phenomona. In: Stark, D. D., Bradley, W. G. (Eds.) *Magnetic Resonance Imaging.* CV Mosby, St Louis, Ch. 7, pp. 108–137.

Gefter, W. B., Hatabu, H., Dinsmore, B. J. et al. (1990) Pulmonary vascular cine MR imaging: a noninvasive approach to dynamic imaging of the pulmonary circulation. *Radiology,* **176**, 761–770.

Gomes, A. S., Lois, J. F., Williams, R. G. (1990) Pulmonary arteries: MR imaging in patients with congenital obstruction of the right ventricular outflow tract. *Radiology* **174**, 51–57.

Haacke, E. M., Masaryk, T. J. (1989) The salient features of MR angiography. *Radiology,* **173**, 611–612.

Mitchell, L., Jenkins, J. P. R., Brownlee, W. C., Isherwood, I. (1988) Case report: Aortic dissection: Morphology and differential flow velocity patterns demonstrated by magnetic resonance imaging. *Clinical Radiology.* **39**, 458–465.

Nyman, R., Hallberg, M., Sunnegardh, J., Thuren, J., Henze, A. (1989) Magnetic resonance imaging and angiography for the assessment of coarctation of the aorta. *Acta Radiologica,* **30**, 481–485.

Parsons, J. M., Baker, E. J., Hayes, A. et al. (1990) Magnetic resonance imaging of the great arteries in infants. *International Journal of Cardiology,* **28**, 73–85.

Posteraro, R. H., Sostman, H. D., Spritzer, C. E., Herfkins, R. J. (1989) Cine-gradient refocused MR imaging of central pulmonary emboli. *American Journal of Roentgenology,* **152**, 465–468.

Rees, S., Somerville, J., Ward, C. et al. (1989) Coarctation of the aorta: MR imaging in late postoperative assessment. *Radiology,* **173**, 499–502.

Solomon, S. L., Brown, J. J., Glazer, H. S., Mirowitz, S. A., Lee, J. K. T. (1990) Thoracic aortic dissection: pitfalls and artifacts in MR imaging. *Radiology*, **177**, 223–228.

Spritzer, C. E., Blinder, R. A., (1989) Vascular applications of magnetic resonance imaging. *Magnetic Resonance Quarterly*, **5**, 205–227.

Underwood, R., Firmin, D. (Eds.) (1990) *Magnetic Resonance of the Cardiovascular System*. Blackwell Scientific Publications, Oxford.

MRI: veins

Erdman, W. A., Jayson, H. T., Redman, H. C., Miller, G. L.,

Parkey, R. W. (1990) Deep venous thrombosis of extremities: role of MR imaging in the diagnosis. *Radiology*, **174**, 425–431.

Spritzer, C. E., Sostman, H. D., Wilkes, D. C., Coleman, R. E., (1990) Deep venous thrombosis: experience with gradient-echo MR imaging in 66 patients. *Radiology*, **177**, 235–241.

Totterman, S., Francis, C. W., Foster, T. H., Brenner, B., Marder, V. J., Bryant, R. G. (1990) Diagnosis of femoropopliteal venous thrombosis with MR imaging: a comparison of four MR pulse sequences. *American Journal of Roentgenology*, **154**, 175–178.

Whitehouse, G. H. (1990) Editorial — venous thrombosis and thromboembolism. *Clinical Radiology*, **41**, 77–80.

CHAPTER 27

THE LYMPHATIC SYSTEM

Graham Cherryman

In this chapter the structure, function and methods of imaging the lymphatic system are discussed. Benign and malignant conditions affecting the lymphatic system are reviewed with the emphasis on the lymphomas.

STRUCTURE AND FUNCTION

The presence of a functioning lymphatic system is essential to health. The lymphatic system consists of a network of lymphatic capillaries that commence in the body tissues, freely anastomose and eventually drain back into the venous system via large lymphatic trunks. There are lymphatics within most body tissues, although lymphatic capillaries are not found in avascular tissues such as articular cartilage. They are also not present in brain, spinal cord, bone marrow and splenic pulp. Within these tissues there are microscopic clefts that have a similar function to lymphatics but, in contrast to lymphatic capillaries, lack an endothelial lining.

The characteristic endothelial wall seen in lymphatic capillaries is permeable to larger molecules than can pass through the endothelial lining of vascular capillaries. This allows the lymphatic system to absorb proteins and particulate matter including cell debris and micro-organisms as well as excess extracellular tissue fluid. The lymphatics draining the gut are also known as *lacteals*. Following a meal the lymph (chyle) within these gut lymphatics appears milky white due to the presence of fat chylomicrons being transported away from the gut wall.

In the body the larger lymphatic trunks accompany the arteries and veins. Almost all lymph in the body eventually passes into the thorax and re-enters the vascular space through either the thoracic duct or the right lymphatic duct. In the retroperitoneum the para-aortic lymphatic trunks empty into the cisterna chyli at the level of the second lumbar vertebra. The cisterna chyli may be recognized on CT sections (Fig. 27.1). Typically the cisterna chyli is a saccular structure about 5 cm long, passing up through the diaphragm to become the thoracic duct, which is smaller in diameter than the cisterna chyli and

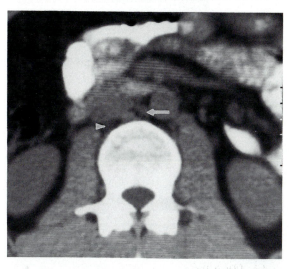

Fig. 27.1 CT section through the upper abdomen of a young male patient shows the cisterna chyli as a small (0.5 cm) low-attenuation structure lying between the aorta and IVC (arrow). The cisterna chyli may be seen on CT examination in almost all patients providing there is sufficient retroperitoneal fat. A smaller lymphatic duct may be seen behind the IVC (arrowhead).

not normally identified on CT examination. The thoracic duct may opacify after lymphography (Fig. 27.2).

The thoracic duct receives all the lymph flow from below the diaphragm as well as that from the left side of the thorax and neck. Typically the thoracic duct terminates by anastomosing with the left subclavian vein. On the right a smaller right lymphatic trunk drains lymph from the right side of the thorax and neck into the right subclavian vein. There are a number of variations in the anatomy of the larger lymphatic ducts.

The typical appearance of peripheral lymphatics at lymphography shows the arrangement of valves allowing movement of lymph in one direction only (Fig. 27.3). Lymph is propelled through the lymphatic system by the combination of filtration pressure in the interstitial spaces, movement of the limbs and muscles, and the contraction

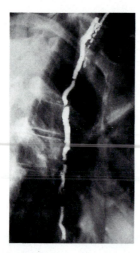

Fig. 27.2 Early phase lymphogram film with contrast medium outlining the thoracic duct.

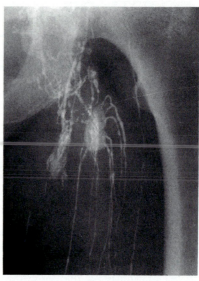

Fig. 27.4 Early phase lymphogram film with opacification of both lymph nodes and lymph vessels. There are several afferent lymphatics feeding into each lymph node. The single efferent lymphatic always leaves the lymph node through the hilum.

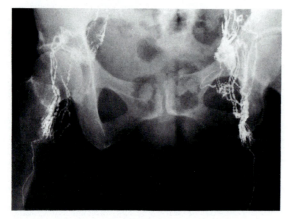

Fig. 27.3 An early phase lymphogram film showing the arrangement of valves in the lymphatic vessels.

of the smooth muscle fibres found within the wall of the larger lymphatic trunks.

Lymph from almost all parts of the body traverses one or more lymph nodes before reaching the venous circulation. Lymph nodes are encapsulated aggregates of lymphatic tissue, normally small and bean-shaped and situated in the path of the lymphatic vessels (Fig. 27.4). The outer surface of the lymph node is covered by a fibrous capsule. Fibrous tissue extends into the lymph node in the form of trabeculae arising from the undersurface of this capsule, so that the lymphoid tissue within the lymph node is supported by a fine meshwork of fibrocellular elements. A slight depression on one side of the lymph node is termed the hilum, and it is through the hilum that blood vessels enter and leave the lymph node. The single efferent lymphatic also leaves from the hilum.

Internally the lymph node contains a central medulla

and a peripheral cortex; the line of demarcation between the two is often indistinct. The cortex is deficient at the hilum so that the efferent lymphatic derives its lymph from the medulla. Afferent lymphatics are usually multiple and pass through the capsule into the cortex. Lymph enters a lymph node through one of these afferent vessels and passes onward into a subcapsular lymphatic plexus. From here the lymph passes into the sinuses of the cortex, then through the sinuses of the medulla, before leaving the lymph node through the efferent vessel. The flow of lymph in the sinuses is slightly retarded and this encourages the deposition of particulate matter. This enables phagocytes to filter off particulate antigenic and other noxious matter from the lymph, prior to drainage of lymph in the venous circulation.

The lymph node has a number of other functions, including a role in both the cellular and the humoral immune responses. Lymphocytes and other antibody-producing cells may be generated in the lymph node, usually within the cortex, where densely packed cells form follicles, often with their own germinal centre. The number and size of the follicles varies and at times of great antigenic stimulation may increase to such an extent that the lymph node itself enlarges. In these circumstances the enlarged lymph node is termed *reactive*.

IMAGING NORMAL AND ABNORMAL LYMPH NODES

Clinical examination is the first step in the evaluation of the lymphatic system. Enlargement of neck, axillary and groin lymph nodes may be palpable and large abdominal

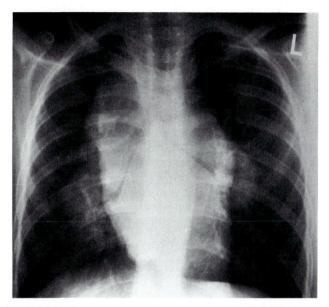

Fig. 27.5 Frontal chest radiograph. A large mediastinal nodal mass in a patient presenting with Hodgkin's disease is seen compressing the major airways.

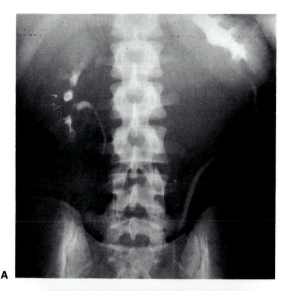

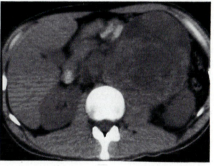

Fig. 27.6 The opacified ureters are seen on the IVU examination to be displaced around a large central abdominal mass (**A**). The presence of this mass is confirmed on the CT section (**B**). The final diagnosis was testicular teratoma.

nodal masses may also be palpated. Smaller volume enlargement of abdominal and pelvic lymph nodes, together with any enlargement of lymph nodes within the thorax, is impalpable. The determination of tumour extent and bulk within the body is only possible after the appropriate imaging tests have been performed.

The presence of adenopathy may be seen on plain-film examination (Fig. 27.5) and inferred from displacement of normal structures. The chest radiograph remains the most important radiological window into the thorax. Enlargement of mediastinal and hilar lymph nodes has a characteristic appearance. In many instances the information available from a chest radiograph is sufficient to plan further management of the patient. Radiographs of the abdomen are less helpful, as only large masses can be confidently recognized and the nodal nature of these masses is difficult to establish. The addition of a contrast medium (especially an IVP) to opacify the ureters is a limited but recognized method of demonstrating mass effect and the displacement of normal abdominal structures by a large abdominal mass (Fig. 27.6).

Lymphography

For many years bipedal lymphography was the standard test for the non-surgical demonstration of lymphadenopathy affecting the abdominal and pelvic lymph nodes. Although lymphography is a sensitive test that may on occasion demonstrate micrometastases in normal-sized lymph nodes, it is only moderately specific, and false positive findings are not infrequent, especially in the elderly, in whom fibrofatty deposits within the lymph nodes may be incorrectly considered metastatic foci. This limits the

value of the lymphogram technique, particularly in the staging of pelvic malignancies.

Successful lymphography depends on several sequential steps: firstly, the visualization of the lymphatics; secondly, the exposure and cannulation of the lymphatic; thirdly, the injection of a contrast material; and finally, the taking of X-rays, both immediately after the procedure, to demonstrate the lymphatics, and again after at least 24 hours delay to demonstrate the lymph nodes (MacDonald 1982). Contrast medium will then remain in the lymph nodes for 6–12 months, and during this time follow-up films can be used to demonstrate changes within the opacified lymph nodes.

Lymphography may be requested when the CT examination is negative, in order to identify small deposits in normal-sized lymph nodes. However the two tests are not complementary. The value of CT is reduced if performed after lymphography. The presence of the dense oily contrast medium within the lymph nodes may cause them to enlarge in reaction, making interpretation of the CT difficult as well as creating artefacts (due to the high density of the oily contrast medium) that may degrade the CT image. There is no doubt that in almost all circumstances CT has obviated the need for lymphography.

There are also practical contraindications to lymphography. These include allergies to contrast agents, vital dyes and local anaesthesia; cardiovascular or pulmonary disease, especially heart failure, angina, pulmonary fibrosis or emphysema; and previous pulmonary irradiation. The latter is a significant risk factor as the arteriovenous shunts opened up at pulmonary irradiation predispose to *systemic oil embolism*. Lymphography is often considered an outpatient procedure, but 24 hours' observation in hospital is prudent (MacDonald 1987).

Technique. The visualization of the lymphatics prior to exposure and cannulation of the lymphatic is generally accepted as helpful. This is accomplished by the injection of 0.5 ml of Patent Blue Violet into the first two web spaces of both feet. (At this time the patient should be warned that blue staining of the skin may persist in this area for several weeks and in addition the urine might appear blue-tinged.) The indicator dye is a large molecular compound that is absorbed into peripheral lymphatics rather than the vascular capillaries. The lymphatic may then be identified as a blue streak under the skin. The optimum time for the cut-down is within a few minutes of the injection of the indicator dye, when the blue streaks of the lymphatics first become visible. After this time the blue dye infiltrates into the skin, making it much harder to identify the opacified lymphatics.

It is easiest to expose and cannulate a single lymphatic on the dorsum of the foot. Lignocaine (1%) is injected into the skin on either side of the exposed lymphatic, making subsequent dissection easier. A longitudinal incision is made over the lymphatic and the vessel exposed under direct vision. Fat and connective tissue is gently stripped off the lymphatic over a distance of a centimetre. The cannulation of the exposed and cleaned lymphatic is a delicate procedure and the simplest approach is the best. A suture (4.0 silk) is loosely tied around the lymphatic proximal to the insertion point. The lymphatic is then stretched between the smooth blades of a pair of forceps, distended, and cannulated, using a purpose-made lymphogram set with a 27 gauge needle. At this time it may be helpful if an assistant can gently inject contrast medium. This, at the appropriate time, will distend the lymphatic, allowing the needle tip to be advanced a further 2–3 mm. The suture is then tightened around the needle and the tubing of the giving set gently fastened to the patient's skin. Second punctures (if required) should be made either in a second vessel or, if that is not possible, then proximal to the initial puncture site.

To opacity the pelvic and abdominal lymph nodes 6–7 ml of Lipiodol is injected into both feet of a typical 70 kg patient. This is usually accomplished by the use of a mechanical injector which can inject the contrast medium at a rate between 0.05 and 0.1 ml/min. Too rapid an injection rate will rupture the lymphatic. Immediately after the injection commences, the lower leg is observed fluoroscopically to ensure that the needle is in a lymphatic and no lymphatico-venous communication is present.

After the injection of approximately 4 ml of contrast medium into each foot an AP radiograph of the pelvis is obtained. This acts as a check for lymphatic obstruction, cross-over or venous communication in the pelvis. After the injection of 7 ml oily contrast medium into each foot, a supine AP radiograph of the abdomen is taken and the injection halted. The feet are then sutured and the standard radiographs obtained: AP abdomen, AP pelvis, RPO and LPO of abdomen and pelvis, lateral abdomen and a chest X-ray to check for possible oil embolism. These radiographs are all repeated after 24 hours and the two series, showing initially the vessels and later the lymph nodes, are compared. Without this precaution normal lymph node hila might be mistaken for pathological filling defects. Lymphographic contrast medium still present in the lymph vessels on the delayed films may indicate lymphatic obstruction, especially if a collateral lymphatic circulation may be identified.

Computed tomography; ultrasound; magnetic resonance imaging

Today the formal staging of malignant disease in patients is undertaken with CT, perhaps supplemented by MRI and US examinations. The cross-sectional imaging capability of these techniques allows the direct demonstration of normal and abnormal lymph nodes. Lymph-node enlargement is the imaging hallmark of metastatic involvement, and a series of size criteria for normal and abnormal lymph nodes have evolved in the different areas of the body (see below). Enlargement of the lymph nodes above these criteria is suggestive but not diagnostic of malignant involvement. The images should always be interpreted in the light of the clinical findings and the known behaviour of the particular tumour. For example, a slightly enlarged right paracaval lymph node is unlikely to be involved in a patient with a left-sided testicular teratoma, but a similarly sized para-aortic lymph node on the left may be the site of metastatic disease following spread of disease from a right testicular tumour. This is because cross-flow in the lymphatic drainage of the retroperitoneum is far more likely to occur from right to left across the midline than from left to right (Dixon et al 1986).

Radionuclide techniques

Injected radiopharmaceuticals may collect in lymph vessels and nodes (McKusick 1985). Circulating radionuclides may be taken up by metastatic lymph nodes. This is best recognized with gallium-67. This is a tumour-avid compound taken up by tumours arising from the lymphatic system liver or lung. Different cell types will take up the isotope differentially. The technique has been applied to patients with lymphoma. The sensitivity of the test to the presence of active lymphoma tissue is related to the volume of the tumour, the location injected, the dose and the instrumentation. Gallium-67 imaging is sensitive to the presence of lymphoma in patients but has proved less effective than CT in determining the extent of disease site by site within individual patients. Approximately 5% of positive results with gallium-67 imaging are incorrect, usually as a result of concomitant or unsuspected infection. At present the clinical role of gallium-67 scanning in patients with lymphoma is best limited to the follow-up of patients with initial positive scans.

Lymphoscintigraphy is at present mainly of research interest. Radiocolloids may be injected intratumour, intradermal, subcutaneous or intramuscular. At present the most commonly used agent is technetium-99m-labelled antimony sulphide and the most common area of investigation is the breast.

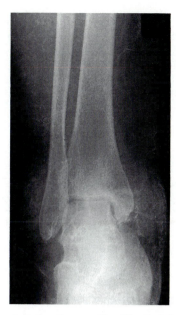

Fig. 27.7 Early phase lymphogram film. The limb is swollen and when lymphography was attempted, lymphatics filled poorly. This is an example of secondary lymphoedema due to filariasis.

IMAGING NORMAL AND ABNORMAL LYMPHATICS

These may be directly opacified at lymphography. The injection of water-soluble radiological contrast media is an acceptable and safe alternative to the injection of oily contrast media but will not opacify the lymph nodes (O'Donnell & Clouse 1985). The technique of lymphography in the oedematous leg is difficult, and prior elevation of the limb for 48–72 hours may help reduce the amount of limb oedema.

On the basis of the lymphographic appearances the **lymphoedemas** may be divided into the *aplasias* with no demonstrable lymphatics, the *hypoplasias* with a reduced number of lymphatics and the *hyperplasias* with an increase in the number of lymphatics present. Allen et al (1946) divided the lymphoedemas into *primary* and *secondary*. The primary type may be further subdivided into *congenital*, *praecox* (before the age of 35 years) and *tarda* (after the age of 35).

Primary lymphoedema is a vascular dysplasia often associated with arterial and venous malformations in the same limb and other congenital defects. Most patients have aplasia or severe hypoplasia of the lymphatics. The oedema may be precipitated by minor trauma or surgery. Peak incidence is seen in girls at puberty and typically involves the left leg. The term *Milroy's disease* is loosely applied to primary lymphoedema but should be limited to those few cases which are both congenital and familial.

The advent of CT has also reduced the need for lymphographic evaluation of the lymphatics as the size and number of lymph nodes parallel the size and number of lymphatics. CT assessment of the size and number of the lymph nodes can objectively classify patients into aplasia, hypoplasia and hyperplasia of the lymphatic system.

Secondary lymphoedema is more common than primary lymphoedema and indicates the presence of obstruction to the normal forward passage of lymph. This may be due to previous surgery or irradiation but may also result from recurrent tumour. Uncommon causes of secondary lymphoedema include infection, especially with *filariasis* (Fig. 27.7). In patients with secondary lymphoedema CT is again the most useful investigation, especially when looking for new or recurrent tumour.

TOPOGRAPHY OF THE LYMPHATIC SYSTEM

The radiologist should have an understanding of the major lymphatic pathways of the body, especially those of the head and neck, thorax, abdomen and pelvis.

Lymphatic drainage of the head and neck

There are approximately 300 lymph nodes in the average adult neck, loosely arranged into several groups (Som 1987). The lymphatics and lymph nodes of the neck make up a collar of lymphoid tissue around the skull base consisting, from posterior to anterior, of the *occipital* lymph nodes, the *mastoid* lymph nodes, the *parotid* lymph nodes (and these may be extra- or intra-glandular (Fig. 27.8)), the *submandibular*, *facial*, *submental* and *sublingual* lymph nodes. These lymphatic chains drain inferiorly through either the anterior or lateral cervical chains into the superior mediastinum. In addition there are also the deep and impalpable *retropharyngeal* lymph nodes (Fig. 27.9)

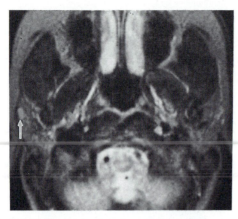

Fig. 27.8 Axial MR examination through the neck shows a small intraparotid lymph node on the right (arrow), an incidental finding. On T₂-weighted MR images lymph nodes appear white.

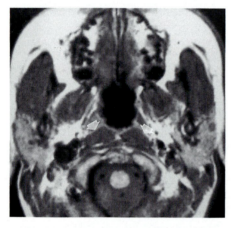

Fig. 27.9 Axial T₁-weighted MR examination through the neck. Bilateral retropharyngeal nodes may be identified (arrows). On T₁-weighted sequences lymph nodes appear darker than the surrounding fat. Note the flow void phenomenon — the great vessels of the neck appear black.

found in the neck lateral to the longus colli and longus capitis muscles which drain lymph from the nasopharynx, oropharynx, sinuses and middle ear to the internal jugular chain. Pathology in the retropharyngeal region is often associated with abnormalities of the 9th–12th cranial nerves.

The *lateral cervical lymph nodes* serve as the common drainage route for all the major head and neck structures. There are superficial and deep groups. The *superficial* group form a chain that runs alongside the external jugular chain. Of greater importance are the lymph nodes of the *deep* group, in three chains forming a triangle. At the apex of the triangle lies the *jugulodigastric* lymph node, seen in the suprahyoid compartment at the anatomical level where the posterior belly of the digastric muscle crosses the anterior jugular vein. Below this the *internal jugular chain* of lymph nodes runs forwards into the anterior triangle of the neck, following the course of the internal jugular vein just behind the anterior border of the sternocleidomastoid muscle. These lymph nodes lie outside the carotid sheath, but on CT and MRI are seen to be close to the structures within the carotid sheath (Fig. 27.10). The *spinal accessory chain* runs posteriorly into the posterior triangle of the neck deep to the sterno-cleidomastoid muscle. The lymph nodes of this group typically lie within fat and in consequence are well seen on CT and MR images (Fig. 27.11). The extremes of the internal jugular and spinal accessory chains are joined by the *transverse cervical chain* of supraclavicular lymph nodes. The most inferior lymph nodes of the internal jugular chain are also known as the *lymph nodes of Virchow* or *Trosier*; enlargement of these lymph nodes may well be secondary to metastatic involvement from a thoracic or subdiaphragmatic primary tumour or lymphoma or from the spread of breast malignancy (Fig. 27.12). Finally an *anterior* chain of cervical lymph nodes accompanies the

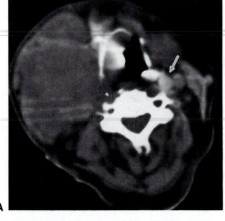

A

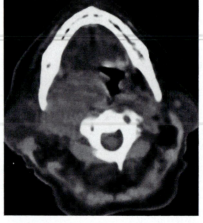

B

Fig. 27.10 A,B Axial CT sections taken during the injection of i.v. contrast medium. A large malignant nodal mass is seen on the right and extending deep to compress the airway. On the left the dynamic injection of i.v. contrast medium has opacified the vessels of the carotid sheath seen in their normal position (arrow).

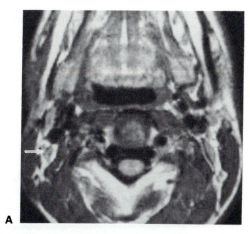
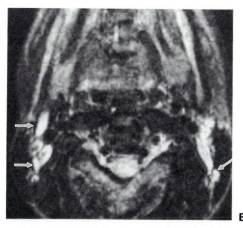

Fig. 27.11 Axial MR examination of a boy presenting with Hodgkin's disease. The T_1-weighted images (**A**) show the posterior triangle nodes as small areas of low signal within the relatively bright signal of the fat (arrows). On the T_2 images (**B**) the fat is of moderate signal intensity and the nodes show increased intensity due to their longer T_2 relaxation time (arrows).

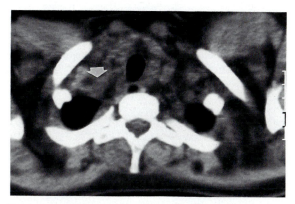

Fig. 27.12 CT scan showing a supraclavicular lymph node (arrow) on the right in this patient with Hodgkin's disease.

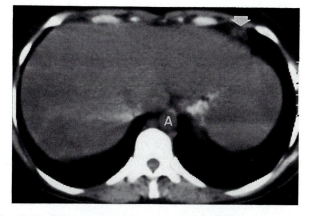

Fig. 27.13 CT scan showing enlargement and almost certain involvement of a diaphragmatic lymph node adjacent to the aorta (**A**). The enlargement of a diaphragmatic or paracardiac lymph node is of great importance in patients with Hodgkin's disease considered for mantle irradiation. Normal-sized lymph nodes in this area are not seen on CT examination.

anterior cervical vein and drains the anterior neck structures, especially the infraglottic larynx and the thyroid.

There is free communication between all the lymph node groups and chains in the neck. Eventually the lymph on the left side of the neck flows into the thoracic duct while that on the right typically enters the venous circulation via the right lymphatic duct. Metastatic involvement of cervical lymph nodes also results in spread of tumour along apparently illogical pathways and this may account for 'skip lesions' often found when assessing the neck for metastatic involvement.

Lymphatic drainage of the thorax

The lymph nodes of the mediastinum consist of a *posterior mediastinal* group of lymph nodes found below the level of the pulmonary veins and in close relationship to the aorta and oesophagus and extending inferiorly to the diaphragm. Above the posterior mediastinal lymph nodes are the *paratracheobronchial* lymph nodes. These consist of a subcarinal lymph node group, the lymph nodes of the pulmonary root, the lymph nodes between the trachea and the bronchi and the paratracheal lymph nodes. Above these lymph nodes are the lymph nodes of the *aortopulmonary window* and the *anterior mediastinum* (Glazer et al 1985, Kiyono et al 1988). These latter lymph nodes are found in front of the great vessels. In addition enlargement of the *internal mammary* and diaphragmatic lymph nodes (Fig. 27.13) should be recognized on CT examination.

The lymphatic drainage of the lungs does not strictly follow the lobar boundaries. The right upper lung drains to right paratracheal lymph nodes, the right middle lung drains to both right paratracheal and right subcarinal lymph nodes, while the lymphatic drainage from the right lower lung goes to right paratracheal, subcarinal and posterior mediastinal lymph nodes. The upper portion of the left lung drains to the paratracheal lymph nodes while both the mid and lower portions of the left lung drain to the paratracheal and subcarinal lymph nodes.

Lymphatic drainage of the abdomen and pelvis

This is best considered (Fig. 27.14) in relation to the appearances seen on the typical lymphogram (Harrison & Clouse 1985). Contrast medium injected into the lymphatic vessels on the dorsum of each foot will opacify the usually large and nonhomogeneous lymph nodes of the *groin*. These are difficult to evaluate radiologically as they are frequently enlarged as a result of previous infection/reaction and often contain numerous fibrofatty filling defects. Occasionally on CT sections pathological enlargement of the groin lymph nodes may be seen, but in such cases the diseased lymph nodes are usually palpable (Fig. 27.15). In the pelvis, lymphographic contrast agent will opacify the *external iliac* and *common iliac* lymph nodes. The *internal iliac* and *obturator* lymph nodes are usually only seen on lymphography if there is derangement of the normal flow pattern, for example, secondary to surgery, but these nodes, if enlarged, may be seen on cross-sectional imaging studies.

In the *retroperitoneum* the lymph nodes as high as L2 typically opacify at lymphangiography. There are lymph nodes *between the aorta and IVC* (Fig. 27.16). *Mesenteric* lymph nodes (Fig. 27.17) and the lymph nodes around the *stomach* and *pancreas* as well as those closest to the *porta hepatis* and *renal* and *splenic hila* may be seen on cross-sectional imaging but these fail to opacify at lymphography (Fig. 27.18).

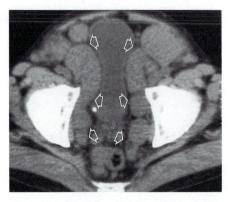

Fig. 27.15 CT section through the pelvis showing bilateral pelvic and groin lymph node enlargement in a patient with NHL.

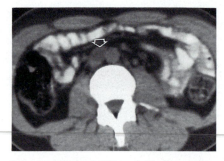

Fig. 27.16 Contrast-enhanced CT study showing enlargement and involvement of an inter-aorticocaval lymph node (arrow) in a patient with a right-sided testicular malignancy. Right-sided testicular tumours frequently spread to the inter-aorticocaval lymph nodes. This is extremely uncommon when the testicular primary is on the left.

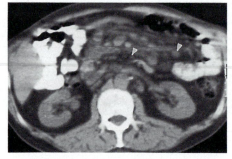

Fig. 27.17 CT section showing mesenteric lymph node involvement (arrowheads) in a patient with NHL. This is common in NHL, but seen in fewer than 5% of patients with Hodgkin's disease.

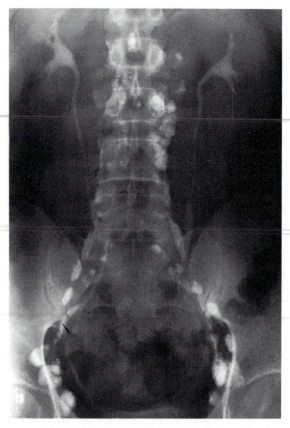

Fig. 27.14 Frontal view of a lymphogram showing opacification of the pelvic and retroperitoneal lymph nodes.

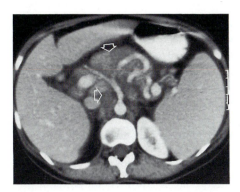

Fig. 27.18 Contrast-enhanced CT showing considerable enlargement of upper abdominal, peripancreatic and portal lymph nodes (arrows). The superior mesenteric artery and the hepatic artery are outlined.

LYMPH NODE ENLARGEMENT

Malignant involvement of a lymph node results in the enlargement of the affected lymph node. This may be considered to involve four stages. *Firstly*, the deposition of a malignant cell within the lymph node and subsequent cell division, resulting in the presence of a micrometastasis within the affected lymph node. At this stage the lymph node remains of normal size and shape and will appear normal on CT and MR examination (Fig. 27.19). *Surgical staging*, with either lymph node sampling or formal lymphadenectomy, will demonstrate malignant involvement of lymph nodes before either the CT/MR scan or the lymphogram become abnormal. Surgery and careful histology is the present 'gold standard' for evaluating lymph-node involvement in patients with malignant disease. This is seen, for example, in the axillary staging of patients with breast cancer.

There is a period in which *lymphography* might demonstrate the presence of a micrometastasis while the lymph node itself remains of normal size. This accounts for the slightly greater sensitivity of lymphography over CT and/or MRI in evaluating the retroperitoneal lymph nodes and is most useful in evaluating slower-growing tumours where this stage is likely to persist longer. The CT demonstration of a micrometastasis within a lymph node is more difficult but may be possible in the neck. A CT density measurement is required to differentiate a small metastasis within a lymph node from a focal deposit of fat. In the neck the incidence of fibrofatty foci within normal-sized lymph nodes is less than in the abdominal, pelvic and axillary lymph nodes, making this a valid technique.

Eventually an involved lymph node will enlarge and become recognizable clinically and/or with cross-sectional imaging. Some tumours result in discrete lymph node metastases (Fig. 27.20) while other tumours rapidly pass onto the next phase, in which the outline of the tumour becomes blurred due to the presence of tumour extending into the perinodal tissues. The final or *fourth* stage of malignant spread of tumour to a lymph node results in a large amorphous tumour mass with infiltration of the tissue planes. At this time it is impossible to identify any residual nodal outline.

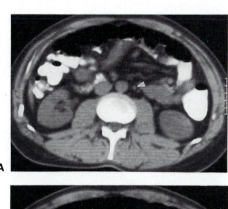

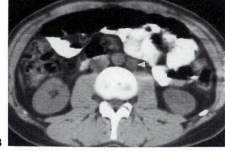

Fig. 27.19 Staging CT on this patient with a testicular primary (**A**) shows no significant adenopathy. Note the 0.25 cm node in the left retroperitoneum (arrowhead). Seven months later (**B**) this lymph node has enlarged (arrowhead), indicating the presence of an occult primary in the lymph node at the time of original staging.

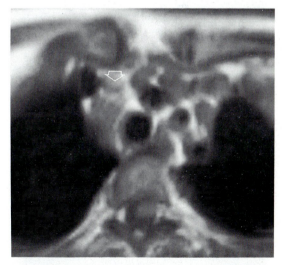

Fig. 27.20 Axial T$_1$-weighted MR scan through the thorax of a patient with Hodgkin's disease showing discrete enlargement of mediastinal lymph nodes. The low-intensity lymph nodes are seen in the high-intensity fat (arrow). Note the vessels give low signal intensity, enabling them to be identified. This is an example of the flow void phenomenon.

BENIGN CONDITIONS AFFECTING THE LYMPH NODES

These are important radiologically as they may result in lymph node enlargement which may be confused with malignant involvement. Benign focal lesions within the lymph nodes can also be mistaken for deposits.

Acute inflammation will enlarge lymph nodes. On lymphograms the texture of the lymph node will become more foamy, an appearance usually associated with lymphoma (Fig. 27.21). Central defects within the lymph node may also be seen. Typically it is the granulomatous or abscess-forming inflammations that produce filling defects in the lymph nodes similar to those seen in secondary deposits (Fig. 27.22). Lymph nodes may be seen to enlarge in a number of *granulomatous diseases* including sarcoid and tuberculosis.

Reactive hyperplasia usually associated with a proliferation of histiocytes is another frequent cause of lymph node enlargement. This may be related to recent surgery (Fig. 27.23).

Fibrofatty deposits are seen within the lymph nodes of older patients and these are most commonly seen in the pelvis. They may be considered a normal finding in the inguinal region, but in the remainder of the pelvis they

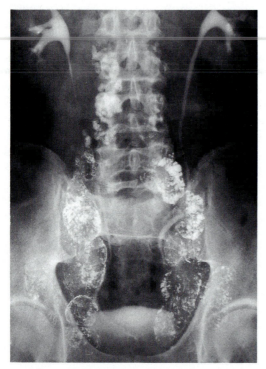

Fig. 27.21 The lymph nodes are generally enlarged and appear foamy in this patient with lymphoma.

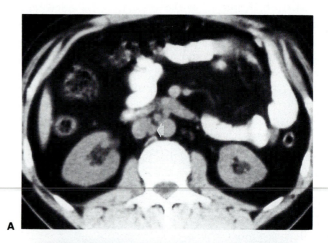

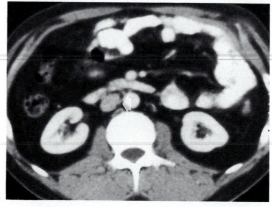

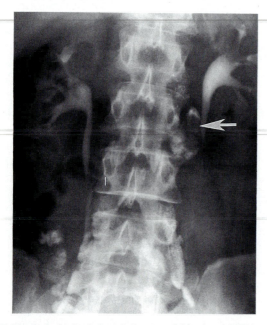

Fig. 27.22 A single focal deposit is seen within the enlarged and opacified lymph node medial to the left ureter (arrow) in this patient with an endometrial cancer.

Fig. 27.23 Staging CT scans in a patient with a recently resected right-sided testicular tumour showed prominent lymph nodes (**A**) between aorta and IVC (arrow). One month later these have resolved without treatment (**B**). Reactive enlargement of lymph nodes is a possible source of error if patients are scanned too close to the date of their surgery. It is better to wait 3–4 weeks.

are a source of confusion, as they may be incorrectly interpreted as secondary deposits in patients with a primary pelvic neoplasm.

MALIGNANT CONDITIONS AFFECTING THE LYMPH NODES

Lymphomas are primary neoplasms of the immune system and arise within lymphoid tissue (Neumann et al 1985). The lymphomas are uncommon, accounting for approximately 4% of the newly diagnosed malignant tumours in the UK. *Hodgkin's disease* accounts for approximately 25% of newly diagnosed lymphomas, i.e. 1% of all malignancies. In children lymphoma is the third most frequent malignancy, following behind leukaemia and CNS neoplasia. As a group the lymphomas vary enormously in outlook but all will reduce life-expectancy if untreated.

The histological subtype of the lymphoma and the anatomical extent of disease at the time of diagnosis have prognostic significance. A practicable histological classification is the key to the appropriate investigation and management of patients with lymphoma (Callihan et al 1980). The first and most important distinction is between *Hodgkin's disease* and the *non-Hodgkin lymphomas* (NHL).

Hodgkin's disease

The aetiology of Hodgkin's disease is obscure. The disease may present at any age, but characteristically has a peak incidence in young adulthood, with a second peak incidence in old age. The disease is slightly more common in males. The histological diagnosis may be difficult and the radiologist should not hesitate to question the diagnosis if the radiological findings are atypical. Fine-needle aspiration cytology is rarely helpful and every effort should be made to obtain an adequate specimen for histological review. This usually requires the surgical excision of enlarged lymph nodes.

The cell of origin for Hodgkin's disease is unknown but the disease is believed to begin within a lymph node. After a time the disease begins to spread by contiguity through the lymphatic system. Haematogenous dissemination is a late phenomenon and almost invariably follows splenic involvement. The orderly spread of disease through the lymphatic system has important therapeutic considerations. Localized disease may be irradiated and cure anticipated. The radiation portals may be chosen to include both the obvious disease sites and the adjacent lymph node groups, which may in turn be the site of occult involvement. This is known as *extended field irradiation* and differs from the more standard involved field techniques commonly employed in other tumours. The use of the extended field technique in

Hodgkin's disease is an example of how knowledge generated by clinical, radiological and surgical mapping of disease can be used to modify treatment successfully.

Lymph nodes involved with Hodgkin's disease will enlarge, and eventually disease will spread extranodally into the adjacent tissues. The four stages of nodal involvement described above may be recognized. True tumour invasion of surrounding organs and structures is a late phenomenon in patients with Hodgkin's disease. CT scanning will initially demonstrate contiguity between the enlarged lymph nodes and adjacent structures but early tumour invasion of contiguous structures is difficult to recognize radiologically.

The histopathological classification of Hodgkin's disease now widely accepted was developed by Lukes et al (1966) and subsequently accepted at the Rye Conference. In essence there are four subgroups of Hodgkin's disease. Three of these are related — at least in part — to the strength of the host reaction, *lymphocyte-predominant* (LP) indicating a strong host response, *lymphocyte-depleted* (LD) indicating a very weak response and *mixed-cellularity* (MC) indicating an intermediate group with an intermediate and moderate immune response (Castellino 1986).

Patients with the LP form almost invariably present with a localized disease, often with palpable supraclavicular lymph nodes. This variety is most frequently seen in young asymptomatic males. On histological review of the excised lymph nodes, the characteristic Reed-Sternberg cells are scanty. This form of Hodgkin's disease has an excellent prognosis and may be treated with local rather than systemic therapy.

The typical patient with the LD form of Hodgkin's disease is older, usually polysymptomatic and on investigation will be found to have advanced disseminated disease. Histological review of excised lymph nodes will show numerous Reed-Sternberg cells. The prognosis is poor.

Mixed-cellularity (MC) Hodgkin's disease is the most frequently seen of these three histopathological subtypes. It may be seen in every age group but is especially frequent in young adults. Patients with MC disease are often symptomatic. Three specific signs and symptoms in patients with Hodgkin's disease, known as the B symptoms (*unexplained weight loss* of more than 10% body weight in the preceding 6 months, *unexplained fever* above 38.4°C, and/or *night sweats*), are an indication that the disease may involve abdominal lymph nodes and/or the spleen. The prognosis of MC Hodgkin's disease lies between that of LP and LD disease. LP or MC variants may progress to LD or even to a non-Hodgkin lymphoma.

The fourth histological subtype of Hodgkin's disease is *nodular sclerosing* (NS). This is the only subgroup more common in female patients. Typically patients present in adolescence or early adulthood, and almost invariably the mediastinal and supraclavicular lymph node groups are involved. Histologically, lymph nodes involved with NS Hodgkin's disease will show a thick fibrous rim. Recent attention has focussed on the contents within this connective tissue reaction and it is now felt that there are subgroups within NS Hodgkin's disease. These depend on the host response and at present are probably best regarded as a *good prognosis* (with a strong host response) and a *poor prognosis* (weak host response) subgroup. Most patients with NS Hodgkin's disease will have a good prognosis, and unlike the LP and MC subtypes, NS Hodgkin's disease rarely progresses to a stage with a less favourable histology.

The presence of fibrous stroma around the lymph nodes is important radiologically. Patients with NS Hodgkin's disease typically have large lymph nodes at presentation. These slowly reduce in size on successful therapy and it is not uncommon for residual soft-tissue masses to persist. Interpretation of radiological findings at this time may be difficult. The temptation to overdiagnose poor response to treatment and/or residual active disease should be resisted.

The second prognostic factor in Hodgkin's disease is the anatomical extent of disease at the time of presentation. The *Ann Arbor staging system* (Table 27.1) has been accepted for many years (Carbone et al 1971). In this system lymph nodes are considered part of clearly defined lymph node-groups, e.g., left neck and left axilla. Involvement of one or more lymph nodes within a group is considered to represent involvement of that group.

Table 27.1 Staging of Hodgkin's disease (Modified from Carbone et al. 1971)

Stage I	Disease confined to a single lymph node group
Stage II	Disease involving two or more lymph node groups on the same side of the diaphragm
Stage III	Disease involving lymph node groups on both sides of the diaphragm
Stage IV	Haematogenous dissemination of disease

Note. Local extension of disease into the extranodal tissues, for example adjacent lung or bone, is recorded by the subscript E rather than changing the stage to IV.

Non-Hodgkin lymphomas (NHL)
Non-Hodgkin lymphomas are a much more heterogeneous group of malignant tumours than the Hodgkin's lymphomas (Bragg et al 1986). They are most frequently seen in the elderly. There have been many attempts to classify the pathological appearances of the tumour, but the terminology unfortunately remains confusing. The National Cancer Institute Working Party (1981) considered all the contemporary classifications and proposed a working formulation dividing the non-Hodgkin lymphomas into low, intermediate and high-grade groups. Radiologists

(along with most clinicians) may find this artificial and still prefer to divide their patients into two groups, the low-grade *nodular* or *follicular lymphomas* and the high-grade *diffuse lymphomas*.

The origin and sub-types of the non-Hodgkin lymphomas may be considered as follows. In fetal life T and B lymphocyte precursors are formed: **T-cells** migrate to the thymus and eventually mature into *helper T-cells* or *suppressor/cytotoxic T-cells* and leave the thymus to circulate around the body. The T-cells antigens on these cells may be recognized by monoclonal antibody techniques. After circulating around the body T-cells accumulate in the lymph nodes and in the spleen.

B-cells are formed in the liver and migrate to bone marrow. Subsequently they may also be found in lymph nodes, but the T-cells and the B-cells are found in different parts of the lymph node. The T-cells remain paracortical while the B-cells are found within the lymphoid follicles. Depending on their nuclear morphology, two subgroups of B-cell types within the follicle may be recognized: B-cells with large round nuclei are known as *centroblasts* (non-cleaved), while those with irregular nuclei are known as *centrocytes* or cleaved cells. B-cells may be found within the circulation, where they are known as *plasma cells*.

Monocytes from the circulation may lodge in the body tissues where they are known as histiocytes. Histiocytes are thought to be a third possible cell of origin for the non-Hodgkin lymphomas but *histiocytic lymphomas* account for fewer than 5% of the non-Hodgkin lymphomas.

The majority of non-Hodgkin lymphomas arise from the follicular cells within the lymph node follicle and may consist of cells that appear cleaved, non-cleaved, or a mixture of the two. Although most non-Hodgkin lymphomas are of B-cell origin and have a tendency to form follicles, they do not all form typical follicles. In practice many show tumour infiltration throughout the affected lymph node. From this simple observation two important subgroups may be recognized — those that tend to remain in the follicles and are *follicular* (or nodular) and those which show the diffusion of tumour cells into the remainder of the lymph node and are called *diffuse*. On occasion both diffuse and follicular features may be seen within the same excised lymph node, or within two lymph nodes excised from the same patient at the same time. Finally, follicular lymphomas may evolve into diffuse large-cell forms as part of their natural history.

Low-grade lymphomas are usually follicular while the intermediate and high grade tumours are usually diffuse. T-cell lymphomas (10% of the total) are found in the skin and thymus from peripheral T-cells.

Non-Hodgkin lymphomas frequently present as painless enlargement of lymph nodes, but the disease may also develop at a number of extranodal sites, leading to a wide variety of presenting features.

Nodal presentations of the non-Hodgkin lymphomas. The most common site is the *neck* and, unlike Hodgkin's disease, the lymphoid tissue of Waldeyer's ring is usually involved. The patient will frequently have nodal enlargement at a number of palpable and radiologically obvious sites. These are often noncontiguous, and if the lymph nodes are followed up without treatment they may be found to spontaneously fluctuate in size. A patient with a non-Hodgkin lymphoma is much more likely to present with enlarged lymph nodes in unusual sites — for example, those of the elbow or knee — than a patient with Hodgkin's disease. The secondary effects of lymph-node enlargement such as limb swelling or SVC obstruction are not uncommon. Backache is suggestive of retroperitoneal lymph-node involvement, and constitutional symptoms, especially weight loss, fever and anorexia, are typical.

Although designed for use in Hodgkin's disease the Ann Arbor approach to staging is frequently used for the non-Hodgkin lymphomas. The majority of patients, especially those with follicular lymphomas, will have widespread disease (Stage III or IV) at presentation. Only about one-third of patients will have clinically localized disease at presentation. Of these fewer than one half will still have limited disease by the time they have been fully staged radiologically. This small subgroup (about one-sixth of the total) is important if local radiotherapy is to be considered as a curative option. With true Stage I diffuse lymphoma there is a 90% chance of long-term disease-free survival. With Stage II disease the proportion of patients free of relapse at five years falls to 40%. For this reason chemotherapy is usually given in Stage II disease unless the patient is elderly or there is some contra-indication to its use. In early-stage follicular lymphomas local radiotherapy will achieve symptomatic control and over 70% of patients may well be alive after ten years. But patients with a follicular lymphoma will relapse and cannot ever be regarded as cured. Unlike Hodgkin's disease, where there is an orderly spread of disease by contiguity through the lymph nodes, the spread of non-Hodgkin lymphoma does not follow a contiguous pattern, and there is no clinical advantage in planning extended rather than involved field irradiation. Palliative local radiotherapy is important, especially in the elderly, and good short-term local control is to be expected. In such patients extensive investigation is not warranted.

Most patients with NHL will have extensive disease and qualify for chemotherapy. In such instances the finer nuances of radiological staging are no longer required for treatment planning. However some idea of tumour extent and bulk is important in assessing response to chemotherapy and for comparison of results. In most patients with diffuse NHL combination chemotherapy is required. There are a number of different drug regimes in use and all will produce a complete response in approximately 75% of patients; of these, three-quarters will still be alive after five years. The prognosis is worse in *men*, in patients with *large abdominal nodal masses*, and in those with *hepatic* or *marrow involvement*. The proportion of complete responders is greatest in those with Stage II disease and falls to 60% in those with Stage III disease and to 35% in those patients with Stage IV disease. The prognosis for incomplete responders is poor, and almost all these patients will be dead in two years. In this group recent attention has focussed on ultra-high dose therapy with autologous bone marrow grafting.

Advanced *follicular (low-grade) lymphomas* are often treated expectantly, as there is little evidence that any treatment alters the outcome. Patients are usually treated symptomatically either with local irradiation and/or chemotherapy. The younger patient may occasionally be given combination chemotherapy more in the hope than anticipation of cure. Long-term chemotherapy has been advocated in patients with low-grade lymphomas. Unfortunately this approach may lead to bone-marrow depression and drug resistance. This may be important if the disease progresses to the diffuse form, and intensive chemotherapy then offers the only hope of disease control.

The majority of *T-cell lymphomas* are seen in younger patients, often with large mediastinal masses. The tumours are aggressive, with short histories, constitutional symptoms, bone-marrow involvement and frequently CNS spread with leptomeningitis, nerve palsy, root compression and increased intracranial pressure. The prognosis is poor and systemic treatment is required.

Extranodal presentations of the non-Hodgkin lymphomas. Extranodal sites of disease are commonly found on detailed staging of patients with a primary nodal presentation (Glazer et al 1983). Nodal disease which has previously been treated may relapse extranodally. The non-Hodgkin lymphomas may also present at an extranodal site without clinically obvious nodal disease. These patients may be difficult to diagnose and to treat.

GASTROINTESTINAL LYMPHOMA

The *small bowel* and *stomach* are the most frequent sites of involvement. In the small bowel the disease is believed to originate within the lymphoid tissue of the mucosal lining. For this reason it is most frequently seen where there is the most lymphoid tissue present. The incidence increases from the duodenum through the jejunum to the ileum. The disease may be single- or multifocal and grows eventually to ulcerate through the mucosa, bowel wall and serosa. Eventually the regional lymph nodes are involved. The disease may progress to bowel obstruction and perforation. Most patients have *diffuse high-grade NHL* of *B-cell origin*. Patients with long standing

Table 27.2 CT staging of primary gut lymphomas (Modified from Blackledge et al. 1979)

Stage	1	Confined to gut
	1A	single tumour
	1B	multiple tumours
Stage	2	Local extension
	2A	adjacent nodes
	2B	adjacent structures
	2C	with perforation and peritonitis
Stage	3	Extra regional nodal spread
Stage	4	Distant dissemination e.g., liver, spleen

coeliac disease may develop *T-cell lymphomas* and these respond poorly to treatment.

The clinical presentation of the bowel lymphomas is varied. Many patients present acutely with abdominal pain and have urgent surgery. The diagnosis may be made after an often incomplete resection and exploration of the abdomen. Complete resection of the tumour with no evidence of spread beyond the bowel is associated with a significantly better prognosis.

NHL of the gut may present subacutely, and the diagnosis is then suggested at barium examination or CT scanning. Blackledge et al (1979) suggested a simple staging system for gastrointestinal lymphoma (Table 27.2) that is useful prognostically. Treatment of gut NHL depends on histology, stage and the presence or absence of residual disease. The present therapeutic trend is towards the use of combination chemotherapy unless the tumour is both low-grade and of limited extent. Small-bowel lymphoma is the most common paediatric bowel tumour, almost invariably involves the terminal ileum and is of intermediate or high grade.

Stomach lymphomas often mimic adenocarcinomas clinically, with nausea and weight loss being the usual presentation symptoms (Fig. 27.24). Treatment is surgical, followed by combination chemotherapy.

The natural history and behaviour of extranodal lymphomas are different from those arising in nodal sites. This may be because of differences in the lymphoid tissue found in the extranodal sites. In the stomach there is mucosa-associated lymphoid tissue (MALT) which is different to the normal somatic lymphoid tissue. MALT is present at a number of sites in the body, including the gastrointestinal tract, the lungs and salivary glands. It would appear that lymphocytes from a MALT site can pass to regional lymph nodes and then to the general circulation before homing back on the mucosa of origin or another MALT site. This may be the explanation of several characteristics of these tumours, including a tendency to remain localized before spreading to regional lymph nodes and finally disseminating throughout the body, typically to other MALT sites. These MALT sites are frequently the site of disease relapse in these patients. Undoubtedly there is a lot to learn about the spread of NHL within the body, and in time it may be that the pattern of dissemination and recurrence will be seen to follow more orderly lines than presently appreciated.

CENTRAL NERVOUS SYSTEM LYMPHOMA

Primary non-Hodgkin lymphoma represents about 1% of primary brain tumours (Fig. 27.25). The incidence is highest in immuno-compromised patients, especially those with AIDS or renal transplants or on long-term immunosuppression for some other reason. Patients rarely develop systemic lymphoma, either at the time of diagnosis or later. Detailed systemic staging is superfluous. Treatment is primarily irradiation and the prognosis is poor. Primary Hodgkin's disease of the brain is rare.

Secondary CNS lymphoma is not uncommon. It is most frequently seen in high-grade tumours, especially in chil-

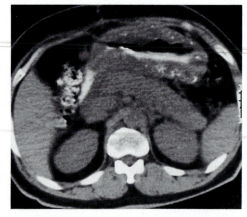

Fig. 27.24 CT scan through the abdomen of a patient with gastric NHL shows thickening of the gastric wall and prominence of the rugal folds. Note how the oral contrast medium is seen to collect in pools between the giant rugal folds.

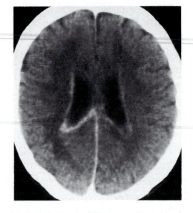

Fig. 27.25 Contrast-enhanced CT brain scan showing periventricular enhancement due to subependymal spread of NHL. This is a common appearance in CNS lymphoma.

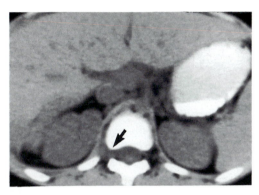

Fig. 27.26 CT scan showing normal fat and soft-tissue densities in the left paravertebral area. On the right the fat in the paravertebral area is obliterated by lymphoma tissue (arrow) which is closely applied to the nerve root exit foramen. The paravertebral tissues should be systematically reviewed when CT scanning any patient with malignant disease, so that lesions may be detected and treated prior to the onset of cord compression.

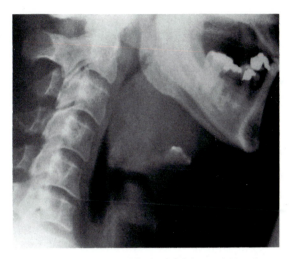

Fig. 27.28 Lateral soft-tissue radiograph of the neck showing abnormal soft tissue from a primary NHL of the neck arising in the epiglottis and presenting with dysphagia.

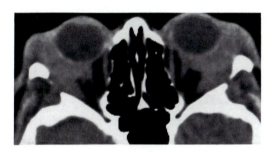

Fig. 27.27 CT scan through the orbits of a patient presenting with orbital NHL. Diffuse thickening of the tissues is seen bilaterally.

dren and those with T-cell disease. Approximately 50% of these patients with CNS involvement will develop *cord compression*, while the other 50% will show evidence of *lymphomatous meningitis* with nerve and root lesions, raised intracranial pressure and mental confusion. CNS involvement is also a feature of testicular, orbital head/neck primary sites. At all times when CT or MR scanning any patient with a known lymphoma, the *paravertebral tissues* should be closely examined; involvement here may portend cord compression (Fig. 27.26).

Orbital lymphomas (Fig. 27.27) almost always disseminate systemically. This is especially true if the disease is bilateral and/or involves neck lymph nodes. CT of the head and neck is the single most useful staging investigation.

HEAD AND NECK LYMPHOMAS

Primary nodal lymphomas arising in the head and neck do not require CT staging of the neck. An experienced clinician should be able to palpate enlarged lymph nodes within the neck. Abdominal CT staging is useful as the

disease often relapses outside the head and neck, typically in the gastrointestinal tract, reflecting the characteristics of a MALT lymphoma. Extranodal NHL of the head and neck is usually associated with disease dissemination in the body and a poor prognosis (Fig. 27.28).

THORACIC LYMPHOMA

Involvement of the lungs is an uncommon feature of both NHL (Fig. 27.29) and Hodgkin's disease. In high-grade NHL pulmonary involvement may be extensive and explosive, the radiological appearances often mimicking those seen in infection. Low-grade NHL may also involve the lungs. Typically, many of these low-grade tumours are indolent, often in the past being described as pseudolymphomas. Some of these arise in the bronchus-associated lymphoid tissue.

In patients with more typical variants of NHL, CT scanning of the thorax is not rewarding, either for the assessment of the lung fields or for detecting mediastinal

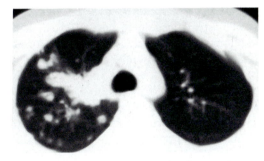

Fig. 27.29 CT scan showing pulmonary involvement in a patient with NHL. A mass of tumour tissue is seen around the right hilum. In addition a number of ill-defined intrapulmonary nodules are seen on the right.

involvement in the presence of a normal chest radiograph. NHL involves the mediastinum less frequently than Hodgkin's disease, and mediastinal involvement in NHL typically reflects widespread disease dissemination.

Bone. Bone-marrow involvement is commonly found in the non-Hodgkin lymphomas. On occasion a patient will present with an apparent primary bone NHL. These are most common in younger patients and involve the appendicular skeleton, especially in the metaphyseal region. *Radiologically*, the most common appearance is a permeative destructive lesion. Pathologically, the lesions are typically high-grade. Full radiological staging of the abdomen and chest should be undertaken and a high percentage of patients will prove to have disseminated disease.

Testis. Testicular lymphomas occur in middle-aged and elderly men. Twenty-five percent will be bilateral. Testicular NHL is aggressive, high-grade and tends to spread not only to the regional lymph nodes in the abdomen but also to lung, the central nervous system and in the neck to Waldeyer's ring.

CT SCANNING OF THE THORAX

CT is the current 'gold standard' for evaluating the extent of thoracic involvement in patients with Hodgkin's disease and, when required, for those with non-Hodgkin lymphoma. The pattern of lymphomatous involvement is different for Hodgkin's disease and non-Hodgkin lymphoma. In addition, the therapeutic implications of any positive findings in these two conditions also differ.

The chest should be scanned in the supine position and in held inspiration. Ideally, a modern scanner with a fast scan time of 3–4 seconds should be used. Contiguous sections are usual and should be obtained at 1 cm intervals. Intravenous contrast enhancement should be dynamic, whenever possible, using at least 100 ml of contrast. Intravenous contrast is helpful in assessing the mediastinum and is crucial to the complete CT evaluation of the lung hila. The presence of i.v. contrast medium is not detrimental to the imaging of the lung fields and when it is to be used pre-contrast studies are not warranted. Normal mediastinal structures and in particular blood vessels should be routinely identified. Normal-sized lymph nodes may on occasion be seen within the mediastinal fat, but this would appear to be a less common observation in the UK than in the USA. CT sections through the mediastinum of a patient with lymphoma should clearly demonstrate the extent of adenopathy. CT identifies abnormal lymph nodes by an abnormal increase in the cross-sectional diameter of the lymph nodes. Typically, mediastinal lymph nodes more than 1 cm in diameter are interpreted as being involved. Hilar nodal enlargement usually follows mediastinal involvement, at least in Hodgkin's disease. Micrometastases occurring in normal-sized mediastinal lymph nodes cannot be diagnosed on CT, and, equally, nodal enlargement for non-malignant reasons may not be discriminated from malignant enlargement.

Hodgkin's disease

The anterior mediastinum is the focus from which Hodgkin's disease of the chest appears to spread (MacDonald et al 1987). It is extremely uncommon to have disease at other sites within the thorax in the absence of anterior mediastinal involvement. Recognition of adenopathy at this site is the first step to successful CT scan interpretation.

Conventional radiographs will only recognize an abnormality in this region when the contour of the mediastinum and its pleural reflections is altered. In general, enlarged lymph nodes on the right side of the mediastinum are easier to identify on plain chest radiography than those on the left side, where the overlying shadow of the aortic arch makes small-volume adenopathy more difficult to recognize.

The typical CT appearance of a nodal mass in a patient with Hodgkin's disease is usually that of an homogeneous soft-tissue mass with sharply defined and often lobulated borders. Occasionally the centre of the nodal mass contains an area of decreased attenuation due to necrosis. If intravenous contrast medium has been given, the lymph node may enhance.

Castellino et al (1986) reviewed the contribution that CT scanning of the thorax made in their Hodgkin's disease practice. From their study it is clear that CT will demonstrate abnormal lymph nodes more readily than conventional X-ray techniques within the thorax.

Primary Hodgkin's disease is managed by chemotherapy or radiotherapy or a combination of both. The most profound impact on management might be expected in those patients being considered for radiotherapy. CT demonstration of the extent of disease at a particular site may influence the size of the proposed fields, and CT demonstration of disease at previously unsuspected sites, particularly in the posterior mediastinum and diaphragmatic area, may lead to a change in management from radiotherapy to chemotherapy. Thus mediastinal CT in Hodgkin's disease is of most value when a high proportion of patients are being considered for radiotherapy. When the patient is to have chemotherapy from the start, then the more precise demonstration of disease extent within the thorax is of no immediate consequence. The value of CT scanning of the mediastinum in these patients is limited to baseline studies for the monitoring of response and assessment of residual changes. In any institution the proportion of patients considered for radiotherapy will vary, and it is this that accounts for differing opinions on the impact of mediastinal CT on the management of patients with Hodgkin's disease. Studies from different institutions confirm that the value of mediastinal CT in patients with Hodgkin's disease is maximal in those who are being considered for radiation therapy.

A decrease in size of previously enlarged lymph nodes also serves as an indicator of response to chemotherapy. In many instances this can be adequately assessed on serial chest radiographs but — especially when the chest radiograph has returned to normal — the CT scan may show residual adenopathy.

CT scanning of the lungs may show evidence of Hodgkin's disease. The most characteristic finding is the presence of one or more nodules within the parenchyma. They are most frequently seen near the lung bases and/or the pulmonary hila, suggesting a haematogenous spread. The demonstration of these would classify the case as Stage IV according to the Ann Arbor convention. As with other small pulmonary nodules, CT has a small advantage over conventional chest radiographs in the demonstration of smaller pulmonary lesions. In lymphoma these small focal changes are often poorly defined.

Lymphoma may involve the lung fields in a variety of other ways. These include patchy pulmonary shadowing, pulmonary consolidation and lobar collapse. Pulmonary involvement is uncommon in the patient with newly diagnosed Hodgkin's disease, being seen at most in 10% of patients. Parenchymal lesions in newly presented patients who have no mediastinal or hilar adenopathy are best considered not to represent Hodgkin's disease. Pulmonary disease is a feature of recurrent Hodgkin's disease, where it may be confused not only with infection but also with the effects of treatment. These include pulmonary consolidation and fibrosis following radiotherapy, drug reactions, and opportunistic infections during or following systemic chemotherapy.

A frequent concern to the clinician is the possibility of early tumour infiltration from enlarged hilar lymph nodes into the surrounding lung tissue. This is well recognized and indicated in the Ann Arbor staging system, as, for example, Stage IIE disease. Although this is a frequent indication for requesting thoracic CT, in practice it is exceptional to detect this infiltration on CT unless the chest radiograph is abnormal.

CT may be helpful in assessing the patency and diameter of airways, especially in children. Over half the children presenting with Hodgkin's disease show significant *airway obstruction* on CT examination and occasionally this may require emergency treatment.

CT is ideally suited to demonstrating pleural and pleurally based lesions. These include *solid plaques* of tumour tissue and *pleural effusions*. It is important to remember that most pleural effusions seen in patients with Hodgkin's disease are benign, and are thought to be a consequence of lymphatic obstruction secondary to

mediastinal and hilar lymph node involvement and enlargement.

Non-Hodgkin lymphomas

The contribution that thoracic CT scanning might make in the management of patients with non-Hodgkin lymphoma is less certain, for several reasons. NHL is more likely than Hodgkin's disease to be widespread and require systemic therapy, the mediastinum is a less frequent site of disease and in many instances the presence of mediastinal involvement will be recognized on a routine chest radiograph. Lung involvement is uncommon, and is seen in fewer than 5% of patients at diagnosis. The presence of a pleural effusion in NHL usually reflects the presence of pleural tumour. This is a reflection of the lower incidence of mediastinal adenopathy seen in NHL than in Hodgkin's disease.

A recent survey concluded that the addition of CT scanning to the diagnostic work-up of patients presenting with a new non-Hodgkin lymphoma may occasionally show additional sites of disease but does not result in a change in management.

CT SCANNING OF THE ABDOMEN

CT is now the standard method of imaging the abdomen in patients with lymphoma. In one study of 168 patients presenting with a non-Hodgkin lymphoma (Pond et al 1989), 29% had abdominal disease detectable only on CT scanning. Typically, CT sections are taken through the abdomen and upper pelvis at 1.5 cm intervals following opacification of the bowel with oral contrast media. Abnormal lymph nodes may be recognized by an increase in size. Retroperitoneal nodes greater than 1.5 cm in diameter are considered abnormal. Particular attention should be paid to the retrocrural region (Fig. 27.30), (where nodes greater than 0.6 cm in diameter are regarded as pathological), the retroperitoneum, the pelvic lymph nodes and (especially in patients with NHL) the mesenteric lymph nodes. Involvement of the spleen or

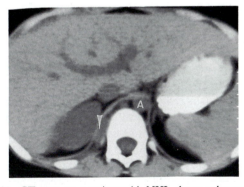

Fig. 27.30 CT scan on a patient with NHL shows enlargement of the retrocrural lymph nodes (arrowhead). A = Aorta.

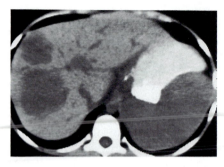

Fig. 27.31 Focal areas of low attenuation are seen in the liver of this boy with recurrent Hodgkin's disease. The spleen is enlarged and inhomogenous.

liver is often difficult to detect. On occasion focal deposits may be seen in the spleen or liver (Fig. 27.31); more typically lymphomatous involvement results in an increase in the size of the affected organ. This may be obvious but in many cases early involvement is especially difficult to diagnose. In addition, in patients with Hodgkin's disease the spleen may enlarge in the absence of direct involvement, leading to possible radiological overstaging.

CT SCANNING OF THE HEAD AND NECK

Enlarged lymph nodes in the neck are usually palpable. CT may demonstrate non-palpable lymph node enlargement and/or *central necrosis* within the lymph node, the latter being a certain sign of a pathological condition. In addition CT imaging may show that a single palpable mass consists of a conglomerate mass of several enlarged lymph nodes, an observation that may alter staging and prognosis of primary head and neck cancers. In general the demonstration of nodal disease in the neck of patients with a primary tumour of the head and neck is of grave prognostic significance. Ipsilateral adenopathy reduces survival by 50% and contralateral adenopathy by a further 50%. CT may also demonstrate extranodal spread of malignancy. This is associated with a further significant reduction in prognosis.

CT examination of the neck is usually performed during the dynamic infusion of intravenous contrast medium, which allows all the vascular structures to be highlighted and in addition may demonstrate ring enhancement in patients with metastatic squamous carcinomas. At present CT remains the method of choice in staging cervical adenopathy, as it may enable small metastatic foci within normal-sized lymph nodes to be recognized — something which cannot yet be achieved with MRI. With MRI, intravenous contrast medium is not required to identify the vessels, and this may be of value in patients who are sensitive to iodine. The MR characteristics of enlarged lymph nodes are nonspecific and do not allow

the cause of the enlargement, or whether the underlying pathology is benign or malignant, to be deduced.

The main criteria for abnormality when imaging the neck with CT and/or MR is an increase in the size. Normally the lymph nodes high in the neck are larger than those lower in the neck, presumably due to benign enlargement secondary to previous recurrent throat infections. It is generally accepted that lymph nodes larger than 1 cm in diameter are abnormal, unless the lymph node is in the jugulodiagastric region, where 1.5 cm is a more reasonable upper limit of normal cross-sectional diameter. Using these criteria, approximately 80% of the lymph nodes considered abnormal at CT and/or MR examination will, under the appropriate clinical conditions, contain tumour.

THE GROWTH AND SPREAD OF SOLID TUMOURS

There are many conventions for the staging of different tumours, and all methods reflect the bulk and distribution of tumour tissue within the body. This is of some prognostic and therapeutic significance, although in many tumours the histological diagnosis and grading is of paramount importance. The TNM system (UICC 1987) is the most widely accepted staging system, although it is inappropriate for patients with lymphoma.

If it is assumed that a primary neoplasm starts as a single malignant cell which has the capacity to replicate itself, then it will take approximately 30 cell divisions for a tumour mass to reach a diameter of 1 cm and become radiologically visible. The doubling time of a tumour varies greatly and may be a few days for a rapidly growing malignancy, or several months for a slow-growing tumour type. From this it may be seen that all tumours will take months or years to become radiologically detectable. For most of their life all tumours are subclinical. Once past the 30-cell division barrier it will require only a few further cell divisions for the tumour burden to become overwhelming and the untreated patient to succumb. Malignant neoplasms may metastasize at the subclinical level. In such patients, by the time the primary tumour has become apparent the patient is already incurable by local methods (surgery and radiotherapy), as these will not treat the distant tumour spread. Metastases result from lymphatic and/or vascular invasion followed by the dissemination of tumour cells within blood or lymph vessels throughout the body. As a result of the nature of vessel wall permeability discussed above, it is probable that malignant cells may be scavenged directly from the interstitial tissues into the lymphatics, passing on through the draining lymphatics into regional lymph nodes prior to any direct vascular invasion by the tumour. The detection of metastatic lymph nodes is an important component of tumour staging, as the presence of tumour within lymph nodes may herald the vascular dissemination of tumour cells.

The primary tumour (T staging)

The size and location of any primary tumour should be assessed clinically and radiologically. Whenever possible objective measurements should be taken. These measurements are invaluable in assessing response. There are recognized criteria for primary tumour or T staging of most common tumours (UICC 1987). Knowledge of the site and extent of the primary tumour mass are valuable in predicting the likely routes of lymphatic and vascular spread.

Lymph node involvement (N staging)

Similarly, criteria have evolved to determine the extent of lymph node involvement at the time of diagnosis. The regional lymph nodes for the common malignancies have been defined and stages of involvement recognized (UICC 1987).

Consider a young man presenting with a testicular teratoma. The primary tumour is removed at orchidectomy and the specimen assessed for evidence of complete resection of the primary tumour and for lymphatic and/or vascular invasion. Teratoma typically spreads initially to to the para-aortic lymph nodes, and these then represent the first-échelon lymph nodes for testicular malignancies. Enlargement of the para-aortic lymph nodes increases the overall staging to Stage II. The subscripts A, B, C reflect the disease bulk in terms of the cross-sectional diameter of the retroperitoneal nodal mass as seen on CT: A represents a cross-sectional diameter less than 2 cm (Fig. 27.32), B a cross-sectional diameter of between 2 and 5 cm, and C a cross-sectional diameter of more than 5 cm (Fig. 27.33). The disease may then progress cephalad through the lymphatic system to involve the lymph nodes of the mediastinum (Stage III disease), although more frequently involvement of the mediastinal lymph nodes in patients with testicular teratoma is associated with evidence of vascular dissemination of tumour to the lungs. The presence of pulmonary or other extranodal metastases would automatically make the disease Stage IV. A further attempt is made to quantify the tumour bulk in the lung fields in terms of both the size and the number of pulmonary metastases.

Distant metastases (M staging)

The M stage of malignancy recognizes the spread of tumour to distant organs. This is a result of haematogenous dissemination, and the most common sites for such involvement are the lungs, liver and brain. These may be diagnosed several ways, but the overall information available from CT examination, often allowing a TNM stage to be assigned to a patient at the one examination, makes this technique supreme.

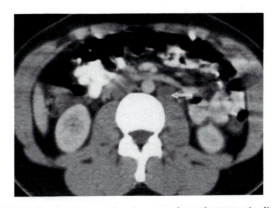

Fig. 27.32 Small-volume (<2 cm) retroperitoneal metastatic disease in a patient with a left-sided teratoma. Left-sided testicular primary teratomas almost always spread initially to a retroperitoneal lymph node under the left renal vein (arrow).

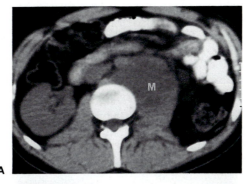

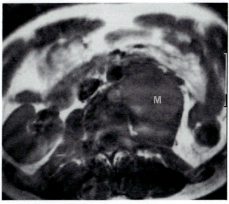

Fig. 27.33 Large retroperitoneal metastasis (M) arising from an ipsilateral testicular teratoma seen both on CT (**A**) and MRI (**B**).

IMAGING THE LYMPHATIC SYSTEM IN PATIENTS WITH MALIGNANT DISEASE

Diagnosis. CT scanning will demonstrate malignant disease within a body structure or viscus as a change in shape and/or a change in attenuation of the affected area. It is possible to propose, from the clinical details and the pattern of disease dissemination seen on CT scanning, the likely primary sites in a patient presenting with lymphadenopathy, but this speculation should never replace formal histological investigation. On occasion the radiologist may help by providing material for pathological examination from percutaneous biopsy.

Staging. As we have seen above, radiological investigation CT is essential in the TNM staging of malignant tumours and may provide information in those tumours (e.g. lymphomas) that are staged by other conventions.

Treatment planning. A patient with a fully treated primary tumour and no evidence of metastatic disease may require no further treatment unless there is evidence of disease relapse. In most circumstances patients are watched clinically and with simple investigations such as serial chest radiographs, but there are certain tumours in which a more aggressive surveillance policy is rewarding. These are usually those tumours for which curative or salvage chemotherapy is available and this includes testicular teratoma. Stage I teratoma patients may be placed on a surveillance protocol which includes regular clinical examination, serum marker estimation, chest radiograph and three-monthly CT examination of the chest, abdomen and pelvis for two years (90% of relapses will occur in the first year).

Radiotherapy planning. In patients whom it has been decided to try to cure by radiotherapy, accurate staging is essential before embarking on a course of treatment. For example, the presence of abdominal adenopathy would preclude the possibility of a cure if the pelvis is to be irradiated for a pelvic primary tumour.

The demonstration of the position, size and extent of a localized primary tumour on CT examination may be used to plan radiotherapy fields. This is usually accomplished with special software packages, and allows dose to the tumour to be maximized while vital structures — e.g., the spinal cord or kidneys — may be partly protected.

The superior soft-tissue contrast of MRI compared to CT, especially when evaluating soft-tissue spread of tumour (e.g., in muscle), suggests that MR depiction of radiotherapy treatment fields will have an application in the future.

The operability of tumours or residual masses may also be assessed at CT or MR examination, and in particular the proximity of vessels and other vital structures to the tumour mass may be determined (Fig. 27.34).

Response to treatment. The treatment of any cancer is limited by the ability of the normal body tissues to withstand the treatment. There is a morbidity and a mortality associated with any treatment. Imaging is an important part of treatment evaluation. A rapid and complete response to treatment may allow a reduction in the number of treatments required, which reduces both the possible side-effects and complications (Oliver et al 1983). Alternatively, a poor or absent response to first-line treatment could lead to either a change of treatment or to a change of approach from a curative to a palliative

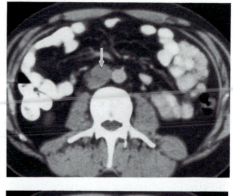

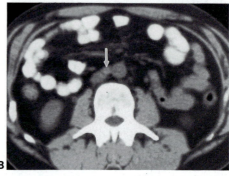

Fig. 27.34 A,B CT scans through the abdomen of this patient with a right-sided teratoma show a reduction in lymph node size (arrow) following treatment (**B**).

one. The objective recording of a response to a particular treatment is also important in the evaluation of treatments and comparative treatment studies. It must be appreciated that like must be compared with like, and CT-staged patients in one arm of the study must be imaged according to the same convention in the other arm of the study. There are at present no satisfactory guidelines on when to measure a response. A reduction in tumour size at any time counts as a partial response (PR), while the objective disappearance of tumour should be regarded as a complete response (CR). On occasion a tumour may enlarge on treatment and yet still respond (Fig. 27.35).

The addition of a more sophisticated imaging modality to the initial staging protocol of a particular tumour type may also appear to alter the outcome. Previously occult metastases will be demonstrated, altering the staging typically from Stage I (no metastases) to Stage IV (distant metastases). This will have the effect of improving survival rates in Stage I disease in the survey as some patients with metastases are now excluded from this group. The survival rate of the group of patients with Stage IV disease will also apparently improve as some of them now will have very small volume metastatic disease. However, the overall survival for the group will not change. This is a further reason why imaging criteria for staging and restaging will need to be standardized.

Residual masses. The radiologist may be asked to

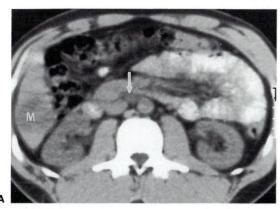
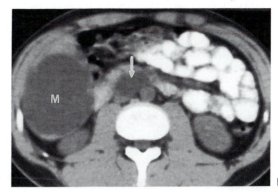

Fig. 27.35 A,B CT scan through the abdomen of this patient with metastatic teratoma show an increase in tumour size, along with a decrease in attenuation following treatment (**B**) for a testicular teratoma. This almost always indicates differentiation of the tumour into a benign variant. The residuum is excised to protect the patient in the future. Note both the residual interaorticocaval lymph node (arrow) and the liver metastasis (M), both of which enlarge on treatment.

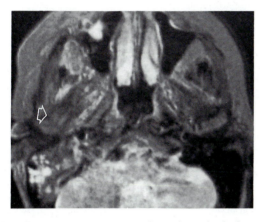

Fig. 27.36 Long-term reassessment of a patient who had previously had a parotid malignancy resected, now with clinical suspicion of recurrence, shows considerable distortion of the architecture, but the low signal intensity on T_2-weighted MR sequences suggested the scar tissue (arrow) to be benign. This was confirmed at subsequent re-exploration.

comment on the possible malignant potential of any residual mass following treatment of a malignancy (Lewis et al 1982). At present it is not possible to deduce residual malignant potential from the appearances. Future possible ways of tackling this problem include functional studies using radionuclides, especially when these may be targeted to the appropriate cell type, and MRI. On MR images it would appear that residual tumour masses that have a low signal on T_2-weighted images — especially when the pretreatment images show a high signal intensity on similar T_2-weighted sequences — are likely to be dormant (Fig. 27.36). Unfortunately the converse — that high signal on T_2-weighted sequences equals activity — is not true.

MAGNETIC RESONANCE IMAGING

Magnetic resonance imaging in oncology is at present of value in assessing the spinal cord, especially in patients with clinical features suggesting cord compression (see Ch. 54). In these circumstances MRI provides a more complete picture of the compressive lesion than may be obtained with myelography. MRI may also prove of value in the assessment of bone-marrow involvement and complement the information available from bone-marrow aspirate and trephine.

In the assessment of nodal disease MRI is a costly and less practical alternative to CT. MRI does not seem reliable in the recognition of splenic and/or hepatic involvement in lymphoma. A possible role for MRI is the assessment of residual masses looking for the low-T_2 signal intensity associated with fibrosis. This is occasionally useful, but, especially in the first year after treatment, high-T_2 signal intensity may persist in the residual tissue due to inflammatory rather than residual neoplastic change.

MR may be used to provide biochemical rather than visual information. This may also be used to assess the response of a tumour to chemotherapy. At present this is of experimental value only.

REFERENCES AND SUGGESTIONS FOR FURTHER READING

Allen, E. V., Barker, N. W., Hines, E. A. (1946) *Peripheral Vascular Diseases.* W. B. Saunders, Philadelphia.

Amendola, M. A. (1986) CT staging of lymphoma. In: Glazer, G. M. (Ed.) *Staging of Neoplasms.* Churchill Livingstone, New York, pp 147–189.

Blake, P. R., Carr, D. H., Goolden, A. W. G. (1986) Intracranial Hodgkin's disease. *British Journal of Radiology,* 59, 414–416.

Blackledge, G., Bush, H., Dodge, O. G., Crowther, D. F. (1979) A study of gastrointestinal lymphoma. *Clinical Oncology,* 5, 209–219.

Bragg, D. G., Colby T. V., Ward J. H. (1986) New concepts in the non-Hodgkin lymphomas: Radiological implications. *Radiology,* 159, 289–304.

Callihan, T. R., Berard, C. W. (1980) The classification and pathology of the lymphomas and leukemias. *Seminars in Roentgenology* 15, 203–218.

Carbone, P. P., Kaplan, H. S., Musshoff, K., Smithers, E. W., Tubiana, M. (1971) Report of the Committee on Hodgkin's Disease Staging. *Cancer Research,* 31, 1860–1861.

Castellino, R. A. (1986) Hodgkin's disease: Practical concepts for the diagnostic radiologist. *Radiology,* 159, 305–310.

Castellino, R. A., Blank, N., Hoppe, R. T., Cho, C. (1986) Hodgkin Disease: contributions of chest CT in the initial staging evaluation. *Radiology,* 160, 603–605.

Dixon, A. K., Ellis, M., Sikora, K. (1986) Computed tomography of testicular tumours: Distribution of abdominal lymphadenopathy. *Clinical Radiology,* 37, 519–523.

Dooms, G. C., Hricak, H., Moseley, M. E., Bottles, K., Fisher, M., Higgens, C. B. (1985) Characterisation of lymphadenopathy by magnetic resonance times: Preliminary results. *Radiology,* 155, 691–697.

Glazer, H. S., Lee, J. K. T., Balfe, D. M., Mauro, M. A., Griffith, R, Sagel, S. S. (1983) Non-Hodgkin lymphoma: Computed tomographic demonstration of unusual extranodal involvement. *Radiology,* 149, 211–217.

Glazer, G. M., Gross, B. H., Quint, L. E., Francis, I. R., Bookstein, F. L., Orringer, M. B., (1985) Normal mediastinal lymph nodes: Number and size according to American Thoracic Society Mapping. *American Journal of Roentgenology,* 144, 261–265.

Harrison, D. A., Clouse, M. E. (1985) Normal Anatomy. In: Clouse, M. E., and Wallace, S. (eds). *Lymphatic Imaging* (2nd edn.). Williams and Wilkins, Baltimore, pp 15–94.

Heron, C. W., Husband, J. E., Williams, M. P., Cherryman, G. R. (1988) The value of thoracic computed tomography in the detection of recurrent Hodgkin's disease. *British Journal of Radiology,* 61, 567–572.

Jack, C. R., O'Neill, B. P., Banks, P. M., Reese, D. F. (1988) Central nervous system lymphoma: Histological types and CT appearance. *Radiology,* 167, 211–215.

Kaplan, H. S. (1980) *Hodgkin's disease.* 2nd edn. Harvard University Press, Cambridge MA.

Khoury, M. B., Godwin, J. C., Halvorsen, R. A., Hanun, Y, Putman, C. E. (1984) The role of thoracic CT in non-Hodgkin's lymphoma. *Radiology,* 158, 659–662.

Kiyono, K., Sone, S., Sakai, F. et al. (1988) The number and size of normal mediastinal lymph nodes: A postmortem study. *American Journal of Roentgenology,* 150, 771–778.

Lewis, E., Barnardino, M. E., Salvador, P. G., Cabanillas, F. F., Barnes, P. A., Thomas, J. L. (1982) Post therapy CT detected mass in lymphoma: Is it viable tissue? *Journal of Computer Assisted Tomography,* 6, 792–795.

Lukes, R. J., Butler, J. J., Hicks, E. B. (1966) Natural history of Hodgkin's disease as related to its pathological picture. *Cancer,* 19, 317–344.

MacDonald, J. S. (1982) Lymphography in lymph node disease. In: Kinmonth, J. B. (Ed.) *The Lymphatics: Surgery, lymphography and diseases of the chyle and lymph systems.* Edward Arnold. London, pp 327–370.

MacDonald, J. S. (1987) Lymphography. In: Ansell, G., Wilkins, R. A. (Eds). *Complications in Diagnostic Imaging.* Blackwell, Oxford, pp 300–309.

MacDonald, J. S., McCready, V. R., Cosgrove, D. O., Cherryman, G. R., Selby, P. (1987) Radiological and other imaging methods. In: Selby, P., McElwain, T. J. (Eds). *Hodgkin's Disease.* Blackwell Scientific, Oxford, pp 126–160.

McKusick, K. A. (1985) Radionuclide lymphography. In: Clouse M. E., Wallace, S. (Eds). *Lymphatic Imaging.* 2nd edn. Williams & Wilkins, Baltimore, pp 95–111.

Meyer, J. E., Linggood, R. M., Lindfors, K. K., McLoud, T. C., Stomper, P. C. (1984) Impact of thoracic computed tomography on radiation therapy planning in Hodgkin disease. *Journal of Computer Assisted Tomography,* 8, 892–894.

National Cancer Institute Sponsored Study of Classifications of Non-Hodgkin's Lymphomas (1981) Summary and description of a working formulation for clinical usage. *Cancer,* 49, 2112–2135.

Neumann, C. H., Parker, B. R., Castellino, R. A. (1985) Hodgkin's disease and the non-Hodgkin lymphomas. In: Bragg, D. G., Rubin, P., Youker, J. E. (Eds) *Oncologic Imaging.* Pergamon, New York, pp 477–501.

O'Donnell, T. F., Jr, Clouse, M. E. (1985) Abnormal peripheral lymphatics. In: Clouse, M. E., Wallace, S. (Eds) *Lymphatic Imaging.* 2nd edn. Williams & Wilkins, Baltimore, pp 142–179.

Oliver, T. W., Bernardino, M. E., Sones, P. J., Jr. (1983) Monitoring the response of lymphoma patients to therapy: correlation of abdominal CT findings with clinical course and histological cell type. *Radiology,* 149, 219–224.

Pond, G. D., Castellino, R. A., Horning, S., Hoppe, R. T. (1989) Non-Hodgkin lymphoma: Influence of lymphography, CT, and bone marrow biopsy on staging and management. *Radiology,* 170, 159–164.

Shiels, R. A., Stone, J., Ash, D. V., Cartwright, S. C., Close, H. J., Worthy, T. S., Robinson, P. J. (1984) Priorities for computed tomography and lymphography in the staging and initial management of Hodgkin's disease. *Clinical Radiology,* 35, 447–449.

Som, P. M. (1987) Lymph nodes of the neck. *Radiology,* 165, 593–600.

UICC (International Union Against Cancer) (1987) *TNM Classification of Malignant Tumours.* 4th edn. Springer-Verlag. Berlin

Williams, M. P., Cherryman, G. R., Husband, J. E. (1989) Magnetic resonance imaging of spinal cord compression. *Clinical Radiology,* 40, 286–290.

Index